Substances Potentially Associated with Hepatic Abnor

Acetaminophen, aflatoxin, carbon tetrachloride, carprofe
(i.e., blue-green algae), diazepam (cat), germander, iron
mothballs, mushrooms, nitrosamines, nonsteroidal anti-i................... .... p.......... .
penitrem A, pennyroyal oil, petroleum hydrocarbons (e.g., diesel fuel, gasoline, kerosene),
phenacetin, phenobarbital, phenol, phenytoin, primidone, pyrrolizidine alkaloids, sago palm
(*Cycas*), sulfonamides, phenol, phosphorus, quinine, *Sassafras* (sassafras), stanozolol, tannic
acid, thiacetarsamide, toluene, trimethoprim sulfas, valium, vitamin A, xylitol, zinc.

Substances Potentially Associated with Hyperthermia

Bromethalin, cocaine, dinitrophenol, disophenol, halothane, hops, pentachlorophenol, seizures
(or muscle tremors).

Substances Potentially Associated with Methemoglobin Production (see Substances Potentially Associated with Heinz Bodies and/or Hemolysis)

Acetaminophen, aniline dyes, benzocaine, chlorate, chloroquine, copper, dibucaine hydrochloride, gallic acid, lidocaine, naphthalene (mothballs), nitric and nitrous oxide, nitrite (nitrate),
nitrobenzene, nitroglycerin, nitroprusside, phenacetin, phenazopyridine, phenol, prilocaine,
primaquine, propitocaine, pyridium, pyrogallol, resorcinol, silver nitrate, sulfonamides, sulfone,
tannic acid.

Substances Potentially Associated with Nervous System Depression

Acetone, amitraz, barbiturates, benzodiazepine, cholecalciferol (and related products), citrus oils,
diethylene glycol, ethanol, ethylene glycol, ice melts (e.g., potassium chloride, magnesium chloride), isopropanol, ivermectin and ivermectin-like parasiticides (e.g., moxydectin, eprinomectin,
selamectin, abamectin), lead, lizard (*Heloderma*), marijuana (*Cannabis*), methanol, mushrooms,
nicotine, opioids, pentobarbital, phenothiazines, pine oil, piperazine, pit viper venom, propylene
glycol, tranquilizers, turpentine, xylitol.

Substances Potentially Associated with Nervous System Excitation

Acetylcholinesterase-inhibiting organophosphate and carbamate pesticides, 4-aminopyridine,
amitraz, amphetamines, antidepressants, *Asclepias* (milkweed), *Atropa* (belladonna), atropine,
bromethalin, *Bufo* (toad), caffeine, camphor, chlorinated hydrocarbons (e.g., aldrin, chlordane,
endosulfan, heptachlor), cholecalciferol, *Cicuta* (water hemlock), citrus oils, cocaine, cyanide,
cyanobacteria (i.e., blue-green algae), *Datura* (jimsonweed), DEET, *Dicentra* (bleedingheart,
Dutchman's breeches), dichloromethane, ethylene glycol, 5-fluorouracil, *Hyoscyamus* (henbane), ice melts (e.g., sodium chloride), *Ipomea* (morning glory), imidacloprid, ivermectin and
ivermectin-like parasiticides (e.g., moxydectin, eprinomectin, selamectin, abamectin), khat, *Latrodectus* spider venom, lead, *Lobelia* (lobelia), LSD, mace, ma huang, melaleuca oil, mercury,
metaldehyde, metronidazole, mushrooms, nicotine, nutmeg, opioids (cat), paintballs, pemoline,
penitrem A, phencyclidine, play dough, potassium bromide, propylene glycol, pyrethrin, pyrethrum, pyrethroids (e.g., allethrin, tetramethrin, resmethrin, permethrin), roquefortine, rote-
none, ricin (*Ricinus*—castor bean), salt (e.g., play dough, ice melts, water deprivation), *Sassafras*
(sassafras), scopolamine, sodium fluoroacetate and fluoroacetamide (Compounds 1080 and
1081), *Sophora* (mescal bean), strychnine, *Taxus* (yew), theobromine (chocolate), theophylline,
tricyclic antidepressants, valproic acid, xylitol, yohimbe, zinc/magnesium/aluminum phosphide.

Substances Potentially Interfering with Oxygen Transport and/or Hemoglobin Binding

Carbon monoxide, cyanide (e.g., mining activity, plants), hydrogen sulfide.

Substances Potentially Associated with Renal Abnormalities

Acetaminophen, antibiotics (e.g., amphotericin B, bacitracin, gentamicin, neomycin, oxytetracycline, paromomycin, polymyxin-B, sulfonamides), *Aristolochia* (birthwort), bismuth, boric
acid, 2-butoxyethanol, cadmium, calcipotriene, calcipotriol, calcitriol, cantharidin, carbamate
fungicides, carbon tetrachloride, cholecalciferol, chromium, citrinin, copper, currants (*Vitis*),

diethylene glycol, diquat, ethylene glycol, grapes, lead, lilies (*Hemerocallis, Lilium*), mercury, mothballs, mushrooms, nonsteroidal antiinflammatory agents, ochratoxin, oxalic acid (e.g., *Oxalis, Rheum, Rumex*), paraquat, petroleum hydrocarbons (e.g., diesel fuel, gasoline, kerosene), phenol, raisins, toluene, uranium, vitamin D–containing plants (e.g., *Cestrum diurnum, Solanum malacoxylon*), zinc.

Substances Potentially Associated with the Respiratory System

Acetylcholinesterase-inhibiting organophosphate and carbamate pesticides, α-naphthyl thiourea, ammonia, chlorinated hydrocarbons (e.g., aldrin, chlordane, endosulfan, heptachlor), formaldehyde, freon, hydrochloric acid, hydrofluoric acid, hydrogen sulfide, iodine, mercury, nitrogen oxide, opioids, overheated Teflon, paraquat, pennyroyal oil, petroleum hydrocarbons (e.g., diesel fuel, gasoline, kerosene), pine oils, selenium, turpentine, zinc/magnesium/aluminum phosphide.

Substances Potentially Associated with Skeletal Muscle Abnormalities/Paralysis

Acetylcholinesterase-inhibiting organophosphates, arsenic, botulism, coral snake venom, ciguatera, cyanobacteria (blue-green algae), curare, ionophores (e.g., laidlomycin, lasalocid, monensin, narasin, salinomycin), macadamia nuts, phenoxy herbicides (e.g., 2,4-dichlorophenoxyacetic acid), roquefortine, saxitoxin, spider (*Latrodectus*—black widow), succinylcholine.

Substances Potentially Associated with Excessive Salivation/Oral Irritation

Acetylcholinesterase-inhibiting compounds (e.g., organophosphate and carbamate insecticides), acids and alkalis (e.g., detergents, disinfectants, soaps), batteries, bleaches, *Bufo* (toads), cationic detergents, citrus oils, corrosives, cyanobacteria (i.e., blue-green algae), DEET, formaldehyde, glow jewelry (dibutyl phthalate), ivermectin and other macrolide antiparasitic agents (e.g., selamectin, moxidectin, doramectin, eprinomectin, abamectin, milbemycin), lizards, metaldehyde, mushrooms, nonionic detergents, insoluble oxalate-containing plants (e.g., *Alocasia* [Alocasia], *Arisaema* [Jack-in-the-pulpit], *Calla* [calla], *Colocasia* [elephant's ear], *Dieffenbachia* [dumbcane], *Monstera* [split leaf philodendron], *Philodendron* [philodendron]), phenol, pine oil, pyrethrins, pyrethroids, spider (*Latrodectus*—black widow), strychnine, superglue, tremorogenic mycotoxins (e.g., penitrem A, roquefortine), turpentine.

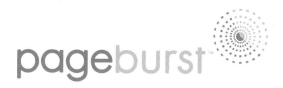

Elsevier Digital Books

What you need, when you need it, how you want it.

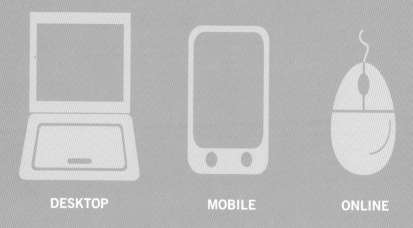

DESKTOP　　　　**MOBILE**　　　　**ONLINE**

Access your entire library of Elsevier textbooks from a simple, smart interface. Pageburst integrates Elsevier's trusted content with powerful interactive tools to help you create a more productive, enjoyable learning experience.

▶ Pageburst offers quick, easy access to the Elsevier content you use and rely on, along with organizational tools to increase your efficiency.

▶ Pageburst makes it easy to search, take notes, highlight content, and collaborate with classmates or colleagues.

3RD EDITION

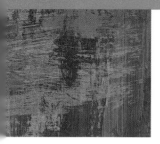

Small Animal Toxicology

Michael E. Peterson, DVM, MS
Reid Veterinary Hospital
Albany, Oregon

Patricia A. Talcott, MS, DVM, PhD, DABVT
Professor
Department of Veterinary Comparative Anatomy,
    Pharmacology & Physiology
Washington State University, College of Veterinary
    Medicine
Pullman, Washington
Veterinary Diagnostic Toxicologist
Analytical Sciences Laboratory
University of Idaho
Moscow, Idaho
Veterinary Diagnostic Toxicologist
Washington Animal Disease Diagnostic Laboratory
Washington State University
Pullman, Washington

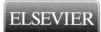

ELSEVIER
SAUNDERS

3251 Riverport Lane
St. Louis, Missouri 63043

SMALL ANIMAL TOXICOLOGY, THIRD EDITION   ISBN: 978-1-4557-0717-1
Copyright © 2013, 2006, 2001 by Saunders, an imprint of Elsevier Inc.

Notices

Knowledge and best practice in this fi eld are constantly changing. As new research and experience broaden our understanding, changes in research methods, professional practices, or medical treatment may become necessary.

Practitioners and researchers must always rely on their own experience and knowledge in evaluating and using any information, methods, compounds, or experiments described herein. In using such information or methods they should be mindful of their own safety and the safety of others, including parties for whom they have a professional responsibility.

With respect to any drug or pharmaceutical products identifi ed, readers are advised to check the most current information provided (i) on procedures featured or (ii) by the manufacturer of each product to be administered, to verify the recommended dose or formula, the method and duration of administration, and contraindications. It is the responsibility of practitioners, relying on their own experience and knowledge of their patients, to make diagnoses, to determine dosages and the best treatment for each individual patient, and to take all appropriate safety precautions.

To the fullest extent of the law, neither the Publisher nor the authors, contributors, or editors, assume any liability for any injury and/or damage to persons or property as a matter of products liability, negligence or otherwise, or from any use or operation of any methods, products, instructions, or ideas contained in the material herein.

Library of Congress Cataloging-in-Publication Data
Small animal toxicology / [edited by] Michael E. Peterson, Patricia A. Talcott.—3rd ed.
    p. ; cm.
  Rev. ed. of: Small animal toxicology / Michael E. Peterson, Patricia A. Talcott. 2nd ed. c2006.
  Includes bibliographical references and index.
  ISBN 978-1-4557-0717-1 (hardback : alk. paper)
  1. Dogs—Diseases—Treatment. 2. Cats—Diseases—Treatment. 3.Poisoning in animals.
4. Veterinary toxicology. I. Peterson, Michael
E. (Michael Edward), 1953- II. Talcott, Patricia A. III. Peterson, Michael E. (Michael Edward),
1953- Small animal toxicology.
  [DNLM: 1. Poisoning—veterinary. 2. Cat Diseases—drug therapy. 3. Dog Diseases—drug therapy.
4. Veterinary Drugs—toxicity. SF 757.5]
  SF992.P64P48 2013
  636.089'59—dc23   2012041928

Vice President and Publisher: Linda Duncan
Content Strategy Director: Penny Rudolph
Content Development Specialist: Brandi Graham
Publishing Services Manager: Gayle May
Production Manager: Hemamalini Rajendrababu
Senior Project Manager: Antony Prince
Design Manager: Teresa McBryan
Designer: Brian Salisbury

Printed in India

Last digit is the print number: 9 8 7 6 5 4

Dedication

I would like to dedicate this edition to my wife Kate and my children Greyson, Rosie, Rube, and Cory. I would also like to express my gratitude to Tim Reid and the staff at Reid Veterinary Hospital for their support of my academic endeavors, and as always thanks to Dr. Talcott.

Michael E. Peterson

I would like to dedicate this book to all of my past and present students who continually challenge me to do my best in the classroom, and who keep my passion in toxicology alive through their interest, support, and humor. I also wish to thank my husband Glenn, daughter Haley, and son Billy for being supportive and patient in my attempts to balance a career and family.

Patricia A. Talcott

Contributors

Rodney S. Bagley, DVM, DACVIM (Neurology)
Professor and Chair
Department of Veterinary Clinical Sciences
College of Veterinary Medicine
Iowa State University
Ames, Iowa
Anticonvulsants

E. Murl Bailey, Jr., DVM, PhD, DABVT
Professor of Toxicology and Emergency
    Medicine
Department of Veterinary Physiology and
    Pharmacology
College of Veterinary Medicine and Biomedical
    Sciences
Texas A&M University
College Station, Texas
Botulism
Ricin

A. Catherine Barr, PhD, DABT
Quality Assurance & Safety Manager
Texas Veterinary Medical Diagnostic Laboratory
College Station, Texas
Household and Garden Plants

Karyn Bischoff, DVM, MS, DABVT
Assistant Professor
Population Medicine and Diagnostic Sciences
Toxicologist
New York State Animal Health Diagnostic Center
Cornell University
Ithaca, New York
Diethylene Glycol
Methanol
Propylene Glycol

Dennis J. Blodgett, DVM, PhD, Diplomate,
    ABVT
Associate Professor Emeritus
Toxicology
Department of Biomedical Sciences &
    Pathobiology
Virginia - Maryland Regional College of
    Veterinary Medicine
Blacksburg, Virginia
Organophosphate and Carbamate Insecticides

Keith Boesen, PharmD, CSPI
Managing Director
Arizona Poison and Drug Information Center
Tucson, Arizona
Toxicologic Information Resources

Kelly Green Boesen, PharmD, BCPS
Clinical Pharmacology Coordinator
University Physicians Hospital
Tucson, Arizona
Toxicologic Information Resources

Cheryl Braswell, DVM
Educational Programs Coordinator
Pet Emergency Clinics & Specialty Hospital
Thousand Oaks, California
Supportive Care of the Poisoned Patient

Ahna G. Brutlag, DVM, MS
Assistant Director of Veterinary Services
Pet Poison Helpline
SafetyCall International, PLLC
Bloomington, Minnesota
Approach to Diagnosis for the Toxicology Case
Metaldehyde

Annie V. Chen, DVM, MS, DACVIM
    (Neurology)
Assistant Professor
Department of Neurology and Neurosurgery
College of Veterinary Medicine
Washington State University
Pullman, Washington
Anticonvulsants

Heather E. Connally, DVM, MS, DACVECC
Head of the Emergency and Critical Care
    Service
Veterinary Specialty Center
Tucson, Arizona
Ethylene Glycol

Alastair E. Cribb, DVM, PhD, FCAHS
Dean
College of Veterinary Medicine
University of Calgary
Calgary, Alberta, Canada
Adverse Drug Reactions

Camille DeClementi, VMD, DABT, DABVT
Senior Director
Animal Health Services
ASPCA
Urbana, Illinois
Instructor
Department of Veterinary Biosciences
College of Veterinary Medicine
University of Illinois
Urbana, Illinois
Arsenic

Linda K. Dolder, DVM
Consulting Veterinarian in Clinical Toxicology
ASPCA Animal Poison Control Center
Urbana, Illinois
Methylxanthines: Caffeine,
Theobromine, Theophylline

Caroline Donaldson, DVM, DABT
Toxicologist
ASPCA
Urbana, Illinois
Paraquat

David C. Dorman, DVM, PhD, DABVT,
DABT
Professor of Toxicology
Department of Molecular Biomedical Sciences
North Carolina State University
Raleigh, North Carolina
Bromethalin

Eric K. Dunayer, MS, VMD, DABT, DABVT
Associate Professor
Department of Veterinary Clinical Sciences
School of Veterinary Medicine
St. Matthew's University
Grand Cayman, Cayman Islands
Small Mammal Toxicology

Tim J. Evans, DVM, MS, PhD, DACT, DABVT
Associate Professor and Section Head
Department of Toxicology
Veterinary Medical Diagnostic Laboratory
University of Missouri
Columbia, Missouri
Toxicokinetics and Toxicodynamics
Reproductive Toxicology of Male and Female
Companion Animals

Kevin T. Fitzgerald, PhD, DVM, DABVP
Associate Veterinarian
VCA Alameda East Veterinary Hospital
Denver, Colorado
Taking a Toxicologic History
Establishing a Minimum Database in Small
Animal Poisonings
Poisonings in the Captive Reptile
Smoke Inhalation
Carbon Monoxide
Cyanide
Insects—Hymenoptera
Metronidazole

Gregory F. Grauer, DVM, MS, DACVIM
(SAIM)
Professor and Jarvis Chair of Small Animal
Internal Medicine
Kansas State University
Manhattan, Kansas
Ethylene Glycol

Sharon M. Gwaltney-Brant, DVM, PhD,
DABVT, DABT
Adjunct Instructor
Department of Comparative Biosciences
College of Veterinary Medicine
University of Illinois
Urbana, Illinois
Toxicology Consultant
Veterinary Information Network
Davis, California
Miscellaneous Indoor Toxicants
Christmastime Plants
Macadamia Nuts
Nonsteroidal Antiinflammatories
Oxalate-Containing Plants
Atypical Topical Spot-On Products

Jeffery O. Hall, DVM, PhD, DABVT
Head, Diagnostic Toxicology
Utah Veterinary Diagnostic Laboratory
Utah State University
Logan, Utah
Ionophores
Iron
Lilies

Dwayne W. Hamar, PhD
Associate Professor
College of Veterinary Medicine and Biomedical
Sciences
Colorado State University
Fort Collins, Colorado
Ethylene Glycol

Steven R. Hansen, DVM, MS, DABT, DABVT
Senior Vice President
Animal Poison Control Center
ASPCA
Urbana, Illinois
Pyrethrins and Pyrethroids

Elizabeth A. Hausner, DVM, PhD, DABT, DABVT
Center for Drug Evaluation and Research
United States Food and Drug Administration
Silver Spring, Maryland
Hazards Associated with the Use of Herbal and Other Natural Products

Lynn Rolland Hovda, DVM, MS, RPh, DACVIM
Director of Veterinary Services
Pet Poison Helpline
SafetyCall International
Bloomington, Minnesota
Effective Use of Veterinary Poison Control Center

Safdar A. Khan, DVM, MS, PhD, DABVT
Senior Director of Toxicology Research
ASPCA Animal Poison Control Center
ASPCA
Urbana, Illinois
Pyrethrins and Pyrethroids

Michael W. Knight, DVM, DABVT, DABT
Senior Toxicologist
ASPCA Animal Poison Control Center
Urbana, Illinois
Zinc Phosphide

Gary R. Krieger, MD, MPH
Associate Professor
Department of Toxicology
School of Pharmacy
University of Colorado
Denver, Colorado
Indoor Environmental Quality and Health

Michelle Anne Kutzler, DVM, PhD, DACT
Associate Professor of Companion Animal Industries
Department of Animal Science
Oregon State University
Corvallis, Oregon
Considerations in Pregnant or Lactating Patients

Jerry J. LaBonde, MS, DVM
Veterinarian and Owner
Avian and Exotic Animal Hospital at Homestead
Centennial, Colorado
Poisoning in the Avian Patient

Justine A. Lee, DVM, DACVECC
Associate Director of Veterinary Services
Pet Poison Helpline
SafetyCall International
Minneapolis, Minnesota
Considerations in the Geriatric Poisoned Patient

Jude McNally, RPh, DABAT
Vice-President, Medical Science Liaison
Rare Disease Therapeutics, Inc.
Franklin, Tennessee
Toxicologic Information Resources
Spider Envenomation: Black Widow
Spider Envenomation: Brown Recluse

Katrina L. Mealey, DVM, PhD, DACVIM, DACVCP
Professor
Veterinary Clinical Sciences
College of Veterinary Medicine
Washington State University
Pullman, Washington
Ivermectin: Macrolide Antiparasitic Agents

Charlotte Means, DVM, MLIS, DABVT, DABT
Senior Toxicologist
ASPCA Animal Poison Control Center
Urbana, Illinois
Organophosphate and Carbamate Insecticides

Matthew S. Mellema, DVM, PhD, DACVECC
Assistant Professor
Department of Surgical and Radiological Sciences
Veterinary Medical Teaching Hospital
University of California – Davis
Davis, California
Initial Management of the Poisoned Patient
Xylitol

Steven Mensack, VMD, DACVECC
Medical Director
Pet Emergency Clinics and Specialty Hospital
Ventura, California
Supportive Care of the Poisoned Patient

Caroline Moore, BS
School of Veterinary Medicine
University of California
Davis, California
Cyanobacteria

Michelle S. Mostrom, DVM, MS, PhD, DABVT, DABT
Veterinary Toxicologist
Deartment of Veterinary Diagnostic Services
North Dakota State University
Fargo, North Dakota
Grapes and Raisins

Motoko Mukai, DVM, PhD, DABT
Senior Research Associate
Animal Health Diagnostic Center
College of Veterinary Medicine
Cornell University
Ithaca, New York
Diethylene Glycol

Lisa A. Murphy, VMD, DABT
Assistant Professor of Toxicology
Department of Pathobiology
University of Pennsylvania
Kennett Square, Pennsylvania
Responding to Mass Exposures

Michael J. Murphy, DVM, PhD, JD, DABVT
Veterinary Medical Officer
Center for Veterinary Medicine
Food and Drug Administration
Rockville, Maryland
Medicolegal Considerations in Toxicology Cases
Anticoagulant Rodenticides

Kristin L. Newquist, BS, AAS, CVT
General and Exotic Practice Technician
VCA Alameda East Veterinary Hospital
Denver, Colorado
Poisonings in the Captive Reptile

Gary D. Osweiler, DVM, MS, PhD, DABVT
Professor Emeritus
Veterinary Diagnostic and Production Animal
  Medicine
Veterinary Toxicologist, Retired
Veterinary Diagnostic Laboratory
Iowa State University
Ames, Iowa
General Toxicologic Principles for Clinicians

Kathy Parton, DVM, MS
Senior Lecturer
Institute of Veterinary, Animal and Medical
  Sciences
Massey University
Palmerston North New Zealand
Sodium Monofluoroacetate (1080)

Michael E. Peterson, DVM, MS
Associate Veterinarian
Reid Veterinary Hospital
Albany, Oregon
Toxicologic Decontamination
Indoor Environmental Quality and Health
Toxicologic Considerations in the Pediatric
  Poisoned Patient
Poisonous Lizards
Snake Bite: North American Pit Vipers
Snake Bite: Coral Snakes
Spider Envenomation: Black Widow
Spider Envenomation: Brown Recluse
Toads

Mathieu Peyrou, DVM, MSc
Faculte de Medecine Veterinaire
University de Montreal
Quebec, Canada
Adverse Drug Reactions

Konnie H. Plumlee, DVM, MS, DABVT, DACVIM
Veterinary Medical Officer
USDA-APHIS-Animal Care
Ozark, Missouri
Citrus Oils
DEET
Nicotine

Robert H. Poppenga, DVM, PhD, DABVT
Professor of Veterinary Clinical Toxicology
California Animal Health and Food Safety
  Laboratory
School of Veterinary Medicine
University of California – Davis
Davis, California
Hazards Associated with the Use of Herbal and
  Other Natural Products

Birgit Puschner, DVM, PhD, DABVT
Professor
Department of Molecular Biosciences
California Animal Health & Food Safety
  Laboratory
School of Veterinary Medicine
University of California
Davis, California
Approach to Diagnosis for the Toxicology Case
Cyanobacteria
Metaldehyde
Mushrooms

Merl F. Raisbeck, DVM, MS, PhD, DABVT
Professor of Veterinary Toxicology
Department of Veterinary Sciences
University of Wyoming
Laramie, Wyoming
Organochlorine Pesticides
Petroleum Hydrocarbons

Jill A. Richardson, DVM
Pharmacovigilance Veterinarian
Department of Pharmacovigilance
Merck Animal Health
Summit, New Jersey
Amitraz
Ethanol

Brian K. Roberts, DVM, DACVECC
Director of Emergency and Critical Care
Veterinary Specialists of South Florida
Cooper City, Florida
Toads

Wilson K. Rumbeiha, DVM, PhD, DABVT, DABT
Professor
Veterinary Diagnostic & Production Animal
 Medicine
College of Veterinary Medicine
Iowa State University
Ames, Iowa
Cholecalciferol

Rance K. Sellon, DVM, PhD, DACVIM
Associate Professor
Veterinary Clinical Sciences
Washington State University
Pullman, Washington
Acetaminophen

John B. Sullivan Jr., MD, MBA
Associate Professor
College of Medicine
University of Arizona
Tucson, Arizona
Indoor Environmental Quality and Health

Patricia A. Talcott, MS, DVM, PhD, DABVT
Professor
Department of Veterinary Comparative
 Anatomy, Pharmacology and Physiology
College of Veterinary Medicine
Washington State University
Pullman, Washington
Effective Use of a Diagnostic Laboratory
Miscellaneous Indoor Toxicants

Miscellaneous Herbicides, Fungicides, and
 Nematocides
Anticoagulant Rodenticides
Copper
Mycotoxins
Nonsteroidal Antiinflammatories
Strychnine
Zinc

John H. Tegzes, MA, VMD, DABVT
Professor of Toxicology
College of Veterinary Medicine
Western University of Health Sciences
Pomona, California
Mercury
Sodium

Mary Anna Thrall, DVM, MS, DACVP
Professor and Section Chief
Department of Pathobiology
School of Veterinary Medicine
Ross University
St. Kitts, West Indies
Ethylene Glycol

Mark D. Van Ert, PhD, CIH
Adjunct Clinical Associate Professor of Public
 Health
Environmental and Occupational Health
 Concentration
Mel and Enid Zuckerman College of Public
 Health
Arizona Health Sciences Center
University of Arizsona
Tucson, Arizona
Indoor Environmental Quality and Health

Petra A. Volmer, DVM, MS, DABVT, DABT
Manager of Pharmacovigilance
Ceva Animal Health, LLCs
Rutherford, New Jersey
"Recreational" Drugs

Katie Von Derau, RN, CPN, CSPI
Supervisor
Washington Poison Center
Seattle, Washington
Use of Human Poison Centers in the Veterinary
 Setting

Tina Wismer, DVM, DABVT, DABT
Medical Director
ASPCA Animal Poison Control Center
Urbana, Illinois
Lead

Preface

This book was originally written with two goals in mind: to provide a valuable aid to the practicing small animal clinician and to supply a textbook for veterinary students that would supplement their classroom instruction. Dr. Peterson approached this text from the viewpoint of an active small animal clinician with an academic background in toxicology and public health. He is also an authority on clinical management of animals envenomated by a variety of zootoxins. Dr. Talcott, a Diplomate of the American Board of Veterinary Toxicology, brings to the book the experience of a practicing veterinary diagnostic toxicologist and as a professor and instructor of 22 years teaching veterinary students at Washington State University College of Veterinary Medicine.

This edition of the book has eight new chapters, which brings the total volume to 85 chapters. All the chapters have been updated with the most recent information available by experts in their fields. The book has also been expanded to four sections from the previous three. The first section, "Toxicologic Concept's" reviews both general toxicologic principles and clinical approaches to diagnosis and initial stabilization of the poisoned patient. This section includes areas such as toxicokinetics and toxicodynamics, effective use of poison centers, taking an adequate history, minimum databases, decontamination, and general supportive care, among other topics. The second section, "General Exposure's" covers large areas of toxicology such as indoor environmental quality, mass exposures, reproductive toxicology, and special classes of intoxicated patients such as pregnant and lactating, pediatric, geriatric, reptile, avian, and small mammals among others. The third section, "Miscellaneous Toxicant Group's" covers large classes of toxicant such as adverse drug reactions, recreational drugs, herbal and natural products, plants, and miscellaneous herbicides among others. The fourth section, "Specific Toxicant's" covers more than 55 specific compounds such as lead, grapes and raisins, copper, and many more. All these chapters have the same format, starting with a brief highlighted outline of critical pieces of information in the chapter, and then followed by sections on sources, toxic dose, toxicokinetics, mechanism of toxicity, clinical signs, minimum database, confirmatory test, treatment, prognosis, gross and histologic lesions, and differential diagnoses.

In addition to the added chapters and updated information, an index inside the book's front cover list toxins by their most likely affected biologic system. The index has been expanded to aid the clinician in finding information quickly and helping to speed identification of the most likely offending toxicant. We hope this textbook will be of assistance to both those students and veterinarians looking for an updated resource on small animal toxicology.

Michael E. Peterson
Patricia A. Talcott

Contents

General Toxicologic Principles for Clinicians

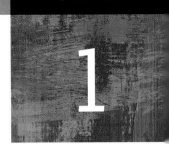

Gary D. Osweiler, DVM, MS, PhD, DABVT

- *Toxicology* is the science and study of how poisons affect organisms.
- Toxicology uses information extensively from medicine, pathology, chemistry, epidemiology, and statistics to reach the best diagnostic and therapeutic outcomes.
- Dosage is the most important factor that determines response to poisons.
- Toxicity is the quantitative amount of toxicant (dosage) required to produce a defined effect.
- Hazard or risk of poisoning depends on toxicity of the agent, characteristics of the animal's biology, and probability of exposure to the toxicant under conditions of use.
- Acute, subacute, and chronic toxicity are different chronological designations of chemical toxicity and are determined by relative dosage and the time and circumstances of exposure.
- LD_{50} values are useful for comparison of toxicity differences among chemicals but do not define the nature of toxicosis produced or the safe dosage for a majority of animals.
- The lowest known clinical toxic dosage is of greatest value for clinical toxicology.
- Many factors alter an animal's response to toxicants, including those inherent in the toxicant (chemical structure, solubility), the animal (metabolism, excretion), the environment (pollutants, natural toxins), and combinations of these major factors.
- Clinical toxicology evaluation depends heavily on determination of exposure, nature of clinical effects, and evidence for interacting factors that can alter toxicity.
- Determination of dosage and concentration are essential for thorough toxicologic evaluation and prognosis.

Dosage Makes the Poison

Toxicology is the study of poisons and their effects on living organisms. In veterinary medicine, this means understanding sources of poisons, circumstances of exposure, diagnosis of the type of poisoning, treatment, and use of management and educational strategies to prevent poisoning.[1-4]

Toxicology is based on the important principle of dose and response. There is a graded and possibly predictable response based on increasing exposure to the toxicant. In the words of Paracelsus, a physician-alchemist of the sixteenth century, "All substances are poisons; there is none which is not a poison. The right dose differentiates a poison from a remedy."[2,4] Paracelsus's principle of dosage and poisoning is still true and relevant in the

1

daily practice of nutrition, therapeutics, and toxicologic analysis. Today, with emphasis on synthetic drugs, natural or alternative therapies, and the rapidly growing fields of nutraceuticals and nanotoxicology, there is continuing interest in evaluating dosage and response principles for both beneficial and detrimental effects in the daily practice of veterinary medicine. Many toxicants discussed in this book provide examples of how dosage determines whether the agent is a nutrient, a remedy, or a poison.

Determinants of exposure that affect dosage may be more than simply the gross amount of material ingested or applied to the skin. Rather, the effective dosage at a susceptible receptor site determines the ultimate response. Thus species differences in metabolism, vehicle differences that promote skin penetration, specific drug or chemical interactions that potentiate response, and organ dysfunction that limits elimination can all influence the ultimate dosage.[2,3,5] Clinicians must consider all of these possibilities when working to diagnose a potential toxicosis or apply therapeutic agents to their patients.

Dosage Is Affected by Animal Systems for Absorption, Metabolism, and Elimination

Toxicology involves the knowledge of poisons, including their chemical properties, identification, and biologic effects, and the treatment of disease conditions caused by poisons. Toxicology shares many principles with pharmacology. The term *toxicokinetics* includes absorption, distribution, storage, metabolism, and elimination; another term, *toxicodynamics*, describes mechanisms of action and effects of poisons on the biochemistry and physiology of animals. These important concepts are more fully described in Chapter 2, "Toxicokinetics and Toxicodynamics."

Every specialty has its important characteristic terminology. Basic terminology is important when reading toxicology literature, reviewing laboratory reports, or describing effects to colleagues. The following are some of the more useful toxicologic terms.

A *poison* or *toxicant* is any solid, liquid, or gas that, when introduced into or applied to the body, can interfere with homeostasis of the organism or life processes of its cells by its own inherent qualities, without acting mechanically and irrespective of temperature. The term *toxin* is used to describe poisons that originate from biologic sources and are generally classified as *biotoxins*. Biotoxins are further classified according to origin as *zootoxins* (animal origin), *bacterial toxins* (both endotoxins and exotoxins), *phytotoxins* (plant origin), *phycotoxins* (from seaweed and algae), and *mycotoxins* (fungal origin).[2,3,5]

Poisons may be categorized as *organic, inorganic, metallic,* or *biologic* and may be synthetic or natural. Synthetic agents may have been designed specifically as toxicants or for other purposes that may have a very broad or very narrow range of toxicity (e.g., drugs for cancer chemotherapy) or may produce effects in very specific targets. Natural products used in nutrition, medicine, or commerce are sometimes believed to be less hazardous than synthetic products. However, natural products are not inherently more or less toxic than synthetic molecules. Indeed, some of the most toxic agents known (e.g., botulinum toxin, tetrodotoxin) are of natural origin. Knowledge of the chemical nature and specific effects of toxicants is the only certain way to assess hazard from exposure.

The terms *toxic, toxicity,* and *toxicosis* are often misunderstood or misused.[3,5] The word *toxic* describes the effects of a toxicant (e.g., the "toxic" effects of organophosphate insecticides are cholinesterase inhibition—lacrimation, salivation, vomiting, dyspnea, and diarrhea). However, *toxicity* is used to describe the quantitative amount or dosage of a poison that will produce a defined effect (e.g., the toxicity of ethylene glycol for cats is 2 to 5 mL/kg body weight). The toxic effects of ethylene glycol are acidosis and oxalate nephrosis; the result of being poisoned by ethylene glycol is ethylene glycol toxicosis. *Poisoning* and *toxicosis* mean essentially the same thing and either may be used.

Dosage Defines Exposure in an Accurate and Reliable Format

Dosage is the correct terminology for toxicity expressed as amount of toxicant per unit of body weight.[2,3,5] The commonly accepted dosage units for veterinary medicine are milligrams per kilogram (mg/kg) body weight. However, toxicity can also be expressed as moles

Table 1-1	Comparison of Body Weight to Surface Area for Animals of Representative Sizes

Body Weight (kg)	Body Surface (m²)
0.5	0.06
1.0	0.10
5.0	0.29
10.0	0.46
20.0	0.74
40.0	1.17

or micromoles of agent per kilogram body weight. In some experimental studies, comparisons of large and small animals relate dosage to the body surface area, which is approximately equal to body weight.[2,3,5] The use of body surface area dosages is advocated by some as a more accurate way to account for very different body sizes in veterinary medicine. Examples in Table 1-1 show that as animals increase in weight, the body surface area increases proportionally less, and this may affect the rate of metabolism, excretion, and receptor interaction with toxicants.[3] For many toxicants, larger animals may be poisoned by relatively lower body weight dosages than smaller mammals.[5] However, other factors, such as species differences in metabolism, excretion, or receptor sites, can alter this generalization.

Dose is a term for the total amount of a drug or toxicant given to an individual organism. In veterinary medicine, the extreme ranges of body weight and surface area, even within species, generally make the term *dose* relatively inaccurate or imprecise.

Characteristics of the LD$_{50}$

A commonly used means to compare the toxicity of compounds with one another is the median lethal dosage, also known as the oral LD$_{50}$ in a standard animal, such as the laboratory rat. The LD$_{50}$ value is usually based on a single oral exposure with observation for 1 to 7 days after the chemical is administered to determine an end point for total deaths. The LD$_{50}$ is a standardized toxicity test that depends on a quantal (i.e., all or none) response to a range of three or more regularly increasing dosages at logarithmic or geometric intervals. In some cases a multiple-dosage LD$_{50}$ is used to show the acute effects (typically up to 7 days) produced by repeated dosages in the same animals. When cumulative deaths are plotted on linear graph paper, the dose-response curve is sigmoid, and the most predictable value is usually around either side of the LD$_{50}$ (Figure 1-1).

The end point of an LD$_{50}$ study is death, and the published LD$_{50}$ value provides no information about severity or characteristics of clinical signs observed in the surviving animals.[2,3,5] Twenty or more animals may be used to arrive at an estimate of the LD$_{50}$, which may limit the use of LD$_{50}$ trials in animals of economic significance. In some species, such as birds and fish, toxicity is often expressed on the basis of the concentration of the substance in air, feed, or water. The acute oral toxicity for birds might be expressed as the LC$_{50}$ (i.e., the lethal concentration for 50% of animals exposed) and may be measured as

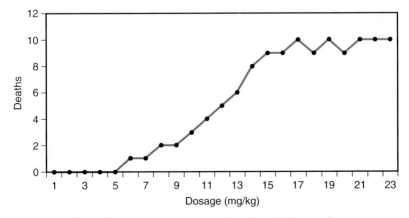

Figure 1-1 Dose-response curve for a typical LD$_{50}$ study.

milligrams of compound per kilogram of the toxic medium (e.g., air, water, feed). For fish, the LC_{50} refers to a concentration of toxicant in the water.

Definition of Response to Toxicant Exposures

Other terms are used in some circumstances (e.g., *safety testing*) to define toxicity of compounds. The highest nontoxic dose, also known as the *no observed adverse effect level,* is the largest dose that does not result in hematologic, chemical, clinical, or pathologic drug-induced alterations. The toxic dose low or the lowest observed adverse effect level is the lowest dose to produce toxicant-induced alterations. The lethal dose low is the lowest dose that causes toxicant-induced deaths in any animal during the period of observation. Various percentages can be attached to the LD value to indicate doses required to kill: 1% (LD_1), 50% (LD_{50}), or 100% (LD_{100}) of the test animals. Another acronym occasionally used is *MTD.* It has been used to note the *maximum tolerated dose* in some situations or *minimal toxic dose.* Thus one should read such abbreviations carefully and look for the specific term defined.

Time Relationships of Poisoning

Acute toxicity is a term usually reserved to mean the effects of a single dose or multiple doses measured during a 24-hour period. If toxic effects become apparent over a period of up to 7 days, it may be considered an acute effect. *Subacute toxicity* may refer to any effects seen between 1 week and 1 month of exposure, whereas *chronic* often refers to effects produced by prolonged exposure of 3 months or longer. The interval between 30 days and 90 days postexposure may be called *subchronic.*

Toxicant Characteristics Can Define Acute or Chronic Response

Duration of exposure to specific toxicants can greatly affect the toxicity. One way to define the effects is the chronicity factor. Chronicity factor is determined by acute LD_{50}/90 day LD_{50}. For warfarin in rats the acute LD_{50} is 1.6 mg/kg, and the 90-day LD_{50} is 0.077 mg/kg, resulting in a ratio of 1.6/0.077, which is a chronicity factor of 21. On the other hand, the single-dose LD_{50} for caffeine in rats is 192 mg/kg and the 90-day LD_{50} is slightly lower at 150 mg/kg, giving an acute to 90-day ratio of 192/150 or 1.3. This demonstrates the chronic or cumulative nature of warfarin versus caffeine.

Animals may also develop tolerance for a compound such that repeated exposure serves to increase the dosage required to produce lethality. The single-dose LD_{50} of potassium cyanide in rats is 10 mg/kg, whereas rats given potassium cyanide for 90 days are able to tolerate a dosage of 250 mg/kg without mortality. Thus cyanide has a very low chronicity factor as a result of tolerance developed with time.

Toxicity Is Different from Risk or Hazard

The concept of *risk* or *hazard* is important to clinical toxicology. Although toxicity defines the amount of a toxicant that produces specific effects at a known dosage, hazard or risk is the probability of poisoning under the conditions of expected exposure or usage. Compounds of high toxicity may still present low hazard or risk if animals are never exposed to the toxicant. For example, ethylene glycol antifreeze is defined as low toxicity (2 to 5 mL/kg body weight), but because it is often readily available in homes, is voluntarily consumed by cats, and is difficult to reverse once clinical signs have developed, it is seen as a high-risk or high-hazard toxicant. By comparison, potassium cyanide is a recognized, very potent poison, but is virtually unavailable in most homes, so risk is low because it is generally not available to pets.

Another way to define risk is to compare the ratio of the lowest toxic or lethal dosage (e.g., the LD_1) with the highest effective dosage, which could be defined as the ED_{99}. The ratio of LD_1/ED_{99} is defined as the standard safety margin, and it is useful for comparing the relative risk of therapeutic drugs, insecticides, anthelmintics, and other agents applied to animals for their beneficial effects.[2,5] For a therapeutic drug or animal insecticide, if the LD_1 is 10 mg/kg and the ED_{99} is 1 mg/kg, then the safety margin is 10 and the likely lethal effect is much higher than the probable use level.

If all animals in an LD_{50} study were the same, then the LD_{50} would actually be a standard toxic dosage for all animals. However, at the same LD_{50} dosage, not exactly 50% of animals will die each time. This biologic variation can be due to many factors, and veterinary clinicians must exercise judgment about the response of animals to a given toxicant.

Even more variability is expected because of the differences in species, age, body size, route of exposure, inherent differences in metabolism, and pregnancy and lactation effects. Remember also that the slope of the LD_{50} curve is important and is not revealed from the LD_{50} value alone. An LD_{50} with a very steep dose-response slope indicates a toxicant or drug has a very narrow margin between no effects and maximal lethal effects.[3,5] Although such compounds may be dangerous to use as therapeutics, they could be very effective pesticides because of lower probability of survival of target animals.

Factors That Influence Toxicity

Many factors inherent in the toxicant, the animal, or the environment can alter a toxicity value determined under defined experimental conditions. The toxicity of a compound varies with the route of exposure. Usual routes of exposure are oral, dermal, nasal, intravenous, intraperitoneal, and subcutaneous. In addition, the most potent routes of exposure are usually the intravenous, intrapulmonary, and intraperitoneal routes. In clinical veterinary toxicology oral and dermal routes of exposure are the most common, and these routes generally delay the absorption and diffuse exposure over a longer period. A daily dosage of toxicant mixed in food and consumed over a 24-hour period may cause much less effect than that same dosage given as a bolus at one specific time. However, retention in the gastrointestinal tract, including enterohepatic cycling, and dermal or hair retention of poisons can significantly prolong the exposure or exposures.[2,3,5] Another factor that can accentuate the toxic effects of a compound is concurrent organ damage as a result of other causes. This is most important for diseases that alter liver or kidney function, leaving the animal with insufficient resources to metabolize and excrete toxicants. Chapter 2 deals with the important aspects of biotransformation, excretion, and toxicodynamics that greatly influence toxicity of many chemicals.

Species and breed differences exert important influences on toxicity. The familiar example of cats and their intolerance to phenolic compounds results directly from their limited glucuronyl transferase activity, which is necessary to produce glucuronides for the excretion of phenolic metabolites. A common example is acetaminophen, which is quite toxic to cats partly as a result of ineffective excretion of the toxic metabolite. In addition, the amino acid and sulfhydryl content of feline hemoglobin and a relative lack of methemoglobin reductase in erythrocytes makes it more susceptible to oxidant damage caused by the acetaminophen metabolite. As a result, the cat is more likely to be poisoned by agents that induce methemoglobinemia.[5] Occasional differences within a species can increase the probability of toxicosis. The anthelmintic ivermectin provides an example of breed susceptibility differences, with collies and individuals in other herding breeds being genetically more susceptible than most other breeds.

Many environmental and physiologic factors can influence the toxicity of compounds, and one should remember that such factors, or possibly other unknown factors, can substantially influence an individual's response to toxicants. Entire publications are devoted to drug and chemical interactions, and the reader is encouraged to be aware of toxicologic interactions that are illustrated throughout this text. Some examples of factors that alter response to toxicants are presented in Table 1-2.

Biologic Variation and Toxicity Data in Veterinary Practice

Biologic variation is a significant factor in interpretation of clinical and diagnostic data used in toxicology. A single toxicity figure will not define the range of toxicity and effects in a given population. Because LD_{50} or other values are usually defined in very similar animals (e.g., laboratory rats and laboratory beagles), the laboratory toxicity figure does not reflect the biologic variation and differences in toxicity that may occur in a diverse group of breeds within the canine or any other species. For animals of veterinary importance, there

Table 1-2	Factors That May Alter Response to Toxicants
Alteration or Change	**Mechanism or Example**
Impurities or contaminants	Recently melamine and cyanuric acid contaminants in cat food caused renal failure. For dogs, aflatoxin contaminated corn in dog foods has caused bleeding and liver failure.
Changes in chemical composition or salts of inorganic agents	Toxicity of metals may be altered by valence state. Trivalent arsenicals are much more toxic than pentavalent arsenic. Specific salts also alter toxicity (e.g., barium carbonate is cardiotoxic, whereas barium sulfate is insoluble and nearly nontoxic).
Instability or decomposition of chemical	Some organophosphate insecticides under adverse storage conditions can decompose to form more toxic degradation products. Zinc phosphide rodenticide decomposes rapidly to release highly toxic phosphine gas.
Ionization	Generally, dependent on pH and pKa, compounds that are highly ionized in the stomach (e.g., strychnine) are poorly absorbed and thus less toxic.
Vehicle effects	Nonpolar and lipid-soluble vehicles usually increase toxicity of toxicants by promoting absorption and membrane penetration. Examples are petroleum products and highly volatile hydrocarbons.
Protein binding	Binding to serum albumin is common for many drugs and toxicants, limiting the bioavailability of the agent and reducing toxicity. Agents displaced from protein binding (e.g., vitamin K responsive anticoagulants) enhance toxicity by allowing more freely available toxicants.
Chemical or drug interactions	Chemicals may directly bind, inactivate, or potentiate one another. One chemical may also induce microsomal enzymes to influence the metabolism of another. Barbiturate drugs stimulate metabolic activation of many toxicants to a more toxic metabolite.
Biotransformation*	Prior exposure to the same or similar chemical may induce increased metabolic activity of microsomal MFOs. Foreign compounds activated by MFOs can then be conjugated by phase II metabolism and be excreted. If toxicants are activated by MFO activity, toxicity may be increased. Liver disease, very young or very old animals, and specific breeds or strains of animal can be factors that lead to altered ability of MFO to begin metabolism followed by phase II detoxification of foreign compounds.
Liver disease	Reduced synthesis of glutathione, metallothionein, and coagulation factors may alter response to acetaminophen, cadmium, and anticoagulant rodenticides, respectively.
Nutrition and diet	Natural dietary compounds, such as calcium and zinc, may affect absorption and response to lead. Vitamin C and vitamin E can aid in scavenging of free radicals and repair of cellular protective mechanisms.

MFO, Mixed function oxidase.
*See Chapter 2 for details on biotransformation.

is usually insufficient information on the variability of effects from low or moderate exposures. Furthermore, individual environmental and husbandry conditions vary widely and can affect the severity of response in any particular group of animals for a specific toxicant and dosage. Therefore thorough clinical and environmental investigation and good laboratory diagnostic procedures are essential to toxicologic evaluation in a suspected exposure.

Calculations for Toxicology

As indicated earlier, the basis for toxicologic effects is the dosage versus response relationship. In a practical clinical situation, the dosage is often not defined. Rather, an animal is ill with clinical signs that suggest toxicosis, and there is potential exposure to a known or suspected amount of poison that is probably at some concentration less than 100% in a commercial product or natural source. Alternatively, the animal owner may have seen an exposure, such as an animal consuming some tablets or a potential toxicant such as chocolate. Sometimes animals with subacute or chronic signs are suspected of consuming some toxicant in the food. Analysis of a food may reveal a concentration in parts per million (ppm), mg/kg, mcg/g, or percentage, and the concentration in the food must be related to a known toxicity based on milligrams per kilogram of body weight. In all these circumstances, the veterinary clinician must first relate a probable amount of toxicant to a body weight dosage and then decide if detoxification therapy or antidotal treatment is necessary. If dosage is low, careful observation with no treatment may be a valid option. Thus the clinician should investigate the probable dosage as part of the decision process for whether therapy or observation is more appropriate.

The ability to accurately convert numbers relating to concentration and dosage and to convert different expressions of exposure or concentration is essential to the practice of medicine, and is equally important in clinical toxicology. The principles of dosage and calculations practiced in pharmacology and therapeutics are similar to those used in toxicology. Of particular importance in toxicology is the need to differentiate between and convert different expressions of concentration as stated on labels or obtained from laboratory analysis. The toxicologist is further challenged to correlate the level of contamination in food, water, or baits to the clinical signs observed in a suspected poisoning. The following examples are intended to clarify some of these calculations and to show how they are used in clinical toxicology.

Table 1-3	Common Comparative and Equivalent Values in Veterinary Toxicology	
Expression or Measurement	**Equivalent Value**
1 ppm	1 mg/kg or 1 mg/L
1 ppm	1 µg/g or 1 µg/mL or 1 mcg/g or 1 mcg/mL
1 ppm	0.0001%
1 ppm	1000 ppb
1 ppm	1,000,000 ppt
1 ppb	0.000001%
1 ppb	1 ng/g
1 ppb	1 µg/kg or 1 mcg/kg
1%	10,000 ppm
(Convert % to ppm by moving decimal point four places to the right)	
1 mg/dL	10 ppm or 10 mg/L
1 ounce	28.35 g
1 pound	453.6 g
1 kg	2.205 lb
1 liter	0.908 qt
1 gallon	3.785 L
1 teaspoon	5 mL
1 tablespoon	15 mL
1 cup	8 oz or 227 mL
1 quart	32 oz or 946 mL

Concentration and Dosage in Veterinary Toxicology

The amount of a toxic agent in feed, water, baits, and solutions is often expressed as a weight/weight relationship (e.g., g/ton, mg/kg, mcg/g), as a weight/volume relationship (e.g., mg/mL, mg/dL, mg/L), or as a proportion of the toxicant to the total medium in which it is held, such as percentage, ppm, parts per billion (ppb), and parts per trillion (ppt). For correct toxicologic evaluation, one must understand the relationships among these expressions. Relationships and equivalencies of common expressions of concentration useful in calculations and interpretation for veterinary toxicology are shown in Table 1-3.

In addition, the clinician may find toxicity data expressed as milligrams per kilogram body weight of animal (dosage), but may receive a label or statement of analysis that expresses the feed, water, or bait concentration as proportional or as weight/weight relationships (concentration). The accurate assessment of toxicologic risk depends on the ability to convert different toxicologic expressions to an equivalent common denominator.

One common clinical situation is the need to convert a feed or bait concentration to body weight basis toxicity. The following clinical problem illustrates this calculation.

Clinical Problem 1   Is This a Toxic Exposure? If the acute toxicity of cholecalciferol rodenticide is 2000 mcg/kg of body weight and the bait concentration is 0.075%, is a 1-oz package of bait likely to be toxic to a 70-lb German shepherd that consumes the entire package at one time?

Solution
To evaluate this risk, one must know or assume the following:
- Amount of food or bait consumed (1 oz)
- Weight of the animal at risk (70 lb)
- Concentration of toxicant in the food or bait (0.75%)

In this case, first convert as much as possible to the metric system:
- 70-lb dog/(2.2 lb/kg) = 31.8 kg
- 0.075% is 750 mg cholecalciferol/kg or 0.75 mg cholecalciferol/g of bait
- One ounce of bait × 28.35 g/oz = 28.35 g bait

Thus total consumption of cholecalciferol is expressed as:
- 28.35 g bait × (0.75 mg cholecalciferol/g bait) = 21.26 mg cholecalciferol consumed
- 21.26 mg cholecalciferol/31.8-kg dog = 0.67 mg/kg or 670 mcg/kg body weight

Thus toxic dosage is not consumed.

From the calculations, it is apparent that this exposure would cause a low risk of toxicosis from cholecalciferol.

If the concentration of vitamin D in a complete pet food is known or assumed, one may also need to calculate the potential for toxicosis based on feed contamination.

Clinical Problem 2   Is There a Cumulative Toxic Exposure? Continuing cholecalciferol to another example, assume that vitamin D at 2000 IU/kg body weight/day for 1 to 2 weeks can cause subacute toxicosis to dogs. If a dog food were accidentally fortified with a concentration of 1000 IU/lb, would long-term consumption likely result in toxicosis in a 35-lb dog?

Solution
In this case, the needed information is expanded from Clinical Problem 1, because we do not know the amount of contaminated material consumed. Also, convert components to the same system (metric units).
- From current knowledge: food intake for a 35-lb dog is 2.5% of body weight.
- Convert a 35-lb dog to kg (i.e., 35 lb ÷ [2.2 lb/kg]) = 15.9 kg; 15.9 kg × 0.025 = 0.3975 kg [amount ingested].
- Vitamin D in feed at 1000 IU/lb: 1000 IU/lb × 2.2 lb/kg = 2200 IU/kg of feed.
- Daily total vitamin D intake = 0.3975 kg/day × (2200 IU/kg feed) = 874.5 IU/day.
- Dosage to the 15.9-kg dog = 874.5 IU/day/15.9 kg = 55 IU/kg/day: Body weight dosage.

Daily body weight dosage at 55 IU/kg is far below the toxic dosage of 2000 IU/kg body weight/day.

In this clinical example, the daily dosage of 55 IU/kg on a body weight basis is approximately twice the recommended requirement but far below the known toxicity of 2000 IU/kg.

Small animal toxicants may sometimes be expressed in blood or body fluids by different units. Most common are ppm, milligrams per deciliter (mg/dL), and milliequivalents per liter (mEq/L). If laboratory results are given in one of these units, but toxicity information is available to the clinician in different units, the ability to convert to comparable units is essential to interpretation. Clinical Problem 3 illustrates this conversion.

Clinical Problem 3   Converting Laboratory Values from ppm to mEq/L In a dog exhibiting neurologic signs and a suspected salt toxicosis, toxicology laboratory results are returned indicating a serum sodium value of 4320 ppm. Expected normal values in your practice are 135 to 145 mEq/L. Is the laboratory analysis indicative of hypernatremia suggesting salt toxicosis?

Solution
In this case, it is necessary to convert the laboratory analysis results to mEq/L for interpretation. There is a common formula for converting mg/dL to mEq/L. To use this formula, do the following:
- Convert ppm to mg/dL.
- Because 1 ppm = 1 mg/L, and 1 mg/dL = 10 mg/L, then dividing ppm by 10 = mg/dL (4320 ppm divided by 10 = 432 mg/dL).
- mEq/L = mg/dL × valence × 10/atomic weight = 432 × 1 × 10/23 = 187.8 mEq/L.

Result provides laboratory confirmation of hypernatremia.

Clinical Problem 3 illustrates the tenfold difference between ppm and mg/dL (1 mg/dL = 10 ppm) and shows that to convert from mg/dL to mEq/L one must know the valence and atomic weight of specific toxicants or metals.

Toxicoses, although difficult clinical problems, can best be managed by using basic principles and calculations to estimate probable exposure to toxicants and the factors that may alter those responses. Adding to this knowledge of the systemic and medical effects of toxicants and the principles of antidotal and detoxification therapy should result in the best possible outcome in response to small animal toxicoses.

Clinical Problem 4   Owners Suspect Acute Aflatoxicosis—Is It Likely? A reported LD_{50} for aflatoxin in dogs is 0.80 mg/kg of body weight. If a beagle dog is exposed to aflatoxin at 200 ppb on a continuing basis, will the toxic dosage be exceeded?

Solution
In this scenario, the toxic body weight dosage must be compared against risk from a known or presumed concentration in the diet. The body weight dosage must be converted to a dietary concentration. In addition, remember the principle that dietary dosage is affected by the amount of food consumed. No weight was given for the dog, but it is a beagle, so one can assume a weight of 22 lb for purposes of calculation.
- First, convert all weights to the metric system. A 22-lb beagle can reasonably be assumed to weigh 10 kg (22 lb/2.2 kg).
- Next, estimate the food intake of the beagle. As in Clinical Problem 2, a reasonable intake is 2.5% of body weight daily.
- Calculate food ingested daily: 10 kg × 0.025 = 0.25 kg food.
- Calculate the amount of aflatoxin in 0.25 kg food: 200 ppb = 200 mg/kg = 0.2 mg/kg or 0.2 ppm; at 0.2 mg/kg × 0.25 kg the food consumed contains 0.05 mg aflatoxin.

- Calculate the dosage of aflatoxin in mg/kg of body weight: 0.05 mg/10 kg body weight = 0.005 mg/kg.
- Alternatively, a formula to convert ppm to mg/kg of body weight is:

$$\text{mg/kg BW} = \frac{\text{ppm in feed} \times \text{kg feed eaten}}{\text{body wt in kg}}$$

$$\text{mg/kg BW} = \frac{0.20 \text{ mg/kg} \times 0.25 \text{ kg}}{10 \text{ kg}} = 0.005 \text{ mg/kg BW}$$

Conclusion: 200 ppb (0.2 ppm) dietary aflatoxin is not an LD_{50} dosage of aflatoxin.

Clinical Problem 5   Express the following concentrations in ppm and in percent

Combination Mixture	Concentration (%)	Concentration (ppm)
a. 17 ounces in 12 liters	4.19	41990
b. 0.25 quarts in 56 gallons	0.1116	1116
c. 9.27 grams in 1 kilogram	0.927	9270
d. 30 lb premix in 2 tons of dog food	0.75	750
e. 34 ounces in 200 gallons	0.1328	1328
f. 54 mg caffeine in 12 oz Mountain Dew	0.0152	152

Solutions

a. Convert to percentage by making a ratio in the same units. (Note: There are 33.81 ounces/L.) Then convert ratio to % and % to ppm (moving decimal 4 places right):

$$\frac{17 \text{ oz}}{12 \text{ L} \times 33.81 \text{ oz/L}} = \frac{17 \text{ oz}}{405 \text{ oz}} = \underset{\text{Ratio}}{0.0419} \text{ ratio} = \underset{\%}{4.19\%} = \underset{\text{ppm}}{41{,}990} \text{ ppm}$$

b. Create ratio in same units (e.g., quarts, then use [ratio × 100 = %] and [% × 4 decimals right]:

$$\frac{0.25 \text{ qt}}{56 \text{ gal} \times 4 \text{ qt/gal}} = \frac{0.25 \text{ qt}}{224 \text{ qt}} = 0.001116 = 0.1116\% = 1116 \text{ ppm}$$

c. 9.27 g in 1 kg (first convert both terms to grams):

$$\frac{9.27 \text{ g}}{1 \text{ kg} \times 1000 \text{ g/kg}} = \frac{9.27}{1000} = 0.00927 = 0.927\% = 9270 \text{ ppm}$$

d. 30 lb of premix in 2 tons of dog food (first convert all terms to pounds, and then calculate ratio, percent, and ppm):

$$\frac{30 \text{ lb premix}}{2 \text{ tons dog food}} = \frac{30 \text{ lb premix}}{4000 \text{ lb food}} = 0.0075 = 0.75\% = 750 \text{ ppm}$$

e. 34 ounces in 200 gallons:

$$\frac{34 \text{ oz}}{200 \text{ gal} \times 128 \text{ oz/gal}} = \frac{34}{25{,}600} = 0.001328 = 0.1328\% = 1328 \text{ ppm}$$

f. 54 mg caffeine in 12 oz soda (convert ounces to milliliters, then grams, then milligrams):

$$\frac{54\ mg}{12\ oz \times 29.6\ mL/oz} = \frac{54\ mg}{355.2\ mL \times 1\ g/mL} = \frac{54\ mg}{355.2\ g \times 1000\ mg/g} = \frac{54\ mg}{355,200\ mg}$$
$$= ratio\ of\ 0.000152113 = 0.0152\% = 152\ ppm$$

• **Quick Guide** Figure 1-2 provides a range of body weight dosages and food consumption for quick reference in estimating equivalent ppm concentrations in the diet without using calculations. Remember that as a higher proportion of food is consumed relative to body weight, then the same dietary concentration will cause increasing dosage of the toxicant per unit of body weight.

		ppm toxicant in diet					
		1	10	50	100	500	1000
% BW Consumed	1	0.01	0.1	0.5	1	5	10
	2	0.02	0.2	1	2	10	20
	3	0.03	0.3	1.5	3	15	30
	4	0.04	0.4	2	4	20	40
	5	0.05	0.5	2.5	5	25	50
	10	0.1	1	5	10	50	100

Equivalent body weight dosage (mg/kg)

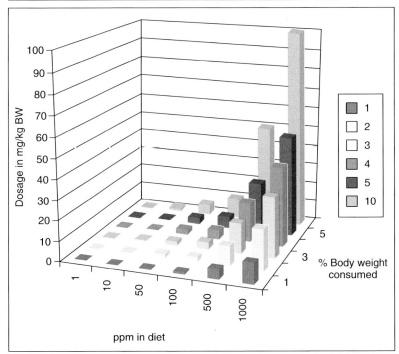

Figure 1-2 Relationships of food intake and body weight dosage.

References

1. Beasley VR, Dorman DC, Fikes JD, Diana SG, Woshner V: *A systems affected approach to veterinary toxicology*, Urbana, Ill, 1999, University of Illinois.
2. Eaton DL, Gilbert SG: Principles of toxicology. In Klassen CD, editor: *Casarette and Doull's toxicology: the basic science of poisons*, ed 7, New York, 2008, McGraw-Hill, pp 11–43.
3. Osweiler GD, Carson TL, Buck WB, Van Gelder GA: *Clinical and diagnostic veterinary toxicology*, ed 3, Dubuque, Iowa, 1985, Kendall Hunt, pp. 3–26.
4. Stine KE, Brown TM: *Principles of toxicology*, ed 2, Boca Raton, 2006, CRC Press: Taylor & Francis Group, pp. 1–13.
5. Osweiler GD: *Toxicology. The National Veterinary Medical Series*, Philadelphia, 1996, Williams & Wilkins, pp. 1–16.

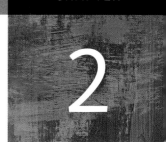

Toxicokinetics and Toxicodynamics

Tim J. Evans, DVM, MS, PhD, DACT, DABVT

Definitions

The basic concepts regarding the toxicokinetics and toxicodynamics of xenobiotics are clinically relevant to veterinary toxicology and need to be understood by veterinary practitioners, professional students, and other personnel who will be participating in the diagnosis and treatment of small animal intoxications. In discussing the aspects of toxicokinetics and toxicodynamics most pertinent to small animal toxicoses, it is first necessary to define several terms. *Xenobiotic* is a general term referring to any chemical foreign to an organism or, in other words, any compound not occurring within the normal metabolic pathways of a biologic system.[1,2] Depending on the compound and the level of exposure, interactions between xenobiotics and animals can be benign, therapeutic, or toxic in nature. The pharmacokinetics and pharmacodynamics of a therapeutic xenobiotic influence the time course and efficacy of that compound in a pharmacologic setting. Likewise, the toxicokinetics and toxicodynamics of a toxic xenobiotic determine the "when," "how long," "what," and "why" for the adverse effects of that toxicant.[2]

The *disposition* of a xenobiotic is what the animal's body does to that compound following exposure. The disposition or fate of a xenobiotic within the body consists of the chemical's absorption, distribution, metabolism (biotransformation), and excretion characteristics (ADME).[2,3] *Toxicokinetics* refers to the quantitation and determination of the time course of the disposition or ADME for a given toxic xenobiotic.[3] There are a variety of specialized toxicokinetic terms, including *bioavailability, volume of distribution (V_d), clearance, half-life, one-compartment model,* and *first-* and *zero-order kinetics,* which are discussed later in this chapter under the separate components of ADME.

The term *toxicodynamics* describes what a toxicant does physiologically, biochemically, and molecularly to an animal's body following exposure. The toxicodynamics of a given toxic xenobiotic depend on the mechanism of action of that toxicant and the relationship between toxicant concentration and the observed effects of the toxicant on biologic processes in the animal (i.e., the dose-response relationship).[1] The disposition and toxicokinetics of a particular xenobiotic also play a role in determining the organs or tissues affected by a toxicant, and the clinical presentation and time course of a toxicosis resulting from excessive exposure to that compound.[1,2]

Toxicokinetics and Disposition

Xenobiotic Absorption

With the exception of caustic and corrosive toxicants that cause adverse effects at the site of exposure, a toxic xenobiotic is generally first "absorbed" or taken up into the body.[3] Absorption involves crossing cellular membranes, which are typically composed of phospholipid bilayers containing various sized pores and embedded proteins.[2] The route of exposure and physiochemical properties of a toxicant, such as its resemblance to endogenous compounds, its molecular size and relative lipid and water solubilities, the magnitude of a molecule's association constant, and whether a compound can be classified as a weak acid or as a weak base, all determine the manner and quantities in which a xenobiotic is absorbed across cell membranes.

Routes of Xenobiotic Exposure and Xenobiotic Bioavailability

The most common routes of exposure for xenobiotics in small animal toxicology are oral (gastrointestinal), dermal (percutaneous), and inhalation (pulmonary). In rare instances of iatrogenic intoxications, xenobiotics can be injected subcutaneously, intramuscularly, intra-peritoneally, or even intravenously.[3] There are unique aspects to the absorption of xenobiot-ics associated with each route of exposure, especially with regard to the bioavailability of potential toxicants.

Bioavailability (often represented by *F* in toxicokinetic equations) represents the fraction of the total dose of a toxic xenobiotic that is actually absorbed by an animal.[2] In intravenous exposures, the bioavailability of a toxic xenobiotic is 100% because the entire dose of the toxicant reaches the peripheral circulation. The absorption of gases and vapors in the respi-ratory tract largely depends on the ratio (blood-to-gas partition coefficient) between the equilibrium concentrations of the toxicant dissolved in the blood and the gaseous phase of the toxicant in the alveolar spaces.[2,3] The size of aerosolized particles determines to a large degree whether a xenobiotic is deposited in the nasopharyngeal region (particles >5 μm) or within the alveoli of the lungs (<1 μm).[2] The stratum corneum and its associated keratinized structures often impede the percutaneous absorption of xenobiotics, and there are varia-tions in the absorptive ability of skin in different anatomic locations.[4] Dermal absorption frequently depends on the vehicle in which a toxicant is dissolved and is generally greater for lipid-soluble compounds as compared with chemicals that are highly soluble in water.[2-4] The bioavailability of toxic xenobiotics that are ingested can be negatively affected by acidic degradation in the stomach and enzymatic breakdown in the small intestine.[2] Decreased gastrointestinal transit time can diminish xenobiotic bioavailability by limiting the access of toxicants to those regions of the digestive tract where rates of absorption are greatest. Some potential toxicants, especially certain heavy metals (e.g., lead and cadmium), resemble essential minerals such as calcium and zinc, respectively. The gastrointestinal absorption of these toxic nonessential metals involves interactions with dietary levels of the correspond-ing essential metals and regulated mechanisms of gastrointestinal uptake designed for these required minerals.

Hepatic biotransformation of xenobiotics, which is discussed in greater detail later in this chapter, can also influence the apparent bioavailability of ingested toxicants. Following oral exposure, xenobiotics absorbed from the gastrointestinal tract are transported to the liver via the hepatic portal circulation. For some xenobiotics, rapid hepatic degradation (and in some instances prior biotransformation in gastrointestinal cells) prevents access of the compound to the systemic circulation, resulting in an apparently decreased bioavail-ability from what is termed the *first-pass effect* or *presystemic elimination*.[3,4] In contrast, the bioavailability of some chemicals is enhanced by a cycle of biliary excretion and subsequent reuptake from the intestines referred to as *enterohepatic recirculation*.[4]

Mechanisms of Xenobiotic Absorption

The passage of xenobiotics through cellular membranes can be either energy-independent (passive transport) or can require the expenditure of energy through specialized or active transport systems. Passive transport of xenobiotics can be accomplished through simple diffusion or filtration. Specialized, energy-dependent, cellular transport systems include the process specifically referred to as *active transport*, along with facilitated transport and pinocytosis.[2,3]

Passive Transport of Xenobiotics

Simple diffusion and filtration are nonsaturable processes, which do not require the expen-diture of energy to transport xenobiotics across cellular membranes.[2,3] Both of these mech-anisms of passive transport depend on the concentration gradient for a given xenobiotic, with the rate of transport being proportional to the difference in that chemical's concentration between the two sides of a particular membrane (Fick's law).[2] Simple diffusion is the most common mechanism by which xenobiotics cross cellular membranes. Uncharged (nonionized), lipid-soluble molecules, especially small molecules, are more readily diffusible across the phospholipid bilayers of biologic membranes than charged (ionized) molecules, which are generally less lipid-soluble.[2,3] The Henderson-Hasselbalch equation can be used to predict whether a particular xenobiotic will be in the nonionized or ionized state in a particular biologic matrix. In this equation, the difference between the association constant (pKa), which is equivalent to the pH at which equal amounts of a xenobiotic are in the nonionized and ionized states, and the pH of the biologic matrix in which the xenobiotic will exist (i.e., pKa – pH) is equal to the common log of the quotient of nonionized xenobiotic divided by ionized xenobiotic for weak acids and the log of the reciprocal quotient (ionized xenobiotic divided by nonionized xenobiotic) for weak bases.[2-4] Filtration involves the passage of xenobiotics through patencies or pores within cellular membranes and is determined, in large part, by the size of the xenobiotic molecule and pore size, which varies in different organs and tissues.[2]

Specialized Transport of Xenobiotics

Active transport is an energy-dependent, saturable process by which xenobiotics are transported across biologic membranes against electrochemical or concentration gradients.[2-4] Specific examples of active transport systems include the ABCB transporters (P-glycoproteins) and members of the organic cation transporter family.[3] Facilitated or carrier-mediated transport can require the expenditure of energy, but, in contrast to active transport, xenobiotic transport by this mechanism is not against a concentration gradient.[2,3] Pinocytotic transport involves cellular engulfment of small amounts of xenobiotics and the transfer of this amount of chemical through the cellular membrane.[2]

Xenobiotic Distribution

Distribution refers to the translocation of a xenobiotic from the site of absorption to various body organs and tissues and involves both transport of the chemical within the circulation and cellular uptake of the xenobiotic.[1-3] The rate of xenobiotic transfer into a particular organ or tissue is determined by the physiochemical properties of the specific xenobiotic (e.g., lipid solubility and molecular weight), the blood flow to the organs or tissues in question, and the rate of diffusion of the xenobiotic across the endothelial walls of the capillary bed into cells within a particular organ or tissue.[2-4] The V_d for a given xenobiotic represents the quotient of the total amount of that chemical in the body divided by the concentration of the xenobiotic within the blood, and is used to describe the extent to which a xenobiotic is distributed within the body.[2,4] The V_d is a clinically relevant indicator as to whether a chemical is primarily contained within the plasma compartment (relatively low V_d) or whether a compound is widely distributed throughout the body within the interstitial or intracellular compartments of various organs and tissues (relatively high V_d).[2,3]

Xenobiotic Storage Depots

Xenobiotics can be stored within a variety of different body organs and tissues. Depending on the anatomic and physiologic relationships between the storage depot and the target organs and tissues for a specific toxicant, storage of toxic xenobiotics can function as either a protective mechanism or as a means by which the toxic effects of a xenobiotic are potentiated. An understanding of the storage sites of toxic xenobiotics can provide additional insight about circumstances that would be expected to exacerbate a particular toxicosis, and can indicate which organs or tissues would be expected to have the highest concentrations for diagnostic sampling. Plasma proteins represent a storage site for many xenobiotics (e.g., salicylates, barbiturates, cardiac glycosides) and important physiologic constituents, including steroid hormones, vitamins, and various essential minerals.[3] Displacement of toxic xenobiotics from plasma proteins can greatly increase the amount of unbound toxicant distributed to target organs or tissue.[3,4] A wide variety of xenobiotics accumulate in the liver and kidneys, making these organs ideal sites for postmortem sample collection in cases of suspected toxicoses.[3] Some toxic metals, such as cadmium, accumulate in the liver and kidneys because of the high endogenous concentrations and induction of metallothionein in these organs. Fat and bone are storage depots for a variety of different xenobiotics, and rapid depletion of body fat stores (weight loss) or increased remodeling of bone during growth or pregnancy have the potential to increase the exposure of target organs or tissue to previously stored toxicants.[3,4]

Potential Tissue Barriers to Xenobiotic Distribution

The blood-brain barrier is frequently mentioned in the current literature with regard to its ability to limit exposure of the central nervous system (CNS) to toxic xenobiotics.[3] Other potential barriers to chemical uptake also occur in the eyes, testes, prostate, joints, and placenta. In these instances only small, nonionized, lipid-soluble molecules are able to cross the membranes and gain access to potential target tissues.[4]

The blood-brain barrier to xenobiotic uptake consists of the relatively nonporous CNS capillary endothelium, which contains multidrug-resistant protein and is surrounded for the most part by glial cells.[3,4] The extremely low protein content of the interstitial fluid within the CNS also contributes to the apparent inability of many protein-bound, toxic xenobiotics to reach clinically relevant concentrations in the brain.[3] Because the blood-brain barrier is not fully formed at birth and is less well-developed in some breeds of dogs (e.g., collies and collie crosses), immature animals and collie-related breeds are more susceptible to the adverse effects of compounds normally blocked by the blood-brain barrier.[3,5]

Xenobiotic Metabolism and Biotransformation

The term *metabolism* can be used to refer to the fate or disposition of a xenobiotic or the sum total of the chemical transformations of normal body constituents, which occur in living organisms.[1,6] *Biotransformation,* on the other hand, is a general term referring to the metabolic conversion of both endogenous and xenobiotic chemicals into more water-soluble forms.[6] For the purposes of this chapter, xenobiotic *metabolism* and *biotransformation* are synonymous and refer to the generally two-phase process by which chemicals are converted to more water-soluble forms for excretion from the body.[1,2] In xenobiotic metabolism or biotransformation, the lipophilic (lipid-soluble) properties of xenobiotics that favor absorption are biotransformed into physiochemical characteristics (hydrophilicity or water solubility) that predispose compounds to excretion in the urine or feces.[6] Although multiple organs within the body have biotransformation capabilities, most xenobiotics are biotransformed in the liver.[2,6]

Phase I and Phase II Xenobiotic Biotransformation

Xenobiotics are usually biotransformed in two phases (I and II), which involve enzymes having broad substrate specificity.[2,6] Phase I reactions generally involve oxidation, hydrolysis, or reduction, and convert apolar, lipophilic xenobiotics into metabolites, which have greater polarity and hydrophilicity.[2] In these instances, hydroxyl, amino, carboxyl, or thiol moieties are usually either exposed or added to increase water solubility.[6] Oxidation reactions, especially those catalyzed by cytochrome P450 enzymes, are the phase I biotransformations most commonly involved in xenobiotic metabolism, and many xenobiotics are able to induce cytochrome P450 activity.[2,5,6] During phase II biotransformation, the xenobiotic or its metabolites are conjugated with a functional group (e.g., glucuronide, sulfate, amino acids, glutathione, or acyl or methyl groups), resulting in a compound with dramatically increased water solubility.[2,6] Not all mammalian species have equal phase II biotransformation capabilities, and the inability of domestic cats to biotransform glucuronidate xenobiotics is especially clinically relevant to veterinary toxicologists.[2,5]

Most xenobiotic biotransformations result in less toxic metabolites. However, there are xenobiotics (e.g., acetaminophen and aflatoxin B_1) for which the products of hepatic phase I metabolism are actually more toxic than the parent xenobiotic.[2,5] In these instances of metabolic activation, bioactivation, toxication, or lethal synthesis, any factors that increase hepatic biotransformation of the parent compound enhance the amount of toxic metabolite to which the animal is exposed.[5,7]

Xenobiotic Excretion

The final step in the disposition of a xenobiotic is excretion, whereby the xenobiotic or its metabolites are removed from the body via a number of different routes.[2] Renal excretion is the most common means by which xenobiotics and the products of their biotransformation are eliminated from the body, but toxicants can also be excreted in the feces (biliary excretion or elimination of unabsorbed xenobiotic), saliva, sweat, cerebrospinal fluid, or even the milk, which is clinically relevant in xenobiotic-exposed bitches or queens nursing offspring.[2,3,5] In instances of exposures to toxic vapors or volatile xenobiotics, exhalation can also be a major route of elimination from the body.[2,3] Xenobiotics and their metabolites can be excreted by more than one route of elimination, and the total excretion is generally broken down into renal and nonrenal routes.

Toxicokinetic Aspects of Xenobiotic Elimination

With regard to toxicokinetics, *elimination* of a xenobiotic generally incorporates both the processes of biotransformation and excretion.[2,8] *Clearance,* which is expressed for the whole body and individual organs in terms of the volume of blood that is cleared of the chemical per unit time, is an indicator of the body's ability to eliminate a given toxicant from the body by processes such as metabolism, excretion, and exhalation.[1,2,8] The toxicokinetic aspects of xenobiotic elimination are clinically relevant to the management and diagnosis of veterinary toxicoses. These quantitative indices can be used to predict the duration of a toxicosis and the period necessary for therapeutic intervention. Toxicokinetic aspects of xenobiotic elimination can also be used to determine the time frame and biologic samples that are best suited for diagnosing a specific toxicosis.

When developing toxicokinetic models, assumptions are often made with regard to whether a given xenobiotic best fits a *one-compartment* or a *multicompartment* model. A one-compartment model is the simplest toxicokinetic model and assumes that changes in xenobiotic concentrations in the blood or plasma are accurate reflections of what is occurring in the tissues.[2] Assuming that a one-compartment model is appropriate for a particular xenobiotic, elimination of this compound is most likely via first-order kinetics, in which the involved processes are most likely nonsaturable and the rate of elimination at any given time point is proportional to the amount of compound that remains in the body at that point in time.[2,4,8] With first-order kinetics in a one-compartment model, it is possible to calculate the elimination half-life of a xenobiotic using the V_d and the clearance for a given xenobiotic.[8] In this instance, *half-life* indicates the time required for the blood or plasma concentration of the xenobiotic to be reduced by one half, with approximately 97% of a xenobiotic being eliminated from the circulation in five half-lives.[5,8] The term *half-life* can also be used in terms of elimination of xenobiotic from body storage depots rather than from the blood or plasma.[5] It is important to know the context in which this particular term is being used and the compartmental model involved to understand what process in the xenobiotic's disposition is actually being discussed.

There are some xenobiotics for which the processes involved in their elimination are saturable and the rate of elimination is independent of the amount of chemical remaining in the body at a given point of time.[2,8] Under these circumstances, the pathways of elimination for a given xenobiotic can be described in terms of zero order kinetics. Only a finite amount of xenobiotic can be eliminated per unit time.

Toxicodynamics

Interactions between Xenobiotic Toxicodynamics and Disposition or Toxicokinetics

In contrast to toxicokinetics, the toxicodynamics of a particular xenobiotic describe what that compound actually does to adversely affect an animal's health rather than how the animal handles the exogenous chemical. However, a xenobiotic's toxicodynamics and toxicokinetics are not mutually exclusive. What a toxicant does physiologically, biochemically, and molecularly to a living organism following exposure not only depends on that xenobiotic's mechanism of action and its dose-response relationship, but also on its disposition or toxicokinetics within an exposed animal.[1,2]

The first step in the development of a toxicosis is the delivery of the "ultimate toxicant" to its site of action or "target."[7] *Ultimate toxicant* refers to the parent xenobiotic, its metabolite, or even a generated reactive oxygen species that actually causes cellular damage. The term *target* is often used to describe a molecule that interacts with the ultimate toxicant, resulting in adversely affected biologic processes within an organism. *Targets* can also be an inclusive term referring to the cell types, organs, or tissues most susceptible to the effects of a toxic xenobiotic.[5,7]

The distribution and biotransformation of a xenobiotic often limit the delivery of the ultimate toxicant to susceptible target cells, organs, or tissues. Distribution of xenobiotics to storage depots that are physically removed from potential target sites is one means by which the disposition of a toxicant can be protective and can limit the adverse effects of a particular xenobiotic on an animal.[3] Presystemic elimination or the first-pass effect prevents toxic xenobiotics from ever reaching the general circulation and therefore many potential sites of action.[4] Most biotransformations produce metabolites that are more water soluble and as a result more readily eliminated from the body.[2,3]

In contrast to circumstances in which the disposition of a xenobiotic decreases the risk of toxicosis, there are also instances in which the distribution and biotransformation of a given toxicant actually increase the likelihood that an ultimate toxicant will be delivered to the site of action. A chemical's toxicity can be enhanced by specialized transport mechanisms and by physiochemical characteristics that facilitate the accumulation of ultimate toxicants within susceptible cells.[7] The toxicity of a xenobiotic can also be facilitated by processes, such as enterohepatic recirculation, that increase its bioavailability.[4,7] Xenobiotic biotransformations that result in lethal synthesis or bioactivation predispose animals to toxicoses and can, in some instances, actually occur within target cells.[5,7] Although some biotransformations result in metabolites that react more efficiently with target enzymes or receptors, it is more common for intoxication to result in chemical species, such as electrophiles, free radicals, nucleophiles, and redox-active compounds that are indiscriminately reactive with endogenous molecules.[7]

General Mechanisms of Xenobiotic Action

The basis for most toxicoses is cellular damage, and this damage is often most dramatic in cells with high rates of metabolism and replication.[5] A toxic xenobiotic's *mode* or *mechanism of action* is the activity of that compound or its metabolites at the molecular or cellular level that results in adverse effects.[1,5] Although most of the chapters of this text review the specific mechanisms of action of toxicants to which small animals are commonly exposed, there are a number of general ways in which toxic xenobiotics adversely affect cellular structure and function.

Although a toxic xenobiotic can adversely affect cells by changing their biologic microenvironment through alterations in pH or occupation of a particular receptor site, as mentioned previously, ultimate toxicants generally interact with target molecules or cells.[7] Some xenobiotics mimic the actions of normal nutrients and endogenous hormones or neurotransmitters. Specific receptors can be stimulated or blocked, and enzymes can be inactivated or inhibited.[5] Electrophiles, free radicals, nucleophiles, and redox-active compounds are often generated through biotransformations, and these chemical species can react indiscriminately with target macromolecules to exert their toxic effects.[5,7] At the cellular level, chemicals can alter cellular maintenance, both internally and externally, by adversely affecting membrane integrity and the ability of cells to regulate their volume and their energy metabolism.[7] Cellular injury and death often result from the impaired cellular synthesis of adenosine triphosphate, uncoupling of oxidative phosphorylation, and the inability of cells to regulate their intracellular calcium concentrations. The cellular production of vital proteins and the regulation of gene expression within cells can also be disrupted by toxicants.[5,7] Ultimately, high enough exposures to toxic xenobiotics cause cellular dysfunction and injury and, sometimes, disrepair, and these adverse effects can be observed clinically as abnormalities in the structure and function of different organs and tissues.[7]

References

1. Hodgson E, Mailman RB, Chambers JE, editors: *Dictionary of toxicology*, New York, 1999, Grove's Dictionaries.
2. Spoo W: Toxicokinetics. In Plumlee K, editor: *Clinical veterinary toxicology*, St Louis, 2004, Mosby.
3. Rozman KK, Klaassen CD: Absorption, distribution, and excretion of toxicants. In Klaassen CD, Watkins III JB, editors: *Casarett & Doull's essentials of toxicology*, New York, 2003, McGraw-Hill.
4. Riviere JE: *Comparative pharmacokinetics: principles, techniques, and applications*, Ames, Iowa, 1999, Iowa State University Press.
5. Osweiler GD: *Toxicology (The National Veterinary Medical Series)*, Philadelphia, 1996, Williams & Wilkins.
6. Parkinson A: Biotransformation of xenobiotics. In Klaassen CD, Watkins III JB, editors: *Casarett & Doull's essentials of toxicology*, New York, 2003, McGraw-Hill.
7. Gregus Z, Klaassen CD: Mechanisms of toxicity. In Klaassen CD, Watkins III JB, editors: *Casarett & Doull's essentials of toxicology*, New York, 2003, McGraw-Hill.
8. Medinsky MA, Valentine JL: Toxicokinetics. In Klaassen CD, Watkins III JB, editors: *Casarett & Doull's essentials of toxicology*, New York, 2003, McGraw-Hill.

Toxicologic Information Resources

Jude McNally, RPh, DABAT

Keith Boesen, PharmD, CSPI

Kelly Green Boesen, PharmD, BCPS

Considering the exponential rate at which the body of toxicology information grows combined with today's improved tools to disseminate this information can easily cause one to feel overwhelmed. The challenge is to recognize the most appropriate resources that will lead the practitioner to the most relevant and current information.

Toxicologic information is available as primary, secondary, and tertiary literature on a variety of media from textbooks to computer databases to portable electronic devices. The purpose of this chapter is to introduce veterinary practitioners to some of the resources found to be beneficial when approaching a toxicologic problem.

Primary Literature

More than 30,000 biomedical journals are published annually. These are the primary literature sources that bring us detailed accounts of research in specialized areas. The level of detail, such as methodology, results, and discussion, exceeds that found in secondary and tertiary resources. This affords readers greater opportunity to determine for themselves the value of the conclusions offered in the study.

There are considerably more toxicologic references written for human medical practitioners than for veterinarians. Any thorough search of a toxicologic topic must query the primary literature in both toxicology and veterinary medicine. Primary literature may be particularly important to the veterinarian practitioner because historically much of the toxicology information is initially elucidated in animal models with the intent to extrapolate this information to the human model.

Primary literature has the advantage of offering the most up-to-date information. However, the conclusions derived are often subject to revision as this research is merged with other work and further scrutinized by the scientific community. A partial list of journals on toxicology is found in Box 3-1. An abbreviated list of veterinary medical journals offering articles pertaining to toxicology is found in Box 3-2.

Secondary Literature

Secondary literature attempts to compile the primary literature through either an index service or an abstracting service. Indexing services are limited to bibliographic information, whereas abstracting services provide brief descriptions of the source cited. In both cases this literature is generally useful as a means, not an end, to a search for information. Today much of the secondary literature has become available online and through applications on portable electronic devises, although CD-ROM formats may also be available. Examples of secondary literature are:

Biosis Previews. These abstracts, which are updated weekly, pertain to biologic research (including biomedical literature) and are available in print and electronic form.

Current Contents. Toxicologic information may be found in Current Contents Life Sciences or Current Contents Clinical Medicine. This abstracting service is available in print, on CD-ROM, and as an online service.

Medline (Ovid [http://www.ovid.com/site/index.jsp] and PubMed [http://www.ncbi .nlm.nih.gov/pubmed/]). Medline is a service of the National Library of Medicine located within the National Institutes of Health in Bethesda, Maryland. This is the world's largest medical library, providing access to primary, secondary, and tertiary literature areas of biomedicine and health care. Both are available online and PubMed is also available for portable electronic devices. It is a large database of literature dating back to 1966. The articles are collected from various countries and include both human- and animal-related issues. Ovid does require a subscription; however, many public and medical libraries provide free access. PubMed provides abstracts at no charge on the Internet.

Box 3-1 **Partial List of Toxicology Journals**

Annual Review of Pharmacology and Toxicology
Archives of Environmental Contamination and Toxicology
Archives of Toxicology
Bulletin of Environmental Contamination and Toxicology
Cell Biology and Toxicology
Chemical Research in Toxicology
Clinical Toxicology
Comparative Biochemistry and Physiology, Part C, Pharmacology, Toxicology and Endocrinology
Critical Reviews in Toxicology
Drug and Chemical Toxicology
Ecotoxicology and Environmental Safety
Experimental and Toxicologic Pathology
Food and Chemical Toxicology
Human and Experimental Toxicology
Immunopharmacology and Immunotoxicology
Journal of Analytical Toxicology
Journal of Applied Toxicology
Journal of Biochemical and Molecular Toxicology
Journal of Environmental Pathology, Toxicology and Oncology
Journal of Pharmacological and Toxicological Methods
Journal of Toxicological Sciences
Journal of Toxicology and Environmental Health
Neurotoxicology
Neurotoxicology and Teratology
Journal of Pharmacology and Toxicology
Regulatory Toxicology and Pharmacology
Reproductive Toxicology
Reviews of Environmental Contamination and Toxicology
Toxicologic Pathology
Toxicological Sciences
Toxicology
Toxicology and Applied Pharmacology
Toxicology and Industrial Health
Toxicology Letters
Toxicon
Veterinary and Human Toxicology (discontinued in 2005)

Search techniques need to be learned before a thorough search can be done on Medline. Using terms like *OR* and *AND* will help broaden and focus the search. For example, *ibuprofen OR Motrin* will locate all articles that contain either of these terms in its text, whereas using *ibuprofen AND Motrin* will only locate the articles that contain both of these terms. An additional technique to achieve a thorough literature search is to include in your search strategy all forms of the toxin and any categories it falls into. For example, a search for Prozac may consist of the terms *Prozac, fluoxetine, selective serotonin reuptake inhibitor,* and *SSRI.* Other terms, such as *truncate, focus,* and *explode,* can be learned from use of the database. Once a search has been completed, the resulting information is either the reference to the article, an abstract, or the complete reference.

VJIndex.com. More than 100,000 major veterinary journals are available via VJIndex.com covering the past 20 years with an average of 5000 added each year. The database is available by CD and is updated with a new CD every 6 months. A subscription fee may be required.

Box 3-2   Partial List of Veterinary Journals with Toxicology Articles

American Journal of Veterinary Research
Animal Genetics
Animal Reproduction Science
Australian Veterinary Journal
Avian Diseases
British Poultry Science
Canadian Journal of Veterinary Research
Canadian Veterinary Journal
Domestic Animal Endocrinology
Experimental Animals
Japanese Journal of Veterinary Research
Journal of the American Animal Hospital Association
Journal of the American Veterinary Medical Association
Journal of Animal Science
Journal of Small Animal Practice
Journal of the South African Veterinary Association
Journal of Veterinary Diagnostic Investigation
Journal of Veterinary Emergency and Critical Care
Journal of Veterinary Internal Medicine
Journal of Veterinary Medical Science
Journal of Veterinary Pharmacology and Therapeutics
Journal of Wildlife Diseases
Journal of Zoo and Wildlife Medicine
Laboratory Animal Science
Laboratory Animals
Preventive Veterinary Medicine
Research in Veterinary Science
Tropical Animal Health and Production
Veterinary Clinics of North America, Small Animal Practice
Veterinary and Human Toxicology (discontinued in 2005)
Veterinary Journal
Veterinary Quarterly
Veterinary Record
Veterinary Research

Tertiary Literature

Tertiary literature refers to textbooks, compendia, and full-text computer databases. These are often the preferred resources of clinicians because they are familiar and contain concise overviews of a wide variety of topics. These resources conveniently cover the most frequently encountered clinical problems. The paucity of tertiary literature focusing on veterinary toxicology was the initial inspiration for the first edition of this text.

Some tertiary references have been scanned electronically and can be accessed via the Internet through various search engines. This provides an economical alternative to purchasing them, but they can be difficult to read and the reference needed may not always be available in this format.

UpToDate is a valuable tertiary reference. Experts in their fields provide evidence-based summaries about clinical issues provided by the health care community. This database is available online and as an application for portable electronic devices. *UpToDate* and a few other tertiary references are updated frequently but this is the exception more than the norm.

Disadvantages inherent in tertiary literature include space limitations requiring priority on selected topics and the risk that the information, however pertinent it was when written, may be outdated by the time it is published. Full-text computer databases may have a better chance of overcoming these problems. Recently published tertiary references are often available for download to portable electronic devices. Although not solely dedicated to animal poisoning, references such as *VetPDA* and *The 5-Minute Veterinary Consult* include chapters on poisoning exposure, which are available for portable electronic devices. Other examples of tertiary toxicology literature are listed in Box 3-3.

Box 3-3	**Partial List of Veterinary and Medical Toxicology Textbooks**

AMA Handbook of Poisonous and Injurious Plants (American Medical Association)
Casarett and Doull's Toxicology: The Basic Science of Poisons (McGraw-Hill)
Clinical Management of Poisoning and Drug Overdose (WB Saunders)
Clinical Toxicology of Commercial Products (Williams & Wilkins)
Clinical Veterinary Toxicology (Mosby)
Ellenhorn's Medical Toxicology—Diagnosis and Treatment of Human Poisonings
   (Williams & Wilkins)
Field Guide to Common Animal Poisons (Iowa State University Press)
Handbook of Mushroom Poisoning (CRC Press, Inc.)
Handbook of Pesticide Toxicology, 3 Volumes (Academic Press)
Handbook of Small Animal Toxicology and Poisonings (Mosby)
Hidden Hazards in House and Garden Plants (Pictorial Histories Publishing Co., Inc.)
Lexi-Tox (Lexicomp, Wolters Kluwer)
POISONDEX (Micromedex, Thomson Reuters)
Merck Veterinary Manual (Merck & Co.)
Natural Toxicants in Feeds and Poisonous Plants (Interstate Publishers, Inc.)
Principles of Clinical Toxicology (Raven Press)
Poisoning and Toxicology Handbook (Lexi-Comp, Inc.)
Poisonous Plants of California (University of California Press)
Small Animal Medicine Therapeutics (Lippincott Williams & Wilkins)
Small Animal Toxicology and Poisonings (Mosby)
Toxicology, The National Veterinary Medical Series (Williams & Wilkins)
Veterinary Drug Handbook (Iowa State University Press)
Veterinary Drug Therapy (Lea & Febiger)
Veterinary Pharmaceuticals and Biologicals (VPB) (Medical Economics Data)
Veterinary Toxicology (Butterworth-Heinemann)

Computer Databases

Computer databases have been compiled to provide rapid access to toxicologic information. Although these databases are not specifically geared to veterinary practice, they often include separate animal poisoning sections and references. The largest such database, Poisondex (Thomson Reuters' Micromedex), is currently used by all U.S. poison control centers as well as the American Society for the Prevention of Cruelty to Animals Animal Poison Control Center (ASPCA-APCC) and the Pet Poison HELPLINE. This database identifies ingredients for hundreds of thousands of commercial, biologic, and pharmaceutical products. The systems link individual products to management recommendations; these often include case reports of animal poisonings. Other databases offering specific information in subspecialty areas of toxicology include Reprorisk (Thomson Reuters' Micromedex), a compilation of reproductive risk information, and Tomes (Thomson Reuters' Micromedex), specializing in hazardous chemicals in the workplace and the environment. These databases can be expensive to subscribe to; alternatively, the information they provide are usually available through your regional poison center.

Lexicomp is also available over the Internet and consists of a variety of medical and pharmaceutical databases covering drug information, dental resources, genomics, calculations, abbreviations, and toxicology. Lexicomp requires a subscription and is available online or can be downloaded to a portable electronic device. Many poison centers also have access to this database.

The introduction and advances in portable electronic devices have allowed for unprecedented access to information resources. Some are available from reputable sources but many have been created by general users and should be used with some caution. Costs vary but are usually less expensive than buying the traditional resource.

Internet Resources

The Internet provides access to a vast array and a prolific volume of information on toxicology topics. As a resource, the Internet, unlike conventional textbooks and journal articles, poses a daunting challenge with regard to its sources' authenticity, reliability, accuracy, and usefulness to the reader. Concern for the quality of the information obtained from a web-based source is a much greater issue when compared with that for the print and broadcast media. The freedom and ease with which authors and contributors of "information" can place and disseminate material online have created a need for the information search to become a more critical and careful process. Critical thinking about and evaluation of web-based sources must be done with considerable skill and discriminating persistence.

To illustrate this point, a study was performed that examined the accuracy of Internet information by searching Google for the terms *aspirin, overdose* or *intoxication,* and *treatment.* Two blinded toxicologists evaluated the first 10 websites that appeared to make treatment recommendations. They concluded that the treatment recommendations of 5 of the 10 sites were "significantly substandard."

Other pitfalls of using websites include the dangers of obtaining information from a site that sells the product about which it is attempting to inform the reader and the danger of obtaining information from a site that has not been updated and is no longer current and accurate. Accurate, reliable websites are often those created and supported by reputable organizations, such as the Centers for Disease Control, the Food and Drug Administration, the World Health Organization, the Environmental Protection Agency, the ASPCA-APCC, the Pet Poison HELPLINE, and local and national organizations recognized as experts in the field (e.g., Veterinary Information Network and the American Board of Veterinary Toxicology [www.abvt.org]). The information obtained from the Internet should not take precedence over the expert knowledge of toxicologists and poison control center specialists. The criteria for evaluating the reliability and validity of authored materials on the web at a minimum should include the following: (1) author's institutional affiliation; (2) author's Internet address; (3) date of information posting; (4) copyright dates; (5) statement of institutional responsibility, sponsorship, or ownership; and (6) clear references to all information sources used. In addition to questioning the purpose and source of a web-based information resource, the following questions about content evaluation and review need to be answered: (1) Is the origin of material clearly stated? (2) Does it seem accurate? (3) Is it comprehensive? (4) Is it current, having a recent update? and (5) Are the hyperlinks relevant and appropriate? A well-designed Internet site enhances the information it offers. You will find good organization, clear and appropriate writing style, and ease of navigation and search capabilities when you pay a visit to such a site.

Poison Control Centers

The concept of a poison control information service began with the collaboration of a pharmacist and a physician at St. Luke's Presbyterian Hospital in Chicago in 1953. The major goal of a poison center is the reduction of morbidity and mortality from poisoning through service as an updated resource for toxicologic information.

Today there are 57 poison centers throughout the United States. All provide treatment advice and referral assistance 24 hours a day, 7 days a week to both the public and health care providers. Most established centers are members of the American Association of Poison Control Centers (AAPCC). In 2009 the AAPCC member centers provided consultation for 116,408 animal-related exposures; this represented 4.5% of all exposure cases called into poison centers.

The AAPCC provides a framework for the development of voluntary standards for poison center operations. Unfortunately, these association guidelines do not specifically address standards for the provision of care in veterinary cases. As a result, the range and level of services available to veterinary caregivers is variable. Some centers deny consultation for animal exposures, whereas others maintain veterinary referrals and establish formal relationships with veterinary consultants. Nurses or pharmacists with additional training in toxicology most often staff poison centers. Upon satisfying criteria established by the AAPCC, these nurses and pharmacists become eligible to sit for an examination that will certify them as poison specialists. A board-certified medical toxicologist provides medical direction in most poison control centers. At a minimum, most poison centers are able to provide veterinarians with specific product information and recommendations for medical management of human patients, necessitating interpretation by the attending veterinarian. Access to regional poison control centers is obtained by calling (800) 222-1222 from anywhere in the United States. Your call will be automatically routed to the poison center designated to provide services in your area. A complete list of AAPCC-certified poison centers can also be found on the Internet at http://www.aapcc.org/.

Animal Poison Control Centers

The APCC was the first animal treatment–oriented poison center in the United States. The APCC is a division of the ASPCA. Specially trained veterinarians staff this emergency hotline. Their collective experience has been gained through handling more than 850,000 animal poisonings to date. Because of their background and training, center veterinarians are prepared to deal with the complexities of animals exposed to poisons. The center is a member of the AAPCC and does work closely with human centers to provide information on animal poisonings. Many human centers refer serious cases directly to the ASPCA-APCC center. The ASPCA-APCC can be contacted by telephone at 888-426-4435. There is a $65 consultation fee for the initial telephone consultation; follow-up calls are free. There is no charge if the product involved is covered by the Animal Product Safety Service. Another nationwide 24-hour service hotline is the Pet Poison HELPLINE (800-213-6680), offered by the Safety Call Pet Poison Control Center. There is an initial $39 consultation fee; all additional follow-up contacts are free.

Effective Use of a Veterinary Poison Control Center

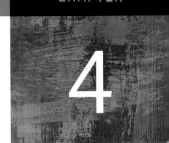

Lynn Rolland Hovda, RPh, DVM, MS, DACVIM

There are currently two veterinary poison control centers in the United States.* Both are staffed by veterinarians and specialists with extensive training in veterinary toxicology. They offer telephone assistance to animal owners and veterinarians 24 hours a day, 7 days a week, and provide legitimate websites related to animal poisoning. Their websites are updated in a timely manner by knowledgeable individuals and provide accurate and comprehensive information involving a number of substances. Although the majority of cases handled by veterinary poison control centers are for small animals, both centers are capable of providing poison information for pocket pets, birds, exotics, aquatics, and large animals (primarily horses and ruminants).

The American Society for the Prevention of Cruelty to Animals Animal Poison Control Center (APCC) is located in Urbana, Illinois. It is staffed by a large number of veterinarians, veterinarians boarded in general toxicology (American Board of Toxicology) and veterinary toxicology (American Board of Veterinary Toxicology), and certified veterinary technicians with specialized training in veterinary toxicology. The APCC has a well-established database incorporating 30 years of veterinary toxicology information that can be used to assist in case management. In addition, the APCC works with a variety of organizations, including human poison control centers, government agencies, animal parks, and zoos, to obtain and disseminate information on current and potential veterinary toxicologic problems. The APCC veterinarians have provided textbook chapters; written articles for veterinary journals; and speak at local, state, and national veterinary meetings. The APCC can be reached by telephone at 1-888-426-4435, with a consultation fee of $65 for most cases. There is no fee for case follow-up and there is no fee in those instances in which the manufacturer has contracted with the APCC to provide services through the Animal Product Safety Division. The website for the APCC is www.aspcapro.org.

The Pet Poison HELPLINE (PPH), located in Bloomington, Minnesota, is a 24-hour poison control center dedicated to animal poisonings. It is staffed by a large group of veterinarians, veterinarians who are board eligible or certified in general toxicology (American Board of Toxicology), veterinary toxicology (American Board of Veterinary Toxicology), emergency and critical care (American College of Veterinary Emergency and Critical Care), and internal medicine (American College of Veterinary Internal Medicine), as well as certified veterinarian technicians with specialized training in veterinary toxicology. They are supported by experts in human poisonings (PharmDs and physicians) and a specialist in snakes and venomous animals. PPH maintains an affiliation with the University of Minnesota. The toxicologists at PPH have more than 30 years of veterinary experience and have managed 2.5 million poisonings. They work closely with the federal government and other agencies to obtain and provide accurate information on emerging veterinary

---

*ASPCA-APCC: 888-426-4435: $65.00 for most cases.
Pet Poison HELPLINE: 800-213-6680: $39.00 for most cases.

toxicologic issues. The veterinarians at PPH have authored a textbook; provided chapters in other textbooks; published in veterinary and medical toxicology journals; and presented at local, state, and national meetings. PPH is a division of SafetyCall International, the world's largest industry poison control center, which provides toxicology information to consumers on a wide variety of substances such as agricultural products, dietary supplements, household goods, personal care products, pesticides, and pharmaceuticals. PPH can be reached by telephone at 1-800-213-6680 with a consultation fee of $39 in most cases. There is no additional fee for follow-up consultations. The website for PPH is www.petpoisonhelpline.com. Recently, PPH now offers a handy iPhone application that contains an extensive database of foods, drugs, chemicals, and plants commonly found in the home and yard that are poisonous to pets—information about this application can be found at their website.

The use of a veterinary poison control center is encouraged for all potential animal-related poisonings. Well-established databases provide invaluable factual and anecdotal poison information that no other centers have access to. The veterinary poison control center staff uses knowledge built on years of experience in the field of veterinary toxicology as well as advanced studies in toxicology to complete a risk assessment for each poisoned animal. Hazards for each toxicant and an assessment of various routes of exposure are considered and evaluated prior to making any recommendations. The detailed understanding of veterinary pharmacokinetics and species-related variations in dose and response provide the caller with the most accurate information available for each individual animal poisoning.

Callers to a veterinary poison control center come from a wide variety of backgrounds and include owners, veterinarians, pesticide control officers, humane society agents, police officers with service dogs, crop agents, and others involved with poisoned animals. Each caller needs to provide an open, honest, and complete history to receive the most effective and comprehensive information regarding a potential poisoning. Although this may seem cumbersome or unimportant, it is in fact essential for a positive outcome. Veterinarians at the center are well trained to ask specific questions that assist with the case management and weed out those answers that are unimportant or mask significant details. This is difficult, however, when an animal has been exposed to illegal or illicit drugs as the caller is often reluctant to offer much information. When this occurs, the referring veterinarian needs to more firmly question the owner and provide this information to the veterinary poison control center specialist.

Providing specific product identification and an estimation of exposure amount is the first step in the risk assessment for a poisoned animal. An accurate animal weight and not just a guess should be obtained so the dose of active ingredients associated with the toxicants as well as dosage of recommended treatment options may be determined. In those instances in which the product cannot be identified by the caller (e.g., bag of unknown pills, torn label, etc.), specialists at the veterinary poison control center are often able to use their databases to assist with identification.

Species and breed identification are commonly provided with small animals but may be lacking in other instances. The toxic dose as well as lethal dose and no effect limit for each individual toxicant are species-dependent, making this an important piece of information to obtain. In addition, ruminants have a more complicated gastrointestinal tract resulting in variable absorption of oral toxicants as well as recommended treatments and antidotes. Many toxicants are metabolized in the liver using pathways limited in some species, and some toxicants, such as lilies, are harmful only to one species (i.e., the cat). Some breeds, such as the collie, collie crosses, and others, exhibit an *ABCB1* delta gene mutation (formerly referred to as *MDR1*), making them susceptible to toxicosis from several substances at much lower doses than other breeds.

Age, reproductive status, and health history are significant parts of the history that should not be overlooked. Very young and old animals may have limited kidney or liver function, thus prolonging metabolism and excretion. These animals may develop a more serious toxicosis than expected or clinical signs may last for an extended period. Preexisting medical conditions, current medications, and any treatments given to the animal prior to contacting a veterinary poison control center should be noted. Not only do they play a role in the current presentation of the animal but become important when formulating a treatment plan.

The presence or absence of clinical signs should be provided as well as the estimated time of exposure to the toxicant. Caution needs to be used when interpreting signs as some, such as those associated with parasympathomimetic or parasympatholytic agents, are very specific and others are very vague. Clinical signs may be used to assist with unknown poisonings but need to be carefully evaluated by an experienced veterinary poison control veterinarian in conjunction with the time of exposure and onset of signs. In these instances, particular attention should be paid to the cardiovascular system and any abnormalities reported as some plants and medications result in specific signs that may be useful in the diagnosis.

Veterinary poison control centers are very effective in providing assistance when there is a suspicious death or legal case. These cases require a much more advanced history to allow the veterinary poison center veterinarian to interpret data and make suggestions for further diagnostic testing. Veterinarians at the center are generally able to provide information on sample collection and submission as well as interpretation of the results. In addition, documentation provided by a veterinary poison control center is normally very thorough and complete. When an unusual poisoning is reported, veterinarians at a veterinary poison control center are able to connect with and gain information from a network of other veterinary toxicologists through a variety of listservs.

Regardless of the caller's ability, veterinary poison control centers are an excellent resource in what is often a stressful situation. They provide a calm, rapid response in an emergency situation and additional support if the case progresses or becomes more difficult. Taking the time to obtain and provide a complete history, including clinical signs, maximizes the effectiveness of the call and provides the caller with concise and comprehensive information needed to treat the animal.

Suggested Readings

Gwaltney-Bramt SM: Toxicology information resources. In Poppenga RH, Gwaltney-Brant SM, editors: *Small animal toxicology essentials*, Sussex, UK, 2011, John Wiley and Sons.

Osweiler GD, Hovda LR, Brutlag AG, et al: *Blackwell's five-minute veterinary consult clinical companion: small animal toxicology*, Ames, IA, 2011, Wiley-Blackwell.

Use of Human Poison Centers in the Veterinary Setting

5

Katie Von Derau, RN, CPN, CSPI

- Human Poison Control Centers (PCC): 800-222-1222
- Open 24-hours a day, seven days a week
- Some, but not all, are free of charge for veterinarians

Despite the differences in the toxicity of substances among species, human poison centers have had a place in treating veterinary poisonings. Unfortunately, this is becoming more difficult as their funding is threatened.[1] Veterinary calls usually take longer for a human poison center to handle than human calls because they require more research into species differences and the necessity to access additional veterinary references. Centers previously managing veterinary calls at no cost can no longer afford to do so, forcing them either to stop handling[2] animal calls or to charge a fee.

The Washington Poison Center (WAPC) chose to charge a fee[3] rather than stop handling these calls. The majority of veterinary exposures reported to WAPC are for household pets, especially dogs and cats, and until the decision to charge for these calls in mid-2009 the veterinary call volume had continually increased (Table 5-1).

The choice to charge a fee has had a double effect: A minimal income is generated for the center and, because of the number of callers declining the fee, the overall call volume has decreased to a manageable level for the center's staff. WAPC anticipated losing approximately 30% to 50% of their animal calls; however, calls dropped significantly more than anticipated (Table 5-2). In 2008, WAPC had 8562 veterinary calls, slightly more than 9% of the total call volume,[4] whereas in 2010 calls dropped to 1021, or approximately 1.4% of the call volume.[4]

WAPC staff were resistant to charging for information they had previously provided for free. Many owners and veterinarians who depended on the center in the past were outraged. Because poisons act fast, there was increased frustration for both staff and callers as a result of the requirement to obtain billing information prior to handling the call. WAPC does offer veterinarians the option to have an open account and to be invoiced for calls. This is not an option for owners.

An unexpected outcome after implementing the fee was that, despite the increased complexity of veterinary calls, the quality of call handling and call length improved. There was also a 7.33% increase in the number of cases that were followed beyond the initial call.[4]

Assessment and Exposure

Animals can be poisoned by human or veterinary medications, plants, chemicals, or cleaning agents as a result of an accidental ingestion, spill, or therapeutic error. Human poison centers receiving calls from owners or veterinarians triage animal exposures just as they do exposure calls from the parents of toddlers. The animal, like the toddler, is unable to convey

Table 5-1		Veterinary Exposure Calls to the Washington Poison Center by Species[4]							
Year	Cat	Dog	Bird	Aquatic	Cow	Horse	Rodent and Lagomorph	Sheep and Goat	Other
1999	1113	4426	80	5	25	18	39	2	53
2000	1122	4671	72	2	33	21	37	12	51
2001	1086	4342	45	3	1	19	38	11	35
2002	1130	4905	46	3	1	17	40	6	26
2003	1011	4805	36	1	0	17	42	8	21
2004	1024	5364	46	4	1	16	28	7	15
2005	964	5543	28	2	0	15	34	14	31
2006	1050	6474	30	5	2	13	33	12	22
2007	1066	6955	29	4	2	16	22	11	16
2008	1017	7443	32	1	0	23	21	8	17
2009	472	3871	13	1	1	9	23	6	11
2010	91	921	2	0	0	1	2	0	4

Table 5-2	All Veterinary Calls to the Washington Poison Center[4]			
Year	Total Number of Animal Exposure Calls	Percent of Animal Exposures Out of Total Exposure Calls	Total Percent of Veterinary Calls (Information and Exposure)	Percent of Exposure Calls Referred to the Poison Center by Veterinarians
1999	5761	6.86	4.36	Tracking began in
2000	6021	7.43	5.18	third quarter
2001	5580	7.21	5.86	of 2005.
2002	6174	8.06	6.53	
2003	5941	8.26	6.7	
2004	6505	8.76	7.16	
2005	6631	8.89	7.27	
2006	7641	10.2	8.26	19.1%
2007	8121	10.7	8.66	17.7%
2008	8562	11.22	9.24	12.5%
2009	4407	6.23	5.24	9.2%
2010	1021	1.6	1.38	3.0%

what happened, and acute poisoning requires as accurate an assessment as possible. The threat is not only related to the potency of the poison, but also to the quantity involved, the duration of the exposure, and the presence of other ingredients, such as propellants and solvents. The degree of danger and the necessity for decontamination or other treatment are able to be determined only after a thorough assessment.

The poison center must seek specific information concerning the exposure. Exact product identification, the estimated amount and concentration of the product involved, the time and route of the exposure, the species and weight of the animal, any signs the animal demonstrates, and any treatment already given are all obtained. Accurate identification of the product or medication involved is essential because of variations in formulations. The specific product name, manufacturer, and ingredients need to be verified by the poison center and confirmed with the original product container, if available. This includes the strength or concentration of the medication or chemical and the form (solid, liquid, etc.) of the product. Tablets, liquids, solids, gases, and granules all pose different risks. Aerosol sprays pose an additional risk from the propellant, which can be more toxic than the active ingredient.

Medication toxicity depends on the species and weight of the animal and the specific dose of ingested medication. Cleaning products can vary from simple irritants to dangerous corrosives; even similarly named products by the same manufacturer can have many different ingredients and thus contrasting management guidelines. Soaps and detergents may be anionic or nonionic, representing little risk, or cationic with the potential for greater harm.

The species, breed, age, gender, weight, and number of animals involved are all part of the history taken. These data are all important in assessing risk factors with regard to increased or decreased sensitivity to various toxic agents and ought to be considered when recommending decontamination, treatment, referral, and follow-up. Differences in physiology and metabolic pathways exist among species, which may alter the range of toxicity, time to onset of signs, and treatment. It cannot be assumed that an exposure that is determined to be nontoxic for humans will also be nontoxic for other animals.

Frequently the amount of toxin in a veterinary exposure is unknown. Together the poison center and the caller try to estimate the amount of product missing or the maximum available to the animal. This is not the toxic amount for the particular animal, but is an estimate of the amount of product actually involved in the exposure. The following questions may be asked to assist the caller in remembering:

- Who used the product last and when?
- Do you remember the level in the container before the animal disturbed it?
- Is this container ever refilled from a larger container, and if so, was it refilled with the exact same product?
- When was the container purchased?
- What was the usual dose or amount used?
- Is there a spill or are there pill fragments around the animal?

If it is possible to calculate a toxic dose, successful questioning can often determine that a toxic amount was not actually available before the exposure. Having the owner reapply the product and measuring what he or she just used or having the owner apply the amount calculated to be toxic and comparing it with what was applied before the exposure are two methods used by the poison center to estimate the amount involved.

It is important to determine if the product was diluted, and if so, how it was diluted. Dilution decreases the concentration or strength and possibly the pH of many toxins, often making the exposure less harmful. A dog lapping full-strength antifreeze from a spilled container is at more risk than a dog lapping diluted antifreeze that was then rinsed off the driveway and collected into a puddle. If the product was mixed with anything, it may be necessary to determine the toxicity of the additive as well.

The time of the call to the poison center can be from minutes to hours after the time of the exposure. Owners may actually witness the exposure and call immediately, they may not realize the exposure is a potential problem and delay calling, or they may return home to discover their pet has been very busy. The time since the exposure may affect treatment advice or the necessity for a veterinary referral.

Any possible benefits of decontamination depend on early detection. With veterinary exposures there are frequently several different routes of exposure with the same incident (Table 5-3). A dermal exposure often becomes an oral exposure as the animal grooms itself, and inhalation of fumes can occur while ingesting a liquid.

The poison center needs to evaluate all possible signs the animal might be exhibiting by asking specific questions about obvious distress, level of activity, signs of irritation, irritability, or any change in the animal's overall behavior. Any unexpected signs need to be assessed for relatedness to another toxin or possible medical conditions unrelated to a poisoning. Animals in distress or those with potentially toxic exposures in which decontamination is either not possible or ineffective need to be referred immediately to the veterinarian.

Many pet owners institute appropriate first aid measures before they call the poison center, and it is important to know what has already been done or not done. They may have provided fresh air or fluids, the two most popular emergency treatments, and may be calling simply for additional decontamination or treatment information. Calls from veterinarians usually come to the poison center after the animal has been given emergency treatment, and additional specific product, antidote, or treatment information is desired (Table 5-4).

In cases in which the ingestion has occurred within 2-3 hours, it is often useful to induce vomiting. It is the job of the poison center to remain in contact with the owner because failure to produce emesis may result in the need for a veterinary referral. Depending on the toxin, if the ingestion is large, even after adequate home decontamination, it is often necessary to refer the animal to the veterinarian for further evaluation because it is impossible to fully empty the stomach. Ingestion of large amounts of some medications (e.g., aspirin, acetaminophen, digoxin) may necessitate a drug level, even though the animal has vomited.

Ocular exposures pose a different threat to animals. Adequate home decontamination is almost impossible, and animals may give no indication of the exposure by their behavior. The risk of injury to both the owner and the animal while trying to rinse the eye is so great, even with the most compliant pet, that these animals need immediate referral to the veterinarian for evaluation and treatment.

Determining risk to the animal requires knowledge of different toxins and their effects on various species. Many reference books list therapeutic doses of medicines used in humans and animals along with usual daily doses, and these may prove helpful as a guide. The animal's weight, past medical history, and a thorough history of the exposure are

Table 5-3   Veterinary Routes of Exposure[4]

Route	1999	2000	2001	2002	2003	2004	2005	2006	2007	2008	2009	2010
Ingestion	5437	5710	5302	5889	5663	6168	6334	7325	7815	8256	4260	987
Inhalation/ Nasal	83	81	73	80	59	87	85	96	105	61	52	15
Aspiration	2	0	2	2	1	1	0	0	1	0	3	1
Ocular	29	31	28	36	30	41	44	39	36	29	19	2
Dermal	448	453	433	459	425	461	391	402	404	395	177	40
Bite or Sting	18	20	17	13	13	18	12	15	9	15	9	1
Parenteral	5	6	9	6	5	18	9	7	11	7	11	1
Rectal	0	4	2	1	0	0	0	0	1	1	1	0
Otic	0	2	1	3	1	1	2	3	1	4	1	0
Vaginal or Other	8	2	2	1	1	4	2	2	1	2	1	0
Unknown	83	47	33	32	42	54	38	39	46	37	13	1

Table 5-4   Calls to the Washington Poison Center from Veterinarians[4]

Year	Animal Exposure Calls	Animal Information Calls	Other Poison Calls	Total Calls
1999	795	82	37	914
2000	821	83	45	949
2001	803	58	31	892
2002	837	61	27	925
2003	844	60	27	931
2004	931	69	27	1027
2005	869	92	21	982
2006	927	95	23	1045
2007	952	113	36	1101
2008	1065	85	7	1157
2009	574	30	5	609
2010	69	5	3	77

reviewed with the owner to try to establish the relative risk to the animal. It is important to discuss the toxicity of the product, along with the expected associated signs, with the owner. A subtoxic ingestion can have mild to moderate signs or normal medication side effects. The management of the animal is determined by the severity of expected signs and the need for observation of the animal over time.

Without specific guidelines to provide the range of toxicity, it is often necessary for the poison center to follow some basic principles in adapting human toxicity information. Several references are available in the poison center to help determine the range of toxicity for a particular ingestion. These include standard human and veterinary textbooks, the Micromedex Healthcare Series,[5] and many books and journals on toxicology.

Examples of Toxicants

More than 37% of the veterinary exposure calls to WAPC in the past 5 years were associated with exposure to medications.[4] Veterinary toxicology books are available to aid the poison center in determining a toxic dose of a medication for a particular species. However, if a toxic dose is not available, veterinary drug handbooks[6] can be used to determine a therapeutic dose and act as a guide. If no veterinary therapeutic dose for the particular medication can be found, then the poison center can assess risk by using the dose of a similar medication.

Benzodiazepines are common hypnotic and sedative drugs. Because of their popular human use, they are frequently available for ingestion by animals, as are antihistamines and decongestants. These patients should be decontaminated when the amount ingested exceeds 1½ times the usual total daily dose for the exposed species.

Antidepressants vary significantly in their degree of toxicity. Selective serotonin reuptake inhibitors are generally safer than other antidepressants and observation may be all that is necessary for an ingestion of up to 1½ times the usual daily dose. Tricyclic antidepressants and monoamine oxidase inhibitors are more of a problem, as are the usual antipsychotic medications, and patients are generally decontaminated when the exposure exceeds 1 time the usual daily dose.

Pain medications containing opioids, with or without acetaminophen, aspirin, or ibuprofen, are also common in many homes. These medications pose a double threat to the animal: Toxicity from the opioid and toxicity from the accompanying analgesic may both result. The signs of opioid ingestion can be either central nervous system depression or central nervous system excitation depending on the species and the time since ingestion.

Acetaminophen, aspirin, and ibuprofen are the most common over-the-counter medications. All can be toxic to animals in small amounts. The range of toxicity for cats versus dogs, the type of toxicity, and presenting signs can differ with these medications. Depending on the species there may not be a usual daily dose because some animals are so sensitive to these medications that they cannot be used therapeutically. Some animals lack the ability to metabolize these medications, or they are so sensitive to the toxic effects that even single doses can be potentially toxic.[7-9] Unless the exact amount of the ingestion can be determined, it is safest to "vomit" the animal. If the time of the ingestion is unknown or the amount of the ingestion is very large, vomit the animal and refer to a veterinarian for follow-up evaluation.

Ingestion of oral hypoglycemic agents and diuretics, as with humans, requires observation, fluids, and foods. If the owner is unable to closely monitor the animal and provide treatment as needed until the medication's effect has peaked, then decontamination or veterinary referral may be required.

Oral ingestion of topical ointments and creams generally requires only observation, but there are always exceptions to this rule. The owner should be warned to expect gastrointestinal signs from the laxative effect of many creams and ointments. Topical medications of concern are those with high methyl salicylate content and products that containing vitamin D–type compounds. One unit of vitamin D is approximately the equivalent of 25 ng of cholecalciferol.[10] Some anticancer ointments can be problematic as well.

Cardiac medications and antihypertensives can usually be tolerated at 1 to 1½ times the usual daily dose. If veterinary doses are not available for the particular medication for the exposed species, it is best to decontaminate the patient.

Hormones and antibiotics are generally well tolerated in cats and dogs and pose no significant risk after a single acute ingestion. Dilution and observation are usually all that is required. Mild gastrointestinal distress may be noted with a very large ingestion, but decontamination is rarely necessary. Hypersensitivity to antibiotics is uncommon in animals.[11]

All homeopathic medications are well tolerated with home observation. It is important not to confuse homeopathic medications with herbal preparations that could potentially contain toxic components. True homeopathic medications contain amounts of active ingredients so small that they are considered nontoxic.

Exposures to iron can be due to ingestion of lawn care products, iron in medications, and even hand and foot warmers. Usually the amount required to cause harm from a lawn care product exceeds the residual amount clinging to a pet after rolling in the yard. Human vitamins with iron, supplemental iron, birth control pills with iron, and now hand and foot warmers continue to be the important sources of iron exposures in small animals. There is even an iron-containing molluscicide on the market.

The most common concern with indoor plants is oral irritation from insoluble oxalate crystals. These exposures usually require only dilution with milk or sugar water and home observation. There are some plants with species-specific concerns (e.g., cats and certain lilies—*Lilium, Hemerocallis*) so the poison center must be diligent in researching. *Dieffenbachia* ingestions can result in significant oral edema and potential airway compromise. Ingestion of this plant should be diluted with milk or sugar water and referred to the veterinarian if there are any signs indicating airway compromise.

Witnessed ingestion of outdoor plants, for which there is some certainty of the amount ingested, can be treated with the same range of toxicity as for a child. An exception to this is plants that are known to cause toxicity in a specific species (e.g., cats and *Chrysanthemum* spp.). In this situation, decontamination and referral to the veterinarian may be necessary. An unwitnessed ingestion of a toxic plant should be treated aggressively according to the toxicity of the plant. Emesis of asymptomatic animals and referral of symptomatic animals, or those with large amounts of plant returned, should be standard policy.

Biologics, such as plants, toads, salamanders, newts, spiders, and snakes, all vary in toxicity depending on their locale and can potentially be problems in different areas of the country. The poison center should know those biologic toxins posing a risk in their area and provide appropriate treatment recommendations. Exact mushroom identification over the telephone is difficult, and the amount of mushroom ingested by animals is usually unknown. Every attempt should be made to remove any amount of a potentially toxic mushroom from the stomach. If emesis fails to bring the mushroom up, activated charcoal in the veterinary setting can be of benefit.

Hydrocarbons and petroleum distillates are surprisingly well tolerated as long as they remain in the gut, are noncaustic, and are not aspirated into the lungs. Dilution with milk to decrease stomach irritation and home observation for at least 4 hours, with referral of any symptomatic animal, are usually all that is required. Respiratory signs, such as repeated coughing and rapid breathing, that persist for longer than 10 minutes can indicate that aspiration has occurred.

Chemical exposures can include products that are low in toxicity, such as fertilizers, to those with a high degree of toxicity, such as rodenticides. Herbicides, insecticides, cleaning products, solvents, and wood preservatives are all chemicals with frequently overlapping management guidelines and varying ranges of toxicity. As in humans, emesis is contraindicated for products that are corrosive (such as acids or alkalis) and burn during ingestion. Dilution with milk, water, or broth is appropriate, with referral of any symptomatic animal to the veterinarian.

Chemical reference texts, Micromedex Healthcare Series with TOMES System5, journals, textbooks, and manufacturer or other appropriate websites are all used in the poison center setting. Many of these references provide species-specific information, including the

LD$_{50}$ for a particular chemical. Using these references makes it possible to more accurately establish relative risk for a particular animal, especially if thorough history taking was done and the amount missing can be precisely estimated.

The responsibility of the poison center to the animal and its owner does not end with the initial call. For those exposures that require induction of emesis or when moderate signs are expected, follow-up calls ought to be made and the owner encouraged to call back to the poison center as necessary. The passage of time can be a helpful diagnostic tool, and these follow-up calls can help guide treatment.

To locate a poison center accredited by the American Association of Poison Control Centers (AAPCC), call the national toll-free number, *1-800-222-1222*, or check the AAPCC website at http://www.aapcc.org/dnn/AAPCC/FindLocalPoisonCenters.aspx.

References

1. American Association of Poison Control Centers: *Poison centers federal appropriations cut by nearly 25 percent in proposed FY 2011 continuing resolution; damaging impact to states' ability to help citizens* [press release]http://www.aapcc.org/dnn/Portals/0/prrel/pressreleasehr1FINAL3.pdf. Retrieved from 2011.
2. Georgia Poison Center: *Poison FAQs: pets,* from http://www.georgiapoisoncenter.org/faq_pets.html. Retrieved 1 Nov 2011.
3. Washington Poison Center: *Noticeable changes to the Poison Center* [Press Release]http://wapc.org/pdf/media/WA%20Poison%20Center%20Changes.pdf. Retrieved from 2009.
4. Washington Poison Center: AAPCC Statistics for 1999 through 2010 (see Tables 5-1 to 5-4).
5. *Micromedex Healthcare Series,* Greenwood Village, CO, Thomson Reuters. (Edition expires 12/2011.)
6. Plumb DC: *Plumb's veterinary drug handbook,* 7th ed, Stockholm, WI, 2011, Pharma Vet.
7. Poisindex Toxicological Managements: *Ibuprofen MICROMEDEX healthcare series,* Vol. 150. (Expires 12/2011.)
8. Poisindex Toxicological Managements: *Salicylates MICROMEDEX healthcare series,* Vol. 130. (Expires 12/2011.)
9. Poisindex Toxicological Managements: *Acetaminophen MICROMEDEX healthcare series,* Vol. 130. (Expires 12/2011.)
10. Poisindex Toxicological Managements: *Vitamin D MICROMEDEX healthcare series,* Vol. 130. (Expires 12/2011.)
11. Poisindex Toxicological Managements: *Penicillin MICROMEDEX healthcare series,* Vol. 130. (Expires 12/2011.)

Taking a Toxicologic History

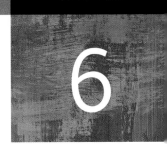

Kevin T. Fitzgerald, PhD, DVM, DABVP

The shortest distance between two points is the truth.

Irish Proverb

History taking is a vital skill. Combined with performing a thorough physical examination, obtaining an appropriate minimum database, and establishing a differential diagnosis, it allows the clinician to potentially arrive at a correct diagnosis. It is a technique that must be continually improved and perfected, both consciously and constantly.

History taking is especially important in cases of suspected animal poisoning. Taking a complete toxicologic history refines and focuses the trajectory of the interview in an attempt to detect the involvement of any potential poison. Let us begin this discussion by reviewing the basic history-taking techniques (Box 6-1).

If any part of veterinary medicine is an art, it is the act of securing from an owner the facts surrounding an animal's clinical signs. The clinician must be sympathetic, gentle, and patient in an effort to quickly establish the trust of the person. Such trust will facilitate spontaneous volunteering of important information by the owner. If a person feels intimidated by the veterinarian, he or she may not offer pertinent observations that are crucial to the case, and valuable time will be lost. If the history is to provide any type of working diagnosis, the veterinarian's interview must be meticulous, caring, and thorough in scope.

For a variety of reasons, owners may give histories that are inaccurate, highly unreliable, and sometimes purposely deceitful. Veterinarians must realize that many owners may feel guilty about the duration a condition has existed, how long it has been since the last veterinary visit, how long an animal is left alone each day, how the animal actually came across a poison, how long it took the owner to realize it, or the level of care with which toxic substances are stored or disposed of in the home. Owners frequently say things they think the veterinarian wants to hear in an attempt to be seen as a more responsible pet owner. Owners often deliberately falsify a history (as in the case of an animal's ingestion of an illicit drug) because of fear of legal repercussions and potential grounds for prosecution. Furthermore, the veterinarian must recognize the fears, anxieties, and emotional distress of many people as they face a potentially devastating health problem in their companion animal. The veterinarian must be a calming influence if a reliable account of events is to be obtained. If it is not possible to obtain an adequate history from the pet owner, it may be necessary to question other family members, neighbors, and friends. Finally, owners have different emotional make-ups, different educational backgrounds, different intellectual levels, and different economic realities. Language differences, physical disabilities, and other barriers may prevent the veterinarian from communicating effectively. If the owner's primary language is not English, there may be a person fluent in the owner's language in the veterinarian's practice. A certified professional interpreter may be available who can act as an interpreter for the deaf or hard of hearing (www.rid.org). Veterinarians must be inventive and flexible in their approach to listening to and communicating with their clients. Clinicians must

Box 6-1	Key Items in the Toxicologic History

- Listen to the client. Avoid any bias or preconceptions.
- At the same time, observe the animal. Although you can't always believe the client, you can believe clinical signs of the animal.
- Identify and treat immediate, life-threatening problems (e.g., arrhythmias, seizures). Do not wait for confirmation of poisons involved to initiate supportive therapy.
- Identify the animal's entire home environment. Could other poisons or other animals or children be involved?
- Identify any current medications, underlying conditions, or pertinent previous medical history for the animal (e.g., heart disease, kidney problems, pregnancy).
- History of the exposure event. How long ago, what toxin, what concentration, how much? Does the occupation or hobby of the owner predispose to the presence of any particular poisons in the home?
- If possible, identify the poison (or poisons). Estimate the mg/kg dose for the exposure and establish a worst-case scenario. Estimate the risk for the animal and the possibility of a toxic or lethal exposure.
- Ask the owner if any treatment was initiated at home. For instance, were they successful in making the animal vomit at home before coming to the veterinary hospital?
- Establish a timeline of exposure and onset of clinical signs. Is the animal getting better, deteriorating, or showing no signs?
- Establish a minimum database.
- Treat the patient, not the poison. Never lose sight of the patient's condition.
- Treat the patient, not the laboratory results. Do not wait for laboratory results to initiate therapy.

consciously strive to eliminate any preconceptions that they may have about owners that will bias the history and affect their diagnostic ability.

The task of the veterinarian is to translate the owner's account into a comprehensive medical history. Remember that clients have not been schooled to give an accurate history in a precise chronologic order and they may have failed to recognize important changes in vital signs or the onset of clinical signs that veterinarians are trained to identify. Just as the clinician must avoid having his or her own preconceptions, incorrect perceptions of owners that their animal has been poisoned must be identified because these can lead veterinarians to search for a toxicologic cause of a problem that is in fact nontoxicologic in origin. **Veterinarians must never suggest that a client's animal has been poisoned unless there is adequate evidence to support such a conclusion.** Last, it is up to the clinician to organize the history in an orderly and logical manner and to establish the exact chronology of events leading up to the animal's clinical presentation. For some veterinarians, a standardized history form is an effective aid in obtaining a complete, thorough, and objective history.

The history and all initial data obtained should be recorded at the time of the original presentation. The animal's record is a medicolegal document that can be subpoenaed, and it should be treated accordingly. Suspected poisoning cases have a particularly high potential for legal action because of possible liability and criminal activity. The recorded history should be organized, legible, and complete. A good rule of thumb is to not take any records that are incomplete or disorganized or that you would be ashamed to have reviewed by your peers or officers of the court.

The history must be organized concisely and logically and must include any and all introductory data. Such data include species; breed; age; sex; reproductive status; vaccine history; previous or current medical problems; current medications; diet; home environment; presence of other animals in the house and any potential appearance of clinical signs in them; recent boarding or kennel history; any recent impoundment and potential exposure to sick or unvaccinated animals; and any recent application of herbicides, pesticides, household cleaners, finishing products, paints or stains (or spills thereof), or use of automotive products or any solvents. Previous or referring veterinarians' notes or any laboratory data outlining previous medical problems or any recent veterinary treatments should be identified, examined, and added to the record. Additional helpful information can be obtained by calling the previous or referring veterinarian. This technique provides an opportunity for the interviewer to obtain supplemental information relevant to the present problem or to underscore the significance of previously obtained data. Next, the chief complaint should be identified, its duration noted, and the physical examination initiated.

Taking a toxicologic history differs a little from the standard clinical history in that it attempts to more specifically establish the time of onset of clinical signs and link them with exposure to a particular toxin. Classically, in suspected poisoning cases, the clinician is faced with one of three scenarios: (1) the animal has been exposed to a known toxin, (2) the animal has been exposed to an unknown substance that may be a toxin, or (3) the animal displays signs of disease of an uncertain or undetermined cause for which toxins must be considered as part of the differential diagnosis. The toxicologic history focuses on the animal. The following questions must be answered: Are there predisposing factors that make the animal more sensitive to exposure? Is the situation compatible with a toxic exposure? Is there a potential source of toxins? Have there been any recent chemical applications?

Despite the often unreliable and possibly unknown nature of the owner's account of events leading to a suspected poisoning, veterinarians must try to obtain as definitive a history as possible. Just as veterinarians must not be misled when owners are convinced that their animals have been poisoned when other causes are actually responsible, clinicians must also never forget that preexisting infections or metabolic, congenital, and neoplastic conditions can mimic the clinical signs of a poisoning or can predispose the animal to a toxicosis. The correlation of an accurate history with the physical examination is crucial. Veterinarians must know the vital signs for the species they care for and must be able to recognize the telltale clinical signs and the characteristic "fingerprints" of specific poisonings.

Despite any possible flaws in the owner's account, the history represents a record of events before and during the onset of the illness. Veterinarians must obtain and organize this information in a logical and orderly manner. Specific criteria characteristic of a toxicologic history include what poison or poisons are involved, when the exposure occurred, how much poison the animal was exposed to, and the route of the exposure (e.g., dermal, oral, inhalation, intravenous, subcutaneous, or intraperitoneal). An important further question is whether other animals at home could also have been exposed.

It is important to review the animal's entire environment. Is the patient an indoor-only cat? An outdoor-only dog? What are the animal's normal daily activities? Is it free to roam? How long is it gone each day? This line of questioning provides helpful information, particularly because many clients may not recognize the potential toxicologic hazards present in their house and yard unless specifically asked. Likewise, information about weather conditions and season and the activities, hobbies, and occupations of the owner may all be important and can provide important clues to the cause of an animal poisoning.

It is of tremendous help if the owner can bring in the original container of the toxic substance. For most suspected poisonings, the exact quantity of toxin ingested is unknown. However, by examining the container in which the poison was stored and questioning the owner, the amount of toxin previously present in the container may be determined. Using this information, the largest amount the animal could have ingested can be estimated. This amount can be compared with the known lethal dosage for an animal of that size. Not only amounts, but also active ingredients, potential antidotes, and related manufacturer information sometimes can be obtained from the package. If the original prescription bottles or containers are not available, the imprint codes from tablets or capsules can be used to identify the substance in question. Imprint codes can be identified in the *Physicians' Desk Reference,* the Internet (e.g., Drugs.com, RxList), regional poison and drug centers, and various pharmacologic sources. Finally, the veterinarian must determine if the owner has initiated

| Box 6-2 | Initial Telephone Contact |

Success or failure in treatment of poisonings can stem from the initial telephone contact. Telephone personnel must establish:

- Name, address, and phone number of person they are speaking with.
- What has been poisoned (e.g., species, breed, age, sex, reproductive status, and weight)?
- What toxin is involved (e.g., amount, concentration; form: liquid, powder, gas, etc.)? Are original containers listing ingredients, concentrations, potential antidotes, or manufacturer's emergency number available?
- When did it happen? (How much time has elapsed since ingestion or exposure? Did the caller see it happen?)
- Route (e.g., ingestion, dermal, inhalation, or ocular)
- Where did it happen (on the owner's premises)?
- How much was ingested? (Original containers allow estimation of how much was consumed and how much remains.)
- What is the animal's present clinical status? (What is the animal doing? Educate the owner about the clinical signs and course of progression for that poisoning.)
- Determine the mg/kg dosage for this exposure. (Compare it with known therapeutic and toxic dose information to establish the risk for this animal; determine a timeline between exposure and onset of clinical signs for this toxin.)
- Other: Find out (1) other toxins the animal could have been exposed to simultaneously, (2) medications the animal is currently taking or other underlying medical conditions (e.g., heart disease, kidney problems, pregnancy), and (3) other animals or children who might have been exposed.
- Determine from this information whether the animal needs to be seen and treated or can be managed conservatively at home and observed. The animal can be observed at home only if a follow-up mechanism is in place (i.e., the owner is familiar with the course of the poisoning and clinical signs and calls frequently [or is called] with progress reports). Final recommendation to treat or observe must rest with the veterinarian.

any treatment before seeking veterinary help. Induction of emesis, bathing to remove dermal toxicants, or administration of any prescription or over-the-counter drugs to offset poisonings are all activities often begun by owners. For example, if the owner has been successful at home in making the animal vomit, this is important. Likewise, well-intentioned owners may unwittingly give medications at home that complicate successful therapy. The first line of defense in the management of poisonings is the telephone. For this reason, all telephone personnel at animal hospitals should be trained as much as possible in the most common small animal poisonings, their relative toxicities, how they are managed, and what to tell people about the treatment (Box 6-2).

Some clinicians and veterinary hospitals use a prepared toxicology history form as a prompt to help them ask the right questions and successfully direct the initial interview in cases of suspected poisoning. Such a standardized document includes the animal's age, weight, environment, and any present medications used. What toxin or toxins are suspected is of course a critical concern. How much poison may have been involved, route of exposure, and when the potential exposure episode occurred are all prominent topics on such a list of questions. If and when clinical signs (and their nature) were first noted is likewise tremendously important. The form also helps determine if other toxins may be implicated and if other animals in the home may also have been exposed. This type of direct-line questioning may help the veterinarian quickly obtain valuable information and aid in more swiftly establishing a diagnosis. An example of such a toxicology history form is included in Box 6-3.

Box 6-3	Sample Toxicology History Form

- What is the animal's name, species, breed, and sex? Is the animal intact or neutered?
- What is the animal's age and weight?
- What medications is the animal presently receiving?
- What other medical history might be pertinent?
- What is the suspected poison involved?
- What is the maximum amount of toxin suspected (worst-case scenario)?
- Was the original container found?
- What is the potential route of exposure suspected?
- When did possible exposure occur?
- When were clinical signs first noted? Describe them.
- Could other poisons be involved?
- Could other animals have been exposed?
- Did the owner initiate any treatment at home (e.g., emesis, baths, etc.)?
- Describe the animal's environment (e.g., where animal is kept, how long left alone, hobbies of owner, anything that might lead to poisoning).

If these history-taking techniques are used and applied in toxicology cases, valuable information can be obtained that will allow the clinician to establish a working diagnosis and determine the most appropriate course of treatment. The toxicologic history is combined with a thorough physical examination, an appropriate minimum database, and a sound list of differential diagnoses. The history is an integral part of the picture in formulating a correct diagnosis and a treatment plan. It is up to the veterinarian to organize it in a logical sequence and then, through correlation with the physical examination, clinical signs, and a complete list of differential diagnoses, identify the diagnosis and undertake an efficacious therapeutic regimen.

Suggested Readings

Carson TL: Taking and interpreting a toxicological history. In Kirk RW, Bonagura JD, editors: *Current veterinary therapy X*, Philadelphia, 1992, WB Saunders.

Galey FD, Hall JO: Field investigation of small animal toxicoses, *Vet Clin N Am Small Animal Pract* 20(2):283–291, 1990.

Lohmeyer C: Taking a toxicological history. In Poppenga RIT, Gwaltney-Brant SM, editors: *Small animal toxicology essentials*, Oxford, UK, 2011, Wiley and Blackwell, pp 27–32.

Approach to Diagnosis for the Toxicology Case

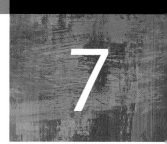

7

Birgit Puschner, DVM, PhD, DABVT

Ahna G. Brutlag, DVM, MS

In small animal practice, intoxications are infrequent, but when they present, extensive diagnostic and therapeutic measures are required. Accurate diagnosis is the key to approaching a potential poisoning case. Such a diagnosis can allow for adequate treatment of poisoned animals and can prevent additional cases. Unfortunately, there is no simple procedure that will test for all toxicants. Rather, these cases require a multifactorial approach that involves assembling and solving a diagnostic puzzle. Information to be compiled includes a complete case history, clinical and clinicopathologic data, postmortem findings, results from chemical analyses, and occasionally bioassay findings.[1] The approach to the toxicology case presented here allows small animal veterinarians to develop a comprehensive diagnostic approach to reach an accurate diagnosis. As clearly illustrated by the tragic outbreak of melamine-cyanuric acid poisoning in dogs and cats in 2007,[2,3] the public expects the veterinary profession to provide professional guidance in the single poisoning case or series of cases with a calm and coherent approach.

Case Presentation and Initial Approach

The small animal practitioner usually must treat one or a few animals, unlike the livestock veterinarian, for whom a toxicology case is more likely to involve large numbers of animals with emphasis on herd health, economics, and food safety in addition to the welfare of an individual. The small animal case presents a further challenge because a wandering animal's recent whereabouts is not always known.

A Poisoning Should Be Suspected If:

- An unexplained death has occurred.
- The animal is sick with no known exposure to infectious disease.
- The animal has been recently exposed to a new environment.
- There has been a recent change in food.
- There has been recent pesticide application in the environment or home.
- There has been recent construction activity in the environment or home.
- An uncommon clinical condition exists.
- There has been a potential threat for a malicious poisoning.

Approach

As mentioned earlier, diagnosis of a toxicology problem involves the assimilation of several classes of data, including the history, clinical signs, clinical chemistry, the presence or absence of lesions, analytical chemistry, and occasionally bioassay.[4,5] Evidence from one class of data rarely provides a definitive diagnosis in the absence of the others. For example, a dog with increased salivation, respiratory distress, vomiting, and diarrhea might have low blood cholinesterase activity. Analysis for an organophosphorus or carbamate insecticide may be negative, yet the animal may have responded to atropine therapy. Historical review of the case might suggest exposure to a short-lived carbamate insecticide (undetectable at sampling), exposure to a pond with neurotoxic cyanobacteria, or exposure to a nicotinic plant, such as tree tobacco (*Nicotiana glauca*) or poison hemlock (*Conium* sp.).

What to Do

- Obtain a complete history.
- Consult with a veterinary toxicologist or animal poison control center (see Chapter 4, "Effective Use of a Veterinary Poison Control Center").
  - Pet Poison Helpline, Minneapolis, MN, 800-213-6680, $39 per case fee
  - American Society for the Prevention of Cruelty to Animals Animal Poison Control Center, Urbana, IL, 888-426-4435, $65 per case fee
- Perform a complete physical examination.
- Perform an exposure assessment.
- Perform a postmortem examination, if an unexplained death has occurred.
- Collect specimens suitable for toxicologic testing (Table 7-1).
- Contact a veterinary toxicology laboratory (www.aavld.org).
- Report a pet food complaint or adverse drug experience to the Food and Drug Administration (http://www.fda.gov/AnimalVeterinary/SafetyHealth/ReportaProblem/default.htm).[6]

History

A thorough review of a case history helps identify possible sources of a toxicant, predisposing factors, situations compatible with exposures, toxicant dose, and clinical signs. The feeding, environmental, and medical histories should be taken along with that of the current problem. The surrounding and immediate areas must be assessed for toxic sources and hazardous conditions. Samples for analysis can be obtained or sought as the investigation proceeds. Potential hazards should be removed as soon as they are identified to prevent additional exposures. Ideally, the entire environment should be inspected for potentially toxic plants, poisonous mushrooms, contaminated water, or household chemicals. When environmental inspection is not possible, the pet owner should be thoroughly questioned about the pet's access to such hazards. Other common hazards include access to garbage; access to a purse or backpack (chewing gum or breath mints with xylitol, cigarettes, medications); recent baking activities (chocolate, raisins, xylitol, or raw dough); over-the-counter and prescription medications in the household; new toys; new cages; or pest control activities with such chemicals as rodenticides, insecticides, or herbicides. Additionally, be sure to inquire about food including human foods such as grapes, macadamia nuts, and sugar-free products with xylitol; pet foods; and dietary supplements and treats. Identify new or different sources. Also inquire about any recent visitors to the home such as friends or relatives. Well-meaning visitors may unknowingly feed the pet harmful foods or have medications stored in their luggage that may be accessible by the pet. Animal husbandry practices, such as types of foods used or outdoor patterns may help identify common sources if multiple animals are affected. The practitioner should discreetly note cultural traits that may yield information about exposure to drugs, herbal medications, or unusual foods. Asking the pet owner about the administration of common human medications such as aspirin, ibuprofen, acetaminophen, and antihistamines with decongestants (e.g., loratadine with pseudoephedrine [Claritin-D] and diphenhydramine [Benadryl-D]) may reveal additional helpful information. Well-meaning but uninformed pet owners may attempt to "treat" their ill animal with drugs such as these. The time of year can also yield important clues. Car radiators are replenished in the autumn, leading to antifreeze exposures; specific plants such as Easter lilies are predominantly sold at certain times during the year.

The signalment of the affected animal should also be identified. The breed of dog may generate information about drug sensitivity. For example, collies, Australian shepherds, and other herding breeds are overly sensitive to the anthelmintic ivermectin and the antidiarrheal loperamide (Imodium). The species and size of animal are also crucial for assessing toxicant exposures. A small cat is more sensitive to a given amount of ethylene glycol than a larger cat or a similar-sized dog. To highlight interspecies differences, consider that,

Table 7-1	Key Specimens for Toxicologic Testing	
Specimen	**Condition**	**Select Possible Tests**
Gastric contents (vomitus, lavage)	Frozen	Comprehensive poison screen for unknowns, strychnine, metaldehyde, insecticides, drugs, anatoxin-a, microcystins, zinc phosphide, plant toxins, metals, ionophores, amanitin; identification of plant parts and seeds
Urine	Frozen	Drugs (amphetamine, cocaine, THC, LSD, ephedrine, methamphetamine, morphine, nicotine, psilocin), anatoxin-a, strychnine, metaldehyde, ethylene glycol, amanitin, paraquat, caffeine
Serum	Separated from clot promptly and frozen	Zinc, copper, iron, sodium, ethylene glycol, diethylene glycol
Blood	Refrigerated	Lead, cholinesterase activity, thallium, mercury
Liver	Frozen	Comprehensive poison screen for unknowns, anticoagulant rodenticides, metals, certain drugs, strychnine, amanitin, organophosphorus and carbamate insecticides, pyrethrins and pyrethroids, vitamins E and A
Kidney	Frozen	Ethylene glycol, melamine and analogues, oxalate, calcium, phosphorus, amanitin, vitamin D
Brain	Frozen	Cholinesterase activity, sodium, bromethalin
Lung	Frozen	Paraquat
Food and source material	Dry material should be kept dry at room temperature; moist material should be frozen	Comprehensive poison screen for unknowns, strychnine, metaldehyde, organophosphorus and carbamate insecticides, pyrethrins/pyrethroids, microcystins, zinc phosphide, plant toxins, metals, ionophores, amanitin, bromethalin, anticoagulants, ethylene glycol, mycotoxins (aflatoxins, vomitoxin, penitrem A), melamine and analogues, vitamins A and E, and plant, mushroom and seed identification
Water	Refrigerated	Microcystins, anatoxin-a, pesticides, poison screen

LSD, Lysergic acid diethylamide; *THC,* tetrahydrocannabinol.

although concentrated pyrethroids are routinely safely applied to dogs for flea and tick control, even a small vial of these products applied to a cat may prove fatal.

Exposure Assessment

The significance of an exposure depends on a great many factors. One of the most significant is the effect on the species in terms of habit and metabolic differences. The toxicity of a xenobiotic may also be affected by its route and rate of exposure and by the animal's age, nutritional status, preexisting disease status, diet, water intake, environment, and management. Considering all factors, the most important is the dose of the xenobiotic that is taken into the system.

Dose-Response Assessment

As Paracelsus instructed, "The dose determines the poison."[7] Almost all compounds, including water, may be toxic if a susceptible animal is exposed to a sufficient quantity. Consideration of dose response involves multiple factors in addition to the animal-related variables previously mentioned. These factors include the magnitude of the dose; the frequency of exposure; and the slope of the dose-response curve for the animal's species, age, nutritional status, disease status, gender, and many other related factors.

The magnitude of the exposure determines toxicity because most poisons act at specific sites or receptors. The action at those sites can usually be related to the magnitude of effect in the patient. Dose-response relationships exist for chemicals that have a wide variety of effects. For example, a small amount of diluted sodium hypochlorite (a few milliliters of bleach in the toilet bowl at greater than 1:23 dilution) probably will not cause damage if ingested. However, if a puppy ingests concentrated bleach, severe damage to the oral mucosa and esophagus may result. A small dog that ingests the tissue of a mouse that suffers from a marginal dose of an anticoagulant rodenticide (<1 ppm in tissue) is not likely to be poisoned. However, if the mouse still has a stomach full of the active rodenticide at approximately 0.005%, or 50 ppm, a mild hazard may exist for the dog. Additionally, some potentially toxic chemicals may be essential nutrients in low concentrations. For example, cats require approximately 10,000 IU/kg of diet of vitamin A for optimal health. Yet chronic toxicosis may result if the diet contains more than 100,000 IU vitamin A per kilogram of food material.

If a sufficient amount of a toxicant is ingested, acute poisoning may occur after one exposure. At lower levels, however, a toxicant may not cause disease until after it has been ingested repeatedly or until a sufficient amount of the chemical has accumulated at the receptor site. For example, repeated daily doses of compounds that can accumulate, such as an anticoagulant rodenticide like brodifacoum or a metal like lead, are toxic at much lower levels than a single acute dose. Additionally, for some compounds, the signs of chronic toxicosis can be different from the acute signs. A bird that has been soaked in an organochlorine insecticide (e.g., dichlorodiphenyltrichloroethane) may develop neurologic signs and die. Daily exposure to low levels of the organochlorine, however, may not cause acute toxicosis. Rather, chronic long-term effects may result, leading to abnormal reproduction, including eggshell thinning and liver degeneration.

It is also important to understand the slope of the dose-response curve. Many texts provide the practitioner with the median lethal dose (LD_{50}) or, in some cases, the median toxic dose. However, that measure simply describes the dose at which 50% of an exposed population may be expected to die or develop toxicosis. More important to the clinician is the dose at which a hazard to any animal may exist. Obviously, that will be a lower value. For toxicants with a steep dose-response curve, the minimum toxic dose will be very close to the median toxic dose. For example, a highly toxic plant, such as oleander (Color Plate 26-2), may kill at almost any dose for which there is an effect. For other toxicants such as organochlorine insecticides, which have a shallow dose-response curve, some effects may be seen at levels that are orders of magnitude (10×) below the median lethal dose.

Exceptions exist to the dose-response relationship in toxicology. For example, hypersensitivity is not generally dose responsive. Once an animal has been sensitized to a xenobiotic (e.g., venom from a bee sting), a very tiny amount later may trigger a massive anaphylactic response. Additionally, some carcinogens may not follow a dose-response curve. For example, one key genetic injury may trigger the formation of a cancer. Nevertheless, for the great majority of toxicants, understanding that the dose determines whether a compound may be toxic to an animal helps the practitioner decide whether an animal has been exposed to a toxic dose of a xenobiotic.

Exposure Assessment Calculations

Given that the dose-response relationship is the major determinant of toxicity, performing basic exposure calculations helps determine the exposure of a potential toxicant in a patient. The practitioner must understand the basic units of concentrations, their sources, and how to convert a source concentration to an exposure level to compare the exposure with known toxicity data.

When conducting an assessment, one must identify the source of the denominator for various concentration units. Additionally, concentration data must be scrutinized to determine whether the level is on an as-is basis or a dry-weight basis. Dry-weight concentrations appear to be much higher than as-is levels for moist samples. The toxicity of a compound is generally expressed in terms of milligrams of toxicant per kilogram body weight. Generally, the practitioner must have information regarding the toxicant concentration in food or source material, and a known toxicity in an animal species (usually obtained from the literature or an animal poison control center). Thus the likely amount of toxicant taken in by the patient is calculated as follows:

Known data:
- Concentration of toxicant in the source material (milligram of toxicant/kilogram of source material)
- Body weight (BW) of patient (in kilograms)
- Toxicity of chemical (milligram of toxicant/kilogram BW)

Estimation: Weight (in grams or kilograms, for example) of source material taken in (or approximate intake of feed or water) or the milligram dose of tablets or capsules; if only an estimate, a good rule of thumb might be to double the estimated intake to be conservative.

Goal: Determine the milligram/kilogram BW taken in to compare with toxic level.

Formula:

$$\text{kg source} \times \text{mg toxicant/kg source} = \text{mg toxicant intake (pure compound ingested)}$$

$$\text{mg toxicant intake/kg BW} = \text{mg/kg (actual exposure)}$$

Interpretation: The calculated value is then compared with the known toxicity value for the compound (e.g., LD_{50}, LD_1, oral lethal dose). Toxicity data is often unavailable or minimal for the toxicant of interest in the species of interest (such as dogs or cats) but may exist for rodents. Conservative advice is to treat exposures within fivefold of an LD_{50} value (i.e., $LD_{50/5}$) determined in the species of interest as potential toxicoses, but not to dismiss those that are tenfold lower than the LD_{50} as innocuous exposures. Uncertainty is greater when dealing with LD_{50} values from other species. It is best to treat exposures within tenfold of an LD_{50} value as potential toxicoses and to not dismiss those that are 50-fold lower than the LD_{50} as innocuous exposures.

Calculations for determining the significance of exposure are a key step in determining the course of action in many potential poisoning cases. These calculations are not difficult, as has been demonstrated, but common sense must be applied to be sure that the estimates and assumptions are as correct as possible.

Example: Brodifacoum Exposure in a Dog

A 20-kg dog was observed to have ingested as much as one 3-oz packet of rodent bait. The remains of the packet revealed that the product contained 0.005% of brodifacoum as-is, a potent "one-bite" formulation of anticoagulant rodenticide. Looking in the literature, you ascertain that the canine oral LD_{50} of brodifacoum may be as low as 0.25 mg brodifacoum per kilogram of body weight. After decontamination, the veterinarian needs to assess whether this dog should be treated with vitamin K_1.

The calculation is as follows:

- First convert to kilograms: kg source: 3 oz × 30 g/oz (approximately) = 90 g = 0.09 kg bait; mg/kg brodifacoum: 0.005% = 50 ppm = 50 mg brodifacoum/kg bait (no adjustment needed for dry weight because toxicity is listed as "as is").

- Next, divide the canine LD_{50} by 5 to determine the treatment threshold: 0.25 mg/kg ÷ 5 = 0.05 mg/kg.
- *Estimation:* 0.09 kg bait × 50 mg brodifacoum/kg bait = 4.5 mg brodifacoum ingested
- *Result:* 4.5 mg brodifacoum/20 kg BW = 0.225 mg/kg (actual exposure)
- *Interpretation:* The patient received up to 0.225 mg/kg BW of brodifacoum. Because this value exceeds one fifth of the LD_{50} (0.05 mg/kg), the safest recommendation is to treat the patient as if it received a toxic dose.

Clinical Signs and Clinical Pathologic Findings

Once the history is understood, the clinical presentation may suggest a toxicant and which organs have been affected. Signs may be specific, like inducible seizures caused by the rodenticide strychnine. Conversely, nonspecific signs, such as vomiting and drowsiness, may indicate anything from ingestion of garbage, a houseplant, or a drug such as an antidepressant or muscle relaxant, to perhaps ethylene glycol. The rate of onset and progression of signs may also be useful to the astute diagnostician. Sudden onset of convulsions may suggest strychnine, metaldehyde, or penitrem A (moldy walnuts or cream cheese) toxicoses. More subtly, insidious bleeding may imply an anticoagulant rodenticide exposure. Development of liver failure following a course of gastrointestinal upset and transient recovery may suggest amanitin (mushroom) toxicosis.

As for other phases of the investigation, it is best to keep an open mind and open eyes. Vomitus should be examined for foreign objects and saved for potential diagnostic testing. Pills or leaves from some plants may be present in recognizable form. Distinct colors and dyes may be due to the ingestion of paintballs, the coating of a medication, or rodenticide baits (Color Plates 7-1 to 7-3). If something is found, the owner can be encouraged to return with source material that might resemble that in the vomitus, giving the practitioner a quick diagnostic comparison.

Assessment of clinical pathologic data may indicate a possible toxicant. Elevations in organ-specific enzymes or metabolites in serum may help to identify affected organs. For example, a dog poisoned by the mushroom toxin, amanitin, likely has very high concentrations of liver-specific enzymes. Animals suffering from ethylene glycol intoxication have a metabolic acidosis, elevated anion gap, increased serum osmolality, and eventually azotemia.

In addition to clinical pathologic testing, samples from the live animal may be useful for analytic toxicology testing and are listed in Table 7-1. The most diagnostically useful samples from an animal presented for a suspect intoxication are vomitus, gastric lavage contents, fecal material, urine, whole blood, serum, and occasionally cerebrospinal fluid. Tissue biopsies may also be useful.

Once obtained, all samples should be frozen, except whole blood (which may be refrigerated). Serum should be separated from the clot as soon as possible before freezing. Some analytes, such as vitamin E or zinc, may be altered by time spent in contact with the clot because red cells continue to metabolize them or release additional material. Because some rubber is hardened with zinc, the use of a rubber plunger syringe or a red-stoppered clot tube invalidates most testing for zinc. If zinc testing is required, all-plastic or special trace element clotting tubes should be used. Vacutainer systems are suggested for the actual collection of the sample. Avoid the use of serum separator tubes for toxicologic testing. All samples should be properly labeled before being shipped to the laboratory.

Testing for ethylene glycol, lead, zinc, cholinesterase, strychnine, metaldehyde, and drugs such as acetaminophen can often be performed on an immediate basis, giving the practitioner a quick answer. Others, like anticoagulant rodenticides or toxic plants, may require a day or longer to allow for extraction and purification before analysis can be completed. In areas where a veterinary diagnostic laboratory is not readily accessible, contacting a local human hospital for immediate testing is recommended.

Postmortem Examination and Sampling

Necropsy of dead animals should be complete. Partial necropsy should be avoided because it could result in missing a pertinent lesion or perhaps a critical sample. Before performing the postmortem examination, inquire about the legal status of the case so that any required sampling (for insurance, legal, or other purposes) can be done. Many suspected toxicoses have turned out to be due to infectious causes and vice versa, so try to keep an open mind during the examination. Also, eyes and nose are often the best diagnostic tools.

Note any external markings and appearance (e.g., bruises or singed fur) before opening the body cavity. Samples needed for diagnosis of infectious diseases (e.g., cultures) should be obtained first to avoid contamination. Next, obtain all the urine from the bladder using a clean syringe before other procedures cause its accidental loss. Transfer the urine to a plastic screw-capped vial for storage or shipping. Despite some myths, urine is still much more useful for testing for drugs than tissue. Next, carefully examine and sample the internal organs and tissues. Inspect the ingesta for unusual material, including plant parts, pills, or chemical granules. The foreign matter should be identified and saved apart from other samples of ingesta. Ingesta are especially useful for chemical testing because many toxicants are metabolized after absorption to such an extent that they may not be detected in other tissues.

Samples of major organs should be placed in fixative for histologic examination. Additionally, samples of appropriate organs, including the brain, should be packaged individually and frozen fresh (not fixed) for toxicologic testing (Table 7-1). Do not combine all organ samples into one bag as this may result in invalid tissue test results.

Lesions from poisoning can be specific, nonspecific, or even absent. For example, birefringent crystals in the renal tubules support the diagnosis of ethylene glycol toxicosis. On the other hand, a hemorrhagic enteritis may suggest a variety of toxic plants (e.g., castor bean plant [*Ricinus*] or an insoluble oxalate containing *Philodendron* spp.), metals (e.g., arsenic, zinc, iron), or pesticides (e.g., anticoagulant rodenticides). Other toxicants, such as organophosphorus and carbamate insecticides, may cause very little postmortem damage except some nonspecific pulmonary edema and serosal reddening. Thus lesions must be interpreted in light of other data collected.

Sample Collection and Toxicology Testing

In-house or bedside tests for certain toxicants such as ethylene glycol and illicit drugs may be useful but should be used with caution. Often, these tests may be quite sensitive but lack specificity. For example, many commercial bedside ethylene glycol tests yield a false positive in the presence of propylene glycol (found in "pet safe" antifreeze and injectable diazepam as well as other drugs),[8] sorbitol (common cathartic in activated charcoal preparations), mannitol, and isopropyl alcohol (do not swab the venipuncture site prior to sampling). Over-the-counter human urine drug screens designed to detect illicit substances such as marijuana, cocaine, methamphetamine, and so on have been used with varied success in pets. In dogs, marijuana is notoriously difficult to detect with such tests and will frequently result in a false negative.[9] Alternatively, other common drugs such as diphenhydramine may yield a false positive result for phencyclidine (PCP) and opioids in humans.[10] It is not yet known if this occurs in veterinary species. Thus results from these tests must be interpreted in light of clinical presentation and should not be relied on for a definitive diagnosis.

A good approach in a case of unknown cause of illness or death is to hold toxicologic samples until the results of other tests (e.g., clinical pathologic, histopathologic, and bacteriologic analysis) are available. Then the involved toxicologic testing can be performed in a focused manner based on the history and available diagnostic data. Recently, new methodologies such as liquid chromatography and mass spectrometry, gas chromatography and mass spectrometry, and direct analysis in real time (DART) mass spectrometry allow for comprehensive screens for unknown toxicants. However, these techniques are not available at all veterinary toxicology laboratories. Key samples for toxicology testing (Table 7-1) should be saved for possible future testing, including samples from the live animal, samples collected during necropsy (if applicable), and samples collected in the animal's environment (e.g., food, water, plants, source material, bait). It is better to toss out an unneeded sample than to wish it were available for a crucial test. Samples should be refrigerated or frozen and stored in separate containers. Dry foods and other sources can be stored in a cool, dark, dry place. Plants to be identified can be submitted fresh to a diagnostic laboratory or other plant expert (including herbaria, local colleges, and plant stores) if the submission can be made quickly. Otherwise, it is best to press the plant carefully in a newspaper between some books and then submit the dried plant. Mushrooms should also be submitted dry for identification or wrapped in paper towels if fresh. Avoid placing mushrooms or moist plants in plastic bags and putting them in the refrigerator as they tend to rot in that environment. Where the specimen was collected is essential information for both plant and mushroom identification, so this information must be included with the specimen (e.g., town, county, under a deciduous tree, near a woodpile, etc.).

Summary

Complaints involving poisoning of pets are not the most common cases presented to veterinarians. When such cases are presented they may be complicated and may involve much emotion. Consultation with personnel in a veterinary toxicology laboratory or animal poison control center can provide significant guidance with respect to establishing a diagnosis and treatment protocol in a suspect poisoning case. It is hoped that the approach presented here can help the practitioner handle these cases with confidence and reach an accurate and confirmed diagnosis.

Acknowledgment

The authors wish to acknowledge the exceptional contribution of Dr. Frank Galey, who co-authored this chapter for the previous edition of the book.

References

1. Galey FD: Diagnostic toxicology for the small animal veterinarian, *Calif Vet* Sept-Oct:7–10, 1994.
2. Puschner B, Poppenga RH, Lowenstine LJ, et al: Assessment of melamine and cyanuric acid toxicity in cats, *J Vet Diagn Invest* 19:616–624, 2007.
3. Brown CA, Jeong KS, Poppenga RH, et al: Outbreaks of renal failure associated with melamine and cyanuric acid in dogs and cats in 2004 and 2007, *J Vet Diagn Invest* 19:525–531, 2007.
4. Galey FD: Diagnostic toxicology. In Plumlee KH, editor: *Clinical veterinary toxicology*, St Louis, 2004, Mosby, pp 22–23.
5. Volmer PA, Meerdink GL: Diagnostic toxicology for the small animal practitioner, *Vet Clin North Am— Small Anim Pract* 32:357, 2002.
6. *Food and Drug Administration: Report a problem.* Retrieved July 14, 2010, from http://www.fda.gov/AnimalVeterinary/SafetyHealth/ReportaProblem/default.htm.
7. Borzelleca JF: Paracelsus: herald of modern toxicology, *Toxicol Sci* 53:2–4, 2000.
8. Acierno MJ, Serra VF, Johnson ME, et al: Preliminary validation of a point-of-care ethylene glycol test for cats, *J Vet Emer Crit Care* 18:477–479, 2008.
9. Teitler JB: Evaluation of a human on-site urine multidrug test for emergency use with dogs, *J Am Anim Hosp Assoc* 45:59–66, 2009.
10. Moeller KE, Lee KC, Kissack JC: Urine drug screening: practical guide for clinicians, *Mayo Clin Proc* 83:66–76, 2008.

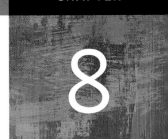

Establishing a Minimum Database in Small Animal Poisonings

Kevin T. Fitzgerald, PhD, DVM, DABVP

Successful diagnosis of a particular poisoning is based on a complete history, a thorough physical examination, and physical parameters and laboratory results obtained through establishment of a minimum database. Identification of the presence of a specific toxin allows the clinician to rapidly initiate a specific treatment that may lead to a successful outcome.

Thousands of different molecules have the capacity to poison living organisms. Unfortunately, less than 5% of all potential toxins have antidotes or effective physiologic antagonists. Nevertheless the public has unrealistic expectations about antidotes and "poison screening" tests available to veterinarians to identify toxicants. Veterinary toxicology laboratories are currently able to detect and quantitate 200 to 300 or so true poisons. Because of the limitations of (1) expense; (2) time necessary to obtain the samples, run the tests, and obtain results; (3) required sample volumes; and (4) the sheer staggering number of potentially poisonous molecules in existence, toxicology screening tests are not commonly pursued in veterinary medicine. However, because only approximately 15 or 20 types of substances account for almost 90% of all small animal veterinary poisonings, if the clinician has a high index of suspicion of a particular toxin, certain screening tests can be very rewarding and should not be overlooked.

Screening tests are maximally effective only if the clinician has good reason (based on the history and clinical signs) to suspect a particular poison and requests a specific laboratory procedure. Just as specific antidotes should not be administered without a definitive diagnosis, the use of toxicology tests as "fishing expeditions" should be avoided if they are to be successful or meaningful. In cases with potential medicolegal consequences, the use of toxicology tests to confirm or deny the presence of a particular poison and its concentration may be recommended. Identification of a poison in toxic levels in appropriate tissues and organs of an animal that is thought to be poisoned is often the only way to confirm a diagnosis. What steps must be taken to obtain samples to provide such information?

Clinical Signs

Following a complete history, a thorough physical examination and assessment of any clinical signs that may be present must be undertaken to arrive at a diagnosis of poisoning. Veterinarians must be thoroughly familiar with the vital signs of the species that they care for so that they can instantly recognize any abnormal signs. Vital signs are the first real physical data the veterinarian receives. Respiratory rate and nature, heart rate and rhythm, pulse rate and rhythm, core body temperature, capillary refill time, mucous membrane color, and any apparent dehydration all reveal clues about an animal's condition. Electrocardiography, pulse oximetry, and Doppler blood pressure monitoring are all readily available methods of documenting an animal's immediate condition more accurately. If the animal is in a life-threatening state, emergency methods must be initiated long before a diagnosis of poisoning can be obtained or therapy started. A final diagnosis is not necessary to stabilize or correct a life-threatening condition. Once the animal is stable, the specific tests and steps necessary to achieve a minimum toxicologic database can be started.

Physical examination and assessment of clinical signs are invaluable and cannot be separated from either the history or laboratory results in the attempt to obtain a definitive diagnosis of poisoning. At the same time, it should be noted that clinical signs for many conditions are stereotyped and similar, and that cells, tissues, and organs can respond in only a limited number of ways that can look much the same, regardless of the cause (e.g., traumatic, toxicologic, infectious, metabolic, or neoplastic). For this reason, poisoning is rarely diagnosed through the physical examination or clinical signs alone. Finally, basing a diagnosis solely on the clinical signs is unreliable because the veterinarian may be seeing only one phase of the disease and may have missed important earlier phases that help to reveal the identity, course, and chronology of the intoxication.

Minimum Database

In developing a minimum toxicologic database, the small animal clinician must keep in mind what diagnostic tests laboratories are capable of running, which toxins can be detected and which cannot be detected, sample types and minimum sample volumes, the turn-around times involved in obtaining results, and the costs. Laboratory results remain a supportive adjunct to a complete history, a thorough physical evaluation of the animal, and recognition of specific clinical signs of certain poisons. To maximize the efficacy of laboratory results, veterinarians must have knowledge of the proper use of each test, a basic grasp of specific laboratory procedures, and an understanding of how to obtain and handle specimens properly. This information can be readily obtained by consulting directly with laboratory personnel. The best guide to the diagnosis, treatment, and selection of the most appropriate laboratory tests is the clinical condition of the animal in question. In addition, the small animal clinician can also check with local human hospitals to see what routine toxicology tests are available.

For every suspected life-threatening poisoning, routine laboratory studies should include a complete blood count and a serum chemistry panel that includes determination of serum electrolytes, glucose, blood urea nitrogen, creatinine, and calcium. A urinalysis should be routinely obtained. Prothrombin time, activated clotting time, or a coagulation panel can be included to identify abnormal coagulation. Pulse oximetry and electrocardiography are performed to assess both hemoglobin saturation (SpO_2) and cardiac irregularities. Liver enzyme tests are usually performed to monitor damage caused by poisons that are directly toxic to or degraded by the liver. Arterial blood gas evaluation is included when available to evaluate respiratory status and acid-base abnormalities. The anion gap should be determined to assist in the diagnosis and management of certain types of poisonings. Finally, radiographs should be taken of both the chest and the abdomen to help identify pulmonary edema, aspiration pneumonia, and any radiopaque toxins in the gastrointestinal tract. Vomitus must be examined as an indicator of recent oral ingestion of any type of poison. Feces should also be collected. Veterinarians need to assist the laboratory by including a list of suspected toxins.

Clinicians must remember to "treat the patient, not the poison." There is no single accurate, rapid, and inexpensive method ("poison screen") that can detect all toxins. Just as specific antidotes should not be used without a narrow index of suspicion based on a matching history, confirming physical examination and clinical signs, and supportive laboratory results, veterinarians must never delay supportive therapy while awaiting a confirmatory laboratory test or positive toxin level in a critically ill animal. The following are the individual components of the minimum toxicologic database.

Complete Blood Count

A complete blood count reveals hemoconcentration; anemia (e.g., possible zinc ingestion); aplastic anemia; platelet deficiency; potential basophilic stippling; and the morphologic characteristics of thrombocytes, erythrocytes, and leukocytes. Blood is also useful for detecting most elements and metals, some pesticides, cholinesterase activity, ethylene glycol, iron, ethanol, methanol, and many drugs (e.g., acetaminophen, salicylates, theophylline, digoxin).

Serum Electrolytes (Sodium, Chloride, Potassium, Magnesium, Phosphorus, Bicarbonate)

Metabolic acidosis results either from the increased production or decreased excretion of nonvolatile acids or from the loss of body alkali. The serum anion gap helps to distinguish between these two types of metabolic acidosis. Most toxins produce an increased anion gap by the accumulation of organic acids. The anion gap is measured by subtracting the measured anions (Cl^- and HCO_3^-) from the measured cations (Na and K). The normal anion gap is 12 to 25 mEq/L. Accumulation of unmeasured anions (e.g., sulfates, phosphates, protein, and organic acids) results in an increased or abnormal anion gap. Most often a high anion gap is associated with metabolic acidosis and is caused by accumulation of organic acids, such as lactate or formate. Toxins that can cause an elevated anion gap and metabolic acidosis include alcohol, methanol, toluene, ethylene glycol, propylene glycol, paraldehyde, iron, salicylates, and any toxin that causes lactic acid build-up. Ethylene glycol should be placed high on the differential diagnostic list whenever an animal presents with a high anion gap of unknown cause. Another electrolyte abnormality that has been seen in dogs is hypokalemia related to albuterol intoxication.

Arterial Blood Gas Analysis

Arterial blood gas analysis is not always available, but if it is, it can be used to evaluate respiratory status and acid-base abnormalities in the poisoned animal. Toxic exposures can cause vomiting, diarrhea, seizures, and respiratory irregularities. As a result, these developments can be responsible for an overall acidosis (metabolic, respiratory, or lactic acidosis) or alkalosis (metabolic or respiratory). Severe metabolic acidosis may require the use of therapeutic sodium bicarbonate. Toxins responsible for respiratory depression and subsequent hypoventilation trigger respiratory acidosis. (See Box 8-1 for a list of toxins affecting respiratory rate.) Substances causing seizures may produce a lactic acidosis as a result of increased muscle activity. (A list of the most common poisons causing seizures [a common toxidrome] is included in Table 8-1.) Severe vomiting and diarrhea can result in a metabolic alkalosis. This will rarely resolve until gastrointestinal losses of metabolites are addressed. Respiratory alkalosis is a side-effect of hyperventilation. Intoxicants that cause excitement and stimulate the respiratory system can result in hypoxemia. Excessive ventilation by mechanically ventilating a patient may lead to respiratory alkalosis, just as patients treated with high dosages of opioids and anticonvulsants may demonstrate hypoventilation and a subsequent respiratory acidosis.

Box 8-1 Common Toxins Affecting Respiratory Rate

Bradypnea (↓)
Barbiturates
Ethanol
Neuromuscular blockers
Opioids
Sedative hypnotics

Tachypnea (↑)
Carbon monoxide
Cyanide
Ethylene glycol
Methanol
Methemoglobin-producing agents
Nicotine
Organophosphates and carbamates
Salicylates
Sympathomimetic agents
Theophylline

Lactate

Monitoring blood lactate has become an important tool in identification of

Table 8-1   Toxins and Specific Toxidromes

Toxin	Vital Signs	Mentation	Signs	Clinical Findings
1. Acetaminophen	Normal (early on)	Normal	Anorexia, vomiting	Jaundice (later)
2. Amphetamines	Tachycardia, tachypnea, hyperthermia, hypertension	Agitation	Anxiety, panic	Mydriasis—hyperactive peristalsis
3. Antihistamines	Hyperthermia, tachycardia, hypotension, hypertension	Agitation, altered mentation, lethargy to coma	Dry mouth, visual problems, difficulty in urination	Dry mucous membranes, mydriasis, urinary retention
4. Arsenic (acute)	Hypotension, tachycardia	Alert to coma	Vomiting, diarrhea, dysphagia, abdominal pain	Dehydration
5. Barbiturates	Hypothermia, hypotension, bradypnea	Altered, lethargy to coma	Stumbling, ataxia	Hyporeflexive, cold, blank stare
6. β-Adrenergic antagonists	Hypotension, bradycardia	Altered, lethargy to coma	Ataxia	Cyanosis, seizures
7. Calcium channel blockers	Hypotension, bradycardia	Altered, lethargic, confused	Anorexic, vomiting	Slow heart rate
8. Carbon monoxide	Often normal	Altered, lethargy to coma	Nausea, vomiting, diarrhea, ataxia	Seizures
9. Cocaine	Hyperthermia, hypertension, tachypnea, tachycardia	Anxiety, agitation, delirious	Anxiety, restlessness, panic	Mydriasis, nystagmus
10. Cyclic antidepressants	Hypotension, tachycardia	Lethargy to coma	Dry mouth, difficulty in urination, confusion, ataxia	Mydriasis, dry membranes, distended bladder, seizures
11. Digitalis	Hypotension, bradycardia	Normal or lethargic	Anorexia, vomiting	None seen
12. Ethanol	Hypotension, tachycardia	Altered	Ataxia, anorexic, vomiting	Ataxia
13. Ethylene glycol (antifreeze)	Tachypnea	Lethargy to coma	Abdominal pain	Ataxia, stumbling, coma
14. Iron	Hypotension, tachycardia	Normal or lethargic	Anorexia, vomiting, diarrhea	Hematemesis

15. Lead	Hypertension	Lethargy to coma	Anorexic, vomiting, constipation, belly pain	Peripheral neuropathy, seizures, gingival pigmentation
16. Mercury	Hypotension (late)	Altered, anxiety	Anorexic, salivation, vomiting	Ataxia, stomatitis, tremors
17. Opioids	Hypotension, bradycardia, bradypnea, hypothermia	Lethargy to coma	Ataxia, confusion	Miosis, decreased peristalsis
18. Organophosphates and carbamates	Hypotension or hypertension, bradycardia or tachycardia, bradypnea or tachypnea	Lethargy to coma	Vomiting and diarrhea, belly pain, visual deficits	Salivation, lacrimation, urination, defecation, miosis, fasciculations, seizures
19. Phenothiazines	Hypotension, tachycardia, hypothermia or hyperthermia	Lethargy to coma	Ataxia, dry mouth, difficulty in urination	Miosis or mydriasis, decreased gut sounds
20. Salicylates	Hyperthermia, tachycardia	Agitation, then lethargy to coma	Anorexia, vomiting	Heart failure
21. Sedative-hypnotics	Hypotension, bradycardia, hypothermia, bradypnea	Lethargy to coma	Ataxia, stumbling	Hyporeflexia
22. Snail bait (metaldehyde)	Hyperthermia, tachypnea, tachycardia	Lethargy to coma	Ataxia, vomiting, diarrhea	Incoordination, muscle tremors, seizures
23. Theophylline (methylxanthine)	Hypotension, hyperthermia, tachycardia, tachypnea	Agitation, anxiety	Anorexia, vomiting	Tremors, seizures, cardiac arrhythmias
24. Pyrethrins and pyrethroids	Variable	Lethargy to coma	Anorexia, vomiting, diarrhea	Salivation, vomiting and diarrhea, muscle fasciculations, tremors, seizures

hypoventilation. In instances of impaired oxygen delivery to tissues and abnormalities or disturbances of normal perfusion, resultant anaerobic metabolism produces lactate. Normal values in adult dogs and cats are less than 2.5 mmol/L; levels greater than 7 mmol/L reveal severe tissue hypoxia. During therapeutic resuscitation, serial measurements of lactate can help evaluate the effectiveness of treatment. Monitoring blood lactate every 2 hours after therapy is initiated can help determine the progress of treatment efforts. Once normalized, monitoring lactate every 8 hours can identify an acute increase in lactate levels, which can signal problems in treatment. For severely compromised animals, lactate may rise after the initial start of fluid therapy as improved tissue perfusion pushes lactate out of the poorly perfused areas. This increase is only transient. As blood supply to compromised tissues increases and fluid therapy continues, lactate values should normalize. A variety of toxins may result in hypoperfusion, thus making lactate measurement an important marker.

Blood Glucose

Numerous toxins and toxin look-alike disease states can affect the blood glucose level. Glucose levels can be rapidly, inexpensively, and accurately assessed by widely available commercial glucometers. Such swift determination allows rapid initiation of therapy.

Blood Urea Nitrogen and Creatinine

A wide variety of toxins can damage the kidneys. This damage can result from a direct insult to the renal tissues by the poison or indirectly through toxic byproducts of the metabolized xenobiotic. Also, decreased renal perfusion can result from various intoxicants or any toxin that causes shock, hypovolemia, or vascular collapse. Initial assessment of kidney measurements reveals the presence of acute injury and can direct rapid therapy, but serial measurements of blood urea nitrogen and creatinine should be taken when poisons are suspected that may have delayed onset of action. Assessment of renal function is discussed in more detail in the later section on urinalysis.

Calcium

Hypercalcemia is most commonly seen in patients with lymphosarcoma, hyperparathyroidism, or a toxicosis caused by vitamin D–containing products. The calcium level should be monitored to help determine whether a poison, neoplasia, or metabolic disease is involved. Hypocalcemia can be seen in cases of ethylene glycol poisoning.

Urinalysis

Urinalysis is necessary in establishing a minimum database for poisonings. When blood levels of toxins are too low to be detected, urine samples may still be revealing. Drugs with rapid elimination or those that have large volumes of distribution can best be screened in the urine. Both qualitative and quantitative methods of detection of toxicants are available (Box 8-2). Antihistamines, phenothiazines, barbiturates, benzodiazepines, sedative hypnotics, and tricyclic antidepressants are examples of such drugs. Urinalysis can confirm the presence of crystals (e.g., calcium oxalate monohydrate crystals specific for ethylene glycol toxicity), casts (which are the hallmark of acute proximal tubule damage and signal

Box 8-2	Urine Color Changes and Causative Agents	
Dipyrone: brown-red		Doxorubicin: pink
Methemoglobin: brown-red		Naphthalene (mothballs): red
Propofol: green		Myoglobin: red
Anticoagulants: yellow-orange		Rhubarb: black-brown
Ibuprofen: pink-red		Carrots: yellow
Metronidazole: yellow-brown		Beets: red
Azulfidine: orange-yellow		Paprika: orange

impending renal failure), blood, bilirubin, and hemoglobin. Urine production should also be monitored to identify either oliguric or anuric states. If urine production falls precipitously, aggressive fluid therapy for renal failure must be initiated. Techniques that use urine specimens to detect toxins have a higher rate of positive findings for many substances compared with analysis of blood or gastric contents.

Liver Enzymes

Measurement of hepatic enzymes is recommended to detect damage to the liver by suspected toxins. Because the liver is the site of metabolism of many molecules, these hepatic measurements are sensitive to any injury suffered by the liver. Serial measurements should be taken when there is a lag time in the metabolism of the suspected substance or when damage to the liver may be ongoing. The animal must be monitored closely because damage to the liver can lead to encephalopathy, coagulation deficits, and other signs of hepatic disease. Ultrasound and ultrasound-directed needle biopsy can be invaluable in determining the extent of liver damage caused by toxicity.

Coagulation Panel

In small animal practice there are some substances (e.g., anticoagulant rodenticides) that can profoundly alter coagulation. The onset of the actual internal bleeding may be delayed, or bleeding into a body cavity may not be evident initially, so prolonged clotting times may be the first abnormality discovered. A finding of this type should prompt the veterinarian to undertake a more thorough evaluation to identify the cause. The test for proteins induced by vitamin K absence or antagonism can be used to test for poisoning with a vitamin K antagonist. Other tests that reveal the animal's capacity for coagulation include the complete blood count and hematocrit, platelet count, prothrombin time, activated partial thromboplastin time, activated clotting time, fibrinogen levels, and fibrin and fibrinogen degradation products. Prolonged clotting times can also occur with any substance that causes hepatotoxicity, such as acetaminophen or certain types of cyanobacteria or bluegreen algae.

Kits

For a few intoxications there are some rapid screening kits commercially available to practitioners (ethylene glycol, a 10-minute test by Kacey Diagnostics; and RapidCheck Pro 5 for illicit drugs by Craig Medical). These tests use blood or urine and can be helpful in obtaining a diagnosis. Nevertheless, for the vast majority of intoxicants, no such quick test exists and for all potentially toxic episodes, the diagnoses of poisoning must continue to be based on evidence obtained from the history, observation of clinical signs, and information obtained from relevant diagnostic tests. For some intoxications, samples can be sent out to human hospitals and laboratories for definitive analysis; however, the clinician must request screening for specific toxicants based upon a high index of suspicion.

Pulse Oximetry and Electrocardiography

The pulse oximeter is a powerful tool that provides information about hemoglobin oxygen saturation in pulsating vessels. From these data, predictions can be made concerning arterial oxygenation and whether supplemental oxygen should be administered. The electrocardiogram can detect arrhythmias caused by toxins and abnormalities caused by shock or hypoxemia. A list of toxins potentially causing arrhythmias is included in Box 8-1. Pulse oximetry and electrocardiography tell the clinician more about the actual state of the animal, and this information can be used to initiate specific therapies to stabilize animals in life-threatening crises. Pulse oximetry units and electrocardiography machines are noninvasive, inexpensive, widely available, and invaluable in handling a variety of emergencies.

Radiographs

Radiographs of the chest and abdomen are useful in diagnosing aspiration pneumonia, pulmonary edema, or the ingestion of radiopaque toxins. Opacities that show up on

Box 8-3	Radiopaque Toxins in Small Animals
Ammonium chloride	Iron
Antivert	Lead (fishing sinkers)
Aspirin (enteric-coated)	Mothballs
Bethanechol	Paradichlorobenzene (highly opaque)
Calcium carbonate	Naphthalene (faintly opaque)
Chloral hydrate	Multivitamins with iron
Compazine	Placidyl
Copper (coins)	Potassium chloride
Crack vials	Sustained-release products
Drug packets	Thorazine
Elavil	Zinc (pennies)

radiographs include chloral hydrate, heavy metals such as zinc (e.g., pennies, toys, cage pieces), lead, iodine, phenothiazines, and enteric-coated tablets (Box 8-3).

Chest radiographs may also supply clues to the source of the problem and should be taken whenever pulmonary edema, aspiration pneumonia, or hypoxemia are suspected. Toxins can cause respiratory complications, including toxic pneumonitis (e.g., metals, phosphine gas, ammonia, smoke, nitrogen oxide), aspiration pneumonia secondary to vomiting, cardiogenic or noncardiogenic shock (e.g., salicylate toxicity, opiates), pulmonary edema, and atelectasis. Radiographs should be taken only if the animal is stable and will not be stressed excessively when the films are obtained.

For some poisonings (smoke inhalation, paraquat), their hallmark pulmonary lesions usually develop more than 24 hours after exposure and initial films may be inaccurate in predicting the extent of the damage. For this reason, for chest radiographs to be effective in documenting the injury, serial radiographs must be taken over time for comparison.

Ultrasound

In the past decade, ultrasound has quietly come into its own as a supporting diagnostic tool for some intoxications. In poisonings as diverse as ethylene glycol toxicity, potentially caustic foreign bodies such as batteries, and the expansive "gorilla" glues, ultrasound can be helpful in obtaining a diagnosis. In cases of tacrolimus ingestion, ultrasound can assist in identifying the medication-induced intussusceptions. Additionally, the tremendous value of ultrasound-directed needle biopsy in determining the extent of tissue damage caused by a toxicity should not be underestimated. Undoubtedly, the future will reveal new uses for ultrasound and other forms of imaging in the diagnoses of poisonings.

The Toxidrome Approach

Veterinarians must attempt to standardize their approach to the evaluation of the poisoned animal. Close monitoring of vital signs can supply important physiologic "fingerprints" implicating the exact toxicologic cause of a condition. Becoming skilled and meticulous observers can increase the likelihood of success of therapeutic intervention and also can help determine when adjustments in the initial therapy may be required.

Clinicians must learn to recognize the most commonly occurring toxic syndromes. Practitioners can readily learn to identify a pattern of changes suggestive of a particular drug or toxin or group of drugs or toxins. A group of signs and symptoms that consistently result from particular toxins are known as *toxidromes* (from toxic syndromes). Some of the more commonly seen toxidromes are listed in Table 8-1. It should be noted that actual clinical manifestations of intoxications can be much more variable than the static list of signs included in a table in a textbook. Clinical signs of poisoning can be full blown, partial, or nonexistent. The absence of clinical signs or partial presentations does not automatically imply less severe conditions and as a result are no less critical to diagnose. Some important typical toxins affecting respiratory rate, body temperature, pulse, and blood pressure are listed in Table 8-1 and Boxes 8-1, 8-4 to 8-6.

Box 8-4 Commonly Seen Toxins Affecting Body Temperature

Hyperthermia ($\uparrow$)
Amphetamines
Anticholinergics
Antihistamines
Bromethalin
Cocaine
Cyclic antidepressants
Hops
Metaldehyde
Monoamine oxidase inhibitors
Pentachlorophenol
Phencyclidine
Pyrethrins and pyrethroids
Salicylates
Thyroxine
Strychnine

Hypothermia ($\downarrow$)
Carbon monoxide
Ethanol
Ethylene glycol
Hypoglycemic agents
Macrolide antibiotics (e.g., ivermectin)
Opioids
Pyrethrins/pyrethroids
Sedative hypnotic agents

Box 8-5 Commonly Seen Toxins Affecting Pulse

Bradycardia ($\downarrow$)
Antiarrhythmic drugs
α- and β-Adrenergic agonists
Baclofen
Calcium channel blockers
Digitalis glycosides
Opioids
Organophosphates
Carbamates

Tachycardia ($\uparrow$)
Amphetamines
Antihistamines
Atropine
Anticholinergics
Arsenic
Caffeine
Carbon monoxide
Cyclic antidepressants
Ethanol
Ephedrine and pseudoephedrine
Epinephrine
Organophosphates and carbamates
Phenothiazine
Theophylline
Thyroxine

BOX 8-6 Commonly Seen Toxins Affecting Blood Pressure

Hypotension ($\downarrow$)
α-Adrenergic antagonists
Angiotensin-converting enzyme inhibitors and antagonists
Antiarrhythmic drugs
β-Adrenergic antagonists
Calcium channel blockers
Cyanide
Cyclic antidepressants
Ethanol
Nitrates and nitrites
Nitroprussides
Opioids
Organophosphates and carbamates
Phenothiazines
Sedative hypnotic agents
Theophylline

Hypertension ($\uparrow$)
Amphetamines
Cocaine
Ephedrine and pseudoephedrine
Epinephrine
Ergot alkaloids
Lead
Monoamine oxidase inhibitors
Nicotine (early)
Phenylpropanolamine

Conclusions

Unfortunately for both veterinarians and poisoned animals, all too frequently the exact identity of the toxic agent involved is unknown. As a result, small animal clinicians must construct a minimum database to establish the condition of the animal and to gain clues about the nature of the poison suspected. Indiscriminate use of antidotes or initiation of specific therapy without confirmatory evidence should be avoided. However, as stated before, supportive therapy should never be withheld while one is awaiting toxicology test results. Support must be the basis of therapy for the animal that is thought to be poisoned, and monitoring of vital signs, cardiac function, and blood oxygen saturation is mandatory. Multisystemic monitoring in conjunction with blood and urine studies should be undertaken, and appropriate supportive treatment should be promptly initiated when any specific system disturbance is detected. It must be remembered that some agents have a latent phase, and subsequent effects may have a delayed onset. Therefore, the patient must be observed for delayed pulmonary, hepatic, renal, and hematologic manifestations of poisoning, and serial tests may have to be performed to monitor for such effects.

Finally, veterinarians must learn the capabilities of the laboratories they deal with and the tests that are available, must understand what is detectable and what is not, and must familiarize themselves with the nature and clinical signs of the most common intoxications that are frequently seen in small animal practice. Once they have accomplished these goals, the diagnosis can be made more effectively and the outcome of these poisoning cases will be more rewarding.

Suggested Readings

Bronstein AE, Spyker DA, Contilena LR, et al: Annual Report of the American Association of Poison Centers' National Data System (NPDS): 27th Annual Report 2010, *Clin Toxicol* 48:979–1178, 2010.

Gfeller RW, Messonnier SP: *Small animal toxicology*, St Louis, 1977, Mosby.

Heliwell M, Hampel G, Sinclair E: Value of emergency toxicological investigations in differential diagnosis of coma, *Br Med J* 2:819–821, 1979.

Petrollini-Rogers E, McNally B: Initial management of acute intoxications. In Poppenga RH, Gwaltney-Brant SM, editors: *Small animal toxicology essentials*, Ames, IA, 2011, John Wiley and Sons.

Osterloh JD: Laboratory diagnoses and drug screening. In Haddad LS, Shannon MW, Winchester JF, editors: *Clinical management of poisoning and drug overdose*, Philadelphia, 1998, WB Saunders.

Osweiler ED: *Toxicology*, Baltimore, 1996, Williams & Wilkins.

Shannon MW, Haddad LS: The emerging management of poisoning. In Haddad LS, Shannon MW, Winchester JF, editors: *Clinical management of poisoning and drug overdose*, Philadelphia, 1998, WB Saunders.

Taylor RL, Cohen SL, White JD: Comprehensive toxicological screening in the emergency department: an aid to clinical diagnosis, *Am J Emerg Med* 3:507–511, 1985.

Teitelbaum DT, Morgan J, Gray G: Nonconcordance between clinical impression and laboratory findings in clinical toxicology, *Clin Toxicol* 10:417–422, 1977.

Volans G, Willop G: Laboratory investigations in acute poisonings, *Br Med J* 289:426–428, 1984.

Initial Management of the Poisoned Patient

Matthew Mellema, DVM, PhD, DACVECC

The 2010 Annual Report of the American Association of Poison Control Centers' (AAPCC) National Poison Data System (NPDS) notes that the NPDS logged 94,823 poison exposures in animal species in that year.[1] This report also demonstrates that animal exposure calls to centers contributing to the NPDS have remained largely static in number for the past decade. Although this information makes it quite clear that real or suspected exposure of companion animals to poisons occurs, the report also highlights the large species differences in the frequency of exposures. The NPDS report makes it clear that poison exposure is reported or suspected far more commonly in dogs than in other species. Of the 94,823 exposures logged by the NPDS, more than 90% were in dogs and 8.4% in cats. No other species made up even 0.3% of the reported exposures. The 2010 report also indicates that the vast majority of exposures occurs via ingestion (75%-90%), and dermal exposure appears to be the next most common exposure route. Inhalational and ocular exposures appear to be much less common. Despite the preponderance of canine ingested-toxin exposures, the small animal clinician needs to be prepared to handle intoxications in other companion animal species and by other routes. Treatment of poisonings can be among the most rewarding and the most frustrating cases in practice. The difference lies largely in establishing both an organized approach and open, forthright communications with the owner.

The aim of this chapter is to provide an overall approach to the acutely poisoned patient in a manner similar to the approach taken to any critically ill patient. Decontamination, general supportive care, antidote administration, and other related topics are covered elsewhere in this text, but are mentioned herein when appropriate to highlight certain key points.

Telephone Triage

The initial contact with the owner or caregiver of an animal is often via the telephone. This initial telephone-based encounter is often termed *telephone triage* despite the technical meaning of *triage*, which is the process of evaluating groups of patients rather than a single patient. Vital information that should be obtained early in the conversation is the species, breed, age, and body weight of the animal. It is largely unknown whether gender or intact or neutered status affects the pathophysiology of most poisonings, and this information should be obtained as well. It is important to note whether the weight given is an owner estimate or a known historical value. Owner estimates of weight differ from actual weight by a considerable margin and this can affect the clinician's assessment of whether a hazardous amount of an agent has been ingested. Historical information that should be obtained early include the following: (1) whether this incidence represents a known, possible, or likely exposure; (2) estimated length of time since the exposure; (3) a summary of any owner contact with poison control hotline personnel; and (4) the form, type, and amount of potential toxicant.

It is impossible over the telephone to fully determine the condition of the animal, but it is important to try to establish the level of consciousness and whether respiratory distress is present. Level of consciousness can be categorized by three levels. *Obtunded* means the animal has a blunted response to its environment. It may appear lethargic, drowsy, or generally disinterested in its surroundings. Owners will typically use the word "depressed" to describe this state, although depression is a symptom, not a clinical sign, and is thus an inappropriate term in regard to veterinary patients. Stuporous mentation indicates that the patient is only responsive to noxious stimuli. Such a patient may not respond to the owner's voice, but may respond when pinched or jostled. Comatose patients are unresponsive to all forms of stimuli. Additional components of altered mental states may include agitation, aggression, inebriation, or fearful or hiding behavior.

If the time before arrival at the hospital will bring the total time elapsed since exposure to more than an hour, it may be of benefit to have the owner induce emesis. Induction of emesis should not be recommended if the animal is significantly mentally compromised, if the level of consciousness cannot be determined, if respiratory distress is evident, or if preexisting diseases that compromise airway protection are known to be present (e.g., laryngeal disease). Induction of emesis is also contraindicated in animals that have ingested caustic substances such as strong acids or alkalis. Owners of animals that have ingested alkali or acid materials should be instructed to give the pet large amounts of water or milk to dilute the material and proceed as quickly as possible to a veterinary hospital for further care.

In alert patients who are not in respiratory distress, emesis may be indicated. Potential emetics available in the home environment include syrup of ipecac, table salt, and 3% hydrogen peroxide. Salt and hydrogen peroxide appear to induce emesis by irritating the pharyngeal and gastric sensory neurons and altered afferent signaling by these neurons stimulates central nervous system (CNS) neuron pools involved in emesis. The use of table salt is never recommended as it may lead to electrolyte and metabolic derangements that are more life-threatening than the ingested toxin itself. One recent case report highlights the risk of inducing emesis with table salt. In this report, a patient that had ingested a dose of chocolate that was unlikely to be toxic ultimately suffered severe complications arising from massive salt ingestion.[2] Hydrogen peroxide ingestion is also not without some degree of risk as its use has been associated with a few cases of fatal air emboli and mucosal erosions in humans.[3] There are indications that inducing mucosal erosions can occur in cats following the use of hydrogen peroxide as an emetic, albeit rare; apparently this is even more rare in dogs. Typical doses of hydrogen peroxide are on the order of 1 teaspoon per 5 pounds of body weight (1 mL per pound) up to a maximum of 3 tablespoons (9 teaspoons) in the largest breeds of dog.

Syrup of ipecac is readily available over the counter despite markedly decreased usage in human medicine. The recommended oral dose is 1-2 mL (dogs) or 3.3 mL (cats) per pound of body weight.[4] Ipecac directly stimulates the gastric mucosal receptors and indirectly stimulates the chemoreceptor trigger zone in the posterior medulla to stimulate emesis. Although ipecac syrup has a high margin of safety, many adverse side effects of its use have been reported, including prolonged vomiting and diarrhea, lethargy, fever, and irritability along with isolated cases of gastric rupture, intracranial hemorrhage, and diaphragmatic hernia in humans.[5] Recently, the AAPCC has issued guidelines for the use of syrup of ipecac for out-of-hospital poison ingestions in humans.[5] Based on an exhaustive review of the literature regarding the use of ipecac syrup in this setting, the authors of the guidelines concluded that the use of syrup of ipecac might have utility in rare settings such as the following: (1) there is no contraindication to the use of ipecac syrup, (2) there is substantial risk of serious toxicity to the victim, (3) there is no alternative therapy available or effective to decrease gastrointestinal absorption (e.g., activated charcoal), (4) there will be a delay of greater than 1 hour before the patient will arrive at an emergency medical facility, (5) ipecac syrup can be administered within 30-90 minutes of the ingestion, and (6) ipecac syrup administration will not adversely affect more definitive treatment that might be provided at a hospital. Such criteria are unlikely to be met in the vast majority of animal poisonings and its routine use is not advised.

If vomiting is induced, it should be in cases of witnessed toxin ingestion and should be performed within 60 minutes of ingestion, and the gastric contents should always be saved and brought to the hospital with the pet for visual and toxicologic examination. Although it is often recommended to repeat the emetic in 15 minutes if no vomiting has occurred, it may be more helpful in the long run if the owners are on their way to the veterinary hospital by that time. One should bear in mind that owners are often quite agitated during potential poisonings of their pet and may be well served by the clinician making several common-sense recommendations such as the following: (1) induce emesis in a location in which it will be easy to collect and clean up the vomitus such as an outdoor patio or balcony or a linoleum-floored area such as the kitchen or bathroom; (2) if no such area is available the owners can lay down a bed sheet and have the animal restrained to that area until vomiting occurs; and (3) line the crate or area of the car that will be used for transport with material such as blankets, sheets, or towels to facilitate cleanup in case emesis occurs or persists during transport.

If the animal is having seizures or muscle tremors, care should be taken to avoid trauma to the owners or self-trauma to the patient during transport to the hospital. Owners should be advised that a pet with an altered mental state, or one that is anxious or uncomfortable, may bite or react unexpectedly and atypically. It should be emphasized that injury to them will only delay effective treatment and they should take all prudent measures to reduce risk in this regard. A heavy blanket can serve multiple roles in this setting, including aiding in restraint and serving as a barrier to bite or scratch injury as well as helping to preserve body heat in recumbent animals.

At the Veterinary Hospital

Management of an acute case of intoxication can be organized into five main areas as follows: (1) the ABCs of critically ill patient stabilization: airway, breathing, and circulation; (2) gaining control of seizures, muscle tremors, or exsanguinating hemorrhage; (3) assessment of medical and metabolic derangements and institution of a plan for their management; (4) gastrointestinal decontamination; and (5) supportive care. The focus of this chapter will be on the first three areas as both decontamination procedures and supportive care are covered elsewhere in this text (see Chapters 10 and 11, respectively). Although the first three areas are often addressed by the clinician simultaneously, for the sake of clarity they are discussed sequentially herein.

On arrival at the veterinary hospital, an initial assessment of vital signs and the six perfusion parameters (i.e., mentation; mucous membrane color; capillary refill time; heart rate; pulse quality; and toe web, ear tip, or other peripheral site temperature). If signs of ineffective breathing are present (e.g., apnea, stertor, stridor, hyperpnea with minimal air flow, hypopnea, marked prolonged inspiration, or agonal breathing) then a patent airway should be established with a cuffed endotracheal tube. Ventilation should be augmented as needed with manual positive pressure breath delivery. Anticonvulsants should be administered as necessary (see later in this chapter), and hydration, effective circulating volume, and metabolic status should be assessed and addressed rapidly. Poisoned patients may have severely altered homeostatic mechanisms and therefore may be hypothermic or hyperthermic. Keep in mind that the clinician needs to treat the whole patient, not just the toxicosis alone. In many cases, the sequelae of the intoxication may present a greater threat to survival than the initial insult. For example, immediate life-threatening concerns need to be addressed prior to moving forward with decontamination procedures despite the undeniable importance of such.

The ABCs of Critical Patient Care

Airway

Any animal that is unconscious, appears to have neuromuscular paralysis or paresis, or is in severe respiratory distress should be evaluated for the need for intubation. If there is no voluntary respiratory effort or if gastric lavage is planned, then intubation is strongly advised.

Anesthesia is required for intubation if the animal is conscious. These patients may or may not also require positive-pressure ventilation. A cuffed endotracheal tube of appropriate size is placed, the cuff is inflated, and the tube is tied securely to the muzzle or around the back of the skull depending on the patients' conformation. When possible, a blood sample is collected for arterial blood gas determination to aid in the determination of the adequacy of alveolar ventilation and the need for oxygen supplementation. Apnea monitors, pulse oximetry, and capnography may all be enlisted to aid in continuous, real-time evaluation of these same parameters.

Breathing

Hypoventilation generally indicates a need for assisted ventilation. In the clinical setting, hypoventilation is defined by the presence of hypercapnia ($Paco_2$ > 45 mm Hg; $Pvco_2$ > 50-52 mm Hg in a hemodynamically stable patient if the sample is drawn from a central vein). If assisted ventilation is contraindicated or is unavailable, a degree of "permissive hypercapnia" may be well tolerated by the patient. Guidelines for permissive hypercapnia state that a $Paco_2$ > 50 mm Hg may be well tolerated if the pH remains above 7.25 and cardiovascular function is adequate.[6] Hypoventilation may be due to reduced respiratory drive, excessive respiratory load, or reduced respiratory capacity and thus may be central or peripheral in nature. Permissive hypercapnia is contraindicated in patients with CNS disease or cerebral edema because the resultant acidosis and cerebral vasodilation may lead to worse outcomes. Supplemental oxygen is advised to avoid hypoxemia; however, hyperoxia (Pao_2 > 300 mm Hg in particular) may also be associated with worse neurologic outcomes in some settings.[7]

Hypoxemia (Pao_2 < 80 mm Hg at sea level) should be treated with supplemental oxygen as required to maintain Pao_2 above 65 mm Hg. If continued increases in the inspired oxygen concentration do not improve the Pao_2 or alleviate excessive respiratory effort needs, then assisted ventilation is indicated. If the toxin was not inhaled (or is not known to cause pulmonary pathologic conditions such as is seen with paraquat intoxication), then the reasons for the hypoxemia should be investigated. Aspiration pneumonia and the presence of preexisting respiratory disease should both be considered, and a diagnostic work-up performed when the patient is suitably stable. The management of patients requiring mechanical ventilation for all but a few hours is complex and requires an organized team of clinicians and technicians. The interested reader is referred to several excellent recent book chapters describing the approaches used at the author's practice.[8,9]

Circulation

Adequate oxygen delivery depends on the volume of blood in the vessels, the pumping function of the heart, the functional integrity of the blood vessels, and the oxygen content of the arterial blood. An early assessment of the electrocardiogram aids in the determination of heart rate and the identification of the cardiac rhythm. Cardiac rhythm as well as pump function may be affected by a wide area of toxins including oleander (Color Plate 26-2), foxglove, other related and unrelated cardiotoxic plant species, organophosphates, albuterol, methylxanthines, and therapeutic drug overdoses. Many hydrocarbons and industrial chemicals have arrhythmogenic properties as well.[10]

The vascular volume status of intoxicated patients varies greatly among individuals. The presence of a deficit in interstitial or vascular volume or both depends on the nature of the intoxication, how acute or severe the insult was, whether the animal has been taking in food and water, whether the patient has been vomiting or having diarrhea, whether the toxin induces a diuresis or increases capillary permeability, and the presence of preexisting medical conditions. As in any emergency situation, tachycardia, cold extremities, pale mucous membranes, and slow capillary refill time indicate a vascular volume deficit and perhaps hypovolemic (vasoconstrictive) shock. A patient with these signs should be resuscitated quickly with isotonic crystalloid solutions (60-90 mL/kg body weight [BW] in dogs; 40-50 mL/kg BW in cats), colloid solutions (10-20 mL/kg BW in dogs; 5-10 mL/kg BW in cats), or a combination of these. If the poison was a vitamin K antagonist, the preferred fluid may be frozen plasma (with or without packed red blood cells) or whole blood depending on availability and needs. In my practice the preferred fluid resuscitation plan for hypovolemic patients secondary to vitamin K antagonist rodenticide poisoning is 10-20 mL/kg intravenous (IV) of fresh frozen plasma (FFP) as a bolus over 20 minutes. Transfusion reactions to plasma are generally mild in nature and represent a far lower risk to the patient than persistent hemorrhagic shock. Frozen plasma (as opposed to FFP) would serve just as well but is not carried in my practice. One point must be made that may be of interest regarding colloids. Although generally considered safe and effective volume expanders, there is growing concern that the current formulations of hetastarch may be themselves nephrotoxic to a degree in some individuals.[11] If such adverse effects are confirmed to be of importance in veterinary species as well as humans, then they may represent an undue risk in the resuscitation of poisoned patients, particularly those in whom a nephrotoxin is considered the most likely agent.

Interstitial deficits are identified by decreased skin turgor, dry or tacky mucous membranes, sunken eyes, and abrupt decreases in body weight. The serum sodium concentration may be high if the patient has had free water losses in excess of solute losses or if table salt has been given as an emetic. Conversely, the serum sodium may be low if the patient has had losses of solute and water via vomiting, diarrhea, or polyuria, but has continued to take in oral water. The percentage of deficit should be estimated and the deficit volume calculated by multiplying the percent deficit by the lean body weight. The deficit can safely be replaced over 24 hours, but I see no advantage to taking more than 4 hours in most cases. In any patient whose cardiovascular system can handle the volume over 4 hours, there seems to be no benefit to allowing the patient to remain dehydrated for a longer period. All but patients with oligoanuric kidney disease, severe sodium abnormalities, or advanced heart disease should well tolerate a 4-hour rehydration approach. An isotonic crystalloid is the appropriate fluid choice to replace extracellular fluid deficits. Maintenance needs and abnormal ongoing losses should also be accounted for in the fluid plan and an isotonic or hypotonic crystalloid serves most patients in this regard. Active diuresis and enhanced renal blood flow may be achieved by providing IV fluids in excess of patient needs. Such a strategy may be employed to enhance toxin elimination or reduce adverse effects of toxins (e.g., nonsteroidal antiinflammatory drugs) or both. Depending on the nature of the toxin, serial evaluation of urine volume and character may be indicated.

If fluid therapy alone does not restore adequate circulatory performance, the heart may be unable to establish adequate cardiac output because of toxin-induced cardiac compromise (heart rate, contractility, diastolic function, or some combination of factors). Inotropic agents may be justified in this setting if adequate monitoring is available. Continuous electrocardiography is always indicated in this setting. Dobutamine may be delivered as a continuous IV infusion at 5-20 mcg/kg/min. Dopamine is an effective first-line vasopressor at an initial dose of 2-10 mcg/kg/min titrated to effect. Higher doses may lead to tachycardia, tachyarrhythmias, and vasoconstriction with no further improvement in cardiovascular performance. Epinephrine may be used if dopamine is unsuccessfully used to address hypotension. Epinephrine is a potent alpha and beta agonist that may increase both cardiac output and systemic vascular resistance (two main determinants of arterial blood pressure). As with dopamine, higher doses may lead to tachycardia, tachyarrhythmias, and vasoconstriction with no further improvement in cardiovascular performance. In addition, the use of high-dose epinephrine may predispose patients to ventricular fibrillation. The IV dose of epinephrine is 0.05-0.3 mcg/kg/min. Norepinephrine is an alternative therapy and is a potent vasoconstrictor. Perfusion to the periphery and the viscera may be compromised while preserving flow to the heart and brain. Infusion doses in the range of 0.05-2 mcg/kg/min are commonly used. It must be noted that all of these sympathomimetic agents may be contraindicated in some poisoned patients even if hypotension is present. In a patient intoxicated with methylxanthines (e.g., theobromine or caffeine), the use of sympathomimetics likely represents an unacceptable risk for the development of severe cardiac arrhythmias, regardless of hypotension. In this setting, the use of alternative agents such as vasopressin may be preferred.

Toxins may affect the vasculature either by direct effects on endothelium and vascular smooth muscle cells or indirectly by altering levels of circulating mediators and autonomic tone. Vascular endothelium is exposed to any blood-borne toxin, and accumulation of toxin in endothelial cells can occur. Toxins can also induce the release of inflammatory mediators from activated cells and these mediators can profoundly influence vasomotor tone. Widespread cellular injury and activation can lead to initiation of multiple inflammatory and other homeostatic cascades and induce systemic inflammatory responses. In this setting the management of arterial blood pressure becomes challenging and maintaining a mean arterial blood pressure of more than 60 mm Hg should remain a goal. Even in settings of markedly abnormal vasomotor tone the augmentation of blood volume remains a primary means of blood pressure support. When hypotension persists in the face of adequate volume loading, systemic administration of vasoactive agents becomes necessary.

Hypertension may also develop in the poisoned patient. If blood pressure is found to be markedly elevated (mean arterial pressure greater than 140 mm Hg) and the patient is volume replete, then vasodilatory agents may be required to reduce systemic vascular resistance and restore adequate blood flow to tissues and ameliorate end-organ damage. Agents such as hydralazine, amlodipine, or nitroprusside are commonly used for this purpose. The use of these agents is best reserved for patients that have adequate myocardial function because their use in patients with myocardial disease may trigger a more profound drop in blood pressure than desired. Hydralazine is primarily an arteriolar vasodilator that is thought to act via a reduction in cytosolic calcium levels. It may be administered by enteral or parenteral routes at doses ranging from 0.5-3.0 mg/kg every 8-12 hours. Onset of action is somewhat slow, taking 10-30 minutes, but the effects are typically evident for several hours. Heart rate may increase and should be monitored. Reflex increases in heart rate may limit the degree to which blood pressure is reduced and concurrent use of β-blockers may be required in rare instances. Amlodipine is a calcium channel blocker with effects largely limited to the vasculature rather than the myocardium or other sites. Doses range from 0.625 mg/cat once daily (increase if needed to 1.25 mg/cat) to 0.1 mg/kg PO q24h for dogs. The onset of action is relatively slow. Nitroprusside is a venous and arteriolar vasodilator. It is given as an IV infusion and its onset of action is nearly immediate. The dosage of nitroprusside is 0.5-1.0 mcg/kg/min. This drug should be used cautiously in patients with renal or hepatic disease. The metabolites of nitroprusside include cyanide-containing compounds and I have witnessed iatrogenically created clinically relevant cyanide toxicity in at least three patients with reduced renal function (i.e., hypertensive dialysis-dependent acute kidney injury patients) when this agent was used in that setting. Administration of any vasoactive agent requires close monitoring of the electrocardiogram, blood pressure, and intravascular volume status. These drugs are all potentially arrhythmogenic and can dangerously alter arterial blood pressure when used incautiously. Their use warrants intensive monitoring.

The oxygen-carrying capability of the blood is affected by several toxins. The blood oxygen content is a sum of the oxygen bound to hemoglobin and that dissolved in the plasma. Toxins may cause reduced oxygen carrying capacity by creating a true or functional anemia. A true anemia may be the result of red blood cell loss (e.g., anticoagulant rodenticides) or chronic bone marrow suppression (e.g., many chemotherapeutic agents). A functional anemia can arise when there is an adequate amount of hemoglobin present, but it is in a form unable to adequately bind oxygen (e.g., carbon monoxide and acetaminophen). When true anemia is present the only effective therapy is to either increase bone marrow output or provide increased red cell mass via transfusions. The treatment of functional anemia caused by agents such as carbon monoxide or acetaminophen is discussed elsewhere in this text (see Chapters 32 and 39). The short-term administration of supplemental oxygen is indicated in nearly every emergency patient, but prolonged administration may also serve to increase hemoglobin saturation, increase dissolved plasma oxygen concentrations to a limited degree, and enhance elimination of some toxins such as carbon monoxide.

Parameters such as heart rate, mucous membrane color, distal extremity temperature, and mentation should be monitored, along with clinical laboratory parameters to aid in adjustment of the fluid plan as the patient's condition changes. Urine output is an important indicator of renal perfusion and blood pressure adequacy. Monitoring urine output accurately requires placement of a urethral catheter and a closed collection system. A urine output of less than 1 mL/kg/hr suggests a vascular volume deficit, hypotension, or a reduction in renal function, and should be evaluated and treated promptly.

Controlling Seizures and Muscle Tremors

Many toxins can lead to seizures, muscle tremors, or both (e.g., metaldehyde). The two may be distinguished by determining whether the patient is conscious. Generalized seizures are associated with an unconscious mental state, whereas muscle tremors are not inherently associated with unconsciousness. Both of these clinical signs must be distinguished from shivering, which generally occurs during the inspiratory phase of respiration alone. Anticonvulsants and muscle relaxants may be required to control seizures and tremors. Initially, IV administration of diazepam is indicated to control seizure activity (dose: 0.5 mg/kg). However, interruptions in the supply of benzodiazepines are frequent in the United States at present and the well-prepared veterinary hospital will have alternatives such as injectable levetiracetam or barbiturates in stock. Repeated administration of diazepam or conversion to a continuous infusion of benzodiazepines approach may be required if seizure activity persists. Pentobarbital (if available) may be used at 2 to 15 mg/kg IV to effect or as a constant rate infusion at 1-6 mg/kg/hr. The use of pentobarbital may anesthetize the patient; if so, intubation is indicated. Propofol can also control gross motor activity during seizures, but without electroencephalography the clinician cannot otherwise be certain that cortical activity is being adequately suppressed. Blood gases, capnography, and pulse oximetry are all indicated for the monitoring of the patient in this setting. If high doses of barbiturates are required for seizure control, respiratory drive may be sufficiently suppressed to warrant mechanical ventilation. Rapidly deteriorating mental status, newly developed anisocoria, or depression of brainstem reflex responses all may be an indication of an elevation of intracranial pressure. Mannitol infusion at 0.5-1 mg/kg over 10-20 minutes is indicated to reduce neuronal volume and reduce intracranial pressure in this circumstance.

An animal poisoned by a tremorgenic toxin may need only diazepam, diazepam combined with an additional muscle relaxant, or barbiturate anesthesia to control tremor activity. Methocarbamol is a centrally acting muscle relaxant. It is a CNS depressant and can itself cause salivation, emesis, ataxia, and sedation, making it difficult to assess these monitoring parameters. The manufacturer's recommended dose in dogs and cats is 44-220 mg/kg IV, generally not to exceed 330 mg/kg/day.

In seizing and tremoring patients, hyperthermia can be a significant clinical concern. Body temperatures exceeding 106° F are not uncommon in this setting. The high temperature need not be treated per se as it will come down when the excessive muscle activity ceases. Sedatives, anesthetics, and muscle relaxants may cause the body temperature to drop quickly and steeply, resulting in hypothermia. Monitoring for temperature fluctuations and heating or cooling as necessary is very important. Rectal temperature probes can be placed for continuous monitoring.

Assessment of Metabolic Status

The availability of inexpensive, rapid tests for blood chemistry and blood gases has made it much easier to provide optimal care for critically ill and poisoned patients. The poisons themselves and the secondary consequences of their ingestion (e.g., vomiting, diarrhea, seizures, and tremors) can induce varied derangements in acid-base and electrolyte values as well as azotemia, and, in some cases, specific organ failure. Mild metabolic acidosis or alkalosis can often be corrected by instituting fluid therapy and treating the underlying disease. For instance, the metabolic acidosis present in seizing or tremoring patients is in large part the result of increased lactic acid production as a result of mismatch of oxygen demand and delivery in the skeletal muscles. Lactic acid quickly resolves once the excessive muscle activity is controlled. Mild changes in bicarbonate and pH usually resolve with fluid therapy and treatment of the underlying disease.

Metabolic acidosis with a pH level less than 7.2 or a base excess more negative than –8 may on rare occasion require treatment with sodium bicarbonate infusion. Although there are formulas for calculating bicarbonate dose, my preferred approach is to infuse 1, 3, or 5 mEq/kg of bicarbonate over 30 minutes for mild, moderate, or severe acidemia, respectively. The serum bicarbonate concentration, pH, and Pco_2 are rechecked after administration of this dose, and treatment is repeated as necessary. It important to note that in hypoventilating patients the administration of bicarbonate will result in increased CO_2 production and CO_2 accumulation in the cellular compartment. Thus the administration of bicarbonate to hypoventilating patients ultimately may just shift an extracellular acid load to the intracellular compartment, which is not desirable.

Respiratory acidosis is a result of hypoventilation and can occur in the acutely poisoned patient either as a result of the direct effects of the toxin on the neuromuscular axis or, as discussed earlier, because of the medications used to control seizure activity and tremors. Respiratory acidosis is identified when the $Paco_2$ is greater than 45 mm Hg. The patient may or may not be concurrently acidemic (low pH) depending on metabolic (nonrespiratory) factors. Respiratory acidosis is the result of alveolar ventilation that is inadequate to keep up the carbon dioxide production. The most (if not only) effective treatment is to increase alveolar ventilation. This may be achieved by reducing respiratory load (e.g., alleviating or bypassing airway obstructions), increasing respiratory drive (e.g., reducing or discontinuing respiratory depressants), or supplementing respiratory capacity with positive pressure ventilation.

Metabolic alkalosis in the poisoned patient is usually a result of excessive losses of chloride ion via gastrointestinal losses. Treating the underlying cause, administering chloride-rich IV fluids, and controlling the underlying disease are usually sufficient to address metabolic alkalosis in this setting. Normal (0.9%) saline may be the preferred fluid type because of its high chloride concentration and acidifying effects. It is rare that metabolic alkalosis requires treatment beyond these interventions in small animal practice.

Respiratory alkalosis is a result of hyperventilation ($Paco_2 < 35$ mm Hg). It usually results from disorders that cause hypoxemia or stimulate the respiratory center (e.g., hypotension, pain, albuterol intoxication). It may also result from excessive mechanical ventilation as well and should prompt an adjustment of the settings. Generally, the identification and treatment of the underlying disorder is sufficient.

Other Metabolic Parameters

It is sometimes useful to calculate the osmolality in an acutely poisoned patient and compare it to the measured value (i.e., the osmolar gap). If the osmolar gap exceeds 15 mosm/kg, the presence of an unmeasured osmole in excessive amounts should be expected. The osmolar gap can be an important tool for detecting the presence of toxins or their metabolites that might otherwise have been missed. Ethylene glycol and its metabolites are important osmoles whose presence or absence should be evaluated in the presence of an increased osmolar gap in an acutely ill patient. There are more than 20 published formulas for the calculation of osmolality, including the following widely used formula:

$$\text{Osmolality} = 2(Na + K) + \text{Glucose}/18 + \text{blood urea nitrogen}/2.8$$

It should be noted that the evidence establishing the "normal" osmolar gap in dogs is extremely limited and nearly nonexistent in cats. The early acquisition of chemistry panel results can be important in the acutely ill patient for many reasons, including obtaining precise values for glucose and blood urea nitrogen so that the osmolar gap may be determined.

Blood glucose, calcium, sodium, potassium, and chloride concentrations can all be altered by various poisons. In the case of specific toxins or overdoses, such as calcium channel blockers, digoxin, and vitamin D–based products, the alterations in these chemical measurements are caused directly by the toxins' effects. In other cases, these abnormalities are a result of the body's response to the disease process (e.g., profuse vomiting). For instance, hypoglycemia may develop with prolonged seizures because of depletion of extracellular carbohydrate sources. Although hypoglycemia, hypercalcemia, and hypocalcemia must be treated quickly and specifically, it is again the treatment of the underlying disorder, withdrawal or elimination of the agent, and restoration of adequate circulation that will provide long-term improvement.

Summary

Poisonings are a frequent cause of acute illness in dogs and cats. The vast majority involve canine ingestion of toxic substances. Telephone triage is an important initial part of patient assessment, but cannot replace the crucial step of physical examination of the patient. Inducing emesis prior to hospital arrival may be indicated in some cases. On hospital arrival, the approach to the acutely poisoned patient differs little from the approach to any other type of acutely injured or ill small animal patient. An organized, thorough approach emphasizing the ABCs of emergency medicine is likely to achieve optimal outcomes compared with other approaches.

Acknowledgments

I consider it a great honor to step in to update this chapter as a proxy for Doctors Drellich and Aldrich (first and second editions). Janet Aldrich is a gifted emergency clinician who developed the emergency medicine service at the University of California–Davis School of Veterinary Medicine and founded the residency program in Small Animal Emergency and Critical Care at that institution. She served as a mentor to both me and Dr. Sharon Drellich while we were residents there many years ago. She is enjoying her richly deserved retirement. Sharon Drellich was a skilled clinician and beloved friend who was taken from us far too early and is dearly missed by all who knew her. Although I have taken over the writing duties at present, this chapter will always belong to them, and every attempt has been made to write it as I feel they would have.

References

1. Bronstein AC, Spyker DA, et al: 2010 Annual Report of the American Association of Poison Control Centers' National Poison Data System (NPDS): 28th Annual Report, *Clin Toxicol (Phila)* 49:10, 2011.
2. Pouzot C, Descone-Junot C, et al: Successful treatment of severe salt intoxication in a dog, *J Vet Emer Crit Care* 17:3, 2007.
3. Henry MC, Wheeler J, et al: Hydrogen peroxide 3% exposures, *J Toxicol Clin Toxicol* 34:3, 1996.
4. DeClementi C: Prevention and treatment of poisoning. In Gupta CG, editor: *Veterinary toxicology*, San Diego, 2007, Academic Press-Elsevier.
5. Manoguerra AS, Cobaugh DJ: Guideline on the use of ipecac syrup in the out-of-hospital management of ingested poisons, *Clin Toxicol (Phila)* 43:1, 2005.
6. Ijland MM, Heunks LM, et al: Bench-to-bedside review: hypercapnic acidosis in lung injury—from "permissive" to "therapeutic," *Crit Care* 14:6, 2010.
7. Kilgannon JH, Jones AE, et al: Relationship between supranormal oxygen tension and outcome after resuscitation from cardiac arrest, *Circulation* 123:23, 2011.
8. Hopper K: Basic mechanical ventilation. In Silverstein DC, Hopper K, editors: *Small animal critical care medicine*, St Louis, 2009, Saunders Elsevier.
9. Hopper K: Advanced mechanical ventilation. In Silverstein DC, Hopper K, editors: *Small animal critical care medicine*, St Louis, 2009, Saunders Elsevier.
10. Ramos RH, Chacon E, Acosta D: Toxic responses of the heart and vascular systems. In Klaassen CD, editor: *Casarett & Doull's toxicology: the basic science of poisons*, New York, 1996, McGraw-Hill.
11. Wiedermann CJ, Dunzendorfer S, et al: Hyperoncotic colloids and acute kidney injury: a meta-analysis of randomized trials, *Crit Care* 14:5, 2010.

Toxicologic Decontamination

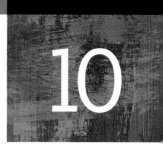

Michael E. Peterson, DVM, MS

This chapter explores multiple decontamination procedures. Other chapters in this text cover the use of specific antidotes, supportive care, and emergency management of the poisoned patient. Owners and staff should be advised to protect themselves from toxic exposure when decontaminating a patient; this principle is particularly true with dermal toxins and toxins that are easily volatilized. An important rule in toxicologic decontamination is not to contaminate the decontaminators. The aim of successful decontamination is to inhibit or cease further toxin absorption and enhance elimination from the body.

Ocular Decontamination

Contaminated eyes should be flushed with copious quantities of water or physiologic saline. The eyes should be flushed for a minimum of 15 minutes; often multiple flushings are required. Mild sedation or a short-acting anesthetic may be necessary to control the patient before flushing. As a first-aid measure, owners should be advised to flush contaminated eyes at least 15 minutes before transporting the patient to the veterinary facility for complete evaluation and specific medical intervention.

Dermal Decontamination

As already mentioned, it is paramount for the veterinarian and paraprofessional staff to protect themselves from dermal exposure when transporting or decontaminating the dermally exposed patient. Rubber gloves and aprons should be used by the attending staff. Toxic dermal exposures allow both transdermal absorption and oral exposure if the patient tries to clean itself by licking.

Long-haired patients may benefit from having the hair clipped before cleaning the skin. Washing with a mild soap or detergent usually removes most toxins. Several washings may be required. Oily substances can often be removed with commercial hand-cleaning degreaser compounds, such as Gojo or Goop. These compounds themselves may be toxic if ingested and should be removed by washing with warm water and soap. Hypothermia is possible, and the patient's overall physical status should be continually evaluated while decontamination procedures are ongoing.

Special care is necessary when decontaminating acid and caustic burns. Toxin-exposed skin should be copiously flushed with tepid water. The damaged tissue is easily traumatized, and extreme care should be taken not to add mechanical injury to the wound when removing the toxin from the skin.

Gastrointestinal Decontamination

Emesis

The effectiveness of vomiting and the percentage of the gastric contents recovered depend on several factors. These factors include the physical properties of the toxin ingested, the time elapsed from toxin ingestion to induction of emesis, the volume of gastric contents, and the emetic agent used.

Emesis is contraindicated when the risk of aspirating vomitus is great. This includes situations in which the patient is stuporous, neurologically depressed, or unconscious or at risk of becoming so before the emetic can work. Additionally, if the animal is having seizures or is at serious risk of a seizure before the emetic works, the risk of aspiration is increased. No emetic should be employed when oil, gasoline, or other petroleum distillates (e.g., volatile compounds) have been ingested. Emesis is contraindicated if vomiting will re-expose the mouth, pharynx, larynx, or esophagus to additional injury from ingested caustic or corrosive compounds.

Studies have indicated that the more rapidly emesis is induced, the greater the percentage of recovery of gastric contents.[1-4] In one study in dogs, the maximum toxin recovery reported was 75% (range, 9% to 75%) with a mean recovery of 49% when emesis was induced within 11 to 30 minutes after toxin ingestion.[1] Generally, gastric recovery in dogs ranges from 17% to 62% if emesis is induced within 60 minutes after toxin ingestion.[1-4] In humans, mean toxin recovery achieved by emesis induction ranged from 21% to 60%.[5,6] In all these studies, the emetic was administered within 60 minutes after toxin ingestion.

Emesis has been successful in removing toxins when it is administered longer than 1 hour postingestion; however, it should be stressed that the volume recovered decreases significantly as time passes. Inducing vomiting more than 4 hours after toxin ingestion is generally of little value.

The usefulness of emetics also depends on the toxic compound ingested. If the toxin has strong antiemetic activity, emetics may be ineffective. As a general rule, if a specific emetic fails to induce vomiting after two doses, it will not be effective. For example, apomorphine, a potent emetic, works by stimulating the chemoreceptor trigger zone in dogs. However, it also directly depresses the emetic center, so if the initial dose fails to induce emesis, subsequent doses are not likely to be effective. Additionally, emetics themselves can be toxic if normal dosages are exceeded.

Emetics are usually classified into two groups—those used by the owner at home as a form of first aid and those used by the veterinarian in the medical facility. Home-use emetics include 7% ipecac syrup, 3% hydrogen peroxide (H_2O_2), liquid dishwashing detergent, and table salt (NaCl). Veterinary emetics include apomorphine, xylazine, and several other less commonly used compounds in cats (e.g., dexmedetomidine, cefazolin, hydromorphone, and midazolam).

I do not routinely advise home induction of emesis. Often the time spent by the owner finding the emetic and then catching and trying to dose the animal usually consumes more time than it would take to drive promptly to the veterinary facility. Generally, home-administered emetics usually succeed only in delaying prompt medical evaluation and specific therapeutic intervention. Additionally, home emetics may not be as successful as clinically available compounds. Owners often miscalculate the weight of the animal and can be either too passive or too aggressive in calculating the dose and administering the compound. The toxin ingested may cause mental depression before the home-administered emetic takes effect, leaving the patient with no airway protection. The risk of aspiration and other secondary side effects of available home emetics is significant. Generally, most owners can transport the animal to a veterinary facility within 30 to 45 minutes. Often the best first aid is rapid transport of the patient and toxin container to the nearest veterinary facility, where prompt induction of emesis is possible.

Home-Use Emetics

7% Syrup of Ipecac

Syrup of ipecac is derived from the dried root of *Cephaelis ipecacuanha,* which is indigenous to South America. The active alkaloids are emetine and cephaeline. This product should not be confused with ipecac fluid extract, which is 14 times stronger. Outdated products can be used, but may be less effective. The mechanism involved is direct gastric irritation and stimulation of the chemoreceptor trigger zone. The dosage for dogs is 1 to 2 mL/kg orally (PO); the dosage for cats is 3.3 mL/kg. Some recommend that the cumulative dosage should not exceed 15 mL in either species. The dose can be repeated once. Effective vomiting should result within 10 to 30 minutes, although it can be delayed for up to 1 hour.

Problems with syrup of ipecac include difficulty in administering the compound to conscious patients because of its bitter taste, which is particularly repugnant to cats. Also, a lack of effectiveness in inducing emesis in 50% of small animal patients has been observed. Additionally, if the patient fails to vomit, the ipecac should be removed from the stomach by lavage because of its potential cardiotoxic arrhythmia-inducing action. In humans the most common complications related to ipecac administration are diarrhea, lethargy, depression, and prolonged vomiting. The use of the emetic is not routinely recommended.

3% Hydrogen Peroxide

Hydrogen peroxide is most effective if it is administered after a small meal. Recommended dosage in dogs and cats is 1 to 5 mL/kg PO (alternatively, 1 mL per pound), generally not to exceed 50 mL for dogs (although many veterinarians exceed this total dose with negligible complications reported) or 10 mL for cats. The mechanism of action is believed to be gastric irritation. There are no significant risks from H_2O_2 ingestion; however, there have been recent concerns regarding the use of this in cats inducing a hemorrhagic gastritis. Because of this, some toxicologists do not recommend the use of hydrogen peroxide as an emetic in cats; and if it is used, it is not recommended to repeat the dose. This risk, albeit low, appears to be even lower in dogs. However, the owner should be careful to prevent the patient from aspirating the hydrogen peroxide when it is being administered. If it is successful, 3% hydrogen peroxide usually induces emesis within 10 minutes. If it is unsuccessful, the dose can be repeated in dogs.

Sodium Chloride (Table Salt)

The recommended dosage in dogs and cats is 1 to 3 tsp PO. Sodium chloride acts as a direct gastric irritant. It usually induces emesis within 10 to 15 minutes. Several negative sequelae are possible with administration of sodium chloride, including hypernatremia, particularly in young animals, if emesis is not induced. Additionally, hematemesis can occur. In children oral sodium chloride administration has produced hypernatremia, cerebral edema, and convulsions. If emesis induction is unsuccessful, lavage should be considered to remove the excess salt. If emesis is successful, water should be available as needed. The use of table salt as an emetic in companion animals is actively discouraged because of the potential for inducing more harm than good.

Liquid Dishwashing Detergent (e.g., Palmolive, Dove, Ivory)

The recommended oral dosage in dogs and cats is 10 mL/kg body weight of a mixture of 3 tbsp detergent to 8 oz of water. Vomiting usually results within 20 minutes after administration. Detergents containing phosphate are most effective. The mechanism of action is primarily gastric irritation. In one human trial, liquid dishwashing detergent appeared to be safe, and emesis was initiated in 83% of patients compared with 97% of controls given ipecac.[7] The effectiveness of liquid detergent in the veterinary population has not been fully elucidated. These detergents should not be confused with caustic detergents, such as electric dishwasher soap or laundry detergent, which are alkaline and are extremely caustic and could induce serious injury to the upper gastrointestinal tract.

Veterinary Emetics

One advantage of "veterinary emetics" is the possibility of using them in conjunction with activated charcoal. Once emesis has been induced, the emetic can be readministered after the patient has received a dose of activated charcoal.

Apomorphine (6.25-Mg Tablets)

Apomorphine acts directly on the chemoreceptor trigger zone to induce emesis. Apomorphine is generally the emetic of choice in dogs because of its rapid onset and the ability to reverse its action. Apomorphine is given at a dose of 0.02 to 0.04 mg/kg intravenous (IV) or intramuscular (IM). It can also be administered by placing it directly behind the eyelid in the subconjunctival sac. Diluting the pill with sterile water minimizes ocular irritation. Apomorphine solutions are not stable and must be made fresh before each administration. Vomiting usually ensues within 4 to 6 minutes. When used conjunctivally, the eye should be flushed copiously once vomiting occurs. Apomorphine can be used in cats but at the lower end of the dosage; however, it appears that apomorphine is much less efficacious in inducing emesis in cats (10% effective by one report) as compared with dogs. Adverse side effects can be reversed with naloxone (0.01 to 0.04 mg/kg IV) in both dogs and cats. Apomorphine administered subcutaneously often has a delayed onset of action, and the duration of action may be prolonged.

Apomorphine can induce central nervous system (CNS) excitability in patients intoxicated with snail bait (metaldehyde), and its use in these patients is not recommended. Apomorphine may also be contraindicated when further CNS depression will significantly alter the patient's condition. Rare adverse side effects include CNS and respiratory depression, excessive vomiting, and occasionally CNS stimulation. "Morphine mania" is also an adverse event that may occur in cats.

Xylazine

Xylazine can be used as an emetic in cats with limited effectiveness (approximately 60% effective by one report) at a dosage of 0.44 to 1 mg/kg IM or subcutaneous (SC). Xylazine has centrally acting α_2-agonist activity. If effective, this drug usually induces vomiting within 10 minutes. A potential adverse effect of xylazine is respiratory depression. The activity of this drug can be reversed with yohimbine, an α_2-antagonist, at a dosage of 0.1 mg/kg IV in both dogs and cats.

Others

It is generally noticed by many veterinarians that inducing vomiting in cats can be a challenge. Some clinicians have suggested the use of cefazolin (300 mg fast IV) or a combination of hydromorphone and midazolam (0.05 mg/kg + 0.2 mg/kg, respectively) as emetics for cats. One drug that seems to be emerging as an effective emetic in cats is dexmedetomidine, an α_2-receptor–specific agent. Many different dosage regimes have been suggested for cats (e.g., 1-2 mcg/kg IV; 40 mcg/kg IM), and the sedative effects can be successfully reversed with atipamezole.

Gastric Lavage

The purpose of gastric lavage is to remove ingested toxins from the stomach by irrigation. The procedure may be indicated if emesis induction is ineffective or contraindicated. The patient must be unconscious or lightly anesthetized, placed in right lateral recumbency. A cuffed endotracheal tube must be in place. A large stomach tube is passed into the stomach no farther caudal than the xiphoid process. The patient is placed in an inclined position with the head down at approximately a 20-degree angle. If the patient is tilted at too great an angle, the weight of the fluid-filled stomach on the diaphragm can impair respiration.

Water or physiologic saline is then instilled by gravity flow at a volume of 10 mL/kg body weight. Physiologic saline is the lavage fluid of choice in smaller patients, which are more prone to fluid and electrolyte abnormalities. Care should be taken to prevent overdistention of the stomach. The degree of gastric distention can be felt by placing a hand on the abdomen. Lavage fluid should be warm to slow gastric emptying and prevent hypothermia of the patient. Manual agitation of the stomach is performed while the lavage fluid is aspirated, and the procedure is repeated until the recovered lavage fluid is clear. Often a bilge or stomach pump is employed to churn the stomach contents and aid in recovering the lavage fluid. Copious amounts of lavage fluid are usually required (often 15 to 20 lavage cycles), and the practitioner should be prepared for disposal of the same volume. The fluid initially recovered should be saved for toxicologic examination. An activated charcoal suspension can be instilled before the stomach tube is kinked and removed.

An increasing trend is to administer activated charcoal before performing lavage to halt further absorption of the toxin. Removal of the toxin-charcoal complex becomes the goal of gastric lavage. Additional activated charcoal is then instilled after the lavage procedure has been completed.

Several studies of lavage have been performed in animals, and none has demonstrated substantial drug recovery, particularly if the procedure was delayed for more than 60 minutes after ingestion of the toxin.[1-3] When lavage was performed within 15 to 20 minutes of toxin ingestion, the mean recoveries were 38% and 29%, respectively. If lavage was delayed until 60 minutes after ingestion of the marker, the mean recoveries were 13% and 8.6%. In the majority of poisoned patients that present to the veterinary hospital nearly 60 minutes have already passed since toxin ingestion, and by the time the mechanics of setting up a lavage procedure are performed and lavage is started, this period has clearly passed. Therefore, the practical clinical success of this decontamination procedure is questionable.

It seems prudent to employ this technique if the ingested material is chunky, and large fragments of material can be expected to be recovered. However, chunky material larger than the diameter of the stomach tube will obviously not be retrieved. Additionally, lavage may be more effective in combating ingestions of toxins that delay gastric emptying, such as salicylates, anticholinergics, and cyclic antidepressants. Concretions may not be recovered. Other examples of anticipated poor recovery are toxins similar to iron tablets, which may adhere to the gastric lining, or large amounts of chocolate, which may melt into a significant ball of material that is difficult to retrieve.

The major complications of gastric lavage are aspiration pneumonia, laryngospasm, hypoxia, hypercapnia, fluid and electrolyte imbalances, and mechanical injury to the throat, esophagus, and stomach. Gastric lavage is contraindicated in patients with an unprotected airway, with ingestions of substances that carry a high risk of aspiration (e.g., hydrocarbons) or that are corrosive, with ingestion of sharp objects, with an underlying pathologic condition that increases the risk of hemorrhage or gastric perforation, and in patients that are postsurgical or have medical conditions that may be compromised by the lavage procedure.

Another version of this technique is enterogastric lavage. This entails gastric lavage combined with retrograde high enema. This technique requires placing a gastric tube and endotracheal tube and then instilling an enema solution until it passes from the stomach tube.

Whole-Bowel Irrigation

In whole-bowel irrigation (WBI), the gastrointestinal tract is cleaned by the enteral administration of large volumes of osmotically balanced polyethylene glycol electrolyte solution (PEG-ES) until a clear liquid stool is achieved. The goal is to physically remove the intraluminal contents of the gastrointestinal tract. The concentration of electrolytes and osmolality in the PEG-ES are balanced so that no net gain or loss of electrolytes or changes in water balance occur.

WBI has a theoretical value in a limited number of toxic ingestions. This technique is indicated in patients with ingestion of toxins that are in a sustained-release or enteric-coated form. It may possibly be of value in cases in which iron pills have been ingested.

Studies in dogs have shown that the average total body clearance of paraquat was increased from 5.67 L/hr to 13.2 L/hr with WBI, which removed 68.9% of the ingested dose.[8,9] Human volunteer studies have reflected mixed results. Studies with ampicillin, delayed-release aspirin, and sustained-release lithium demonstrated toxin reductions of 67%, 73%, and 67%, respectively.[10-15] However, in a study in which coffee beans were used as the marker, no significant improvement was demonstrated in the rate of removal from the gastrointestinal tract with WBI.[16]

WBI requires a nasogastric tube, a type of nasogastric feeding bag, a large quantity of PEG-ES, and an easy-to-clean location in the hospital. The nasogastric tube is necessary because the patient will not willingly consume an adequate volume of PEG-ES at a sufficient rate. Force feeding an adequate volume of PEG-ES is difficult to manage over a 24-hour period. If the patient is in an upright position, the incidence of emesis is decreased because gravity aids in moving the solution into the intestinal tract. The solution is usually administered at a rate of 500 mL/hour. If vomiting occurs, it is best controlled with metoclopramide because of its antiemetic and gastric emptying effects. If this does not work, the flow rate of PEG-ES should be reduced by 50% for 60 minutes and then returned to the original infusion rate. This procedure should be continued until the fecal effluent is clear. The technique may take several hours.

WBI is contraindicated in patients with an obstructed or perforated bowel; ileus; significant gastrointestinal hemorrhage; hemodynamic instability; uncontrollable vomiting; and an unprotected, compromised airway. PEG-ES interactions with activated charcoal are unclear. The charcoal does not significantly alter the osmolality of the solution. The binding capacity of the charcoal may be decreased if it is administered concurrently with the PEG-ES. Complications of WBI generally include nausea and vomiting (particularly in patients receiving emetics before the irrigation procedure). Human patients occasionally complain of abdominal cramps and bloating.

Ion Exchange Resins, Cathartics, and Activated Charcoal

Ion Exchange Resins

Ion exchange compounds are used to bind the toxin to a carrier, thereby trapping it in the gastrointestinal tract until it is passed in the stool. Cholestyramine and activated charcoal are the two most commonly used compounds. Cholestyramine (Questran) and to a lesser extent colestipol (Colestid) are anion exchange resins that bind with lipoproteins and bile acids, thereby preventing intestinal absorption of toxic compounds taken up through these systems. Additionally, cholestyramine can interrupt enterohepatic recirculation of substances excreted through the bile. Some examples of susceptible compounds include phenobarbital, tetracycline, penicillin G, anticoagulants, thyroxine, chlorothiazide, digitalis, β-blockers, some pesticides, any highly lipophilic compound, and heat-stable *Escherichia coli* enterotoxin.

Cholestyramine is packaged as a powder, containing either 444 mg or 800 mg of dried cholestyramine resin per gram of powder. An oral suspension is made by mixing the powder with 60 to 180 mL of water, milk, fruit juice, or other noncarbonated beverage. The recommended dose is 50 to 75 mg/kg PO. Patients should be well hydrated during therapy. Cholestyramine has a wide margin of safety. The potential side effects include nausea, hypoproteinemia, constipation, steatorrhea, and loss of fat-soluble vitamins.

Cathartics

Another decontamination approach is the use of cathartic solutions to speed the transit time of the toxicant through the gastrointestinal tract, thereby decreasing the time allowed for toxin absorption. Saline cathartics work by altering the physical-chemical forces within the intestinal lumen. Osmotic forces increase the fluid volume within the gastrointestinal tract, which stimulates motility and speeds expulsion of the gastrointestinal contents. Cathartics are especially useful in aiding the elimination of ingested solid toxicants and enteric-coated or timed-release compounds.

The two primary types of osmotic cathartics administered to poisoned patients are saline solutions and saccharide solutions. Saline cathartics include sodium sulfate, magnesium sulfate, and magnesium citrate. The most common saccharide cathartic is sorbitol. Mineral oil (paraffin oil) is generally not recommended for use as a cathartic in dogs and cats. Mineral oil has a higher risk of pulmonary aspiration than other cathartics and is no longer recommended for use in organic compound ingestions or organochlorine insecticide intoxications. Mineral oil has been advocated in the past as an adsorbent for lipid-soluble toxins. Mineral oil should not be used concurrently with dioctyl sodium sulfosuccinate because emulsification could occur that could cause hepatic accumulation of the indigestible oil.

Animal studies that measured the effectiveness of cathartics used alone showed no statistically significant difference in toxin clearance between controls and treatment groups.[17-20] These results are remarkable because the doses of cathartic administered were greater than the recommended therapeutic levels and the intervals between toxin ingestion and cathartic administration were less than those expected in an actual toxicosis.

The most rapid and potent cathartic is sorbitol, which is administered as a 70% solution at a dosage of 1 to 2 mL/kg. If catharsis is to be attempted it should be instituted within 60 minutes after toxin ingestion. Multiple doses can be dangerous and can intensify side effects, such as vomiting, nausea, abdominal cramps, dehydration, and possible hypotension. Many veterinarians use sorbitol-containing activated charcoal products, which appear to be very safe with few side effects (but may be less effective at binding toxin).

Contraindications to cathartic administration include a lack of bowel sounds, ingestion of a corrosive substance, presence of diarrhea, recent abdominal trauma, or intestinal obstruction or perforation. Additionally, patients with hypotension, volume depletion, or electrolyte abnormalities should not receive a cathartic. Based on current data, there are no definitive indications for the use of cathartics alone in the management of the poisoned patient.

Activated Charcoal

Activated charcoal, the most commonly used adsorbent, is often called the *universal antidote.* The large surface area of the charcoal adsorbs the toxicant, thus reducing or preventing systemic absorption (Box 10-1). The quality of the various charcoal products depends on the size and surface area per gram of charcoal. On average, 1 g of activated charcoal has approximately 1000 square meters of surface area. Activated charcoal is produced by heating wood pulp to 900° C and, then washing it with inorganic acids and drying it. The resulting small charcoal particles are "activated" with steam or strong acids. The final adsorptive surface contains several carbon moieties that adsorb compounds with varying degrees of affinity. In vitro adsorption to activated charcoal in aqueous solutions is a nonspecific process that reaches equilibrium in less than 30 minutes. Once equilibrium is reached, some desorption can occur. For this reason, some individuals advocate using activated charcoal in conjunction with a cathartic, most commonly sorbitol, to speed gastrointestinal transit and thereby decrease the time available for desorption to occur.

Activated charcoal has an undisputed role in the treatment of acutely poisoned patients. The earlier it is administered after toxin ingestion, the more effective it is. Activated charcoal is particularly effective against large nonpolar compounds. Neutral molecules are more adsorptive than ionized toxins. Activated charcoal interferes with endoscopic visualization. In human volunteers an average of 62 hours elapsed after administration before stools were no longer black.[21]

The dosage of activated charcoal to be used varies with the individual product and other contributing factors, such as the amount of food present in the gastrointestinal tract. However, the dose-response curve indicates that higher doses are more effective. If the volume of toxicant is known, the general rule is to administer the activated charcoal in a dose of 10 times the dose of toxicant. Activated charcoal tablets and capsules are not as effective as activated charcoal slurries.[22,23]

For animals, the recommended dose of powdered activated charcoal and water is 2 to 5 g/kg of body weight (1 g activated charcoal in 5 mL water). If sorbitol is added as a cathartic, it is given at a dose of 3 mg/kg and mixed with the activated charcoal. If the intoxicant is subject to significant enterohepatic recirculation, repeat administration of activated charcoal every 4 to 6 hours for 2 to 3 days may be indicated. When multiple doses of activated charcoal are used, it is important that the patient be adequately hydrated to prevent constipation (kaolin-containing products can enhance the probability of causing constipation). Additionally, repeat dosing with sorbitol may cause significant hypotension or hypovolemic shock, particularly in small patients or those with underlying cardiovascular instability.

As mentioned, cathartic use in conjunction with activated charcoal has been advocated. Several cathartics have been used; however, sorbitol seems to have the fewest drawbacks and enhances the flavor of the suspension. Other cathartics used are sodium sulfate (Glauber's salts) and magnesium sulfate (Epsom salts). Magnesium sulfate is not recommended

Box 10-1	Partial List of Compounds That Bind to Activated Charcoal
Acetaminophen	Meprobamate
Amphetamines	Methyl salicylate
Antibiotics	Methylene blue
Anticoagulant rodenticides	Morphine
Anthelmintics	Muscarine
Aspirin	Narcotics
Atropine	Nicotine
Barbiturates	Nortriptyline
Camphor	Organic iodine
Cantharides	Organic metal compounds
Carbamates	Organochlorine insecticides
Carbamazepine	Organophosphorus insecticides
Chlordane	Phenobarbital
Chloroquine	Phenothiazine
Chlorpheniramine	Phenylbutazone
Cocaine	Phenylpropanolamine hydrochloride
Diazepam	Phenytoin
2,4-D (dichlorophenoxy acetic acid)	Quinacrine hydrochloride
Digitalis	Quinidine
Digitoxin	Quinine
Ethylene glycol	Salicylamide
Fungicides	Salicylates
Hexachlorophene	Strychnine
Ipecac	Sulfonamides
Isoniazid	Theophylline
Mefenamic acid	Tricyclic antidepressants

in patients exhibiting CNS depression. Mineral oil should not be used in conjunction with activated charcoal because it coats the activated charcoal, blocking its ability to adsorb gastrointestinal toxicants.

Activated charcoal is contraindicated in patients with a compromised airway (without intubation), with hydrocarbon ingestion (because of an increased risk of aspiration), or with a gastrointestinal tract that is not anatomically intact. Activated charcoal should not be used in patients that have ingested caustic substances nor in those that are vomiting, having seizures, or are comatose unless endotracheal intubation has been accomplished to protect the compromised airway. The major complication of activated charcoal administration is emesis. Those patients receiving concurrent sorbitol cathartics are at higher risk of vomiting. In dogs administration of a sorbitol-containing solution in concentrations greater than 30% sorbitol frequently induces emesis.[19]

Care should be taken when using activated charcoal as it is very osmotically active and the potential exists to induce a clinically significant hypernatremia that might be difficult to control (more commonly seen in small breed animals, less than 30 lb). If possible a baseline sodium level should be obtained, and if the toxicant is known its ingredients should be reviewed. Hypernatremia can occur in patients with preexisting hypernatremia (e.g., dehydrated) or if the toxicant has excess sodium chloride (e.g., sodium bicarbonate, modeling clay, play dough) or osmotically active substances (e.g., gummy candies, sugar-free candies, sorbitol, paintballs, glycerol, bulk artificial sweeteners).

Cathartic and Activated Charcoal Combinations

Administration of a cathartic and activated charcoal combination has been advocated with the rationale that the charcoal binds the toxicant and the cathartic speeds expulsion of the charcoal-toxicant moiety from the gastrointestinal tract before significant desorption of the toxicant from the activated charcoal occurs. Several manufacturers of activated charcoal supply it in a 10 to 20% sorbitol slurry solution. This combination is administered at a dose of 10 mL/kg. The earlier this combination is administered, the more effective it is. Administration of activated charcoal with a sorbitol cathartic may be beneficial even as late as 6 hours after toxin ingestion. Studies have shown that the addition of sorbitol to activated charcoal does not affect the adsorption of acetaminophen and actually increases the adsorption of aminophylline.[24,25] However, salicylate elimination was slowed with administration of an activated charcoal–sorbitol combination compared with charcoal use alone.

When treating patients that have ingested sustained-release or enteric-coated toxins or toxins with delayed absorption or marked hepatic biliary recirculation, "pulse" dosing of the activated charcoal is advocated (every 6 hours for 2 to 3 days). There is a risk of dehydration if all doses of activated charcoal are mixed with a cathartic. It is recommended that subsequent doses of activated charcoal not be mixed with a cathartic solution unless the clinician is confident that the patient's fluid balance will not be compromised.

Forced Diuresis

Forced diuresis is induced by administering a fluid overload and a diuretic concurrently. The patient must not be anuric or significantly oliguric. The object is to increase urine flow rates to 3 to 5 mL/kg/hr to force renal clearance of the toxicant. The most common diuretics employed are furosemide (5 mg/kg every 6 to 8 hours) and mannitol (1 to 2 g/kg IV every 6 hours). Intoxications that are most likely to respond to forced diuresis are those with a high level of renal excretion of the primary toxicant (e.g., bromide, lithium, amphetamine, phenobarbital, and salicylate). Protein-bound toxins are not cleared efficiently by diuresis.

The primary problems associated with forced diuresis include potential fluid overload and electrolyte abnormalities. The practitioner should monitor for hyponatremia, hypokalemia, water intoxication, pulmonary edema, and cerebral edema. Additionally, some toxins such as tricyclic antidepressants and many sedative-hypnotics increase the patient's susceptibility to interstitial pulmonary edema. Forced diuresis is contraindicated in these intoxications.

Ion Trapping

Ion trapping alters the urine pH to inhibit reabsorption of toxins across the renal tubular membranes. The principle behind this approach is to "trap" the toxin in its ionized form in the urine where it can be excreted. Most nonionized molecules diffuse across membranes because of their high lipid solubility (i.e., nonionic diffusion). Ionized molecules usually cannot diffuse across cellular lipid membranes. The toxic compounds most successfully trapped are weak acids and bases.

Ion trapping can be successful only in the presence of the following conditions: the compound is excreted predominantly unchanged through the kidneys, the compound is a weak electrolyte with a suitable pKa, and the toxicant is primarily distributed to the extracellular space and is not protein bound. Ion trapping is contraindicated when the toxicant has a large volume of distribution, is strongly protein bound, is highly lipid soluble, and is cleared primarily by tissue or hepatic metabolism. Any attempt to alter urine pH requires monitoring of baseline urine pH, serum sodium and potassium levels, and blood pressure. Urine pH should be reevaluated hourly and sodium and potassium levels every 1 to 2 hours as indicated by the patient's condition and trends in serial laboratory values.

Acid diuresis is most commonly employed in patients intoxicated with compounds such as amphetamines and phencyclidine. Acidification is achieved by the administration of ammonium chloride at a dose of 100 mg/kg every 12 hours PO. A problem with urinary acidification is that many intoxicated patients already have a preexisting metabolic acidosis. Acidification may also affect the excretion rates of other drugs being used to treat the patient.

Alkaline diuresis is achieved with sodium bicarbonate administered at a dose of 1 to 2 mEq/kg of body weight added to intravenous fluids infused over 6 hours. Complications of alkaline diuresis include volume overload, hypernatremia, decreased serum ionized calcium, decreased oxygen delivery to tissue, paradoxical CNS acidosis, and hypokalemia. Contraindications for alkaline diuresis include any existing metabolic alkalosis (especially if the patient is concurrently receiving furosemide), hypokalemia, or hypocalcemia.

Gastrotomy

Gastrotomy and actual physical removal of toxins may be necessary if these toxins are refractory to other methods of decontamination. One example is ingestion of iron tablets that adhere to the gastric lining and have to be physically scraped off the gastric wall.

Lipid Emulsion

Intravenous fat emulsions usually composed of triglycerides and phospholipids can be used therapeutically for some toxicities with fat-soluble compounds (e.g., pyrethrins, permethrin, ivermectin, ionophores, marijuana). These fat emulsions theoretically form chylomicron-like droplets in the patient's serum, which may act as a "sink" for highly lipid-soluble xenobiotics. Compounds pulled into this "sink" are then unavailable for binding at their sites of action or to their target organs. The use of lipid emulsion therapy is new and its effectiveness against a growing list of lipid-soluble toxic compounds is being studied. Authors of individual chapters in this text highlight the effectiveness of this therapy against a variety of toxic xenobiotics.

References

1. Arnold FJ, Hodges JB Jr, Barta RA Jr: Evaluation of the efficacy of lavage and induced emesis in treatment of salicylate poisoning, *Pediatrics* 23:286–301, 1959.
2. Abdallah AH, Tye A: A comparison of the efficacy of emetic drugs and stomach lavage, *Am J Dis Child* 113:571–575, 1967.
3. Corby DG, Lisciandro RC, Lehman RW, et al: The efficiency of methods used to evacuate the stomach after acute ingestions,, *Pediatrics* 40:871–874, 1967.
4. Teshima D, Suzuki A, Otsubo K, et al: Efficacy of emetic and United States Pharmacopoeia ipecac syrup in prevention of drug absorption, *Chem Pharm Bull* 38:2242–2245, 1990.
5. Neuvonen PJ, Vartiainen M, Tokola O: Comparison of activated charcoal and ipecac syrup in prevention of drug absorption, *Eur J Clin Pharmacol* 24:557–562, 1983.
6. Tenenbein M, Cohen S, Sitar DS: Efficacy of ipecac-induced emesis, orogastric lavage, and activated charcoal for acute drug overdose, *Ann Emerg Med* 16:838–841, 1987.
7. Gieseker DR, Troutman WG: Emergency induction of emesis using liquid detergent products: a report of 15 cases, *Clin Toxicol* 18:277–282, 1981.
8. Mizutani T, Yamashita M, Okubo N, et al: Efficacy of whole bowel irrigation using solutions with or without adsorbent in the removal of paraquat in dogs, *Hum Exp Toxicol* 11:495–504, 1992.
9. Burkhart KK, Wuerz RC, Donovan JW: Whole bowel irrigation as adjunctive treatment for sustained-release theophylline overdose, *Ann Emerg Med* 21:1316–1320, 1992.
10. Tenenbein M, Cohen S, Sitar DS: Whole bowel irrigation as a decontamination procedure after acute drug overdose, *Arch Intern Med* 147:905–907, 1987.
11. Rosenburg PJ, Livingstone DJ, McLellan BA: Effect of whole bowel irrigation on the antidotal efficacy of oral activated charcoal, *Ann Emerg Med* 17:681–683, 1988.
12. Olsen KM, Ma FH, Ackerman BH, et al: Low volume whole bowel irrigation and salicylate absorption: a comparison with ipecac-charcoal, *Pharmacotherapy* 13:229–232, 1993.
13. Kirshenbaum LA, Mathews SC, Sitar DS, et al: Whole bowel irrigation versus activated charcoal in sorbitol for the ingestion of modified-release pharmaceutical, *Clin Pharmacol Ther* 46:264–271, 1989.
14. Mayer AL, Sitar DS, Tenenbein M: Multiple-dose charcoal and whole-bowel irrigation do not increase clearance of absorbed salicylate, *Arch Intern Med* 152:393–396, 1992.
15. Smith SW, Ling LJ, Halstenson CE: Whole-bowel irrigation as a treatment for acute lithium overdose, *Ann Emerg Med* 20:536–539, 1991.
16. Scharman EJ, Lembersky R, Krenzelok EP: Efficiency of whole bowel irrigation with and without metoclopramide pretreatment, *Am J Emerg Med* 12:302–305, 1994.

17. Gaudreault P, Freidman PA, Lovejoy FH Jr: Efficacy of activated charcoal and magnesium citrate in the treatment of oral paraquat intoxication, *Ann Emerg Med* 14:123–125, 1985.
18. Van de Graaff WB, Thompson WL, Sunshine I, et al: Adsorbent and cathartic inhibition of enteral drug absorption, *J Pharmacol Exp Ther* 221:656–663, 1982.
19. Picchioni AL, Chin L, Gillespie T: Evaluation of activated charcoal-sorbitol suspension as an antidote, *Clin Toxicol* 19:433–444, 1982.
20. Chin L, Picchioni AL, Gillespie T: Saline cathartics and saline cathartics plus activated charcoal as antidotal treatments, *Clin Toxicol* 18:865–871, 1981.
21. Minocha A, Herold DA, Bruns DE, et al: Effect of activated charcoal in 70% sorbitol in healthy individuals, *Clin Toxicol* 22:529–536, 1985.
22. Otto U, Stenberg B: Drug adsorption properties of different activated charcoal dosage forms in vitro and man, *Svensk Fram Tids* 77:613–615, 1973.
23. Tsuchiya T, Levy G: Drug adsorption efficacy of commercial activated charcoal tablets in vitro and in man, *J Pharm Sci* 61:624–625, 1972.
24. Van de Graaff WB, Thompson WL, Sunshine I, et al: Adsorbent and cathartic inhibition of enteral drug absorption, *J Pharmacol Exp Ther* 221:656–663, 1982.
25. Scholtz EC, Jaffe JM, Colaizzi JL: Evaluation of five activated charcoal formulations for the inhibition of aspirin adsorption and palatability in man, *Am J Hosp Pharm* 35:1355–1359, 1978.

Supportive Care of the Poisoned Patient

11

Cheryl Braswell, DVM

Steven Mensack, VMD, DACVECC

The poisoned patient will almost always require broad-based monitoring and supportive care to guard against direct and collateral organ damage. Organ injury may result from the direct effects of the poison/intoxication or secondary consequences, such as hypoperfusion, hypoxemia or ischemia, and subsequent reperfusion. Poisoned patients may have respiratory, cardiovascular, neurologic, gastrointestinal, renal, hepatic, or hematologic abnormalities. The potential for multiorgan dysfunction necessitates vigilant monitoring and appropriate supportive care. There are important nursing care considerations in patients that are recumbent, stuporous, or comatose.

Within the text, the authors have provided numerical parameters for various organ systems to help guide the assessment of the poisoned patient and direct therapy. Readers are cautioned to remember that in any illness, as one respected colleague cogently remarked, "Tests measure what they measure and they don't measure anything else" (Steve Haskins, *ACVECC Review,* Jan 2011, San Diego) One should always treat the patient in light of the numerical data and not just the numbers themselves.

Respiratory

Breathing Rate, Rhythm, Nature, and Effort

Breathing rate can vary widely in normal animals and, except for extreme variations, is of limited value as a respiratory monitor. A change in breathing rate, however, is a sensitive indicator of a change in the underlying status of the patient. Bradypnea may be a sign of respiratory center depression secondary to intracranial or extracranial disease. The underlying cause should be identified and treated if possible. Irregular breathing patterns usually indicate a problem within the central pattern generator in the brainstem, and such a finding suggests a poor prognosis. A weak breathing effort may be caused by central or peripheral neurologic impairment or neuromuscular dysfunction, depending on the specific poison or toxin. Bradypneic, arrhythmic, and weak breathing patterns may be associated with hypoventilation, and such patients should be intubated and assisted ventilation should be instituted. Tachypneic breathing is usually a sign of hypoxemia, hypercapnia, hyperthermia, hypotension, sepsis, pain, or opioid administration, and seldom should be treated specifically, but the underlying cause should be investigated and addressed if possible, as in the case of opiate toxicity.

Body postures and extrapulmonary signs also may be noted in patients that are having respiratory difficulty. These may include extension of the head and neck to decrease upper airway resistance, reluctance of the patient to lie down, flaring of the nostrils, abduction of the elbows, sucking of skin over the thoracic inlet, and/or an abdominal component to breathing.

Audible Sounds

Low-pitched, snoring, or high-pitched, squeaky inspiratory noises heard without the aid of a stethoscope suggest an upper airway obstruction. Such patients should receive oxygen therapy and may need general anesthesia to gain access to the airway. Large airway obstructions must be removed or bypassed (by intratracheal oxygen insufflations, endotracheal intubation, or temporary tracheostomy). Mid-pitched, wheezing, asthmatic sounds heard during inspiration and expiration suggest a fixed, large airway obstruction or narrowed lower airways, as would occur in bronchospasm or with the accumulation of airway exudates (pneumonia). Bronchodilators should be used if bronchospasm is thought to be the problem; positive pressure ventilation may be required if there is airway fluid.

Auscultation of crepitation or bubbling is indicative of small airway fluid, as would occur in pulmonary edema (transudate), pneumonia (exudate), or hemorrhage. Such patients may require positive pressure ventilation if oxygen therapy alone does not remedy the hypoxemia. Aspiration is a common problem in obtunded patients that vomit or regurgitate. The aspirated material may cause airway obstruction and sets the stage for pneumonia. Aspirated gastric fluid with a pH of less than 2 is also associated with epithelial necrosis and inflammation.

Diminished, muted, or absent lung or heart sounds may indicate a pleural space disorder, such as pneumothorax or hemothorax. Thoracic radiography may be a useful diagnostic tool for intrathoracic abnormalities but should only be attempted if the respiratory distress is not considered life threatening at the moment. The focused assessment by sonography in trauma of the thorax (t-FAST) examination has been developed in canine and feline patients and validated in canine patients. The t-FAST scan is a noninvasive, rapid, and repeatable examination that can be performed within minutes of a patient's arrival while the technical staff is initiating resuscitative measures. The t-FAST procedure has good sensitivity and specificity for detection of free fluid and/or air within the pleural and/or pericardial space. With this scan, fluid and/or air can be localized and samples collected with ultrasound guidance or treatment of life-threatening pleural effusions, pericardial effusions, or pneumothoraces can be initiated very shortly after presentation. In some instances, injuries or other pathology to the lungs or other thoracic structure also may be detected during a t-FAST examination. If ultrasound is not immediately available, life-threatening pleural space disease is suspected, and the patient is too unstable for radiography, a diagnostic/therapeutic thoracocentesis may be indicated before any imaging studies.

If pneumonia is detected radiographically, it should be treated with broad-spectrum antibiotics (empiric initially, later supported by airway secretion culture and sensitivity testing), nebulization and coupage, postural drainage, and early ambulation (to the extent possible). Cough suppressants should be avoided.

Ventilometry

Ventilation volume can be estimated by visual observation of the chest wall and can be measured by ventilometry. Normal tidal volume ranges between 8 and 20 mL/kg. Normal total minute ventilation ranges between about 150 and 250 mL/kg per minute for dogs. The arterial partial pressure of carbon dioxide ($Paco_2$) defines alveolar minute ventilation and the measured minute ventilation should be appropriate. A large minute ventilation in combination with a normal (or high $Paco_2$) is indicative of dead space ventilation, as might occur in hypovolemia and pulmonary thromboembolism.

Partial Pressure of Carbon Dioxide

The arterial Pco_2 ($Paco_2$) is a measure of the ventilatory status of the patient and normally ranges between 35 and 45 mm Hg. A $Paco_2$ in excess of 60 mm Hg may be associated with excessive respiratory acidosis and often represents sufficient hypoventilation to warrant positive pressure ventilation. $Paco_2$ values below 20 mm Hg are associated with respiratory alkalosis and a decreased cerebral blood flow, which may impair cerebral oxygenation and negatively impact mentation.

There are additional ways to estimate $Paco_2$ without arterial blood sampling. Venous Pco_2 ($Pvco_2$) is usually 3 to 6 mm Hg higher than $Paco_2$ in stable states, and generally can be used as an approximation of $Paco_2$. $Pvco_2$ is variably higher in transition states and during hypovolemic or anemic states. An increased arterial-venous Pco_2 gradient (larger difference between measured $Paco_2$ and $Pvco_2$) suggests decreased tissue perfusion. $Paco_2$ also may be estimated by measuring the carbon dioxide in a sample of gas taken at the end of an exhalation. End-tidal CO_2 ($ETCO_2$) values are typically 2 to 10 mm Hg less than that of $Paco_2$, so $ETCO_2$ readings can give relatively accurate reflections of $Paco_2$ in dogs and represents a good estimate of ventilatory status in the intubated patient.

Hypoventilation

Hypoventilation is treated with positive pressure ventilation. Whether manually ventilating or using a mechanical ventilator, the general guidelines for positive pressure ventilation are the same. Peak proximal airway pressure should be about 10 to 15 cm H_2O; tidal volume should be about 10 to 15 mL/kg; inspiratory time should be about 1 second (or just long enough to achieve a full tidal volume); ventilation rate should be about 8 to 12 times per minute.

Diseased lungs and some lungs in older patients are stiffer (less compliant) than normal lungs and therefore are much more difficult to ventilate. It is a common finding that the preceding guidelines are insufficient to adequately ventilate a patient with diffuse pulmonary parenchymal disease or significant age-related changes. To improve ventilation in these patients, the proximal airway pressure could be increased in a slowly progressive manner up to 60 cm H_2O (or to the limit of the ventilator) and the ventilatory cycle rate could be increased in a slowly progressive manner up to 60 breaths per minute. The tidal volume should be decreased in a patient with diffuse lung disease because such lungs have a reduced vital capacity; a normal tidal volume could overdistend the reduced number of remaining lung units, leading to rupture and potential pneumothorax. Protective lung strategies currently aim for very small tidal volumes (i.e., 4-6 mL/kg) with a higher ventilator frequency. If blood oxygenation must be improved, (1) the inspired oxygen could be increased up to 100% for short periods of time or up to 60% for prolonged periods of time; (2) positive end-expiratory pressure (PEEP) can be added or increased ($\leq$20 cm H_2O); or (3) the inspiratory time or the inspiratory plateau could be increased. Use of inspired oxygen concentrations of greater than 60% (FIO_2 >60%) for longer than 6 to 24 hours (the higher the FIO_2, the shorter the time) has been associated with oxygen-induced lung injury. Positive end-expiratory pressure increases transpulmonary pressure and functional residual capacity and keeps small airways and alveoli open during the expiratory phase and improves ventilation and oxygenation, thus potentially decreasing the FIO_2. Positive end-expiratory pressure also minimizes the repetitive collapse and reopening of small airways, a process that contributes to ventilator-induced lung injury. The inspiratory/expiratory (I/E) ratio must allow sufficient time for exhalation of all of the last breath; otherwise air trapping will occur. However, positive pressure ventilation can lead to hemodynamic alterations. By increasing transthoracic pressure, there can be significantly decreased venous return, especially when supraphysiological airway pressures are used.

Cyanosis

A blue to gray hue to the mucous membranes is caused by the presence of unsaturated hemoglobin in the capillaries. Cyanosis is most often caused by hypoxemia and always should be considered to be a late sign of severe hypoxemia. Because 4 mg/dL of unsaturated hemoglobin is necessary to observe cyanosis, cyanosis is not a reliable sign of hypoxemia in the anemic patient. Cyanosis may also be caused by sluggish capillary circulation. Methemoglobinemia, as can be noted with acetaminophen toxicity, can cause a brownish to bluish discoloration of the blood and mucous membranes.

Partial Pressure of Oxygen

The arterial Po_2 (Pao_2) measures the tension of oxygen dissolved in the plasma, irrespective of the hemoglobin concentration. The Pao_2 is a measure of the oxygenating ability of the lungs. The normal PaO_2 is considered to range between 80 and 110 mm Hg when an animal is breathing room air at sea level (FIO_2 = 21%), and greater than 500 mm Hg when breathing 100% oxygen ($FIO_2 = 100\%$). Hypoxemia could be caused by low inspired oxygen, hypoventilation while breathing 21% oxygen, and lung disease such as pulmonary hemorrhage, edema, or pneumonia. A PaO_2 less than 60 mm Hg is commonly selected as a trigger for supplemental oxygen therapy.

Venous PO_2 (PvO_2) reflects tissue PO_2 and bears no correlation to PaO_2. Mixed or central venous PvO_2 ranges between 40 and 50 mm Hg. Values below 30 mm Hg may be caused by anything that decreases the delivery of oxygen to the tissues (e.g., hypoxemia, anemia, low cardiac output, vasoconstriction); values greater than 60 mm Hg suggest reduced tissue uptake of oxygen (e.g., septic shock, metabolic poisons, shunting). Venous blood for such evaluations must be taken from a central vein, such as the jugular, anterior vena cava, or pulmonary artery; peripheral venous PO_2 values are highly variable and difficult to interpret.

Hemoglobin Saturation with Oxygen

When red to infrared light is transmitted through a blood sample, the various forms of hemoglobin present in the blood sample will absorb a certain proportion of light as oxyhemoglobin, methemoglobin, carboxyhemoglobin, and reduced hemoglobin. A benchtop co-oximeter measures and displays values for the first three. The displayed oxyhemoglobin is functional (i.e., it is expressed as a percentage of the amount of hemoglobin available for oxygen binding [total hemoglobin minus methemoglobin and carboxyhemoglobin]), as opposed to fractional oxyhemoglobin, which is expressed as a percentage of total hemoglobin irrespective of methemoglobin or carboxyhemoglobin. Normally, methemoglobin and carboxyhemoglobin are less than 1% each and so usually functional and fractional oxyhemoglobin measurements are quite similar. To the extent that either methemoglobin or carboxyhemoglobin is present in large concentrations, fractional oxyhemoglobin will be variably lower than functional.

Hemoglobin saturation (SO_2) measures the percent saturation of the hemoglobin and is related to PaO_2 by a sigmoid curve (Fig. 11-1). In general, a PaO_2 of 100 mm Hg is equivalent to an SO_2 of about 98%; a PaO_2 of 80 mm Hg is equivalent to an SO_2 of about 95%; a PO_2 of 60 mm Hg is equivalent to an SO_2 of about 90%; and a PO_2 of 40 mm Hg is equivalent to an SO_2 of about 75%. This oxyhemoglobin equilibrium curve is not a stationary line and can be influenced by acid-base status, blood CO_2 levels, and temperature. Hypoventilation/increased CO_2, increased temperature, and metabolic acidosis all shift the curve to the right, meaning that hemoglobin will not bind oxygen as avidly. Conversely, hyperventilation, hypothermia, and metabolic alkalosis will all shift the curve to the left, implying that hemoglobin will bind more avidly to oxygen. The clinical information derived from the measurement of arterial SO_2 (SaO_2) is similar to that obtained from a PaO_2 measurement in that they both are a measure of the ability of the lung to deliver oxygen to the blood.

Pulse oximeters estimate oxyhemoglobin saturation in the pulsatile blood of peripheral tissues (SpO_2). The probes are commonly attached externally to a patient (via tongue, lips, tail, ear, or vulva). The accuracy of a pulse oximetry reading is greatest within the range of 80% and 95% and is determined by the accuracy of the empirical formulas that are programmed into the instrument. Tissue, venous and capillary blood, nonpulsatile arterial blood, and skin pigment also absorb light. A pulse oximeter must differentiate this background absorption from that of pulsatile arterial blood. It does this by measuring light absorption during a pulse and subtracting from that the light absorption occurring between the pulses. If the pulse oximeter cannot detect a pulse, it will not make a measurement. One of the common reasons for poor instrument performance is peripheral vasoconstriction. Other reasons for inaccurate pulse oximetry readings include heavily pigmented membranes, patient motion, venous pulsation caused by right-sided heart disease or the probe being too tight around the area of measurement, ambient light, sensor slippage, tissue edema, and severe anemia.

When a low SpO_2 measurement is obtained, particularly when it seems incongruous for the patient's condition at the time, retry the measurement in several different locations and then either take the average of the readings or the highest reading and, if possible, confirm the reading with a PaO_2 measurement. Methemoglobin and carboxyhemoglobin absorb

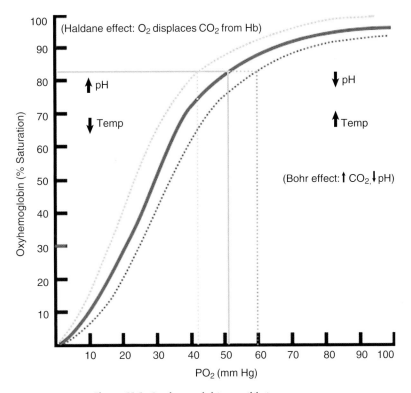

Figure 11-1 Oxyhemoglobin equilibrium curve.

light and impact the measurement made by a two-wavelength pulse oximeter designed to measure only oxyhemoglobin. Because of the biphasic absorption of methemoglobin at both 660- and 940-nm wavelengths, abnormal accumulations tend to push the oximeter reading toward 85% (underestimating measurements when Sao_2 >85% and overestimating it when <85%). Carboxyhemoglobin absorbs light like oxyhemoglobin at 660 nm, but hardly at all at 940 nm. When present in increased concentrations, it increases the apparent oxyhemoglobin measurement.

Oxygen Therapy

Oxygen therapy may be beneficial when the predominant cause of the hypoxemia is ventilation-perfusion mismatching or diffusion impairment. Oxygen therapy may not be substantially beneficial if the predominant cause of the hypoxemia is hypoventilation or small airway and alveolar collapse; positive pressure ventilation is preferred in these situations. High inspired oxygen concentrations can be attained via multiple methods (Table 11-1). A facemask is a quick and easy way to provide supplemental oxygen therapy. If the animal does not tolerate the facemask, the oxygen outlet should be held as close to the animal's nose as possible (within 3-4 cm). Oxygen cages and hoods are commercially available or can be homemade. Oxygen tents and infant incubators are available from used medical equipment suppliers. Enclosed oxygen environments should not be used during the initial stabilization stages but are useful afterward when the patient needs to be maintained in an oxygen-enriched environment. In any enclosed environment, it is important to measure and control the oxygen concentration, eliminate the carbon dioxide produced by the animal, and control the temperature. High humidity is acceptable as long as the temperature is controlled at a comfortable level.

A convenient way to increase the inspired oxygen concentration is via insufflation. Commercially available nasal prongs can be used or a soft, flexible catheter can be inserted into the nasal cavity, to about the level of the medial canthus of the eye. The catheter is sutured as it passes through the lateral alar notch and again at points along the side of the face or the top of the head to keep the catheter out of the patient's view (Fig. 11-2). An oxygen flow rate of 100 mL/kg per minute is initially recommended; flow rates should be subsequently adjusted to the needs of the patient. Medical oxygen is anhydrous and should be humidified by bubbling it through warm water.

The effectiveness of the oxygen therapy, however it is applied, should be evaluated shortly after beginning therapy. If therapy is not judged to be effective, positive pressure ventilation may be indicated.

Table 11-1 Inspired Oxygen Concentrations Obtainable for Different Oxygen Delivery Devices at Various Oxygen Flow Rates

Device	Flow Rate	F_{IO_2}
Flow-by	6-8 L/min	35%
Mask	6-10 L/min	35%-55%
Nasal prongs	100 mL/kg/min	50%-60%
Nasal cannula(s)	100 mL/kg/min	30%-50%
	300 mL/kg/min	50%-75%
Cages		50%
Hood	0.2-0.5 L/min	30%-40%
Tracheal insufflation	50 mL/kg/min	40%-60%
Tracheostomy	100 mL/kg/min	100%

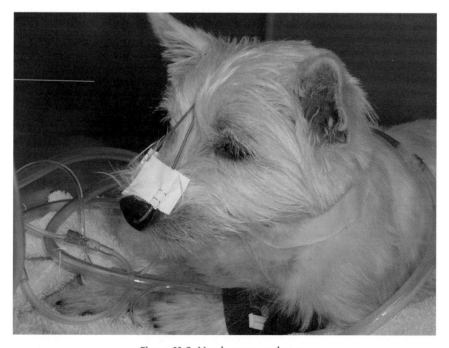

Figure 11-2 Nasal oxygen catheters.

Cardiovascular

Heart Rate and Rhythm

Heart rate and stroke volume are important to cardiac output. Slower heart rates are normally associated with larger end-diastolic ventricular volumes and consequently, larger stroke volumes. Up to a point, larger stroke volumes preserve cardiac output. Heart rate is too slow when it is associated with low cardiac output, hypotension, or poor tissue perfusion. This may occur when the heart rate falls to less than 60 beats/minute in the dog or 90 beats/minute in the cat. Common causes for bradycardia are excessive vagal tone secondary to visceral inflammation, distention, or traction; hypothermia, hyperkalemia, atrioventricular (AV) conduction block, end-stage metabolic failure, hypoxia, acetylcholinesterase inhibitors, organophosphate and carbamate poisonings, rapid administration of hypertonic saline, and digitalis overdose.

Sinus tachycardia is primarily a sign of an underlying problem (e.g., hyperthermia, hypoxemia, pain, parasympatholytics [e.g., atropine], sympathomimetics, or supraventricular or ventricular ectopic pacemaker activity). In people, because of coronary artery narrowing, sinus tachycardia can increase myocardial oxygen consumption beyond oxygen delivery capabilities. In animals, in whom coronary artery disease is rare, tachycardia only becomes a problem for the patient when there is not enough time for diastolic filling, which results in a decrease in cardiac output. Specific treatment of sinus tachycardia may be indicated when the heart rate is greater than 180 in dogs or the high 200s in cats.

Supraventricular tachyarrhythmias (SVTs) may be caused by certain toxins (e.g., digitalis glycosides, bufotoxins), sequelae to the effects of the toxin (e.g., anemia, hypoxemia, electrolyte, and acid-base imbalances), or comorbid disease (e.g., cardiomyopathy). They originate in the atria or AV node or are secondary to a re-entrant circuit. Ablation of the SVT may occur after performing a vagal maneuver, such as carotid sinus massage. If this is ineffective in resolving the SVT, then drug therapy is indicated (Table 11-2). Other treatment options include direct current cardioversion or cardiac pacing; these therapies are more effective for re-entrant SVT rather than accelerated automaticity of the atria or AV node.

Ventricular dysrhythmias may be caused by sympathomimetics, hypoxia, hypercapnia, myocarditis, electrolyte disturbances (e.g., potassium, calcium, magnesium), arrhythmogenic

Table 11-2	Injectable Antiarrhythmic Drugs		
Drug	**Mechanism**	**Indication**	**IV Dosage**
Lidocaine	Sodium channel blocker	VPCs	1.0-4.0 mg/kg; 25-80 mcg/kg/min
Procainamide	Sodium channel blocker	VPCs; SVPCs	2.0-10.0 mg/kg; 25-50 mcg/kg/min
Quinidine	Sodium channel blocker	VPCs; SVPCs	6.0-20.0 mg/kg
Amiodarone	Sodium channel blocker and other effects	VPCs	5.0 mg/kg over 20 min
Atenolol	β-blocker	SVPCs; VPCs	0.2-1.0 mg/kg
Esmolol	β-blocker	SVPCs; VPCs	0.2-0.5 mg/kg; 10-200 mcg/kg/min
Propranolol	β-blocker	SVPCs; VPCs	0.01-0.02 mg/kg
Diltiazem	Calcium channel blocker	SVPCs	0.05-0.25 mg/kg
Verapamil	Calcium channel blocker	SVPCs	0.025-0.05 mg/kg; 2-10 mcg/kg/min

SVPCs, Supraventricular arrhythmias; *VPCs*, ventricular arrhythmias.

factors released from various debilitated abdominal organs, intracranial disease, or digitalis intoxication. Ventricular dysrhythmias become a problem for the patient when they interfere with cardiac output, arterial blood pressure, and tissue perfusion. Ventricular tachyarrhythmias are also of concern when they threaten to convert to ventricular fibrillation when (1) the minute-rate equivalent exceeds the high 100s for dogs and the low 200s for cats; (2) the complexes are multiform; or (3) the ectopic beat overrides the T wave of the preceding depolarization. Total elimination of ventricular dysrhythmia is not necessarily the goal of therapy because large dosages of antiarrhythmic medications (Table 11-2) have deleterious cardiovascular and neurologic effects. A simple decrease in the rate or severity of the dysrhythmia may be a suitable end point to the titration of the antiarrhythmic medications.

Ventricular dysrhythmias can be caused by several mechanisms that are not readily apparent from the ECG appearance of the arrhythmia, especially in lead II. A given antiarrhythmic may be effective in one mechanism and ineffective or potentiate the dysrhythmia in another. Antiarrhythmic therapy is always a clinical trial. Lidocaine is usually a first choice antiarrhythmic for ventricular dysrhythmias because it selectively affects abnormal cells without affecting automaticity or conduction in normal cells.

Pulse Quality

Assessment of pulse quality by digital palpation involves an evaluation of both the height and width of the pulse pressure compared with normal. The pulse pressure is largely a reflection of stroke volume and vessel size. It is not a measure of arterial blood pressure per se, although in a general way, vessels with low pressure are easier to collapse and vice versa. Peripheral pulse quality (e.g., the dorsal metatarsal artery in the dog) decreases and disappears earlier than do larger, more central pulses (e.g., the femoral artery) with progressive hypovolemia. The relative pulse quality of more peripheral versus more central arteries may provide a rough index to the magnitude of the hypovolemia. Small stroke volumes occur with hypovolemia, poor heart function, tachycardia, and ventricular arrhythmias.

Central Venous Pressure

Central venous pressure (CVP) is the luminal pressure of the intrathoracic vena cava. Peripheral venous pressure (PVP) is slightly higher than CVP and may provide some useful information but is subject to unpredictable extraneous influences. Central venous pressure (or PVP) is the relationship between venous blood volume and venous blood volume capacity. Venous blood volume is determined by venous return and cardiac output. For CVP, verification of a well-placed, unobstructed catheter can be ascertained by observing small fluctuations in the fluid meniscus within the manometer, synchronous with the heartbeat, and larger excursions synchronous with ventilation. Large fluctuations synchronous with each heartbeat may indicate that the end of the catheter is positioned within the right ventricle.

The normal CVP is 0 to 10 cm H_2O; PVP would be on average 2 to 3 cm H_2O higher. Venous pressure is a measure of the relationship between blood volume and blood volume capacity and could be measured to help determine the end point for large fluid volume resuscitation. Below-range values suggest hypovolemia and that a rapid bolus of fluids should be administered. Above-range values indicate relative hypervolemia and that fluid therapy should be stopped. Venous pressure is also a measure of the relative ability of the heart to pump the venous return and should be measured whenever heart failure is a concern. Venous pressure measurements are used to determine whether there is "room" for additional fluid therapy in the management of hypotension.

Arterial Blood Pressure

Arterial blood pressure is the pressure of the blood against the inner walls of the arteries. It is determined by flow and the resistance to flow. It needs to be sustained from the arteries to the capillaries to ensure that enough blood reaches vital organs and tissues. This perfusion ensures nutrient supply to organs and tissues, exchange/excretion of metabolic waste, and delivery of oxygen to the tissues.

Blood pressure measurement consists of three components: the systolic arterial pressure (SAP), diastolic arterial pressure (DAP), and mean arterial pressure (MAP). The systolic blood pressure is the pressure produced on the arteries with each contraction of the heart. The DAP is the pressure produced on the arteries while the heart is at rest. It is determined by duration of the resting phase of the heart (diastole), amount of circulating blood volume, and degree of arterial elasticity. Mean arterial pressure is physiologically the most important because it represents the mean driving pressure for organ perfusion. Mean arterial pressure is a value of the average pressure on the arteries throughout duration of one complete cycle of the heartbeat (contraction and relaxation). The relationship between SAP and MAP is variable, depending on the shape and duration of the pulse pressure waveform; systolic blood pressure should always be assessed with this in mind. The formula for estimating the mean blood pressure is:

$$\frac{(SAP + 2 \times DAP)}{3}$$

The regulation of blood pressure involves complex interactions among multiple sensors of blood pressure and multiple organs that respond to the sensors to adjust cardiac output, blood volume, and vascular diameter and tone. The sensors of blood pressure are found in the major arteries and kidneys. The major effector organs include the kidneys, the central and peripheral nervous system, and the heart.

Arterial blood pressure can be measured indirectly by sphygmomanometry or directly via an arterial catheter attached to a transducer system. Sphygmomanometry involves the application of an occlusion cuff over an artery in a cylindrical appendage. The width of the occlusion cuff should be about 40% of the circumference of the limb to which it is applied. A cuff that is too small will measure the blood pressure erroneously higher than normal and a cuff that is too large will measure the blood pressure erroneously lower than normal. The occlusion cuff should be placed snugly around the limb. If it is applied too tightly, the pressure measurements will be erroneously low because the cuff itself, acting as a tourniquet, will partially occlude the underlying artery. If the cuff is too loose, the pressure measurements will be erroneously high because excessive cuff pressure will be required to occlude the underlying artery. Inflation of the cuff applies pressure to the underlying tissue and will totally occlude blood flow when the cuff pressure exceeds systolic blood pressure. As the cuff pressure is gradually decreased, blood will begin to flow intermittently. When the cuff pressure falls below systolic pressure: (1) systolic blood pressure can be estimated as the manometer pressure at which needle oscillations begin to occur during cuff deflation (caused by the pulse wave hitting the cuff); (2) systolic blood pressure can be estimated also as the manometer pressure at which one can digitally palpate a pulse distal to the cuff; (3) systolic blood pressure can be estimated as the manometer pressure at which the first blood flow sounds are heard via a Doppler ultrasound crystal placed over an artery distal to the occluding cuff; and (4) oscillometry analyzes the fluctuation of pressure in the cuff as it is slowly deflated and provides a digital display of systolic, diastolic, mean blood pressure, and heart rate. Most of these instruments can be set to recycle at discrete time intervals. Small vessel size and motion can interfere with measurements. Most external techniques are least accurate when vessels are small, the blood pressure is low, and the vessels are constricted. However, newer technology using high-definition oscillometric measurement can reduce the inaccuracies associated with motion, high heart rates, arrhythmias, and low blood pressures.

Direct measurements of arterial blood pressure are more accurate and continuous compared with indirect methods, but require the introduction of a catheter into an artery by percutaneous or cutdown procedure. The dorsal metatarsal, tibial, femoral, and ear arteries are commonly used in dogs and cats. The subcutaneous tissues around dorsal metatarsal and ear arteries are tight and hematoma formation at the time of catheter removal is rarely a problem. Once the catheter is placed, it is connected to a monitoring device. The catheter must be flushed with heparinized saline at frequent intervals (hourly) or continuously to

Table 11-3	Blood Pressure Ranges and Level of Risk of End-Organ Damage		
Risk Level	Systolic Pressure	Diastolic Pressure	Risk of End-Organ Damage
Hypotension	<80	<50	
I	<150	<95	Minimal
II	150-159	95-99	Mild
III	160-179	100-119	Moderate
IV	≥180	≥120	Severe

prevent blood clot occlusion. The measuring device could be a long fluid administration set suspended from the ceiling. However, different fluid administration sets have different compositions and thus are slightly softer or harder. This difference in distensibility of the fluid administration set can artificially increase or decrease the pressure measurement (stiffer tubing gives higher readings than softer tubing). Therefore, monitoring of trends in blood pressure measurement by this method can provide more information than single measurements. Fluid is instilled into the tubing via a three-way stopcock to a very high level and then allowed to gravitate into the artery until the hydrostatic pressure of the column of water is equalized with the mean arterial blood pressure of the patient. Because blood pressure oscillates, the system should be closed between measurements to prevent blood from entering into, and clotting, the end of the catheter. The arterial catheter also can be attached to a commercially available transducer and recording system. The extension tubing between the catheter and the transducer should not be excessively long and should be constructed of nonexpansible plastic to prevent damped signals. The transducer should be "zeroed" periodically. With computerized patient monitors, the transducer can be placed anywhere with reference to the patient. The monitor will compensate internally with an "offset pressure" for any vertical differences between the patient and the transducer. If the relative vertical position between the patient and the transducer changes, the transducer must be "zeroed" again.

Normal systolic, diastolic, and mean arterial blood pressures are approximately 100 to 140, 60 to 100, and 80 to 120 mm Hg, respectively. In general, one should be concerned when the SAP falls below 100 mm Hg or the MAP falls below 80 mm Hg (Table 11-3). In general, one should be *very* concerned when the SAP falls below 80 mm Hg or the MAP falls below 60 mm Hg. Hypotension may be caused by hypovolemia, poor cardiac output, or vasodilation. Hypertension (high MAP), when it occurs, is generally attributed to vasoconstriction. High SAP, not associated with a high MAP, is generally attributed to an inappropriate frequency response of the measuring system (for that patient and that time). Hypertension can cause increased hemorrhaging, retinal detachment, increased intracranial pressure, and high afterload to the heart and should be treated when MAP exceeds 140 mm Hg. High MAP may be caused by a light level of anesthesia, hyperthermia, sympathomimetic drugs, hyperthyroidism (thyroxine-catecholamine synergy), renal failure (renin-angiotensin), pheochromocytoma (epinephrine), and increased intracranial pressure. With increased intracranial pressure, the hypertension is most likely caused by Cushing's response to maintain an adequate cerebral perfusion pressure and should not be treated.

Cardiac Output

Cardiac output can be measured by a variety of techniques in clinical patients, but in veterinary medicine it is usually not measured. The concept of cardiac output must be on the forefront of one's monitoring and therapeutic considerations; it is after all the whole point of adequate cardiovascular function. Poor cardiac output is implied when preload parameters (CVP or PVP, pulmonary artery occlusion pressure, jugular vein distention, postcaval distention on chest radiograph, and large end-diastolic diameter on cardiac ultrasound image) are high and the forward flow parameters (pulse quality, arterial blood pressure, signs of vasoconstriction, urine output, and physical and laboratory measures of

Table 11-4	Cardiovascular Drugs				
		INDICATION			
Drug	Contractility	Heart Rate	Vasomotor Tone		IV Dosage
Dobutamine	↑↑↑	↑↑	↓		5-15 mcg/kg/min
Dopamine	↑↑↑	↑↑	↑↑		5-15 mcg/kg/min
Epinephrine	↑↑↑	↑↑↑	↑↑↑		0.1-1 mcg/kg/min
Norepinephrine	↑	NC	↑↑↑		0.2-2 mcg/kg/min
Phenylephrine	0	↓	↑↑↑		1-5 mcg/kg/min
Vasopressin	0	↓	↑↑		0.5 units/kg
			Arterial	**Venous**	
Hydralazine	0	↑↑	↓↓	0	0.5-1 mg/kg
Nitroprusside	0	↑↑	↓↓↓	↓↓↓	1-5 mcg/kg/min
Acepromazine	0	↑	↓	↓	0.01 mg/kg
Morphine	0	↓	↓	↓↓	0.1-0.5 mg/kg
Diltiazem	↓↓	↓	↓	↓	0.05-0.25 mg/kg; 0.05-0.3 mg/kg/hr
Enalaprilat	0	NC	↓	↓	0.01-0.02 mg/kg

tissue perfusion) are abnormal. Cardiac output is a flow parameter and can be low even when arterial blood pressure is normal.

Cardiac output may be reduced by poor venous return and end-diastolic ventricular filling (e.g., hypovolemia, positive pressure ventilation, inflow occlusion); ventricular restrictive disease (e.g., hypertrophic or restrictive cardiomyopathy, pericardial tamponade, pericardial fibrosis); decreased contractility; excessive bradycardia, tachycardia, or arrhythmias; regurgitant atrioventricular valves; or outflow tract obstruction. Poor cardiac output should be improved by correcting the underlying problem when possible. Preload should be optimized. When poor contractility is thought to be the problem, sympathomimetic therapy (Table 11-4) may be indicated.

Oxygen Delivery

Oxygen delivery (DO_2) is the product of cardiac output and arterial oxygen content (Fig. 11-3). Oxygen content is determined by hemoglobin concentration (most important) and PO_2. Oxygen delivery must be adequate to meet metabolic requirements (oxygen consumption). Excessive anemia, hypoxemia, bradycardia, arrhythmias, reduced stroke volume, poor heart contractility, valvular lesions, tamponade, and hypovolemia may cause inadequate oxygen delivery. Combinations of these abnormalities can compound the oxygen delivery deficit. Excessive oxygen consumption can occur with hyperthermia and intense muscular activity, such as seizures. A disparity between oxygen delivery and oxygen requirement results in an increased oxygen extraction, low venous oxygen, metabolic (lactic) acidosis, and an increased arterial-mixed venous PCO_2 gradient. Treatment of an oxygen delivery deficit should be directed at the underlying cause(s). If hypovolemia is thought to be the primary problem, fluids should be administered to re-establish an effective circulating volume. If contractility is thought to be the primary problem, dobutamine should be administered (dopamine if the patient is also hypotensive).

Fluid Therapy

Poisoned patients are commonly dehydrated and hypovolemic, and such issues must be addressed early in the course of their management. Hypovolemia is defined as a low circulating blood volume. Dehydration is defined, for the purposes of this discussion, as a low extracellular volume caused by the loss of a crystalloid solution (sodium and water). The clinical signs of hypovolemia and extracellular dehydration are different. Hypovolemia is identified

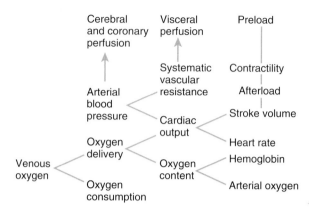

Figure 11-3 Overview of cardiopulmonary function.

by low preload (e.g., low CVP, PVP, or pulmonary artery occlusion pressure; collapsed jugular veins; radiographic appearance of a small postcava; and cardiac ultrasound appearance of a small end-diastolic diameter) and low forward flow (e.g., poor pulse quality, hypotension, vasoconstriction, oliguria in a patient that does not have renal disease, increased oxygen extraction, low venous oxygen, metabolic [lactic] acidosis, and an increased arterial-mixed venous Pco_2 gradient). Dehydration is identified by an acute loss of body weight, a decrease in skin elasticity, dry mucous membranes in a patient that is not open-mouth breathing and has not received an anticholinergic, and high urine specific gravity and high sodium concentration in a patient that does not have renal disease and has not recently received a bolus of colloids or a diuretic. Hemoconcentration may occur, depending on the nature of the fluid loss. By definition, dehydrated patients have lost extracellular fluid and therefore all dehydrated patients are to some extent hypovolemic. However, the magnitude of the dehydration and hypovolemia do not necessarily correlate; therefore each should be evaluated independently. Animals with evidence of subcutaneous edema may be associated with hypervolemia (e.g., heart failure, renal failure, and iatrogenic fluid overload) or hypovolemia (e.g., hypoproteinemia/hypocolloidemia and increased vascular permeability). In general, hypovolemia requires an initial, rapid fluid therapy plan (over a period of 10-60 minutes), whereas dehydration requires a slow fluid plan (over a period of 4-24 hours).

The crystalloid fluids are the mainstay of fluid therapy. Crystalloid fluids consist primarily of water with a sodium or glucose base, plus the addition of other electrolytes and/or buffers. The concentration of these different solutes dictates their indication in various clinical situations. Within the crystalloid group are four different types of fluids: replacement solutions, maintenance solutions, hypertonic solutions, and dextrose in water. Replacement crystalloid solutions contain dissolved solutes that approximate the solute concentration found in plasma water (Table 11-5). These solutions are indicated for the rapid replacement of intravascular volume and electrolytes, as seen with shock and hemorrhage or severe volume depletion secondary to the losses associated with vomiting, diarrhea, third body spacing, or excessive diuresis. With replacement crystalloid fluids, only 20% to 25% of the infused volume of fluid remains within the intravascular space 1 hour after infusion. Therefore large volumes of replacement crystalloids need to be administered to replace intravascular volume. The commonly available replacement solutions include normal saline (0.9% NaCl), Ringer's solution (lactate or acetate), Normosol R, and Plasmalyte. Each type of replacement fluid listed above has a specific composition that makes its use in certain situations preferential.

Maintenance solutions are also composed of dissolved solutes but their concentrations approximate the solute concentration found in extracellular fluid. The difference in these solutions compared with replacement solutions is that maintenance solutions are designed to

	Feline Normal Values	Canine Normal Values	0.9% NaCl	Lactated Ringer's Solution	Normosol R or Plasmalyte A	Lactated Ringer's + Dextrose
Na$^+$ mEq/L	155	145	154	130	140	130
K$^+$ mEq/L	4	4	0	4	5	4
Ca^{2+} mg/dL	9	10	0	3	0	3
Mg$^+$ mg/dL	2.5	3	0	0	3	0
Cl$^-$ mEq/L	120	110	154	109	98	109
Buffer			None	Lactate	Acetate/ Gluconate	Lactate
pH	7.35-7.45	7.35-7.45	4.5-7.0	6.0-7.5	6.5-8.0	4.0-6.9
Osm	310	300	308	273	294	525

Table 11-5   Canine and Feline Extracellular Fluid Normal Values and Replacement Crystalloid Composition

fulfill the electrolyte requirements of patients with normal daily electrolyte losses that are unable to maintain adequate fluid or electrolyte intake. Because these solutions are hypotonic, they can cause hyponatremia and hyperkalemia, and less than 10% of the infused volume remains within the vascular space 1 hour after infusion. Therefore they are rarely infused at rates greater than that necessary to meet the patient's maintenance needs. Commercially available maintenance fluid solutions include half-strength saline (0.45% NaCl), half-strength saline + dextrose, lactated Ringer's + dextrose, and Plasmalyte 56. Commonly, potassium supplementation is added to maintenance solutions and/or replacement solutions to further balance them for the patient's electrolyte requirements, especially if a replacement solution is being used to meet maintenance needs.

Hypertonic saline (7.2%-23% NaCl) is commonly used to rapidly increase intravascular volume. This fluid is used where severe hypovolemia is present that may lead to impending death, when low-volume resuscitation is appropriate, such as with cerebral edema, or when large volumes of crystalloids cannot be infused fast enough to have the rapid desired effect. Because of the sodium rapidly diffusing out of the vasculature, the effect of hypertonic saline is very transient (lasts up to 30 minutes). To prolong this effect, hypertonic saline is often combined with a colloidal fluid to help keep the fluid that has shifted from the extravascular space into the vascular space. Replacement crystalloid fluids should be administered after hypertonic saline infusion to replace the fluid that was translocated into the vasculature. Contraindications for hypertonic saline include patients that are dehydrated (inadequate fluid to draw into intravascular space), hyperosmolar, hypokalemic, those that may develop problems with hypervolemia (preexisting heart or lung disease), or that have uncontrolled hemorrhage (intraabdominal hemorrhage or pulmonary contusion).

Five percent dextrose in water (D$_5$W) is not commonly used in veterinary medicine. This fluid contains no active solute; therefore it readily redistributes throughout the body. The most common indications for D$_5$W are as a vehicle for infusion of other medications and to provide free water in acute (<6 hours) severely hypernatremic states. Infusion of large volumes of this fluid can lead to dilution of serum electrolytes and/or the development of edema.

Colloids are fluids with high-molecular-weight compounds in a crystalloid base that do not readily leave the intravascular space. They exert their effect of expanding intravascular volume by holding and potentially drawing water into the vasculature. Colloid fluid solutions are indicated for the treatment of hypovolemia, sepsis, and other inflammatory conditions such as pancreatitis. They are also used to improve colloid oncotic pressure in patients with low albumin from protein loss secondary to renal or gastroenteric disease, vasculitis, or burns. Colloid solutions include plasma, human serum albumin (5% and

25%), canine- and feline-specific albumin concentrates, and synthetic compounds such as hydroxyethyl starch, dextrans, and modified gelatin solutions. Contraindications for the use of colloidal fluids include coagulopathies, potential for volume overload (heart disease, pulmonary disease, oliguric renal failure), and anaphylactic reactions.

When choosing a fluid type for your patient, an important question to think about is, "What am I trying to accomplish?" The most common reasons for administration of supplemental fluid therapy include replacing deficits of intravascular volume (relative or absolute) to improve tissue perfusion, replacing deficits of tissue volume (dehydration), meeting the maintenance fluid needs of patients that are not consuming sufficient quantities of fluid, and replacing ongoing losses resulting from vomiting, diarrhea, pneumonia, burn or wound exudates, and third body spacing. In most of these situations, crystalloid fluid therapy is all that is required, although colloids can be very beneficial in providing intravascular volume.

At certain times a fluid diuresis is required, such as in patients with renal disease or to hasten the elimination of toxins that are excreted by the kidneys. In these situations, replacement crystalloid fluids are the fluid of choice. Rates required to induce a sufficient diuresis can be as high as 2.5 to 4 times a patient's maintenance requirements.

In situations in which the patient is anemic, whole blood (fresh or stored) or packed red blood cells can be administered to provide oxygen-carrying molecules. In situations in which the patient is coagulopathic, fresh-frozen or frozen plasma can provide certain clotting factors. Fresh-frozen plasma provides all clotting factors and frozen plasma provides all clotting factors except the most labile (factors V and VIII). When a patient has low plasma proteins such as protein-losing disease, prolonged starvation, or vasculitis, fluids with osmotically active particles such as colloids (preferred) or plasma (fresh frozen or frozen) should be administered for colloidal oncotic support. Finally intravenous nutritional solutions are indicated when the patient is not able to consume sufficient food for a prolonged period of time.

Fluid therapy is administered as subcutaneous therapy, a rapid intravenous bolus, or an intravenous constant rate infusion. Fluid therapy also can be administered intramedullary in small patients in which venous access is not able to be obtained. A regular hypodermic needle works well in the very young patients (neonates), whereas a bone marrow aspirate needle or power-driven IO system such as the EZ-IO works well in the older animal. The bony prominence at the proximal humerus and proximal tibia and the trochanteric fossa of the femur are common sites for needle introduction.

Subcutaneous fluid therapy is indicated for the replacement of deficits, for maintenance needs, or to counteract ongoing losses. It is usually used on an outpatient basis, as intravenous fluid therapy has proved more effective in the hospital setting. Because only a limited amount of fluid can be administered subcutaneously, it has the limitation of possibly not being able to fully account for the patient's needs in a single treatment. A contraindication for subcutaneous fluid therapy is a severely volume-depleted patient. In this situation, blood is shunted away from the cutaneous vasculature, leading to poor and inconsistent absorption of fluids.

In the hospitalized setting, intravenous is the preferred route of fluid therapy administration. Although convenient, the use of fluid therapy via a multiple of "maintenance needs" is inappropriate because most patients do not lose or require fluid therapy in these multiples. Fluids may be administered as a bolus or constant rate infusion. Bolus fluid therapy is indicated in the severely volume-depleted patient (absolute or relative) and the dehydrated patient. In the intravascular volume-depleted patient, the volume of the bolus is determined based on resolution of the clinical signs known as perfusion parameters (e.g., slower heart rate and respirations, improved pulse quality, improved mucous membrane color). Therefore frequent reassessment of the volume-depleted patient is required. Bolus fluid therapy for intravascular volume replacement that should be administered is approximately 20-mL/kg aliquots for dogs and 10-mL/kg aliquots for cats until the signs of hypovolemia are not severe. Complete normalization of cardiovascular signs is not necessarily the objective of this initial rapid fluid plan. This may require fluid doses in the range of 90 mL/kg in the dog and 55 mL/kg in the cat. The immediate objective is to achieve an acceptable circulating volume; fine tuning to normal should be accomplished more slowly. Colloids also can be administered as boluses to rapidly improve intravascular volume. The patient should be re-assessed after each bolus of crystalloid or colloid to determine if the bolus has been effective in resolving the volume-depleted state or additional boluses are indicated. Crystalloid fluids are often administered along with colloids to augment their vascular volume–expanding effect. Smaller doses of crystalloids are necessary with the concomitant use of colloid to improve intravascular volume. In the dehydrated patient, the quantity of a fluid bolus is based on part of the estimated degree of dehydration.

Constant rate fluid administration is indicated in several situations. As described, it is used to replace dehydration deficits. It is also necessary to account for a patient's mainte-nance fluid requirements if the patient is not consuming sufficient quantities of fluid on its own. Daily maintenance needs for patients varies on the age and size of the patient. Most of us were taught that the maintenance crystalloid fluid needs of a patient are approximately 54 to 66 mL/kg per day (lower end in large dogs and higher end in small dogs and cats). This may lead to under- or over-administration of fluids. The volume of fluids required to fulfill the maintenance needs of a patient can be assumed to be between 50 mL/kg per day for large dogs or 75 mL/kg per day for small dogs and cats. In pediatric patients, the require-ments may be as high as 90 mL/kg per day. With the use of colloid fluid therapy, infusions at rates of up to 20 mL/kg per day (dog) or up to 10 mL/kg per day (cat) have been used to provide continuous intravascular volume support. With the use of infusions of colloid fluids, lower infusion rates of crystalloid fluids are necessary. If a patient has ongoing losses because of vomiting, diarrhea, third spacing (ascites, pleural effusion), or diuresis (postob-structive diuresis, glucosuria, diseases that produce polyuria such as hyperadrenocorticism or renal failure), these losses should be replaced by 2 to 3 mL per estimated 1 mL lost. When the fluid therapy plan is being constructed, it is usually not known how much fluid will be lost over the day beyond the patient's maintenance needs. One could either leave this category blank for the time being or add fluid to the plan as losses occur. If the patient has a disease or effects of a toxin, which is known to be associated with unrelenting fluid losses, an estimated volume could be factored in at the time of the construction of the initial fluid plan and then adjusted upward or downward as the patient progresses.

Just as with any other administered medication, monitoring for the desired effect as well as potential adverse effects is necessary for successful fluid therapy. Proper moni-toring of the patient receiving fluid therapy is a hands-on endeavor. Much of the infor-mation we need is gained through serial examinations. No single parameter evaluated will necessarily provide all the information required to guide fluid therapy. Physical examination parameters that should be evaluated include a patient's weight, mentation, skin turgor, pulse rate and quality, respiratory rate and effort, serial lung auscultation for rales, mucous membrane color, and capillary refill time. If an indwelling urinary catheter is in place, serial evaluation of fluid input and urine output can provide sig-nificant information regarding whether too little or too much fluid therapy is being administered. Renal chemistry parameters (blood urea nitrogen [BUN], creatinine) in conjunction with urine specific gravity measurement provide additional information. Serum lactate measurement and/or acid-base status can provide information regard-ing tissue perfusion. The gold standard in veterinary medicine for evaluating adequacy of fluid therapy is serial CVP measurement. This method allows the clinician to make adjustments to fluid type and rate based on the ability of the patient's heart to handle the infused volume.

There are several situations in which fluid therapy is not necessarily in the best interest of the patient. The most common situation occurs when a patient has congestive heart dis-ease. In this situation, the patient develops congestion because the heart is not able to pump its current volume. However, heart disease is not an absolute contraindication. In some situations, there may be concomitant dehydration or the need for medications infused at a constant rate of infusion to treat the heart disease and judicious use of fluid therapy may be warranted. In these patients, hypotonic fluids such as the maintenance crystalloids or D_5W

are indicated. Meticulous monitoring of vital parameters, urine output, and central venous pressure is necessary for successful use of fluid therapy in this patient population.

The other situation in which fluid therapy may not be necessary occurs when the patient is consuming adequate volumes of water and is adequately hydrated. In this situation, fluid therapy may lead to dilution of blood cell or plasma volume, medullary washout, or development of pulmonary edema if occult heart disease is present. However, even in this situation, fluid therapy may be warranted if fluid diuresis is necessary because of toxic ingestion or a medication needs to be administered via constant rate infusion.

Discontinuing fluid therapy is as important as initiating fluid therapy. In most instances, fluid therapy should not be abruptly discontinued, especially if the patient is receiving high flow rates. During fluid therapy, the solute gradient in the kidneys may be changed because of the fluid therapy (medullary washout). If the fluid therapy is abruptly discontinued, the patient may not be able to concentrate urine well and may continue to lose excessive fluid in the urine for several days. This can be a serious problem if the patient is not ingesting adequate amounts of water, leading to dehydration. The patient should be gradually weaned off fluid therapy. In the ideal situation, the fluid therapy should be tapered to a submaintenance rate for at least 24 hours before the discontinuation of fluid therapy. However, this is not always possible. In this situation, the patient should consume adequate quantities of water and the owner informed of the patient's increased water requirements over the next several days.

Neurologic

The neurologic status of the patient should be characterized as part of the initial examination. Mental awareness and cranial nerves should be evaluated. Muscle weakness, twitching, tremors, or hyperexcitability should be noted. Continued re-evaluation at frequent and regular intervals to detect declining neurologic status is imperative.

Mental Awareness and Cranial Nerves

Consciousness is maintained by the ascending reticular formation (in the midbrain and pons of the brainstem) and the cerebral cortex. Dysfunction of either area causes decreased mentation. Degrees of mental unawareness (when not asleep) may be classified as (1) normal, alert; (2) mildly obtunded but spontaneously aware; (3) moderately obtunded: does not spontaneously care about its environment but responds to loud or brusque external stimuli—responses may be inappropriate (disoriented, confused) or erratic (delirium); (4) severely obtunded and responds only to deep pain stimulation (stuporous); and (5) comatose—no conscious responses (reflexes are present). A loss of vision, menace, and the presence of obtundation while maintaining subcortical reflexes (e.g., pupillary light reflex [PLR], dazzle reflex, vestibulo-ocular nystagmus, corneal reflex, eyeball retraction, and palpebral reflex) are suggestive of cerebral disease.

The menace reflex is done by pretending to poke the eye with a finger; the animal should blink and may move the head away from the danger. When performing this test, one must take care not to touch or stimulate the whiskers because this may result in a false-positive response. The menace reflex tests the ability of the animal to see the danger (optic n.), interpret it (cortical), and react to it (blink, facial nerve [n.] VII). Cerebellar lesions can also interfere with the menace reflex (unilateral cerebellar lesions cause ipsilateral loss of menace) via the corticotectopontocerebellar pathway in the rostral colliculi of the midbrain, without loss of vision. Corticocerebellar disease may result in the loss of the menace reflex, whereas the subcortical corneal and dazzle reflexes remain.

Normal ocular position should have both eyes looking ahead in the same direction at the same time. Strabismus is caused by lesions of the oculomotor n. (ventrolateral), abducens n. (medial), or trochlear n. Strabismus may also occur in some positions with vestibular disease. Strabismus may also be caused by retrobulbar masses. Gaze deviation, when both eyes are looking in the same direction but off to the side, is attributed to severe cerebral injury.

Mydriasis is caused by adrenergic stimulation of the iris dilator muscle and simultaneously inhibition of cholinergic stimulation of the sphincter muscle. Miosis is caused by cholinergic stimulation of the sphincter muscle and inhibition of adrenergic stimulation of the dilator muscle. Direct examination of each eye, including the fundus, must be made to rule out ocular causes such a uveitis, which causes miosis, or glaucoma or retinal disease/atrophy, which cause mydriasis. Asymmetrical or bilateral miotic pupils may represent either cerebral or brainstem disease. Mydriatic, non–light responsive pupils represent irreversible brainstem disease. In general, in order of increasing severity of lesion and decreasing prognosis: (1) normal pupil size and PLR; (2) slow PLR; (3) anisocoria; (4) bilateral miosis, responsive to light; (5) pinpoint, unresponsive; and (6) bilateral mydriasis, unresponsive. Anisocoria is caused by an imbalance between the parasympathetic and sympathetic influences (oculomotor nerve) and several intraocular diseases.

The pupils should dilate in the dark (or when the eyelid is closed) and should constrict in the light (or when a bright light is shined on the retina). Both eyes should be checked for both direct and indirect responses. Observe (1) latency of the response; (2) the speed of the response; and (3) the magnitude of the contraction. The intensity of the light stimulus is important; use the same bright light source each time. Diseases such as iris atrophy, glaucoma, posterior synechia, high sympathetic tone or sympathomimetic therapy, or anticholinergic therapy cause mydriasis, anisocoria, and diminish the pupillary light reflex. Retinal or preoptic chiasmal disease is suspected if pupillary dilation occurs when that retina is exposed to light at the same time that light is removed from the contralateral retina ("swinging flashlight test" or the "cover-uncover test").

The dazzle reflex occurs when one or both eyelids blink in response to the bright light shined on the retina. It is a subcortical reflex.

The oculovestibular reflex (physiologic nystagmus; "doll's eyes") is normal. It occurs only when the head (or head and body) is being rotated; its absence indicates vestibular n., brainstem, medial longitudinal fasciculus, or oculomotor/abducens n. dysfunction. If the nystagmus continues after the head motion is stopped, vestibular disease should be suspected. Unilateral absence suggests ipsilateral oculomotor or abducens nerve lesion. Absence of the oculovestibular reflex in association with coma suggests brainstem injury.

Pathologic nystagmus (spontaneous; positional, occurring when the head position is static) indicates inner ear, vestibular n., brainstem or cerebellar dysfunction. Horizontal nystagmus when the head is in a normal position is commonly seen in peripheral vestibular dysfunction (fast phase is usually away from the side of the lesion within the brain). Vertical nystagmus when the head is in an abnormal position, such as lateral or dorsal recumbency, is more commonly seen in central vestibular, brainstem, or cerebellar dysfunction. Rotary nystagmus is not localizing.

The corneal blink reflex is a blink when the cornea is stimulated. To prevent injury to the cornea, stimulate the cornea with a puff of air from a syringe rather than direct digital stimulation. An animal that blinks spontaneously but not in response to corneal stimulation has a sensory problem but not a motor problem. Head withdrawal requires conscious perception of the stimulus. A blink or head withdrawal before actually touching the cornea is the menace test and requires both vision and conscious perception.

The palpebral reflex (blink) when the medial canthus is touched is mediated by the trigeminal n. (sensory) and the facial n. (motor). Its absence suggests brainstem disease.

The nasal sensation is assessed by passing a cotton-tipped swab into the nose; it should evoke an avoidance response. Its absence suggests brainstem disease.

Swallowing and gagging are mediated by the glossopharyngeal and vagus nerves (both are both afferent and efferent). Their absence suggests brainstem disease.

Irregular breathing patterns (tachypnea, Cheyne-Stokes, apneustic, cluster-breathing, bradypnea, or apnea) suggest brainstem injury.

Brainstem involvement carries a very poor prognosis. It is heralded by a constellation of signs: unconsciousness; bilaterally unresponsive miotic or mydriatic pupils; absent gag,

> **Box 11-1   Toxic Etiology of Muscle Weakness**
>
> Aminoglycoside antibiotics
> Botulism
> Cationic detergents (fabric softeners, sanitizers)
> Ionophores
> Ivermectin (and similar compounds)
> Lead
> Macadamia nuts
> Myasthenia gravis
> Polyradiculoneuritis
> Spinal cord disease
> Tick paralysis

swallow, and laryngeal reflexes; strabismus; absent physiologic nystagmus; spontaneous or positional nystagmus; irregular breathing rhythms/apnea; decerebrate posturing (extensor rigidity of all four limbs and opisthotonus). Compression of the brainstem can result in abrupt changes in respiration, heart rate, and blood pressure, which are often the immediate cause of death.

Neuromuscular Status

Toxic etiologies of muscle weakness can be found in Box 11-1. The symptomatic therapy of muscle-weak patients is first to protect them from self-induced injury if they are "flopping around" because they have enough muscle strength to be active but not enough to do it in a coordinated fashion. If they are mostly immobile, they should be managed as per the recumbent care protocol discussed later in the chapter. If the muscle weakness is so severe that it interferes with ventilation, the patient must be intubated and ventilated until such time that adequate ventilatory muscle strength returns. Toxins associated with muscle tremors, twitching, and hyperexcitability are listed in Box 11-2. These patients also must be protected from self-induced injury. If the hyperexcitability is not too bad and the patient does not appear to be too uncomfortable, and if the poison/toxin is short acting, perhaps the best option would be no therapy but rather hospitalization and observation to assure resolution of the modest clinical signs in a timely fashion. Sedatives or tranquilizers, however, are often required for these patients to facilitate their management. Almost any sedative or anesthetic except ketamine can be used; however, there are some important caveats. First, almost all sedatives or anesthetics have been associated with seizure activity in the human literature. Etomidate and propofol occasionally cause muscle twitching. Phenothiazines have a reputation for paradoxical hyperexcitability but are therapeutic at least for phencyclidine-induced hyperexcitability. Opioids cause central nervous system (CNS) excitation (delirium) in modest dosages in cats and in high dosages in dogs, but the threshold for this side effect may be lowered in the face of hyperexcitable poisons and toxins. Benzodiazepines are not reliable sedatives in normal patients, causing hyperexcitability. They are more reliable in patients with preexisting CNS disease or sedation. The benzodiazepines diminish the hyperexcitable effects of ivermectin intoxication but are GABA-receptor agonists and might potentiate the CNS depressant effects of the ivermectin (which is also a GABA agonist). Unfortunately, barbiturates, propofol, and etomidate also have GABA-receptor agonist activity; therefore it is a difficult problem to escape. Inhalational anesthetics could be used to anesthetize such patients, but they must be intubated to minimize environmental pollution with the anesthetic and protect the patient's airway. The goal of sedation is simply to take the "edge" off of the hyperexcitability, not necessarily to make it go away entirely or anesthetize the patient. To this end and specifically because an advantageous effect without a disadvantageous effect of the anesthetic cannot be predicted, it is recommended to start with very small dosages and titrate to effect. Comatose or anesthetized patients have lost any ability to take care of themselves (Box 11-3). These patients require the care described for the unconscious patient discussed at the end of this chapter.

Management of Deteriorating Neurologic Status

The intracranial contents consist of the brain (cellular structures, neurons and interstitium), cerebrospinal fluid (CSF), and blood encased in a nonexpandable vault of bone (Monro-Kellie doctrine). An increase in the volume of one must be accompanied by either a decrease in volume of another (usually CSF or blood volume) or an increase in

Box 11-2	Toxins Associated with Twitching, Tremors, and Hyperexcitability

4-Aminopyridine
Amphetamines
Benzodiazepines (small dose)
Blue-green algae
Bromethalin
Cationic detergents (fabric softeners, sanitizers)
Chocolate
Cocaine
5-Fluorouracil
Hypocalcemia
Hypomagnesemia
Herbal ephedra, ma huang, or guarana root
Ivermectin (and similar compounds)
Lead
Marijuana
Metaldehyde
Methylxanthines (caffeine)
Moldy foodstuffs (mycotoxins— penitrem A)
Mushrooms
Nicotine
Opioids (large dose)
Organophosphates and carbamates
Organochlorine insecticides
Paraquat
Permethrins
Pseudoephedrine
Phencyclidine
Pyrethrins and pyrethroids
1080 — sodium monofluoroacetate
Strychnine
Tricyclic antidepressants
Vitamin D rodenticides
Zinc phosphide

Box 11-3	Toxins Associated with Obtundation to Coma

Barbiturates
Benzodiazepines (large dose)
Phenothiazines
Opioids
Ivermectin (and similar compounds)
Amitraz
Marijuana
Ethanol
Xylitol
Methanol
Ethylene glycol
Propylene glycol
Mushrooms
Metabolic disease (hepatic encephalopathy, hypoglycemia, uremia, hypoxia, hypoosmolality or hyperosmolality, heat stroke)
Neoplasia
Infectious or inflammatory disease
Thromboemboli
Coagulopathies

intracranial pressure. The normal brain has some margin for safety in this process (intracranial compliance), because early changes in volume are not associated with much of an increase in pressure. This is accomplished by fluid shifts in the cerebral vasculature and CSF. However, the limit can be reached rapidly such that additional, small, incremental increases in intracranial volume are associated with logarithmic increases in intracranial pressure. As intracranial pressure increases, cerebral perfusion is decreased. Increases in intracranial volume can accrue with cellular swelling (cytotoxic cellular edema); interstitial edema (vasogenic); an increase in cerebrospinal fluid (hydrocephalus); an increase in blood volume (venous outflow obstruction, arterial vasodilation, hypertension); hematoma formation; or neoplasia. Elevated intracranial pressure can subsequently result in: (1) interference with neuronal function; (2) diminished cerebral blood flow; and eventually (3) subtentorial herniation of the cerebrum or foramen magnum herniation of the cerebellum; causing brainstem compression.

Cerebral perfusion pressure (CPP) is the difference between mean arterial blood pressure and intracranial pressure. For reasons of maintaining adequate CPP, it is commonly recommended to maintain the mean arterial blood pressure greater than 60 mm Hg in patients with normal intracranial pressure (ICP) and greater than 90 mm Hg in patients with suspected elevated ICP. The cerebral ischemic reflex (Cushing's reflex) is a late clinical sign reflecting severe increases in intracranial pressures. The decrease in cerebral blood flow from increased intracranial pressure triggers an elevation in systemic blood pressure.

The resulting systemic hypertension causes a reflex bradycardia. The recognition of this reflex mandates immediate therapy.

Support of respiration and circulation is the first priority in the patient with deteriorating neurologic status. Good physiologic management of the patient is of paramount importance. Avoid events and drugs that increase intracranial blood flow (aggressive fluid therapy, drugs such as alpha$_2$-agonists, ketamine), cause cerebral vasodilation (hypercapnia, hypoxemia, hyperthermia, or inhalational anesthetics), or decrease outflow (jugular vein obstruction, aggressive positive pressure ventilation, head-down positioning). The blood-brain barrier of the cerebral capillaries prevents the movement of most particles, including sodium, from the vascular to the interstitial spaces as long as it remains intact. Isotonic replacement crystalloid solutions are effective in supporting cerebral blood flow without increasing cerebral interstitial volume. The benefits of rapid, adequate fluid resuscitation in patients suffering from brain trauma have been demonstrated. Although fluid overload is to be avoided, the practice of keeping head trauma patients "on the dry side" is not supported by current clinical and experimental evidence. Hypertonic saline and mannitol are both effective in decreasing intracranial pressure because they create osmotic gradients from the intracellular to the vascular space. The rheologic effects of mannitol and its beneficial effects on cerebral blood flow (CBF) and CPP make it a useful part of the overall fluid therapy plan. Mannitol is currently the first choice hyperosmotic for increased intracranial pressure. However, hypertonic saline has been found to be neuroprotective as well as hyperosmotic and is currently being investigated as a preferred therapy for increased intracranial pressure. The usual dose of hypertonic saline is 4 mL/kg of a 7.2% solution, as a bolus over 5 minutes; rapid bolus administration of hypertonic saline can cause reflex bradycardia. The duration of effect (for cerebral edema) is 15 to 75 minutes. The dose of mannitol is controversial (0.5-1.5 g/kg), usually 0.5 g/kg administered over 20 minutes. Mannitol should be administered as intermittent 20-minute infusions and not as a continuous infusion. The duration of the rheologic effect is approximately 75 minutes. The goal with mannitol is to achieve a serum osmolality, which exceeds calculated osmolality [2(Na + K) + BUN/2.8 + glucose/18] by about 20 mOsm/kg. The actual measurement of plasma osmolality can only be ascertained with appropriate laboratory equipment (osmometer). Administration of mannitol should be in conjunction with adequate crystalloid therapy to prevent dehydration. Concurrent administration of furosemide with mannitol is no longer recommended.

Glucose-containing solutions should be avoided unless they are specifically indicated to treat hypoglycemia. Hyperglycemia and the administration of glucose-containing solutions (whether or not they produce hyperglycemia) have both been associated with worse neurologic outcome in brain-injured patients.

Corticosteroids have only been found to be beneficial in vasogenic cerebral edema secondary to neoplasia. Not only have they not been found to be useful in cytotoxic cerebral edema or traumatic brain injury, but also the use of these drugs increases mortality in human studies. The potential sequela of hyperglycemia, immunosuppression, delayed wound healing, and gastric ulceration contraindicates corticosteroid administration.

Deep barbiturate anesthesia reduces cerebral blood flow and metabolic oxygen consumption and may be protective in some instances of traumatic or hypoxic brain damage but is not generally recommended for the poisoned patient. Deep barbiturate coma, in the case of traumatic brain injury, is only considered when other methods of managing increased intracranial pressure have failed.

Hyperventilation (to a Paco$_2$ of about 25 mm Hg) results in vasoconstriction and reduces cerebral blood flow to areas of the brain with intact reactive vasoactivity. This effectively compromises brain oxygenation. Damaged vessels lose the ability to respond to carbon dioxide and blood flow to these regions may actually increase when the patient is hyperventilated secondary to a decrease in blood flow to the normal regions. Hyperventilation is not normally recommended but may represent a temporary adjunct for the acute management of patients with deteriorating neurologic function suspected to result from increased intracranial pressure. However, any beneficial effect of hyperventilation is transient as the brain adjusts its internal pH after just a few (4) hours.

Systemic or regional cooling has been experimentally demonstrated to reduce the magnitude of neuronal degeneration associated with traumatic or hypoxic brain injury. Hypothermia is currently thought to decrease metabolic brain demands, reduce release of excitatory neurotransmitters, inhibit posttraumatic inflammatory response, and preserve the blood-brain barrier. Intentional systemic cooling has a significant array of problems (coagulopathy, hypotension, bradycardia, and dysrhythmias) and is not currently recommended for veterinary patients. These complications usually occur at temperatures of 30° C or lower. In human medicine, induced moderate hypothermia (32° C-34° C) is considered in the therapy of traumatically brain-injured patients and post-CPR resuscitation. Hyperthermia should be avoided.

Reactive oxygen metabolite inhibitors (calcium channel blockers, allopurinol, superoxide dismutase and catalase, deferoxamine), scavengers (mannitol, dimethylsulfoxide), and membrane protectants (corticosteroids, 21-aminosteroids, vitamins E and C) have been demonstrated to have beneficial effects in the laboratory models of traumatic and hypoxic brain damage, but clinical efficacy remains to be determined. There is not enough known about the mechanisms of excitotoxic or inflammatory cascade–mediated neuronal damage to provide therapeutic recommendations.

Temperature

Hypothermia

Hypothermia is commonly encountered in the critically ill poisoned patient. Severity of the secondary effect is commensurate with the patient's temperature and can include cardiovascular, respiratory, electrolyte, nervous system, acid-base, and coagulation abnormalities. The cardiovascular effects of clinically relevant hypothermia include bradycardia, hypotension, dysrhythmias, decreased cardiac output, and asystole. The pulmonary consequences include decreased respiratory rate and depth, pulmonary tissue injury, and oxygen dissociation disturbances. Neurologically, patients have decreased mentation that can progress to unconsciousness. The initial renal response to hypothermia is inappropriate diuresis, which may result in dehydration and azotemia. With progressive decrease in body temperature, renal blood flow and consequently glomerular filtration rate decreases and can result in acute renal failure. With progressive hypothermia, hepatic enzyme activity decreases, which can lead to decreased metabolism of medications such as anesthetics. Metabolic acidosis (lactic acidosis) can occur as a result of decreased tissue perfusion and increased muscle activity (shivering). Primary immune functions (chemotaxis of and phagocytosis by granulocytes, macrophage movement, oxidative killing by neutrophils) are impaired in hypothermic patients. Both primary and secondary hemostatic mechanisms (decreased) as well as the fibrinolytic equilibrium (impairment of intrinsic inhibitors of fibrinolysis) are affected.

Rewarming technique is dictated by the degree of hypothermia and patient stability. Core body temperatures down to 36° C (96° F) are not associated with detrimental effects to the patient; if the patient is protected from further heat loss (passive rewarming through wrapping in insulated blankets), it should rewarm spontaneously. Active rewarming can be achieved by circulating warm water or air blankets, infrared heat lamps (optimal distance 75 cm), or radiant heat warmers or hot water bottles placed under the drapes (avoid contact with the skin if the water temperature exceeds 42° C). These measures should be applied to the trunk of the patient, not the extremities. If extremities are warmed first, peripheral vasodilation can lead to "rewarming shock" and hypotension. Severe hypothermia requires active core warming such as administration of warmed IV crystalloid fluids, flushing the abdominal cavity or colon with warm, sterile, isotonic, polyionic fluids, or by extracorporeal techniques. The rewarming rate should be limited to about 1° C per hour.

Hyperthermia

Fever is a reset thermostat and is caused by the release of endogenous pyrogens (interleukin-I) from monocytes in response to infection, tissue damage, or antigen-antibody reactions.

Mild degrees of hyperthermia (<40° C or 104° F) are not per se harmful to the patient and may represent an appropriate response to an underlying disease. True fever rarely exceeds 106° F. Hyperthermia, without a reset thermostat, is pathologic. It is usually caused by inadequate heat dissipation secondary to exposure to high environmental temperatures, excessive muscular activity (seizures, eclampsia, metaldehyde toxicity), excessive exercise (in humid climate, obese dog or those with brachycephalic syndrome) or certain metabolic conditions (malignant hyperthermia, hyperthyroidism, pheochromocytoma). Direct thermal injury to cells occurs at body temperatures greater than 42° C (108° F) when oxygen delivery can no longer keep pace with the racing metabolic activity and increased oxygen consumption. Severe hyperthermia causes multiple organ dysfunction and failure; renal, hepatic, and gastrointestinal failure; myocardial and skeletal muscle damage; cerebral edema, disseminated intravascular coagulation, hypoxemia, metabolic acidosis, and hyperkalemia. True fever always should be ruled out before active cooling measures are initiated.

Surface cooling techniques are most effective with room temperature fluids; it is the evaporation of the water from the skin surface that causes the cooling. The haircoat should be soaked to the skin. Ice water should be avoided because it causes vasoconstriction, which can impede heat loss from the core until skin temperature is less than 10° C, at which time vessel paralysis and vasodilation occur and core temperatures decrease precipitously. Convective heat loss can be enhanced with fans. Conductive heat loss can be enhanced with ice packs. Antipyretic drugs are not recommended in hyperthermic patients.

Gastrointestinal

Many poisons and toxins are associated with vomiting and diarrhea. Diarrhea may be caused by irritant or corrosive intoxicants, dietary indiscretion (moldy foodstuffs), arsenic, detergents, paraquat, heavy metal intoxication (iron, lead, zinc), mushroom poisoning, and a host of other diseases not associated with poisoning or intoxication (e.g., infections, food allergies, foreign bodies). Symptomatic therapy often includes activated charcoal (toxins), sucralfate, and appropriate fluid and electrolyte restoration. Diarrhea is associated with an alkaline, crystalloid loss containing variable amounts of albumin and red blood cells. The gastrointestinal irritation/inflammation may be associated with abdominal pain and the translocation of bacteria and bacterial endotoxin into the systemic circulation. Often therapy with antibiotics against gram-negative and anaerobic bacteria is indicated. Motility modifiers (opioids and anticholinergics) and antisecretory drugs are not generally indicated.

Vomiting

Vomiting is the active, forceful elimination of stomach contents caused by contraction of the abdominal muscles. The "vomiting center" in the reticular formation of the brainstem is stimulated by the chemoreceptor trigger zone (CRZ), ascending vagal or sympathetic influences, the vestibular apparatus, or cerebral cortex influences. The CRZ is primarily stimulated by humoral substances such as uremia and toxemias; digitalis, opioids, and other drugs; infections; and motion sickness. Mechanical stimulation/inflammation of the gastrointestinal tract, peritoneum, genitourinary tract, heart and lungs, and liver activates ascending vagal and sympathetic afferent nerves. Vomiting is associated with antiprostaglandins, ethylene glycol, mushrooms, organophosphates, carbamates, pyrethrins, permethrins, arsenic, iron, lead, zinc, phenols, detergents, disinfectants, bleach, chlorinated hydrocarbons, crayons, and organic solvents.

Vomiting sets the stage for the aspiration of material into the airways, especially in obtunded patients. This may be associated with physical obstruction of the airway, tracheobronchitis, and bronchopneumonia secondary to bacterial contamination of the respiratory tract. If the pH of the aspirant is less than about 2, an immediate contact necrosis of the airway epithelium occurs. If the vomiting is prolonged, it will cause dehydration and electrolyte abnormalities. Animals vomiting only gastric fluids tend to be hypernatremic, hypochloremic, hyperbicarbonatemic, and hypokalemic. Most dogs and cats, however, reflux considerable amounts of duodenal secretions into the stomach and lose a net alkaline solution. These animals are generally hypernatremic, hyperchloremic, hypobicarbonatemic, and hypokalemic. These "duodenal vomiters" are by far the most common and can be verified by observing greenish or yellowish coloration in the vomitus or measuring the pH of the vomitus. Animals that have been drinking water in association with the vomiting are commonly hyponatremic.

When the cause of the vomiting is not known and it is protracted, symptomatic therapy is indicated. Antiemetics should be administered on a trial basis and in sensible combinations until an effective therapy is established. Central and peripheral receptor activity responsible for mediating vomiting includes D_2-dopaminergic, alpha$_2$-adrenergic, 5-HT_3-serotonergic, M_1-cholinergic, $H_{1\&2}$-histaminergic, and ENK-enkephalinergic. Many antiemetic drugs exhibit multiple receptor activity and therefore have multiple mechanisms (and sites) of potential effectiveness. An empty stomach and forward gut motility are important aspects of therapy. Drugs that encourage gastric emptying include metoclopramide, erythromycin, domperidone, and bethanechol.

Metoclopramide is a D_2-dopaminergic and 5-HT_3-serotonergic receptor antagonist that inhibits vomiting induced by gastrointestinal irritation and the chemoreceptor trigger zone stimulation. The drug has some sedative effects and may cause extrapyramidal signs, disorientation, and excitement (especially in high dosages). It should, perhaps, not be used in patients with seizure disorders. Metoclopramide also enhances gastric emptying by peripheral cholinergic sensitization and does so without stimulation of gastric, pancreatic, or biliary secretions. The drug increases lower esophageal sphincter tone (inhibiting gastric reflux), relaxes the pyloric sphincter tone, and increases duodenal and jejunal peristalsis (but not colonic). It may cause abdominal pain and diarrhea and it should not be used in patients with intestinal obstruction. The dosage is 0.2 to 0.5 mg/kg q 6 to 8 hours, PO, SC, IM, slowly IV, or 1-2 mg/kg/day as a CRI (constant rate infusion).

Prochlorperazine is a D_2-dopaminergic, alpha$_{1\&2}$-adrenergic, M_1-cholinergic, and $H_{1\&2}$-histaminergic receptor antagonist with tranquilizer, antiemetic, and vasodilatory effects. It may cause hypotension, sedation, and extrapyramidal signs (tremors, incoordination). It is generally considered to be a very effective antiemetic. The dose is 0.2 to 0.4 mg/kg q 8 hours, SC or IM.

Diphenhydramine is an H_1-receptor antagonist with sedative, anticholinergic, antitussive, and antiemetic effects. It may cause drowsiness, dry mouth, and excitation. The dosage is 2 to 4 mg/kg q 8 hours, PO or IM.

Ondansetron and dolasetron are 5-HT_3-serotonergic antagonists that inhibit vomiting by actions on the chemoreceptor trigger zone and the vagal afferents. Side effects include sedation and head shaking. The dosage for ondansetron is 0.1 to 0.5 mg/kg IV or PO q 12 to 24 hours. Dolasetron is only available in the injectable form. The dosage is 0.6 mg/kg IV/SQ q 24 hours for nausea and 1 mg/kg IV/SQ q 24 hours for vomiting.

Domperidone is a D_2-dopaminergic antagonist that inhibits vomiting by actions on the gastrointestinal (GI) smooth muscle. It has both prokinetic and antiemetic activity (chemoreceptor trigger zone). It does not cross the blood-brain barrier and is therefore devoid of other CNS effects (drowsiness, excitation, extrapyramidal signs). It has no cholinergic activity and is not inhibited by atropine. The dosage is 2 to 5 mg (total dose) PO q 8 to 12 hours for vomiting due to gastritis (dogs only) or 0.05 to 0.1 mg/kg PO q 12 to 24 hours as a prokinetic (dogs and cats) 0.1 to 0.3 mg/kg q 12 hours.

Scopolamine is an M_1-cholinergic antagonist that inhibits vomiting by actions in the vestibular apparatus and chemoreceptor trigger zone. It also is an antagonist for $M_{2\&3}$ and therefore inhibits gastric emptying and gut peristalsis. Side effects include dry mouth, GI stasis, and drowsiness. The dosage is 0.03 mg/kg q 6 hours SC or IM.

Yohimbine is an alpha$_2$-adrenergic antagonist that inhibits vomiting by actions in the chemoreceptor trigger zone and emetic center. It may cause excitation and sedation. The dosage is 0.1 to 0.5 mg/kg q 12 hours, SC or IM.

Sucralfate reacts with hydrochloric acid to form a complex that binds to proteinaceous exudates at ulcers and protects the site from further damage by pepsin, acid, or bile. It may also stimulate prostaglandin E_2 and I_2 activity and therefore have a cytoprotective effect similar to misoprostol. It does not alter acid, trypsin, or amylase secretion. Sucralfate decreases the bioavailability and absorption of other drugs and may cause constipation. The dosage is between 0.25 and 1 g q 6 to 8 hours PO for a small dog or cat to a large dog, respectively.

Cimetidine, ranitidine, and famotidine block the H_2 receptor on the basolateral membrane of the parietal cells of the stomach. They decrease acid production and do not alter gastric emptying time or lower esophageal or pyloric sphincter tone or pancreatic or biliary secretion. Cimetidine inhibits P-450 microsomal enzyme function in the liver and may alter the metabolic rate of other commonly used drugs (β-blockers, calcium-channel blockers, diazepam, metronidazole, acetaminophen). Cimetidine binds H_2 receptors on red cells and platelets and may be associated with anemia and thrombocytopenia. Cimetidine crosses the blood-brain barrier and may be associated with mental confusion and depression. All agents, by virtue of increasing gastric fluid pH, may allow repopulation of the stomach and mouth with potentially pathogenic organisms, which in turn predispose to nosocomial pneumonia. The dosage of cimetidine is 5 to 10 mg/kg PO, IV, IM q 6 to 8 hours; the dosage of ranitidine is 0.5 to 2 mg/kg PO IV, IM q 8 to 12 hours; and the dosage of famotidine is 1 to 2 mg/kg PO, IV, SC, IM q 12 hours.

Omeprazole is a gastric acid proton pump inhibitor. In an acid environment, it is activated to a sulfonamide derivative that binds irreversibly to the H+/K+ exchange ATPase enzyme on the secretory surfaces of the parietal cells. Recovery from the drug's effects depends on the synthesis of new H+/K+ ATPase protein (3 days). The drug also inhibits the cytochrome P-450 mixed function oxidase system in the liver and therefore inhibits metabolism of a variety of other drugs, such as sedatives and anesthetics. It may cause abdominal cramping, vomiting, or diarrhea. The dosage is 0.5 to 1 mg/kg PO q 24 hours. The current assessment is that proton pump inhibitors are more beneficial than H_2 receptor antagonists; however, it may take up to 72 hours for the full effect. Consequently, famotidine is often started concurrently and discontinued after 72 hours.

Antacids have largely been supplanted by sucralfate and H_2-blockers because the latter work better and have fewer side effects. Antacids neutralize gastric acid, inhibit the proteolytic activity of pepsin, and have a local astringent effect. They may be used as a supplement to the other drugs and are still recommended for the therapy of hyperphosphatemia in renal failure; they may cause hypophosphatemia in patients without renal failure. Magnesium products should not be used in renal failure. Some products contain significant amounts of sodium and potassium and should be used with caution in patients with hypernatremia or hyperkalemia. Aluminum products may delay gastric emptying and should be used with caution in renal-compromised patients. Aluminum and calcium products may cause constipation, whereas magnesium products may cause diarrhea. These drugs should also be given remote to other oral medicants. The dosage of aluminum, calcium, or magnesium hydroxide is 1 to 10 mL, depending on the size of the animal.

Misoprostol directly inhibits gastric parietal cell acid secretion and is cytoprotective by increasing secretion of gastric mucus and bicarbonate. The drug also enhances mucosal defense mechanisms and healing of acid-induced injuries. It is specifically therapeutic for the GI complications of antiprostaglandin therapy but does not interfere with the antiinflammatory/analgesic effects of those drugs. Misoprostol enhances uterine contractions and specifically should not be used in the pregnant animal. It also enhances GI motility; cramps, diarrhea, or vomiting may be a problem. The dosage of misoprostol is 2 to 5 mcg/kg PO q 8-12 hours.

Renal

Acute renal failure can occur as a direct result of some poisons and intoxications (e.g., ethylene glycol, vitamin D rodenticides, some mushrooms, grapes, lilies, some snake or spider envenomation, lead, zinc) or as an indirect consequence of the systemic hemodynamic and inflammatory effects of other poisons. Urine flow is an indirect measure of renal blood flow and renal blood flow is an indirect measure of visceral blood flow. Maintaining visceral blood flow and urine output is an important aspect of managing the poisoned or intoxicated patient. Renal blood flow is optimized by restoring and maintaining an effective circulating blood volume. Urine output can be assessed by serial palpation of the urinary bladder, weighing bedding/litter boxes, or by actual measurement following aseptic placement of a urinary catheter. Normal urine output should be about 1 to 2 mL/kg per hour. If oliguria or anuria persists after restoration of an effective circulating volume, a diuretic should be administered: furosemide (0.5 to 5 mg/kg IV bolus ± 0.1 to 0.5 mg/kg per hour) or mannitol (0.5 g/kg IV bolus ± 0.1 g/kg per hour). Statistically, diuretic therapy does not prevent acute renal failure, but it does facilitate the medical management of the case. Oliguria (<1 mL/kg per hour) or anuria (0 mL/kg per hour) lead to fluid and electrolyte retention (edema, hyperkalemia, metabolic acidosis) and failure to excrete normal metabolic products (azotemia) as well as the poison or toxin.

Many poisons and toxins are weak acids or bases. Modification of urine pH, by increasing the ionized component of the product, can facilitate its elimination. Acidification of the urine can enhance the excretion of weak bases such as amphetamine, phencyclidine, and strychnine. Oral ammonium chloride is administered at a dosage of 200 mg/kg/day divided q 6 hours to enhance renal elimination of certain toxins or drugs in dogs and 20 mg/kg q 12 hours in the cat for urine acidification. Urine pH should be monitored to assure adequate urine acidification and plasma ammonia should be monitored to prevent hyperammonemia. Alkalinization of the urine can enhance the excretion of weak acids such as salicylates, ethylene glycol, and barbiturates. Sodium bicarbonate is administered (depending on the size of the patient and pretreatment pH) at a dosage of 650 mg to 5.85 g PO per day (dog and cat). Potassium citrate may also be used at 40 to 75 mg/kg q 12 hours or 50 to 100 mg/kg q 12 hours (dog and cat, respectively). Urine and plasma pH should be monitored.

Hepatic

The liver plays an important role in the detoxification of exogenous and endogenous poisons and toxins. It is also a primary target of several poisons and toxins (e.g., acetaminophen, mothballs, mushrooms, cycads, xylitol, cyanobacteria). Hepatocellular damage and cholestasis can be ascertained by routine measures of hepatic enzymes and function tests (alanine aminotransferase, aspartate aminotransferase, alkaline phosphatase, and bilirubin). There are several important consequences of acute liver failure. Hypoglycemia, hypoproteinemia, and coagulopathy are discussed in the following. Hyperammonemia may be associated with an encephalopathy. Acute renal failure may occur secondary to acute liver failure (hepatorenal syndrome). Significant reversible renal vasoconstriction is considered the etiology of the renal component in this syndrome; however, the exact mechanism is unknown.

General hepatosupportive measures include the administration of glutathione donors (*N*-acetyl cysteine, *S*-adenosyl methionine), silymarin, vitamins C and E, carnitine, ursodeoxycholic acid, and low doses of vitamin K.

Hematological

Hemoglobin

Anemia is associated with a number of poisons and toxins resulting from intravascular hemolysis (bee stings, some snake or spider envenomation, anionic detergents, zinc), extravascular hemolysis (mothballs, onions, garlic), gastrointestinal blood loss (antiprostaglandins, iron, arsenic, phenols, detergents, disinfectants, bleach, chlorinated hydrocarbons, and organic solvents) or the lack of red cell production. Anticoagulant rodenticide intoxication and disseminated intravascular coagulation can be associated with bleeding anywhere. Historically, in humans, the trigger for a hemoglobin transfusion has been a hemoglobin concentration of 10 g/dL (a packed cell volume [PCV] of 30%). Recent studies in humans have suggested that a more relaxed trigger of 7 g/dL (PCV = 21%) is associated with at least as good, and perhaps better, morbidity and mortality statistics. In veterinary medicine, in animals with immune-mediated hemolytic anemia, it is well accepted to withhold blood transfusions until the hemoglobin concentration is less than 5 g/dL (PCV = 15%). There are many examples of human and veterinary patients surviving much greater levels of anemia.

It may not actually be possible to define a minimum hemoglobin concentration, given the complexities of cardiac output and oxygen extraction compensatory mechanisms. An animal can tolerate greater degrees of anemia if it has the wherewithal to increase cardiac output. Metabolic markers of tissue oxygenation may help guide the need for hemoglobin transfusions. Blood may need to be administered in volumes of 10 to 30 mL/kg in the dog, depending on the magnitude of anemia. Cats have a smaller blood volume (50-55 mL/kg), and bolus dosages of all fluids should be approximately 50% of canine recommendations. The amount of blood to administer also can be calculated: (desired PCV – current PCV) × BW (kg) × 2 mL whole blood (or 1 mL packed red blood cells).

Oncotic Pressure

Plasma oncotic pressure is an important vascular fluid retention force. When depleted, there is an increased risk of interstitial edema, but because of an off-setting decrease in perimicrovascular oncotic pressure, hypoproteinemia is not as edemagenic as might be expected. An increased capillary hydrostatic pressure and vascular permeability are, in contrast, potent causes of edema. Colloid oncotic pressure (COP) can be measured; values in normal animals are 20 to 25 mm Hg. Values of 15 to 20 mm Hg are common in critically ill patients but are not thought to be of important concern. Values in the low teens should trigger therapy and values in the single digits should cause great concern. Colloid oncotic pressure can be qualitatively approximated from an albumin measurement (albumin normally accounts for about 70% of the COP). Albumin values in normal dogs and cats are 2.9 to 4.2 and 1.9 to 3.9 g/dL, respectively. A 50% decrease in albumin is associated with about a 50% reduction in COP.

One cost-effective way to augment COP is the administration of an artificial colloid such as dextran 70 or hetastarch in bolus dosages (if volume augmentation is also desirable) of 10 to 20 mL/kg or continuous infusions of 1 to 2 mL/kg per hour. Recently canine lyophilized albumin has been made available. A total of 5 to 6 mL/kg of canine albumin (16%) is recommended for the correction of hypoalbuminemia with a maximum of 200 mg/kg per day. The maximum rate of administration in normovolemic patients or patients with preexisting conditions resulting in volume overload is 1 mL/minute. Dogs with anemia or extreme dehydration should not receive canine albumin unless concurrent red blood cell products or appropriate fluid therapy is first administered. Plasma is not considered an acceptable replacement modality for hypoalbuminemia primarily because of cost and volume required; however, plasma may be indicated if there are concurrent coagulation issues, and whole blood may be indicated if there are concurrent hemoglobin issues.

In the face of normal liver function, providing appropriate caloric intake is another method of increasing albumin levels. Nutrition may be delivered via enteral or parenteral routes, although enteral is usually preferred.

Coagulation

Coagulopathies can be primary (platelets), secondary (clotting factors), or tertiary (fibrinogen). Platelet numbers can be assessed with a platelet count or a platelet screen on a blood smear (normal = 12 to 25 per oil immersion field, in a good blood smear without platelet clumping; platelet count is estimated at 15,000 × number of platelets per oil immersion field). Platelet function can be assessed by examining for petechia or a buccal mucosal bleeding time (normal, <4 minutes). Coagulation factors are assessed by in vitro tests such as prothrombin time (PT, normal values are laboratory dependent), partial thromboplastin time (PTT, normal values are laboratory dependent), activated clotting time (ACT <120 seconds at 37° C), and whole blood clotting time (<4 minutes at 37° C; 8 minutes at room temperature). Elevated fibrin degradation products represent activation of the clotting/fibrinolytic cascades; elevated d-dimer represents fibrinolysis. Decreased antithrombin levels (normal, 80%-140% in the dog) may be indicative of a protein-losing "-opathy" and prothrombotic state or may represent consumption and disseminated intravascular coagulation (DIC). Thromboelastography provides an integrated assessment of clot formation that can be used to assess for hypercoagulopathy or hypocoagulopathy.

Coagulopathies may or may not need to be treated. If bleeding is minor (not into a vital organ), and blood can easily be replaced by transfusion, specific therapy may not be necessary. Specific treatment with fresh-frozen plasma is used if platelets are not required, but labile factors such as von Willebrand's factor, factor 8, or antithrombin are required. For vitamin K antagonist poisoning, any plasma will suffice (fresh or frozen). The goal of plasma therapy is to stop the bleeding. Laboratory tests can be improved, but it is not the objective of therapy to push them to normal. Thrombocytopenia cannot be markedly improved with plasma therapy, is very expensive, and probably would not be possible because of hypervolemia. Platelet concentrate is available; however, it is also expensive and requires significant volumes. Spontaneous bleeding from thrombocytopenia is not anticipated until platelet counts are less than 30,000/μL.

Glucose

An adequate level of blood glucose is important for cerebral metabolism. Hypoglycemia might occur during hepatic failure or sepsis; hyperglycemia is also a common nonspecific hormonal response to stress hormones. Blood glucose less than 60 mg/dL should be treated with a 2.5% to 5% glucose infusion. Severe hypoglycemia should be treated, in addition, with a bolus of glucose (0.1-0.25 g/kg). There is growing evidence that persistent moderate hyperglycemia (>200 mg/dL; >11 mM/L) in the intensive care setting is associated with significantly poorer outcomes. In this setting, it has been recommended to enforce glycemic control with insulin in quantities sufficient to maintain the blood glucose concentration below 150 to 200 mg/dL (8-11 mM/L).

Metabolic Acid-Base Status

Lactic metabolic acidosis results from inadequate tissue oxygenation. The marker for metabolic acidosis is a decreased bicarbonate concentration (normal = 20-24 mEq/L in the dog; 18-22 mEq/L in the cat); a decrease in total carbon dioxide concentration (normally 1-2 mEq/L higher than bicarbonate); or an increase in the base deficit (normal = 0 to −4 mEq/L in the dog, −3 to −7 in the cat). Lactate is the marker for lactic acidosis (normal = <2 mM/L), which is usually presumed to represent inadequate tissue oxygenation but also can be elevated as a result of other abnormalities, such as catecholamine-stimulated Na-K-ATPase activity.

Mild to moderate metabolic acidosis does not need to be treated specifically; correction of the underlying problem should suffice. Severe metabolic acidosis (pH <7.20) in the face of adequate effective circulating volume may benefit from therapy with sodium bicarbonate:

$$\text{desired base deficit} - \text{measured base deficit} \times \text{body weight (kg)} \times 0.3$$

These dosages of bicarbonate should be administered over a period of at least 20 minutes.

Sodium

Sodium concentration is an expression of the relative numbers of sodium molecules to water molecules in the extracellular fluid (ECF). Sodium concentration is important to transcellular fluid flux. Abnormalities in sodium concentration (hyponatremia <140 mEq/L dog, <149 mEq/L cat; and hypernatremia >150 mEq/L dog, >162 mEq/L cat) may occur in any combination with abnormalities in ECF sodium and water content (dehydration, edema). Abnormalities in sodium concentration usually can be attributed to changes in free water. Free water must be added to reduce a sodium concentration (hypernatremia = free water deficit) and taken away to increase it (hyponatremia = free water excess). Free water may be gained by drinking water, may be administered in the form of 5% dextrose in water, or may occur secondary to high levels of antidiuretic hormone. Free water may be lost via evaporation (lungs and skin) or losing fluids, which are low in sodium compared with normal ECF (diarrhea, vomitus, urine). Abrupt changes of sodium concentrations of more than about 15 to 17 mEq/L (in either direction) should be avoided because they may be associated with untoward transcellular water shifts and unfavorable neurologic consequences.

The combination of hypernatremia and hypervolemia can be caused by impermeant solute gain (excessive sodium intake or administration) or hyperadrenocorticism. The combination of hypernatremia and normovolemia can be caused by diabetes insipidus (central or nephrogenic), reset osmostat, fever, or high environmental temperatures, or may be iatrogenic (inadequate access to water). The combination of hypernatremia and hypovolemia (dehydration) can be caused by water loss in excess of sodium through extrarenal routes (vomiting, diarrhea, third space, burns) or via renal routes (osmotic or chemical diuresis, chronic renal failure, postobstructive diuresis). Hypernatremia causes ECF hyperosmolality and intracellular dehydration. The cells first manifesting signs of dehydration are those of the CNS (depressed mentation, restlessness, irritability, muscle twitching/tremors, hyperreflexivity, muscle rigidity/spasticity, ataxia, myoclonus, tonic spasms, coma). Tissue shrinkage can cause intracranial hemorrhage. Acute hypernatremia (<6 hours) should be treated by the rapid administration of free water (in the form of 5% dextrose in water). In acute hypernatremia, the plasma sodium level may be corrected more quickly. In time the intracellular compartment increases its intracellular osmoles to offset the effects of the extracellular sodium aberration and restore intracellular water volume toward normal. Chronic hypernatremia (>24 hours) must be treated with caution to lower the sodium no faster than 1 mEq per hour to avoid water intoxication. The clinical signs of water intoxication are acute obtundation. Rapid volume replacement in the hypernatremic patient initially should be treated with a solution with a sodium concentration that is close to that of the patient (within 6 mEq of the patient's plasma sodium level). The sodium concentration is then slowly decreased by administering 5% dextrose in water at the rate of about 3.7 mL of water/kg body weight per hour.

The combination of hyponatremia and normal plasma osmolality is referred to as *pseudohyponatremia* and is most often associated with hyperlipidemia or hyperproteinemia. Hyponatremia with high plasma osmolality is usually the result of hyperglycemia or mannitol infusion. Patients with hyponatremia and low plasma osmolality are further divided based on volume status. Causes of hyponatremia, low plasma osmolality and hypervolemia include congestive heart disease, severe liver disease, nephrotic syndrome, or advanced renal failure. If the patient is normovolemic (with hyponatremia and low plasma osmolality) antidiuretic drugs, myxedema coma of hypothyroidism, or hypotonic fluid therapy should be considered as possible etiologies. Hypovolemic patients (with hyponatremia and low plasma osmolality) may have renal (hypoadrenocorticism, diuretic administration) or extrarenal causes (vomiting, diarrhea, third space, cerebral salt wasting, syndrome of inappropriate antidiuretic hormone secretion).

Hyponatremia causes intracellular edema and has been associated with obtundation, anorexia, muscle weakness and wasting, and GI signs. Common coexisting electrolyte problems include hypochloremia, hyperkalemia, and hyperphosphatemia. Mild hyponatremia requires no special consideration beyond therapy directed to the underlying disease process and volume restoration with any ECF replacement solution. Acute severe hyponatremia (<6 hours) should be treated by the rapid administration of saline. In time the intracellular compartment decreases its intracellular osmoles to offset the effects of the extracellular sodium aberration and restore intracellular water volume toward normal. Chronic hyponatremia (>24 hours) must be treated with caution so as to raise the sodium no faster than 0.5 mEq per hour to avoid myelinolysis. Initially, volume problems should be treated with a solution having a sodium concentration that is close to that of the patient. The sodium concentration is then slowly increased by administering a hypertonic saline solution at a rate of about 0.3 mEq of sodium/kg per hour. The clinical signs of myelinolysis occur 2 to 7 days after inappropriate correction of severe hyponatremia and include spastic quadriparesis, facial palsy, dysphagia, vocal dysfunction, and mental confusion to coma.

Potassium

Most of the potassium in the body is located in the intracellular fluid compartment (140 mEq/L), whereas very little of it is located in the extracellular fluid compartment (4 mEq/L). Repolarization of electrically excitable cells is largely attributed to the rapid efflux of potassium. Resting membrane potential is determined by the equilibrium between potassium moving out of the cell in response to the intracellular to extracellular potassium gradient, and potassium moving back into the cell in response to the extracellular to intracellular electronegativity.

Hyperkalemia is primarily caused by decreased urinary excretion (oliguric/anuric renal disease, hypoadrenocorticism, ruptured bladder, urethral obstruction, selected GI disease, or certain drugs such as ACE inhibitors, ACE receptor antagonists, cyclosporine, potassium sparing diuretics, nonsteroidal antiinflammatory drugs, heparin, or trimethoprim). Hyperkalemia also may be caused by translocation from intracellular to extracellular such as insulin deficiency (diabetic ketoacidosis, DKA), acute tumor lysis syndrome, reperfusion after aortic thromboembolism, rhabdomyolysis, metabolic (inorganic)/respiratory acidosis, periodic familial hyperkalemia, infusion of lysine or arginine in total parenteral nutrition, or certain drugs such as nonspecific beta-blockers and cardiac glycosides. It also can be iatrogenic from rapid infusion of potassium-containing fluids at excessive rates. *Pseudohyperkalemia* can occur if the blood sample is not analyzed for a period of time because of hemolysis, or from platelet or white cell degradation (only in severe thrombocytosis or leukocytosis).

Hyperkalemia causes membrane hypopolarization, which may result in extrasystoles/fibrillation if the resting membrane potential is slightly more negative than threshold potential or asystole when resting membrane potential is slightly less negative. Hyperkalemia also increases potassium permeability, which augments the repolarization phases of the electrocardiograph (tall, tented, narrow T wave) and diminishes the depolarization phases (small P waves, prolonged PR intervals, bradycardia, and widened QRS complexes). Hyperkalemia also may be associated with peripheral muscle weakness, decreased contractility, and weak pulse quality. Finally there is a blending of the QRS and T waves (a sinusoidal pattern), hypotension, and either ventricular asystole or fibrillation. Calcium is cardioprotective in patients with clinically relevant dysrhythmia attributed to hyperkalemia (1.0-1.5 mL of 10% calcium gluconate), administered intravenously. By virtue of its effect on membrane threshold potential, calcium antagonizes the effect of hyperkalemia and immediately returns the electrical performance toward normal. The effects of calcium, however, are short-lived, lasting only until the calcium is redistributed. Therapies to specifically address hyperkalemia include a dextrose bolus (stimulating endogenous insulin), administration of exogenous insulin and dextrose (0.25-0.5 units/kg of regular insulin/kg administered as an intravenous bolus and 2 g of glucose per unit of insulin, administered as an intravenous infusion over 2 hours) and sodium bicarbonate (1-2 mEq/kg slow IV bolus). In human medicine the administration of beta agonists, such as terbutaline, has been shown to redistribute potassium intracellularly.

Hypokalemia is primarily attributed to excessive abnormal gastrointestinal (vomiting, diarrhea) or renal (chronic failure, aldosterone-mediated, hyperadrenocorticism) losses or secondary to drugs such as diuretics (loop or thiazide) and amphotericin B. Hypokalemia may be caused by a lack of intake such as potassium free fluids or severely aberrant diet. It may also be caused by translocation in catecholamine administration, insulin- or glucose-containing fluids, alkalosis, bicarbonate therapy, beta$_2$-agonist administration, and familial periodic hypokalemia. Hypokalemia causes membrane hyperpolarization (electrical paralysis) and decreases potassium permeability (diminishes repolarization processes and enhances the depolarization processes). Hypokalemia is associated with general muscle weakness (skeletal, gastrointestinal, and myocardial) and may be associated with electrocardiographic changes opposite to those of hyperkalemia (although the changes are not as characteristic as they are with hyperkalemia): flattened T wave, U waves (a positive deflection following the T wave), elevated P wave, increased R wave amplitude, and depressed ST segment. Hypokalemia is also associated with CNS depression and an impaired ability of the nephrons to concentrate urine. A severely hypokalemic patient needs to be potassium loaded. As a general rule, potassium can be administered at rates up to 0.5 mEq/kg per hour. Moderately hypokalemic patients should be treated by supplementing the potassium concentration in the administered fluids to 20 to 50 mEq/L, depending on the magnitude of the hypokalemia.

Calcium

Plasma calcium exists in three forms: ionized (55%), nonionized chelated (10%), and albumin-bound (35%). The ionized is physiologically the most important and the form that is regulated by the body. Normal total calcium concentrations in the dog and cat are about 9 to 11 mg/dL (2.2-2.8 mM/L); ionized calcium concentrations are about 1.1 to 1.4 mM/L (4.4-5.6 mg/dL).

Hypercalcemia impairs the function of most cells in the body by decreasing threshold potential (less negative transmembrane potential) for excitable cells (making them less excitable and slowing conduction), increasing the contractile state of smooth and skeletal muscle, increasing ATP use by cell membrane and endoplasmic reticulum membrane calcium pumps, and interfering with ATP production associated with the mitochondrial accumulation of the calcium. This is manifested clinically by obtundation, poor diastolic heart function, increased arteriolar vasomotor tone, impaired nephron concentrating ability, lethargy and muscle weakness, arrhythmias, muscle twitching, and seizures. Chronic hypercalcemia is also associated with gastric hyperacidity and vomiting, and calciuresis, urolithiasis, and renal failure. Pathologic hypercalcemia is caused by hyperparathyroidism, hypervitaminosis D (rodenticides, calcitriol glycoside plants, antipsoriatic creams, iatrogenics), hypervitaminosis A, lymphoid and anal sac apocrine gland malignancy, hematologic malignancy (multiple myeloma), granulomatous disease (blastomycosis, dermatitis, panniculitis), diuretic phase of acute renal failure, chronic renal failure, and idiopathic hypercalcemia of felines. The mainstay of hypercalcemia treatment is effective therapy of the underlying disease process. Hypercalcemia should be symptomatically treated with volume support and saline diuresis. The latter can be augmented by furosemide; thiazides should be avoided. Sodium bicarbonate therapy decreases the ionized calcium concentration via alkalinization and increased protein binding. Corticosteroids may lower serum calcium if it is elevated because of neoplasia, hypoadrenocorticism, or granulomatous disease. Corticosteroids also decrease intestinal reabsorption, increase renal excretion of calcium, and decrease bone demineralization. Life-threatening hypercalcemia could be treated with chelating agents such as sodium or potassium phosphate (0.25-0.5 mM/kg IV over 4 hours), EDTA (50 mg/kg per hour IV to effect), sodium citrate, or calcium-channel blockers. Bisphosphonate therapy also has been used to treat hypercalcemia in dogs and cats. This therapy has been associated with the development of renal impairment, which appears to be dependent on the rate of infusion and bisphosphonate chosen. Pamidronate, at 1.3 mg/kg in 150 mL of 0.9% saline given over 2 hours IV, rapidly decreases serum calcium with minimal side effects. Peritoneal or hemodialysis also could be used to remove calcium from the body.

Hypocalcemia lowers (more negative) threshold transmembrane potential and increases the excitability of the nervous system and muscles. This may be manifested by muscle tremors, fasciculations, and twitching; muscle contractions, cramps, and tetany; disorientation, restlessness, hypersensitivity to external stimuli, paresthesias, and facial rubbing; panting and hyperthermia; prolapse of the third eyelid; and arrhythmias and hypotension. Hypocalcemia commonly may be attributed to hypoalbuminemia, acute or chronic renal failure, eclampsia, or acute pancreatitis. Conditions occasionally associated with hypocalcemia are soft tissue trauma or rhabdomyolysis, ethylene glycol poisoning, hypoparathyroidism, phosphate enema, and after $NaHCO_3$ administration. Other less common conditions are intestinal malabsorption, severe starvation, hyperphosphatemia, the administration of citrated blood products or EDTA, hypomagnesemia, nutritional secondary hyperparathyroidism, tumor lysis syndrome, and laboratory error. There is no broad agreement as to when hypocalcemia should be treated, but as a general guideline, ionized concentrations less than 0.75 mM/L should be treated. Calcium gluconate can be administered as a slow IV bolus (0.5-1.5 mL of the 10% solution) and if needed, an IV constant rate infusion (5-15 mg/kg of the 10% solution/ kg per hour) to maintain normal calcium. Patients should be monitored for bradycardia.

Magnesium

Magnesium is a cofactor for many intracellular enzyme systems and metabolic pathways, including formation and degradation of ATP and as a cofactor with ATP in driving intracellular ion pumps such as Na/K-ATPase, HCO_3-ATPase, and Ca-ATPase. Because Mg-ATP is required to maintain ionic gradients, magnesium is important to maintain intracellular potassium concentration and sequester cytosolic calcium. By virtue of its pivotal role in the handling of intracellular calcium, magnesium is important in cardiac excitability, contraction, and conduction as well as the smooth muscle of peripheral vasculature. Magnesium is vital in DNA synthesis and transcription, nucleic acid polymerization, and production of intracellular second messengers. Magnesium exists in plasma in three forms: ionized (55%); nonionized, chelated (15%); and bound to albumin (30%). The ionized fraction is the biologically active form. Normal total magnesium concentrations in the dog and cat are about 1.7 to 2.5 mg/dL (0.7-1.0 mM/L); ionized magnesium concentrations are about 0.8 to 1.3 mg/dL (0.3-0.55 mM/L).

Hypermagnesemia is associated with diminished neuromuscular transmission: skeletal muscle weakness and paralysis, respiratory depression, vasodilation, and hypotension. It may also be associated with heart block and coma. Hypermagnesemia can be iatrogenic by the administration of magnesium-containing antacids, cathartics, or magnesium-supplemented fluid therapy. Hypermagnesemia may be treated with aggressive fluid and diuretic therapy, and can be antagonized with 0.5 to 1 mL of 10% calcium gluconate/kg per hour (4.65-9.3 mg/mL).

Hypomagnesemia lowers the threshold potential (more negative) for excitable cells, which increases their excitability, enhances the release of calcium from stores in the endoplasmic reticulum, facilitates the release of neurotransmitters, inhibits the Na-K-ATPase membrane pump, and enhances the leakage of potassium from the cell (eventually raising resting membrane potential toward or beyond threshold potential), and is generally associated with widespread impaired cellular function. Hypomagnesemia is manifested by neural and neuromuscular excitability: hyperexcitability and noise hypersensitivity, muscle twitching, fasciculations, spasms, tetany, and eventually coma and muscle paralysis. Hypomagnesemia may be associated with refractory hypokalemia, hypophosphatemia, hyponatremia, and hypocalcemia. It also may be associated with ventricular arrhythmias; ECG changes may be similar to those of hyperkalemia. Hypomagnesemia may be caused by malnutrition and malabsorption, chronic diarrhea, colonic neoplasia, diabetes mellitus/ DKA, diuresis (loop diuretics, osmotics, thiazides, saline, polyuric renal failure, hyperaldosteronism, hyperthyroidism), renal tubular acidosis, concurrent electrolyte abnormalities (hypokalemia, hypercalcemia, hypophosphatemia), aminoglycoside and penicillin antibiotics, cisplatin, cyclosporine, citrate-anticoagulated blood, and lactation. Hypomagnesemia should be treated if the patient is symptomatic, serum magnesium concentrations are less than 1.0 mg/dL (0.4 mM/L) total or less than 0.2 mM/L (0.45 mg/dL) ionized. An initial dose of magnesium sulfate (0.2 mEq/kg) can be slowly administered to see if clinical signs improve. Magnesium sulfate can be administered at a daily dosage of 0.75 to 1.0 mEq/kg per day administered as a continuous-rate infusion. There are many oral magnesium supplements available for longer-term supplementation.

General Principles in the Care of Critically Ill Poisoned Patients

Infection Control

All critically ill poisoned patients should be considered susceptible to nosocomial infections; that is, those acquired during hospitalization and not present or incubating at the time of admission. There are many factors that may lead to this increased susceptibility. These patients are nonspecifically stressed by their disease process; they may have comorbid diseases such as viral infections, diabetes mellitus, hyperadrenocorticism, or uremia, which lower their resistance to infection; they have high levels of immunosuppressive endogenous or perhaps exogenous corticosteroids. They are often subjected to invasive surgical, diagnostic, or therapeutic procedures and/or indwelling devices and often suffer varying degrees of malnutrition. These patients may concurrently be receiving antibiotics, which predispose them to resistant bacterial or fungal overgrowth. They are surrounded by other patients with possible infections and environments contaminated with virulent organisms; and they are minimally mobile.

The emphasis of nursing care protocols should be in maintaining asepsis. Precautions should be taken to prevent the spread of infections to other patients. Precautions should include both personal protection as well as environmental decontamination. Personal protection is needed to prevent the spread of infectious organisms that may contaminate the caretaker and be transmitted to the critically ill poisoned patient. Personal protection should include clean disposable gloves and proper hand decontamination at the completion of any interaction with any patient. Any soiled clothing should be changed immediately.

As important as personal protection is, environmental decontamination is even more important. Because of this, the hospital environment can be a reservoir for infection to naïve dogs. Environmental decontamination should include the area where the critically ill poisoned patient is located and any objects that come in contact with the patient or caretaker who handles the patient. Soiled bedding and bandages should be placed in designated receptacles and not on the floor or counter. Floors, counters, and kennels should be regularly cleaned and decontaminated. Also, stethoscopes, thermometers, and writing implements should be routinely cleaned and decontaminated. Effective sanitation requires applying a germicidal agent to a basically clean surface. This requires use of both detergent and disinfectant products. Detergents in themselves do nothing to kill germs. Their purpose is to remove any organic matter before disinfection. Although some disinfectants can also act as detergents, many (e.g., bleach) do not. The majority of disinfectants used in veterinary hospitals are inactivated by organic material, so they are less effective when applied to surfaces that have not been thoroughly cleaned first. Periodically, a stronger degreaser should be used to remove body oils and other grunge that builds up on surfaces over time and can also inactivate disinfectants.

All surgical, diagnostic, or therapeutic procedures should be completed under strict aseptic conditions using properly sterilized equipment. All indwelling devices should receive regular insertion site care. All fluids administered to the patient should be sterile; all fluids drained from the patient should be collected in sterile containers, which are completely closed to the atmosphere. All administration and collection apparatus should be changed at regular intervals. All mechanical therapeutic equipment to which the patient is attached should be properly sterilized and changed at regular intervals. Immobile patients should be repositioned regularly (every few hours), and convalescing patients should be encouraged to ambulate early to minimize the accumulation of respiratory secretions in lower lung regions that predispose to pneumonia.

Insertion and Maintenance of Indwelling Vascular Catheters

The incidence of catheter-related infection increases with duration. A catheter-related infection should be suspected if an otherwise unexplainable fever or leukocytosis develops or if there is any evidence of inflammation (pain, redness, heat, or swelling) at the skin puncture site. The ideal treatment for a catheter-related infection is to remove it, culture the tip of the catheter, culture the blood, and aseptically replace a new catheter in another location. When there is no other location to place the new catheter, an over-the-wire catheter exchange is the compromise.

Catheters should be aseptically placed and then taped (on appendages) or sutured (on flat surfaces) close to the skin puncture site to prevent it from sliding in and out of the vessel. Antibiotic/antifungal ointments (chlorhexidine and povidone iodine) at the skin puncture site can be used but are not universally recommended. The site should be wrapped occlusively. Indwelling catheters should be redressed and inspected every 24 to 48 hours. All soiled bandage material should be discarded. The puncture site should be cleaned with antiseptic solutions and the occlusive wrap reapplied.

Infusion fluids and administration tubing must be sterile. Connections should not be disconnected unless absolutely necessary and then must be done aseptically. All injection caps should be cleaned well with an antiseptic solution before needle insertion. The fluid bottles and all administration tubing should be changed every 24 to 48 hours. Tubing should be changed after blood or colloid infusion. A peripheral over-the-needle-type catheter should not be used for the collection of blood samples except in emergencies. Peripherally inserted central catheters or central venous catheters can be used safely for blood collection, as long as strict aseptic protocol is followed.

Insertion and Maintenance of Indwelling Urinary Catheters

An indwelling urethral catheter is indicated if the urinary bladder cannot be easily expressed, urine needs to be quantified, or to maintain the cleanliness and comfort of recumbent or neurologically inappropriate patients. Urinary catheters should be soft, flexible, and made of the least reactive material available to lessen irritation of the urethral mucosa. Urinary catheters must be placed aseptically and attached to a closed drainage system; all joints should be firmly attached or taped to prevent accidental disconnection. The collection system should be positioned so that urine drains downhill with gravity. The collection system also should be kept from direct contact with the floor. Draining the collection reservoir or needle puncture of the collection tube to obtain a urine sample for analysis must be accomplished aseptically. The collection tubing should be taped to the tail, a hind limb, or abdomen to prevent accidental traction on the catheter and suture sites. Enough slack should be provided in the tubing to allow the patient a full range of hind limb motion. Antibiotic flushes have not been shown to prevent urinary infections, only to delay them and select for resistant infections. The bag should be drained only every 8 to 12 hours unless more discrete output measurements are desired.

The prepuce or vestibule should be flushed with a dilute chlorhexidine or povidone iodine solution three times daily to prevent migration of infectious agents into the bladder along the outside of the catheter. The urinary catheter should be removed when it is no longer necessary.

Patient Comfort

The patient should always be clean and dry. Urine, feces, and other secretions are irritating to the skin and predispose to dermatitis. The emotional needs of the patient also must be addressed frequently. Critically ill patients must be allowed time to sleep. Make sure that some of the caregiver interactions are pleasant and not associated with poking, prodding, and injecting. Owner visitations are almost always helpful to the patient's sense of well-being; only an occasional animal gets very upset because of separation anxiety when an owner leaves. In human patients, this contact has been shown to improve patient comfort and to shorten hospital stays.

The Recumbent Patient

Positioning

Immobility and positional stasis for prolonged periods of time (1) predispose to tissue necrosis and decubitus over bony protuberances, (2) are associated with the accumulation of secretions and atelectasis in the lower regions of the lung, (3) are associated with contracture and stiffening of muscles and ligaments, and (4) may be associated with regional appendage edema because of poor lymphatic drainage.

The recumbent or debilitated poisoned patient should be kept in a well-padded cage or kennel, especially when the patient does not move around much. Pressure sores, or decubital ulcers, are open wounds that develop over bony prominences when a patient lies in the same position for a prolonged period of time. In people, these sores are known as bed sores. To prevent the development of decubital ulcers, patients should be placed on soft bedding, be kept clean and dry, and be turned periodically. Special bandages may be needed to keep pressure off bony prominences, especially after surgical procedures. If decubital ulcers do develop, pressure must be kept off the area that has ulcerated to allow it to heal. This is another instance in which special bandages may be beneficial. These wounds may have to be surgically addressed and antibiotics are warranted.

Prolonged recumbency can also cause the lung to collapse on the bottom, a condition called atelectasis. During breathing, air follows the path of least resistance, which is the upper lung. Over time, all the air will be removed from the alveoli of the lower lung because of normal gas exchange and pressure of the weight of the tissues on top of the lung. When the lung collapses, fluid secretions can accumulate in the air spaces and/or the air space collapses. These patients are also prone to aspiration pneumonia or secondary bacterial pneumonia. To help prevent this, patients should be turned frequently. Alternating among right lateral, left lateral, and sternal recumbency can help with lung lobe expansion. Supplemental oxygen therapy sometimes is needed in animals with cardiovascular or respiratory compromise until the lung recovers. Postural drainage techniques help move respiratory secretions from small airways to larger airways. Minimally, this is performed by putting the patient's head down from the remainder of the body by around 20 degrees from horizontal for at least 5 to 10 minutes. Thoracic percussion (coupage) may promote clearance of large airway secretions. Coupage is performed by clapping cupped hands on the thoracic wall over the affected lung. Correct technique and positioning are more important than the amount of force used. Coupage should not be performed over normal lung because it will cause atelectasis. Coupage may be performed after a session of nebulization. Using saline for nebulization helps keep the respiratory secretions hydrated, making them easier to be "coughed up." Poisoned patients that are cardiovascularly unstable or those with pleural space disease, severe thrombocytopenia, open wounds, thoracic tumors, and pain should not receive coupage.

In the recumbent poisoned patient, the body and all appendages should be padded, positioned comfortably, and repositioned every 4 hours. The critically ill patient commonly requires some form of physical therapy, preferably every 4 hours. The goals of physical therapy are preventing limb edema, preserving joint range-of-motion, and preventing contracture and atrophy of muscles because of inactivity. Massage and range-of-motion exercises are the most common forms of therapy. These procedures should be considered early in the course of hospitalization to be most effective. There are five components to massage for it to have its desired effect: rhythm, rate, pressure, direction, and frequency. Obtaining some training in massage techniques is important for massage to be effective and to prevent injury or pain to the patient. Massage is most effective if it is combined with range-of-motion exercises. Because critically ill patients are commonly very weak, passive range-of-motion and active-assisted range-of-motion exercises are used. The time spent performing all of this therapy helps the healing process and has been shown to increase patient comfort and shorten hospital stays.

Optimizing Fluid Therapy

The moistness and mobility of airway secretions depends on adequate systemic hydration. With exudative secretions (pneumonia), patients should be maintained in the upper range of normal hydration to keep the fluid secretions moist and able to be expectorated. Patients with transudative secretions (pulmonary edema) should be maintained in the lower range of normal hydration to minimize fluid flux into the lungs. Patients that are being mechanically ventilated tend to retain sodium and water because of high aldosterone levels. Fluid ins and outs, body weight, and physical evidence of edema should be evaluated frequently as part of the normal assessment of a patient's hydration status.

The Unconscious, Heavily Sedated, or Anesthetized Patient

Many toxins have undesired effects on the neurologic, neuromuscular, or respiratory system. Some patients present comatose, or require heavy sedation or anesthesia to manage the neurologic or neuromuscular manifestations, or require anesthesia to manage the airway or provide mechanical ventilation for those patients that display significant respiratory compromise because of toxic exposure.

Endotracheal Intubation

Unconscious patients should have airway access via endotracheal intubation or temporary tracheostomy to (1) assure an open airway, (2) protect the airway should the patient vomit or regurgitate, and (3) provide a means of positive pressure ventilation should the need arise.

Avoiding traction on the tube when the patient is moved or rotated prevents accidental tube dislodgment. Tubes should be secured by tying around the maxilla, mandible, or back of the head (for orotracheal tubes) or around the neck (for tracheostomy tubes). These ties should be snug enough to prevent the tube from dislodging or moving excessively if the patient suddenly regains consciousness. Ties around the muzzle should be moved every 4 hours to minimize pressure points and lip necrosis.

The endotracheal or tracheostomy tube cuff should not be inflated unless positive pressure ventilation is being performed or frequent vomiting or regurgitation is occurring in these unconscious patients. Keeping the cuff deflated allows the patient to move some air around the tube if it becomes obstructed. If the endotracheal or tracheostomy tube cuffs are to be inflated, remember that these cuffs are round but the trachea is not. To seal some portions of the circumference, other portions are likely to be subjected to excessive cuff pressure. Asymmetrical tube cuffs and overinflated cuffs magnify the problem. Because the endotracheal or tracheostomy tube may be in place for several days, prevention of pressure-induced tracheal damage by the inflated cuff is of paramount importance. Use high-volume, low-pressure cuffs for long-term intubations. Inflate the cuff with just enough air to barely stop the flow of air around the tube (auscult over the larynx) when positive pressure is applied to the airway. The pilot balloon should not be used to gauge the degree of cuff inflation; it is used only to indicate that there is air in the cuff, and it bears no correlation whatsoever with the amount of pressure being applied to the tracheal wall.

It may be advantageous to periodically change the cuff pressure point. This can be accomplished with endotracheal tubes by deflating the cuff every 4 hours and moving the tube slightly inward or outward. The cuff is then carefully reinflated. Before cuff deflation, flush the mouth, pharynx, and the lumen of the trachea rostral to the cuff with saline. All fluid should be removed by suctioning before deflating the endotracheal tube cuff.

Mucus and debris elevated from the depths of the airways and being produced secondary to the presence of the tube accumulate at the end of the tube. Intubated animals cannot cough and accumulated secretions can dry and obstruct the tracheal tube. The inner cannula of a double-cannulated tracheostomy tube can be easily removed and cleaned every 4 hours. Tracheal tubes without inner cannulas and endotracheal tubes must be suctioned and should be exchanged every 24 to 48 hours (depending on the quantity and viscosity of the secretions).

Tracheal suctioning should be performed every 4 hours irrespective of the tube type and more frequently if there are a lot of secretions. There are always some secretions; tracheal suctioning should never be ignored. Suction catheters should be soft and flexible and should have more than one hole in their tip to prevent sucking an epithelial plug into a single hole, which would then be ripped away when the catheter is withdrawn. The suction catheter should have a proximal thumb hole so that suction can be applied in a controlled manner. The inside diameter of the catheter should be as large as possible to facilitate the removal of thick secretions. The outside diameter of the catheter should be no larger than 50% of the diameter of the endotracheal tube or tracheostomy tube adapter. The air that is suctioned through the catheter must come from the room and must be able to flow freely down around the outside of the suction catheter to prevent excessive reduction in airway pressure and small airway and alveolar collapse.

The suctioning procedure must be atraumatic and aseptic. The airway should be well humidified just before the suctioning. The animal should breathe 100% oxygen for 5 minutes before suctioning to minimize the inevitable hypoxemia. Secretions can be mobilized into the central airways by chest coupage just before suctioning. Inject 0.2 mL/kg of saline into the tracheal tube and then manually hyperinflate the lungs several times. Gently insert the suction catheter into the trachea as far as it will advance without any suction applied to the suction catheter. Suction is applied with a rotating and winding motion while the catheter is being withdrawn. Suction should not be applied to the airways for more than about 5 seconds to minimize small airway and alveolar collapse. The suctioning procedure should cease immediately if discomfort, restlessness, or changes in cardiac or respiratory rhythm occur. The patient should be manually hyperinflated with oxygen after suctioning to alleviate the small airway and alveolar collapse. The entire procedure should be repeated several times if it is productive.

Tracheal suctioning should always net some airway secretions. If not, it is because they are too dry. Better humidification and secretion liquefaction are necessary. The presence of blood in the aspirant indicates an excessively traumatic procedure. Try a gentler aspiration technique with less pressure and lower flow rates and perhaps a smaller suction catheter if blood is seen in the aspirate.

Airway Humidification

Humidification is the provision of water vapor to dry air or supplemental oxygen to help prevent the drying of airway secretions. Endotracheal intubation and temporary tracheostomy bypass the upper nasal passages, which are very efficient at humidifying inspired air.

For patients receiving mechanical ventilation, in-line humidifiers should be heated and sealed by a semipermeable membrane so that there is no water-air interface (warm water supports growth of infectious organisms, which are a source of nosocomial pneumonia). Unsealed humidifiers should be exchanged with sterile equipment every 24 hours. Cooling between the heated humidifier and the patient causes water to condense in the inspiratory tubing; it will need to be periodically drained. As an alternative to a commercial humidifier, sterile distilled water can be instilled into the inspiratory tubing and endotracheal/tracheostomy tube about every 2 hours. There are commercial condenser/humidifiers that attach to the tracheal tube and function as an artificial nose.

For patients receiving oxygen insufflation, the supplemental oxygen provided is anhydrous, and when insufflated, it must be humidified to prevent mucous and epithelial desiccation. This is usually accomplished with a bubble humidifier.

Systemic hydration is of paramount importance in ensuring airway hydration. In a dehydrated patient, airway humidification procedures are not very effective in keeping the airways and secretions moist, as the fluid is systemically absorbed.

Nebulization is the provision of particulate water droplets to therapeutically moisten desiccated secretions. This is usually accomplished with an ultrasonic nebulizer, which produces a dense mist of appropriately sized water droplets, which is then inhaled by the patient. The nebulization treatment is generally applied for about 20 minutes at about 4-hour intervals. This procedure may be followed by coupage to mobilize the now-hydrated secretions.

Oral Care

Unconscious patients do not eat, drink, or swallow. The mouth and pharynx accumulate secretions, which soon become colonized with resident bacteria and predispose the animal to nosocomial infections. The mouth and pharynx should be washed with sterile saline and suctioned at about 4-hour intervals. It is important to prevent torque or traction on the tracheal tube during this procedure. The pharynx and mouth should then be rinsed with a commercial chlorhexidine-based oral antiseptic solution.

The tongue will dry out if it is allowed to protrude from the oral cavity for any significant length of time and may develop pressure-induced ulcers if it is allowed to drape across teeth or if a pulse oximetry clip is left in one place for too long. The tongue should be cleaned along with the mouth. It should be left wholly within the mouth between cleanings. It can be wrapped in a saline and glycerin-soaked gauze sponge to keep it moist and minimize sublingual edema.

Ocular Care

Some patients may be so debilitated from their toxic exposure or under the influence of heavy sedation or anesthesia that they are unable to blink their eyes. Blinking allows the eye to spread tears over the cornea, preventing it from drying out. When the cornea dries out, corneal ulcers can develop. This can be prevented by placing a tear-like lubricant (drops or ointments) in the eyes at 2- to 4-hour intervals. If corneal ulceration is suspected, a fluorescein stain should be applied to the eye to check for corneal damage, and if corneal damage is noted, broad-spectrum antibiotic ophthalmic ointments or drops should be applied to the injured eye.

Bladder Care

Unconscious patients often do not urinate normally and when they do, the urine soils the skin. Human infant absorbent diapers, properly positioned, work very well for collecting the urine and preventing it from soaking the skin. The diapers can be weighed to quantitate the urine output. If the patient does not urinate regularly, the bladder should be expressed; however, a urinary catheter is often placed to facilitate urine collection, sanitation, and patient comfort and to quantitate urine output. The catheter must be inserted and maintained in an aseptic manner as described.

Colon Care

Comatose, heavily sedated, or anesthetized patients often do not defecate normally. The colon should be palpated daily to check for constipation. A warm saline enema, sometimes with the addition of an osmotic stool softener such as dioctyl sodium sulfosuccinate may be indicated. Long hair in the perineal region should be clipped to facilitate the cleaning of feces. If diarrhea develops, clipping of perineal fur and wrapping of the tail will help keep the area clean and lessen the chance of developing dermatitis.

Nutrition

Nutritional supplementation is vital to the recovery process for many poisoned patients. However, many of these patients do not receive sufficient nutrition during this recovery process. Over time, this lack of proteins, minerals, and energy substrates can lead to a state of general illness, malnutrition, and profound disability, a condition defined as cachexia. A cachectic patient has the potential to develop anemia, reduced cardiac mass and function, decreased pulmonary function and respiratory drive, and altered intestinal morphology and impaired absorptive ability. By providing nutrition to a patient unable to consume sufficient food, we can improve immune function, improve tissue synthesis and repair, improve intermediary drug metabolism, suppress the body's hypermetabolic response, reverse any carbohydrate imbalance, and reduce protein catabolism.

The first key in assessing whether a patient requires supplemental nutrition is to determine which patients are at risk for malnutrition. These patients may include those with a recent weight loss greater than 5% of body weight resulting from incidental comorbidity, those with partial or complete anorexia of more than 3 days' duration, or those unable to take in food because of neurologic deficit, toxic neuromuscular effects, or heavy sedation or anesthesia. For some patients, proactive nutritional intervention is beneficial. These are the patients we suspect will not eat for 3 to 5 days, as well as neonatal and juvenile puppies and kittens and obese cats. Unfortunately, there are no current biochemical markers that help to consistently determine which patients will benefit from supplemental nutrition.

Once those patients who may benefit from supplemental nutrition are identified, the next key to a nutritional program is determining what type of nutrition will suit them best. When all or part of the GI tract is available and functional, it is best to attempt to provide at least a portion of the patient's nutritional needs via the enteral route. This route has advantages because there are more options for nutritional supplementation and the cells lining the GI tract derive their nutrition via direct absorption from the intestine rather than through the blood. If the GI tract is not functioning sufficiently, then the parenteral or intravenous route is preferred. In some instances, there is some function to the GI tract but still a reason that not all nutritional requirements can be provided through enteral routes. In these situations, a combination of enteral and parenteral nutrition can be given.

The easiest options for feeding patients include offering food and coercion feeding. However, there are potential drawbacks to these methods, including stress and insufficient or inconsistent caloric intake, and they are not practical in mentally inappropriate, unconscious, heavily sedated, or anesthetized patients. Because of these issues, assisted feeding through tubes may have to be used. Options for feeding devices include nasogastric or nasoesophageal feeding tubes, gastrostomy tubes, and enterostomy tubes.

Many different calculations for determining caloric requirements are available. Most of these methods of calculating nutritional requirements are based on a patient's ideal body weight. Some of these methods also incorporate an "illness factor," although these are falling out of favor. The reason behind this is that studies are now showing that these illness factors tend to lead to oversupplementation of nutrients and calories, which also can have detrimental effects. Commonly accepted formulas for determining caloric requirements in patients receiving supplemental nutrition are given in Figure 11-4.

Resting Energy Requirement

$$70 \times (\text{body weight in kg})^{0.75} = \text{kcal/day}$$

or

$$30 \times (\text{body weight in kg}) + 70 = \text{kcal/day for patients with body weight 2.0 to 45.0 kg}$$

In some patients that are not able to tolerate full nutritional requirements by an enteral route, providing microenteral nutrition may still be of benefit. Microenteral nutrition is the

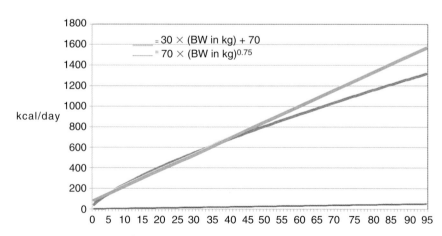

Figure 11-4 Resting energy requirements.

delivery of small amounts of water, electrolytes, and readily absorbed nutrients directly to the GI tract to maintain mucosal cell integrity. Patients that are candidates for microenteral nutrition include those that are predisposed to or already have developed stress gastric ulceration or direct GI injury because of the toxin. Microenteral nutrition may assist these patients by allowing gastric decompression, improving regional GI blood flow, providing protection against GI bacterial and endotoxin absorption, and promoting progressive gastric motility.

The GI tract receives its nutrients from intraluminal absorption. Food within the GI tract serves as a direct source of nutrients to the mucosa. There are specific "gut fuels" that are preferentially used as energy substrates by enterocytes, colonocytes, and immune cells that may be present depending on the composition of the diet. The enteral route of feeding also stimulates mesenteric blood flow, the autonomic nervous system, secretion of various digestive enzymes, hormones, and growth factors; increases GI mucus production and helps prevent ileus. Finally, the sources and processing of nutrients in a diet can influence the makeup of the GI microflora. When the GI tract does not receive sufficient nutrients, several pathologic consequences can occur. These include villous atrophy leading to increased mucosal permeability, decreases in gut-associated lymphoid tissue, and decreased surface area for absorption of nutrients for systemic use.

When gut barrier failure occurs in critical illness secondary to shock, trauma, or sepsis, it allows translocation of bacterial and endotoxin into the portal and, sometimes, systemic circulations. This gut-derived sepsis may lead to a systemic inflammatory response, which can alter the function of distant organs, possibly leading to multiorgan failure and death.

Patients that are candidates for microenteral nutrition include those that are predisposed to or already have developed stress gastric ulceration, patients with orofacial or cervical injury, patients that are actively vomiting, and those that are early in recovery from severe GI disease or GI surgery. Microenteral nutrition is commonly delivered by nasoesophageal or nasogastric feeding tubes. Nasoesophageal and nasogastric tubes are among the easiest and least expensive forms of feeding tubes available for use. Argyle infant feeding tubes are ideal. They are soft and pliable and are well tolerated by most patients after placement. Red rubber feeding tubes are a viable alternative, although they can be more reactive with the nasal mucosa.

Microenteral feedings are accomplished at a low, continuous rate infusion. Feedings are started at rates of 0.25 to 0.5 mL/kg per hour to assess the patient's tolerance for feeding. If tolerated, rates can be increased to 1 to 2 mL/kg per hour. The patient is monitored for deleterious effects of administering large volumes of fluid/food, including vomiting and potential aspiration, worsening of pancreatitis, and diarrhea. Gastric decompression of both air and residual fluid is beneficial, if indicated. The removal of residual air can decrease gastric distention, making the patient more comfortable, decreasing the chance of emesis, and increasing gastric motility. The removal of residual food or fluid also decreases gastric distention and prevents food from stagnating within the stomach if limited motility is present. The volume of fluid should be quantified to help monitor fluid balance (ins/outs), and electrolytes should be monitored because gastric secretions are being removed along with the introduced food or fluid.

Gastric stasis resulting in the accumulation of previous feedings is a common problem and with continued feeding results in gastric distention and regurgitation. Gastric residuals must be checked before each feeding and should not be allowed to exceed approximately 10 mL/kg. Gastric motility may require augmentation by metoclopramide, cisapride, bethanechol, or the use of microenteral nutrition.

Just because patients start eating does not mean an abrupt end should be brought to supplemental enteral nutrition. Gradual discontinuation of assisted feeding should be performed when the patient voluntarily consumes at least half of its resting energy requirements. Unfortunately, there are no good tests to determine when assisted feeding is no longer needed. These clinical decisions should be based on when the patient has achieved good electrolyte balance and blood sugar control. Depending on the type of assisted feeding device placed, removal might not be warranted at the discontinuation of feeding by the tube. Removal of the tube is appropriate once assisted feeding is discontinued for a short period in patients receiving nutrition via a nasogastric, nasoesophageal, or esophagostomy tube. However, patients receiving supplemental nutrition via a gastrostomy or enterostomy tube should only have their feeding tube removed after assisted feeding is discontinued for several days or after 7 to 10 days after tube placement, whichever is later. This will lessen the likelihood of leakage from the stoma in the stomach or intestine.

Effective Use of a Diagnostic Laboratory*

12

Patricia A. Talcott, MS, DVM, PhD, DABVT

Veterinary toxicology laboratories offer a wide range of testing by using highly specific and sensitive analytical methods. Most toxicology laboratories are integrated within full service veterinary diagnostic laboratories, which also provide pathology, histopathology, microbiology, serology, virology, endocrinology, electron microscopy, parasitology, and other diagnostic services. Combining results from analyses from all diagnostic "sections" will provide a high probability of establishing an accurate diagnosis, especially if the "diagnostic puzzle" is used to narrow the search. Toxicologists and their analytical staff work closely with other personnel within the diagnostic laboratory from the other sections to fine tune the diagnostic approach to maximize the use of the submitted samples and hopefully achieve a successful diagnosis. Many veterinary diagnostic laboratories have close established contacts and working relationships with clinical experts present in associated teaching hospitals. This close working relationship helps the toxicologist narrow down or sometimes expand the list of potential toxins that may be involved in the case at hand.

Getting Started

Your first contact with a veterinary diagnostic laboratory should start with a telephone consultation. In most veterinary diagnostic laboratories a veterinary toxicologist provides differentials for a case, and assists in choosing appropriate diagnostic testing and proper sample collection. Good communication in the early stage of a suspected poisoning case between the practitioner and the diagnostic toxicology laboratory personnel is one of the most useful tools in an investigation and will guarantee proper sample collection and accurate selection of initial tests. The veterinary toxicologist also can provide recommendations for the initial treatment of a potentially poisoned animal. Consulting with laboratory personnel to determine the laboratory's analytical capabilities, costs of analyses, turn-around times, and interpretation abilities is critical so that everyone involved is kept thoroughly informed. The toxicologist can help expand or narrow down the focus of the investigation, so that the clinician is not asking for the "toxicology screen," but rather focusing on some select differentials to target for testing. This also can be the appropriate time for a practitioner to pass along critical pieces of history regarding the case that may be too cumbersome to write on the accession forms. The telephone consult also can provide necessary information regarding packaging, preserving, and shipping the samples of interest. Some laboratories are open for Saturday deliveries, but many are not. You might need to know this in case samples arrive later than expected and are potentially perishable. Many laboratories have much of this information on Internet websites, but often it is a good idea to contact the laboratory directly to make sure that all information on the website is current and correct. Box 12-1 lists the American Association of Veterinary Laboratory Diagnosticians (AAVLD)-accredited veterinary diagnostic laboratories located in the United States and Canada.

*http://www.aavld.org/accreditation.

| Box 12-1 | AAVLD-Accredited Veterinary Diagnostic Laboratories—2011 |

State or Province	Laboratory Information
United States	
Arizona	Arizona Veterinary Diagnostic Laboratory Tucson, AZ 85705 520-621-2356
Arkansas	Veterinary Diagnostic Laboratory Arkansas Livestock and Poultry Commission Little Rock, AR 72205 501-907-2430
California	California Animal Health and Food Safety Laboratory System University of California, Davis Davis, CA (Main lab) 95617-1770 530-752-8709
Colorado	Colorado State University Veterinary Diagnostic Laboratory Fort Collins, CO 80523 970-297-1281
Connecticut	Connecticut Veterinary Medical Diagnostic Laboratory Storrs, CT 06269-3089 860-486-4000
Florida	Bronson Animal Disease Diagnostic Laboratory Kissimmee, FL 34741 321-697-1400
Georgia	University of Georgia Athens Veterinary Diagnostic Laboratory Athens, GA 30602-7383 706-542-5568 University of Georgia Veterinary Diagnostic and Investigational Laboratory Tifton, GA 31793 229-386-3340
Illinois	Veterinary Diagnostic Laboratory University of Illinois, College of Veterinary Medicine Urbana, IL 61802 217-333-1620
Indiana	Animal Disease Diagnostic Laboratory Purdue University West Lafayette, IN 47907 765-494-7440
Iowa	Veterinary Diagnostic Laboratory Iowa State University Ames, IA 50011 515-294-1950
Kansas	Veterinary Diagnostic Laboratory Kansas State University Manhattan, KS 66506 785-532-5650
Kentucky	Veterinary Diagnostic Laboratory Lexington, KY 40511 859-253-0571 Breathitt Veterinary Center Murray State University Hopkinsville, KY 42240 270-886-3959

Louisiana	Louisiana Animal Disease Diagnostic Laboratory Baton Rouge, LA 70803 225-578-9777
Michigan	Diagnostic Center for Population and Animal Health Michigan State University Lansing, MI 48910-8104 517-353-0635
Minnesota	Veterinary Diagnostic Laboratory University of Minnesota St. Paul, MN 55108 612-625-8787
Mississippi	Mississippi Veterinary Research and Diagnostic Laboratory System Pearl, MS 39208 601-420-4700
Missouri	Veterinary Medical Diagnostic Laboratory University of Missouri Columbia, MO 65211 573-882-6811
Montana	Montana Veterinary Diagnostic Laboratory Bozeman, MT 59718 406-994-4885
Nebraska	Veterinary Diagnostic Center University of Nebraska Lincoln, NE 68501-2646 402-472-1434
New York	Animal Health Diagnostic Center Cornell University Ithaca, NY 14853 607-253-3900
N. Carolina	Department of Agriculture & Consumer Services Raleigh, NC 27607 919-733-3986
North Dakota	Department of Veterinary Diagnostic Services North Dakota State University Fargo, ND 58105 701-231-8307
Ohio	Animal Disease Diagnostic Laboratory Reynoldsburg, OH 43068 614-728-6220
Oklahoma	Animal Disease Diagnostic Laboratory Oklahoma State University Stillwater, OK 74078 405-744-6623
Oregon	Veterinary Diagnostic Laboratory Oregon State University Corvallis, OR 97331 541-737-3261
Pennsylvania	Pennsylvania Veterinary Laboratory System Pennsylvania Department of Agriculture Harrisburg, PA 17110-9408 (Main lab—others located in University Park and Kennett Square) 717-787-8808

Continued

Box 12-1	AVLD-Accredited Veterinary Diagnostic Laboratories—2011—cont'd
S. Carolina	Clemson Veterinary Diagnostic Center Clemson University Columbia, SC 29229 803-788-2260
South Dakota	Animal Disease Research and Diagnostic Laboratory South Dakota State University Brookings, SD 57007-1396 605-688-5171
Tennessee	CE Kord Animal Disease Diagnostic Laboratory Nashville, TN 37220 615-837-5125
Texas	Veterinary Medical Diagnostic Laboratory (TVMDL) – College Station; others located in Amarillo, Gonzales, Center College Station, TX 77843 979-845-3414
Utah	Veterinary Diagnostic Laboratory Logan, UT 84341 435-797-1895
Washington	Washington Animal Disease Diagnostic Laboratory Washington State University Pullman, WA 99164-7034 509-335-9696
Wisconsin	Wisconsin Veterinary Diagnostic Laboratory Madison, WI 53706 608-262-5432
Wyoming	Wyoming State Veterinary Laboratory University of Wyoming Laramie, WY 82070 307-742-6638
Canada	
BC	Animal Health Centre Abbotsford, BC V3G 2M3 604-556-3003
Ontario	Animal Health Laboratory University of Guelph Guelph, ON N1G 2W1 519-824-4120

Filling out the paperwork to accompany the samples is sometimes time consuming, but essential to the case. It allows the consultant to refresh his or her memory of any previous telephone contacts and may provide additional pieces of information that were not apparent at the time of initial contact. The laboratory accession sheet also provides the laboratory with critical pieces of information that are necessary for internal tracking and appropriate billing. A typical laboratory accession sheet requests the following pieces of information: owner and submitting veterinarian's name, address, and contact information (including telephone and facsimile numbers and e-mail address); number of animals affected and/or dead (age, breed, sex, and weight); animals at risk; numbers and types of animals on the premises; duration of problem; location of lesion(s); clinical history; disease conditions suspected; date the samples were collected; amount and types of specimens collected; and tests desired. The information provided on the paperwork should be complete and legible, and placed in a ziplock baggie in case accompanying tissue specimens leak in transit.

Samples submitted to the toxicology unit should be individually packaged and labeled so as to avoid any confusion about specimen identification and type. Some analyses require unique specimen handling; this is why initial contact with the laboratory is essential to make sure that all samples are submitted appropriately. For example, some samples should be wrapped in foil to protect light-sensitive compounds from degrading; some samples should be frozen to prevent volatile compounds from escaping; and some samples should be wrapped in foil instead of using traditional plastic bags to prevent potential contamination by organic chemicals. All specimens should be double-bagged, and submitted in appropriate shipping containers to prevent leaking and that comply with the shipping standards of the shipping carrier you are using. A typical selection of tissues for toxicology testing is listed in Table 12-1.

It is also imperative that the clinician not forget that many toxicology diagnoses are made by sections of the laboratory other than toxicology (e.g., pathologists can diagnose ethylene glycol poisoning from fixed kidney sections). For this reason one should consider collecting as complete a selection of tissues as possible, particularly during postmortem examinations. Both fixed and fresh tissues should be collected, in case tissues need to be examined elsewhere in the laboratory system. Many times toxicology testing is used to confirm a diagnosis that is initially made by examination of fixed tissues. Do not limit your tissue selection to those systems only deemed abnormal by clinical examination or gross postmortem inspection; the laboratory may pick up interesting and perhaps important changes or lesions in tissues or systems that were thought to be unaffected. Many cases labeled as potential toxicology cases turn out to be something entirely different, so it is useful to have as complete a tissue selection as possible so as not to limit the diagnostic laboratory's capabilities. A complete set of tissues collected from postmortem examination should include, but is not limited to, the brain, eyeball, thymus, thyroid, heart, lung, spleen, kidney, liver, urinary bladder, pancreas, lymph nodes, skin, adrenal glands, various sections of the gastrointestinal tract, ovaries, placenta, testes, and skeletal muscle. In a multiple animal outbreak, submitting samples from more than one animal is advised.

Capabilities

Toxicology test methods range from simple visualization (e.g., identification of plant parts) to the use of modern analytical chemistry techniques. In many cases, several analyses have to be performed to reach a diagnosis. The techniques used in a toxicology laboratory are very specific and potentially very time consuming and expensive. Most veterinary toxicology laboratories provide routine testing for the most commonly encountered toxins in small animal practice, such as insecticides, rodenticides, avicides, molluscicides, herbicides, metals, drugs, and mycotoxins. Some laboratories also provide testing for unusual or less frequently encountered toxins, such as blue-green algae (cyanobacteria) toxins or mushroom toxins. Because of intensive networking between the veterinary diagnostic laboratories worldwide, a veterinary toxicologist can identify a suitable laboratory that can offer analytical and technical support and therefore provide the best advice regarding diagnostic workup of a particular case.

Analysis of metals, such as lead or zinc in blood, serum, plasma, tissue, or source material, is typically achieved through the use of spectroscopy. Spectroscopy employs absorption or emission of characteristic light waves following atomization (superheating) of samples. Spectroscopy is rapid and accurate and allows analysis of liquids, such as blood for lead, within a few hours. Tissue analyses requires additional time for digestion of the sample to free the metals before they can be analyzed, and therefore these types of analyses can take several hours to a few days.

Analyses for drugs, pesticides, and other organic toxins are usually performed using chromatography methods. Chromatography is the separation of compounds based on their chemical properties in liquid (high-performance liquid chromatography), solids (thin-layer chromatography), or gas (gas chromatography). After chromatographic separation, chemicals are detected by analysis for chemical properties, including absorption of ultraviolet

Table 12-1	Samples That May Be Needed for Analytical Toxicology Testing*		
Sample	Amount	Condition	Examples of Toxicoses
Antemortem			
Whole blood	1-3 mL	EDTA or heparin anticoagulant	Lead, arsenic, mercury, selenium, pesticides, anticoagulants
Urine	10-50 mL	Plastic screw-capped vial	Drugs, some metals, paraquat, alkaloids
Serum	5 mL	Remove from clot; element tubes	Trace metals (no rubber contact if testing for zinc), some drugs, ethylene glycol, pesticides
Cerebrospinal fluid	1 mL	Clot tube	Sodium
Gastrointestinal contents	100 g	Obtain representative sample	Pesticides; plant-, metal-, and feed-related poisons
Body fluids	10-20 mL	Clot tubes	Anticoagulants
Hair	1-5 g	Rarely useful	Call laboratory; chronic selenosis
Postmortem			
Urine, serum, body fluids	1-50 mL	Same preparation and tests as for antemortem samples; get serum from heart clot	Drugs, metals, pesticides
Liver	100 g	Plastic (foil for organics)	Pesticides, metals
Kidney	100 g	Plastic (foil for organics)	Metals, compound 1080 (sodium monofluoroacetate), ethylene glycol, cholecalciferol
Brain	50%	Cut sagittally; put half in plastic for analysis (fix other half for histopathologic examination)	Organochlorines, sodium, bromethalin
Fat	100 g	Foil in plastic	Organochlorines
Lung	100 g	Plastic	Paraquat
Pancreas	100 g	Plastic	Metals (zinc)
Gastrointestinal contents	100 g	Obtain representative sample	Pesticides/baits; plant-, metal-, or feed-related toxicants
Bone	100 g	One long bone	Fluoride
Miscellaneous		Injection sites, spleen	Some drugs (barbiturates in spleen)
Environmental			
Baits/sources	200 mL	Clean mason jar (liquid); plastic vial (write chemical name if available)	Unidentified chemicals, organics

Table 12-1	Samples That May Be Needed for Analytical Toxicology Testing*—cont'd		
Sample	Amount	Condition	Examples of Toxicoses
Feed	1 kg	Plastic, box; must be representative	Mycotoxins, feed additives, plants, pesticides
Plants	Entire plant	Fresh or pressed, send all parts	Identification, chemical assay
Water	1 L	Clean mason jar; foil under lid for organics, plastic lid for metals	Metals, nitrates, pesticides, cyanobacteria, organics

Modified with permission from Galey FD: Effective use of an analytical laboratory for toxicology problems. In Kirk RW, Bonagura JD, editors: *Current veterinary therapy, small animal practice XI*, Philadelphia, 1992, WB Saunders.

*Submit samples frozen except for blood and brain, or if very dry. Amounts given are optimum amounts; smaller samples may be accommodated (call laboratory about testing for smaller-sized samples). Appropriate tissue samples should be fixed in formalin for histologic analysis as well. Do not submit material in syringes.

light, fluorescence, oxidation/reduction, electron transfer, and mass weight. Chromatography is often more labor intensive and time consuming than spectroscopy because extraction of the chemical from the sample by means of solvent and purification is frequently required before testing can proceed. If a chromatography screen has detected a suspicious compound, additional testing may be required to confirm and quantify that substance.

Some analytical methods, such as that for cyanide, rely on the use of characteristic chemical reactions for analysis. Assays of cholinesterase enzyme activity in brain or blood can be done within hours to assess exposure to compounds, such as organophosphorus and carbamate insecticides.

Pitfalls

There may be many reasons that a diagnostic laboratory cannot confirm a clinician's suspicions. However, there are some common problems that toxicologists routinely face. Many times the wrong sample is collected for the test requested. This can be minimized by making sure you have collected a complete set of specimens or by calling the laboratory in advance. Another common problem that hampers a toxicology service is low sample volume being submitted for the test(s) requested. Most toxicology tests are designed to be run on a minimum sample volume; below this volume there is decreased sensitivity and accuracy. It is always better to submit too much than submit too little.

Reporting

The veterinary toxicologist typically interprets analytical findings to determine their significance in light of the historical, clinical, and pathological findings. For example, a variety of types of information are necessary to prove the presence of chronic chlorpyrifos (organophosphate) toxicosis in a cat. Clinical signs may include vomiting, anorexia, and depression, all of which are fairly nonspecific abnormalities. Identification of the compound in vomitus or blood confirms exposure. Depressed cholinesterase activity in blood or brain (if the test is performed postmortem) indicates that the exposure to chlorpyrifos was significant. A veterinary toxicologist can also provide consultation about possible toxic differential diagnoses for a case, treatment of affected animals, and steps to take to prevent additional animals from being poisoned. If a poisoning case results in a legal investigation, the veterinary toxicologist can provide specific advice necessary for documentation, testing, and data collection.

Two types of bioassays are useful for toxicology diagnostics. The most common bioassay is monitoring patients for response to treatment with known antidotes. For example, a dog suffering from an organophosphorus insecticide toxicosis may be given a test dose of atropine at a preanesthetic dose (0.02 mg/kg). Failure to develop the typical evidence of atropinization (e.g., changes in heart rate, mydriasis) suggests exposure to an organophosphorus or carbamate insecticide. Following that, successful alleviation of clinical signs with therapeutic doses of atropine (approximately 0.2 to 0.5 mg/kg IV, IM, or SC) is further evidence of exposure to one of those insecticides.

The second type of bioassay is performed only if all other analytical methods are negative. This assay involves feeding or otherwise administering sources suspected of being toxic to animals in the laboratory to demonstrate a toxic effect. The need for such testing is very rare, but is occasionally necessary to protect other pets or livestock from toxicants. If a toxic source is identified, further research can be done in an attempt to identify a new toxin and perhaps at some future date a chemical assay of diagnostic use.

Very few toxicology diagnoses are reportable diseases. However, in cases involving malicious poisonings, a multiple animal outbreak, potential risks to the public, or misuse of pesticides, it might be judicious to report your findings to an appropriate regulatory agency (e.g., state or federal department of agriculture or local law enforcement agency). The toxicologists can assist and direct you to the appropriate agency or individual in these cases.

Conclusion

Your approach to using a diagnostic facility should be thoughtful, logical, and insightful. There is no such test as the "poison screen" that can test for all toxicants (because *everything is toxic in the right dose*). You should refine your approach so that it is systematic and reasonable, and employs all aspects of the diagnostic laboratory so as to maximize your efforts at an affordable price to achieve a successful resolution to the case.

Medicolegal Considerations in Toxicology Cases

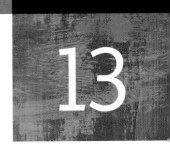

Michael J. Murphy, DVM, JD, DABVT, PhD

- Most pet poisonings are accidental; sometimes they are intentional. In some states this intent may make the poisoning a crime.
- There have been several high profile cases during the last few decades involving poisoning of hundreds of companion animals from consumption of commercial pet food contaminated with toxic levels of compounds (e.g., melamine and cyanuric acid, aflatoxin, vitamin D, deoxynivalenol).
- The pet owner and/or veterinarian can find information about pet food recalls involving chemical contamination, along with the steps required to report a pet food complaint, at the following website: http://www.fda.gov/AnimalVeterinary/default.htm.
- With suspected contaminated pet food, the owner should save the original container/bag and maintain a record of the exact product name, date purchased, location purchased, lot number, and bar code. The food material should be double-bagged in ziplock baggies and frozen until it is decided what tests should be run.

Companion animal practitioners may hear from a client that "the neighbor poisoned my pet" with varying frequency throughout a career. Although in many cases the pet has not been poisoned, or the poisoning is accidental, intentional pet poisoning does occur. Pet poisoning cases may involve the legal system in insurance claims, civil claims, or criminal prosecution. This chapter presents some areas to consider when a pet poisoning case becomes a "legal" case. These areas are medical records, client confidentiality, and animal cruelty.

Medical Records

The medical records of the veterinarian(s) making or supporting a diagnosis of pet poisoning are likely to be reviewed in a medicolegal setting. The medical records may include "registration forms, consent forms, radiographs, estimate sheets, billing records, telephone consultations, controlled drug logs, laboratory results, surgery reports, discharge records, imaging recordings, patient history, treatment records, and consultation reports."[1]

The content of veterinary medical records may be defined by the state. For example, the Minnesota Board of Veterinary Medicine has established, by rule, the minimum standards for medical records for veterinary practice in Minnesota. Some of these record-keeping requirements are:

A. A veterinarian performing treatment or surgery on an animal or group of animals, whether in the veterinarian's custody at an animal treatment facility or remaining on the owner's or caretaker's premises, shall prepare a written record or computer record concerning the animals containing, at a minimum, the following information:

(1) name, address, and telephone number of owner;
(2) identity of the animals, including age, sex, and breed;
(3) dates of examination, treatment, and surgery;
(4) brief history of the condition of each animal, herd, or flock;
(5) examination findings;
(6) laboratory and radiographic reports;
(7) tentative diagnosis;
(8) treatment plan; and
(9) medication and treatment, including amount and frequency.

Minnesota Rule 9100.800 sub. 4, A

Practitioners may choose to consult their state licensing board to determine if rules or guidelines exist in that state for veterinary medical records.

Documenting telephone consultations in the medical record, including the results of specific toxin testing, the owner's decision to decline such testing, and any consultation reports obtained, may strengthen the final diagnosis reached in a specific case. The veterinarian may consider consulting a veterinary toxicologist (http://www.abvt.org), a veterinary diagnostic laboratory (http://www.aavld.org), or veterinary teaching hospital to receive advice on which samples and what testing may be desirable. Notation of the rationale used to rule in the toxicosis and rule out other differential diagnoses is extremely useful.

Updating a medical record may be necessary at times. However, the record should be updated only in a way that allows the original record to be read. "Entries that are completely blacked out or obliterated always raise suspicion when records are viewed by a third party.... The corrected entry should be signed and dated by the person making the correction."[1]

Client Confidentiality

Client confidentiality should be considered whenever a veterinarian considers reporting an animal's condition to one who is not the client. Balancing client confidentiality with mandatory reporting requirements may be more difficult if the veterinarian suspects that the animal was intentionally poisoned by the client. Briefly, some states have mandatory animal cruelty reporting requirements or immunity from liability if animal cruelty is reported. Specifically, Arizona, California, Illinois, Kansas, Minnesota, Oregon, West Virginia, and Wisconsin have laws requiring the reporting of animal cruelty.[2] Arizona, California, Colorado, Georgia, Idaho, Illinois, Florida, Kansas, Maine, Maryland, Massachusetts, Michigan, Mississippi, New Hampshire, New York, Oregon, Rhode Island, South Carolina, Vermont, Virginia, and West Virginia offer some immunity from liability for reporting suspected animal cruelty.[2] See *Requirements for Mandatory Reporting of Animal Cruelty* for an expanded discussion of this issue.[1] Veterinarians should consult their state licensing board for guidance before concluding that animal poisoning is animal cruelty that requires reporting to entities other than the client.

Are Drugs of Abuse Considered Poisons?

Alcohol, marijuana, cocaine, or other human drugs of abuse occasionally are encountered by veterinarians in emergency clinics or practices. Animals may certainly experience adverse effects after exposure to alcohol or these drugs. Many practitioners may not equate alcohol with "poison" in the routine veterinary practice. The Maine animal cruelty statute includes the phrase "gives poison or alcohol to an animal," apparently distinguishing alcohol from poison.

Screening a pet's urine can be done to detect drugs of abuse using over-the-counter kits. The kits are often used as a practical way to indicate to concerned pet owners that such drugs are not detected in the urine of their animals when the tests give a negative result (though false positives are known to occur). Any positive results should probably be confirmed with analytic chemistry testing because most human kits have not been validated for use in animal urine. See http://www.aavld.org for laboratories that may be able to perform such analytical chemistry testing. It may be wise to consult the state licensing board to determine if positive findings for alcohol or human drugs of abuse identified in the urine of pets requires reporting to anyone other than the client.

Animal Cruelty

Most pet poisonings are accidental; sometimes they are intentional. In some states this intent may make the poisoning a crime. In some states this element of intent may support an argument that a crime of animal cruelty has been committed. Animal cruelty statutes that include a version of the term "poison" are found in Arkansas, California, Hawaii, Maine, Michigan, Minnesota, North Carolina, New Mexico, Nevada, Ohio, Pennsylvania, Texas, Utah, and Vermont at the time of this writing. Statutes may use the terms "knowingly," "willfully," "intentionally," or "maliciously." Animal cruelty may be a misdemeanor or a felony. In most states animal cruelty may be a felony.[1] For example, in Texas a person may be found guilty of a state jail offense if the person intentionally or knowingly:

(5) kills, seriously injures, or administers poison to an animal, other than cattle, horses, sheep, swine, or goats, belonging to another without legal authority or the owner's effective consent….

(Tex. Penal Code Ann. § 42.09)

As an example, a criminal case is presented to highlight some of the issues that may arise when an animal toxicosis involves the legal system.

Celinski v. State

The criminal application of the Texas animal cruelty statute was reviewed in the case of *Celinski v State*.[3] Mr. Celinski was found guilty of cruelty to animals in part for poisoning two cats with acetaminophen. He appealed the conviction. The conviction was upheld by the Texas court of appeals based on the evidence. The evidence cited by the Texas court of appeals in upholding Mr. Celinski's conviction was:

(1) The cats were in good health when Jones [the owner] left; they were very sick when he returned the following day. They had diarrhea, were foaming at the mouth, and were too weak to stand.
(2) The veterinarian who treated the cats concluded that they were suffering from acetaminophen poisoning, based upon his observation of their physical symptoms and upon the results of a blood test.
(3) The veterinarian was unable to reverse the results of the poisoning with an antidote. He estimated that the cats had ingested the equivalent of five to six tablets apiece some time during the afternoon of February 21, 1994.
(4) Texas A&M laboratory results confirmed that Sugar Ray and Bonnie died of acetaminophen poisoning.
(5) The veterinarian had seen a dozen cases of feline acetaminophen poisoning in his 14 years of practice, but had never heard of a cat voluntarily ingesting acetaminophen, nor had he ever seen a case of multiple cats simultaneously ingesting acetaminophen.
(6) Appellant testified there were no pills lying about the apartment the day the cats became sick—pills they could have accidentally ingested. He was the only person present in the apartment with the cats on that day.

(Celinski v. State)

Celinski demonstrates the importance of medical records in legal cases. The first four points above may have been useful to determine whether the cats had previous illnesses, whether the cats were exposed to a potentially toxic dose of acetaminophen, and whether the previously known adverse effects of acetaminophen were observed in the cats. The last two points reviewed by the court of appeals were more directly aimed at determining whether the exposure was accidental or intentional. The veterinarian's medical record may contain important facts in a legal case.

Commercial Pet Food Contamination Issues

There have been several high profile cases during the last few decades involving poisoning of hundreds of companion animals from consumption of commercial pet food contaminated with toxic levels of compounds (e.g., melamine and cyanuric acid, aflatoxin, vitamin D, deoxynivalenol). As veterinary toxicologists, we receive telephone queries routinely from pet owners who are highly suspicious because, "their pet became ill following ingestion of newly acquired/newly opened pet food." The veterinarian must always be aware of the fact that a temporal relationship almost always exists between the pet eating and the client observing adverse clinical signs—this is because most pets, like ourselves, eat daily and many illnesses that pets succumb to cause abrupt onset of ill effects. It is the responsibility of the veterinarian to obtain a very thorough history to determine whether this temporal relationship between eating and onset of ill effects is truly a cause and effect relationship. And the reverse may be true: pet owners may not relate their pets' illness to consumption of contaminated pet food because of a delay between time of ingestion and onset of initial clinical signs.

Once it is established that there might be an issue with food contamination, it is absolutely essential that the veterinarian perform a complete physical examination of the patient, including running appropriate diagnostic tests. It is important that veterinarians not get tunnel vision, and make sure that they keep an extensive list of differential diagnoses that can elicit similar clinical signs and laboratory abnormalities that mimic toxins that may be found in the pet food. The pet owner and/or veterinarian can find information about pet food recalls involving chemical contamination, along with the steps required to report a pet food complaint, at the following website: http://www.fda.gov/AnimalVeterinary/default.htm. In addition to the veterinarian performing a thorough diagnostic workup on the patient based on history and clinical signs, all steps must be accurately documented in the medical record. In addition, the pet owner should save as much of the remaining suspect pet food as possible. The owner should save the original container/bag and maintain a record of the exact product name, date purchased, location purchased, lot number, and bar code. The food material should be double-bagged in ziplock baggies and frozen until it is decided what tests should be run.

With the easy access and availability of the Internet to pet owners, concerns about pet food contamination can quickly "go viral" on the Internet. On a positive note, when these pet food contaminations have been proved to be valid, this has provided a medium to rapidly disseminate accurate information to warn pet owners and prevent further poisonings of pets. However, there have been instances where Internet postings of pet food poisoning have been inaccurate, which led to "Internet hysteria" and further led to erroneous claims by pet owners that their pets' illnesses were associated with consumption of the suspect pet food. Some veterinarians became so focused, like their clients, on the suspect pet food problem that they failed to perform adequate medical history taking, as well as failing to perform a thorough diagnostic workup to rule out other differential diagnoses. When it was discovered that there was no contaminant in the pet food, veterinarians were put in an uncomfortable position of having to defend their inaccurate working diagnosis.

As an example, a pet food contaminant that has been the cause of several recent pet food recalls is the mycotoxin, aflatoxin. Aflatoxin, at toxic doses, can lead to liver disease. Pets poisoned with aflatoxin will present with many vague and nonspecific clinical signs of general lethargy and depression, abdominal pain, and vomiting. However, pets suffering from hepatic disease associated with a cholangiohepatitis, chronic-active copper storage disease, or hepatic tumors may present with a very similar cluster of clinical signs. It is important that the veterinarian separate out those pets with true aflatoxicosis from all the other pets with abdominal neoplasia or copper storage disease that are receiving the same pet food.

In summary, veterinary medical records may be useful when cases of pet poisoning involve the legal system. These records may contain differential diagnoses and the results of examination, laboratory testing, consultation, and specific diagnosis. It may be wise for veterinarians to consult their state licensing board to determine if (1) standards for medical records exist in their state, (2) poisoning an animal could be considered animal cruelty, and (3) their state requires the reporting of animal cruelty.

References

1. Scott JF: Veterinary Medical Records, Proceedings of the American Veterinary Medical Law Association, *AVMLA*, 2006 CE Program.
2. Babcock SL, Neihsl A: Requirements for mandatory reporting of animal cruelty, *J Am Vet Med Assoc* 228(5):685, 2006.
3. Celinski v. State 911 S.W.2d 177 (Tex. App. 1995).

Indoor Environmental Quality and Health

14

John B. Sullivan Jr., MD, MBA

Mark D. Van Ert, PhD, CIH

Gary R. Krieger, MD, MPH

Michael E. Peterson, DVM, MS

O f the 71 million employees who work indoors in the United States, the Bureau of Statistics estimates that more than 21 million are exposed to some degree of poor indoor air quality.[1] The Occupational Safety and Health Administration (OSHA) estimates that 69,000 persons reporting severe headaches and 105,000 persons reporting respiratory problems in the workplace may be suffering from poor indoor environmental quality.[1] Similar environmental quality problems exist in homes, possibly at a more severe degree, because no regulatory agency monitors indoor home environments. The impact of these indoor home conditions on the companion small animal population is unknown. However, it is reasonable to hypothesize that the impact may be greater in that group than in their human counterparts, particularly in view of the fact that many animals never leave the indoor environment in which they live and in certain instances may come into closer contact with specific sources, such as flooring contaminated with biologic agents like mold or chemical agents including pesticides and cleaning products.

The goal of this chapter is to familiarize the veterinary practitioner with the conditions and issues involved in indoor environmental quality problems. The magnitude of the problem in human medicine has not yet been fully elucidated, and the field has been practically unaddressed by the veterinary community. It is hoped that information shared in this chapter may begin to define a possible problem that the veterinary practitioner may consider in patients with nebulous clinical signs. It is not the purpose of this chapter to make the veterinarian an indoor air specialist but only to make him or her conversant in the field. Any attempts to characterize the suspected environmental problem and to remedy the problem should be left to a trained environmental specialist, such as an industrial hygienist.

Sources and Causes of Poor Environmental Quality

Changing energy use strategies in the 1970s resulted in construction of buildings with improved energy efficiency and tighter sealing to prevent energy loss. As a consequence, human health complaints relating to indoor environments began to increase, and the terms *tight building syndrome* and *sick building syndrome* (SBS) were adopted to describe this problem. Complaints relating to the environment had previously been attributed to either poor working conditions or psychological factors. It soon became apparent, however, that health complaints could also be attributed to inadequate ventilation, mold overgrowth, lack of fresh air exchange, excess biological and chemical contaminants, and dampness or inadequate dilution of indoor contaminants.[1-9] The phrase *poor indoor air quality* is used to describe indoor environmental conditions that can result in clinical signs attributable to the buildup of airborne contaminants. Illnesses, however, are often multifactorial. Increased incidences of allergic diseases, coughing, wheezing, shortness of breath, asthma, bronchitis,

---

Box 14-1   Symptoms Commonly Expressed in Cases Involving Poor Environmental Air Quality

---

Mucous Membrane Irritation
Eye irritation
Nasal symptoms
Throat irritation
Drying of mucous membranes
Drying of skin
Rashes
Sinus congestion
Respiratory symptoms
Cough
Chest tightness
Sore throat
Voice changes and hoarseness
Asthma
Difficulty in breathing
Bronchial hyperresponsiveness

Constitutional
Nausea
Abdominal complaints
Myalgia
Arthralgia

Neurological and Neurobehavioral
Headache
Fatigue
Dizziness
Lethargy
Difficulty in concentrating
Memory problems

---

headaches, eye irritation, muscle aches, fever, chills, nausea, vomiting, and diarrhea are reported among children and adults exposed to indoor biological contaminants; these substances encompass a wide array of contaminants and biochemical byproducts.

The World Health Organization (WHO) characterized SBS in 1983. Since then health complaints associated with poor indoor air quality have been classified as either SBS or building-related illness (BRI). This classification, although lacking refinement, serves to categorize this type of illness as traceable or untraceable to a defined cause or source.

The term *SBS* defines a set of clinical signs and, in humans, symptoms whose origin is uncertain or is related to ill-defined factors in the environment (Box 14-1). Affected individuals experience multiple and sometimes vague health complaints. In such cases, health complaints tend to cease when the individual leaves the site and recur when the individual reenters the site.

The term *BRI* applies to a definable medical condition that can be traced to a single source and is documented by specific signs consistent with a known disease. Examples include *Legionella pneumophila* pneumonia, hypersensitivity pneumonitis caused by organic dusts and bioaerosols, carbon monoxide (CO) poisoning, and allergy-mediated asthma caused by identifiable allergens.

The seriousness of BRI became apparent in the infection of 182 members of the American Legion who attended a convention in 1976 in Philadelphia; they were infected with *Legionella pneumophila,* which resulted in 29 fatalities. Dissemination of these bacteria from contaminated ventilation systems emphasizes the contribution of the multiple factors of humidity, biological growth, and ventilation in the cause of illness.

Vague complaints relating to mucous membrane irritation, respiratory signs, and headache commonly occur in indoor environments.[3,4,9,10] But sources and causes of such health complaints are multiple and can be difficult to identify. Investigations of the sites involved show that deterioration of indoor environmental quality is most often because of problems with airborne contaminants that are chemical, biological, or physical in nature.

A dynamic mixture of chemical, biological, and particulate pollutants arising from a variety of sources circulates in indoor air (Box 14-2). These pollutants are influenced by air movement, ventilation, temperature, and humidity. Most of the chemical sources of indoor contaminants are volatile organic chemicals (VOCs). Analyses of indoor air samples have demonstrated that between 50 and 300 different VOCs can be present at low levels in nonindustrial environments, such as offices, homes, shopping centers, and malls.[11-13]

| **Box 14-2** | Sources of Common Indoor Air Contaminants |

Chemical Sources
Chemicals emitted from building materials and furnishings
Cleaning materials and disinfectants
Chemicals emitted from office machines and materials
Pesticides
Tobacco smoke
Combustion products from cooking and fireplaces

Physical Sources
Ventilation problems
Dust
Particulates
Fibers, such as asbestos or fiberglass

Biological Sources
Pollen
Mold and fungi
Biological byproducts of microbes
Bacteria
Viruses
Dander from pets
Insects and insect parts
Human skin particles
Dust mites

Biological sources of indoor pollution include mold, fungus, pollen, spores, bacteria, viruses, and insects, such as dust mites and roaches. Water reservoirs and damp areas provide nutrient sources for the growth of microorganisms. Relatively high levels of humidity and moisture allow biological agents to increase to levels that, when disseminated indoors, can trigger illness and allergies. Reports indicate that indoor dampness and mold growth are associated with increased respiratory illness in adults and children.[5,7,8] High relative humidity also encourages growth of the dust mite population, which can cause allergies and asthma. More attention is being focused on biochemical products of microorganisms as potential causes of indoor-related respiratory illness. These include endotoxin, 1,3-β-glucan, mycotoxins, peptidoglycan, and VOCs emitted from fungi.[9]

Physical factors, the third source of indoor-related illness, include dusts, fibers, particulates, and overall comfort factors, such as ventilation, lighting, temperature, humidity, noise, and vibration. Dust and particulate matter are always present indoors. Each cubic meter of air contains small concentrations of millions of particulates, of which 99% are invisible to the eye.[9]

Energy conservation strategies dating from the 1970s have contributed to declining indoor air quality. Building design and operational changes have focused on decreasing energy consumption to comply with the goal of reducing American dependency on foreign energy sources. But energy-efficient buildings may sacrifice ventilation effectiveness to reduce overall energy costs.[14-17] Such efforts may result in better insulated buildings but reduced performance of ventilation systems. The overall result is often inadequate fresh air exchange for building occupants that allows concentration of airborne chemical contaminants and pollutants.

Building Materials and Furnishings

Products used in construction contain chemicals that can off-gas into the indoor environment. Building materials are constantly changing, and new products are entering the

Table 14-1	Common Sources of Volatile Organic Chemicals
Source	**Volatile Organic Chemicals (VOCs)**
Building Materials	
Plywoods	Formaldehyde, terpenes, methylacetate, *n*-butanol, tetrachloroethylene, toluene, nonanol, *n*-undecane, tetradecane, naphthalene, *p*-dichlorobenzene, xylenes
Polystyrene foam	Styrene, ethylbenzene, aromatics
Rubber-backed nylon carpet	Toluene, benzene, *n*-decane, 4-phenylcyclohexane
New vinyl flooring	Isoalkanes, methylbenzenes, xylenes, ethylbenzene, toluene, 2-ethylhexanol, formaldehyde
Rubber floor covering	1,1,1-Trichloroethane, styrene, indane, 1,3/1,4-diisopropylbenzene, isodecane, acetophenone
Solvents and Adhesives	
Solvent-based adhesives	Toluene, styrene, *n*-decane, *n*-undecane, cyclohexane, methylcyclopentane, alcohols
Water-based adhesives	Nonane, decane, undecane, octane
Wall/flooring adhesives	Toluene, benzene, ethyl acetate, styrene, ethylbenzene
Sealants	Methylethyl ketone, butyl propionate, 2-butoxyethanol, butanol, benzene, toluene
Wood stains	Nonane, decane, undecane, methyloctane, dimethylnonane, trimethylbenzene
Polyurethane varnish	Nonane, decane, undecane, methylethyl ketone, ethylbenzene, xylene
Solvent-based waxes/detergents	Alkanes, alkenes, terpenes
Water-based waxes/detergents	Alcohols, esters, alkoxy alcohols, terpenes, alcohols/acetates
Deodorizers	Nonane, decane, undecane, ethylheptane, limonene
Liquid cleaners/disinfectants	Limonene, *p*-cymene, undecane, α-pinene, heptene, decane, nonane, heptanes

market, so it is difficult to keep track of the large variety of volatile chemicals contained in these products. Building products ranging from structural materials to coatings contain chemicals that are emitted indoors.[11-13,18] Emissions of VOCs from building materials depend on the nature of the material, the chemicals involved, and the location of the material in the structure (Table 14-1). Emission rates can vary from an initial high release in minutes or hours to long-term off-gassing that occurs over weeks, months, or even years. Such products include wood, insulation, plastics, sealers, caulking, adhesives, paints, varnishes, waxes, finishes, lacquers, fabrics, and carpets.

Wood furnishings purchased for use in homes are rarely solid wood anymore; rather, they may have a wood facing on a product mainly composed of particleboard or plywood. Formaldehyde and other contaminants that are "outgassing" from these products into energy-efficient "tight" homes can result in significantly elevated indoor air exposures.

Furnishings and fabrics can act as "sinks" that absorb airborne chemicals, releasing them slowly back into the indoor environment depending on temperature, humidity, and ventilation. In general, warmer temperatures and higher humidity increase the rate of emission of VOCs.

Human Factors

Human activity contributes to indoor contamination by introducing irritating cleaning agents, pesticides, solvents, tobacco smoke, particulates, dust, fibers, mold, and allergens.

Humans also shed millions of skin particles and microbes indoors. Cooking and other combustion sources introduce carbon dioxide (CO_2), CO, nitrogen dioxide (NO_2), sulfur dioxide (SO_2), and particulates into indoor air.[19,20] Computers, copiers, fax machines, laser printers, and other office machines emit volatile chemicals and ozone (O_3).

Smokers contribute to the indoor chemical and particulate pollutant load, with many of the ingredients of cigarette smoke adsorbing to porous surfaces such as fabrics and carpeting. Although environmental tobacco smoke (ETS) has previously been considered a nuisance by most nonsmokers, the Environmental Protection Agency (EPA) considers it a substantive risk factor for cancer and heart disease.[21,22] The EPA classifies ETS as a group A carcinogen, meaning that it causes human cancer. Although the EPA's cancer conclusions are being questioned, ETS remains a prime contributor to cough, shortness of breath, and chest tightness in exposed human asthmatics.[23] ETS also contributes to significant formaldehyde exposure indoors.[24,25]

Ventilation System

Up to 50% of cases involving poor indoor air quality can be traced to a ventilation problem.[16,17] A properly functioning ventilation system provides adequate fresh air and dilutes and removes pollutants. It also balances indoor air quality with comfort. Ventilation is a dominant cost of building maintenance and energy use, and decreasing ventilation is sometimes employed as a cost-saving measure. However, such approaches can lead to the buildup of pollutants indoors. Improperly maintained ventilation systems can also serve as a source of indoor contaminants. Air ducts contaminated with dirt, dust, and moisture can provide sources for microbial growth that may cause illness. The 1976 discovery of legionnaires' disease in Philadelphia underscores the fact that serious illness and death can result from a contaminated ventilation system.

Breathing produces CO_2 as a byproduct, and its concentration indoors is a useful measure of air freshness. Accumulation of CO_2 concentrations above 800 parts per million (ppm) of air indicates an inadequate fresh air supply and in humans can be associated with health complaints, such as fatigue, headache, lethargy, and general discomfort. The American Society of Heating, Refrigeration, and Air-Conditioning Engineers (ASHRAE) recommends that indoor CO_2 concentrations not exceed 1000 ppm.[16,26,27] However, elevated CO_2 concentrations of more than 800 ppm may signal the buildup of other indoor pollutants caused by their inadequate removal or dilution. Direct reading instruments are available to track CO_2 levels in various environments to ensure that adequate fresh air is available to occupants.

Temperature

Thermal comfort is usually achieved between a temperature range of 68° F to 79° F (20° C to 26° C). Illness caused by airborne chemicals can be exacerbated by higher temperatures.[78] Warmer temperatures also enhance chemical emissions from building materials and furnishings. Formaldehyde release from particleboard or other sources increases in warm, humid environments. Copier machines release more volatile chemicals into the air in warmer temperatures. Turning the thermostat down about 5° F to 10° F can help to alleviate some of the irritant symptoms caused by poor indoor air quality.

Humidity

In humans excessive dampness indoors increases the risk of childhood asthma and other respiratory symptoms.[5,7,8] Relative indoor humidity values more than 60% are associated with overgrowth of fungus and bacteria that can contaminate ventilation systems, carpet, wall spaces, insulation, ceiling tiles, window seals, and other areas of the indoor environment. Humidity below 20% can cause drying of skin and mucous membranes, leading to irritation. High relative humidity increases upper airway moisture, allowing dusts and water-soluble toxic chemicals to dissolve more easily, thus contributing to upper airway irritation, inflammation, and cough. A humidity range of 45% to 50% is recommended by ASHRAE and the EPA.[21] Properly functioning ventilation systems help to maintain the relative humidity between 20% and 60%.[17]

Biological Mechanisms of Indoor Environment-Related Illness

Pollutants, thermal comfort, humidity, adequacy of ventilation, and air movement play interacting roles in the quality of home environments. Health complaints, such as headache, sinus congestion, and fatigue may be difficult to separate from general symptoms experienced by the overall population. Establishing a cause-effect relationship between the indoor environment and illness is often difficult because of the numerous variables involved.[28] However, there are patterns of illness that can be correlated with environmental clues. Poor indoor environmental quality should at least be considered if typical clinical signs occur in a site characterized by one or more of the following: presence of chemical odors, recent remodeling, newly constructed building, presence of moisture or water damage, heavy use of cleaning agents, indoor combustion sources, mold contamination and discoloration of walls and ceilings, musty or stale odors, excess dust or particulates on walls or other surfaces, new carpet odors, recent indoor pesticide treatment, and office machines in unventilated areas or in direct sunlight.

Affected persons or animals show improvement of signs when they are away from the suspected indoor environment and recurrence of signs when they return. In humans, the duration of exposure seems to be important in determining how quickly symptoms resolve in anecdotal cases. The longer the exposure, the slower the resolution of symptoms. The search for biological models to explain the causes of these signs and symptoms has focused on the following mechanisms: inflammation involving upper and lower airways, mucous membrane irritancy, neurobehavioral and neurological effects of VOCs, allergic reactions and hypersensitivity to chemicals and biological agents, stress and psychological reactions, infections, and effects of chemicals and biological toxins on the immune system.[11-13,19,20,28-33]

Inflammation and irritation of mucous membranes are primary mechanisms at the root of many indoor air quality–related health problems. Underscoring the complexity of the problem, environmental factors, such as temperature and humidity, can interact with airborne contaminants to trigger illness.[29,34] Also, the reason why some individuals are more susceptible than others may be partially explained by their atopic status and their heightened susceptibility to inflammation.[30,35] Still, clinical signs associated with poor indoor air quality are sometimes difficult to distinguish from those caused by common allergies because allergens and nonallergens share similar pathways of inflammation and illness production.

Because humans and animals breathe thousands of liters of air daily with most passing through the nose, upper airway, and respiratory tract, exposure to airborne contaminants is unavoidable.[29] Thus, those with a predisposition to inflammation by either nonimmune stimuli or immune stimuli may be more prone to respiratory irritation and inflammation caused by airborne contaminants.[30-32]

Xenobiotic-Induced Inflammation and Immune Responses

A xenobiotic is any substance foreign to the body. Xenobiotics include chemicals, infectious agents, bioaerosols, dusts, and other agents, such as proteins and allergens, to which the body responds.[33] Host defenses against airborne toxins, low-molecular-weight chemicals, and allergens include nonspecific (passive) and specific (immune-mediated) defenses. Once the passive airway defense barriers are breached by a chemical or allergen, subsequent respiratory defense is either immune mediated or nonimmune mediated or a combination of these. Mast cells are central to a type I hypersensitivity reaction, and their sudden degranulation is a hallmark of IgE-mediated response and allergic-mediated asthma. The next line of defense following the breaching of passive barriers includes nonspecific phagocytosis by macrophages and tissue monocytes or specific immune responses (e.g., antibodies and cell-mediated immune mechanisms).

Activation of a specific immune response requires processing of an antigen by antigen-presenting cells (APCs). The airways contain efficient APCs that can process antigens by endocytosis, digest them, and associate the digested antigen with the major histocompatibility complex (MHC) before transporting the antigen-MHC combination to the cell's surface to present it to lymphocytes.[31,36] Naive T lymphocytes can be activated by the antigen-MHC complex to differentiate into specific T cells that express cell surface markers. Chemicals, especially those of low molecular weight, can be allergenic when they serve as haptens via binding to proteins or amino acids.

Irritation and Pungency Caused by Airborne Contaminants

Airborne contaminants include particulates, bioaerosols or chemicals, and respirable airborne particles of 10 μm in diameter or less that can penetrate the airways. Detection of airborne chemicals and particulates by the nasal passages and upper airways involves the common chemical senses (CCS), a specialized network of nerves emanating from the trigeminal nerve with endings located in the face, eyes, and nasal passages.[32,37,38] Activation of these chemical sensory pathways by airborne hazards serves to warn of danger by producing an irritancy reaction. If this CCS interaction with irritants is unregulated or if a constant activation occurs, inflammation can result.

The CCS responds quantitatively and qualitatively to stimulation by chemical vapors and airborne particulates.[32,34,39] Small changes in molecular structure among VOCs lead to large differences in chemical potencies. The nerve receptors in the membranes of the nose and mouth are very close to the surface, separated only by a thin film of moisture. Airborne chemicals can penetrate this moisture layer to react with the nerve endings. It may be significant that small companion animals often have much larger nasal surface areas and therefore an increase in the size of the CCS apparatus.

VOCs and low-molecular-weight chemicals can activate the CCS nerve receptors by either physical or chemical reactions. Those that bind chemically produce a more potent reaction.[33,37] Examples of such chemicals are formaldehyde, acrolein, chlorine, ozone, sulfur dioxide, and aldehydes.

The nerves of the CCS release neuropeptides in response to environmental irritants. This type of inflammatory response is termed *neurogenic inflammation*. Neuropeptides (also called neurokinins) are found in nerve fibers of the nose, dental pulp, and eyes and can be released by lung tissue. Therefore, volatile chemicals can produce irritant effects and release inflammatory neuropeptides at nerve sites in various locations in the body and throughout the nasal mucosa, lungs, and other sites that store such mediators.[32,34,35] Neuropeptide release results in a cascade of events leading to more inflammation, swelling, pain, and release of other inflammatory mediators from tissue, amplifying the effects and producing clinical signs. Desensitization of these sensory nerves may also occur, causing the irritation response to fade. No single predictor dictates which response may occur in a given individual.

Disorders in the regulation of neurogenic inflammation can lead to prolonged and more intense responses to environmental stimulants. Neurogenic inflammation is controlled through neural endopeptidase, which degrades neuropeptides. Conditions that decrease neural endopeptidase activity may increase neurogenic inflammatory responses. Irritant chemicals and respiratory viral infections that inhibit neural endopeptidase regulatory activity therefore can contribute to an individual's sensitivity to airborne pollutants. This mechanism may explain some individuals' symptomatic reaction to indoor air pollutants.

Respiratory Irritation, Bronchial Hyperreactivity, and Asthma

The lungs also respond to airborne chemicals and hazards through inflammation. The surface epithelial cell layer of the lungs forms a physical barrier against inhaled toxins and hazards. These cells secrete a thin, sterile moisture barrier over the surface of the lungs and bronchioles. Other specialized cells secrete a thick mucous layer on top of the water layer. Together, these layers form a gel phase that traps chemicals, particles, and dusts. The surface lining of the lower airway is made up of ciliated epithelial cells, forming a brush border that constantly pushes trapped substances toward the mouth, where they can be expectorated or swallowed.

Besides epithelial cells that can release cytokines and other mediators of inflammation, nerve endings can be stimulated by irritants to cause bronchoconstriction. If the cell layer lining the airway is damaged by an inhaled hazard, nerve endings can react by constricting the airway. This reaction may result from a high-level acute exposure or chronic low-level exposure. Also, pulmonary macrophages and epithelial cells release mediators in response to stimuli by irritants, causing an inflammatory cascade that results in an acute or chronic response.

Because the tissue of the airways forms an interactive protective mechanism, irritants and toxins that affect one cell or tissue type affect others. Toxins and particulates that damage the protective mechanism and result in inflammation of the airway (referred to as toxic inflammation) can cause cough, shortness of breath, chest tightness, wheezing, and asthma. Once an inhaled hazard induces the inflammatory process, chemical mediators of inflammation are released by epithelial cells and macrophages.[40] Once released these chemical mediators activate other cells, causing a cascade of inflammation.

Acute exposures produce an inflammatory response that differs from that of chronic exposures. Also, chronic exposures that produce ongoing inflammation may result in pathologic alterations in airway tissue, including fibrosis and increased production of mucus.

The term *reactive airways* or *nonspecific bronchial hyperresponsiveness* is used to describe nonimmune-mediated asthma caused by inhaled respiratory irritants. Once an individual has developed reactive airways, exposure to chemically unrelated airborne irritants may trigger the onset of symptoms through inflammation.[41] In humans an entity termed *reactive airways dysfunction syndrome* (RADS) has been described following a high-level exposure to irritant chemicals. Signs and symptoms of respiratory irritation occur quickly following such an exposure with coughing, chest tightness, and a burning sensation in the throat. Reexposure to irritating vapors or fumes can precipitate signs of cough, wheezing, and shortness of breath. Pulmonary function test results may be abnormal but are usually reversible on treatment with a bronchodilator.

Another inflammatory syndrome in humans of a nonallergic nature attributed to airborne pollutants is *reactive upper airways dysfunction syndrome* (RUDS). It too has been described following an acute high-level exposure or following chronic low-level exposure to airborne contaminants.[39] This syndrome is manifested by signs and symptoms of rhinitis (runny nose), nasal stuffiness, eye burning, sinus congestion, facial pain, and severe headache almost of a migraine nature.[30,32,37,39]

Irritant-Associated Vocal Cord Dysfunction

Irritant-associated vocal cord dysfunction (IVCD) is a newly recognized human medical disorder that is often misdiagnosed as asthma.[42] Cases of IVCD have occurred following acute high-level occupational or environmental exposures. Vocal cord dysfunction is a disorder of the larynx in which the vocal cords adduct inappropriately during inspiration or expiration. Signs and symptoms of IVCD include wheezing, cough, shortness of breath, throat tightness, and chest pain. The abnormality can occur during inspiration or expiration or in both phases of the respiratory cycle. Patients with IVCD report a significant increase in chest complaints.

Indoor Pollutants

Chemical Emissions from Office Products

Concern about the impact of manufacturing processes and product waste streams on the outdoor environment has resulted in a wide variety of innovations dedicated to the development of sustainable manufacturing and consumption processes. However, this emphasis on manufacturing and waste stream environments ignores an important environmental niche between manufacture and disposal. This unique niche is the indoor environment surrounding product use. Concern about the outdoor environment has caused many companies to spend more resources attempting to understand how a product will affect a sanitary landfill than how that same product will affect the indoor environment and its occupants. Although traditional product safety is a major concern for most manufacturers, the impact of a product on the indoor environment is complex.

Although efforts in the United States to minimize air and water pollution have met with measurable success, there is increasing public concern about a new generation of pollution-related human illnesses in the office, home, and transportation environments. High-speed printers, copiers, visual display terminals, duplicators, and microfiche and blueprint machines are point sources of indoor contaminants that cannot be disregarded, especially when they are used in inadequately ventilated locations. Most modern electronic products emit low levels of volatile organic compounds into the indoor environment. These fugitive emissions arise from the plastics, solvents, coatings, adhesives, and encapsulants associated with manufacture of the product and from consumable supplies, such as toners, inks, paper, transparency films, and labels. The newer an item of electronic equipment, the higher its potential rate of chemical emissions. Whether a product's emissions will affect an indoor environment significantly depends on two opposing factors: (1) the type and rate of chemical emitted and (2) the rate and effectiveness of that environment's ventilation (Table 14-2).

Home office and clerical work environments are common sites of poor indoor air quality. In these offices computers, copiers, fax machines, laser printers, and paper products are used. They also depend on centrally controlled ventilation systems. Laser printers and copiers located in unventilated rooms contribute to elevated levels of ozone and volatile irritant chemicals.

Chemical Emissions from Building Materials

Materials used for building, remodeling, and construction vary from wet to dry. Most building products contain chemicals that can be emitted indoors (Table 14-2). Building products emit VOCs indoors at varying rates that are affected by volatility, temperature, and humidity. The distribution and persistence of these VOCs in the indoor environment are influenced by air exchanges per hour, air circulation, the presence of reabsorbing "sinks" (other materials in the environment that reabsorb the chemicals and then slowly release them over time), and air filtration.

Many other variables affect mammalian responses to low-level volatile chemicals, such as exposure duration, time of day, temperature, and humidity. Temperature and humidity act additively with the total volatile chemical load indoors to initiate symptoms. Most outgassing of VOCs occurs when a building is new and slowly declines over time with a variety of half-lives depending on the chemical, environmental factors, and the building material. In addition there may be odors associated with VOCs in a closed environment.

Building materials, such as self-leveling mortar containing casein, have been shown to release trace amounts of 2-ethyl-1-hexanol, ammonia, isopropylamine, ethylamine, triethylamine, dimethylamine, trimethylamine, and dimethyl sulfide. In addition to the irritant effects of these chemical emissions, an objectionable odor results from the casein content of the mortar and possibly texturing materials for ceilings and outgassing of sulfhydryl compounds into the indoor environment.

Vapor emissions from building materials can persist for days to months and even years for formaldehyde emissions from particleboard and pressed wood products.[43] Sources of formaldehyde emissions are sealants, mortar, caulking compounds, paints, woods composites, plastics, vinyl products, foams, paper products, and insulation materials. New homes release VOCs over a period of months, with the highest concentration occurring immediately and then tapering off over a few months; low levels may persist for years. Formaldehyde concentrations, however, tend to fluctuate, with higher indoor emissions occurring in the warmer months.

New Carpet

A variety of chemicals may be emitted from new carpets and the adhesives used to attach carpet to floors. The distinctive new carpet odor has been traced to the chemical 4-phenylcyclohexene (4-PC).[44,45] The source of 4-PC is styrene-butadiene rubber (SBR) latex

Table 14-2	VOC Emissions from Building Materials, Interior Furnishings, and Office Equipment	

Material	Volatile Organic Chemicals Emitted	
Adhesives	Alcohols	2-Methylnonane
	Amines	Nonane
	Benzene	Pinene
	Decane	n-Propylbenzene
	Dimethylbenzene	Terpenes
	Dimethyloctane	Toluene
	Formaldehyde	Undecane
	Limonene	Xylenes
Caulking compounds	Acetic acid	Diethylbenzene
	Alkanes	Ethylbenzene
	Amines	Formaldehyde
	Benzene	Methylethyl ketone
	Butanol	Nonane
	2-Butoxyethanol	Toluene
	Butyl propionate	Xylenes
Carpeting	Alcohols	4-Phenylcyclohexene
	Formaldehyde	Styrene
	4-Methylethyl-benzene	
Ceiling tiles	Acetone	Hexanol
Chipboard	Alkanes	Isopropanol
Paneling	Amines	Limonene
Plywood	Benzaldehyde	Methylethyl ketone
Gypsum board	Benzene	3-Methylpentane ethanol
Fiberboard	Butanone	Pinene
	3-Carene	Propanol
	Ethylbenzene	n-Propylbenzene
	Formaldehyde	Terpenes
	Hexane	Toluene
Floor and wall coverings	Acetates	3-Methylpentane
	Alcohols	4-Methyl-2-pentanone
Wallpaper	Alkanes	Methyl styrene
Linoleum floor covering	Amines	Nonane
	Benzene	n-Propylbenzene
Vinyl coatings	Dodecane	Toluene
	Ethyl acetate	1,2,3-Trimethylbenzene
	Ethylbenzene	1,2,4-Trimethylbenzene
	Formaldehyde	Undecane
	Heptane	Xylene
	Methylethyl ketone	
Wood stains and varnishes	Acetates	Ethylbenzene
	Acrylates	Formaldehyde
Latex paints	Alcohols	Hexanol
Polyurethane floor finishes	Alkanes	Limonene
	Amines	Methyloctane
Floor lacquers	Benzenes	Nonane
	Butanone	1,1'-Oxybisbutane
	n-Butanol	Polyurethane

Table 14-2   VOC Emissions from Building Materials, Interior Furnishings, and Office Equipment—cont'd

Material	Volatile Organic Chemicals Emitted	
	Butyl propionate	2-Propanol
	Decane	Propylbenzene
	Dimethylnonane	Toluene
	Dodecane	Trimethylbenzene
	2-Ethoxyethyl acetates	Undecane
		Xylene
Appliances	Carbon monoxide	Polyaromatic hydrocarbons
	Nitrogen dioxide	Sulfur dioxide
Computers/video display terminals	*n*-Butanol	Dodecamethyl cyclosiloxane
	2-Butanol	Ethylbenzene
	2-Butoxyethanol	Hexanedioic acid
	Butyl-2-methylpro- pylphthalate	2-Ethoxyethyl acetate
	Caprolactam	Toluenez
	Cresol	Xylene
	Diisooctyl phthalate	
Duplicating machines	Ethanol	1,1,1-Trichloroethane
	Methanol	Trichloroethylene
Electrophotographic printers	Ammonia	Styrene-acrylate copolymer
	Ammonium salts	
Photocopiers and related supplies	Benzaldehyde	Terpene
	Benzene	Toluene
Microfiche developers and blueprint machines	Butyl methacrylate	1,1,1-Trichloroethane
	Carbon black	Trichloroethylene
	Nonane	Xylenes
	Ozone	Zinc stearate combustion products
	Polyolefin wax	
	Styrene	
Carbonless copy paper	Ammonia	Diethylethane
	Chlorobiphenyl	Formaldehyde
	Cyclohcxanc	Kerosene
	Dibutylphthalate	Naphthalene
Preprinted paper forms	Acetaldehyde	Heptane
	Acetic acid	Hexamethyl
	Acetone	Hexanol
	Acrolein	Hydroxy-4-methyl pentanone
	Benzaldehyde	Isopropanol
	Butanol	Paper dust
	Cyclosiloxane	Propionaldehyde
	1,5-Dimethylcyclopentene	1,1,1-Trichloroethane
	2-Ethyl furan	
Typewriter correction fluid	Acetone	1,1,1-Trichloroethane
Artificial essences	Aromatic fragrances	Limonene
Fragrances	Decane	Nonane
	Ethylheptane	Undecane

continued

Table 14-2 VOC Emissions from Building Materials, Interior Furnishings, and Office Equipment—cont'd

Material	Volatile Organic Chemicals Emitted	
Room deodorants, air fresheners	Acetaldehyde	Isobutyl acetate
	Acetols	Isopropane/isobutane
	Alcohols	Isopropyl alcohol
	Aldehydes	Lactones
	Benzylacetate	Methylchloroform
	n-Butanol	Nonylphenol
	Brucine sulfate	Paradichlorobenzene
	Cyclomenaldehyde	Pinene
	Essential oils	Propyl acetate
	Esters	Propylene glycol
	Ether	Resins
	Ethyl acetate	Terpenes
	Hexanol	Tertiary butyl alcohol
	Hexylene glycol	Triethylene glycol
Sealants	Acetic acid	Petroleum hydrocarbons
	Aliphatic hydrocarbons	Toluene
	Hexane	Xylene
	Methylethyl ketone	
Cleaning agents	Ammonium	Hydroxide
Detergents	2-Butoxyethanol	Isobutane/Isopropane
	Diethylene glycol methyl ether	Isopropanol
	Dipropylene glycol methyl ether	Phosphates
	Ethyl alcohol	Phosphoric acid
	Ethylenediamine tetraacetic acid (EDTA)	Pine oil
	Ethylene glycol monobutyl ether	Polyalkoxylated alcohol
		Sodium carbonate
		Sodium hydroxide
		Sodium metasilicate
Glazing compounds	Acetic acid	
Dry cleaning fluids	Tetrachloroethylene	Trichloroethylene
	1,1,1-Trichloroethane	
New clothing	Formaldehyde	
Resins	Butyl acrylate	
Polymers		
Textile and leather finishes		
Carpet shampoos	Pentachlorophenol	
Disinfectants		
Wood preservatives	Hexachlorobenzene	Tetrachlorophenol
Fungicides	Pentachlorophenol	
Insulation materials	Formaldehyde	n-Propylbenzene
	Pinene	Styrene
Floor waxes	Decane	o-Ethyltoluene
	Dimethyloctane	Nonane

Table 14-2 VOC Emissions from Building Materials, Interior Furnishings, and Office Equipment—cont'd

Material	Volatile Organic Chemicals Emitted	
	Ethylmethyl benzene	α-Terpene
	Ethyltoluene	1,2,3-Trimethylbenzene
	m-Ethyltoluene	Trimethylcyclohexane
	m,p-Ethyltoluene	Undecane
Paint removers	Carbon tetrachloride	Trichloroethylene
Grease cleaners	Ethylbenzene	Undecane
Cleaning fluids	Methylene chloride	Xylene
	1,1,1-Trichloroethanol	
Paint and lacquer solvents	Acetone	Naphtha
	n-Butyl benzene	Toluene
	Chlorobenzene	Trichloroethylene
	Cyclohexane	Xylene
Deodorizers	m-Dichlorobenzene	p-Dichlorobenzene
Moth balls	o-Dichlorobenzene	
Molding tape	n-Butanol	Toluene
Edge sealing	Isobutanol	
Joint compounds	n-Butanol	Styrene
	Ethylbenzene	Toluene
	Formaldehyde	1,2,4-Trimethylbenzene
	Isobutanol	Xylene
	Nonane	
Heaters	Carbon monoxide	Formaldehyde
Unvented gas heaters		
Unvented gas ovens		
Carpet (latex backed)	Formaldehyde	Xylene
	4-Phenylcyclohexene	
Plastics	Dibutylphthalates	Propyl acetate
Carbon paper	Carbon black	Oleic oil
	Crystal violet	Stearic oil
	Methyl violet	Victoria blue
	Mineral oil	Waxes
	Nigrosine	
Paints	Butyl acrylate	N-Methylol-acrylamide
	Epoxy acrylate	Pentaerythritol triacrylate
	Ethoxyethanol	Titanium dioxide
	Ethoxyethylacetate	Trimethylpropane triacrylate
	Ethyl acrylate	Tripropylene glycol triacrylate
	2-Ethylhexyl acrylate	
	Latex	

Box 14-3	Irritant Chemicals in Disinfectants and Cleaning Agents

Benzalkonium chloride	Ethyl alcohol
Benzoyl peroxide	Ethylenediaminetetraacetic acid (EDTA)
Isopropanol	Quaternary ammonium chlorides
Formaldehyde	Cationic detergents
Glutaraldehyde	Octyl decyl dimethyl ammonium
Phenol	chloride
Alcohols	Dioctyl dimethyl ammonium
Chlorine compounds	chloride
Potassium permanganate	Didecyldimethyl ammonium
Free iodine	chloride
Povidone iodine	n-Alkyl dimethylbenzyl ammonium
Thimerosal	chloride
Gentian violet	Nonionic surfactants
Hexachlorophene	Sodium metasilicate
Chlorhexidine	Fragrances
Phenylphenol	Colorant

used to bind the backing of new carpet. Analysis of carpet pieces demonstrated that 4-PC was a common contaminant in several environments reported to cause health effects after new carpet had been installed. In humans acute and subacute exposure to low parts per billion of 4-PC may be responsible for symptoms of headache, lethargy, and skin and mucous membrane irritation.[46] In commercial lays of carpet, adhesives are frequently employed to adhere carpet directly to floors. These adhesives are either water or solvent based. The latter can serve as significant sources of volatile organic compounds that contribute to indoor air pollution.

Cleaning Agents, Disinfectants, and Pesticides

Many cleaning agents, disinfectants, and pesticides can contribute to poor indoor air quality. Cleaning agents and disinfectants contain a variety of irritating and sensitizing chemicals that can cause ocular and respiratory irritation, exacerbate reactive airway symptoms, cause dermatitis, and may cause asthma (Box 14-3). The use of these agents in poorly ventilated areas or on large surfaces in enclosed spaces may result in exposure of occupants to moderate to high levels of irritants or sensitizers, such as quaternary ammonium compounds, surfactants, and alkyl benzyl ammonium chloride. Contact and allergic dermatitis may occur following exposure to some chemicals in these products. Also, chronic exposure may cause bronchial hyperreactivity and airway inflammation.

Disinfectants, cleaning products, and pesticides can be responsible for chemical odors and respiratory irritation. Chemicals in these products are amines, surfactants, cationic and anionic detergents, ammonia, acids, hypochlorites, phenols, alcohols, and caustic agents. When such products are used in confined spaces, significant pulmonary irritation and potential permanent damage can occur. Substituting less irritating agents for these cleaning agents can be helpful in eliminating indoor pollution sources. Indoor application of pesticides should be avoided or used with considerable caution. Both the active ingredients and "inert" diluents, which may be organic solvents, can contribute to indoor odors and contamination. Because these products are generally applied to flooring surfaces, pets especially are likely to come into repeated contact, increasing their dose and potential for toxicity. Exterior applications are generally safe provided exterior air handler rooms are not treated. If unintended liquid intrusions from the outside occur during a treatment, appropriate cleanup will prevent any potential adverse effects.

Indoor Combustion Sources

Pilot lights and cooking and gas appliance use contribute to nitrogen dioxide, a respiratory irritant. Natural gas is used by almost 50% of households in the United States, potentially exposing occupants to byproducts of combustion such as carbon monoxide, carbon dioxide, and oxides of nitrogen. Besides gas appliances, other combustion sources are fireplaces, tobacco smoke, cooking appliances, internal combustion machines, and charcoal fires. If wood stoves or coal stoves are not airtight, pollutants can escape indoors. Airflow patterns indoors may be altered, causing backdrafting of combustion byproducts. Faulty design of fireplace flues can also result in backdrafts of emissions. Burning treated wood products may lead to particularly toxic emissions and should be avoided.

Formaldehyde

Formaldehyde is a common indoor contaminant and a known upper airway, eye, and skin irritant. Formaldehyde has many sources: fabrics, pressed wood products such as plywood and particle boards incorporating phenol- and urea-formaldehyde resins, binders in fiber glass insulation, cosmetics, food, and combustion byproducts. Formaldehyde is a colorless gas at room temperature but is also found in liquid and solid forms. Low concentrations of formaldehyde are present in ambient air, primarily caused by burning of petroleum fuels and automobile exhaust. Formaldehyde emissions from building materials indoors occur in the following materials (listed in order by decreasing emission rate): chipboard, plywood, plasterboard, bituminized fiberboard, 15-mm plywood, mineral wool insulation, and curtains.[43]

Formaldehyde releasers are used as preservatives in many commercial products including cleaning agents, shampoos, soaps, paints, lacquers, cutting oils, cosmetics, coloring agents, skin care products, toilet cleaners, automotive cleaning agents, disinfectants, dishwashing liquids, and descaling agents. In most cases, the levels are sufficiently low as to be of no concern, although skin reactions can occur in susceptible individuals.

Health effects from formaldehyde include upper airway irritation and eye irritation. Some individuals experience asthma exacerbations on exposure to formaldehyde. Patch testing can determine whether an individual has an allergic hypersensitivity skin reaction to formaldehyde.

Environmental Tobacco Smoke

The burning of tobacco indoors introduces chemical pollutants and particulates. Tobacco smoke is made up of more than 4000 toxic substances including carcinogens. The EPA has classified environmental tobacco smoke (ETS) as a group A carcinogen, meaning that there is sufficient evidence to prove that it causes cancer in humans.

Nitrogen Oxides

Nitrogen oxide sources are fossil fuels, industrial processes, and motor vehicles. Nitrogen dioxide (NO_2), the most common of the oxides of nitrogen, has an acrid irritating odor. Nitrogen oxides are involved in the photochemical generation of ozone. Indoor exposure to nitrogen oxides occurs from gas-burning appliances, unvented furnaces, stoves, hot water heaters, tobacco smoke, kerosene space heaters, and influx of outdoor air contaminated by vehicle exhaust. Gas stoves are a principal source of nitrogen dioxide indoors, and when a gas stove is used for cooking, the peak nitrogen dioxide concentration in a kitchen can be 1 ppm or higher.

Nitrogen oxides are insoluble in water and therefore can penetrate to the lower respiratory tract. Pediatric patients are particularly susceptible to NO_2 because of their developing respiratory systems. Studies have linked NO_2 exposure and increased respiratory illness in children.[19,20] Low levels of NO_2 cause rhinorrhea, throat irritation, eye irritation, and cough. Asthmatics are sensitive to low NO_2 levels. Mild exposure causes shortness of breath, headache, cough, fatigue, nausea, and dizziness that can persist up to 2 weeks after exposure. Exposure to massive concentrations of nitrogen oxides can produce severe lung damage, asphyxiation, laryngospasm, and death. The irritant effects of NO_2 do not occur until concentrations reach about 13 ppm.[20]

Sulfur Dioxide

The main source of sulfur dioxide (SO_2) is burning of sulfur-containing fuels. Sulfur dioxide is a component of both indoor and outdoor pollution arising from automobile exhaust.

It is found in lower concentrations indoors than outdoors. The use of kerosene space heaters can generate significant concentrations of indoor SO_2.

Sulfur dioxide is very soluble in water and tends to be absorbed in the upper respiratory tract. Nasal breathing filters out most inhaled SO_2, preventing its passage into the more sensitive areas of the lungs. Mouth breathing tends to increase the amount of SO_2 that reaches the lungs.

Sulfur dioxide is highly irritating to the eyes and airways. Its odor is detectable at 0.5 ppm. Concentrations above 6 ppm induce clinical signs of irritation including eye irritation, tearing, runny nose, coughing, shortness of breath, bronchospasm, chest tightness, and a choking sensation. Prolonged and chronic exposure to SO_2 can produce chronic bronchitis, airway inflammation, chronic cough, increased mucous secretions, and clearing of the throat. Massive exposure to sulfur dioxide can result in severe permanent pulmonary damage.

Ozone

Ozone (O_3) is a naturally occurring, colorless or light blue gas with a very repugnant electrical-type odor. It is a potent chemical respiratory tract irritant and is the principal oxidant in photochemical smog. Exposures occur more commonly in urban and suburban environments, particularly during air pollution alerts. Ozone is a common outdoor pollutant and is consumed in the transformation of nitrogen monoxide into nitrogen dioxide.

Ozone concentrations are higher outdoors than indoors, but indoor levels can increase when windows or doors are open. Ozone is found in disinfectants and bleaching agents. Copiers, laser printers, electrostatic air filters, and some negative ion generators are other sources of ozone indoors.

Ozone has a short half-life, and consequently interaction with mammals is limited to an air-fluid interface, such as the mucous membranes of the upper airway, the respiratory tract, or the eye. Because ozone is not very water soluble, it can penetrate to deep areas of the respiratory tract. Fifty percent of ozone is taken up in the upper airway and nasal passages. Ozone that reaches the lower airways can actually be absorbed into the blood to a small degree. Because ozone contains a potent oxidizing agent, it can damage tissue.

Signs and symptoms of ozone exposure include cough, headache, chest pain, chest tightness on deep inspiration, shortness of breath, a dry throat, wheezing, and difficulty in breathing. Ozone significantly impairs the ability to perform sustained exercise, probably through the discomfort that it produces on inspiration during intensive periods of exercise. Other human symptoms include extreme fatigue, somnolence, dizziness, insomnia, decreased ability to concentrate, acrid taste and smell, and eye irritation.

Biology of the Indoor Environment

Biological contamination of the indoor environment has increasingly become a major focus of indoor environmental quality investigations. Biological contaminants are complex mixtures of microorganisms and particulates that may circulate indoors as bioaerosols or contaminate moisture-damaged areas. Biological contaminants consist of one or a combination of the following: bacteria, fungi, spores, hyphal elements, viruses, amoebae, insects, dust mites, insect droppings, plant particles, pollens, chemical byproducts of microorganisms (β-glucan, enzymes, ergosterol, and mycotoxins), and animal proteins.[47]

Concern about biological contamination has escalated since studies have linked indoor dampness and mold growth with increased respiratory symptoms in adults and children.[5,7,48-51] Excessive moisture promotes mold growth and is associated with an increased prevalence of symptoms caused by irritation, allergy, and infection.[49] Besides asthma, bronchitis, rhinitis, and allergies, some individuals exposed to indoor biological contaminants complain of fatigue, headache, myalgia, fever, nausea, vomiting, and arthralgia. Common sites of microorganism overgrowth indoors are areas where moisture damage to a structural element provides a nutrient source, such as in kitchens, bathrooms, window frames, mattresses, carpets, wood and other flooring, wallpaper, cellars, insulation, crawl spaces, soil of indoor potted plants, stagnant water, basement surfaces, moisture-damaged walls, and ventilation systems. Relative to mold, proximity to the source of contamination can enhance the health impact for an individual or pet.

Fungi and bacteria are the most common biocontaminants found indoors; in addition dust mites and animal dander are found in homes. *Penicillium, Cladosporium, Stachybotrys,* and *Alternaria* species are the most prevalent fungi found normally in indoor environments.[52] However, because a wide variety of bacteria and fungi are normally found both outdoors and indoors, numbers and taxa of suspected indoor contaminants must be compared with those found outdoors or in other reference environments to determine whether a true contamination situation exists. A history of water intrusions or visible staining may be useful in determining that a source of hidden mold contamination exists in an indoor environment.

To promote microbiological growth leading to indoor contamination, three required conditions must be combined: (1) temperature, usually between 2° C and 43° C (35° F to 109° F); (2) appropriate humidity, usually greater than 80%; and (3) nutrients for growth and amplification, such as moisture and organic material. For biological agents to become a health hazard, they must be respirable in size. When fungal or bacterial overgrowth is disturbed by airflow or mechanical disruption, high concentrations of bioaerosols that can be inhaled are generated.

Indoor bacterial populations originate primarily from human and animal activity. High airborne concentrations of gram-positive bacteria (*Bacillus subtilis*) may indicate overcrowding and inadequate ventilation. High levels of gram-negative bacteria in the indoor environment suggest contamination sources such as sewage (black water) contamination. Gram-negative bacteria may be associated with respiratory diseases when they contaminate heating, ventilation, and air conditioning (HVAC) systems or humidification systems in buildings. The presence of pathogens, such as the actinomycetes, *Legionella pneumophila, Pseudomonas,* or endotoxins usually indicates a source of contamination. Actinomycetes, which can cause hypersensitivity pneumonitis, are unusual in nonagricultural indoor environments, and their presence is a health concern.

Ventilation and Indoor Environmental Quality

The ventilation system or air-handling unit of a home is frequently referred to as the HVAC system. The HVAC system consists of the mechanical and functional components of duct work, air filter, air conditioning, and heating unit. The primary functions of the HVAC system are cooling, heating, and humidification; maintenance of overall comfort, odor control; and maintenance of oxygen and carbon dioxide levels at acceptable concentrations. HVAC systems in some homes are installed to service zones. As the number and size of zones increase, so does the cost of ventilation. A zone is typically defined by the presence of a thermostat.

The HVAC system is frequently cited as a cause of indoor air quality problems, typically because of insufficient fresh air and/or contamination. The National Institute for Occupational Safety and Health (NIOSH) identified the following major concepts of ventilation-related health problems in studies of more than 1300 cases of poor indoor air quality:

- Fifty percent of cases were related to deficiencies in ventilation, lack of outside fresh air, poor air distribution, uncomfortable temperature, or uncomfortable humidity.
- Thirty percent of cases were related to indoor chemical or biological contaminants.
- Ten percent of cases were attributed to an outdoor pollutant introduced to the indoors.
- Forced ventilation was common in sites with health problems.
- Health complaints increased as the density of people indoors rose.
- Problem buildings were energy efficient, thus creating a tight envelope.

Understanding HVAC functioning is critical to indoor air quality evaluations. HVAC systems for commercial and industrial operations often have an outside air intake on the top or side of a building that brings outdoor air inside. The outdoor air is then mixed with recirculated air from the occupied area. The mixed air usually passes through a filter to remove gross contaminants. This filtered air then passes through a fan, which creates a positive pressure, forcing the air through coils that either cool or heat. A drain pan beneath the coils collects water that condenses on the cooling coil. Air leaving the coil may be humidified or dehumidified depending on the circumstances. This conditioned air then moves through a ventilation duct at a speed of 10 to 20 mph to a distribution box. The supplied air then travels from the distribution box through small ducts to terminal ducts and diffusers and from there into the rooms. The supplied air migrates throughout the room and eventually enters an air return vent, also called a plenum, where it is recirculated or exhausted outdoors.

Inadequately functioning or maintained HVAC systems allow indoor contaminants to accumulate, contributing to stale and stagnant air and may even introduce outdoor pollutants and allergens into the indoors, especially if the air is unfiltered. A frequently occurring problem is an imbalance between the flow of fresh air and the outflow of stale air. This can create "dead zones" in which there is an absence of air movement or circulation indoors. HVAC systems can be sources of moisture, which allows mold and other microorganisms to grow and then be circulated indoors. Moisture can be supplied by plugged condensate drains and leaks in roofs, water and sewer lines, and chiller systems. Over time, dust, dirt, and debris build up in the ventilation system serving as potential sources of nutrients for mold growth. Proper maintenance can help prevent accumulated dirt and dust from being circulated indoors.

Evaluating Indoor Environment–Related Health Problems

Evaluation of indoor environmental quality–related illness requires a systematic approach because of the complexity of the potential causes. The objectives of the investigation are to gather information about the building, identify the signs and symptoms of those with health complaints, locate and identify potential causes, determine the work-relatedness of any illness, and remedy the cause by removing or isolating the source. For these reasons, a qualified environmental specialist, such as a trained industrial hygienist, should be used to evaluate the indoor environment. An evaluation of the building includes:

1. *Building inspection.* On concluding the building inspection, the investigators should provide a preliminary assessment of their findings, recommendations for changes, and recommendations for any further evaluations and monitoring. Easily identified causes of health complaints should be addressed immediately. At this phase, more in-depth investigation of particular problem areas may be conducted with appropriate monitoring.
2. *Health audit.* A health questionnaire can be useful in determining the health status of the building occupants and can help identify individuals who manifest symptoms associated with poor indoor environmental quality. After completing the questionnaire, symptoms can be tabulated so that the actual incidence and prevalence of illness can be determined and the location associated with the symptoms identified. Often, a detailed history examining the temporal relationship between an activity (e.g., pesticide treatment, a new floor stripper, appearance of water stains or mold on ceilings, musty odor) and the onset of symptoms will reveal the likely cause of a reported health problem. Symptoms can be generated by the buildup of low concentrations of multiple indoor contaminants, including outgassing from building materials, emissions from office machinery, and solvents and other chemicals used in office work and building maintenance. This synergy of low-level multiple pollutants is accentuated by a suboptimally performing HVAC system.

Monitoring strategies for pollutants are based on the environmental assessment and health survey. Decisions about monitoring for VOCs and biological contaminants are driven by what is found on the inspection and the pattern of illness of the occupants. Monitored variables may include the following:

1. Presence of carbon dioxide (should be <800 ppm)
2. Relative humidity: winter, 30% to 50%; summer, 40% to 60%; plenum and ductwork, <70%
3. Ambient air temperature
4. HVAC system function and condition
5. Total number and concentrations of VOCs
6. Specific volatile chemicals
7. Combustion products, such as CO, NO_2, SO_2, and O_3
8. Biological contaminants, bioaerosols, and chemical byproducts
9. Lighting level
10. Airflow: supply diffusers, return grills, and local exhaust systems
11. Airflow between spaces
12. Vertical air temperature
13. Air filtration
14. Noise and vibration

References

1. U.S. Department of Labor: Occupational Safety and Health Administration: Indoor air quality, *Federal Register* 59(65):15968–16039, 1994.
2. Dales R, Burnett R, Zwanenburg H: Adverse health effects among adults exposed to home dampness and molds, *Am Rev Respir Dis* 143:505–509, 1991.
3. Amalkin R, Martinez K, Marinkovich V, et al: The relationship between symptoms and IgG and IgE antibodies in an office environment, *Environ Res A* 76:85–93, 1998.
4. Norback D, Wieslander G, Bjornsson E, et al: Eye irritation, nasal congestion, and facial skin itching in relation to emissions from newly painted indoor surfaces, *Indoor Build Environ* 5:270–279, 1996.
5. Dales R, Zqanenburg H, Burnch R, et al: Respiratory health effects of home dampness and molds among Canadian children, *Am J Epidemiol* 134:196–203, 1991.
6. Menzies D, Bourbeau J: Building related illness, *N Engl J Med* 337(21):1524–1531, 1997.
7. Verhoeff A, VanStrien R, VanWijnen J, et al: Damp housing and childhood respiratory symptoms—the role of sensitization to dust mites and molds, *Am J Epidemiol* 141:103–110, 1995.
8. Waegemaekers M, VanWageningen N, Brunckreef B, et al: Respiratory symptoms in damp homes, *Allergy* 44:1–7, 1989.
9. Seltzer JM, et al: Effects of the indoor environment on health, *Occup Med State Art Rev* 10(1):229–244, 1995.
10. Middaugh A, Pinney S, Linz D: Sick building syndrome: medical evaluation of two work forces, *J Occup Med* 34(12):1197–1203, 1992.
11. Lagoudi A, Loizidou M, Asimakopoulos D: Volatile organic compounds in office buildings: presence of volatile organic compounds in the indoor air, *Indoor Build Environ* 5:341–347, 1996.
12. Lagoudi A, Loizidou M, Asimakopoulos D: Volatile organic compounds in office buildings: identification of pollution sources in indoor air, *Indoor Build Environ* 5:348–354, 1996.
13. Holcomb L, Seabrook B: Indoor concentrations of volatile organic compounds: implications for comfort, health and regulation, *Indoor Environ* 4:7–26, 1995.
14. Mendell M, Smith A: Consistent pattern of elevated symptoms in air conditioned office buildings: a reanalysis of epidemiologic studies, *Am J Pub Health* 80:1193–1199, 1990.
15. Diasty R, Olson P: Improving indoor air quality through healthy building envelope design and systems selection, *Indoor Environ* 2:285–290, 1995.
16. Rolloos M: HVAC systems and indoor air quality, *Indoor Environ* 2:204–212, 1993.
17. Burton J: General ventilation of nonindustrial occupancies. In Plog B, Niland J, Quinlan P, editors: *Fundamentals of industrial hygiene*, ed 4, Itasca, IL, 1996, National Safety Council.
18. Girman JR: Volatile organic compounds and building bake-out. In Cone JE, Hodgson MJ, editors: *Occupational medicine: state of the art reviews*, vol 4, Philadelphia, 1989, Hanley & Belfus.
19. Linaker C, Chauhan A, Inskip H, et al: Distribution and determinants of personal exposure to nitrogen dioxide in school children, *Occup Environ Med* 53:200–203, 1996.
20. Strom J, Alfredsson L, Malmfors T, et al: Nitrogen dioxide: causation and aggravation of lung diseases, *Indoor Environ* 3:58–68, 1994.

21. Steenland K: Passive smoking and the risk of heart disease, *JAMA* 7(1):94–99, 1992.
22. Humble C, Croft J, Gerber A: Passive smoking and 20-year cardiovascular disease mortality among non-smoking wives, *Am J Pub Health* 80:599–601, 1990.
23. Stankus R, Menon P, et al: Cigarette smoke-sensitive asthma: challenge studies, *J Allerg Clin Immunol* 82(3 Pt 1):331–338, 1988.
24. Godish T: Formaldehyde exposure from tobacco smoke: a review, *Am J Pub Health* 79:1044–1045, 1989.
25. Hodgson MJ: Environmental tobacco smoke and the sick building syndrome. In Cone JE, Hodgson MJ, editors: *Occupational medicine: state of the art reviews*, vol 4, Philadelphia, 1989, Hanley & Belfus.
26. Stricker S, et al: Physiological responses to elevated carbon dioxide levels in buildings, *Indoor Build Environ* 6:301–308, 1997.
27. Turner W: Ventilation in occupational medicine, *Occup Med State Art Rev* 10(1):41–57, 1995.
28. Molhave L: Controlled experiments for studies of the sick building syndrome, *Acad Sci* 641:46–55, 1992.
29. Molhave L, Liu Z, et al: Sensory and physiological effects on humans of combined exposures to air temperatures and volatile organic compounds, *Indoor Air* 3:155–169, 1993.
30. Bascom R, Kesavanathan J, Swift D: Human susceptibility to indoor contaminants, *Occup Med State Art Rev* 10(1):119–132, 1995.
31. Frew J: The immunology of respiratory allergies, *Toxicol Lett* 86:65–72, 1996.
32. Damgard G: Mechanisms of activation of the sensory irritant receptor by airborne chemicals, *Toxicology* 21(3):183–208, 1991.
33. Schook L, Laskin D, editors: *Xenobiotics and inflammation*, San Diego, 1994, Academic Press.
34. Dusser D, Djokic T, Borson D, et al: Cigarette smoke induces bronchoconstrictor hyperresponsiveness to substance P and inactivates airway neutral endopeptidase in the guinea pig, *J Clin Invest* 84:900–906, 1989.
35. Mygind N, Dahl R, Nielsen L: Effect of nasal inflammation and of intranasal anti-inflammatory treatment on bronchial asthma, *Respir Med* 92:547–549, 1998.
36. Hirsch F, Kroemer G: The immune system and immune modulation. In Kresina T, editor: *Immune modulating agents*, New York, 1998, Marcel Dekker.
37. Cometto-Muniz J, Cain W: Relative sensitivity of the ocular trigeminal, nasal trigeminal, and olfactory systems to airborne chemicals, *Chem Senses* 20(2):191–198, 1995.
38. Cometto-Muniz J, Cain W: Thresholds for odor and nasal pungency, *Physiology Behav* 48:719–725, 1990.
39. Meggs WJ: RADS and RUDS - The toxic induction of asthma and rhinitis, *Clin Toxicol* 32(5):487–501, 1994.
40. Farley J: Inhaled toxicants and airway hyperresponsiveness, *Annu Rev Pharmacol Toxicol* 32:67–88, 1992.
41. Lemanske R, Busse W: Asthma, *JAMA* 278(22):1855–1873, 1997.
42. Perkner J, et al: Irritant associated vocal cord dysfunction, *J Occup Environ Med* 40(2):136–143, 1998.
43. Crump D, Squire R, Yu C: Sources and concentrations of formaldehyde and other volatile organic compounds in the indoor air of four newly built unoccupied test houses, *Indoor Build Environ* 6:45–55, 1997.
44. Harving H, Dahl R, Molhave L: Lung function and bronchial reactivity in asthmatics during exposure to volatile organic compounds, *Am Rev Respir Dis* 143:751–754, 1990.
45. Van Ert MD, Clayton JW, Crabb CL, et al: *Identification and characterization of 4-phenylcyclohexene, an emission product of new carpeting.* Presented at the American Industrial Hygiene Conference, San Francisco, May, 1988.
46. Vogelman I, Clayton JW, Crutchfield CD, et al: *Evaluation of 4-phenylcyclohexene concentrations in home and chamber environments.* Presented at the American Industrial Hygiene Conference, San Francisco, May, 1988.
47. Burge H: Aerobiology of the indoor environment, *Occup Med State Art Rev* 10(1):27–40, 1995.
48. Andrae S, et al: Symptoms of bronchial hyperreactivity and asthma in relation to environmental factors, *Arch Dis Childh* 63:473–478, 1988.
49. Jaakkola M, et al: Indoor dampness and molds and development of adult-onset asthma: a population-based incident case-control study, *Envir Hlth Persp* 110(5):543–547, 2002.
50. Gent F, et al: Levels of household mold associated with respiratory symptoms in the first year of life in a cohort at risk for asthma, *Envir Hlth Persp* 110(12):A781–786, 2002.
51. Stark P, et al: Fungal levels in the home and lower respiratory tract illness in the first year of life, *Am J Respir Crit Care Med* 168:233–237, 2003.
52. Smith J, Anderson J, Lewis C: Cytotoxic fungal spores in the indoor atmosphere of the damp domestic environment, *FEMS Microbiol Lett* 100:337–344, 1992.

Responding to Mass Exposures

15

Lisa A. Murphy, VMD, DABT

This chapter explores disaster situations that may necessitate the evacuation and decontamination of large numbers of people and their pets (Color Plate 15-1). Common natural disasters include hurricanes, floods, tornadoes, and earthquakes. Other incidents may be related to human activities such as transportation or power plant accidents or intentional terrorist activities. All of these events could potentially result in the dispersion of chemical contaminants into the environment, and sometimes even biological agents or radioactive substances. When this occurs, both humans and animals may need to be decontaminated as they evacuate the scene of the incident. In large-scale emergencies the availability of trained personnel and the necessary resources for the decontamination of large numbers of pet animals may be very limited, particularly in the early stages of the incident. Other chapters in this text cover the decontamination and care of individual animals. Universal standards for the decontamination of large numbers of domestic animals do not currently exist. This chapter will discuss the challenges of animal decontamination, and aspects such as planning and triage, that are critical to ensuring the health, safety, and well-being of humans and companion animals affected by mass catastrophes.

Initial Considerations

Human Safety and Animal Welfare

Human safety will be the first and most important consideration when making decisions about decontaminating large numbers of animals. Only personnel with appropriate hazardous materials training should participate in animal decontamination operations.[1] An incident's safety officer will assess the hazards and risks to responders, determine what kinds of activities can occur within the disaster area, and formulate personal safety plans to protect the health of all on-scene personnel. Hazards associated with the care of domestic animals include bites and scratches, exposure to bodily fluids and zoonotic diseases, and injuries related to lifting.[2] All personnel who intend to be involved in the decontamination and care of animals at a disaster site should obtain prior medical clearance and prophylaxis against likely biological hazards.

The main role of veterinarians at a disaster scene will be assisting with an assessment of the number of animals affected by an incident and the current status of their condition, making a plan to decontaminate animals and provide veterinary care when indicated, and requesting appropriate resources for the subsequent care and medical treatment of recovered animals. In situations where veterinary personnel are unable to directly access the disaster site, remote communications may enable recommendations to be made from a safe distance.[1]

Making the Decision to Decontaminate

Establishing Control Zones

Control zones—hot, warm, and cold—are established around dangerous areas to limit access and contain the hazard.[3] The hot zone is where the actual hazard is located and only essential personnel wearing appropriate personal protective equipment (PPE) will be allowed to enter.

The hot zone is immediately surrounded by the warm zone, where contaminants are expected to be present though at lower levels than in the hot zone. This is where some veterinary triage and all animal decontamination activities will take place. Only animals and personnel that have been decontaminated in the warm zone's contamination reduction corridor will be permitted into the cold zone.[2]

The cold zone surrounds the warm zone. Multiple incident-related activities will occur in this location, including at least initial medical care, and sheltering of animals. Even though risk of exposure to contaminants should be minimal or nonexistent in this area, access by nonessential personnel should still be prevented.

Minimizing Further Animal Contamination

As detailed decisions regarding animal decontamination are being determined, actions to minimize direct contact with known or suspected toxicants will benefit both humans and animals.[4] If a disaster site can be made safer by stopping or removing a point source of contamination such as a leaking chemical container or vehicle, and adequate supplies of food and water are either in place or can be provided, it may be reasonable to have people and their pets remain in place until decontamination teams are in place. This also assumes that all companion animals are safely confined or under the control of their owners or another responsible party. Depending on the nature of the incident or the potential hazard involved, it may instead be necessary to evacuate human and animal populations to a safe staging area until decontamination operations can begin. Ideally this site should be located in the warm zone and be staffed by medical and veterinary personnel that can triage patients upon arrival.

Decontamination of Live Animals

Technical Decontamination

Technical decontamination is a thorough and time-consuming decontamination process that may involve dermal, ocular, and possibly even gastrointestinal or internal decontamination that are discussed elsewhere in this text. For the external decontamination of companion animals, large volumes of water will be needed and liquid dishwashing detergents are recommended for the removal of most chemicals.[5] Eyes, ears, and noses should also be cleaned and inspected. All of these can be decontaminated by gently flushing with copious amounts of tepid water, though some debris may need to be manually removed from ear canals and nasal passages using soft toothbrushes, cotton swabs, or gauze.[4] Under most circumstances more involved gastrointestinal and internal decontamination procedures should be performed beyond the decontamination line in the cold zone.

Mass Decontamination

Mass decontamination may be used rather than technical decontamination in events involving the contamination of large numbers of people.[3] Tents and trailers have been designed for the mass decontamination of people, because of necessity alternatives such as fire hoses and hydrants, locker rooms, and swimming pools have also been utilized. Although similar techniques have been described using chutes and corrals for groups of livestock and horses,[4] it is unlikely that individual companion animals could be safely comingled and adequately contained to facilitate this type of decontamination without significant risk of injury or escape. Because this essentially limits the companion animal decontamination process to several people working on one individual at a time, the entire process will require significant time, personnel, and resources if many animals are affected by a large-scale event.

Emergency Decontamination

Emergency, or gross, decontamination is a life-saving measure that involves the rapid removal of as much contamination as possible, and is typically restricted to decontamination of the haircoat and skin.[4] Emergency decontamination can facilitate the rapid transfer of a critically injured or gravely ill animal from a contaminated area to a location where immediate veterinary care can be provided. Examples of conditions that may require emergency decontamination include airway obstruction, pneumothorax, shock, arterial hemorrhage, and unconsciousness.[3,6] Because these animals may still retain contaminant residues either on the outside of their bodies or internally, they should ideally be treated and housed in a warm zone location that is isolated from other decontaminated animals.

Medical Decontamination

Once companion animals have passed through the decontamination line, additional treatments such as intravenous fluids, activated charcoal, specific antidotes, and gastric lavage to limit absorption of toxic substances may be indicated[4] and are discussed in detail elsewhere in this text.

Euthanasia

Humane euthanasia may need to be considered for animals that are unlikely to survive the decontamination process because of injuries or illness, either preexisting or associated with the incident. When large numbers of companion animals are impacted by an incident or decontamination personnel or resources are limited, decontamination and additional treatments should be performed on the animals that are most likely to live.[1] These decisions will be very stressful for both owners and the emergency personnel working with the animals, so the presence of a veterinarian will be critical for determining the course of action that best addresses the human-animal bond, public health and safety, and animal welfare.

Special Considerations
Animal Identification and Documentation

Whether an animal is brought to a decontamination line by a family member or is presented by a rescuer or other individual, adequate identification and documentation procedures must be in place to best ensure that pets and owners are later reunited. Ideally, medical and veterinary personnel would be processing people and their pets in parallel decontamination lines, and then transporting them together to a pet-friendly shelter, but this will not always be possible. Because leashes, collars, and harnesses will generally have to be removed as hazardous waste during the decontamination process, these unique items should either be photographed or otherwise preserved or documented in a way that will later assist in the positive identification of individual animals, especially when these items contain owner names and addresses.[2] Animals themselves should also be individually photographed and a unique identifier should be assigned to each pet until it can be returned to its proper owner.

Physical Restraint

Although under normal circumstances many companion animals, particularly dogs, may not object to routine bathing, pets that are stressed and brought into an enclosed location for decontamination by unfamiliar people may not be as easy to handle. In addition, it is important to expect that emergency personnel wearing PPE will frighten many animals.[1] PPE worn during the decontamination of animals should ideally protect against common injuries such as bites and scratches, but these same injuries could also damage the PPE itself, jeopardizing the health and safety of emergency responders. An adequate supply of clean leashes, harnesses, collars, and muzzles should be available to facilitate the safe and secure handling of animals during decontamination.

To minimize the risk of injury to both animals and people, it may be helpful to place a frightened or fractious animal inside a portable plastic or metal animal carrier of an appropriate size with adequate drainage and openings that are large enough to visually monitor the animal's well-being (Color Plate 15-2). If the carrier can then be securely placed on an elevated surface it should be possible to at least grossly decontaminate the animal without having to directly restrain it.

Chemical Restraint

Some companion animals may be either too stressed or aggressive to be safely decontaminated using physical restraint techniques alone. Although the administration of sedatives is commonly performed in veterinary hospitals, it should not be considered a routine procedure during an emergency evacuation. Stressed, injured, debilitated companion animals or those with preexisting medical conditions may potentially develop hypotension or arrhythmias, or become ataxic or otherwise unstable.[4] Some aggressive animals become more unpredictable when sedated. Should complications arise, animal safety may be compromised by the lack of immediate access to emergency care. Human personnel may be at increased risk of accidental needle sticks and other injuries because of the decreased dexterity and mobility and limited field of vision typically experienced when working in PPE.

Wastewater Management

Contaminated wastewater generated during the decontamination of animals should be managed in such a way that prevents animals from ingesting it and keeps the water from being dispersed into the surrounding area.[1] Environmental officials should be consulted before decontamination operations begin and again after they are completed, in order to determine the best method for disposal of wastewater, along with accumulated urine, feces, and hair.

Decontamination of Deceased Animals

Not all companion animals may survive a large-scale disaster. Even though pets are family members and owners may want to bring their remains with them when they evacuate, environmental concerns and legal/jurisdictional issues may preclude this. If access to water, personnel, and other decontamination resources is limited, decontamination of live people and animals will have to take precedence. In addition, if the nature of the incident is potentially the result of either human error (such as a transportation accident) or an intentional malicious act, the affected area will be considered a crime scene. As part of their investigation, local, state, or federal law enforcement officials may need any deceased animals as evidence. Also the presence of chemical, biological, or radiologic contaminants may necessitate handling of dead animals as hazardous waste under the direction of local, state, or federal environmental authorities.[4]

Laws and Regulations Related to Animal Decontamination

The Pets Evacuation and Transportation Standards Act was signed into federal law and requires that pets and service animals be included in disaster and emergency plans;[4] however, there are few laws that would require emergency personnel to decontaminate animals. Local, state, and federal authorities may have jurisdiction over other issues related to animal decontamination operations, such as disposal of wastewater (environmental protection), worker health and safety (OSHA, EPA, public health), and disposition and care of domestic animals (agriculture).

Working and Service Animals

Working animals typically include dogs and horses.[4] Working dogs are commonly used for police operations, detection of explosives and narcotics, and search-and-rescue. These animals must be afforded the same rights and protections as their handlers, including access to decontamination and veterinary care during emergency deployments.

Most jurisdictions also afford special privileges to animals that are specially trained to assist their disabled owners.[4] In addition to dogs, other service animals such as monkeys and pigs may present for decontamination following a disaster. Because many of these animals must remain in close proximity to their owners at all times, not only is it imperative that they be adequately decontaminated so they do not transfer contaminants to people, but it may also be necessary to adapt procedures so service animals and their disabled owners can be decontaminated together (Color Plate 15-3).

Luckily most working and service dogs are accustomed to frequent bathing; however, certain animals, particularly police dogs, may be most easily and safely decontaminated with the assistance of a familiar person. Because many working dog handlers may themselves be emergency responders with hazardous materials training, they may be able to significantly assist with the decontamination of their animals.[1]

Commonly Encountered Contaminants

Although an incident involving a point-source release may make identification of the specific agent involved relatively simple, larger-scale natural and manmade disasters can result in the vast dispersion of unknown quantities of a variety of toxic and hazardous contaminants. Floodwaters are known to contain heavy metals such as lead;[7] household, agricultural, and industrial chemicals; and fecal coliforms.[2] Contaminants associated with urban disaster areas include automotive fluids, polychlorinated biphenyls, pesticides, molds, hazardous metals, asbestos, toxic gases, cleaning products, and solvents.[1,8] Intentional criminal acts may involve chemical, biological, radiological, nuclear, and explosive materials, or merely conveniently available hazardous substances.[4]

Personal Protective Equipment

Level D

Level D personal protective equipment (PPE) consists of everyday attire and equipment that is needed to safely conduct a specific activity.[3] When working around animals this should include coveralls or other durable clothing, protective gloves, protective footwear, and safety glasses. This level of protection is only appropriate if there is minimal risk of exposure to contaminants and zoonotic diseases, so it may be best suited to personnel caring for animals in the cold zone.

Level C

Level C PPE includes all of the elements of level D, with the addition of an outer layer that is chemical- and splash-resistant, and a National Institute of Occupational Safety and Health (NIOSH)-approved air-purifying respirator.[3,4] Prior medical clearance and certification are needed before personnel can be cleared to wear most air-purifying respirators. Level C PPE provides a good level of protection against many diseases and contaminants, and would likely be the most common type of PPE worn by personnel performing animal triage and decontamination. Because of the potential for bites and scratches when working with companion animals, all PPE should be thoroughly inspected for leaks or other damage before, during, and after routine use.

Levels A and B

Levels A and B PPE incorporate everything used at level C; however, they derive their air supply from an air line or tank rather than an air-purifying respirator.[3] Level A provides a higher level of protection than level B because everything is enclosed in a totally encapsulating chemical protective suit. This level of protection is reserved for environments that pose the highest risks to human safety, because of the presence of either unknown contaminants or known agents in dangerously elevated concentrations. Level B PPE still provides the highest level of respiratory protection that is achieved with level A, but less skin protection against splashes.[4] Because of the advanced training and frequent recertifications needed to work in levels A and B PPE, it is unlikely that most veterinary personnel will be qualified or permitted to work in such highly contaminated locations. In reality, few or no animals would be expected to survive under such overwhelmingly hazardous environmental conditions.

Post-Decontamination Monitoring and Aftercare

Sheltering of Decontaminated Animals

Many human evacuation shelters do not admit animals, except for working or service animals. With this in mind, animal decontamination planning should include the identification of designated locations that can temporarily house otherwise healthy animals that have been decontaminated. Most local jurisdictions have some sort of animal sheltering facility; however, these sites may become either inaccessible or otherwise unusable if directly impacted by the emergency situation. Conventional facilities immediately outside the disaster zone such as animal shelters, kennels, and veterinary hospitals may quickly fill to capacity, and following a large-scale incident alternative locations such as schools, gymnasiums, stadiums, and fairgrounds may already be in use for human evacuees. National-level animal sheltering groups and local and state animal response teams may be able to assist with the establishment of temporary sheltering operations, and preparations should be made to transport animals to other suitable nearby locations.

Short-Term Monitoring and Care of Hospitalized Animals

Following decontamination, symptomatic animals or those that are otherwise at risk for developing adverse clinical signs associated with exposure to contaminants should receive symptomatic and supportive care, including the administration of specific antidotes when indicated as discussed throughout this text.

In addition to problems related to toxicant exposures, animals emerging from disaster sites may also require veterinary care for other injuries and health problems. Acute injuries and illnesses documented in dogs that deployed in response to the September 11, 2001, terrorist attacks included fatigue, conjunctivitis, respiratory problems, dehydration, cuts and abrasions, gastrointestinal signs, skin problems, urinary tract problems, and lameness.[9,10]

Long-Term Surveillance

There are no uniform protocols or procedures for the long-term monitoring of companion animals that have been affected by large-scale releases of contaminants; however, some monitoring data is available from the assessments of working dogs that responded to the September 11, 2001, disaster sites and were extensively exposed to environmental contaminants.[10,11] Initial collection of blood samples for a complete blood count and serum biochemistry profile should be part of a complete physical examination. Depending on the known or suspected toxicants associated with a specific incident, thoracic and abdominal radiographs and collection of additional samples for toxicologic analysis may also be warranted.

Long-term care should consist of physical examinations at least yearly, and more frequently if health problems arise that are suspected to be associated with a previous exposure to contaminants.

References

1. Murphy LA: Basic veterinary decontamination: who, what, why? In Wingfield WE, Palmer SB, editors: *Veterinary disaster response*, Ames, Iowa, 2009, Wiley-Blackwell.
2. Soric S, Belanger MP, Wittnich C: A method for the decontamination of animals involved in floodwater disaster disasters, *JAVMA* 232(3):364–370, 2008.
3. Wenzel JGW: Awareness-level information for veterinarians on control zones, personal protective equipment, and decontamination, *JAVMA* 231(1):48–51, 2007.
4. Murphy L, Slessman D, Mauck B: Decontamination of large animals. In Gimenez R, Gimenez T, May KA, editors: *Technical large animal emergency rescue*, Ames, Iowa, 2008, Wiley-Blackwell.
5. Wismer TA, Murphy LA, Gwaltney-Brant SM, et al: Management and prevention of toxicoses in search-and-rescue dogs responding to urban disasters, *JAVMA* 222(3):305–310, 2003.
6. Otto CM, Franz MA, Kellogg B, et al: Field treatment of search dogs: lessons learned from the World Trade Center disaster, *J Vet Emerg Crit Care* 12(1):33–42, 2002.
7. Marris E: First tests show flood waters high in bacteria and lead, *Nature* 437:301, 2005.
8. Murphy LA, Gwaltney-Brant SM, Albretsen JC, et al: Toxicologic agents of concern for search-and-rescue dogs responding to urban disasters, *JAVMA* 222(3):296–304, 2003.

9. Slensky KA, Drobatz KJ, Downend AB, et al: Deployment morbidity among search-and-rescue dogs used after the September 11, 2001, terrorist attacks, *JAVMA* 225(6):868–873, 2004.

10. Fox PR, Puschner B, Ebel JG: Assessment of acute injuries, exposure to environmental toxins, and five-year health surveillance of New York Police Department working dogs following the September 11, 2001, World Trade Center terrorist attack, *JAVMA* 233(1):48–59, 2008.

11. Otto CM, Downend AB, Serpell JA, et al: Medical and behavioral surveillance of dogs deployed to the World Trade Center and the Pentagon from October 2001 to June 2002, *JAVMA* 225(6):861–867, 2004.

Reproductive Toxicology of Male and Female Companion Animals

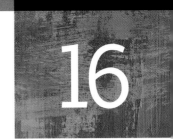

Tim J. Evans, DVM, MS, PhD, DACT, DABVT

Although reproduction is required for species survival, it is essentially a "luxury" function, with respect to individual animal longevity. This is especially true in companion animals, in which a relatively small proportion of animals are maintained exclusively for breeding purposes and millions of unwanted animals are euthanized each year. In fact, reproductive toxicants or the potential toxic effects of nonreproductive toxicants on reproductive performance in small animals often receive very limited attention in toxicology texts. However, there are many instances in which optimal individual canine and/ or feline reproductive efficiency is critical for owner or caretaker satisfaction. Many of these animals were not selected for breeding purposes based on criteria related to fertility, and some of these animals might even be older and have age-related health problems. As a result of this selection process, a subpopulation of these animals chosen for breeding might be inherently more susceptible to subtle, xenobiotic-induced effects on reproductive function. Although impaired reproductive function can have a single toxic etiology, the causes of diminished reproductive performance are often multifactorial, involving various predisposing factors and/or stressors, including toxicants. The purpose of this chapter is to provide the basic facts concerning canine and feline reproduction and briefly discuss xenobiotics, meaning any chemicals foreign to the body, such as drugs or toxicants, not only as the primary causes of observed reproductive abnormalities, but also in the context of other variables, including physiology, genetics, nutrition, infectious disease, environmental factors, and management, which can also impact reproductive performance. Selected toxins of fungal and plant origin, as well other xenobiotics are listed and briefly reviewed. The recognition and prevention of the potential adverse reproductive effects of these toxic stressors and their interactions are essential for optimal canine and feline reproductive performance.

Introduction

The major objective of this chapter is to provide a quick and practical review of (1) canine and feline reproductive physiology; (2) the basics of what is currently known regarding small animal reproductive toxicology and the ways in which xenobiotics, meaning any chemicals foreign to the body, such as drugs or toxicants, might pose a risk to reproductive function in companion animals; and (3) specific xenobiotics, especially potential pet food and environmental contaminants, as well as common medications, which can adversely affect spermatogenesis, estrous cycles, and embryonic and fetal development, in females (Tables 16-1 to 16-3).

Table 16-1	Summary of Essential Facts Pertaining to Small Animal Reproduction*	
Reproductive Parameter	**Dog**	**Cat**
Peak breeding age	2-6 years of age	1.5-7 years of age
Postnatal testicular descent	Completed by 6-8 weeks Prepubertal mobility	Completed by 6-8 weeks Prepubertal mobility
Onset of male puberty	7-10 (up to 12) months Range of 5-12 months	7 to 10 months
Duration of cycle of seminiferous epithelium	~13.2 ± 0.7 days	~10.4 ± 0.3 days
Duration of spermatogenesis	~62 days	~46.8 days
Epididymal transit time	~12 days	10+ days?
Threshold semen parameters	≥300 × 10^6 sperm/ejaculate ≥70% progressive motility	≥30 × 10^6 sperm/ejaculate ≥70% progressive motility
Onset of female puberty	6 to 14 months Larger dogs by 18 to 24 (30?) months	Range of 5 to 12 months Most by 6 to 9 months
Frequency of estrous cycles	Monestrous	Polyestrous
Seasonality of estrous cycles	Possible seasonal influences/ whelping year-round?	Seasonal long-day breeder
Average duration of proestrus	~9 days (6-11 days) Range of 3-25 days	~0-2 days Might not be exhibited
Average duration of estrus	~9 days (5-9 days) Range of 2-20 days	~7 days Range of 1-21 days
Follicular phase: estrus ratio	1:1	Possibly ≥1:1
Type of ovulation	Spontaneous	Induced or "reflex"
Average duration of diestrus	~60 days ± pregnancy	~60 days with pregnancy ~40-45 days if not pregnant
Average duration of anestrus	Minimum of 7-8 weeks Usually 18-20 weeks	~3-4 months Range of 30-90+ days
Type of oocyte ovulated	Primary	Secondary
Interestrous interval/period+	5-11 months Range of 3.5-13 months	Interestrus or "postestrus" Range of 8-15 days
Gestational length	65 ± 1 days after LH surge 63 ± 1 days after ovulation	63-66 days after P$_4$ ↑
Entry into uterus	10-13 days after ovulation	5-6 days after ovulation
Beginning of fetal stage	~33 days after ovulation	~28 days after ovulation
Sources of gestational progesterone	Corpora lutea Prolactin is luteotrophic	Corpora lutea Placenta after 40+ days
Type of placentation	Zonary/endotheliochorial/ deciduate	Same as dog
Biochemical alterations during canine pregnancy	Normocytic, normochromic anemia/↓calcium 7-9 weeks after estrus ↑Cholesterol, total protein, clotting factors, 3-8+ weeks after estrus	

*Information is adapted from the text of this chapter, based on References 4-12.

+Interestrous interval does not mean the same thing in the dog as it does in the cat (see text).

Table 16-2 Summary of Reproductive Effects of Selected Predisposing Factors and Stressors*

Predisposing Factors and Stressors	Adverse Effects on Reproduction
Physiological factors: Stress/fever	Stress and ♂/♀ infertility Fever damages sperm and germ cell precursors
Genetic factors: Lack of hybrid vigor/disease predisposition	↓ ♂/♀ fertility with these predisposing factors Some breeds predisposed to diseases/ conditions
Nutritional factors: ↓ Body condition/nutritional deficiencies	Delayed onset of puberty Stress and ♂/♀ infertility from malnutrition
Environmental factors: Heat/microwaves/radiation/stray voltage	Heat- and radiation-damaged gametes ↓ ♂/♀ fertility with these stressors
Infectious diseases and parasitism: Bacteria/viruses/parasites	Brucellosis and ↓ ♂/♀ fertility/Pyometra prevents pregnancy. Bacteria, viruses, and parasites cause abortions/neonatal death.
Xenobiotic Stressors	
Mycotoxins: Aflatoxins/vomitoxin/zearalenone/ ergot	Aflatoxins are hepatotoxic/Vomitoxin affects GI. Zearalenone is estrogenic/Ergot toxins ↓ prolactin.
Phytotoxins: Phytotoxins/phytoestrogens	Stress and ♂/♀ infertility from systemic disease Phytoestrogens have been associated with ↓ fertility.
Heavy metals: Cadmium/lead/mercury	↓ Testosterone and ↓ sperm number with Cd ↓ Sperm quality and teratogenesis in CNS with Pb and Hg
Rodenticides: Anticoagulants/strychnine/zinc phosphide	Stress and ♂/♀ infertility from systemic disease/other effects Teratogenesis/neonatal coagulopathies with anticoagulants
Insecticides and molluscicides: OPs/carbamates/pyrethroids/ metaldehyde	Stress and ♂/♀ infertility from systemic disease Pyrethrins/pyrethroids can be antiandrogenic.
Fungicides: Dibromochlorpropane (DBCP)/ vinclozolin	DBCP is testicular toxicant. Vinclozolin has antiandrogenic activity.
Herbicides: 2,4-D/diquat and paraquat	Testicular degeneration reported with 2,4-D Diquat and paraquat alter sexual differentiation
Organic pollutants: HAHs: Dioxins/PCBs/PBDEs/others	Systemic effects with high doses; also endocrine disruptors ↓ Number of normal gametes and teratogenesis
Plasticizers and plastic byproducts: Bisphenol A/phthalates	Endocrine disruption BPA is estrogenic and phthalates cause testicular effects.

*Information is adapted from the text of this chapter, based on References 1, 4, 5, 7, 8, 9, 14.

Table 16-3 Potentially Adverse Reproductive Effects of Selected Commonly Used Medications*

Xenobiotic	Effect on Males	Safety During Pregnancy+
Anticancer Drugs		
Cyclophosphamide	↓ Sperm number and teratogenesis	C: ↓ Fertility and teratogenesis
Doxorubicin	Assume abnormal spermatogenesis	C: Embryotoxic, teratogenic, abortifacient
Vincristine	↓ Sperm number Possible reversibility	C: Safety not established in dogs and cats Assume fetotoxic and teratogenic effects
Methotrexate	Assume abnormal spermatogenesis ↑ Abnormal sperm	C: Abortifacient, teratogenic, mutagenic
Anticonvulsant Drugs		
Diazepam	Impotence and ejaculatory failure	C: Teratogenesis in rodents and humans
Phenobarbital	Chronic low-dose exposure: ↓ Sperm motility	B: Possible teratogenesis Bleeding tendencies in neonates
Phenytoin	Chronic exposure: ↓ Sperm motility	C/D: Teratogenesis in rodents and humans Fetal hydantoin syndrome
Primidone	Converted to phenobarbital Same risks and ↑ hepatotoxic risks	C: Same risks as phenobarbital ↑ Hepatotoxicity
Valproic acid	Chronic exposure to high doses: ↓ Sperm number and motility	C: Teratogenesis Neural tube defects in humans
Anti-inflammatory Drugs		
Acetaminophen	Delayed spermiogenesis ↑ Abnormal sperm	C: Toxic in cats Safety not established in dogs
Nonsteroidals (NSAIDs)	↓ Seminal prostaglandins? ↓ Sperm motility and fertilization?	C: Embryotoxic in rodents Safety not established in dogs and cats
Glucocorticoids	↓ Testosterone and libido ↓ Sperm number and motility	C: ↑ Incidence of cleft palate Premature labor or abortion
Antifungal Drugs		
Ketaconazole/ miconazole	↓ Testosterone and libido ↓ Sperm number and motility	B/C: Antiandrogenic? ↑ Stillbirths? "Safe" in dogs and cats
Griseofulvin	No adverse effects with routine usage	D: *Teratogenic in rats Feline skeletal/brain malformations*
Antimicrobial Drugs		
Aminoglycosides	Possible spermatogenic effects Routinely used in semen extenders	C: Crosses the placenta easily 8th nerve toxicity/ nephrotoxicity

Table 16-3 Potentially Adverse Reproductive Effects of Selected Commonly Used Medications*—cont'd

Xenobiotic	Effect on Males	Safety During Pregnancy+
β-Lactams	No adverse effects with routine usage	A: Crosses placenta easily No harm to fetus demonstrated
Cephalosporins	No adverse effects with routine usage	A: Crosses the placenta easily No harm to fetus demonstrated
Fluoroquinolones	High doses: ↑ Abnormal sperm and ↓ sperm number	D: *Articular cartilage defects* *Avoid use during pregnancy*
Xenobiotic	Effect on male	Safety during pregnancy+
Metronidazole	High doses: ↑ Abnormal sperm and ↓ sperm number	C: Teratogenic in lab animals Safety not established in dogs and cats
Sulfonamides	High doses or long-term treatment: ↓ Sperm number and motility	B/C: Teratogenic in lab animals "Safe" in dogs and cats
Tetracyclines	Very high doses: ↓ Sperm number and capacitation	D: *Maternal toxicity* *Bone and teeth malformations*
Trimethoprims ± sulfas	Long-term treatment: ↓ Sperm numbers by 7%–88%	B/C: Folate and bone marrow effects? "Safe" in dogs and cats
Antiparasitic Drugs		
Avermectins	No adverse effects with routine usage	A: No adverse effects demonstrated
Benzimidazoles	No adverse effects with routine usage	A: Safe according to reproductive studies B: Thiabendazole and toxemia in ewes?
Organophosphates	No information available Avoid use because safer alternatives	B/C: Little information available Congenital intoxications in some species
Piperazine	No adverse effects with routine usage	A: No adverse effects demonstrated
Praziquantel	No adverse effects with routine usage	A: Safe when tested in dogs
Pyrantel pamoate	Safe with routine, approved usage	A: Safe in pregnant and nursing pets Class C in pregnant women
Praziquantel/ Pyrantel pamoate/± Febantel	Conflicting information on testing in breeding dogs?	Safety of Praziquantel/Pyrantel pamoate? *DO NOT give Febantel during pregnancy*
Thenium closylate	No adverse effects with routine usage	A: No adverse effects demonstrated Use in young puppies contraindicated?

continued

Table 16-3	Potentially Adverse Reproductive Effects of Selected Commonly Used Medications*—cont'd	
Xenobiotic	Effect on Males	Safety During Pregnancy+
Cardiovascular Medications		
ACE inhibitors	Testicular effects with chronic use Possible alterations in sperm motility	C: Embryotoxic in lab animals and goats
Cardiac glycosides	Testicular effects with chronic use Altered testosterone secretion?	A: Safe when tested in dogs No adverse effects in humans or rodents
Dopamine	No adverse effects with routine usage	B: Probably safe at therapeutic doses
Furosemide	Chronic exposure: Possible effects on testicular function	B: Probably safe at therapeutic doses No adverse effects reported
Heparin	Probably no effect with routine usage ↑ Bleeding might affect fertility	B: Probably safe at therapeutic doses Does not appear to cross placenta
Isoproterenol	Probably no effect with routine usage Testicular effects with chronic usage	C: Possible fetal tachycardia β-adrenergics inhibit uterine contractions
Lidocaine/Procainamide	Probably no effect with routine usage ↓ Sperm motility in vitro	A/B: Probably safe in dogs and cats Possible fetal bradycardia
Thiazide diuretics	Chronic exposure: Possible effects on testicular function	C: Possible ↑ incidence in perinatal death
Warfarin	Probably no effect with routine usage ↑ Bleeding might affect fertility	D: Crosses placenta rapidly Abortions/stillbirths from ↓ clotting
Xenobiotic	Effect on male	Safety during pregnancy+
Gastrointestinal Drugs		
Antacids/Sucralfate	Safe with routine, approved usage	A: Safe when tested in dogs Not absorbed systemically
Diphenhydramine Dimenhydrinate	↓ Sperm motility	B: Safe if used short term
Cimetidine/Omeprazole	↓ Sperm number	B/C: "Safe" in dogs and cats
Hormones		
Androgens/Anabolics	↓ Sperm number, quality, and motility Testicular degeneration	D: Masculinization of female fetuses
Estrogens/DES	↓ Sperm number Behavioral feminization	D: Feminization of male fetuses Cancer in daughters of treated women
Progestogens	↓ Sperm number and quality	D: Masculinization of female fetuses

Table 16-3 Potentially Adverse Reproductive Effects of Selected
Commonly Used Medications*—cont'd

Xenobiotic	Effect on Males	Safety During Pregnancy+
Preanesthetic and Anesthetic Drugs		
Atropine	↓ Ejaculated sperm and seminal fluid	B/C: Crosses placenta easily Fetal tachycardia and ↓ gonadotropins?
Glycopyrrolate	↓ Ejaculated sperm and seminal fluid?	B: Crosses placenta less than atropine No teratogenesis in rats and rabbits
Phenothiazine derivatives	Priapism and impotence ↓ Spermatogenesis	C: Nervous disorders and jaundice in humans CNS depression if given near term
Xylazine	Retrograde flow of sperm into bladder	D: *No information on teratogenesis* *Premature labor or abortion*
Ketamine	Possible ↓ sperm number and motility	B/C: Premature labor/neonate depressed "Safe" in dogs and cats
Barbiturates	↓ Testosterone? ↓ Sperm motility?	C/D: *Pentobarbital high fetal mortality* All barbiturates depress neonates
Opiates/Butorphanol	↓ Hormone production? ↓ Sperm number and motility	B: Possible neonatal depression Safe in dogs and cats
Propofol	No adverse effects with routine usage	B: Useful for cesarean section induction in dogs ↓ Possible apnea/hypoxia with O_2
Sevoflurane/ Isoflurane	Possible ↓ sperm number and motility	B: Possible neonatal depression Safe in dogs and cats
Halothane/ Methoxyflurane	Possible ↓ sperm number and motility Polyspermy in female?	C: Neonatal depression ↑ Bleeding with halothane

*Information is adapted from this chapter, based on References 1, 4, 5, 8, 9, 49, 50, and 51.

+Definition of categories [both categories listed (e.g., B/C), if information is conflicting]:

A: Probably safe. No specific studies have proved the safety of all drugs in dogs and cats, but no reports of adverse effects in laboratory animals or women.

B: Safe for use if used cautiously. Studies in laboratory animals might have discovered some risk, but these drugs appear to be safe in dogs and cats or are safe if not administered near term.

C: These drugs might have potential risks. Studies in people or animals have discovered risks. These drugs should be used cautiously, as last resort, *if benefits outweigh risks.*

D: Contraindicated. *These drugs cause congenital malformations or embryotoxicity.*

Furthermore, the author's experiences as a theriogenologist and toxicologist suggest several other basic concepts and possible misconceptions that this chapter should address within the context of these objectives:

1. Dogs and cats selected for breeding based on nonreproductive criteria and older canine and feline breeding animals might be predisposed to subfertility.
2. Xenobiotics can either directly affect reproductive organs or functions or indirectly affect reproductive function by having adverse effects on other organs or body systems.
3. Reproductive abnormalities can be the first direct or indirect xenobiotic effects observed, and changes in canine and feline reproductive performance might serve as biomarkers for similar effects in humans.
4. Xenobiotics can play a primary role in causing reproductive inefficiency or, because of interactions with other factors or stressors, a secondary role in causing subfertility.
5. Synthetic as well as natural xenobiotics can adversely affect reproduction.

The Relevance of Reproduction in Small Animals

Reproduction is a critical biological process in all living systems and is required for species survival. Reproduction is also essential for the production of such important agricultural commodities as milk and meat for human and companion animal consumption. However, on an individual animal basis, reproduction can be essentially viewed as a luxury function, or even in some cases a nuisance, unless of course fertility is among the criteria used for culling animals from livestock production systems or breeding colonies. Most aspects of sexual reproduction in domestic mammalian species, including embryonic and fetal development, actually can be suppressed or impaired by stress, which implies excessive stimulation of the hypothalamic-pituitary-adrenal (HPA) axis and the release of large amounts of endogenous glucocorticoid.[1,2] Reproductive processes, in particular those associated with pregnancy, also can be adversely affected by diseases, including intoxications, which affect other organ systems and not the reproductive tract directly. The mechanisms for those adverse effects might be stress-related or might involve other interactions between those organ systems and various aspects of pregnancy and fetal development. Furthermore, with respect to companion animal species, it is rarely essential to use an individual pet for breeding purposes, especially when one considers that three to four million unwanted dogs and cats are euthanized each year.[3] In fact, it can be argued that most dogs and cats are perhaps too fertile, and companion animal population control, rather than propagation, is a primary focus of the majority of small animal practices.

With the exception of the previous edition of this book, reproductive toxicants or the potential toxic effects of nonreproductive toxicants on reproductive performance in small animals often receive very limited attention in small animal toxicology textbooks.[4,5] However, there are many instances in which individual canine and/or feline reproductive efficiency is critical for the livelihoods of owners or caretakers and their satisfaction with the veterinary services being provided. Cats and especially dogs of particular specialized lineages can be desired as pets or used for purposes of exhibition, service to individuals with disabilities, security and protection of military or law enforcement personnel, detection of illicit drugs and explosives, search and rescue, and/or participation in hunting and other sporting activities. There are also dogs and cats carrying selected gene mutations, which are used for biomedical research, as well as species of endangered canids and felids, in which gene pool conservation and/or expansion (particularly in instances of relatively closed breeding colonies) are very worthwhile objectives. Additionally it should not be forgotten that companion animals live in environments and consume foodstuffs very similar to those of their owners and caretakers.

Overview of Breeding Selection and Reproduction in Small Animals

Selection of Dogs and Cats for Breeding Purposes

Before going into greater detail about potential negative reproductive outcomes and the variables that can adversely affect reproductive function in small animals, including potentially toxic xenobiotics, it is appropriate to briefly review how dogs and cats might be selected for breeding purposes and what is considered normal reproductive function in dogs and cats.[1,2] Reproduction encompasses the wide range of physiologic processes and the associated behaviors and anatomical structures necessary for the birth of the next generation of animals.[1,2,6] As shown in Figure 16-1, reproduction is a dynamic continuum involving precise coordination and integration of the functions of multiple organs, within and between both male and female animals, as well as the conceptus or, in litter-bearing or polytocous species (e.g., dogs and cats), conceptuses.[1,2] The efficient production of viable and functional gametes and their transport and union to form a zygote or zygotes that

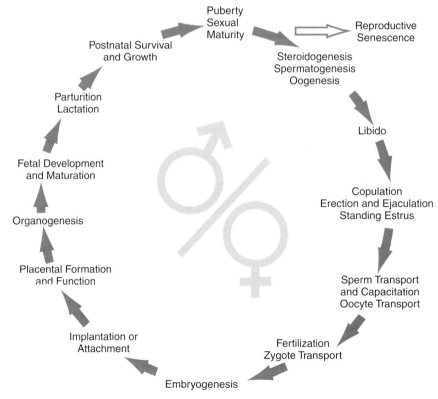

Figure 16-1 The continuum of developmental stages and reproductive functions taking place in males and/or females, as well the embryo and fetus, are shown schematically and illustrate the complexity of reproduction in companion animal species. (Borrowed with permission from Evans TJ: Reproductive toxicity and endocrine disruption. In Gupta RC, editor, *Reproductive and developmental toxicology*, New York, 2011, Academic Press/Elsevier. The artwork is courtesy of Don Connor and Howard Wilson.)

develop into a healthy and fertile individual or a litter of such individuals require that stringent physical, physiologic, and metabolic needs be met in at least three distinct animals (i.e., two parents and their offspring).[1,2,6] Companion animals that are selected for breeding do not always represent the subpopulations that are most likely to reproduce effortlessly. An understanding of which dogs and cats are chosen to breed and what might constitute normal reproductive function for a given species (see Table 16-1) is invaluable in discerning what truly represents abnormal reproductive performance and whether xenobiotics might play a role in decreased reproductive efficiency.

Either because of their own or their offspring's accomplishments, many dogs and cats are likely to be bred when they are older. There is usually some point at which fertility decreases with advancing age (i.e., >6 years in dogs and >7 years in cats).[2,7] Exposures to potential stressors are more likely to be chronic in nature in older animals, and they are also more likely to have preexisting health conditions, the treatment of which can require the administration of medications associated with adverse reproductive effects. In addition, unlike livestock species selected for breeding soundness, many dogs and cats selectively bred by their owners or caretakers often have not had to meet any minimum requirements associated with reproductive performance. These animals are often selected based on their individual qualities, most of which have little to do with potential reproductive performance. Although many of the dogs and cats being selectively bred are very likely to be extremely fertile, non-reproductively based culling and inbreeding have the potential to result in breeding animals predisposed to certain breed-specific conditions and with less than optimal fertility. In addition, many of the primary uses of these animals might not be conducive to reproductive efficiency or are associated with procedures or environments that can diminish fertility. Therefore, although the vast majority of dogs and cats appear to be able to reproduce, or rather overproduce, with amazing efficiency, a subpopulation of these high-performing companion animals from which progeny are desired might actually already be potentially subfertile, resulting in an inherent, increased susceptibility to the adverse effects of various stressors, including certain xenobiotics.[1,2] These individual animals are also more likely to require some form of assisted reproduction or more intensive reproductive management, very likely requiring consultation with a boarded theriogenologist, so as to ensure optimal reproductive performance and the production of offspring. Possible preexisting subfertility, combined with sophisticated reproductive techniques, might remove the cushion provided by surplus sperm in normal ejaculates or the possibility of multiple, potentially fertile ovulations, which can mask subtle xenobiotic-induced abnormalities in reproductive function.

Review of Canine and Feline Reproductive Physiology

Familiarity with canine and feline reproductive physiology is necessary for the early recognition, treatment, and/or prevention of abnormal reproductive function, as well as subtle changes in optimal reproductive efficiency in dogs or cats with traits considered worthy of reproducing.[1,2,6] A full appreciation of the major take-home points of this chapter, with regard to potential negative reproductive outcomes and the primary or secondary role of specific xenobiotics in causing subfertility, requires some familiarity with additional background information specific for these species. It is important to recognize that certain stages of reproduction are more susceptible to the effects of stressors, including xenobiotics, than others (see Fig. 16-1). Early postnatal development, and especially those events leading to puberty, can be adversely affected by exposures to xenobiotics and other stressors, and the multiple replications and differentiation steps inherent to spermatogenesis increase its sensitivity to various toxicants, medications, and thermal stress.[6] The developing embryo and fetus are particularly susceptible to certain types of chemical exposures and infections, both of which are characterized by rapidly multiplying and differentiating populations of cells.[1,2,6] Detailed species-specific information is also valuable if one is using or considering the use of assisted reproductive technologies, which require more intensive reproductive management, especially if the animals they are working with are in less than optimal health and/or already experiencing reproductive difficulties. Furthermore, subtle changes in companion animal reproductive parameters might be the first early indicators of xenobiotic-related risks posed to humans. The essential canine and feline reproductive facts briefly discussed in the sections that follow are summarized in Table 16-1 and are covered in detail in references cited extensively in this chapter.[7-9]

Puberty in the Male Dog and Cat

The testes are generally descended within the scrotum by 6 to 8 weeks of age in both species, but there is usually free mobility within the inguinal canal until the early stages of puberty (see Table 16-1).[8] Species, photoperiod (cats), nutritional status, and environmental factors, as well as stress and disease, can all influence the onset of puberty in male dogs and cats.[6-9] Mature spermatozoa can first appear in the lumina of the seminiferous tubules where they are produced by 6 to 7 months of age in both male dogs and cats.[7] Spermatozoa are usually first noted in the ejaculate by 7 to 9 months of age.[9] However, puberty in the male, most often defined by the ejaculation of threshold amounts of potentially fertile sperm, accompanied by adequate libido and the ability to copulate, and generally takes place during the range of ages shown in Table 16-1 or just slightly earlier in smaller dogs and tom cats.[7,9] There should not be undue concern if some large breed dogs do not satisfy these criteria until after 12 months of age.[9] It also should be remembered that male reproductive performance is not maximized until after puberty, most likely corresponding with peak reproductive performance in females.[6-9]

Compared with the relatively dramatic differences in female reproductive physiology between the bitch and queen, discussed later in this chapter, spermatogenesis and other reproductive processes in the male dog and tom are relatively similar to one another, with more being known about sperm production in the male dog than the tom cat. Spermatozoa are highly specialized haploid cells equipped with a self-powered flagellum to facilitate motility, as well as an acrosome to mediate penetration of the zona pellucida.[6] Spermatogenesis in the male, unlike oogenesis in the female, begins around the time of puberty and continues throughout the lifetime of the male, with possible seasonal influences observed in cats.[6,8] The preovulatory hypothalamic gonadotropin-releasing hormone (GnRH) surge center, which is well developed in the female, is diminished in the male, and the tonic release of GnRH allows for multiple daily gonadotrophic pulses, which facilitate the androgen-dependent endocrine milieu necessary for the maintenance of a population of stem cells and continuous spermatogenesis, as well as the stimulation of typical male sexual behavior.[1,6] Testosterone and its more potent metabolite, 5α-dihydrotestosterone (DHT), are androgenic hormones and the primary gonadal steroids that regulate spermatogenesis.[1,2,6,7] Testosterone is produced by Leydig cells in the interstitium of the testes in response to anterior pituitary luteinizing hormone (LH), as early as 6 months of age.[1,2,6,7,9] Serum concentrations of testosterone increase to adult concentrations by 8 months of age in male dogs, but circulating testosterone concentrations are highly variable because of episodic secretion in the male cat.[9] It also should be noted that the primary role of androgens, normal male reproductive function, including sexual behavior and epididymal sperm maturation and transport, does not occur completely independent of estrogenic influences.[2,7] Sertoli cells, stimulated by follicle-stimulating hormone (FSH), provide the basic architecture for the structure of the seminiferous tubules, and junctional complexes between adjacent Sertoli cells form the blood-testis barrier.[1,6,9]

Canine and Feline Spermatogenesis

Spermatogenesis can be subdivided into three phases or stages referred to as *proliferation* (also called spermatocytogenesis or mitosis), *meiosis*, and *differentiation* (also called spermiogenesis).[1,2,6-9] Each phase involves a different type of germ cell precursor undergoing a different developmental process, and as such these phases have the potential to differ in their susceptibility to the mechanisms of action of various reproductive toxicants.[1,2] The proliferation phase involves mitotic divisions of several generations of spermatogonia (beginning with type A_1 spermatogonia derived from spermatogonial stem cells) to form primary spermatocytes, followed by primary and secondary spermatocytes undergoing meiosis (i.e., division that results in haploid sperm precursors referred to as *round spermatids*) during the meiotic phase.[1,2,6,9] Differentiation is a very specialized stage of spermatogenesis. The haploid round spermatids formed during the meiotic phase are dramatically transformed into elongate spermatids and, subsequently mature spermatozoa or sperm, with newly formed acrosomes, limited cytoplasm, and specialized flagella.[1,2,6,7] Mature spermatozoa are released into the lumen of the seminiferous tubules by a process referred to as *spermiation*, and are transported within the testicular parenchyma, from the seminiferous tubule to the rete testis (rete tubules) and mediastinum, eventually reaching the excurrent or extragonadal duct system for each testis, which consists of the efferent ductules, epididymidis duct, and ductus deferens (vas deferens).[1,6,7,9]

Various distinct associations of spermatogonia, spermatocytes, round, and/or elongate spermatids or mature spermatozoa are referred to as *stages* of the seminiferous epithelium, for which there are eight in both the dog and cat.[1,9,10] These stages repeat in a cyclic manner along a seminiferous tubule, and the earliest type A spermatogonium progresses and transforms through approximately four and a half cycles of the seminiferous epithelium before undergoing spermiation as a mature spermatozoa.[1,6,9,10] The length of each cycle of the seminiferous epithelium dictates that canine spermatogenesis lasts 62 days (i.e., 4.5 × 13.6 = 62 days) and the duration of spermatogenesis in the cat is 46.8 days (i.e., 4.5 × 10.4 = 46.8 days).[7,9,10]

Postgonadal Sperm Maturation and Transport Before and During Copulation

Mature spermatozoa leaving the testis are actually neither motile nor capable of fertilization and undergo further maturation to acquire at least the potential for these capabilities, as well as transport and storage, within the various segments of the epididymal duct (i.e., initial segment, head, body, and tail) before ejaculation.[1,6,7] Epididymal transit is estimated to be approximately 12 days in the male dog, but this length of time is subject to variation, based on frequency of ejaculation, in particular the duration of storage in the tail of the epididymis (see Table 16-1).[7,8] Both male dogs and cats have prostate glands, with cats also having bulbourethral glands, and these accessory sex glands are considered to be primarily androgen dependent.[1,6] The secretions of these glands, as well as those of the epididymal duct or epididymis, are important components of seminal fluid and are required for optimal reproductive performance in the male.[6-9] Adequate libido and female sexual receptivity, as well as sufficient concentrations of testosterone, are necessary for penile erection, which facilitates intromission and ejaculation during copulation.[1,6] Erection of the penis is generally considered to be dependent on parasympathetic neuronal stimulation, whereas the events that lead to emission of the secretions of the accessory sex glands and ejaculation of spermatozoa generally involve both tactile stimuli and stimulation by sympathetic neurons.[1,6,8]

Normal Canine and Feline Ejaculates and Their Evaluation

Although most canine ejaculates contain more than 300×10^6 spermatozoa (see Table 16-1), some references suggest that ejaculates from male dogs can contain slightly fewer spermatozoa (i.e., 200×10^6) and still be quite normal.[7-9] Certainly this is the case with male cats (see Table 16-1), for which there appears to be less information than there is for dogs and in which normal ejaculates, depending on the method of collection, usually contain greater than or equal to 30 (electroejaculation) or greater than or equal to 50×10^6 spermatozoa (artificial vagina).[9] In addition to the information presented in Table 16-1, it should be remembered that usually more than 70% to 80% of ejaculated sperm should be morphologically normal.[5,8,9] However, although baseline information for the "average" male is liable to be very useful, there might be fertile males for which the measured semen parameters fall slightly below these thresholds. In these instances, it is important to know what is normal for that individual and to be aware when there are alterations from those normal thresholds for that particular male.

Appropriately performed assessments of fertility, using semen parameters ± bacterial cultures, hormone concentrations ± gonadotropin response tests, ultrasound examinations, and evaluations of testicular biopsies (initially fixed in Bouin's or modified Davidson's solution), as well as confirmed pregnancy rates and numbers of live offspring born, are critical for monitoring male reproductive function.[1,6-8] Sperm precursors and spermatozoa are extremely sensitive to thermal stress, and testicular thermoregulatory mechanisms and the absence of fever are critical for optimal male reproductive performance (see Table 16-2).[1,6] The approximate duration of less severe, reversible stressor exposures affecting the testes, including those involving thermal stress, and the populations of sperm precursors most susceptible to those exposures, can be evaluated by observing changes in the relative numbers of normal and abnormal spermatozoa in serial ejaculates collected over time.[1,7-9] For severe but reversible thermal or toxic insults to the testes, the duration of both spermatogenesis and epididymal sperm transport (i.e., total of ~74 days in dogs and ~60 days in cats; see Table 16-1) can be used to reasonably estimate when normal spermatozoa might be expected to reappear in ejaculates.[1,7,8] Diminished numbers of normal, motile spermatozoa or the complete absence of any spermatozoa in serial ejaculates from a given male dog or tom cat, persisting beyond this time frame, which is inclusive of spermatogenesis and epididymal transit, are indicators of the severity and irreversibility of stressor-induced damage to the testes.[1,7-9]

Puberty in the Female Dog and Cat

The onset of puberty in the female dog or cat signals the maturation of the hypothalamic preovulatory GnRH surge center, which, as mentioned, is diminished in the male hypothalamus, as well as the final stages in the development of the hypothalamic-pituitary-gonadal (HPG) axis. The mature GnRH surge center and HPG axis both play a role in the initiation and regulation of the cyclic pattern of FSH and LH release from the anterior pituitary gland, which is typical for the female of each of these species.[4] As in the male, animal species, photoperiod, nutritional status, size, breed, and individual variation, as well as stress and disease, can be major determinants of when these endocrine events begin in canine or feline females.[6,8] In female dogs, the occurrence of the first proestrus is the primary indicator of puberty. Puberty generally does not occur until the female reaches at least 80% of mature body weight.[7-9] Females belonging to smaller breeds of dogs generally experience their first proestrus earlier than larger breed females.[6,8] It is not uncommon for some large breed bitches to experience their first proestrus between 18 and 24 months of age and, in some cases, as late as 30 months of age (see Table 16-1).[6-9] Some bitches can experience "silent" heats, especially when they are younger, and the occurrence of these "silent" or unobserved heats can erroneously increase the female's age at what is thought to be the "first" proestrus.[8] The onset of puberty in the queen is similarly influenced by body condition and the attainment of at least 80% of adult body weight.[6,8] However, the occurrence of proestrus is very variable in the queen, and the queen is also dependent on photoperiod (i.e., sufficient day length for the occurrence of her first estrus).[6-9] In most instances, female dogs are not evaluated for cyclicity until 24 months of age and queens not until they are at least 12 months old, unless one is involved in clinical circumstances dealing with multiple smaller dogs or cats, when photoperiod is not a determining factor (see Table 16-1).[9]

Canine and Feline Estrous Cycles and Their Evaluation

Unlike the male, in which gametogenesis begins during the pubertal process and spermatogenesis increases until sexual maturity (peak reproductive age) and remains an ongoing and continuous process, the female is born with all the primary oocytes she is ever going to have in her lifetime.[4,6] These oocytes, which are undergoing nuclear arrest and have not completed the first meiotic division, actually decline in numbers between birth and the onset of puberty.[6] A female's oocytes are arranged in follicles, surrounded by granulosa and thecal cells that are responsible for the synthesis of the gonadal steroids, estradiol (preovulation) and progesterone (postovulation).[1,2,6] In contrast with the general similarities between the reproductive function of the males of these two species, there are notable differences in the reproductive physiology between the bitch and queen.[6] Canine and feline estrous cycles each consist of proestrus, estrus, diestrus, and anestrus, but unlike the bitch, the queen is a seasonally polyestrous, induced or reflex ovulator, with coitus required for, but not guaranteeing, sufficient LH secretion for ovulation of secondary oocytes.[6,7] Because ovulation might not necessarily occur and, unlike the bitch, because another estrus will be occurring in a matter of days rather than months, some references have assigned the queen another stage of the estrous cycle referred to as *postestrus* or the nonestrous or interestrous interval, which is distinct from the interestrous interval described for dogs.[6-9] Estrogen (estradiol) is the primary gonadal steroid produced by ovarian follicles during proestrus and estrus, and progesterone is the primary gonadal steroid produced following ovulation and during diestrus, when the female is neither attractive nor receptive to males.

Most dog breeds, unlike cats, are not seasonal breeders. Most dogs can have their annual estrus and produce puppies throughout the year, with subtle peaks in cyclicity and whelping noted during the late winter/early spring and possibly fall.[8] Following puberty and depending on the breed of dog, proestrus generally occurs every 7 months in most females (4 to 4.5 months for German shepherds; every 12 months for Basenjis).[6,8] The time between the end of one estrus and the start of the next proestrus is referred to as the *interestrous* interval, and its duration is extremely variable among individuals.[6-9] Similarly, the lengths of the various stages of the canine estrous cycle differ a great deal among individual dogs, but are often consistent for a given bitch during her period of optimal reproductive function, between 2 and 6 years of age.[9] The durations of these various stages are shown in Table 16-1.[6,8,9] The female dog is unique in that, unlike females of other species, such as the queen, the bitch ovulates primary rather than secondary oocytes (preovulatory LH surge very early in estrus), and there is a longer than usual interval between the completion of ovulation and fertilization (~2 or 3 to possibly almost 6 days after ovulation; almost immediately to 1 day after ovulation in most other species), as well as the beginning of diestrus, based on vaginal cytology.[6,7,9] In addition, the female dog is, surprisingly, usually in standing heat and being bred in an unusual endocrine milieu, where circulating concentrations of estradiol are decreasing and those of progesterone are increasing above 1.5 ng/mL^{-1}, coincident with the preovulatory LH surge.[6,7-9] Diestrus in the bitch usually lasts about 60 days with or without pregnancy, followed by several months of anestrus.[6,8,9] Changes in female behavior, the gross appearance of any vaginal discharge, hormone concentrations, the results of vaginoscopic and digital examinations, as well as cultures, and especially, cytologic characteristics of vaginal smears can be used to distinguish the stages of the estrous cycle from one another to evaluate any suspected irregularities.[7-9] General trends for delayed onset of puberty, especially in smaller breeds of dogs, and excessively short or long interestrous intervals in multiple females might warrant evaluation of factors, such as management, animal health, genetics, nutrition, and/or possible xenobiotic exposures that might influence the occurrence or detection of normal estrous cycles.

Feline reproductive physiology is obviously very different from that of dogs. Cats are polyestrous, long-day breeders. Estrous cycles in the average queen, between the optimal breeding ages of 1.5 and 7 years, occur between February and October in the Northern hemisphere.[7,8] Likewise, cats in the Northern hemisphere generally experience anestrus from October through December or, occasionally, January.[7-9] Males are attracted to nonreceptive females during proestrus.[6,8] However, many cats do not clearly exhibit this stage of the estrous cycle.[8,9] It is simplest to view the queen as having polyestrous breeding seasons, in which repeating periods of estrus characterized by sexual receptivity are associated with recurring follicular phases.[8] However, the association between periods of sexual receptivity and follicular activity does not necessarily represent a 1:1 ratio in the queen.[7-9] On the average, estrus behavior lasts longer than the corresponding follicular phase.[8] In fact, distinct waves of follicular development, maturation, and degeneration, as indicated physiologically by elevated blood estradiol concentrations, might occur during what appears to be only one estrus.[6-9] Estrous behavior usually lasts 7 days (range of 1-21 days) and, somewhat counterintuitively, is actually usually of longer duration (8.5 vs 6 days) if there is coitus, plus or minus ovulation, than in the absence of coital contact.[8] As mentioned, feline ovulation of secondary oocytes (not primary, as in the dog) requires sexual contact for the preovulatory LH surge and formation of progesterone-secreting ovarian luteal structures or corpora lutea.[6-9] Unlike the female dog, the duration of diestrus in the queen is dependent on the presence or absence of at least one conceptus and the secretion of progesterone of most likely placental origin (see Table 16-1).[8,9] Postestrus or interestrus, which occurs when there is estrus without ovulation, lasts 8 to 10 or 8 to 15 days.[7,9] It also should be noted that pregnant queens frequently experience lactational anestrus, which generally resolves 14 to 60 days after weaning.[7] The onset of reproductive abnormalities can be difficult to monitor and rather insidious, especially when owners and caretakers are inexperienced in breeding cats. It is important to recognize that general trends for estrous cycle irregularities in multiple queens might warrant evaluation of factors such as photoperiod, management, animal health, genetics, nutrition, and/or possible xenobiotic exposures, which might influence the occurrence or detection of normal estrous cycles. As in the bitch, changes in blood hormone concentrations and especially cytologic characteristics of vaginal smears and culture results can be used to distinguish the stages of the queen's estrous cycle from one another and evaluate any suspected irregularities.[7-9]

Canine and Feline Gestational Length

Pregnancy begins at the time of fertilization in the uterine or fallopian tubes of the female, and ends at the time of parturition. Progesterone is necessary for pregnancy maintenance, and gestational sources of progesterone are summarized in Table 16-1.[6-9] Because the female dog ovulates primary oocytes, which can be viable for approximately 9 to 10 days, and canine spermatozoa are usually viable for as long as approximately 7, and for some male dogs, up to 9 to 11 days (fresh semen) in the female reproductive tract, the length of gestation in the bitch, if calculated from the first mating, can vary widely (i.e., 56-72 days).[7-9] Likewise, in the queen gestational length can range from 56 to 69 days (some references suggest 52-74 days) after the first breeding because coitus does not necessarily guarantee ovulation.[8,9] Therefore, it should be evident that gestational length, as defined using the first, potentially fertile mating, is not a consistent parameter on which to evaluate changes in canine or feline reproductive efficiency.[7,8] On the other hand, knowing the precise timing of the canine preovulatory LH surge, ovulation, and/or the first day of diestrus, the due date for a given bitch can be predicted fairly accurately as 65 ± 1 days after the preovulatory LH surge, 63 ± 1 days after ovulation, 60 ± 1 days after fertilization, and 56 to 58 days after the first day of diestrus (see Table 16-1).[7-9] Similarly, feline gestation lasts 63 to 66 after the initial rise in blood progesterone concentration, which correlates fairly well with ovulation.[7]

Canine Prenatal Development

In the dog, prenatal development of what begins as a zygote, after fertilization of an oocyte by a single sperm, can be divided into three distinct periods, denoted as the *period of the ovum* (days 3-17 after ovulation), the *period of the embryo* (days 18-32 after ovulation), and the *period of the fetus* (days 33 to ~63 after ovulation; see Table 16-1).[11] During the *period of the ovum*, an actively dividing cluster of cells reaches the uterotubal junction (~days 10 to 13 after ovulation; ~7-10 days after fertilization) and enters into the uterus at the 16-cell, morula, or possibly, the blastocyst stage of development (see Table 16-1).[6,11] From days 10 to 15 postovulation, free-floating blastocysts migrate within the uterus, including the uterine horn on the opposite side of the uterine tube from which they emerged.[11] Before fixation and implantation (not the same as "true" implantation described in primates and rodents) approximately 15 to 17 days after ovulation, these blastocysts distribute themselves uniformly within the uterine horns.[1,2,6,8,11] The *period of the embryo* corresponds to germ layer formation, a cephalocaudal sequence of organogenesis (which is particularly susceptible to the effects of nonendocrine disrupting teratogens), and finally, the development of the extraembryonic membranes and zonary, endotheliochorial placentation.[6,7,9,11] Other than a heartbeat detectable by postovulatory days 21 to 22, there is little discernible canine anatomy before the 28th day after ovulation. However, by the beginning of the *period of the fetus* on day 33 after ovulation, the conceptus is clearly recognizable as being canine.[7-9,11] Many of the key events occurring during the fetal stage have to do with sexual differentiation (which is very sensitive to the teratogenic effects of endocrine-disrupting xenobiotics), fetal growth, and the initiation of parturition.[6,11] By approximately the 34th day after ovulation of multiple primary oocytes, the Y chromosome–controlled testis determining factor has facilitated the transformation of a sexually indifferent gonad into a testis.[1,6,11] Secretion of Müllerian inhibiting substance by differentiated Sertoli cells in the testis cause the regression of the precursors of the female tubular genitalia.[1,6] Testosterone production by fetal Leydig cells, as well as the subsequent synthesis of DHT from testosterone, results in the sequential, androgen-induced formation of the epididymides and ductus deferentes (testosterone) and finally the prostate, penile urethra, penis, and scrotum (DHT).[1,6,11]

Feline Prenatal Development

Although overly simplistic to some investigators, who prefer to view mammalian gestational development in terms of 10+ stages (up to 22 in some references), prenatal life in the cat, like that in the dog, can be also subdivided into the *period of the ovum*, the *period of the embryo*, and finally, the *period of the fetus*.[11,12] Likewise, much of what occurs in feline prenatal development is very similar to what is observed in dogs; however, there are several notable exceptions, particularly with respect to timing of several specific events.[8,12] Fertilized feline ova or zygotes usually can be observed within the oviducts by 20 to 28 hours after coitus.[12] Unlike canine blastocysts, which take longer to develop after ovulation of primary oocytes and fertilization, feline embryos generally enter the uterus, as morulae or even blastocysts, approximately 5 (morulae) to 6 days (blastocysts) after ovulation of secondary oocytes and fertilization, which generally occur within hours of each other in this species if sperm are present (see Table 16-1).[7-9,12] Feline blastocysts (8+ days) are assumed to be free-floating and mobile until approximately 13 to 14 days after ovulation and fertilization, when they appear uniformly spaced within the uterine horns and fixation and trophoblastic attachment (i.e., implantation) take place.[6,8,12] The embryo proper is identifiable by high resolution ultrasonography at this stage of embryogenesis. Formation of the fetal heart (with a detectable heartbeat) and neural tube development can be noted by approximately day 17 after fertilization.[7] By day 28 after ovulation/fertilization the developing embryo has completed organogenesis and is clearly identifiable as a fetal feline (see Table 16-1).[7,12] Between 32 and 38 days after ovulation, the Müllerian duct regresses in the male feline fetus, with the testicular formation well under way, and a penis is identifiable in these individuals by days 44 to 48 days postovulation.[12]

Physiology of Parturition and Lactation

Although less well-defined than in ruminants, maturation of the fetal HPA axis and the appropriately timed release of cortisol by the fetus play key roles in initiating the cascade of events leading to parturition, under normal physiologic circumstances.[1,2,6] This cascade of physiologic events essentially involves a cortisol-induced decline in the placental progesterone/estrogen ratio (i.e., progesterone converted to estrogen) and the release of prostaglandins $F_{2\alpha}$, leading to myometrial contractions, luteolysis, cervical stimulation, and the release of oxytocin and relaxin.[4,7] It should be evident that pregnancy maintenance and parturition can both be dramatically affected by any factors that affect circulating concentration of cortisol. The fetal membranes are deciduate in both dogs and cats, and they are either shed soon after the delivery of each fetus or as several sets of fetal membranes shed together after the delivery of their corresponding fetuses.[6-9] Litter size is highly variable in dogs and cats (i.e., range of 1 to 16+ in dogs; range of 1-10 in cats) and is generally dependent on the size of the mother (i.e., larger females and larger breeds having larger litters).[7-9] It is advisable for owners and caretakers to know what is normal for a given breed of dog or cat, as well as for a given female that has previously given birth. Lactogenesis or the initiation of lactation (i.e., milk synthesis and secretion by the mammary glands) occurs in two stages and is essential for neonatal survival in all mammalian species in the absence of human intervention. The first stage of lactogenesis involves cytologic and enzymatic differentiation within the mammary glands. The second stage of lactogenesis corresponds to copious secretion of all the components of milk and is dependent on changes in blood concentrations of progesterone, estrogen (estradiol), and especially, prolactin. Unlike ruminants, pregnant dogs and cats do not secrete placental lactogens, which have growth hormone- and prolactin-like effects. Prolactin synthesis and secretion by adenohy-pophysial lactotropes is regulated in large part by hypothalamic dopamine-mediated tonic inhibition. Decreasing blood progesterone concentrations, especially with increasing concentrations of estradiol, act on the hypothalamus and adenohypophysis to overcome the tonic inhibition of prolactin secretion, resulting in elevations in blood concentrations of prolactin. The maintenance of milk synthesis and secretion, also referred to as *galactopoiesis*, is dependent on prolactin secretion in dogs and cats, as opposed to growth hormone in cattle.[1,2]

Diagnosis and Evaluation of Pregnancy and Fetal Health

Canine and feline pregnancies can be diagnosed and monitored by a number of different methods, including abdominal palpation and various forms of ultrasound, endocrine assays, and radiographs.[7-9,11,12] Although progesterone concentrations likely will not be different between pregnant and non-pregnant animals during diestrus (depending on the circumstances, referred to as physiological or clinical pseudopregnancy), relaxin is pregnancy-specific in the bitch and queen.[7] Real-time, B-mode ultrasonography can be very useful in assessing embryonic loss and fetal viability and growth, as well as movement and even fetal stress, and tocodynamometry can be used to monitor premature myometrial contractions.[7-9,11,12] It also should be remembered that puppies and kittens, unlike the offspring of domestic livestock species, are not precocious and are completely dependent on their mothers and, in some breeds of dogs and cats, their owners and caretakers to ensure the delivery and survival of offspring.[7] Instances of fetal or neonatal death should be investigated in an extremely timely manner on, ideally, fetuses or neonates kept refrigerated or on ice packs (not frozen, if possible). Necropsy examinations (gross and microscopic) should include the fetal membranes from abortions or stillbirths and should be performed by a veterinarian or ideally a board-certified pathologist. Appropriate ancillary testing for infectious and parasitic diseases, as well as possibly exposures to toxicants also should be performed on properly collected and stored samples.

Negative Reproductive Outcomes and Potential Xenobiotic-Related Mechanisms of Action

Delayed puberty and estrous cycle abnormalities, impaired gametogenesis, inability to copulate, anovulatory follicles, cystic endometrial hyperplasia, pyometra, conception failure, embryonic death, teratogenesis, abortions and stillbirths, and agalactia are all negative reproductive outcomes that can have devastating effects on the various key steps involved in companion animal reproduction (see Fig. 16-1).[1,4,5,7-9,13] All of these negative reproductive outcomes can arise either from direct effects of the xenobiotic on the reproductive tract or, probably more likely, indirectly where impaired reproductive function arises from adverse effects on other organs or functions initially targeted by xenobiotics.[13]

Pathogenesis of Xenobiotic-Induced Negative Reproductive Outcomes

Direct Effects of Xenobiotics on Reproduction

An attempt to understand the basic mechanism of xenobiotic exposure-related reproductive abnormalities can be extremely useful in improving reproductive management and, ultimately, reproductive performance.[1,13] Sexual reproduction requires copulation at the appropriate time and the union of a normal ovum of female origin with a functionally mature sperm cell produced by the male. In natural breeding situations, male animals must be able to detect sexually receptive females in estrus and successfully introduce adequate numbers of spermatozoa into the female reproductive tract, generally before ovulation.[1,6,13] These accomplishments on the part of the male are necessary for induced ovulation to occur in felines and to ensure that enough normal motile sperm cells are transported to the female's uterine tubes for one healthy spermatozoa to be available and able to fertilize each viable ovum, which is transported to the site of fertilization.[1,2,4-6,13] Many xenobiotics have

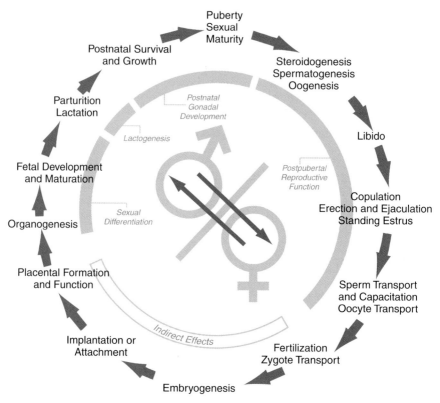

Figure 16-2 The continuum of developmental stages and reproductive functions, which or directly or indirectly susceptible to the effects of endocrine disrupting chemicals or compounds (EDCs), are shown schematically. (Borrowed with permission from Evans TJ: Reproductive toxicity and endocrine disruption. In Gupta RC, editor, *Reproductive and developmental toxicology*, New York, 2011, Academic Press/Elsevier. The artwork is courtesy of Don Connor and Howard Wilson.)

the potential to mimic or antagonize the effects of estrogens or androgens or, in some other way, including alterations in hormone synthesis and secretion, metabolism, and excretion, interfere with or disrupt normal endocrine function (i.e., endocrine disruption).[1,13,14] Reproduction, by its very nature, is dependent on normal biologic signaling mechanisms, including neurologic and endocrine or hormonal functions. As shown in Figure 16-2, the onset of puberty, female cyclicity, oogenesis and spermatogenesis, libido, conception, uterine function and placental formation, normal embryonic and fetal development, parturition, and lactation are all directly or indirectly susceptible to the effects of endocrine disrupting chemicals (EDCs) or compounds, which also can be referred to as hormonally active agents (HAAs).[1,14] Hormonally active xenobiotics, which alter the normal endocrine events associated with oogenesis, spermatogenesis, and the development and function of the tubular genitalia in females and the epididymal ducts and accessory glands in males, can adversely affect reproductive function.[1,2,4,5,13] Sperm transport within the female reproductive tract can be impaired by exposure to xenoestrogens of plant origin (i.e., phytoestrogens), and normal lactogenesis can be inhibited by the D_2 dopamine receptor agonists found in ergotized grains, both of which are examples of naturally occurring endocrine disruption.[1,2,13-16]

Some of the most devastating negative reproductive outcomes in dogs and cats involve abnormal fetal development, as well as prenatal and/or neonatal mortality. It is generally recognized that the embryo and fetus are the stages of life that are most sensitive to the adverse effects of most xenobiotics.[1,2,13,14] Although the placenta has traditionally been represented as an effective "barrier" to harmful chemicals and infectious agents, many if not most xenobiotics and microorganisms can cross the placenta by simple diffusion, which is primarily dependent on molecular size and solubility.[1,2,6,14] Teratogenesis can be characterized by embryonic or fetal mortality, structural or functional abnormalities, and/or alterations in birth weight.

Indirect Effects of Xenobiotics on Reproduction

Optimal reproductive function is dependent on overall animal well-being. Therefore, it should not be surprising that xenobiotics can indirectly cause adverse effects on reproductive performance by directly "targeting" other, nonreproductive organ systems or functions that affect reproduction. Induction of stress is one way in which xenobiotics can indirectly cause adverse effects on several reproductive processes. In many species, the amplitude of the pulsatile release of LH can be greatly reduced by glucocorticoids.[1,2,6,13,17] If prolonged, this effect has the potential to impact the release of gonadal steroids (i.e., estrogens and androgens) in sexually mature animals.[1,2] In addition, as mentioned, appropriately timed release of cortisol by the fetus plays an important role in initiating the cascade of events leading to parturition, under normal physiologic circumstances.[1,2,6] "Systemic" intoxications interpreted as life threatening by homeostatic mechanisms within the dam and/or fetus, such as maternal and/or fetal hypoxia, can trigger a stress response, activating the maternal and/or fetal HPA axis, and contribute to premature parturition or abortion in dogs and cats.[7-9]

Xenobiotic exposures also can indirectly affect reproductive function by decreasing body condition, which is another determinant of reproductive performance.[1,2] Male and female animals generally must be healthy and not debilitated and have sufficient fat stores to ensure adequate libido and successful copulation between fertile males and sexually receptive females.[1,2,6] Puberty in both males and females and normal female estrous cycles are extremely dependent on sufficient energy stores and body condition.[6] Initial adverse effects on reproductive function related to decreasing body condition will most likely reflect that there are not adequate energy reserves for optimal reproductive efficiency. Severe depletion of fat stores and drastic changes in body condition can have additional negative effects on reproductive function by inducing stress through the activation of the HPA axis. Any of the aforementioned factors that influence exposure to sufficient artificial or natural light can also dramatically diminish reproductive efficiency in cats because of effects involving photoperiod.

It should be evident by now how xenobiotic-related effects on nonreproductive organs or functions can manifest themselves as abnormal reproductive outcomes. In fact, in some instances, impaired reproductive performance in dogs and cats regularly used for breeding might be the first indicator of altered well-being and health in these individual animals. This will be especially true if a particular xenobiotic's direct effects on the primary target organ are subclinical because they are not obvious or have not been diagnosed. Stress can diminish the numbers of extra spermatozoa present in an ejaculate, and likewise decrease the number of potentially fertile ovulations. Excessive endogenous or exogenous glucocorticoids can also negatively affect the survivability of some neonates, thereby removing factors that might mask subtle changes in reproductive performance.

Single Etiology/Multifactorial Causes of Negative Reproductive Outcomes

Primary versus Contributory Roles of Xenobiotics in Abnormal Reproductive Function

One of the purposes of this chapter is to discuss the possible primary and secondary roles (or, alternatively, sole and contributory involvement) of xenobiotics in diminished reproductive performance in small animal species. Although impaired reproductive function can have a single, diagnosable, toxic etiology (i.e., the proverbial smoking gun), the precise causes of diminished reproductive efficiency in dogs and cats, like those in livestock species, are more often nutritional, environmental, or infectious in nature or, alternatively, extremely difficult to distinguish and therefore probably multifactorial in many instances.[1,13] This seems to be particularly true in clinical situations in which the observed reproductive abnormalities are indirect effects of stress arising from metabolic diseases, failures of major organs, or malnutrition caused by xenobiotics in combination with a variety of other possible etiologies. Consequently, cases of subfertility, especially those without any known or apparent etiology, very likely have multiple causes involving various predisposing factors and/or stressors, including potentially toxic xenobiotics.[13] It is important to understand how these factors and stressors might interact with one another to cause reproductive inefficiency.

Predisposing Factors and Stressors

Enzootic Physiologic or Genetic Factors

A number of predisposing factors and stressors are generally enzootic in nature because they are inherent to a given individual, a particular animal species or breed, a given use, and/or a specific geographical location (Fig. 16-3). Enzootic physiologic or genetic predisposing factors can influence reproductive function or interact with each other and/or with various types of stressors to impact reproduction (see Table 16-2).[13] Certain individuals, because of physiologic factors, might be predisposed to a disease or syndrome, such as Cushing syndrome, hypo- or hyperthyroidism, or diabetes mellitus, which in some ways negatively affects reproduction.[8] Certain stages of embryonic and fetal development, when key structures are forming or important functions are being acquired, are much more susceptible to stressor-induced alterations than other aspects of embryonic or fetal development.[1,2,11,12,14] Physiologic or species-specific predispositions to certain intoxications in dogs and cats might also include the potentially indiscriminant eating habits of many dogs, the relative lack of Phase II metabolism in an animal, glucuronidation conjugation pathways in cats (e.g., enhanced acetaminophen toxicity), and the potential for cystic endometrial hyperplasia and, potentially, pyometra in both dogs and cats.[1,7-9] Non-purebred dogs and cats exhibit hybrid vigor, which can be observed in some reproductive traits and overall fertility.[7,9] Some breeds of dogs and cats are more susceptible to certain metabolic diseases and neoplasias, and brachycephalic breeds in particular are frequently bred with the intent of delivering the puppies or kittens by elective cesarean section.[7-9]

Enzootic Nutritional, Environmental, Infectious, and/or Toxic Stressors

Similar to the aforementioned physiologic and genetic predispositions, a variety of nutritional, environmental, infectious, and/or toxic stressors can also, either alone or through multifactorial interactions, influence reproductive performance (see Table 16-2 and Fig. 16-3). As mentioned, it is well recognized that inadequate nutrition can delay puberty, cause irregular estrous cycles, and/or adversely affect pregnancy rates (see Table 16-2).[1,6-9] Nutritional deficiencies can also impair immune function, making animals more susceptible to infections that can affect reproduction.[4,13] Spermatogenesis and, to a lesser degree, oogenesis are sensitive to elevations in body temperature.[1,6,13] Suboptimal environmental conditions can affect reproductive function in multiple ways by impairing sperm production or decreasing libido in both males and females. Environmental factors can also predispose animals to exposures to various infectious agents or parasites, which can negatively affect canine and feline reproduction. The mechanisms by which bacteria, viruses, and parasites can impair reproduction include stress, physical debilitation, and the release of pyrogens (e.g., endotoxin), as well as specific effects on the reproductive tract, including the conceptus (e.g., pyometra, orchitis, and/or colonization or infection of the developing embryo, fetus, or placenta).[1,7-9,13,17]

As discussed, various xenobiotics, some of them enzootic in nature, can diminish reproductive performance either directly or indirectly. Mycotoxins, which are secondary fungal metabolites produced within cereal grains or other substrates, under specific growth

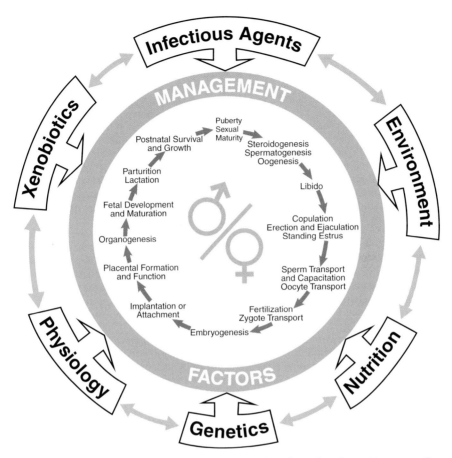

Figure 16-3 The possible influences of genetic and physiological predispositions, as well as nutritional, environmental, infectious, and, especially, toxic stressors, on decreased reproductive performance, are shown schematically. The role that management can play in modulating those influences on reproductive function is also illustrated. (Borrowed with permission from Evans TJ: Diminished reproductive performance and selected toxicants in forages and grains. *Vet Clin North Am Food Anim Pract* 27(2):345, 2011. The artwork is courtesy of Don Connor and Howard Wilson.)

conditions, can contaminate pet foods and cause many of the same direct or indirect adverse reproductive effects in dogs and cats as they do in livestock species and possibly humans. These mycotoxins might play a primary role or, probably more likely with lower concentrations, contribute to multifactorial causes of impaired reproductive function (see Table 16-2 and Fig. 16-3).[1,13] Similarly, by virtue of the way small animals are often selected for breeding purposes, offspring might be desired from older animals with chronic diseases, including neoplasia or metabolic diseases, which require treatment with xenobiotics known to adversely affect reproduction.

The relative role of mycotoxins, medications, and other xenobiotics in decreased reproductive efficiency is often determined in large part by the size of the dose and the duration of exposure.[1,13] Exposure to a high dose of a given xenobiotic suggests that the xenobiotic might very likely play a potentially primary role in causing the observed adverse reproductive effect, even if organ systems other than those immediately involved in reproductive function are more severely or directly affected by a given xenobiotic. On the other hand, an exposure involving a lesser but still potentially relevant dose of the xenobiotic could suggest the possibility that the xenobiotic most likely played a contributory role in the observed negative reproductive outcome. In this instance, other stressors also played a part in impairing reproductive performance, regardless of whether reproductive function was directly or indirectly targeted.[13] Somewhat more challenging for interpretation is the role played by a xenobiotic in an observed reproductive problem when the dose of the xenobiotic is relatively low but the duration of exposure is chronic in nature. The reproductive tract might be directly targeted by a given xenobiotic. On the other hand, there might very likely be a target organ or function other than the reproductive tract that is affected directly by a given xenobiotic. Under these circumstances, the direct toxic effects on the primary target organ might be subclinical in nature, already resolved, or simply not of major interest and, therefore not obvious at first glance. The first observed abnormalities caused by a particular xenobiotic exposure might actually be subfertility, as evidenced by abnormalities in semen quality, decreased diagnosed pregnancy rates, or number of live offspring delivered per litter, and/ or other negative reproductive outcomes. Alternatively, there might be multiple stressors involved in this scenario, with each playing some part in either specifically targeting various aspects of reproductive function (i.e., direct effects on reproductive organs or function) or debilitating the exposed animal (i.e., indirect reproductive effects because of stress, malaise, decreased body condition, or systemic illness), or even possibly a combination of direct and indirect reproductive effects caused by multiple predisposing factors and/or stressors.

The estimated exposure dose for a given xenobiotic exposure always must be taken into consideration when determining the cause or causes of a reproductive problem. On the other hand, it is important when there is no smoking gun or an obvious single cause of diminished reproductive performance to take an integrated approach and objectively evaluate the relative contributions of a wide variety of variables to the apparent reproductive problems. Multiple predisposing factors and stressors, including toxicants, plus possible contributions of interactions involving these variables and even management can all have adverse effects on fertility (see Fig. 16-3).[1,13]

The Importance of Management Factors to Optimize Reproductive Efficiency

Management constitutes an important interface between enzootic predisposing factors and/ or stressors and the ultimate goal of optimal reproductive performance (see Fig. 16-3).[13] Management can maximize reproductive efficiency or, conversely, augment the adverse reproductive effects of the predisposing factors and stressors inherent to a given situation.[1,7-9,13] Artificial insemination (AI) of chilled semen and cryopreserved semen has become relatively routine in canine reproduction. Although semen collection in cats is not nearly as easy as the method of digital manipulation commonly used in dogs, electroejaculation, artificial vaginas, and urethral catheterization techniques are all means by which adequate numbers of spermatozoa can be collected for AI in felines.[7-9] Vaginal deposition and nonsurgical transcervical or surgical insemination directly into the uterus or, with surgery, the uterine horns or uterotubal junctions, using chilled or cryopreserved semen, involve relatively low numbers of sperm already stressed by cooling and especially freezing and thawing, as well as limited opportunities for insemination.[7-9,13] In addition, in vitro fertilization (IVF) and cloning techniques have also been used successfully in dogs and cats.[7] In all of these assisted reproductive technologies, the large room for error or tolerance for errors or exposures to stressors, which are inherent to companion animal breeding when healthy males deposit millions of surplus, normal, progressively motile spermatozoa into the reproductive tract of fertile females ovulating multiple viable ova, can be greatly diminished by the use of advanced reproductive methods without appropriate training and attention to detail. This observation is especially true when individual animals with preexisting suboptimal fertility are selected for breeding purposes by relatively inexperienced owners or caretakers.

Management Factors

The following management factors can have the greatest impact on reproductive efficiency:[13]

1. Type of breeding colony, breeding selection criteria, and owner and/or caretaker expectations
2. Knowledge and experience with animal husbandry, health care, and reproductive management
3. Understanding of causes of suboptimal reproductive performance in small animals
4. Quality of nutrition relative to physiologic demands
5. Supervision and veterinary participation in health and reproductive management
6. Prophylactic measures for common infectious agents and contagious diseases and parasites
7. Structure and hygiene of facilities, especially during prenatal and neonatal periods
8. Pre-breeding examinations of males and females and semen evaluation at each collection
9. Appropriately timed breeding, insemination, pregnancy diagnosis, and monitoring
10. Adequate surveillance and assistance during parturition and early neonatal period

Implications of Management Factors 1 to 5

Just as in large animal production systems, small animal breeding colonies must be of a size and scope of operation that is appropriate for the levels of knowledge and experience and infrastructure available to adequately manage the individual animals that have been selected for reproductive purposes. Within reason and practicality, it can be argued that the reproductive efficiency and ultimate success of a breeding colony depend on Management Factor 1 to set the bar for what is required for Management Factors 2 to 5, which in turn are the major determinants of Management Factors 6 to 10. In other words, the type of breeding colony (i.e., size, location, species, breed, animal use), along with breeding selection criteria and owner/caretaker expectations, determine the necessary levels of knowledge and practical husbandry skills as well as the amount of participation by a veterinary professional, which essentially dictate the requirements for facilities and hygiene, pre-breeding screening procedures, reproductive management, pre- and post-parturient husbandry considerations for the bitch and queen, and neonatal and postnatal puppy and kitten care.[13]

Stated somewhat differently, all of the Management Factors for a specific breeding colony *must* be consistent with and compatible for one another for that particular operation to be successful in the eyes of the owner or caretakers. For example, a very large breeding operation, with high breeder/caretaker expectations, will require more expertise and supervision, as well as intense health and reproductive management and ongoing veterinary involvement, than a small breeding colony. High levels of expertise, supervision, and intense management, in turn, will necessitate up-to-date prophylaxis for common puppy and kitten diseases, well-managed and pristine facilities, routine pre-breeding examinations, including semen evaluations for males, and carefully monitored pregnancies and parturitions. All of the preceding steps, which essentially represent the ideal situation for large-scale production scenarios, should result in a maximum number of weaned, healthy puppies or kittens, *and*, especially if these offspring meet expectations, owner/caretaker satisfaction. This particular model, particularly if state-of-the-art assisted reproductive techniques are used, is obviously going to require individuals with extensive training and experience, possibly even animal reproductive specialists (i.e., theriogenologists), and potentially significant capital investment and labor costs, to meet the attendant high expectations.[13]

Although the aforementioned large-scale example is undoubtedly a bit unrealistic for most situations, it nevertheless illustrates several principles that are most commonly discussed in the context of large animal production settings. The general tendency to think that bigger, newer, and more modern always equate to improved reproductive function and greater breeding success can lead to poor management decisions that can precipitate animal health concerns and subfertility, as well as unfulfilled expectations and owner/caretaker frustration. The scale of a breeding operation must be compatible with the amount of management expertise necessary *and* available to ensure that basic animal husbandry requirements are met and animals selected for breeding can successfully produce sufficient numbers of satisfactory progeny.[13] Small animal owners and caretakers accustomed to the almost effortless procreation associated with most dogs and cats in a casual and more natural setting can be unprepared for the efforts sometimes required to produce offspring from certain exceptional individuals. Advanced assisted reproductive techniques and the skills of reproductive specialists are best used when there is appropriate management and supervision to compensate for the diminished wiggle room attendant to the reduced numbers of sperm and fewer opportunities for insemination associated with these methods.[7-9,13] Owners and caretakers also need to have realistic expectations for potential reproductive success, given the age and health of animals being bred and husbandry-related factors, such as nutritional status, parasite control, and facility cleanliness.

Management Practices to Identify and/or Prevent Impaired Reproductive Function

Subtle abnormalities in male reproductive performance, possibly related to xenobiotic exposures, will be more evident and caught earlier in well-managed colonies in which male dogs or even cats are being collected regularly for AI using fresh, chilled, or frozen-thawed semen. These assisted reproductive procedures require routine semen evaluations to quickly detect unsatisfactory collections which do not meet specific criteria and generally use lower numbers of sperm for insemination doses, thereby increasing the likelihood that decreased reproductive efficiency will be evident. Suboptimal semen quality can result in collections unsuitable for further use, decreased diagnosed pregnancy rates, or fewer than anticipated puppies or kittens per litter. Adequate management of breeding males should not only involve appropriate health care, including pre-breeding tests (e.g., *Brucella canis* in dogs), vaccinations, and deworming, routine semen evaluations, and proper semen handling procedures, but also satisfactory health and semen collection records.

Likewise, diminished female reproductive efficiency associated with exposures to various xenobiotics is most evident in well-managed colonies when bitches or queens are being bred, either naturally or by AI, on a regular basis. Similar reproductive problems observed in multiple females, which are managed in the same breeding colony environment or in close proximity, give added credence to the possibility of xenobiotic-related subfertility. Suspect xenobiotics might be contaminants in the diet, an administered medication, or even some chemical in the animals' immediate surroundings, which directly or indirectly play a primary or secondary causative role in less than optimal female reproductive efficiency. Each female's general health and well-being (e.g., *Brucella canis* testing for dogs; vaccination and deworming histories), stage of each female's estrous cycle, timing and frequency of breeding, subsequent pregnancy status, litter size, and birth weights should be appropriately determined and/or monitored and recorded to optimize female reproductive performance.

Adequate reproductive management of companion animals also requires satisfactory record keeping pertaining to health, as well as to reproduction. Depending on the size of the breeding colony, special emphasis should be given to recording any observed changes in individual animal attitude or behavior, any suspected illnesses, all medications administered and chemicals used for environmental pest control or disinfection, shipments or purchase of pet food diets fed to breeding animals (including tags with lot numbers), and most important, variations in routine semen evaluation parameters, estrous cyclicity, pregnancy rates, and numbers of live offspring born. All of this recorded information can be used to evaluate alterations in indices of reproductive performance and temporally related changes in health status, diet, and other factors or even stressors in the animal's environment.

Xenobiotics that temporarily impair spermatogenesis can affect semen quality for up to the total length of spermatogenesis and epididymal sperm transport (see Table 16-1). One-time exposure to teratogens at any one of multiple critical points during especially embryonic or fetal development can have devastating consequences (see Table 16-1). Nonessential xenobiotic exposures should be avoided, if at all possible, when animals are being bred or collected on a regular basis or when they are pregnant or lactating. Deworming procedures to minimize prenatal or perinatal parasitic exposure that can be very detrimental to the neonatal health would definitely be considered *essential*, particularly if such infections have historically been a problem. Breeding facilities should not contain lead-containing pipes or paint. Medications should be administered only if they are absolutely necessary to maintain animal health and survival. Pesticides must only be used in areas and for purposes for which they are explicitly labeled. If applicable, dilution and spraying instructions should be strictly followed. Regardless of whether the chemical is considered safe, if the person using the pesticide is required to wear specialized personal protection equipment (PPE), then animals and containers used for feeding and watering should be removed from the areas that are being treated. Owners and caretakers, particularly those responsible for larger numbers of animals, in which commercial diets are more likely to be bought in larger quantities and consist of a single lot, also should be informed regarding pet food recalls. Large-scale pet food recalls are frequently reported in the popular media, but there are also governmental, veterinary, and animal poison control websites that report these events in an objective and accurate manner.[3,18-20]

The Adverse Reproductive Effects of Specific Xenobiotics

Tables 16-2 and 16-3 are brief summaries of predisposing factors and stressors, including selected xenobiotics, which can negatively impact reproduction, and these topics are covered in additional detail in several other texts.* As is apparent from reviewing Tables 16-2 and 16-3, there are many xenobiotics that can directly or indirectly influence reproductive performance. These xenobiotics can adversely affect male and/or female fertility, as well as prenatal development, either alone or in combination with some of the various predisposing factors and/or stressors, including other xenobiotics, listed in Table 16-2.

Although some of the xenobiotics listed in Table 16-2 represent classes of compounds with well-documented adverse effects on dogs and cats, several chemicals are listed, such as bisphenol A and phthalates, for which potential adverse effects on companion animals have not yet been clearly demonstrated. However, these and other environmentally relevant xenobiotics are mentioned for completeness, because their effects on wildlife, rodents, and potentially humans have been publicized extensively and are of great interest to the general public, their manufacturers and principal users, and government regulatory agencies.

For most of the chemicals listed in Table 16-2, the precise exposure dose for a given xenobiotic is very difficult to evaluate. In the case of large-scale food contaminations or environmental catastrophes, the levels of acute, subacute, or perhaps even subchronic exposure are likely to be relatively high and toxic in nature in vague terms. However, it is still challenging, especially in mycotoxin contaminations, to determine precisely how long and how much a specific individual animal was exposed to a given mycotoxin. Secondary fungal metabolites generally are unequally distributed within the contaminated grain matrix, and sufficient samples of raw ingredients and finished product might not have been retained by some manufacturers. Low-level exposures to common environmental contaminants are more likely to be chronic in nature, but will be even more difficult to evaluate with respect to exposure dose and toxic dose. Many of these xenobiotics are ubiquitous in the environment at very low concentrations, and there are even very likely yet-to-be-determined differences in the bioavailability, metabolism, and/or toxic effects of different forms or metabolites of these chemicals, especially with respect to nonrodents.

Table 16-3 lists several classes of common medications used in small animal practice, and the potential adverse effects of these therapeutic agents on male reproduction and pregnancy are summarized. In stark contrast to the xenobiotics listed in Table 16-2, the drugs and therapeutic agents listed in Table 16-3 are intentionally given to dogs and cats

---

*References 1, 2, 4, 5, 7-9, 13.

at well-defined, therapeutically effective doses. Therefore, the magnitude of the exposures to these medications is generally pharmacologic in nature and relatively easy to estimate. Although analyses can be performed, for many of these medications analytical results are only useful in confirming exposure to a given therapeutic xenobiotic in most instances.

Mycotoxins

Aflatoxins, Vomitoxin, and Zearalenone

Commercially prepared pet foods continue to be the best sources of safe and nutritionally balanced diets for companion animals. That said, in recent years, several manufactured pet food products have been associated with mycotoxin contamination, in particular those mycotoxins that can contaminate corn used in these products.[21] In most cases, the root causes of these contaminations have been lapses in normally stringent mycotoxin surveillance programs, and most recent mycotoxin-related pet food recalls have been primarily precautionary in nature.[18]

Aflatoxin-induced hepatic dysfunction or decreased immunity associated with exposure to aflatoxin or vomitoxin can interfere with an animal's optimal reproductive function (see Table 16-2). However, the adverse reproductive effects of these toxins should be considered collateral damage of the direct effects on their primary target organs, even if those effects might be subclinical or possibly resolved when the observed subfertility is being investigated. Unlike the indirect reproductive effects of aflatoxins and vomitoxin resulting from stress and altered nutrition, zearalenone is a naturally occurring xenoestrogen that can directly affect reproductive function by virtue of its estrogenic or antiestrogenic effects, even in dogs, depending on its concentration relative to that of endogenous estradiol (see Table 16-2).[22-24]

The simplest approach to preventing mycotoxin-related problems in companion animals is elimination of these xenobiotics from pet food products. Unfortunately, it is probably neither possible nor economically feasible to eliminate *all* measurable mycotoxins from pet diets. The number of mycotoxins that have currently been identified probably represents just the tip of the iceberg of all of the potentially toxic secondary fungal metabolites that exist. Even if none of the presently recognized toxic secondary fungal metabolites were present in a given pet food diet, other currently unknown xenobiotics of fungal origin *could be* present in that product. Certain uncontrollable, agronomic conditions continue to induce unavoidable fungal contaminants in grain to produce mycotoxins. In addition, analytical capabilities keep improving their abilities to detect lower concentrations of known fungal metabolites and identify new fungal metabolites.

However, although low-level mycotoxin contamination is inevitable, there is also absolutely no nutritional requirement for mycotoxins, including aflatoxins, vomitoxin, and zearalenone in pet foods. It is definitely a very *bad* idea to consider small animals—in particular, those intended for show, sporting, service, military/police, or breeding purposes—as the ultimate destination for grains deemed unsatisfactory for consumption by humans. A reasonable management approach to possible mycotoxin contamination in rations fed to potential or current breeding animals (and one used by most pet food manufacturers) is at least maintaining concentrations at or below current Food and Drug Administration guideline levels applying to aflatoxin and vomitoxin in food intended for human consumption (i.e., <20 mcg/kg of aflatoxins and 1 mg/kg of vomitoxin) and less than 0.5 mg/kg of zearalenone.[18] Although admittedly, clinical signs would most likely *not* be observed if these thresholds were exceeded slightly, particularly with short-term exposures, these concentrations take into consideration sampling differences, heterogeneous distributions of mycotoxins in feedstuffs, and the possibility of more chronic exposures to mycotoxins. Ideally these current threshold concentrations for mycotoxins should provide a cushion or safety net to prevent undue concern, but they could conceivably be modified if new information came to light concerning health risks associated with lower concentrations of these contaminants. Almost all veterinary diagnostic laboratories and many grain elevators, pet food manufacturers, regulatory agents, and independent analytical laboratories have some means to measure these particular common mycotoxins, as well as possibly other currently identifiable fungal contaminants in diets manufactured for consumption by companion animals.

Ergot and Ergopeptine Alkaloids

Ergopeptine alkaloids produced by *Claviceps purpurea* are not routinely tested for in pet foods, and elevated concentrations of these compounds only occur sporadically in small grains (*not* corn), including wheat, rye, triticale, oats, and barley.[15] However, their direct hypoprolactinemic effects could present as agalactia in dogs and cats or potentially as premature labor, abortion, stillbirths, or even dystocia in female dogs, which depend on prolactin for the maintenance of corpora lutea and the secretion of progesterone (see Table 16-1).[1,15] Although fewer laboratories perform analyses for ergopeptine alkaloids than for aflatoxins, vomitoxin, and zearalenone, it is possible to have suspect pet foods evaluated for the presence of these xenobiotics, particularly if canine abortions have been observed.

Phytotoxins

Similar to aflatoxins and vomitoxin, which initially have systemic effects, many toxins of plant origin, including ricin in *Ricinus communis* (i.e., castor bean plant), cardiac glycosides in *Digitalis* species (i.e., foxgloves), and the unknown nephrotoxin in *Lilium* or *Hemerocallis* species of "true" lilies, are much more likely to affect systems other than the reproductive tract (see also Chapters 54 and 74).[25] Exposures to these phytotoxins, unlike those to aflatoxins and vomitoxin contaminating corn or other cereal grains incorporated into pet foods, would be much less common in larger breeding colonies than in household settings. However, similar to the systemic effects of aflatoxins and vomitoxin, these plant toxins affect nonreproductive organs, inducing the release of glucocorticoids or creating enough maternal or fetal stress to initiate parturition and, if too early in gestation, abortion and stillbirths.[4-7,15] Diagnosis of plant intoxications usually depends on clinical circumstances and a history of phytotoxin exposure, which is usually based on plant identification or rarely measurement of a specific toxic plant metabolite.

Phytoestrogens

Unlike the aforementioned plant toxins in castor bean plants, foxglove and "true" lilies, phytoestrogens, such as the isoflavones found in soybeans (*Glycine max*) have direct effects on the reproductive tract. These isoflavones, such as the estrogenic mycotoxin zearalenone, are naturally occurring xenoestrogenic endocrine disruptors.[1,2,13,14] Phytoestrogens and zearalenone can also function as antiestrogens when high enough concentrations of these xenoestrogens are present to compete with endogenous estrogens for estrogen receptor binding.[13,14] Therefore, the phenotypic effects of either of these natural xenoestrogens vary from estrogenic (e.g., enlargement of mammary glands and external genitalia) to antiestrogenic (e.g., prevention of the preovulatory LH surge), depending on the exposure dose, an exposed individual's stage of sexual development or where they are in the estrous cycle at the time of exposure and the reproductive outcome being evaluated.[1,2,13,14] In fact, the term *selective ER modulators* which refers to synthetic antiestrogenic xenobiotics that can also function as estrogen receptor agonists, recently has been applied to several common phytoestrogens.[14] Recent reports of phytoestrogen-related effects in canids and felids demonstrate the range of adverse effects that can occur in these animal species.[26-28] It also should be taken into consideration that phytoestrogen and zearalenone contamination, although present in different grains, are not mutually exclusive of one another and in fact their combined estrogenic effects could be additive in nature. Reproductive problems involving phytoestrogens should be suspected when estrous cycle irregularities and conception rates occur in companion animals consuming diets known to contain soybeans or their byproducts or "secret" natural ingredients. Some laboratories can test for dietary concentrations of some of the more common phytoestrogens. There are even in vitro testing systems that can measure estrogenic activity of feedstuffs using breast cancer cells or other cell lines stimulated by estrogenic compounds, and these analyses might be helpful under certain circumstances of observed subfertility.

Heavy Metals

Heavy metals, such as cadmium, lead, and mercury, can all be either directly or indirectly associated with sperm abnormalities (see Table 16-2).[1,5,29] Exposures to these metals and metalloids, such as arsenic, always should be minimized, especially in pregnant females.[1,29,30] However, unfortunately humans are still routinely at risk for exposures to toxic heavy metals or metalloids. Cigarettes remain a major source of human exposure to inhaled cadmium, and there are still human occupational exposures to very high concentrations of lead, arsenic, cadmium, zinc, aluminum, and beryllium.[5,29]

Lead and Mercury

Similarly, prenatal exposures to lead and mercury continue be a problem in humans, as well as potentially small animals living in the same environments.[1,2,29,30] Inhalation or ingestion of soils highly contaminated by previous mining and/or smelting operations is one potential source of lead exposure that might not always be taken into consideration.[1,2,29] Consumption of water from lead-containing pipes and the ingestion of the remnants of lead paint are two other ways that chronic exposure to lead can occur in older houses or animal husbandry facilities (see Chapter 53).[1,29] Transplacental lead transport most likely makes use of calcium-binding proteins and other mechanisms used to preferentially supply calcium to the growing fetus.[31] Pregnant mammalian species, particularly humans and cats, can be exposed to methylmercury by eating contaminated fish, and this small molecule is rapidly transported across the placental barrier (see Chapter 57).[1,2,30] Both lead and methylmercury, which is the cause of Minamata disease, are teratogenic because of their direct adverse effects on prenatal development of the nervous system.[1,2,29,30] Certain clinical histories, husbandry environments, and diets might be suggestive of potential exposures to lead and methylmercury. *Whole* blood samples or even semen samples from males can be monitored for lead, with concentrations greater than 10 mg/dL lead in the blood suggesting excessive exposure to this element.

Pesticides

Fungicides, herbicides, molluscicides, insecticides, and rodenticides all represent classes of compounds that are considered pesticides. Obviously direct exposures to *any* of these compounds are to be avoided, but it is especially important to prevent direct animal contact with these xenobiotics, by males within 60 days of collections or breeding, cycling females, bred or pregnant bitches or queens, and neonates or growing puppies and kittens, if at all possible. These products and disinfectants should *always* be used in exact accordance with label instructions. Use of products in secondary containers labeled only as weed killer, bug killer, or rat killer should not be used. Furthermore, the "Less is good; more is better" principle should definitely *never* be applied to the use of these classes of xenobiotics. Although the most common reproductive problems associated with exposure to toxic amounts of these pesticides can be attributed to toxicosis-related stress and its effects on male and female fertility and gestational length, both dibromochloropropane and vinclozolin are fungicidal chemicals that have fairly well-defined, direct effects in males of various species, at various stages of development (see Table 16-2).[1,2,5] There are also specific considerations that should be taken into account, with regard to the use of pyrethrin and pyrethroid insecticides as well as anticoagulant insecticides around facilities in which breeding animals, pregnant females, and neonatal puppies and kittens are being housed.

Pyrethrins and Pyrethroid Insecticides

Fly control is always a concern in facilities housing animals, but appropriate sanitation and design of facilities can be used to minimize the need for excessive use of insecticides. Pyrethrins and pyrethroid-type compounds are some of the most common insecticides used and generally are considered to be extremely safe. However, it is important to consider that the term *safe* in this context generally is used with respect to the severe neurologic signs associated with excessive pyrethrin and pyrethroid exposures, especially those observed in cats (see Chapter 73).[32] Data in the recent literature suggest that some of these types of insecticides also have the potential for antiovulatory, antiprostaglandin, and especially antiandrogenic activities in vitro as well as in vivo, resulting in subtle alterations in fertility.[5,33-36] Given the frequency of their use, the possibility of pyrethrin- or pyrethroid-associated subfertility is surprising to many people who have used these insecticides uneventfully for many years. However, it is extremely likely, under normal conditions of use in animals bred infrequently or bred only under natural breeding conditions, that the effects of any minor changes in semen quality in exposed males would be masked by the safety net of millions of extra sperm present in each ejaculate and the multiple healthy, secondary oocytes usually available for fertilization in dogs and cats. This would be particularly true with animals producing exceptionally high-quality semen, which greatly exceeds the threshold of normal parameters outlined in Table 16-1. On the other hand, subtle changes in semen quality resulting from the inappropriate use of these and other related insecticides in breeding facilities in which semen is being evaluated regularly before insemination or cryopreservation, would be much more likely to be detected under these circumstances, dictating the rejection of affected ejaculates. Based on recent experimental results, the direct adverse reproductive effects of pyrethrins and pyrethroids generally would be expected to be short term and reversible in nature and would be anticipated to be more likely with high levels of exposure.[33-36] That said, because exposures to pyrethrins and pyrethroids are most likely to be repeated and chronic in nature, it is not unreasonable to prevent direct contact with these compounds, if at all possible, by valuable breeding and developing animals. This approach is particularly appropriate when considering the use of new unfamiliar products that have not been previously used on a given premises. Diagnosis of such problems would require a close temporal relationship between a recent pyrethrin or pyrethroid exposure and sudden declines in semen quality and/or less than optimal post-thaw sperm motility or viability, as well as possibly detection of pyrethrins or pyrethroids, especially in semen or other biologic samples collected from exposed individuals.

Anticoagulant Rodenticides

Anticoagulant rodenticides, particularly the newer coumarin derivatives, which have half-lives up to 10 times more than that of warfarin (~14 hours), are ubiquitous around animal husbandry facilities.[37-39] In fact, the serum half-life of brodifacoum, a second-generation coumarin anticoagulant, which is the xenobiotic most commonly involved in rodenticide toxicoses in the United States, has a reported serum half-life of 6 ± 4 days.[38] In addition, exposure doses of commercially available baits containing brodifacoum, which have been associated with acute lethality, especially in dogs, are extremely low (i.e., 0.06 oz of bait/lb of body weight in dogs; much higher in cats).[37] The coumarin class of anticoagulants antagonize the vitamin K 2,3-epoxide reductase enzyme (also referred to as vitamin K_1 epoxide reductase or vitamin K epoxide reductase) and cause coagulopathies because of the depletion of clotting factors II, VII, IX, and X, which require active vitamin K_1 for activation of their precursors.[37-39]

Coumarin derivatives can cross the placenta, resulting in placental hemorrhage and vaginal bleeding, abortions, stillbirths, and neonatal mortality.[38,39] Fetuses and neonates are much more susceptible to coumarin anticoagulant intoxication than adult animals (e.g., possibly no clinical signs in a mother with a high rate of stillbirths and neonatal mortality). Fetal and neonatal susceptibility to the adverse effects of coumarin derivatives are enhanced by the absence of alternative vitamin K_1 reactivation pathways present in adults, the slow transplacental transfer of vitamin K_1 to fetuses, and the lower concentrations of active clotting factors in fetuses and neonates.[38] With respect to the presence of coumarin derivatives in the milk from exposed females, there are conflicting reports, with individual compounds probably varying in their ability to be excreted in the milk.[37-39] Some references have stated that coumarin anticoagulants are generally not excreted in the milk.[38] However, other references have expressed concerns about the lactational transfer of coumarin derivatives because of what has been observed with warfarin in humans.[37,39]

Treatment of anticoagulant rodenticide intoxication is covered in detail in several references, including the current and previous editions of this text, but it is necessary to address several specific points related to intoxications involving pregnancy and lactation.[37,39] Obviously, antidotal therapy with vitamin K_1 should start in the pregnant female as soon as anticoagulant rodenticide exposure and/or intoxication are confirmed or, at least, are highly suspect. Whole blood or plasma transfusions can be used to prevent hypovolemia and fetal hypoxia. Although some coumarin derivatives are teratogenic, there is a reasonable chance that normal, viable neonates will still be born when coumarin anticoagulant intoxication is diagnosed and treated during the first half of pregnancy.[4,7,9,38] However, even though the pregnant female herself might respond to antidotal vitamin K_1 therapy, multiple stillbirths and neonatal deaths of her offspring might still occur and be attributed to vitamin K_1–related coagulopathies, when anticoagulant rodenticide exposures are not diagnosed and treated until late pregnancy.[38] Care of offspring exposed to coumarin derivatives, either prenatally or neonatally, poses some additional challenges to owners, caretakers, and veterinarians.[37] The need for postnatal treatment of previously exposed neonates depends on several factors, including the coumarin derivative involved in the exposure (might not be known), the timing of the anticoagulant exposure (possibly unknown), and the severity of the mother's and neonates' clinical signs, as well as when the diagnosis was made and vitamin K_1 treatment was initiated (all of which should be known). Vitamin K_1 is fat soluble and and concentrates in human breast milk; therefore if the lactating mother is being treated with vitamin K_1, postnatal treatment of prenatally exposed fetuses is most likely not necessary. However, it is also important to know whether prenatally or postnatally exposed offspring are nursing their exposed and treated dam and how well the female is actually lactating. The health status of the puppies or kittens and, unfortunately, under some circumstances, their monetary value can be additional parameters that come into play in the decision-making process about neonatal treatment. Decreased body weights of neonates can indicate impaired postnatal growth, hemograms can reveal anemia, and blood clotting profiles can be used to monitor the abilities of the mother's and prenatally exposed neonates' blood to clot. Analyses of blood from live animals or unfixed liver collected during postmortem examinations of dead animals for the presence of anticoagulant rodenticides can be used to confirm the diagnosis and identify the specific coumarin derivative involved. However, the results of these analyses are not available immediately, therefore necessitating the initiation of antidotal vitamin K_1 therapy almost always before the diagnosis is confirmed (unless consumption was witnessed or bait was discovered in vomitus, gut contents, or feces).

Despite the debate in the current literature, there are likely to be specific circumstances, such as confirmed exposures occurring during late gestation or especially those taking place during lactation, where there is added concern about possible milk transfer of a specific anticoagulant—in particular, newer, more potent, and longer-lasting anticoagulant formulations—to nursing offspring.[37-39] Some references have alluded to the ability of coumarin anticoagulants to be excreted in the milk, and early weaning of puppies or kittens has been suggested as one way to address this concern about lactational exposure to coumarin derivatives (see Chapter 32).[37,39] If this conservative early weaning approach is followed, then neonates being treated with vitamin K_1 that are no longer nursing their mothers most likely should be treated for 2 to 3 weeks with oral vitamin K_1.[37] The decision to feed and care for neonates should take into consideration multiple factors, including the specific anticoagulant rodenticide suspected in the exposure, the age of the offspring, and the owner's and/or caretaker's desire and capabilities to provide such care in an appropriate manner, as well as in many instances the perceived value of the puppies or kittens. Based on the timing of the anticoagulant exposure and/or evaluation of the potential for adequate foster care, early weaning and feeding of neonates might not seem necessary or practical. Under these circumstances, the post-partum mother can still be treated with vitamin K_1, and neonatal health and clotting ability can be monitored, with postnatal vitamin K_1 therapy ± blood transfusion used as indicated.[37,39]

Organic Environmental Contaminants

Aryl Hydrocarbon Receptor-Mediated Endocrine Disruption

Xenobiotics, including dioxins, polychlorinated biphenyls (PCBs), and polybrominated diphenyl ethers (PBDEs), and related chemicals are common environmental contaminants and, in large enough concentrations, have been associated with potentially devastating systemic health effects.[1,2,5,14] As shown in Table 16-2, a number of these organic compounds, classified collectively as halogenated or polyhalogenated aryl hydrocarbons (HAHs or PAHs), can also cause endocrine disruption by interacting with the aryl hydrocarbon receptor (AhR). The antiandrogenic and antiestrogenic properties HAHs arise from their ability, even in low concentrations, to directly induce enzymes involved in androgen and estrogen metabolism. Adverse reproductive effects mediated by the AhR can interfere with the biosynthesis of testosterone and disrupt testosterone signal transduction pathways. Many of these chemicals have been associated with adverse reproductive effects in wildlife species and/or laboratory animals.[1,14] In addition, there are epidemiologic data indicating that environmental spills of dioxins, such as 2,3,7,8-tetrachlorodibenzo-p-dioxin (TCDD) and PCBs can have long-term effects on reproductive functions in exposed humans.[2,12,40-43] More recently, the importance of pets as sentinels for human populations for exposures to these types of compounds has been recognized, with respect to an apparent relationship between hyperthyroidism in cats and exposure to PBDEs.[44] It is important to be aware of the environmental history or previous use of the geographical locations and facilities selected for breeding colonies. It is also important that individuals understand that adverse effects noted in animals might also be important to humans. Although not possible in all laboratories, exposures to some of these compounds can be confirmed by analyzing serum, urine, or especially, fat samples from potentially exposed animals.

Endocrine Disruption Associated with Bisphenol A and Phthalates

Bisphenol A (BPA) and phthalates are both ubiquitous environmental contaminants, which have had well-documented (and highly publicized) endocrine-disrupting effects on wildlife species, as well as laboratory rodents.[14] However, the potential for these xenobiotics to have real-life adverse effects on larger mammalian species, especially humans and their pets, has been the subject of numerous acrimonious discussions, both within and without the scientific community.[1,2,14] These contentious debates, in particular those focused on the societal impact of chronic exposures to low-level environmentally relevant concentrations of BPA and phthalates, are ongoing, and the possible causative roles of BPA and phthalates, along with a multitude of other endocrine disruptors, in human and animal health problems are still being studied.[1,2,14,45,46]

The primary uses of BPA are the manufacture of polycarbonate plastics and epoxy resins used to line metal cans.[45,46] Although BPA interacts with estrogen receptors, its phenotypic effects, like those of other SERMs, can be estrogenic or antiestrogenic, depending on a number of factors (i.e., exposure dose, sexual maturity of exposed individual, and the reproductive effect being evaluated).[1,14,45,46] Phthalates are used as plasticizers and have a unique antiandrogenic mechanism, which involves alterations in fetal Leydig cell function.[14,47] A recent study suggests that nonhuman primate species and adult rodents might actually eliminate BPA much more efficiently than immature rodents, especially mice.[45] It has also been recently reported that a small sampling of canned pet foods contained extremely low concentrations of BPA.[46]

Although the aforementioned results should be reassuring, several practical steps can be taken by those owners and caretakers still wishing to further minimize their animals' exposures to BPA and phthalates.[18,48] It is useful to be aware of which types of plastics are likely to be involved in unintentional exposures to BPA and phthalates. Exposures to BPA are often associated with polycarbonate plastics (recycling code 7), and polyvinyl chloride (PVC) plastics can be potential sources of phthalates (recycling code 3).[1,2,14,18,48] Owners and caretakers concerned about BPA and phthalates should select products made from polyethylene,non-polycarbonate,ornon-PVC,phthalate-freeplastics(recyclingcodes1,2,4,or5), especially for water and food conatainers.[18,48] Alternatively, stainless steel containers, without plastic liners, also can be used for these purposes.[48] Polycarbonate- or PVC-containing plastics, if used around pregnant females and neonatal puppies and kittens, should not be exposed to excessive heat (i.e., microwaves or dishwashers) or trauma, to prevent leaching of BPA and exposure to phthalates.[18,48] For those owners and caretakers who are extremely concerned about BPA exposures arising from cans containing epoxy resins, some consideration might be given to avoiding canned diets when selecting diets for breeding animals and neonatal puppies and kittens. However, high concentrations of BPA have yet to be demonstrated in these specific types of canned products, and there might be prescription pet food diets that can only be purchased in cans.[46] In these instances, the benefits of using those prescription diet products for an individual animal with a specific health condition or nutritional needs should definitely take precedence over concerns associated with animal exposures to BPA and phthalates. Depending on the findings of ongoing investigations, it is possible that analyses for BPA concentrations in serum and urine samples might become more available in the future to confirm companion animal exposures to this xenobiotic.

Medications

Table 16-3 is intended to be a quick guide to classes of therapeutic agents or specific xenobiotics within a given class of medications that are most likely to impair spermatogenesis and/ or harm a developing conceptus. Although the female estrous cycle and ovarian function are not immune to adverse drug reactions, these aspects of reproductive function are generally less susceptible to nonendocrine disrupting effects than the rapid cellular replications and differentiations during gametogenesis in the male and prenatal development. Accurate interpretation and prudent application of the information provided in Table 16-3 requires consideration of the essential reproductive facts presented in Table 16-1 and a thorough understanding of why a given animal needs to be medicated and for how long. While Table 16-3 is based on an A, B, C, D classification system to characterize the safety of administering certain medications during pregnancy, other recent references have also provided similar information based on an A, B, C, D, X system for describing the potential risks associated with the administration of selected medications to pregnant animals.[49] Xenobiotics classified as "D" in Table 16-3 or as "X" using the alternative classification scheme should not be given to pregnant females.[1,4,8,9,49] Furthermore, xenobiotics classified in Table 3 as "C" are similar to those compounds in Category D in the other reference and should only be administered during gestation IF ABSOLUTELY NECESSARY.[4,49] However, regardless of what specific classification systems are used to characterize the relative safety of medications in animals used for breeding purposes, the overall guiding principles for administering therapeutic xenobiotics to breeding animals, pregnant females, and neonates are fairly straightforward:

1. NO medications are without potentially toxic effects, BUT the anticipated benefits of a therapeutic approach MUST outweigh its associated risks.
2. HIGHER doses and/or CHRONIC administration of medications are MORE likely to be "TOXIC" than lower doses and/or one-time use.
3. Medications should be administered to valuable breeding stock, especially during pregnancy and lactation, ONLY in accordance with product LABEL INSTRUCTIONS AND PRECAUTIONS.
4. Animals used for breeding should be treated long enough to produce desired THERAPEUTIC EFFECTS, WITHOUT COMPROMISING reproductive function.
5. When possible/practical, REPRODUCTIVE PARAMETERS should be MONITORED over the course of a treatment regimen to minimize adverse reproductive effects.

However, it is naïve to think that reproductive complications arising from drug therapy can always be avoided. This is particularly true when hormonally active xenobiotics are intentionally used at pharmacologic concentrations to mimic the beneficial effects of gonadal steroids or endogenous glucocorticoids, which obviously also play key roles in reproduction and its associated feedback mechanisms (see Table 16-3). Likewise, medications that affect abnormally replicating cells (i.e., anticancer drugs) or those that counteract the inflammatory effects of prostaglandins (i.e., NSAIDs and glucocorticoids) cannot be expected to not have some potential negative impact on normal cellular replications and prostaglandin-mediated signaling pathways that are inherent to sexual reproduction.[1,4,5,8,9]

On the other hand, some therapeutic xenobiotics can, *if necessary*, be used safely during pregnancy. Careful review of Table 16-3 will point out that *MOST* antiparasitic drugs are relatively safe for use in breeding animals and pregnant females. In addition, within most of the other classes of drugs listed, there are some therapeutic alternatives that are more appropriate for use in breeding males, females during gestation, and neonates than others.[4,5,8,9] For instance, phenobarbital is a better alternative as an anticonvulsant than valproic acid in pregnant females, and cephalosporins and β-lactams (i.e., penicillins) are considerably safer for the fetus than aminoglycosides or fluoroquinolones (quinolones).[4,8,9] Of particular interest to veterinarians performing canine cesarean sections, especially those considered elective, are which anesthetic drugs are likely to be safest for both the pregnant female and her puppies. A variety of anesthetic protocols have been used successfully to minimize maternal and neonatal mortality. Propofol induction of anesthesia, in combination with supplemental O_2 and anesthetic maintenance with isoflurane (via endotracheal tube) has been found to be preferable to similar canine anesthetic protocols using barbiturates or other anesthetics, such as ketamine, for anesthetic induction.[7,50,51] Mask induction using isoflurane and anesthetic maintenance with isoflurane (via endotracheal tube) has also been used successfully for cesarean sections, but the incidence of maternal and fetal hypoxia is greater under these circumstances than with propofol induction.[7] Additionally, sevoflurane and isoflurane generally are thought to be safer than halothane and methoxyflurane for use as inhalation anesthetics (via endotracheal tube) during cesarean sections (see Table 16-3).[4,7-9] Epidural anesthesia with opioids or lidocaine also has been found to be useful ± inhaled anesthetics, especially in severely compromised pregnant patients, when it is particularly desirable minimize anesthetic depth.[7,51]

Reproductive Safety of Selected Medications for Which Chronic Administration Might Be Necessary

A growing number of treatable veterinary diseases require chronic administration of selected medications. As is evident from Table 16-3, long-term treatment with antineoplastic medications, anticonvulsants, steroidal as well as nonsteroidal antiinflammatory drugs, and therapeutic xenobiotics mimicking the effects of various gonadal steroids will, in most instances, have direct, adverse effects on reproductive function in small animals.[1,4,5,8,9] On the other hand, chronic administration of thyroxine, cardiac glycosides, and the 5α-reductase inhibitor finasteride reportedly can be administered with some degree of safety for the treatment of hypothyroidism, congestive heart failure, and benign prostatic hypertrophy (BPH), respectively.[1,4,5,8,9,52] It is interesting to note with finasteride therapy that DHT synthesis can be decreased enough to diminish the size of the prostate without adversely affecting testosterone production and the quality of semen. However, this observation emphasizes a basic therapeutic principle. With these chronic treatment regimens it is important to limit the total xenobiotic dose to that associated with the lowest approved dosage of a drug which is effective in treating or managing a specific disease. It is also critical to carefully monitor any changes in reproductive parameters over the course of therapy. Using these observations and the information provided in Table 16-1 will help dictate the possible need to discontinue treatment and will assist in determining the aspects of reproduction most sensitive to a specific medication. Such information also can be used to predict when these most sensitive reproductive parameters might return to normal relative to the cessation of xenobiotic administration.

Reproductive Safety of Herbal Medicinal Preparations

Given the information presented in Table 16-3, it is important to remind the reader that manufactured medications can have very beneficial effects when used appropriately, according to label instructions. However, that said, there is growing interest in the use of "natural" herbal preparations to enhance health and even reproductive function in humans as well as companion animals. Natural is not necessarily synonymous with safe, and many xenobiotics of plant origin, such as phytoestrogens, have the potential to alter reproductive efficiency while potentially having seemingly positive health effects on other organ systems or physiologic functions.[1,53] In addition, various extracts of several plants, including papaya (*Carica papaya*), cottonseed (*Gossypium hirsutum*), and chaste tree (*Vitex agnus-castus*) have been used for reproductive purposes, including "natural" contraception.[52]

Botanical preparations, unlike purified synthetic medications, are often complex mixtures of secondary plant metabolites, with variable active ingredients and biologic effects. One might not necessarily always know exactly what they are getting with a specific product, especially if they are not familiar with the manufacturer's level of quality assurance. Herbal medicines should be used very cautiously in animals intended for reproductive purposes, particularly breeding males and pregnant females. Owners, caretakers, and veterinarians should be familiar with *all* of the ingredients of a given herbal preparation (even those not of plant origin) as well as the potential effects of each of those constituent xenobiotics before administering a given botanical medicine to their breeding animals or even potentially their pets not used for reproductive purposes. Historically some herbal preparations have been found to contain high concentrations of arsenic or even adrenal or pituitary extracts from slaughtered cattle. There is a growing number of manufacturers of herbal medicines that provide guaranteed analyses of the products they are selling, and it is probably worthwhile to preferentially purchase these types of preparations from these manufacturers if one desires to use natural therapeutic xenobiotics.

Conclusions

This chapter was written from the perspectives of a clinical and diagnostic toxicologist and theriogenologist, with the intent of taking a somewhat novel yet practical integrated approach to reproductive toxicology in companion animals. Although this is an area that generally receives limited attention in most veterinary toxicology textbooks, many veterinarians and dog breeders are concerned about the possible roles of xenobiotics—in particular, mycotoxins in dog food, environmental contaminants, and even various therapeutic agents—in observed cases of reproductive failure. Companion animals also have the potential to act as sentinel populations for possible human exposures to many xenobiotics. Health and fertility trends in dogs and cats might be indicative of xenobiotic-related effects that are also applicable to susceptible human subpopulations, particularly pregnant women and infants.

It should be evident that xenobiotics can directly or indirectly (i.e., by stress-, nutrition-, or other body/organ system–related effects) impact the reproductive function of breeding animals within these species, many of which are selected for reproductive purposes based on nonreproductive criteria. It also should be apparent that potential reproductive toxicants can have primary as well as contributory roles in causing observed reproductive abnormalities in companion animals. The contributory roles of xenobiotics in diminished reproductive performance most likely involve interactions among various predisposing factors and/or stressors also associated with subfertility. Although it is much more convenient to think of impaired reproductive function having a single, obvious toxic etiology (i.e., a smoking gun), the causes of diminished reproductive performance in small animals are most likely multifactorial in nature, as shown in Figure 16-3. Management plays a critical role as an interface among various predisposing factors and stressors and normal reproductive function. It is important that the size, location, and type of breeding operation, as well as breeding selection criteria and owner/caretaker expectations, are always consistent with the levels of management, veterinary support, and animal husbandry infrastructure provided.

Table 16-1 provides a helpful review of essential facts associated with canine and feline reproduction. Tables 16-2 and 16-3 contain information pertinent to the potential adverse reproductive effects of certain predisposing factors and enzootic stressors (see Table 16-2), as well as medications commonly used in companion animal medicine (see Table 16-3). It is hoped that this chapter will help in the future recognition, diagnosis, management, and, ultimately, prevention of xenobiotic-related subfertility in companion animals.

References

1. Evans TJ: Reproductive toxicity and endocrine disruption. In Gupta RC, editor: *Veterinary toxicology: basic and clinical principles*, New York, 2007, Academic Press/Elsevier.
2. Evans TJ, Ganjam VK: Reproductive anatomy and physiology. In Gupta RC, editor: *Veterinary toxicology: basic and clinical principles*, New York, 2011, Academic Press/Elsevier.
3. http://www.aspca.org/.
4. Wilker CE, Ellington JE: Reproductive toxicology of the female companion animal. In Peterson ME, Talcott PA, editors: *Small animal toxicology*, ed 2, St Louis, 2006, Elsevier-Saunders.
5. Ellington JE, Wilker CE: Reproductive toxicology of the male companion animal. In Peterson ME, Talcott PA, editors: *Small animal toxicology*, ed 2, St Louis, 2006, Elsevier-Saunders.
6. Senger PL: *Pathways to pregnancy and parturition*, rev ed 2, Moscow, ID, 2005, Current Conceptions.
7. England G, von Heimendahl A, editors: *BSAVA manual of canine and feline reproduction and neonatology*, ed 2, Gloucester, UK, 2010, British Small Animal Veterinary Association.
8. Feldman EC, Nelson RW: *Canine and feline endocrinology and reproduction*, ed 3, St Louis, 2004, Saunders.
9. Johnston SD, Root Kustritz MV: *Olson PNS: Canine and feline theriogenology*, Philadelphia, 2001, Saunders.
10. França LR, Godinho CL: Testis morphometry, seminiferous epithelium cycle length, and daily sperm production in domestic cats (*Felis catus*), *Biol Reprod* 68(5):1554, 2003.
11. Pretzer SD: Canine embryonic and fetal development: a review, *Theriogenology* 70(3):300, 2008.
12. Knopse C: Periods and stages of the prenatal development of the domestic cat, *Anat Histol Embryol* 31:37, 2002.
13. Evans TJ: Diminished reproductive performance and selected toxicants in forages and grains, *Vet Clin North Am Food Anim Pract* 27(2):345, 2011.
14. Evans TJ: Endocrine disruption. In Gupta RC, editor: *Reproductive and developmental toxicology*, New York, 2011, Academic Press/Elsevier.
15. Evans TJ, Rottinghaus GE, Casteel SW: Ergot. In Plumlee KH, editor: *Clinical veterinary toxicology*, St Louis, 2004, Mosby.
16. Cheeke PR: *Natural toxicants in feeds*, ed 2, Danville, IL, 1998, Interstate Publishers.
17. Gulati K, Ray A: Stress: its impact on reproductive and developmental toxicity. In Gupta RC, editor: *Reproductive and developmental toxicology*, New York, 2011, Academic Press/Elsevier.
18. http://www.accessdata.fda.gov/scripts/newpetfoodrecalls/.
19. http://www.avma.org/petfoodsafety/recalls/default.asp.
20. http://www.petpoisonhelpline.com/.
21. Dereszynski DM, Ceneter SA, Randolph JF, Brooks MR, et al: Clinical and clinicopathologic features of dogs that consumed foodborne hepatotoxic aflatoxins: 72 cases (2005-2006), *JAVMA* 232(9):1329, 2008.
22. Minervini F, Dell'Aquila ME: Zearalenone and reproductive function in farm animals, *Int J Mol Sci* 9(12):2570, 2008.
23. Gajecka M, Janowski T, Jakimiuk E, et al: Histopathological and immunohistochemical examinations and changes in proliferation activity of the uterus in bitches following zearalenone mycotoxicosis, *Polish J Vet Sci* 10(3):143, 2007.
24. Gajecka M, Obremski K, Jakimiuk E, et al: Histopathological examination in bitches after zearalenone mycotoxicosis, *Polish J Vet Sci* 11(4):363, 2008.
25. Burrows GE, Tyrl RJ: *Toxic plants of North America*, Ames, IA, 2001, Iowa State University Press. 2001.
26. Setchell KD, Gosselin SJ, Welsh MB, et al: Dietary estrogens: a probable cause of infertility and liver disease in captive cheetahs, *Gastroenterology* 93(2):225, 1987.
27. McClain RM, Wolz E, Davidovich A, et al: Subchronic and chronic safety studies with genistein in dogs, *Food Chem Toxicol* 43(10):1461, 2005.
28. Mostrom M, Evans TJ: Phytocstrogens. In Gupta RC, editor: *Reproductive and developmental toxicology*, New York, 2011, Academic Press/Elsevier.
29. Flora SJS, Pachuari V, Saxena G: Arsenic, cadmium, and lead. In Gupta RC, editor: *Reproductive and developmental toxicology*, New York, 2011, Academic Press/Elsevier.

30. Ni M, Mareilha dos Santos AP, Farina M, et al: Mercury. In Gupta RC, editor: *Reproductive and developmental toxicology*, New York, 2011, Academic Press/Elsevier.
31. Evans TJ, James-Kracke MR, Kleiboeker SB, et al: Lead enters Rcho-1 trophoblastic cells by calcium transport mechanisms and complexes with calcium-binding proteins, *Toxicol Appl Pharmacol* 186:77, 2003.
32. Boland LA, Angles JM: Feline permethrin toxicity: retrospective study of 42 cases, *J Feline Med Surg* 12(2):61, 2010.
33. Zhang J, Zhu W, Zheng Y, et al: The antiandrogenic activity of pyrethroid pesticides cyfluthrin and β-cyfluthrin, *Reprod Toxicol* 25:491, 2008.
34. Liu J, Yang Y, Yang Y, et al: Disrupting effects of bifenthrin on ovulatory gene expression and prostaglandin synthesis in rat ovarian granulosa cells, *Toxicology* 281(1-2):47, 2011.
35. Ji G, Xia Y, Gu A, et al: Effects of non-occupational environmental exposure to pyrethroids on semen quality and sperm DNA integrity in Chinese men, *Reprod Toxicol* 31(2):171, 2011.
36. Ahmad M, Hussain I, Khan A, et al: Deleterious effects of cypermethrin on semen characteristics and testes of dwarf goats (*Capra hircus*), *Exp Toxicol Pathol* 61(4):339, 2009.
37. Murphy MJ, Talcott PA: Anticoagulant rodenticides. In Peterson ME, Talcott PA, editors: *Small animal toxicology*, ed 2, St Louis, 2006, Elsevier-Saunders.
38. Munday JS, Thompson LJ: Brodifacoum toxicosis in two neonatal puppies, *Vet Pathol* 40:216, 2003.
39. Osweiler GD, Hovda LR, Brutlag AG, et al: *Blackwell's five-minute veterinary consult clinical companion small animal toxicology*, Ames, IA, 2011, Wiley-Blackwell.
40. Safe SH, Khan S, Wu F, et al: Chemical-induced estrogenicity. In Gupta RC, editor: *Veterinary toxicology: basic and clinical principles*, New York, 2007, Academic Press/Elsevier.
41. Warner M, Eskenazi B, Mocarelli P, et al: Serum dioxin concentrations and breast cancer risk in the Seveso Women's Health Study, *Environ Health Perspect* 110:625, 2002.
42. Mocarelli P, Gerthoux PM, Patterson DG Jr, et al: Dioxin exposure, from infancy through puberty, produces endocrine disruption and affects human semen quality, *Environ Health Perspect* 116:70, 2008.
43. Eskenazi B, Warner M, Samuels S, et al: Serum dioxin concentrations and time to pregnancy, *Epidemiology* 21:224, 2010.
44. Dye JA, Venier M, Zhu L, et al: Elevated PBDE levels in pet cats: sentinels for humans? *Environ Sci Technol* 41(18):6350, 2007.
45. Doerge DR, Twaddle NC, Vanlandingham M: Pharmacokinetics of bisphenol A in neonatal and adult CD-1 mice: inter-species comparisons with Sprague-Dawley rats and rhesus monkeys, *Toxicol Letts* 207(3):298, 2011.
46. Schecter A, Malik N, Haffner D, et al: Bisphenol A (BPA) in U.S. food, *Environ Sci Technol* 44(24):9425, 2010.
47. Mahood IK, McKinnell C, Walker M, et al: Cellular origins of testicular dysgenesis in rats exposed in utero to di(*n*-butyl) phthalate, *Int J Androl* 29(1):148, 2006.
48. http://www.niehs.nih.gov/.
49. Wiebe VJ, Howard JP: Pharmacologic advances in canine and feline reproduction, *Top Companion Animal Med* 24(2):71, 2009.
50. Funkquist PM, Nyman GC, Löfgren AJ, et al: Use of propofol-isoflurane as an anesthetic regimen for cesarean section in dogs, *J Am Vet Med Assoc* 211(3):313, 1997.
51. Luna SP, Cassu RN, Castro GB, et al: Effects of four anaesthetic protocols on the neurological and cardiorespiratory variables of puppies born by caesarean section, *Vet Rec* 154(13):387, 2004.
52. Papich MG: *Saunders handbook of veterinary drugs*, ed 3, St Louis, 2011, Elsevier, pp 1–858.
53. Van Wyk BE, Wink M: *Medicinal plants of the world*, London, 2004, Timber Press, pp 1–478.

Considerations in Pregnant or Lactating Patients

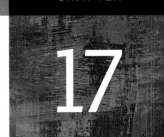

17

Michelle Anne Kutzler, DVM, PhD, DACT

Pregnant animals are a unique population with respect to their response to xenobiotic exposures, either therapeutic or accidental. The dynamic physiologic changes that occur within the maternal-placental-fetal unit during pregnancy influence the pharmacokinetic processes of xenobiotic absorption, distribution, metabolism, and elimination. In lactating patients, the xenobiotic concentration in milk is directly proportional to the corresponding concentration in maternal plasma. For most xenobiotics, the amount ingested by neonates rarely attains toxic concentrations. However, xenobiotic toxicity can develop in the pregnant or lactating animal, fetus, or neonate when sufficient compound is present to exert a damaging effect on cells. Conversely, subtherapeutic concentrations of xenobiotics may lead to treatment failures in the pregnant or lactating animal.[1] There is a scarcity of data on specific pharmacokinetic measurements during pregnancy and lactation in dogs and even less in cats. Most specific information on pharmacokinetics presented in this chapter is based on comparative data from humans and laboratory animals (Box 17-1).

Pregnant Patients

General Considerations

In dogs, apparent serum concentrations of progesterone and estradiol are similar in pregnant and nonpregnant cycles except for the abrupt decrease of both at parturition. However, if corrections are made for the hemodilution that occurs during pregnancy, both steroid hormone concentrations are significantly higher in the last half of gestation.[2] This is supported by increased fecal estradiol and progesterone concentrations during the second half of pregnancy.[3] Increased hepatic clearance and increased metabolism by the uterus and mammary gland also contribute to the absence of obvious increase in estradiol and progesterone concentrations during pregnancy.[4] In addition, thyroxine and adrenocortical hormones are increased during the latter half of gestation. The combined effect of increased hormone secretion during pregnancy results in alterations in dermal, pulmonary, cardiovascular, renal, gastrointestinal, and hepatic function (Table 17-1). Although these changes are necessary for a successful pregnancy, unique absorption, distribution, metabolism, and clearance of xenobiotics must be considered when using drugs to treat or prevent disease or in response to accidental toxin exposures.

Absorption

Gastrointestinal

The site of absorption for most xenobiotics is the small intestine because of its large surface area and the fact that the oral route is a common route of administration. Xenobiotic

---

| Box 17-1 | Did You Know That Xenobiotics ... |

Xenobiotics are chemical compounds (e.g., medications, other organic substances) that are found in animals but are not normally produced or expected to be present (or present at that concentration).

Table 17-1   Physiologic Changes during Pregnancy That Alter Pharmacokinetics

Physiological Parameter	Change
Absorption	
Gastric pH	Increased
Gastric emptying time	Increased
Intestinal motility	Decreased
Pulmonary function	Increased
Cardiac output	Increased
Blood flow to the skin	Increased
Absorption from IM-administered xenobiotics	Increased
Distribution	
Plasma volume	Increased
Total body water	Increased
Plasma proteins	Decreased
Body fat	Increased
Metabolism	
Hepatic metabolism	Increased or decreased*
Extrahepatic metabolism	Increased or decreased*
Intestinal wall metabolism	Increased
Excretion	
Protein binding	Decreased
Glomerular filtration rate	Increased
Renal blood flow	Increased
Pulmonary blood flow	Increased
Tidal volume	Increased

*Changes to metabolism depend upon whether the xenobiotic agent is hydrophobic (increased metabolism) or hydrophilic (decreased metabolism).

absorption across the small intestine is similar between dogs and humans, and is often faster than the rate of gastric emptying, such that gastric emptying is a rate-limiting role in xenobiotic absorption.[5] In dogs, gastric emptying after a meal is 90 minutes.[6] For many therapeutically useful drugs, the biological half-time is long enough to ensure that stomach emptying is not a critical parameter. However, a slower intestinal transit time can significantly increase xenobiotic absorption. High progesterone concentrations during pregnancy result in delayed gastric emptying and reduced small intestinal motility, with the net effect of orally administered compounds spending a longer time in both the stomach and small intestine.[7] As a result of prolonged intestinal transit time, there is an increase in absorption of poorly water-soluble (hydrophobic) xenobiotics and an increase in metabolism of xenobiotics by the intestinal wall. These modifications may affect (increase or decrease) the oral absorption of a drug.[8,9] Gastric pH is also increased during pregnancy as a result of reduced gastric acid secretion and increased gastric mucous secretion. The increase in gastric pH increases the ionization of weak acids within the stomach, which reduces their absorption.

Pulmonary

Respiratory rate is unchanged during pregnancy, but tidal volume (the amount of air per breath) and pulmonary blood flow are increased, which alters the kinetics of inhaled xenobiotics in favor of alveolar uptake and elimination by exhalation.[10,11] Aerosol (bronchodilator compounds) absorption is increased. Highly lipid-soluble anesthetic agents would be absorbed more rapidly and cleared more rapidly during pregnancy. Although the rate of anesthetic induction with volatile agents is not faster, the dose requirements for volatile anesthetic drugs (e.g., halothane, isoflurane, methoxyflurane) are reduced.[12] Volatile anesthetics also have been shown to delay intramuscular absorption of ketamine (Box 17-2).[13]

| Box 17-2 | Did You Know That During Pregnancy ... |

During pregnancy, dose requirements for inhaled anesthetics are reduced.

| Box 17-3 | Did You Know That During Pregnancy ... |

During pregnancy, topical administration of compounded pharmaceuticals or insecticides are more likely to result in toxicity.

Skin

In humans, substantial changes in blood flow to the skin occur during pregnancy, such that circulation to the hand increases by sixfold.[14] Alterations in dermal blood flow may have a significant impact on the pharmacokinetics of transdermal xenobiotic exposure (e.g., fentanyl), although this has not been studied in pregnant domestic animals.[15,16] Topical administration of compounded pharmaceuticals or insecticides may result in toxicity during pregnancy.[17,18] Xenobiotic absorption following intramuscular administration is also enhanced during pregnancy because of increased tissue perfusion secondary to vasodilation (Box 17-3).

Distribution

During pregnancy, increases in body weight, total body fat, cardiac output, total body water, extracellular water, and intravascular volume can influence xenobiotic distribution (Fig. 17-1). Increases in body fat allow for a larger volume of distribution for lipophilic xenobiotics. Cardiac output increases by greater than 20% in sheep, guinea pigs, goats, and rabbits and about 40% in humans during pregnancy. However, in dogs, cardiac output increases by approximately 60% during pregnancy.[19,20] It has been suggested that the pregnancy-associated increase in progesterone concentration leads to increased aldosterone secretion and results in increased renal fluid retention. During pregnancy in most species, the resting concentration of plasma angiotensin-2 is increased.[21] The concentration of vasopressin is also increased relative to plasma osmolality in humans and rats.[21] Despite an increase in blood volume, mean arterial pressure is decreased.[21] Increased total body water results in an increased hydrophilic xenobiotic distribution.[22] For example, pharmacokinetic parameters calculated from the results of the intravenous administration of lidocaine in pregnant ewes showed that the volume of distribution was increased, resulting in an increase in half-life.[23] Beginning in midgestation and lasting 1 to 2 months after parturition, hemodilution occurs as reflected in a decrease in hematocrit and plasma albumin concentration.[2] In humans, the size of the fetus and number of fetuses influence the increase in plasma volume, but this relationship has not been studied in domestic animals.[24] As a result of this pregnancy-associated dilutional hypoalbuminemia, there is a decrease in total plasma concentration of a protein-bound xenobiotic substances. In addition, steroid and placental hormones and serum lipids (from increased body fat) will displace xenobiotics from protein-binding sites, resulting in a rise in free (active) xenobiotic concentration of agents that would normally be protein-bound and potentially result in an increased physiological (toxic) effect. This is most noticeable for acidic xenobiotics that are highly protein-bound.

Almost all xenobiotics cross the placenta and reach pharmacologic concentrations in the fetus after exposure of the mother. Drugs administered to the mother may cross the placenta by passive diffusion, facilitated transport, and active transport. Lipophilic, nonionized molecules less than 500 Da can cross the placenta by passive diffusion.[25,26] In women undergoing elective cesarean sections, rapid placental transfer of ketamine,[27] propofol,[28] diazepam,[29,30] and atropine[31] occur such that fetal cord vein concentrations are several times higher than maternal. To date, these pharmacokinetic studies have not been done

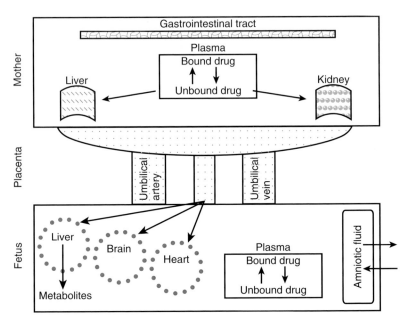

Figure 17-1 Xenobiotic distribution in the maternal-placental-fetal system. Factors affecting the pharmacokinetics and xenobiotic effects on mother and fetus are (1) altered maternal absorption; (2) increased maternal unbound xenobiotic fraction; (3) increased maternal plasma volume; (4) altered hepatic clearance; (5) increased maternal renal blood flow and glomerular filtration rate; (6) placental transfer; (7) placental metabolism; (8) placental blood flow; (9) maternal-fetal blood pH; (10) preferential fetal circulation to the heart and brain; (11) undeveloped fetal blood-brain barrier; (12) immature fetal liver enzyme activity; and (13) increased fetal unbound xenobiotic fraction.

in domestic animals but inferences have been made based on the use of these anesthetics and neonatal survival in dogs. Alpha-2 agonists (e.g., xylazine, metdetomidine), ketamine, thiobarbiturates (e.g., thiopental, thiamylal) and methoxyflurane should be avoided.[32,33] The current recommended anesthetic protocol for canine and feline patients undergoing cesarean sections is hydromorphone or fentanyl premedication, propofol induction and inhalant anesthetic maintenance.[34] If premedicating with an anticholinergic, glycopyrrolate has limited placental passage compared with atropine with significantly lower maximum fetal to maternal serum concentration (0.04-1, respectively).[35]

Maternal and fetal blood pH and plasma protein binding also influence the rate of passive diffusion across the placenta. The fetal plasma pH is slightly more acidic than the maternal. Consequently, xenobiotics that are weak bases are nonionized and able to easily penetrate the placental barrier. However, after crossing the placenta and making contact with the relatively acidic fetal blood, these molecules become more ionized, leading to "ion trapping." Protein-bound xenobiotics do not cross the placenta. In general, fetal plasma proteins bind xenobiotics with less affinity compared with those of the dam (e.g., ampicillin), with the exception of a few xenobiotics (e.g., salicylates) that have a greater affinity for fetal plasma proteins than maternal. Compounds that become bound to fetal proteins represent a depot of xenobiotic exposure in the fetus that would prolong fetal exposure after cessation of maternal exposure. Although hydrophilic compounds cannot cross the placenta by passive diffusion, they cross via aqueous diffusion through the water-filled pores between the cells (paracellular pathway) (Box 17-4).[25]

Box 17-4	Did You Know That During Pregnancy ...

During pregnancy, almost all xenobiotics reach pharmacologic concentrations in the fetus after exposure of the mother and umbilical vein concentrations are typically several times higher than maternal.

Metabolism

Alterations in the hormonal milieu of pregnancy are associated with changes in xenobiotic metabolism. In most cases, xenobiotic metabolism occurs primarily in the liver. Decreased protein binding during pregnancy results in greater xenobiotic availability for hepatic biotransformation, a process that renders a xenobiotic more water soluble and thus readily excreted by the kidneys. Hepatic metabolism during pregnancy has been well investigated in rats and to a much lesser extent in domestic animals. Changes in xenobiotic metabolism may have an impact on the first-pass effect of drugs given orally during pregnancy. Some microsomal enzymes of the hepatic cytochrome P-450 system are induced by progesterone, resulting in a higher rate of xenobiotic metabolism by the liver.[36] For example, it has been found clinically that the phenytoin dosage needs to be increased during pregnancy to maintain plasma concentrations that are adequate to control epileptic seizures in women.[37] However, the capacity for hepatic biotransformation is six times greater in dogs compared with humans.[38] Some microsomal enzymes are competitively inhibited by progesterone and estradiol, resulting in impaired xenobiotic metabolism.[39] Because of hormonal inhibition of hepatic microsomal oxidases, theophylline degradation is delayed during pregnancy.[40] Elevated progesterone during pregnancy also inhibits hepatic glucuronidation and extrahepatic cholinesterase activity.[41] However, in a pharmacokinetic study involving dogs treated with lamotrigine during and after pregnancy, the authors concluded that pregnancy has little or no effect on glucuronidation.[42]

Pregnancy may enhance a drug's biotransformation by increasing the access of the drug to the site of metabolism (e.g., liver) and by increasing the activity of the enzymatic system (e.g., hepatic cytochrome P-450 family).[1] However, during pregnancy, there may be decreased expression of genes encoding for hepatic cytochrome P-450.[43,44] Most biotransformation reactions present in the liver have also been described within the placenta, although placental biotransformation capacity is many times less than that of the liver.[45] The placenta contains several enzymes that are capable of metabolizing xenobiotics via oxidation, reduction, hydrolysis, and conjugation pathways. For example, the placental cytochrome P-450 enzyme 1A1 is induced following exposure to aromatic hydrocarbons found in tobacco smoke.[46] Alternatively, toxic intermediate formation may result from the placental oxidative biotransformation system. Xenobiotics that are not metabolized by the placenta enter the fetal hepatic circulation via the umbilical vein. However, approximately 50% of umbilical venous blood flow will bypass the liver via the ductus venosus, contributing to a possible accumulation of xenobiotics within the fetus. The near-term dog fetus shows evidence of a functioning enterohepatic circulation of bile salt, and xenobiotics can be found in meconium. Because of the small bile salt pool, apparent limited capacity of the gallbladder to concentrate bile, and evidence of a functional hepatic bypass, fetal hepatic metabolism is immature compared with that of the adult.[47]

Elimination

As a general rule, lipophilic compounds will be cleared mainly by metabolism, whereas hydrophilic compounds will be subjected to renal and/or biliary clearance. Xenobiotic clearance from plasma is generally faster in dogs than in humans (lidocaine: 14 vs 30 mL/minute per kg;[48,49] metoclopramide: 8 vs 25 mL/minute per kg;[50] domperidone: 10 vs 20 mL/minute per kg;[51] and pentobarbital: 1 vs 2 mL/minute per kg[52,53]). In dogs, renal blood flow and glomerular filtration rate are increased during pregnancy.[54,55] In humans, renal blood flow is increased by 60% to 80% and glomerular filtration is increased by 50% during

Box 17-5	Did You Know That During Pregnancy ...

During pregnancy, the amount of ampicillin necessary to maintain antimicrobial drug concentrations doubles and the elimination half-life for cephalosporins is reduced.

pregnancy.[56] Decreased protein binding during pregnancy results in more unbound xenobiotics available for renal excretion. As a result of increased glomerular filtration rate, the rate of elimination for compounds cleared by the kidney is enhanced (e.g., resulting in a reduced half-life), which can have a significant impact on drug treatment. For example, the amount of ampicillin necessary to maintain antimicrobial drug concentration doubles during pregnancy because of the combined effect of increased volume of distribution and rate of elimination.[57] The elimination half-lives are also reduced for cephalosporin and some anticonvulsants. Opposite results were described for gentamicin because increased clearance and decreased half-life occur in women[58,59] and ewes[60] during pregnancy but did not change for mares.[61] The fetus relies largely on the maternal system for elimination of xenobiotics. Elimination from the fetus to the mother via the placenta is by diffusion. However, because most xenobiotic metabolites are polar and not capable of simple diffusion, they can accumulate within the fetal compartment. Placental efflux transporters (e.g., P-glycoprotein) actively remove xenobiotics from the fetal circulation into the maternal circulation for elimination (Box 17-5).[38,62-65]

Lactating Patients

General Considerations

During lactation, estrogen and progesterone concentrations are at baseline, whereas prolactin concentrations are elevated. Milk is produced in mammary alveolar cells from which it is expelled by contractile myoepithelial cells into the duct system. Prolactin stimulates the synthesis of milk proteins such as α-lactalbumin. Milk proteins are synthesized within ribosomes in the rough endoplasmic reticulum and transported to the Golgi region of the mammary alveolar cells, where the protein is packaged into vacuoles. The milk protein vacuoles are pinched off and fuse with the alveolar cell membrane to become released into the alveolar lumen. The major proteins found in the milk are casein, lactoferrin, α-lactalbumin, and IgA. α-Lactalbumin, along with galactosyltransferase, uridine diphosphogalactose, and glucose form lactose.[66] Lactose is the principal osmotically active compound in milk. Although water is the principal component of milk, the amount of water within milk is regulated by the quantity of lactose. A reciprocal relationship among lactose and sodium, potassium, and chloride concentrations is maintained to keep the total osmolality of milk similar to that of blood.[67] Fat is delivered to mammary tissue from serum chylomicra of gastrointestinal origin and from endogenous low-density lipoproteins. Triglycerides are hydrolyzed at the capillary level, whereupon glycerol and free fatty acids enter the mammary alveolar cells by passive diffusion. Unlike plasma, canid milk contains on average 9.5% of emulsified fat.[68] Milk fat can concentrate lipid-soluble xenobiotics, causing the total amount of xenobiotic in milk to increase. For highly lipid-soluble drugs (e.g., diazepam and chlorpromazine), well more than half of the total amount of drug in milk is found in milk fat.[69]

Xenobiotics enter and exit the alveolar lumen by passive diffusion through the lipid portion of the alveolar membrane or via active transport through protein channels in the membrane. Passive diffusion is the most common route in which xenobiotics enter milk. Xenobiotics pass through the mammary epithelium by passive diffusion down a concentration gradient on each side of the membrane. With passive diffusion, the xenobiotic concentration in milk is directly proportional to the corresponding xenobiotic concentration in maternal plasma. The higher the dose administered to the mother, the more xenobiotic that will pass into the milk. Milk concentrations are the highest following intravenous administration compared with other routes of administration.

| Box 17-6 | Did You Know That During Lactation ... |

During lactation, milk concentrations of xenobiotics are the highest following intravenous administration compared with other routes of administration.

| Box 17-7 | Did You Know That During Lactation ... |

During lactation, xenobiotics that are weak bases (e.g., erythromycin and antihistamines) are more likely to pass into milk than weak acids (e.g., barbiturates and penicillins).

Table 17-2 Milk to Plasma (M:P) Ratios Relating to the Ratio between the Area Under the Curve of the Drug in Women

Drug	M:P Ratio
Amoxicillin[74]	0.014-0.043
Penicillin[75]	0.02-0.2
Prednisolone[76]	0.078-0.221
Diazepam[77]	0.08-0.13
Cephalothin[74]	0.14
Metronidazole[78]	1.7
Fentanyl[79]	2.45
Morphine[80]	2.46
Acyclovir[81]	2.94

For those drugs excreted in milk, lactation can markedly increase drug clearance.[70] The physicochemical characteristics of the xenobiotic (i.e., molecular size, plasma protein binding, lipophilicity, and ionization) also determine how much of the compound will be transferred into milk. The mammary epithelium membrane acts as a semipermeable lipid barrier. Small pores permit xenobiotics with a low molecular weight (<200 kDa) to pass through the alveolar membrane. Larger xenobiotic molecules must dissolve in the outer lipid membrane of the epithelial cells, diffuse across the aqueous interior of the cells, dissolve in and pass through the opposite cell membrane, and then pass into the milk. Only unbound xenobiotics in maternal plasma can diffuse across the alveolar membrane and accumulate in milk. High plasma protein binding decreases the amount of xenobiotic excreted into milk, whereas high milk protein-binding results in the sustained presence of a xenobiotic in milk. Casein is the major xenobiotic-binding protein found in milk.[71] However, as a general rule, milk proteins do not bind xenobiotics well.[72] As milk (pH 7.2) is slightly more acidic than plasma (pH 7.4), compounds that are weak bases (e.g., erythromycin and antihistamines) are more likely to pass into milk than weak acids (e.g., barbiturates and penicillins). The degree of xenobiotic ionization, determined by the xenobiotic pKa (ionization constant) and the pH of the plasma and the milk, plays a role in determining the amount of xenobiotic excreted in the milk in a process called "ion or xenobiotic trapping," similar to the fetal circulation. A good example of ion trapping can be seen with orbifloxacin because, like other fluoroquinolones, it is amphoteric with its carboxylic acid group and basic amine functional group and it extensively passes from blood into milk (Boxes 17-6 and 17-7).[73]

Although water-soluble xenobiotics must cross through pores within the alveolar membrane, lipid-soluble xenobiotics dissolve into the lipid bilayer of the alveolar membrane. The more lipid-soluble the xenobiotic, the greater the quantity and the faster the transfer into milk. Another factor that comes into play is the retrograde diffusion of xenobiotics from the milk back into maternal plasma. Studies in cattle indicate that compounds instilled directly into the udder pass out of the milk and are detectable in the plasma. The milk-to-plasma ratio (M:P) compares milk with maternal plasma xenobiotic concentrations and serves as an index of the extent of xenobiotic passage into milk to estimate a neonate's exposure to xenobiotics through milk (Table 17-2). The milk xenobiotic concentration usually does not exceed the maternal plasma concentration but even when M:P is greater than 1, the amount of xenobiotic ingested by a neonate is rarely sufficient to attain therapeutic or toxic concentrations. Peak drug concentrations after oral administration occur 1 to 3 hours after the dose.

Analgesics and Anesthetics

Ibuprofen, naproxen, and diclofenac do not cross into milk (M:P = 0.01).[82] However, the former two are known to cause toxicity in dogs and should therefore be avoided in both lactating and nonlactating canids. On the other hand, aspirin crosses into breast milk (M:P = 0.3) and is slower to be eliminated from milk than the plasma. A cumulative effect from aspirin could have adverse consequences on suckling neonates. In addition, the elimination half-life of aspirin is considerably longer in neonates than mature animals, which increases the likelihood of drug accumulation and adverse effects. As a general rule, nonsteroidal antiinflammatory drugs should be avoided during lactation.[83]

Meperidine (pethidine) also crosses into breast milk (M:P ~1). The half-life of pethidine (13 hours) and its hepatic metabolite, norpethidine (63 hours), in the neonate can lead to high neonatal plasma concentrations over time. Neonates nursing from mothers who were treated with intravenous pethidine following a cesarean section were neurologically and behaviorally depressed.[84] Dipyrone and its metabolites are passed into milk and have resulted in cyanosis in a human nursing neonate.[85] Benzodiazepines with long-acting metabolites can accumulate in infants, especially neonates, because of their immature excretory mechanisms and have caused adverse effects in infants.[86] Milk halothane concentrations equal or surpass concentrations in maternally inhaled air.[87]

Antibiotics

Penicillins appear in milk in amounts that could lead to disruption of neonatal gastrointestinal flora. Similar to penicillins, cephalosporins could lead to disruption of neonatal gastrointestinal flora.[74] First- and second-generation cephalosporins are considered to be safer in neonates compared with third-generation agents because of their activity against normal flora.

Following oral administration, clavulanic acid is transferred into the milk but no harmful effects have been reported.[88] Sulfamethoxazole is secreted into milk and has a long elimination half-life in neonates (36 hours for human neonates).

Xenobiotics Affecting Lactation

In addition to the effects of xenobiotics on the neonate, the potential effects of xenobiotics on lactation should be considered. Many xenobiotics affect prolactin secretion centrally. Cyproheptadine, bromocriptine, cabergoline, and metergoline lower maternal plasma prolactin concentrations and should be avoided unless cessation of lactation is desired. Sympathomimetics can also decrease milk production, probably by centrally decreasing suckling-induced oxytocin and prolactin release and peripherally reducing mammary blood flow.[89] Metoclopramide, a dopamine agonist, is used to stimulate lactation and is concentrated in milk because of ion trapping. Neonatal plasma prolactin concentrations may be elevated after maternal administration of metoclopramide.[90] Like oxytocin, prostaglandin $F_2\alpha$ administered intranasally increases milk ejection.[91] Fenugreek is an herbal product used in human medicine[92-94] and has been shown to have oxytocin-like activity in animals.[95] Although the use of herbal products seems to be increasing because they are viewed as safer or more natural alternatives to pharmaceutical products, the potential exists for herbal products to have all of the properties of pharmaceuticals, ranging from clinical usefulness to toxicity.

Conclusion

Although the majority of pregnant or lactating patients are healthy and drug administration can be avoided, acute disorders such as infection may require short-term medical treatment. The results of one veterinary survey indicate that the possibility of pregnancy was rarely considered when prescribing medications to companion animals.[96] Within veterinary medicine, pharmacokinetic data are typically generated in small groups of normal healthy animals, and it is often assumed that these data will reflect the drug's kinetic properties across the intended patient population. Few pharmacokinetic studies of drug absorption, metabolism, distribution, and elimination during pregnancy or lactation exist specifically for canids and felids. Information to modify dose schedules to ensure efficacy and minimize the risk of toxicity is definitely necessary. Whenever drugs are used in pregnant and lactating patients, the prescribing clinician must explain the relative benefits and risks associated with the treatment and obtain informed consent from the owner.

References

1. Rebuelto M, Loza ME: Antibiotic treatment of dogs and cats during pregnancy, *Vet Med Int* 2010: 385640, 2010.
2. Concannon PW, Powers ME, Holder W, et al: Pregnancy and parturition in the bitch, *Biol Reprod* 16:517, 1977.
3. Gundermuth DE, Concannon PW, Daels PF, et al: Pregnancy-specific elevations in fecal concentrations of estradiol, testosterone and progesterone in the domestic dog (*Canis familiaris*), *Theriogenology* 50:237, 1998.
4. Concannon PW: Canine pregnancy, *J Reprod Fertil Suppl* 57:169, 2001.
5. Clark B, Smith DA: Pharmacokinetics and toxicity testing, *CRC Crit Rev Toxicol* 12:343, 1984.
6. Theodorakis MC: External scintigraphy for gastric emptying in beagles, *Am J Physiol* 239:G39, 1980.
7. Davison JS, Davison MC, Hay DM: Gastric emptying time in late pregnancy and labour, *J Obstet Gynaecol Br Commonwealth* 77:37, 1970.
8. Dawes M, Chowienczyk PJ: Drugs in pregnancy. Pharmacokinetics in pregnancy, *Best Pract Res Clin Obstet Gynaecol* 15:819, 2001.
9. Qasqas SA, McPherson C, Frishman WH, et al: Cardiovascular pharmacotherapeutic considerations during pregnancy and lactation, *Cardiol Rev* 12:201, 2004.
10. Kerr MG: Cardiovascular dynamics in pregnancy and labour, *Br Med Bull* 24:19, 1968.
11. Metcalf J, Stock MK, Barron DH: Maternal physiology during gestation. In Knobil E, Neil J, editors: *The physiology of reproduction*, New York, 1988, Raven Press.
12. Palahniuk RJ, Shnider SM, Eger EI: Pregnancy decreases the requirement for inhaled anesthetic agents, *Anesthesiology* 41:82, 1974.
13. Wood M: Pharmacokinetic drug interactions in anaesthetic practice, *Clin Pharmacokinet* 21:285, 1991.
14. Mattison DR: Transdermal drug absorption during pregnancy, *Clin Obstet Gynecol* 33:718, 1990.
15. Wilson D, Pettifer GR, Hosgood G: Effect of transdermally administered fentanyl on minimum alveolar concentration of isoflurane in normothermic and hypothermic dogs, *J Am Vet Med Assoc* 228:1042, 2006.
16. Cohen RS: Fentanyl transdermal analgesia during pregnancy and lactation, *J Hum Lact* 25:359, 2009.
17. Barr DB, Ananth CV, Yan X, et al: Pesticide concentrations in maternal and umbilical cord sera and their relation to birth outcomes in a population of pregnant women and newborns in New Jersey, *Sci Total Environ* 408:790, 2010.
18. McGready R, Hamilton KA, Simpson JA, et al: Safety of the insect repellent N, N-diethyl-M-toluamide (DEET) in pregnancy, *Am J Trop Med Hyg* 65:285, 2001.
19. Williams JG, Ojaimi C, Qanud K, et al: Coronary nitric oxide production controls cardiac substrate metabolism during pregnancy in the dog, *Am J Physiol Heart Circ Physiol* 294:H2516, 2008.
20. Williams JG, Rincon-Skinner T, Sun D, et al: Role of nitric oxide in the coupling of myocardial oxygen consumption and coronary vascular dynamics during pregnancy in the dog, *Am J Physiol Heart Circ Physiol* 293:H2479, 2007.
21. Keller-Wood M: Reflex regulation of hormonal responses during pregnancy, *Clin Exp Pharmacol Physiol* 22:143, 1995.
22. Carlin A, Alfirevic Z: Physiological changes of pregnancy and monitoring, *Best Pract Res Clin Obstet Gynaecol* 22:801, 2008.
23. Bloedow DC, Ralston DH, Hargrove JC: Lidocaine pharmacokinetics in pregnant and nonpregnant sheep, *J Pharm Sci* 69:32, 1980.
24. Rovinsky JJ, Jaffin HM: Cardiovascular hemodynamics in pregnancy 1. Blood and plasma volumes in multiple pregnancy, *Am J Obstet* 93:1, 1965.
25. Schneider H, Sodha RJ, Progler M, et al: Permeability of the human placenta for hydrophilic substances studied in the isolated dually perfused in vitro perfused lobe, *Contrib Gynecol Obstet* 13:98, 1985.
26. Wiebe VJ, Howard JP: Pharmacologic advances in canine and feline reproduction, *Top Companion Anim Med* 24:71, 2009.

27. Ellingson A, Haram K, Sagen N, et al: Transplacental passage of ketamine after intravenous administration, *Acta Anaesthesiol Scand* 21:41, 1977.
28. Dailland P, Cockshott ID, Lirzin JD, et al: Intravenous propofol during cesarean section placental transfer, concentrations in breast milk, and neonatology effect: a preliminary study, *Anesthesiology* 71:827, 1989.
29. Gamble JAS, Moor J, Lamki H, et al: A study of plasma diazepam levels in mother and infant, *Br Journal Obstet Gynaecol* 84:588, 1977.
30. Idanpaan-Heikkila JE, Jouppila PI, Puolakka JO, et al: Placental transfer and foetal metabolism of diazepam in early human pregnancy, *Am J Obstet Gynecol* 109:1011, 1971.
31. Kivalo I, Saarikoski S: Quantitative measurements of placental transfer and distribution of radioactive atropine in fetus, *Ann Chir Gynaecol Fenn* 59:80, 1970.
32. Moon PF, Erb HN, Ludders JW, et al: Perioperative risk factors for puppies delivered by cesarean section in the United States and Canada, *J Am Anim Hosp Assoc* 36:359, 2000.
33. Moon-Massat PF, Erb HN: Perioperative factors associated with puppy vigor after delivery by cesarean section, *J Am Anim Hosp Assoc* 38:90, 2002.
34. Traas AM: Surgical management of canine and feline dystocia, *Theriogenology* 70:337, 2008.
35. Proakis AG, Harris GB: Comparative penetration of glycopyrrolate and atropine across the blood-brain and placental barriers in anesthetized dogs, *Anesthesiology* 48:339, 1978.
36. Tabei T, Heinrichs WL: Hepatic steroid hydroxylase and aminopyrine N-demethylase activities in pregnant rats and rabbits and the effect of phenobarbital, *Biochem Pharmacol* 25:2099, 1976.
37. Eadie MJ, Lander CM, Tyrer JH: Plasma drug level monitoring in pregnancy, *Clin Pharmacokinet* 2:427, 1977.
38. Unadkat JD, Dahlin A, Vijay S: Placental drug transporters, *Curr Drug Metabol* 5:125, 2004.
39. Kardish R, Feuer G: Relationship between maternal progesterones and the delayed drug metabolism in the neonate, *Biol Neonate* 20:58, 1972.
40. Davis M, Simmons CJ, Dordini B, et al: Induction of hepatic enzymes during normal pregnancy, *J Obstet Gynaecol Br Commonwealth* 80:690, 1973.
41. Hsia DY, Riabov S, Dowben RM: Inhibition of glucuronosyl transferase by steroid hormones, *Arch Biochem Biophys* 103:181, 1963.
42. Matar KM, Nicholls PJ, Tekle A, et al: Effects of pregnancy on the pharmacokinetics of lamotrigine in dogs, *Epilepsia* 40:1353, 1999.
43. Mondragon JA, Ocadiz-Delgado R, Miranda C, et al: Expression of P450-aromatase in the goat placenta throughout pregnancy, *Theriogenology* 68:646, 2007.
44. Dickmann LJ, Tay S, Senn TD, et al: Changes in maternal liver Cyp2c and Cyp2d expression and activity during rat pregnancy, *Biochem Pharmacol* 75:1677, 2008.
45. Juchau MR: Drug biotransformation in the placenta, *Pharmacol Ther* 8:501, 1980.
46. Pasanen M: The expression and regulation of drug metabolism in human placenta, *Adv Drug Deliv Rev* 38:81, 1999.
47. Smallwood RA, Lester R, Piasecki GJ, et al: Fetal bile salt metabolism, *J Clin Invest* 51:1388, 1972.
48. Branch RA, Shand DG, Wilkinson GR, et al: The reduction of lidocaine clearance by dl-propranolol: an example of hemodynamic drug interaction, *J Pharm Exp Ther* 206:431, 1978.
49. Tucker GT, Wiklund L, Berlin-Wahlen A, et al: Hepatic clearance of local anaesthetics in man, *J Pharmacokinet Biopharm* 5:11, 1977.
50. Bakke OM, Segura J: The absorption and elimination of metoclopramide in three animal species, *J Pharm Pharmacol* 28:32, 1976.
51. Heykants J, Knaeps A, Meuldermans W, et al: On the pharmacokinetics of domperidone in animals and man, *Eur J Xenobiotic Metab Pharmacokinet* 6:27, 1981.
52. Davis LE, Baggot JD, Davis CAN, et al: Elimination kinetics of pentobarbital in nephrectomized dogs, *Am J Vet Res* 34:23, 1973.
53. Ehrnebo M: Pharmacokinetics and distribution properties of pentobarbital in humans following oral and intravenous administration, *J Pharm Sci* 63:114, 1974.
54. Davis JO, Lindsay AE, Southworth JL: Mechanisms of fluid and electrolyte retention in experimental preparations in dogs. I. Acute and chronic pericarditis, *Bull Johns Hopkins Hosp* 90:64, 1952.
55. Robb CA, Davis JO, Johnson JA, et al: Mechanisms regulating the renal excretion of sodium during pregnancy, *J Clin Invest* 49:871, 1970.
56. Dawes M, Chowienczyk PJ: Pharmacokinetics in pregnancy, *Best Pract Res Clin Obstet Gynaecol* 15:819, 2001.
57. Jeffries WS, Bochner F: The effect of pregnancy on drug pharmacokinetics, *Med J Austral* 149:675, 1988.
58. Locksmith GJ, Chin A, Vu T, et al: High compared with standard gentamicin dosing for chorioamnionitis: a comparison of maternal and fetal serum drug levels, *Obstet Gynecol* 105:473, 2005.

59. Lazebnik N, Noy S, Lazebnik R, et al: Gentamicin serum half-life: a comparison between pregnant and non-pregnant women, *Postgrad Med J* 61:979, 1985.
60. Oukessou M, Toutain PL: Influence of the stage of pregnancy on gentamicin disposition in the ewe, *Ann Rech Vet* 23:145, 1992.
61. Santschi EM, Papich MG: Pharmacokinetics of gentamicin in mares in late pregnancy and early lactation, *J Vet Pharmacol Ther* 23:359, 2000.
62. Ganapathy V, Prasad PD: Role of transporters in placental transfer of drugs, *Toxicol Appl Pharmacol* 207:381, 2005.
63. Ceckova-Novotna M, Pavek P, Staud F: P-glycoprotein in the placenta: expression, localization, regulation and function, *Reprod Toxicol* 22:400, 2006.
64. Aye IL, Paxton JW, Evseenko DA, et al: Expression, localisation and activity of ATP binding cassette (ABC) family of drug transporters in human amnion membranes, *Placenta* 28:868, 2007.
65. Vähäkangas K, Myllynen P: Drug transporters in the human blood-placental barrier, *Br J Pharmacol* 158:665, 2009.
66. Noel GL, Suh HK, Frantz AG: Prolactin release during nursing and breast stimulation in postpartum and nonpostpartum subjects, *J Clin Endocrinol Metabol* 38:413, 1974.
67. Nichols BF, Nichols VN: Lactation, *Adv Pediatr* 26:137, 1979.
68. Oftedal OT: Lactation in the dog: milk composition and intake by puppies, *J Nutr* 114:803, 1984.
69. Syversen GB, Ratjke SK: Drug distribution within human milk phases, *J Pharm Sci* 74:1071, 1985.
70. Martinez M, Modric S: Patient variation in veterinary medicine: part I. Influence of altered physiological states, *J Vet Pharmacol Ther* 33:213, 2010.
71. Stebler T, Guentert TW: Binding of drugs in milk: the role of casein in milk protein binding, *Pharm Res* 7:633, 1990.
72. Atkinson HC, Begg EJ: Prediction of drug concentrations in human milk from plasma protein binding and acid-base characteristics, *Br J Clin Pharmacol* 25:495, 1988.
73. Marín P, Escudero E, Fernández-Varón E, et al: Pharmacokinetics and milk penetration of orbifloxacin after intravenous, subcutaneous, and intramuscular administration to lactating goats, *J Dairy Sci* 90:4219, 2007.
74. Kafetzis DA, Siafas CA, Georgakopoulos PA, et al: Passage of cephalosporins and amoxicillin into the breast milk, *Acta Paediatr Scand* 70:285, 1981.
75. Greene HJ, Burkhart B, Hobby GL, et al: Excretion of penicillin in human milk following parturition, *Am J Obstet Gynecol* 51:732, 1946.
76. Ost L, Wettrell G, Bjorkhem I, et al: Prednisolone excretion in human milk, *J Pediatr* 106:1008, 1985.
77. Wesson DR, Camber S, Harkey M, et al: Diazepam and desmethyldiazepam in breastmilk, *J Psychoactive Drugs* 17:55, 1985.
78. Erickson SH, Oppenheim GL, Smith GH: Metronidazole in breast milk, *Obstet Gynecol* 57:48, 1981.
79. Steer PL, Biddle CJ, Marley WS, et al: Concentration of fentanyl in colostrum after an analgesic dose, *Can J Anaesth* 39:231, 1992.
80. Findlay JW, DeAngelis RL, Kearney MF, et al: Analgesic drugs in breast milk and plasma, *Clin Pharmacol Ther* 29:625, 1981.
81. Bork L, Benes P: Concentration and kinetic studies of intravenous acyclovir in serum and breast milk of a patient with eczema herpeticum, *J Am Acad Dermatol* 32:1053, 1995.
82. Townsend RJ, Benedetti TJ, Erickson, et al: Excretion of ibuprofen into human milk, *Ann J Obstet Gynecol* 49:184, 1984.
83. Sallami S, Ben Rhouma S, Ben Rais N, et al: Renal colic in pregnancy and lactation: diagnostic and therapeutic approaches, *Tunis Med* 89:593, 2011.
84. Wittels B, Glosten B, Faure EA, et al: Postcesarean analgesics with both epidural and intravenous patient-controlled analgesia: neurobehavioral outcomes among nursing neonates, *Anesth Analg* 85:600, 1997.
85. Rizzoni G, Furlanut M: Cyanotic crises in a breast-fed infant from mother taking dipyrone, *Human Toxicol* 3:505, 1984.
86. Kanto JH: Use of benzodiazepines during pregnancy, labour and lactation, with particular reference to pharmacokinetic considerations, *Drugs* 23:354, 1982.
87. Coté CJ, Kenepp NB, Reed SB, et al: Trace concentrations of halothane in human breast milk, *Br J Anaesth* 48:541, 1976.
88. Matsuda S: Transfer of antibiotics into maternal milk, *Biol Res Pregnancy Perinatol* 5:57, 1984.
89. Thomas GB, Cummins JT, Doughton BW, et al: Direct pituitary inhibition of prolactin secretion by dopamine and noradrenaline in sheep, *J Endocrinol* 123:393, 1989.
90. Kauppila A, Arvela P, Koivisto M, et al: Metoclopramide and breast feeding: transfer into milk and the newborn, *Eur J Clin Pharmacol* 25:819, 1983.
91. Toppozada MK, El-Rahman HA, Soliman AY: Prostaglandins as milk ejectors: the nose as a new route of administration, *Adv Prostaglandin Thromboxane Leukotriene Res* 12:449, 1983.

92. Betzold CM: Galactogogues, *J Midwifery Womens Health* 49:151, 2004.
93. Gabay MP: Galactogogues: medications that induce lactation, *J Hum Lact* 18:274, 2002.
94. Tiran D: The use of fenugreek for breast feeding women, *Complement Ther Nurs Midwifery* 9:155, 2003.
95. Fleiss P: Herbal remedies for the breastfeeding mother, *Mothering Summer 68*, 1988.
96. Landsbergen N, Pellicaan CH, Schaefers-Okkens AC: The use of veterinary drugs during pregnancy of the dog, *Tijdschr Diergeneeskd* 126:716, 2001.

Toxicologic Considerations in the Pediatric Patient

18

Michael E. Peterson, DVM, MS

A relatively unexplored area in veterinary medicine is that of age-related responses to toxic xenobiotics. The majority of differences between adult and pediatric patients exposed to toxicants are developmental. These differences can markedly affect the four components of drug disposition: absorption, distribution, metabolism, and excretion. The information contained in this chapter is designed to illustrate these differences and how they may affect the toxin-exposed pediatric patient.

Physiologic Considerations in the Pediatric Patient

Pups and kittens may be exposed to xenobiotics through several routes—ingestion (including the ingestion of mother's milk), topical exposure, inhalation, and ocular contact. In dogs and cats the term *pediatric* generally refers to the first 12 weeks of life.[1] Further division into neonatal (0 to 2 weeks), infant (2 to 3 weeks), and pediatric (6 to 12 weeks) stages is justified because of the significant developmental changes that occur during this 12-week period. Physiological alterations associated with these maturation stages can predispose the pediatric patient to be more susceptible to adverse reactions.

Differences between adult and pediatric physiology can significantly impact a victim's response to xenobiotic exposure, both toxic and therapeutic. Pediatric patients have differences in regional organ blood flow that may alter toxin disposition. Proportionally greater blood flow to the heart and brain in pediatric patients increases the risk of adverse effects resulting from exposures to lower concentrations of cardiac and central nervous toxins.[1]

Pediatric patients have no significant blood-brain barrier until 3 months of age. This protects the brain from deficiencies in nutritional fuels in stressful states because oxidizable substrates such as lactate can pass from the blood into the central nervous system.[2] However; this mechanism also increases the potential for central nervous system exposure to toxins, particularly because pediatric patients have an increased central nervous system (CNS) blood flow relative to adults. Most xenobiotics will have equivalent plasma and CNS concentrations. Brain cells normally protected in adults are at higher risk of exposure to toxins in the neonate.

Pediatric patients have decreased blood pressure; arterial pressure approaches adult levels by 6 weeks to a few months of age dependent on the breed maturation rate. Also decreased are the stroke volume and vascular resistance. The heart rate, cardiac output, and plasma volume are increased in these patients. Central venous pressure approaches adult levels by 7 months. The autonomic nervous system is incomplete in the heart and blood vessels. This limits the ability to increase cardiac output by altering contractility or affecting preload, making the neonate less responsive to either xenobiotics or therapeutics that target the autonomic nervous system. Preservation of cardiac output is dependent on increased heart rate and preserving low vascular resistance.

Pediatric patients also have minimal glycogen stores and limited capacity for gluconeo-genesis or glycogenolysis. Additionally, nephrogenesis is not complete until 3 weeks. Cortical blood flow alterations and maturation of nephrons cause various regions of the kidney to be very vulnerable to drug toxicities. Protein, glucose, and amino acid levels are normally higher in pediatric urine than in the adult.

Packed red cell volume is approximately 47% at birth and drops to a nadir of approximately 24% at 6 weeks of age. Hematopoiesis does not begin until about 6 to 12 weeks of age. Prothrombin time, partial thromboplastin time, and antithrombin levels are increased compared with adults until approximately 1 week of age. Hemoglobin concentrations are less than those for adults.

Following is a review of aspects of drug disposition—absorption, distribution, metabolism, and excretion—affected by these dramatic developmental changes as the neonate matures[3,4] (Box 18-1).

Absorption

Following oral exposure, toxin absorption occurs primarily in the small intestine. The pediatric patient has a decreased gastric emptying time and irregular peristalsis because motility is more controlled by distention than electrical activity until 40 days of age, causing a slower rate of absorption resulting in lower peak plasma toxin levels.[5,6] This decreased rate of absorption may actually protect against toxic drug concentrations. However, in neonates before colostrum is absorbed these protective mechanisms may not be present. Before colostrum absorption the permeability of the intestinal mucosa is increased, which also increases the rate of toxin uptake including the uptake of compounds that normally would not reach the systemic circulation. Intestinal permeability rapidly decreases after colostrum ingestion.[6,7] This closure may well be induced by endogenous release of hydrocortisone or adrenocorticotropic hormone. Exogenous supplementation of these hormones to the mother within 24 hours prepartum prevents the increase in permeability and uptake of colostrum.

Several other factors may affect small intestinal drug absorption in pediatric patients. Newborns have a neutral gastric pH, and the rate of progression to adult levels depends

Box 18-1	Altered Xenobiotic Disposition in Pediatric Patients
Alteration	**Impact**
Increased intestinal permeability	Increased oral uptake; toxic plasma concentrations
Increased gastric pH	Increased oral uptake of weak bases and acid-labile compounds; prolonged and elevated plasma levels; toxic plasma concentrations
Altered peristalsis (decreased gastric emptying time)	Decreased absorption; lower plasma levels of toxin
Decreased plasma proteins	Toxin may accumulate, leading to more unbound compound and thus a potentially longer half-life
Decreased body fat	Increased plasma levels; decreased accumulation of lipid-soluble toxins
Increased total body water (more extracellular fluid)	Decreased plasma concentrations; longer half-life
Increased uptake of volatile gases	High plasma concentrations; increased response and toxicity
Increased dermal absorption	Higher or prolonged plasma exposure levels; toxicity increased
Immature P-glycoprotein system	Poor ability to clear toxins

on the species involved.[5,7] Achlorhydria (increased gastric pH) may cause decreased absorption of many compounds that require disintegration and dissolution or that need to be ionized in a more acidic environment (e.g., weak acids). Milk diets can interfere with absorption of toxic compounds by reducing gastric motility or interacting directly with the toxins. The "unstirred water layer" adjacent to the surface area of the mucosal cells is thicker in the neonate compared with the older pediatric patient, and this may limit the rate of absorption of some compounds.

Newborns have decreased bile flow and lower bile acid concentrations until 8 weeks of age. Absorption of fat-soluble compounds increases as biliary function develops. Both extrahepatic metabolism and enterohepatic circulation may be altered as microbial colonization of the gastrointestinal tract occurs.[8,9] Absorption from the rectal mucosa is rapid in neonates.

Absorption of xenobiotics administered parenterally to pediatric animals varies from that in adults. As muscle mass develops, with its accompanying increase in blood flow and maturation of the vasomotor response, the rate of absorption following intramuscular administration of xenobiotics is altered.[8] Subcutaneous administration of potentially toxic drugs may exhibit variable absorption rates relative to the patient's age. Smaller amounts of body fat but greater water volume may result in quicker absorption of xenobiotics compared to that in adults.[10]

Ambient temperature directly affects physiologic responses in the neonate. As an example a normal neonatal body temperature is 96° F with a normal heart rate of 200 to 250 bpm. A drop of body temperature to 70° F results in a heart rate of 40 bpm. Body temperature of less than 94° F induces gastrointestinal ileus and decreased lymphocyte function. It is suspected that environmental temperature influences subcutaneous absorption. This is especially true in neonates whose thermoregulatory mechanisms are poorly functional. If the neonate is in a cold environment, subcutaneous xenobiotic absorption tends to be reduced.

Percutaneous absorption of xenobiotics may be greater in pediatric patients. Percutaneous absorption is directly related to skin hydration, which is highest in neonates. Topical exposure to potentially toxic lipid-soluble compounds (e.g., hexachlorophene and organophosphates) places the pediatric patient at higher risk of significant absorption.

Volatile gases are absorbed rapidly from the pediatric respiratory tract owing to greater minute ventilation. Pediatric patients have two- to threefold higher oxygen tissue demand relative to their body weight compared to adults. This results in a higher respiratory rate. Tidal volumes are similar to those in adults; however, pediatric patients have a lower functional residual capacity. The respiratory system approaches that of the adult by 3 weeks of age. If normal environmental temperatures are present, panting is almost always an indicator of respiratory distress.

Distribution

The two major differences between adult and pediatric patients relative to xenobiotic distribution are those of body fluid compartments and toxin or drug binding to serum proteins. Body fluid compartments undergo tremendous alterations as the neonate grows. As the neonate matures, significant changes occur in both the percentage of total body water and the ratio of compartmental volumes. Although both the percentage of total body water and the volume of the extracellular versus the intracellular compartment decrease as the animal ages, the change in the ratio of extracellular to intracellular volume is significantly greater.[11] Daily fluid requirements are greater in neonatal and pediatric patients because a larger proportion of their body weight is represented by body water. The net effect on xenobiotic distribution depends on these differences in body compartments. Most water-soluble compounds are distributed into extracellular fluids. Plasma concentrations of these compounds are lower in pediatric patients compared with adults, because the volume into which the compound is distributed is greater in the young. Unbound lipid-soluble compounds have the same type of distribution because they are distributed into total body water. Changes in xenobiotic distribution directly alter the half-life of that xenobiotic. Increases in distribution directly decrease the plasma concentration, a fact that may potentially protect the pediatric patient from toxic xenobiotic concentrations.[12]

Distribution of lipid-soluble compounds that accumulate in the fat (e.g., some organophosphates and chlorinated hydrocarbons) may be decreased owing to a smaller proportion of body fat in the pediatric patient. Xenobiotic plasma concentrations may be higher, but the half-life is shorter. The movement of many fat-soluble compounds may be facilitated by their high tendency to bind to plasma proteins. This binding decreases their ability to be distributed to target tissues.

Predicting the distribution of highly protein-bound compounds is complicated in the pediatric patient. Most compounds are bound to serum albumin, and basic toxins have a high affinity for alpha-1-glycoproteins. Both of these proteins are available in lower concentrations in pediatric patients.[13] Albumin levels reach adult values at approximately 8 weeks of age and exposure before this age can be an issue, with protein-bound drugs resulting in an increase in active compound or increased t½. Additionally, differences in albumin structure and competition with endogenous substrates (e.g., bilirubin) for binding sites may decrease protein binding.[6,14] If bound toxins are displaced, the risk of toxicity increases as the concentration of free pharmacologically active compound rises. When a compound has a narrow therapeutic index and is highly protein bound, these age-related changes are significant. Xenobiotic half-life may rise owing to increased amounts of compound that are unbound, allowing free distribution to the tissues and decreasing the plasma concentration.[14] Despite the increased volume of distribution, the half-life of a compound may be "normalized" by the increased clearance of free toxin.

Metabolism

Pediatric metabolism is significantly different from that of the adult. Hepatic and renal excretion is limited in neonatal and pediatric animals, thus decreasing toxin elimination. Intoxication by xenobiotics in young animals may be induced by decreased clearance.[3,6]

Pediatric patients have decreased protein synthesis and immature hepatic enzyme systems until 5 months of age, including microsomal cytochrome P450, which directly results in incomplete hepatic metabolism affecting reduction, hydroxylation, and demethylation of xenobiotics. Both phase I (e.g., oxidative) and phase II (e.g., glucuronidation) reactions are reduced.[15-17] Maturation of various metabolic pathways occurs at different rates. Neonatal puppies may not manifest phase I activity until the ninth day of life; this activity steadily increases after day 25 until it reaches adult levels at day 135.[16] Because hepatic xenobiotic metabolism is decreased, plasma clearance of toxins is decreased, plasma half-life is increased, and toxic plasma compound concentrations may result.

The oral bioavailability of compounds with a significant first-pass metabolism is probably greater in pediatric patients. Xenobiotics whose toxicity is generated from toxic metabolites may be less hazardous because there is decreased formation of active components. For example, children less than 9 to 12 years of age have a lower incidence of hepatotoxicity following overdose of acetaminophen than adults.[18] Pediatric hepatic metabolizing enzymes (e.g., cytochrome P450) do appear to be inducible by phenobarbital and other drugs.

Excretion

Alterations in toxin excretion are manifest in several ways. Significant differences in renal blood flow can result in alterations in toxin excretion.[19,20] Pups have reduced renal excretion, which decreases the clearance of renally excreted parent compounds and the products of hepatic phase II metabolism. As pups age glomerular filtration and renal tubular function steadily increase.[20,21] The total number of glomeruli remains constant. Adult levels of glomerular filtration and tubular function are attained by 2½ months of age. If normal levels of body fluids and electrolytes are maintained, pediatric renal tubular resorption is equivalent to that in adults.[22,23] In this pediatric renal environment water-soluble toxins have decreased clearance and extended half-lives. Decreased urine blood flow results in decreased glomerular filtration rate (GFR). Water soluble compounds have decreased clearance and increased elimination half-lives ($t\frac{1}{2}$). GFR and tubular function is at adult function levels by 3 months of age. Normal pediatric urine specific gravity generally is in the 1.006 to 1.017 range for the first 8 weeks of life.

An example of this phenomenon is the recommendation that pediatric patients require higher doses (because of the increased volume of distribution) and longer dosing intervals (because of increased distribution and decreased clearance) of gentamicin. One can anticipate alterations in excretion in sick or dehydrated pediatric patients.

Maternal Transfer of Toxin

Almost all xenobiotics cross the placenta and reach pharmacologic concentrations in the fetus after exposure of the mother. (See Chapter 17, "Considerations in Pregnant or Lactating Patients.") Drugs administered to the mother may cross the placenta by passive diffusion, facilitated transport, and active transport. Protein-bound xenobiotics do not cross the placenta. Factors affecting the pharmacokinetics and xenobiotic effects on mother and fetus are (1) altered maternal absorption, (2) increased maternal unbound xenobiotic fraction, (3) increased maternal plasma volume, (4) altered hepatic clearance, (5) increased maternal renal blood flow and glomerular filtration rate, (6) placental transfer, (7) placental metabolism, (8) placental blood flow, (9) maternal-fetal blood pH, (10) preferential fetal circulation to the heart and brain, (11) undeveloped fetal blood-brain barrier, (12) immature fetal liver enzyme activity, and (13) increased fetal unbound xenobiotic fraction.

Passive diffusion is the most common route in which xenobiotics enter milk. Xenobiotics pass through the mammary epithelium by passive diffusion down a concentration gradient on each side of the membrane. The higher the dose received by the mother, the more xenobiotic will pass into the milk. Generally, milk proteins do not bind xenobiotics well. Because milk (pH 7.2) is slightly more acidic than plasma (pH 7.4), compounds that are weak bases are more likely to pass into milk than weak acids. The more lipid soluble the xenobiotic, the greater the quantity and the faster the transfer into milk.

Most Common Inquiries to Poison Centers for Pediatric Patients

Common exposures in pediatric canine and feline patients are listed in Box 18-2.

Rodenticides

Rodenticides (e.g., bromethalin, anticoagulants) are commonly available and dogs are intoxicated more frequently than any other domestic animals. The veterinarian should read the product label to identify the exact compound involved. The majority of anticoagulant rodenticides inhibits the recycling of vitamin K_1, blocking the victim's ability to clot. More than half of the victims exhibit anorexia, weakness, coughing, epistaxis, and dyspnea. Laboratory tests show prolonged clotting times and possibly thrombocytopenia. Administration of vitamin K_1 is therapeutic but may take several hours to have a therapeutic effect.

Nonsteroidal Antiinflammatory Drugs

Nonsteroidal antiinflammatory drugs (NSAIDs) (human and animal products) are a common cause of toxicity in puppies and kittens. These animals have extensive enterohepatic recirculation of NSAIDs, increasing their toxicity. NSAIDs are a particular problem for cats because they are deficient in glutathione hepatic pathways, thereby prolonging the half-life of these compounds. The most common clinical manifestations are gastrointestinal. Clinical signs include vomiting, depression, diarrhea, anorexia, ataxia, bloody stool, polyuria, polydipsia, and tachypnea. There is no specific antidote and treatment is largely supportive.

| **Box 18-2** | The Most Common Groups of Toxicants (Both Serious and Not So Serious) for Animals under 1 Year of Age |

Dogs
Rodenticides (bromethalin, anticoagulants, and unknown) were the top category
NSAIDs (human and animal products)
Antidepressants
Herbicides
Mushrooms
Silica gel
Cleaning products
Chocolate
Amphetamines (prescription and illicit)
Birth control pills
Cats
Flea products (sprays, spot-ons, collars, dips) far and away the #1 category
NSAIDs
Silica gel
Insoluble calcium oxalate plants
Liquid potpourri

Courtesy Tina Wismer, ASPCA Animal Poison Control Center.

Antidepressants

Antidepressant exposures generally involve the tricyclic antidepressants or serotonin reuptake inhibitors or monoamine oxidase inhibitors. Once ingested, clinical signs usually develop within 60 minutes initially but their anticholinergic activity can inhibit gastrointestinal motility, slowing further uptake. These drugs are highly protein bound. Several compounds have toxic metabolites. Life-threatening clinical signs are related to the compounds' effects on the central nervous system and cardiovascular aberrations. Clinical signs include ataxia, lethargy, hypotension, disorientation, vomiting, dyspnea, mydriasis, hyperactivity, urine retention, ileus, seizures, and cardiac arrhythmias.

Herbicides

Herbicide exposure from pesticide-treated plants is unlikely to result in intoxication in puppies and kittens. Exposure to concentrates can induce clinical signs and treatment is supportive. Acute exposures rarely induce altered biochemical profile data, unlike long-term feeding trials. Vomiting is a common nonspecific clinical sign.

Mushrooms

Mushroom ingestion can occur year round. Common clinical signs are those of gastrointestinal distress including abdominal pain, vomiting, and diarrhea. A wide variety of toxins are available in mushroom ingestion. These compounds can affect the gastrointestinal tract, nervous system (excitation, hallucinogenic, and muscarinic), kidneys, red blood cells, and liver. A confirmed diagnosis is difficult to obtain, and clinicians should become familiar with the mushroom species available in their geographic region.

Silica Gel

Silica gel is used as a desiccant and often come in paper packets or plastic cylinders. They are used to absorb moisture in a variety of packaging. Silica is considered "chemically and biologically inert" upon ingestion. Clinical signs, though rare, would consist of gastrointestinal upset manifested as nausea, vomiting, and inappetence.

Home Cleaning Products

The list of home cleaning products is extensive, highlighting the need for the owner to bring in the toxin container if possible.

Methylxanthines

The active (toxic) agents in chocolate are methylxanthines, specifically theobromine and caffeine. Methylxanthines stimulate the CNS, act on the kidney to stimulate diuresis, and increase the contractility of cardiac and skeletal muscle. The relative amounts of theobromine and caffeine will vary with the form of the chocolate (see Chapter 60).

The lethal dose of 50% theobromine and caffeine are 100 to 300 mg/kg, but severe and life-threatening clinical signs may be seen at levels far below these doses. Based on Animal Poison Control Center experience, mild signs have been seen with theobromine levels of 20 mg/kg, severe signs have been seen at 40 to 50 mg/kg, and seizures have occurred at 60 mg/kg. Accordingly, less than 2 ounces of milk chocolate per kg is potentially lethal to dogs. Clinical signs occur within 6 to 12 hours of ingestion. Initial signs include polydypsia, bloating, vomiting, diarrhea, and restlessness. Signs progress to hyperactivity, polyuria, ataxia, tremors, seizures, tachycardia, PVCs, tachypnea, cyanosis, hypertension, hyperthermia, and coma. Death is generally caused by cardiac arrhythmias or respiratory failure. Hypokalemia may occur later in the course of the toxicosis. Because of the high fat content of many chocolate products, pancreatitis is a potential sequela.

Amphetamines

Amphetamines (prescription and illicit) have a minimum oral lethal dose of 20 to 27 mg/kg for amphetamine sulfate and 9 to 11 mg/kg of methamphetamine hydrochloride in dogs. Victims generally manifest hyperactivity, restlessness, mydriasis, hypersalivation, vocalization, tachypnea, tremors, hyperthermia, ataxia, seizures, and tachycardia.

Birth Control Pills

Birth control pills generally come with each packet containing 21 tablets of estrogen and/or progesterone and possibly 7 placebo pills. Estrogen could cause bone marrow suppression at levels greater than 1 mg/kg in adult dogs. Some oral contraceptives also contain iron. Decontamination is not necessary unless the level of estrogen is greater than 1 mg/kg or the level of iron is greater than 20 mg/kg.

Flea Products

Flea products (sprays, spot-ons, collars, dips) are still a major problem for inducing toxicity although much less now that organophosphates are no longer the mainstay of treatment for flea control. These compounds reversibly alter the activity of sodium ion channels in nervous tissue. Clinical signs result from allergic, idiosyncratic, and neurotoxic reactions. The majority of toxicities are from pyrethrin and pyrethroid flea products applied to cats. Cats are much more sensitive than dogs and the dog products have several times higher concentration of the active ingredient (cat products often 2%, dog products often 45%–65%). The most common problem is misapplication of dog products onto the cat or splitting a large dog product onto several cats.

Calcium Oxalate Plants

Insoluble calcium oxalate plants are generally overrated as a toxic exposure. The calcium oxalate contained in the plant is an irritant to the mucous membranes, which generally inhibits ingestions of large volumes.

Liquid Potpourri

Liquid potpourri may contain essential oils and cationic detergents; because product labels may not list ingredients, it is wise to assume that a given liquid potpourri contains both ingredients. Essential oils can cause mucous membrane and gastrointestinal irritation, central nervous system depression, and dermal hypersensitivity and irritation. Severe clinical signs can be seen with potpourri products that contain cationic detergents. Dermal exposure to cationic detergents can result in erythema, edema, intense pain, and ulceration. Ingestion of cationic detergents may lead to tissue necrosis and inflammation of the mouth, esophagus, and stomach. Treatment is symptomatic and supportive.

References

1. Robinson EP: Anesthesia of pediatric patients, *Compend Cont Educ* 5(12):1004–1011, 1983.
2. Hellmann J, Vannucci RC, Nardis EE: Blood-brain barrier permeability to lactic acid in the newborn dog: lactate as a cerebral metabolic fuel, *Pediatr Res* 16:40–44, 1982.
3. Green TP, Mirkin BL: Clinical pharmacokinetics: pediatric considerations. In Benet LZ, Massoud N, Gambertoglio JG, editors: *Pharmacokinetic basis for drug treatment*, New York, 1984, Raven Press.
4. Boothe DM, Tannert K: Special considerations for drug and fluid therapy in the pediatric patient, *Compend Cont Educ* 14:313–329, 1991.
5. Heimann G: Enteral absorption and bioavailability in children in relation to age, *Eur J Clin Pharmacol* 18:43–50, 1980.
6. Rane A, Wilson JT: Clinical pharmacokinetics in infants and children. In Gibaldi M, Prescott L, editors: *Handbook of clinical pharmacokinetics*, New York, 1983, ADIS Health Science Press.
7. Gillette DD, Filkins M: Factors affecting antibody transfer in the newborn puppy, *Am J Physiol* 210(2):419–422, 1966.
8. Morselli PL, Morselli RF, Bossi L: Clinical pharmacokinetics in newborns and infants: age-related differences and therapeutic implications. In Gibaldi M, Prescott L, editors: *Handbook of clinical pharmacokinetics*, New York, 1983, ADIS Health Science Press.
9. Jones RL: Special considerations for appropriate antimicrobial therapy in neonates, *Vet Clin North Am Small Anim Pract* 17(3):577–602, 1987.
10. Shifrine M, Munn SL, Rosenblatt LS, et al: Hematologic changes to 60 days of age in clinically normal beagles, *Lab Anim* 23(6):894–898, 1973.
11. Sheng HP, Huggins RA: Growth of the beagle: changes in the body fluid compartments, *Proc Soc Exp Biol Med* 139:330–335, 1972.
12. Davis LE, Westfall BA, Short CR: Biotransformation and pharmacokinetics of salicylate in newborn animals, *Am J Vet Res* 34(8):1105–1108, 1973.
13. Poffenbarger EM, Ralston SL, Chandler ML, et al: Canine neonatology. Part I. Physiological differences between puppies and adults, *Compend Cont Educ* 12(11):1601–1609, 1990.
14. Ehrnebo M, Agurell S, Jalling B, et al: Age differences in drug binding by plasma proteins: studies on human fetuses, neonates and adults, *Eur J Clin Pharmacol* 3:189–193, 1973.
15. Reiche R: Drug disposition in the newborn. In Ruckesbusch P, Toutain P, Koritz D, et al: *Veterinary pharmacology and toxicology*, Westport, CT, 1983, AVI Publishing.
16. Peters EL, Farber TM, Heider A, et al: The development of drug-metabolizing enzymes in the young dog, *Fed Proc Am Soc Biol* 30:560, 1971.
17. Inman RC, Yeary RA: Sulfadiamethoxine pharmacokinetics in neonatal and young dogs, *Fed Proc Am Soc Biol* 30:560, 1971.
18. Rumack BH: Acetaminophen overdose in young children: treatment and effects of alcohol and other additional ingestants in 417 cases, *Am J Dis Child* 138:428–433, 1984.
19. Horster M, Kemler BJ, Valtin H: Intracortical distribution of number and volume of glomeruli during postnatal maturation in the dog, *J Clin Invest* 50:796–800, 1971.
20. Horster M, Valtin H: Postnatal development of renal function: micropuncture and clearance studies in the dog, *J Clin Invest* 50:779–795, 1971.
21. Cowan RH, Jukkola AF, Arant BS: Pathophysiologic evidence of gentamicin nephrotoxicity in neonatal puppies, *Pediatr Res* 14:1204–1211, 1980.
22. Bovee KC, Jezyk PF, Segal SC: Postnatal development of renal tubular amino acid reabsorption in canine pups, *Am J Vet Res* 45(4):830–832, 1984.
23. Kleinman LI: Renal bicarbonate reabsorption in the newborn dog, *J Physiol* 281:487–498, 1978.

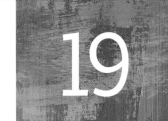

Considerations in the Geriatric Poisoned Patient

19

Justine A. Lee, DVM, DACVECC

Geriatric Patients

In veterinary medicine there is a growing population of geriatric patients, which may be due to advances in the quality of medicine. With this increase in the geriatric patient population, age-related considerations in pharmacology must be considered. Physiologic changes seen in geriatric patients include organ-related dysfunction (e.g., age-related hepatic changes, age-related nephron loss),[1,2] changes in body composition,[1,2] changes in cardiac output (resulting in changes in regional and organ blood flow),[1] decreased compensatory physiologic responses,[2] and other miscellaneous effects on the body (e.g., decreases in metabolic rate, diminished receptor response, underlying diseases).[1,3] Concurrently, oxygen consumption is decreased while there is a decline in physiologic functions (Box 19-1).[3] All these changes may markedly affect the pharmacokinetics (i.e., altered drug concentration at the site of action),[1] pharmacodynamics (i.e., altered drug action),[1] and the four components of drug disposition: absorption, distribution, metabolism, and excretion (Box 19-2). These changes directly affect the body's ability to dispose of drugs and how the body (or tissues) will respond to drugs.[4-6] This chapter will review geriatric pharmacology and how it applies to the geriatric poisoned patient.

The definition of a geriatric patient is one that has reached 75% of the expected lifespan.[2] When a patient reaches geriatric age, approximately 30% of body cells are permanently lost.[3] In human medicine, this is generally defined as 80 years of age.[3] In veterinary medicine, the definition of "geriatric" is not well defined, and is more subjective due to variability in species, breed, and overall size. For example, a 5- to 7-year-old Great Dane may be considered geriatric, whereas for a Chihuahua this may be at 9 to 15 years of age.

Organ-Related Dysfunction

Age-Related Hepatic Changes

As the liver plays a key role in the metabolism of xenobiotics, age-related changes in hepatic function can result in increased potential toxicity of these compounds. Age-related hepatic changes include decreases in hepatic function, decreases in hepatocyte numbers (with a resultant decrease in overall liver mass), decreases in hepatic and splanchnic blood flow, and an overall reduction in the liver's intrinsic activity of drug-metabolizing enzymes.[1,2] Decreases in the ability of the liver to produce sufficient protective compounds (e.g., oxygen radical scavengers), along with alterations in hepatic function, nutrition, and oxygenation, may further contribute to xenobiotic-induced hepatotoxicity in the geriatric patient.[3] All these changes result in a net decrease in both hepatic oxidation and the primary xenobiotic metabolizing enzyme cytochrome P450, resulting in changes in the liver's ability to metabolize compounds that require either capacity-limited or flow-limited hepatic metabolism.[3] For example, nonsteroidal antiinflammatories (NSAIDs) are compounds that

223

Box 19-1 **Age-Induced Physiologic Alterations**

Hepatic
Decreased protein synthesis
Decreased numbers of hepatocytes
Phase I xenobiotic metabolism altered
Decreased liver size

Renal
Creatinine clearance decreased, serum
　creatinine normal
Decreased tubular absorption
Decreased glomerular filtration rate
Decreased renal blood flow

Body Composition
Increased body fat
Decreased total body water
Decreased plasma volume
Decreased plasma albumin
Decreased lean body mass

Gastrointestinal Tract
Increased gastric pH
Decreased active transport
Decreased rate of gastric emptying
Decreased esophageal peristalsis
Decreased gastric secretions

Cardiovascular
Heart
Decreased cardiac output
Cardiac hypertrophy
Decreased stress response

Vascular
Decreased tissue perfusion
Decreased vascular elasticity
Increased systolic blood pressure
Increased vascular wall thickness

Box 19-2 **Factors That Affect Xenobiotic Disposition**

Pharmacologic Factors
Pharmaceutical interactions
Therapeutic inequivalence
Direct drug-drug interactions
Drug-diet interactions
Pharmacokinetic interactions
Pharmacodynamic interactions

Pathologic Conditions Modifying Drug Action
Gastrointestinal disease
Hepatic disease
Renal disease
Cardiovascular disease
Pulmonary disease
Neurologic disease

Metabolic disease
Other disease
Drug protein binding

Physiologic Factors
Route of exposure
Species variations
Genetic (breed) factors
Age
Sex
Body weight/surface area
Pregnancy/lactation
Diet/nutrition
Temperament
Environment
Circadian rhythms

---

require primarily capacity-limited hepatic metabolism, and geriatric patients may exhibit prolonged hepatic clearance.[3] Likewise, drugs like opioids are compounds which undergo flow-limited metabolic hepatic clearance; geriatric patients typically have an increased response that requires 60% to 75% less drug than that needed in younger patients, primarily because of reduced drug elimination.[3,5,7,8]

Hepatic clearance (Cl_H) is determined by the liver's intrinsic ability to extract the drug (hepatic extraction ratio [ER_H]) and the hepatic blood flow (Q_H).[1] High-clearance drugs such as lidocaine, propranolol, morphine, isoproterenol, and verapamil have a high ER_H (approaching 1), meaning that their hepatic clearance is almost equal to hepatic blood flow.[1] Therefore, drugs with a high ER_H are highly influenced by changes in hepatic blood flow.[1] However, when these drugs are given orally, they undergo high "first-pass effect" and typically do not reach high systemic concentrations because of high clearance of the drug. In the geriatric patient, the first-pass effect is diminished; therefore, in drugs with a high ER_H, systemic toxicity may occur because of increased oral bioavailability of the drug:

$$Cl_H = (Q_H)(ER_H)$$

Conversely, drugs with a low ER_H (<0.2) such as phenobarbital, benzodiazepines, chloramphenicol, and phenylbutazone are not significantly affected by hepatic blood flow.[1] These drugs with a low ER_H are not typically affected by the first-pass effect. Rather, changes in protein binding and hepatic microsomal enzyme systems may affect drug clearance.[1] In the geriatric patient, the level of albumin decreases relative to the increase in globulins (therefore maintaining normal total protein values).[3] If a geriatric patient is exposed to highly protein-bound toxicants, the portion of the xenobiotic that is free (versus protein-bound) may then be increased.[3] For example, most NSAIDs are close to 99% protein bound; even a small decrease of 1% (e.g., 99% to 98% binding) results in a doubling of the concentration of the pharmacologically active drug.[3] Some protection against this elevated plasma concentration may occur with the increased clearance of unbound compound by both the liver and kidneys.[3]

Age-Related Nephron Changes

Also in the geriatric patient, age-related nephron loss occurs along with reductions in renal blood flow. As a result both the glomerular filtration rate and the active secretory rate of the nephron unit are diminished,[3] resulting in a decline in renal xenobiotic clearance. Because most xenobiotics are renally excreted, age-related nephron changes and alterations in renal clearance can lead to increased blood concentrations of the parent or metabolite(s) of the xenobiotic, along with prolonged elimination,[3] placing the geriatric patient at increased risk of toxicosis. For example, the use of certain xenobiotics that are known to be nephrotoxic (e.g., NSAIDs, angiotensin-converting enzyme inhibitors, and aminoglycosides) should be judiciously considered in the geriatric patient.[3] Again, because of the decreased nephron population and increased filtering load per nephron,[3,9] increased plasma concentrations and prolonged exposure per nephron may occur, resulting in nephrotoxicity.

Changes in Body Composition

In the geriatric patient, decreases in total body and interstitial water, decreases in muscle mass, and increases in fat content occur. For example, in human geriatric males, body fat content is typically 50%, whereas in young males, body fat content is typically 18%.[5] Although this has not been evaluated in veterinary medicine, these changes in body composition can result in altered pharmacokinetics and pharmacodynamics. For example, geriatric patients with decreased muscle mass may have increased plasma concentrations of drugs that distribute normally to skeletal tissue (e.g., digoxin).[2] Likewise, in geriatric patients with decreased total body water, increased plasma concentrations of water-soluble drugs (e.g., aminoglycosides, digoxin) can occur.[2] Because these water-soluble drugs have poor fat distribution, dosing should ideally be performed on lean body weight.

Changes in Cardiac Output

In geriatric humans, cardiac output decreases by 30% to 40% over time (typically at a rate of approximately 1% a year). In veterinary medicine, a decrease in cardiac output also occurs in our geriatric pets, resulting in decreases in regional and organ blood flow[1] and a resultant increase in circulatory transit time.[3] Alternations in these cardiovascular dynamics likely affect the disposition (e.g., absorption, distribution, metabolism, and excretion) of drugs.[3] Xenobiotic plasma or tissue concentrations can be affected in either direction—decreased absorption and distribution or increased metabolism and excretion.[5,10] As a result of decreased cardiac output, blood is preferentially shunted to key organs (e.g., heart, brain), which can result in increased risk of toxicity to these organs receiving more blood flow.[1,3] Likewise, decreased cardiac output can result in a prerenal azotemia, which can affect renally cleared drugs (e.g., furosemide, enalapril, digoxin).

Decreased Compensatory Physiologic Responses

In geriatric humans, response to catecholamines is diminished. As a result, compensatory responses to hypotension or cardiac arrhythmias may be blunted, resulting in poor response to drug-induced hypotension or hypovolemia. As geriatric patients often have underlying cardiac (e.g., chronic valvular heart disease) or metabolic (e.g., hyperthyroidism) disease, further ability to compensate may be affected. Geriatric patients also have age-related alterations in GABA receptors and decreased dopamine concentrations; this may make geriatric patients more sensitive to excessive sedation and adverse events (e.g., tremoring from metoclopramide) to drugs, respectively.[2]

Miscellaneous Changes (e.g., Decreases In Metabolic Rate, Diminished Receptor Response, Underlying Diseases)

Geriatric patients have reduced gastrointestinal motility (including pharyngeal and esophageal),[3] decreased salivation and deglutition,[3] decreased absorptive capacity, and diminished gastric acid secretion (resulting in secondary increased gastric pH). In addition, age-related atrophy of intestinal villi may occur, increasing the potential for risk of bacterial overgrowth.[3] As a result, geriatric patients exposed to xenobiotics may be at greater risk of adverse gastrointestinal effects by certain compounds (e.g., chemotherapeutic agents, NSAIDs).[3]

Age-related changes are also seen in the pulmonary system. Decreases in residual lung volume, vital capacity, and overall respiratory function occur in the geriatric patient, resulting in low arterial partial pressure of oxygen (PaO_2).[3] Higher than normal alveolar-arterial gradients are seen in geriatric patients. Finally, geriatric patients have diminished central nervous system responses to hypoxemia or hypercapnea, making them less likely to compensate for xenobiotics that potentially affect ventilation (e.g., opioids, baclofen).

Geriatric patients have diminished immune system function as compared with young patients, which may increase the risk of toxicosis from immunosuppressive agents (e.g., 5-fluorouracil, chemotherapeutic agents, steroids).[11] Lastly, geriatric patients are more likely to have underlying metabolic disease (e.g., hepatic, renal, neoplasia), which may affect xenobiotic disposition.

Conclusion

Geriatric patients may have alterations in pharmaokinetics and pharmacodynamics because of age-related changes. Geriatric patients exposed to toxicants should be carefully assessed for underlying organ-related dysfunction (e.g., age-related hepatic changes, age-related nephron loss),[1,2] changes in cardiac output (resulting in changes in regional and organ blood flow),[1] changes in body composition,[1,2] decreased compensatory physiologic responses,[2] and other miscellaneous effects on the body which may affect the patient's response.[1,3] Because geriatric patients are often receiving multiple drugs for underlying medical conditions, there is potential for increased risk of drug-drug or drug-toxin interactions.[3] Aggressive therapy (including decontamination) and evaluation of underlying metabolic disease is imperative in geriatric poisoned patients for the best outcome.

References

1. Trepanier LA: Neonatal and geriatric pharmacology, *Proceedings of International Veterinary Emergency and Critical Care Symposium*, 2007.
2. Dowling PM: Geriatric pharmacology, *Vet Clin North Am* 35:557–569, 2005.
3. Boothe DM, Peterson ME: Considerations in pediatric and geriatric poisoned patients. In Peterson ME, Talcott PA, editors: *Small animal toxicology*, St Louis, 2006, Saunders.
4. Massoud N: Pharmacokinetic considerations in geriatric patients. In Benet LZ, Massoud N, Gambertoglio JG, editors: *Pharmacokinetic basis for drug treatment*, New York, 1984, Raven Press.

5. Ritschel WA: *Gerontokinetics: The pharmacokinetics of drugs in the elderly*, W. Caldwell, NJ, 1988, Telford Press.
6. Feely J, Coakley D: Altered pharmacodynamics in the elderly, *Clin Pharmacol* 6:269–283, 1990.
7. Enck RE: Pain control in the ambulatory elderly, *Geriatrics* 46:49–60, 1991.
8. Workaman BS, Ciccone V, Christophidis N: Pain management for the elderly, *Aust Fam Physician* 18:1515–1527, 1989.
9. Frazier DL, Dix LP, Bowman KF, et al: Increased gentamicin nephrotoxicity in normal and diseased dogs administered identical serum drug concentration profiles: increased sensitivity in subclinical renal dysfunction, *J Pharmacol Exp Ther* 239:946–951, 1986.
10. Aucoin DP: Drug therapy in the geriatric animal: the effect of aging on drug disposition, *Vet Clin North Am Small Anim Pract* 19:41–48, 1989.
11. Schultz RD: The effects of aging on the immune system, *Compend Cont Educ* 6(12):1096–1105, 1984.

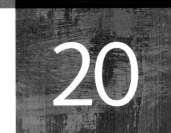

Poisonings in the Captive Reptile

Kevin T. Fitzgerald, PhD, DVM, DABVP

Kristin L. Newquist, BS, AAS, CVT

- Exotic animals are increasingly being kept as pets in American homes.
- Exotic animals present special diagnostic challenges to veterinarians when they become ill.
- Because of captivity, reptiles can become accidentally poisoned in a number of ways.
- The basic tenets of emergency medicine are the same for all animal species, despite their rare or exotic nature.
- Veterinarians seeing small animal emergency cases must make an attempt to familiarize themselves with the large body of literature and resources that is developing regarding nontraditional companion species.

"Gentle mercy even to the snakes."

SHAKESPEARE

Introduction

Increasing numbers of exotic species are being kept as household pets. Reptiles, in particular, are enjoying a huge rise in popularity in American homes. These exotic species present a special challenge when they become ill. Veterinarians are often not familiar with rare or less frequently encountered exotic species and may not recognize particular syndromes or know how to effectively treat them. In this discussion we will look at the care and management of the poisoned reptile.

Emergency Management of the Poisoned Reptile

Emergency situations in reptiles are not always obvious for veterinarians and certainly not for average reptile owners. Many veterinarians are not familiar with the anatomy, physiology, and vital signs of captive reptile species. In addition, like other wild animals, exotic reptiles do much to mask outward signs of disease. However, the basic tenets of emergency medicine remain the same regardless of species.

Emergency care begins with a sound history. How long has the reptile been in the home, what is its origin, are cage mates involved, what type of cage setup is employed, and heat and light sources (how long a photo period and how warm is the cage setting) are all pertinent questions. How often is the animal fed and watered, what type of diet is used, and how often is the environment cleaned and with what chemicals? A thorough physical examination is performed next. Heart rate, respiration, hydration status, neurological condition, and mentation are all critical cues to both diagnosis and prognosis. However, physical examination and clinical signs are only part of obtaining a successful diagnosis. Laboratory parameters will also help determine what treatment modalities are necessary. Reptiles injured or seriously ill nearly always benefit from administration of fluids. Various methods of fluid administration are touted, but actual intravenous fluid therapy is not practical for most reptiles. Many reptiles (particularly desert species) can tolerate dramatic degrees of dehydration. Lizards, snakes, and turtle relatives all show sunken eyes and changes in skin if dehydrated. Intraosseous catheters are a legitimate alternative to intravenous types. Enteral, intracoelomic, and subcutaneous fluids are also available to support the poisoned reptile.

Reptiles are ectothermic and dependent on environmental temperature for their warmth. Reptilian species have their own preferred body temperature and optimum thermal zone. For most reptiles, range is dependent on the species. Debilitated reptiles can be so weak that they cannot move away from heat sources and may end up overheating or even being burned. Use only safe heat sources, such as heating small rooms, overhead heat lights, and under-tank heating pads. Cage thermometers must be diligently monitored to ensure that animals are kept within a safe thermal range. Rigorous, persistent nursing care can often help save severely poisoned reptiles.

Common Toxicants

Vitamin A Toxicity

Vitamin A is necessary for the health of normal skin and periocular tissue. Chelonians (turtles and tortoises) are particularly sensitive to vitamin A deficiency. Turtles with hypovitaminosis typically show ocular discharge, palpebral edema and blindness, hyperkeratosis of skin and mouth parts, and aural abscesses. Patients can improve with vitamin A supplementation (2000 IU/kg IM q 7 days) and improved dietary management.[1]

Excessive iatrogenic administration of vitamin A can cause a separate set of problems. Hypervitaminosis A can cause inappetence, full-thickness skin sloughing, secondary bacterial infection, discoloration of the skin, and extreme lethargy. Generally this occurs at doses of 10,000 IU/kg or higher given IM as a single injection. Treatment involves ceasing vitamin A administration, antibiotics, fluid therapy, wound management, and nutritional support. Skin lesions may heal slowly, but animals managed supportively can recover completely.

Vitamin D Toxicity

Excesses of water-soluble vitamins can be excreted into the urine. This makes their margin of safety very large. For fat-soluble vitamins, such as vitamin A and vitamin D, this is not the case. Owners, breeders, and veterinarians often oversupplement captive reptiles with disastrous results. Doses of 50 to 1000 times the minimum daily requirement are often given for weeks to months. This can be insidious, particularly when the minimum daily requirement of most vertebrates for vitamin D is only 10 to 20 IU/kg body weight.[2]

The mechanism of action of the toxicity of vitamin D is related to the hypercalcemia and hyperphosphatemia it induces. This prolonged hypercalcemia and hyperphosphatemia causes dystrophic calcification of the gastrointestinal tissue, the kidneys, lungs, heart, blood vessels, and joints.[3] Complete removal of vitamin D–containing supplements and administration of cortisone may help control hypercalcemia, but resolution of soft-tissue calcification may not be successful.

In light of the inherent calcium problems of captive reptiles, it is incumbent on veterinarians to counsel clients about proper husbandry, nutrition, and dietary requirements and to ensure that *no* supplements are given to animals without veterinary approval.

Antimicrobial Toxicity

Selection of antibiotics should be made judiciously. Selection depends on experience of the clinician; empirical considerations; the type of infection present based on culture and sensitivity and Gram stains; and, last but not least, the size, age, species, and condition of the reptilian patient. There is no antibiotic that can be relied on to be effective for all situations.

In addition, antibiotics are no substitute for good wound management, nursing care, nutrition, or husbandry.

Gentamicin

Gentamicin is an aminoglycoside antibiotic. Other aminoglycosides include amikacin, tobramycin, neomycin, streptomycin, and kanamycin. Gentamicin is bactericidal and is a broad spectrum antibiotic (except against streptococci and anaerobic bacteria).[4] Its mechanism of action involves inhibition of bacterial protein synthesis by binding to 30S ribosomes. Gentamicin is indicated for acute serious infections, such as those caused by gram-negative bacteria. Amikacin is more consistently active against resistant strains of bacteria.

Nephrotoxicity of gentamicin in reptiles is well documented.[5-8] Patients must have adequate fluid and electrolyte balance during therapy. Ototoxicity in reptiles has also been reported. Recommended dosage for gentamicin varies from 2.75 to 6 mg/kg IM q 72 hours given no sooner than every third day.

Amikacin

Amikacin is also an aminoglycoside, bactericidal, broad spectrum in activity, and operates on bacteria through the same mechanism of action as gentamicin. It is indicated particularly against gram-negative organisms in which it may have greater activity than gentamicin.

Like gentamicin, nephrotoxicity is the most dose-limiting effect of amikacin. Patients must be maintained in fluid and electrolyte balance during therapy. Ototoxicity has also been reported. If used together with anesthetic agents, aminoglycosides may show neuromuscular blockade. Dosages for amikacin range from 2.25 to 5 mg/kg IM given no more frequently than every third day.

Chloramphenicol

Chloramphenicol is an antibacterial agent with a broad spectrum of activity against gram-positive bacteria, gram-negative bacteria, and *Rickettsia*. Its mechanism of action is by inhibition of bacterial protein synthesis by binding with ribosomes.

The major toxicity of chloramphenicol is hematological.[9] In all vertebrates studied, it produces direct, dose-dependent bone marrow depression resulting in reductions in red blood cells, white blood cells, and platelets. This manifestation is aggravated by inappropriate doses, extended treatments, and repeated use of the drug. Treatment of chloramphenicol intoxication is supportive and may require blood transfusions. The drug has also been reported to be appetite suppressive. Like gentamicin, chloramphenicol is being used less frequently as safer antibiotics become available. The recommended dosage for chloramphenicol is 50 mg/kg IM (SC in snakes) administered once daily or every other day.

Enrofloxacin

Enrofloxacin is a fluoroquinolone antibacterial drug. It is bactericidal with a broad spectrum of activity. Its mechanism of action involves inhibition of deoxyribonucleic acid (DNA) gyrase, thus inhibiting both DNA and ribonucleic acid (RNA) synthesis.[4] Sensitive bacteria include *Staphylococcus, Escherichia coli, Proteus, Klebsiella,* and *Pasteurella. Pseudomonas* is moderately susceptible but requires higher doses. In most species studied, enrofloxacin is metabolized to ciprofloxacin. Damage to cartilage has been seen in growing animals treated with fluoroquinolones. Doses of enrofloxacin range from 5 mg/kg IM or PO q 24 hours. There are other choices of antibiotics for use in reptiles, based on Gram staining, culture and sensitivity, and age of the animal. We have seen many species of reptiles (e.g., lizards, snakes, and turtles) develop lesions after enrofloxacin injections.

Metronidazole

Metronidazole is used as an antibacterial, an antiprotozoal, an antiparasitic, and an appetite stimulant in reptiles. It is formulated as a suspension, as an injectable, and as tablets.

The activity of metronidazole is specific for anaerobic bacteria and protozoa. It is specific, particularly for *Giardia* organisms. Metronidazole disrupts DNA in target microbes through reaction with intracellular metabolites.[10]

The most severe side effect of metronidazole is dose-related central nervous system (CNS) toxicity. High doses can cause ataxia, inability to walk, nystagmus, opisthotonos, tremors of the lumbar muscles and hindlimbs, seizures, and death.[11,12] Treatment is symptomatic and supportive.

Metronidazole has been recommended for a variety of conditions in reptiles. Particular care must be given when this drug is used regarding dose, duration, and size of the animal.

Antifungal Toxicity

A variety of fungal infections have been documented in reptiles. Ranging from dermatophytes to systemic mycotic infections, these conditions are treated with a variety of antifungal medications. Treatment with antifungals can lead to serious intoxications, based on the small size of the reptilian patient, the mechanisms of action of these drugs, and idiosyncrasies of reptilian physiology.

Amphotericin B

Amphotericin B is a macrolide class antibiotic unrelated to erythromycin. This antifungal inhibits ergosterol synthesis.[13] Ergosterol is a component of the cell membrane unique to fungal organisms. Amphotericin B is a potent nephrotoxin.[14] It produces signs of renal toxicity in 80% of patients that receive it. Its action causes renal vasoconstriction, reduces glomerular filtration rate, and has direct toxic effects on the membranes of the renal tubule cells. Through these mechanisms, amphotericin B causes acute tubular necrosis. Hypokalemia develops in almost 35% of human patients treated with amphotericin B, which is sufficient to warrant potassium supplementation.

Clinical signs mimic acute renal failure: anorexia, lethargy, weight loss, and other signs. Elevated blood urea nitrogen (BUN) and creatinine with decreased potassium and sodium are commonly seen.[15]

Treatment includes discontinuing the drug, aggressive fluid therapy to prevent further kidney damage, and diminishing renal effects with sodium chloride-containing fluids. Treatment with mannitol may help increase the elimination of amphotericin B.

Prognosis after amphotericin B toxicity depends upon the severity of the renal damage. Amphotericin B is still listed as a treatment for aspergillosis in reptiles (1 mg/kg intracoelomically once daily for 2 to 4 weeks).[16] There may be safer drugs available. A less toxic, new formulation of amphotericin B is available for humans and may soon be available for veterinary use. Amphotericin B should not be used in animals that already have renal disease.

Griseofulvin

This antifungal works by inhibiting fungal spindle activity and leads to distorted, weakened fungal hyphae.[17] It has also been shown to cause bone marrow suppression in mammals, although the mechanism of this action is unknown.

Anorexia, lethargy, diarrhea, and anemia have been reported in intoxicated animals. In reptiles the recommended dosage for fungal dermatitis is 20 to 40 mg/kg given orally every third day for five treatments. It is available as a tablet and a topical ointment.

Treatment includes discontinuing the drug and treating the patient supportively. There is no specific antidote. Griseofulvin has been shown to be teratogenic in pregnant animals of many species. Topical treatments can be removed with tepid water and gentle hand soap. Antifungal overdoses can be best avoided by preventing fungal infection through good husbandry.

Imidazoles (Ketoconazole) and Triazoles (Fluconazole and Itraconazole)

These antifungal drugs inhibit fungal replication by interfering with ergosterol synthesis. Ketoconazole also has direct effects upon the fungal membrane. The liver metabolizes these fungistatic drugs. Itraconazole is more potent than ketoconazole and is better tolerated by patients.

Clinical signs of intoxication include anorexia, lethargy, weight loss, and diarrhea. Elevated liver enzymes may be present in intoxicated animals. Dosages recommended for reptiles include 2 to 5 mg/kg orally daily for 5 days for fluconazole, 15 to 30 mg/kg given orally daily for 3 weeks for ketoconazole, and 5 to 23.5 mg/kg orally once daily for itraconazole.[18] There seems to be little problem with miconazole preparation applied topically.[19]

There is no specific antidote for toxicity by these antifungals. Treatment involves stopping the drug, decontaminating any topical material remaining, and supportive therapy (fluids, warmth). For ketoconazole, treatment includes countering the hepatotoxicity. Mild intoxications usually improve with simple cessation of the drug.

The safest, most effective drugs must be selected for use in fungal infections in reptiles and must reflect the severity of the infection, the size of the animal, and the condition of the animal before treatment. Doses must be meticulously checked, particularly for topicals and dips to be used on reptiles. Finally, reptiles must *never* be left alone in any bath or medicated dip.

Organophosphates and Carbamates

Organophosphates are the most commonly used insecticide worldwide. In the United States alone, 250 million pounds of organophosphates are used annually.[20] They are found in agriculture, in the home, and on or around various domestic animals. Some organophosphates are meant to stay on surfaces to which they are applied, and others are absorbed and become systemic in animals. They are the active ingredients in a long list of products. For animal use as insecticides, they are formulated as dips, sprays, topical medications, systemic parasitic agents, and flea collars. This group of insecticides includes chlorpyrifos (Dursban), dichlorvos, diazinon, cythioate (Proban), fenthion (ProSpot), malathion, ronnel, parathion, metrifonate, and vapona. Their cousins, the carbamates, include aldicarb, carbaryl (Sevin), bendiocarb, methiocarb, propoxur, and carbofuran. As newer, safer insecticides are marketed, these two groups are involved in fewer accidental poisonings but still account for a large number of intoxications.

Organophosphates and carbamates interfere with metabolism and breakdown of acetylcholine at synaptic junctions.[21] Acetylcholinesterase is the enzyme responsible for breaking down the neurotransmitter at these sites. Acetylcholinesterase is inhibited by organophosphates and carbamates at these cholinergic sites. As a result, acetylcholine accumulates at the synapses, which at first excites and then paralyzes transmission in these synapses, giving it the characteristic "nerve gas" signs associated with organophosphate toxicity.[22] This inhibition of the synapse is irreversible with organophosphates and reversible with carbamates. Organophosphates are readily absorbed by all routes: dermal, respiratory, gastrointestinal, and conjunctival. Overdose with organophosphates may happen more readily if given together with imidothiazoles, such as levamisole.

Clinical signs seen in reptiles include salivation, ataxia, muscle fasciculations, inability to right themselves, coma, and respiratory arrest. Death results from massive respiratory secretions, bronchiolar constriction, and effects on respiratory centers in the medulla leading to the cessation of breathing.

Animals with dermal exposure should be washed with a mild dishwashing detergent and copious amounts of water. Animals should be dried after rinsing to prevent further uptake of the insecticide. The need for fluid therapy to counter dehydration and electrolyte imbalances should be considered. The specific physiological antidote, the muscarinic antagonist atropine, should be given (0.4 mg/kg IM). This should help with salivation, bronchospasm, and dyspnea. Diazepam may be given as needed for seizures. Use of antihistamines to treat insecticide poisonings is controversial and most likely not that effective. Prognosis is dependent on dose, duration of exposure, and size of the animal. Therapies both more effective and safer than organophosphates and carbamates exist for treatment of parasites in captive reptiles. These therapeutic regimens are outlined in detail elsewhere in various sources dealing with reptilian parasitology.

Pyrethrins and Pyrethroids

Pyrethrin is the oldest used botanical insecticide. It is made from the dried and ground flowers of *Chrysanthemum cinerariifolium* (Color Plate 20-1). Pyrethroids are synthetic derivatives of pyrethrin and are widely available. Pyrethroid insecticides have enhanced stability, potency, and half-life compared with the parent molecule. A variety of dilute pyrethrin- and pyrethroid-containing sprays have been recommended for reptiles.

The mechanism of action of both pyrethrins and pyrethroids is the same. These molecules affect parasites by altering the activity of the sodium ion channels of nerves. These poisons prolong the period of sodium conductance and increase the length of the depolarizing action potential.[23] This results in repetitive nerve firing and death. With the right conditions or at higher doses, these compounds can intoxicate host animals. Because of the potential for transcutaneous absorption, pyrethrin and pyrethroid sprays must be thoroughly rinsed from the animal immediately after their application. Rinsing with lukewarm water is usually sufficient.

Like ivermectin, organophosphates, and carbamates, pyrethrins and pyrethroids should *never* be given concurrently with cholinesterase-inhibiting compounds.

Clinical signs have been reported for pyrethrins and pyrethroids, particularly if sprays used also contain insect growth regulators (e.g., methoprene). Signs can develop in animals within 15 minutes of application. Signs include salivation, ataxia, inability to right themselves, and muscle fasciculations.[24] Idiosyncratic reactions to pyrethrins can happen at much lower doses than expected. A small percentage of animals appear to be extremely sensitive to pyrethrins and pyrethroids.

If caught early enough, treatment for pyrethrin and pyrethroid toxicity involves dermal decontamination (bathing in copious amounts of water), isotonic fluids, and diazepam for seizures. Care must be taken to keep pyrethrin and pyrethroid sprays away from the reptile's eyes and mouth to prevent intoxication. Prognosis depends on the strength of the agent used, the duration of the exposure, and the size of the animal involved. Animals that are treated early do best.

A variety of pyrethrins and pyrethroids have been recommended for use against reptile parasites. If used prudently, they are both safe and effective. Animals are sometimes saturated with the spray. As soon as the parasiticide is applied, it should be rinsed off. Gently running lukewarm tap water should be used to wash off the insecticide. This very brief exposure is enough to kill the parasites. Pyrethrin and pyrethroid sprays should not be left on to prevent absorption and systemic toxicity in host animals. In smaller animals that have larger surface-to-volume ratios, most sprays should be diluted to the smallest effective dose to prevent accidental intoxication from transcutaneous absorption.

Ivermectin

Ivermectin is an antiparasitic from a family of chemicals called avermectins. These are macrocyclic lactones made from the fermentation broth of the fungus *Streptomyces avermitilis*.[25] The macrolide ivermectin is available as an injectable, a spray, and an oral formulation. It has activity against a variety of parasites including nematodes, arthropods, and arachnids.

Avermectins work by potentiating the effects of the inhibitory neurotransmitter, γ-aminobutyric acid (GABA). They stimulate release of GABA by presynaptic sites and increase GABA binding to postsynaptic receptors. This causes neuromuscular blockage. Avermectins also open chloride channels in membranes of the nervous system and further depress neuronal function. These actions cause paralysis and death of susceptible parasites. Ivermectin is absorbed systemically by host tissue. When parasites bite the host they then absorb the ivermectin. Ivermectin is active against intestinal parasites, mites, microfilaria, and developing larvae. Concurrent treatment with diazepam, which also works through GABA potentiation, may heighten deleterious effects.

Ivermectin can cause depression, paralysis, coma, and death in chelonians.[26] Species susceptible to ivermectin toxicosis may have a blood-brain barrier more permeable than in nonsensitive species. This greater permeability may be due to p-glycoprotein mutation in membranes of the CNS. Another theory postulates the existence of a specific protein receptor only present in the brains of ivermectin-sensitive species. This has not yet been demonstrated. Ivermectin toxicity has also been reported in several species of lizards and snakes.[27] Ball pythons (*Python regius*) in particular may show mild neurological signs when treated. As a result, if there is any question regarding safety, it may be more prudent to use ivermectin only as a topical.

There is no known antidote or physiological antagonist for ivermectin. Treatment is supportive and should include decontaminating any topical sprays with soap and water, providing fluid therapy, nutritional support, monitoring electrolytes, and respiratory support. Recovery may take days to weeks. One debilitated tortoise recovered fully after 6 weeks. We have seen two box turtles completely recover in 4 weeks. IV lipid therapy has been used to treat ivermectin poisoning successfully in many animal species other than reptiles.

Ivermectin, and similarly related compounds, should *never* be given to chelonians, pregnant animals, or neonatal individuals. Also, for particularly tiny species, other therapies should be investigated. If there is any question, use it only as a topical or find an alternative.

Fenbendazole

Fenbendazole is a benzimidazole type of antiparasitic drug.[28] It is safe and effective against many helminth parasites in animals. Fenbendazole inhibits glucose uptake in the parasites. Because of its wide range of activity, its high degree of efficacy, and its broad margin of safety, this anthelmintic is frequently prescribed by veterinarians. Fenbendazole has a good margin of safety and has been reported to be well tolerated, even at six times recommended dose and three times recommended duration.[29] It has been extensively used as an anthelmintic therapy in reptiles at a dosage of 50 to 100 mg/kg PO once (repeated in 2 weeks) or 50 mg/kg PO q 24 hours for 3 to 5 days.[30,31]

Toxic effects have been reported in birds, rats, cats, and dogs.[32-36] Recently, evidence of fenbendazole overdose has been reported in individuals of a small snake species given an exceedingly large dose of the drug. Four adult Fea's vipers (*Azemiops feae*) died after being administered single doses of fenbendazole ranging from 428 mg/kg to 1064 mg/kg.[29] Necropsy findings were suggestive of intestinal changes consistent with fenbendazole toxicity. Fenbendazole is regarded as a safe anthelmintic drug at recommended therapeutic doses.

Chlorhexidine Toxicity

Soaking living animals in any solution can be potentially life threatening. Recently, turtles soaked for 1 hour in chlorhexidine scrub were shown to become intoxicated.[37] Cutaneous absorption of the solution and possible oral ingestion of these soaks have been postulated as the cause of the problem. Before using any substances as a soak, review the literature for preferred usage, dose, and duration of the soak. Affected animals should be removed from the soak, rinsed, and supported with warmth and fluids. Remember to *never* leave any reptile unattended in a bath. Animals can drown much faster than anticipated. Also, particular attention must be paid to the depth of fluids reptiles are bathed and soaked in.

Bleach

Various hypochlorite bleach solutions can be found in most households. Typically, these are 3% to 6% hypochlorite solutions in water.[38] Bleaches are moderately irritating. If contact with skin is prolonged, the damage is worsened. Bleaches can be very effective in treating cage parasites of reptiles, but should *never* be applied to live animals. Bleach can cause alkali burns if splashed in the eyes of lizards and turtles. Immediate irrigation of the eye with copious amounts of water minimizes the damage done by the bleach. Skin exposed to bleach should be washed with a mild soap and lukewarm water. Animals should be kept out of recently bleached cages a minimum of 24 hours to prevent respiratory tract irritation. Cages should be allowed to air out, and residual disinfectant removed by wiping with a clean cloth or towel.

Zinc Toxicosis

Zinc is an essential trace element. It is necessary for the synthesis of more than 200 enzymes required for cell division, growth, and gene expression. Chronic zinc deficiency from improper diet is more commonly seen than acute zinc poisoning from excessive zinc intake. Zinc toxicosis may result from overzealous administration of supplements, ingestion of galvanized metal objects, zinc oxide ointment, or from ingestion of pennies. Before 1982 U.S. pennies were more than 90% copper; since that time they are 97% zinc. We have seen two iguanas and one snake with gastrointestinal tracts full of pennies exhibiting signs of zinc toxicity.

The precise mechanism of action of zinc toxicosis is not known. However, the red blood cells, kidneys, pancreas, and liver are affected most. Intravascular hemolysis is the most consistent abnormality seen. It is thought that zinc causes oxidative damage that leads to lysis of the red blood cell membrane, which leads to anemia.[39]

Clinical signs of zinc toxicosis depend on the amount and form of the zinc ingested. Signs are delayed if coins are the source of the zinc. As few as one or two pennies can cause toxicity. First, the animal may be anorexic and lethargic, and the zinc ingestion may mimic gastrointestinal enteritis. This is followed by intravascular hemolysis, hemoglobinemia, yellow discoloration of the skin and mucous membranes, and weight loss. Palpation may be positive for coins, but in larger animals radiographs may be necessary to reveal the pennies. Elevated zinc levels can be confirmed on a serum sample antemortem and liver, kidney, and pancreas postmortem.

Treatment consists of removing the zinc-containing foreign object. Surgery may be required, but we have been very fortunate with removal of the coins via endoscopy. Additional supportive therapy involves fluid treatment to maintain hydration, possible blood transfusion to control anemia, and in severe cases use of a zinc chelator (e.g., ethylenediaminetetraacetic acid, penicillamine).

Prognosis depends on the amount of zinc ingested, the duration of the toxic exposure, and the severity of the resulting anemia. Reptiles must be kept in environments free of potential sources of zinc ingestion.

Smoke Inhalation

Dangerous fires are still a daily occurrence in the new millennium. In the continental United States alone, every 17 seconds a fire department responds to a fire call.[40] Depending on the source, it is estimated that 50% to 80% of fire deaths are the direct result of smoke inhalation rather than injuries from burns or trauma.

When compared with the rest of the world, the United States has one of the highest death rates caused by fire. This may be attributable to wider use of synthetic materials for building and furnishings. These synthetic substances generally produce much more toxic combustion substances. In addition, the nature of our buildings, and more high rises, skyscrapers, and multifloor dwellings, all make it much harder to escape from the effects of a disastrous fire and much harder to quench these fires once started.

The pathophysiology of smoke inhalation is dealt with in Chapter 29. Suffice it to say that a toxic combustion product (i.e., smoke) exerts its poisonous effects by filling enclosed vital airways with gases other than oxygen and by inducing local chemical reactions in the respiratory tract; chemical asphyxiants elicit toxic changes in tissue distant from the lung. Water solubility of toxic inhalants is the most important factor in determining the level of injury. Injury from water-soluble molecules occurs in the upper airways. Chemical toxicants with low water solubility reach the lungs, where they then exert their damaging effects. In addition, duration of exposure, concentration of the combustion products, and toxin particle size all contribute to the overall severity of the injury. Pathological changes in the lungs and respiratory tissues may progress over hours to days.

In our practice, several captive reptiles have come in after being exposed to the damaging smoke of house fires. Two young Ball pythons arrived after a particularly aggressive apartment fire. Direct laryngoscopy of the animals revealed the accumulation of soot and carbonaceous debris, copious secretions, and edematous laryngeal tissue. Both snakes were in severe respiratory compromise. Their breathing was weak and rapid, and the airways became increasingly edematous. The animals were treated by intubating and administering 100% oxygen, supportive fluids, and antibiotics. Despite our aggressive efforts, the smaller snake continued to deteriorate and expired. After 2 days of therapy, the larger snake survived. A box turtle presented after a residential fire. The reptile displayed no burns, was nonresponsive, and never regained consciousness despite our efforts, which included supplemental oxygen, fluid therapy, antibiotics, and suctioning of airways. The turtle died roughly 2 hours after exposure. Effective management of smoke inhalation must include establishing airway patency, administration of supplemental oxygen, frequent airway suctioning and removal of both debris and secretions, and cardiovascular support. Early intubation is often more beneficial than watching for the animal to decompensate.

Smoke inhalation patients are labor intensive to manage but may result in successful outcomes if animals are managed early and aggressively.

Rodenticides

Each year rodents destroy crops in the field, eat food in storage, serve as vectors for human diseases, bite people, and cause material damage by gnawing. As a result, a variety of rodenticides are ubiquitously employed in an attempt to control populations of these animals. These substances prove to be nearly as dangerous to humans and nontarget species as they are to rodents. Rodenticide intoxication has been documented in a variety of species, reptiles included. It is certainly worth the effort if the original container housing the poison is brought in with the animal so that active ingredients can be positively identified and appropriate treatment can be initiated.

Anticoagulants

The long-acting anticoagulants are responsible for 80% of rodenticide poisoning in humans and animals in the United States.[41] The long-acting agents have the same mechanism of action as warfarin. However, they are more potent and their half-life is longer. They are effective in single or very limited feedings when compared with older rodenticides. They act by decreasing the activity of the vitamin K–dependent blood-clotting factors (II, VII, IX, and X). When clotting factors are sufficiently reduced, bleeding occurs. The most common and most toxic second-generation anticoagulants in use are brodifacoum and bromadiolone.

Clinical signs depend on the site and extent of hemorrhage. The majority of intoxicated animals show anorexia, weakness, and lethargy.[42] The most common clinical sign is dyspnea. Typically animals bleed into body cavities, abdomen, thorax, and joints. Most of these poisons are packaged as molasses-soaked grain laced with the anticoagulants. These various plant materials can attract herbivorous or omnivorous reptiles. Newer formulations of these baits are dyed turquoise.

We have seen one iguana and one box turtle intoxicated by anticoagulant bait ingestion. Baseline determinations of one-stage prothrombin time (PT) are helpful in animals suspected of consuming anticoagulant poisons. One antidote for anticoagulant poisoning, vitamin K_1, should be administered in animals if the PT is increased. The daily dose recommendation for vitamin K_1 is 2.5 mg/kg. Therapy with this antidote must be maintained until toxic amounts of the poison are no longer present in the animal. Length of treatment depends on the dose and type of anticoagulant ingested, but may be as long as 3 to 4 weeks. A PT test should be run 48 hours after cessation of vitamin K_1 treatment. If clotting time is normal, therapy is discontinued. If the clotting time is increased, therapy is continued for another week. Vitamin K_1 treatment can be given by subcutaneous injection or orally. Intravenous injections have a high incidence of anaphylactic reaction. Other treatment options include possible oxygen support and plasma transfusions.

Bromethalin

Bromethalin is one of the "newer" rodenticides. It is formulated in baits of pelleted grain and may be dyed green or turquoise. Bromethalin is a neurotoxin, but because of its name it can be confused with the long-acting anticoagulants bromadiolone and brodifacoum. Clients should be encouraged to bring in original containers to obtain valuable label information concerning ingredients.

The mechanism of action of bromethalin is the uncoupling of oxidative phosphorylation. The brain is the primary target for bromethalin because of its unique dependence on oxidative phosphorylation. The drug causes brain electrolyte disturbances and results in the development of cerebral edema.[43]

Clinical signs include hindlimb paralysis, abnormal postures, fine muscle tremors, and seizures. Severely poisoned animals are comatose. Clinical signs are usually seen within 24 hours of ingestion.

Bromethalin is a nonselective vertebrate poison. No antidote exists, and treatment is initially directed at reducing gastrointestinal absorption and providing supportive care. Treatment must also aim at controlling cerebral edema seen in severe poisonings. Administration of dexamethasone and mannitol has been recommended to control bromethalin-induced cerebral edema. Unfortunately the efficacy of these diuretic agents in controlling bromethalin-poisoned animals is not very successful. Animals showing severe signs, such as seizures, paralysis, or coma, generally have a grave prognosis.

Cholecalciferol

Cholecalciferol (vitamin D_3), a "newer" rodenticide, exploits the fact that rodents are extremely sensitive to small percentage changes in the calcium balance in their blood. Cholecalciferol causes hypercalcemia through mobilization of the body's calcium stores, predominantly found in bone.[44] This dystrophic hypercalcemia results in calcification of blood vessels, organs, and soft tissue. It leads to nerve and muscle dysfunction and cardiac arrhythmias.

The rodenticide is formulated in pelleted baits of grain or seed. Accidental ingestion of human medication containing vitamin D_3 or its analogues by animals is also possible. Iatrogenic over supplementation of vitamin D_3 to reptiles is likewise possible.

Clinical signs include depression, weakness, and anorexia. Eventually signs of renal disease become evident as the glomerular filtration rate decreases.

Treatment usually involves corticosteroid and diuretic therapy. Corticosteroids suppress bone resorption and intestinal calcium absorption and promote calciuresis. Prednisone (6 mg/kg PO) and furosemide (1 to 4 mg/kg PO) have been recommended.[44,45] Supportive fluids (physiological saline) are essential. Calcitonin therapy has been recommended, but its efficacy is questionable. Pamidronate disodium (Aredia), a biphosphonate, has been recommended in dogs, with 1 to 2 mg/kg given slowly (over 2 hours).[45]

Prognosis is poor for animals in which dystrophic mineralization has already occurred.

Metaldehyde

Metaldehyde is the active ingredient in most slug and snail baits. It is formulated in granules, powder, pellets, and a liquid. Protein-rich material, such as bran or grain, is usually added to the bait to make it more attractive to snails. Unfortunately, other animals find it more palatable as a result. Metaldehyde poisoning has been reported in a wide range of species ranging from dogs to livestock. This is not a common intoxication in reptiles; however, the authors did see one captive tortoise fatality after encountering the poison in a household backyard garden.

The mechanism of action of metaldehyde poisoning was once thought to be a result of the degradation of the compound to acetaldehyde. Recent studies suggest metaldehyde itself may be the agent that affects the CNS.[46] GABA levels are decreased by metaldehyde, and this decrease can lead to depression, seizures, and coma.

Clinical signs include ataxia, incoordination and locomotor signs, muscle spasms, abnormal postures, and convulsions.[47] The tortoise involved presented as comatose, nonresponsive, and with the head and legs rigidly extended. Clinical signs develop within a few hours of ingestion.

There is no specific antidote for metaldehyde poisoning. Instead, animals are treated supportively. Fluids should be given and oxygen administered to counter respiratory depression. Mammals may display the "shake and bake" syndrome and are treated with diazepam or other appropriate anticonvulsants and steps are taken to counter the hyperthermia. Prognosis is generally better if the animal survives the first 36 hours.

Mushrooms

Confirmed mushroom toxicities are relatively rare, but the potential for such poisonings remains constant (see chapter 62). For humans poisoned by mushrooms in the United States, in more than 95% of the cases the exact species is never identified.[48] Furthermore, for humans known to have ingested toxic mushrooms, the individuals show no symptoms more than 50% of the time. Far and away the most toxic North American mushrooms are members of the *Amanita* species. The next most dangerous are hallucinogenic mushrooms.

This relative rarity of mushroom poisoning, the sparsity of lethal or even serious ingestions, and the inability of most physicians and veterinarians to correctly identify mushroom species involved all contribute to complicating the successful diagnosis of such toxicities. Nevertheless, a successful strategy and treatment plan for suspected mushroom poisoning is necessary.

Veterinarians must strive to learn the toxic varieties of mushrooms in their region and their general incidence. Successful diagnosis includes gross identification of the mushroom specimen and a microscopic spore assessment ("spore-prints") by trained mycologists. Investigation and confirmation of species by such collaboration is crucial to distinguishing toxic mushrooms from those mistakenly believed to be edible.

Captive reptiles can be exposed to mushrooms in yards and greenhouses, in household terrariums, and as additives to their diet. Owners witnessing potential toxic mushroom ingestions in small animals must be instructed to bring portions of the culprit mushroom in for identification. We have seen one case where a pet iguana ingested *Amanita pantherina* in a backyard. Within 30 minutes of ingestion, the approximately 1-kg lizard became lethargic and ataxic. The owners brought parts of the remaining mushrooms along with the lizard.

A. pantherina can occur throughout the United States and usually exists singly. It has a brilliant red cap and is often photographed by naturalists because of its dramatic appearance. These mushrooms contain ibotenic acid and muscimol, its decarboxylated metabolite. Ibotenic acid is related structurally to the stimulatory transmitter agent, glutamic acid.[48,49] Muscimol is very similar to the neurotransmitter, GABA, and acts as a GABA agonist with typical GABA signs and manifestations.

Treatment is supportive. Most GABA manifestations respond solely to supportive care, and the animals completely recover. Benzodiazepines, such as diazepam, may be required for the management of seizures.

The iguana involved in our hospital responded within a few hours to fluids, warmth, and tube feeding. No long-lasting effects were noted, and the animal was released after 24 hours. This case represents the value of owners bringing in the mushroom involved for correct identification. Veterinarians must establish solid contacts with other local health professionals, such as human toxicologists, university mycologists, and laboratories well versed in toxicologic analysis.

Plant Poisonings

Some plants can produce very powerful poisons. For many years veterinary toxicology largely dealt with livestock suffering from plant poisonings. The last 20 years have seen a tremendous growth in our understanding of small animal intoxications.[50] Because many reptiles are either partially or entirely herbivorous, the potential for the accidental ingestion of toxic plants is very real (Box 20-1). Although consideration of all plants potentially toxic to reptiles is beyond our present discussion, this section will examine the more frequently encountered plant poisonings and those commonly reported in the literature.

Heaths

The heath family plants (e.g., azaleas, laurel, rhododendrons) are commonly planted in the United States as ornamental shrubbery (Color Plate 20-2). These plants contain

---

Box 20-1   Factors Affecting the Potential Toxicity of Poisonous Plants

Geographical and Seasonal Variables
- Plants known to be poisonous in one part of the world may not be so toxic in other areas.
- Season may also affect toxicity of plants.

Plant Part Ingested
- Not all parts of poisonous plants are always toxic.
  - Example: tomato—a very edible fruit, but the stems and leaves contain toxic alkaloids
  - Example: apples, peaches, and apricots possess cyanide-containing seeds; the fruit itself is edible

Absorbability of Toxins
- Apples, peaches, apricots—cyanide not released unless seeds are broken
- Castor bean—poison (ricin) not released unless seeds are chewed

Species Ingesting the Plant
- Much of poisonous plant intoxication depends directly on which species has done the ingesting.

---

grayanotoxins (diterpenoids) that interfere with membrane-based sodium channels.[51] The toxin is found in the stem, leaves, flower, and nectar. Dogs and people may develop bradycardia. Ingestion of small amounts can lead to gastrointestinal signs; larger amounts can cause depression, ataxia, and convulsions. No antidote exists, and treatment is supportive. We have seen two iguanas stricken after eating azalea, and one of the lizards subsequently died. The editor was aware of a case where three tortoises ingested rhododendron leaves; all three died.

Yews

Ground hemlock, Florida yew, English yew, Pacific yew, and Japanese yew are all members of a group of shrubs and trees that contain taxine, a cardiotoxic alkaloid. This substance is a sodium channel blocker that can cause both cardiac and neurological toxicity.[52] The bark, leaves, and seeds are poisonous but not the red fruit surrounding the seeds of these ornamental shrubs. No antidote exists. Poisonings have been reported in livestock, dogs, and caged birds.

Lilies

Easter lily, tiger lily, day lily, Japanese show lily, and Asiatic lily are known to be poisonous to cats by causing renal toxicosis (Color Plate 20-3).[53] All parts of the plant are poisonous. In addition, lily of the valley contains a potent cardiac glycoside. In our experience, toxic plant ingestion by reptiles is more than possible; captivity exposes animals to a wide variety plants. We have administered activated charcoal to an iguana that ingested Easter lilies. In general, treatment is supportive.

Fruit Seeds

The seeds of apples, apricots, cherries, peaches, plums, and the jetberry bush contain cyanogenic glycosides. The seeds are dangerous if the seed capsule is broken. In humans as few as 5 to 25 broken seeds can cause cyanide toxicosis.[54] Cyanide disrupts the ability of cells to use oxidative phosphorylation by poisoning mitochondria. The net effect is tissue hypoxia. The onset of clinical signs may be very rapid, and death can occur suddenly. Treatment for cyanide toxicosis is often not successful, but does include 100% oxygen administration, supplemental fluids, and perhaps sodium nitrite or sodium thiosulfate.

Avocado

Avocado (*Persea americana*) has been shown to be toxic to rabbits, mice, and caged birds.[55] All above-ground parts of the plant are toxic. Persin, a compound isolated from the leaves, is believed to be the toxin responsible for avocado toxicity. Intoxicated mammals display cardiac arrhythmias, necrosis of the myocardium, and acute death. Caged birds show respiratory distress. Until more is known concerning the nature of avocado poisoning, they should not be included in the diet of herbivorous captive reptiles.

Ricin (Castor Bean Intoxication)

Castor bean plants contain ricin, a potent toxin that inhibits protein synthesis. The poison is present in the whole plant, but most concentrated in the seed.[56] Chewing or breaking of the seed coat is necessary before intoxication can take place. For mice, rats, rabbits, and dogs, as few as one seed can be fatal. In dogs clinical signs involve the gastrointestinal tract, but can lead to kidney failure and convulsions. No known antidote is available. All ingestions of castor beans should be taken seriously because of the high toxicity of ricin. However, seed coats are not always chewed or broken when animals ingest seeds.

Cycad (Sago) Palms

These plants are used as houseplants and occur naturally in tropical and subtropical regions (Color Plate 20-4). All parts of the plant are toxic. The nuts (seeds) are most toxic and only produced by female plants. The toxins induce gastrointestinal and hepatic signs (cycasin), neurological signs (B-methylamino-L-alanine), and an unknown toxin causes additional neurological signs.[57] Gastrointestinal signs generally appear within 24 hours of ingestion. No antidote exists, and treatment is supportive. Clients should be encouraged to bring in the chewed plant to help identify the species.

Holly, Mistletoe, and Poinsettia

During the holiday season, several potentially toxic plants are brought into the home. Although their toxicity is exaggerated, reptiles may blunder into them. Here is an overview of the most common holiday plants.

Mistletoes (*Phoradendron* species) are evergreen parasitic plants that grow on trees (Color Plate 20-5). Human exposures usually involve the berries either eaten by small children or the berries brewed into tea.[58] Attempts to reproduce clinical signs in animals have been unsuccessful. In humans the most common clinical signs are gastrointestinal. No antidote is available, and treatment is supportive.

Holly (*Ilex* species) includes the English or Christmas holly, American or white holly, and winterberry. Berries contain the saponin, ilicin, which is a potent gastrointestinal irritant.[58] In humans and companion mammalian species, the most common sign is upset of the digestive tract. No antidote exists, and treatment is symptomatic.

Poinsettia (*Euphorbia pulcherrima*) possesses a milky sap rich in diterpenoids. These molecules are fairly irritating to the skin, mucous membranes, and gastrointestinal tract. Reports of toxicity stem from a single account.[58] Poisoning is rare, and treatment is supportive.

Cardiac Glycosides

Several plants contain cardiac glycosides, including oleander *(Nerium oleander)*, foxglove (*Digitalis purpurea*), and lily of the valley (*Convallaria majalis*).[59] For oleander (Color Plate 26-2), all parts of the leaf are poisonous; a single well-chewed leaf has been reported to be lethal. Foxglove leaves and seeds are toxic. Lily of the valley poisoning occurs from ingestion of the leaves, flowers, or roots. The cardiac glycosides are gastrointestinal irritants, may be responsible for a variety of cardiac arrhythmias (e.g., irregular pulse, bradycardia, rapid thready pulse, ventricular fibrillation), and can be fatal. With plant ingestions, the exact amount of toxin involved is never known.

Ivy

Ivy (*Hedera* species) is used in greenhouses, as a houseplant, and as a ground cover. English ivy, Irish ivy, Persian ivy, Atlantic ivy, and others are all potentially toxic (Color Plate 20-6). These plants, particularly the berries, contain terpenoids. These molecules can cause salivation, gastrointestinal irritation, and diarrhea. Most ingestions are not serious, and treatment is supportive.

Nicotine

Tobacco products including pipe tobacco, cigarettes, cigars, chewing tobacco, and snuff contain the alkaloid nicotine. Nicotine is a stimulant of the central nervous and cardiovascular systems. It stimulates sympathetic ganglia and increases heart rate and blood pressure.[60] High-dose exposures can cause paralysis of the chest muscles and lead to respiratory compromise and cardiac arrest. Cigarettes average from 15 to 25 mg of nicotine depending on the brand. Cigars have four to five times the nicotine content of cigarettes. Chewing tobacco is even more palatable to animals because of flavors added (e.g., honey, sugar, molasses, cinnamon, licorice, various syrups). Aids to stop smoking can also be a source of accidental nicotine ingestion. Nicotine "patches" usually contain between 7 and 25 mg, and nicotine gum contains 2 to 4 mg per piece.[61] Some garden spray insecticides contain 40% nicotine (Black Leaf 40).

Captive reptiles may ingest cigar and cigarette butts, pipe tobacco, chewing tobacco, or nicotine patches and gums. We have seen death in one tortoise and one iguana after eating cigarette butts. Clinical signs of high-dose nicotine intoxication include excitement followed by depression, diarrhea, seizures, coma, and respiratory or cardiac arrest. There is no known antidote. Treatment includes frequent monitoring of heart rate, and animals may benefit from fluid therapy and oxygen administration. Prognosis is poor for high-dose intoxications. As few as two cigarettes have been shown to cause lethal poisonings. No data exists for secondary cigarette smoke intoxication, but an association between chronic respiratory conditions in captive reptiles and households with one or more smokers has been suspected.

Oak Poisoning

Oak trees are found almost worldwide. Acorns, buds, twigs, and leaves have been implicated, but most incidents of intoxication involve either immature leaves in the spring or freshly fallen acorns in the spring.

Toxicosis from oak is produced by high concentrations of tannic acid and its metabolites, gallic acid, and pyrogallol.[62] Ingestion of toxic amounts of oak has been shown to cause ulcerative lesions in the upper and lower gastrointestinal tract, liver lesions, and necrosis of proximal renal tubular epithelial cells.

A fatal episode of oak intoxication has been reported in a tortoise. An African spurred tortoise *(Geochelone sulcata)* was found dead in an outdoor enclosure possessing numerous oaks hanging over and into the area.[63] Necropsy of the tortoise revealed a markedly distended stomach with partially digested oak leaves. Extensive necrosis was found in the oral cavity, esophagus, stomach, and kidneys. The proximal renal tubules showed 45% necrosis.

Marijuana

Marijuana continues to be by far the most used illicit drug in the United States.[64] *Cannabis sativa* has been used for centuries for its hemp fiber, as rope, and for its psychoactive resins. Totally or partially herbivorous captive reptiles may encounter growing marijuana plants or ingest dried stems, leaves, and flowers.

The main active ingredient of marijuana is tetrahydrocannabinol (THC).[65] The highest concentration of this psychoactive constituent is found in the leaves and the flowering tops of plants. Hashish is the dried resin of flower tops. The precise mechanism of action of THC is unknown, but the psychoactive effects of this drug are thought to stem from a number of sites within the CNS, including cholinergic, dopaminergic, serotoninergic, noradrenergic, and GABA receptors. Ingested marijuana induces clinical signs much more slowly than the inhaled smoke; however, the effects of ingested THC last much longer.

Clinical signs after ingestion of marijuana include mydriasis, weakness, ataxia, brady-cardia, hypothermia, and stupor. The extent of clinical signs following marijuana ingestion is almost totally dose related.

Treatment for marijuana ingestion is primarily supportive and symptomatic. Marijuana intoxications are rarely fatal because of the wide margin of safety of THC. Activated char-coal administration is recommended to decrease enterohepatic recirculation. Despite its relative safety margin, recovery following ingestion may be prolonged and take up to 3 to 4 days. Fluids and monitoring body temperature may be beneficial.

We have seen two reptiles ingest fairly large amounts of marijuana. A 10-pound Sulcata tortoise showed no effects after eating four marijuana cigarettes. However, a 6-pound male green iguana was stuporous after eating into a "baggie" of marijuana. Both animals recovered completely.

Undoubtedly, reptiles have blundered across other "under-the-counter" drugs. Various over-the-counter drugs kept on nightstands, kitchen counters, or bathroom shelves may be encountered by captive reptiles given free range in the house. For their own safety, captive animals should be confined and *all* medications kept in their original containers in child- and animal-proof cabinets.

Venomous and Poisonous Animals

Snake Envenomation

Snake venoms are complex mixtures of enzymatic and nonenzymatic proteins.[66] Derived from modified salivary glands, snake venoms immobilize prey and predigest their tissue. Hyaluronidase is present in most snake venom and works by catalyzing the cleavage of internal glycoside bonds and mucopolysaccharides. This action potentiates the activity of many of the other toxic agents. Phospholipase A, which causes hydrolytic breakdown of membrane phospholipids, is common to many snake venoms.[67] This molecule displays cytotoxic, anticoagulant (prevents activation of clotting factors), and neurotoxic activities. Collagenase is also found in snake venom, leading to the digestion of collagen and breaking down of connective tissue.

Snake venoms are incredibly complex, diverse combinations of toxins and may vary even between closely related species.[68] Many of the toxic principals in snake venom have yet to be precisely identified. Snake venom toxins are usually named either after the snake venom that they were first identified in or after their primary pharmacological effect on the victim.

Snake venoms are approximately 90% water and, in addition to enzymatic and nonen-zymatic proteins, can contain lipids, carbohydrates, and biogenic amines. The actual toxins, which compose the "killing fraction," are referred to as *venins*. The entire mixture is called *venom*. Not only is there much variability in venom composition among snake species, there is also tremendous variability in susceptibility to different snake venoms by potential prey species.[69]

It has been proposed since ancient times that venomous snakes are more resistant or even immune to their own venom. Venomous snakes do appear to be relatively more resis-tant to their own venom. Neutralizing antibodies have been documented in the serum of many snakes to the toxins of their own venom. However, the authors have seen fatalities in venomous snakes bitten by conspecifics. The severity of the response appears to be depen-dent on the location of the bite, the volume of venom injected, and the size of the bite recipient. It should also be mentioned that we have seen bites between conspecifics and self-inflicted bites that were nonfatal.

Certain nonvenomous snake species that prey on other snakes (including venomous ones), such as the king snake, *Lampropeltis getulus,* also appear to have some resistance to venom.[70]

Effective antivenins exist for some venomous snake venoms.

Poisonous Lizards

Out of the approximately 3000 species of lizards, there are only two known poisonous species.[71] The Gila monster *Heloderma suspectum* (with two subspecies) and the Mexican beaded lizard *Heloderma horridum* (with three subspecies) make up the venomous lizards and are only found in the Americas. Their venom is only used in defense.[72]

The venom of these lizards is antigenically unrelated to snake venom.[73] The venom glands are in the lower jaw, and the venom is delivered to the gums at the base of the teeth. Delivery of the venom is dependent on intense chewing action.

Heloderma venom consists of multiple enzymatic proteins including hyaluronidase, phospholipase, arginine hydrolase, and kallikrein-like enzymes. Other proteins have been identified in this venom, including gilatoxin and helothermine.

Hyaluronidase acts as a spreading factor, decreases the viscosity of connective tissue, and catalyzes the cleavage of acid mucoglycosides. Arginine hydrolase causes hydrolysis of peptide linkages, and the kallikrein-like enzymes cause vasodilation, increase capillary permeability, lead to edema, and affect the contraction or relaxation of extravascular smooth muscle.

Phospholipase has been documented in many types of venom and contributes by releasing other enzymes leading to membrane destruction. It also stimulates histamine, kinin, and serotonin release. Gilatoxin is a neurotoxic protein. Helothermine has been shown to depress the body temperature in mice subjected to this poison.[74] Bites of these lizards in people have been reported as very painful. Currently, there is no specific antivenin available for venomous lizard bites, and treatment is supportive. Gila monsters appear to be relatively resistant to the effects of their own venom.

Amphibian Toxins

Certain amphibians are poisonous and can cause intoxications. In the United States two toad species (genus *Bufo*) are the source of the majority of toad poisonings. The cane or marine toad (*Bufo marinus*) and the Colorado River toad (*Bufo alvarius*) are the two species most implicated.[75,76]

All *Bufo* species of toads have parotid glands that release toxic substances when the animals are threatened. These toxic substances are biologically active compounds, such as dopamine, norepinephrine, epinephrine, serotonin, bufotenine, bufogenin, bufotoxins, and indolealkylamines. Severe toxicosis has been seen in small animals that bite, masticate, or hold these toads in their mouths. The active compounds secreted from the toad's parotid gland are rapidly absorbed by the mucous membranes of the predator and enter the systemic circulation.

Once these compounds have entered the circulation, the greatest effects are seen on the peripheral vascular system, the CNS, and the heart. Bufotenine has pressor effects on blood vessels, but may act as a hallucinogen as well. Bufogenin has digitalis-like effects.[77] It causes alterations in heart rate and rhythm. Bufotoxins are vasoconstrictors and add to the pressor effects. Indolealkylamines have activity similar to the hallucinogen LSD.

Dogs are the animals most commonly affected by amphibian parotid toxins. However, cats and ferrets have been reported to be affected. Exposure in reptiles has not been documented; however, it is logical to assume predatory reptiles that include amphibians in their diet might encounter and ingest poisonous toads. No specific antidote is available, and treatment is basically supportive. Therapy includes thoroughly flushing the oral cavity with running water. Severely affected animals may require seizure intervention and medications to stabilize heart rhythms. Supportive care involving fluids may be necessary in badly debilitated animals. Many other toxicoses and conditions can lead to neuropathies, and cardiac arrhythmias can present with signs very similar to those of toad poisonings.

Fire Ants

In the early 1900s the imported fire ant reached the United States from South America. The black fire ant, *Solenopsis richteri,* has remained in a small area of central Alabama and Mississippi. The red imported fire ant, *Solenopsis invicta,* has now reached 13 southern states from Texas to North Carolina. They are highly adaptive insects that have both supplanted and interbred with local ant species. New fire ant hybrids display a greater tolerance against cold and drought, which enables their spread much farther into the continental United

States. In some areas as many as 60% of local humans report being stung at least once annually.[78]

The fire ants and hybrids are small and are similar in appearance to native house and garden ants. These fire ants bite *and* sting. First the ant uses powerful mandibles to bite and anchor itself to the skin of the victim; then it uses its abdominal stinger to inject venom in a series of stings rotating in a circle around the head. Unlike the venom of most stinging insects, ant venom is composed primarily of alkaloids, particularly piperidine. Ant venoms have local necrotic and hemolytic effects.[79]

The authors have seen several small reptiles victimized by these predatory ants in Louisiana and Florida. Neonatal reptiles are especially vulnerable to these aggressive insects. In Florida we saw several small snakes fall prey to them.

No antidotal therapy exists; however, the use of antihistamines, topical steroid ointments, topical alcohol, and warm water baths may provide symptomatic relief.

Fire ants generally build mounds in warm, sunny areas, places similar to where reptiles typically bask. We can expect more reptile species to fall victim to the bites of these ants as these predatory insects continue to expand their range. Efforts to control the spread of these ants so far have not been effective.

Firefly Toxicosis

Reptile caretakers often supplement the diet of captive animals with freshly caught insects. Fireflies of the genus *Photinus* have been shown to contain steroidal pyrones (lucibufagins) that are poisonous.[80] The pyrones are structurally similar to cardenolides of plants and bufodienolides of toads, both of which are well-studied toxins.[81] These two compounds cause nausea and vomiting at low concentrations and can be potentially cardiotoxic at higher doses. If extrapolations from mammals are correct, less than one half of a firefly could be lethal to a 100-g lizard.

Bearded dragons (*Pogona vitticeps*) have shown fatal intoxication after ingestion of fireflies.[82] In both cases documented the lizards showed signs 30 to 60 minutes postingestion. Clinical signs included pronounced oral gaping, intense color change in the neck area, and dyspnea. Both animals died within 90 minutes of eating the fireflies. At present no effective therapy is known.

Lucibufagins protect fireflies from predators.[83] Spiders, birds, and several species of lizards have been shown to avoid fireflies.[84,85] Like many lizards, bearded dragons show indiscriminate eating strategies and may ingest toxic substances. Furthermore the bearded dragon, an Australian native, has no natural contact with *Photinus* species of fireflies and thus may exhibit no self-protective avoidance behavior.

Keepers must be advised to feed only safe food items. Any questions should be referred to a veterinarian. Fireflies should not be fed to reptiles or additionally any insects that sequester cardenolides, such as monarch butterflies (*Donaus plexippus*), queen butterflies (*Donaus gilippus*), and lygaeid bugs (*Oncopeltus fasciatus*). Other lizard species and other captive reptiles may be susceptible to intoxication following firefly ingestion, and they should not be offered as food.[86]

Dioctyl Sodium Sulfosuccinate

Dioctyl sodium sulfosuccinate (DSS) is an anionic surfactant substance that traditionally has been recommended as a laxative and stool softener for a variety of vertebrates ranging from humans to rodents. DSS has been advocated for the same use in reptiles.

DSS generally is regarded as a relatively safe pharmaceutical agent with a low toxicity, but reports of toxic effects exist in the literature for horses, dogs, monkeys, rats, rabbits, guinea pigs, and mice after either oral or topical administration.[87-93] Furthermore, fatalities in reptiles after oral use of DSS have been reported.[94] One study documents severe changes in gastric and esophageal mucosa in Gopher snakes (*Pituophis melanoleucus*) given oral DSS at a dosage of 250 mg/kg.

A specific dose of DSS has not been established for reptiles, but dosages for other species range from 50mg for dogs and 40mg for cats to 200 mg/kg for horses.[92,95] Concentrations (dilutions) of 1:30 have been recommended for reptiles.[96] A DSS dosage of 15 mg/kg PO has been recommended.

The study in the gopher snakes and the several reports in various other species indicate that DSS may not be as innocuous as once popularly believed. These studies demonstrate that DSS can have adverse effects, and, in reptiles, levels greater than 250 mg/kg can cause caustic changes to epithelial surfaces. In addition, the potential for overzealous administration of DSS leading to aspiration pneumonia clearly exists in captive reptiles. Extreme care must be taken if DSS is to be used, and the use of other laxatives, stool softeners, and enhancers of gastric motility should be explored.

Diets to Avoid

Although some foods may be relished by reptiles, nevertheless, many of these same foods have potentially toxic components and should only be fed in small quantities. Spinach, rhubarb, and beets contain the chelating agent oxalic acid, which binds with calcium ions in the blood to form calcium-oxalate crystals. This can lead to a decrease in calcium levels and predispose to bladder stones.

Broccoli, brussels sprouts, and cabbage contain mustard oil glycosides, which have been shown to contribute to the formation of goiter. Fagopyrine found in buckwheat can cause photosensitivity. Iguanas fed buckwheat may develop blepharitis and conjunctivitis when exposed to sunlight. This condition is self-limiting and can be remedied without treatment if animals are kept in the dark and out of the sun for 48 hours.[97]

References

1. Rossi JV: Dermatology. In Mader DR, editor: *Reptile medicine and surgery*, Philadelphia, 1996, Saunders.
2. Frye FL: *Biomedical and surgical aspects of captive reptile husbandry.* vol 2, ed 2, Melbourne, FL, 1991, Krieger Publishing.
3. Lewis LD, Morris ML Jr, Hand MS, et al: *Small animal clinical nutrition*, Topeka, KS, 1987, Mark Morris Assoc.
4. Papich MG: *Handbook of veterinary drugs*, Philadelphia, 2002, Saunders.
5. Montali RJ, Bush M, Smeller JM: The pathology of nephrotoxicity of gentamycin in snakes, *Vet Pathol* 16:108–115, 1979.
6. Bagger-Sjoback D, Wesall J: Toxic effects of gentamycin on the basilar papilla in the lizard Calotes versicolor, *Acta Octolaryngol* 81:57, 1976.
7. Funk RS: A formulary for lizards, snakes, and crocodilians, *Vet Clin of North Amer Exot Pract* 1:333–358, 2000.
8. Klingenberg RJ: Therapeutics. In Mader DR, editor: *Reptile medicine and surgery*, Philadelphia, 1996, Saunders.
9. Holt D, Harvey J, Hurley R: Chloramphenicol toxicity, *Adverse Drug React Toxicol Rev* 12:83–95, 1993.
10. Papich MG: Metronidazole. In Papich MG, editor: *Handbook of veterinary drugs*, Philadelphia, 2002, Saunders.
11. Bennett RA: Neurology. In Mader DR, editor: *Reptile medicine and surgery*, Philadelphia, 1996, Saunders.
12. Lawton MPC: Neurological disease. In Benyon PH, editor: *Manual of reptiles, British Small Animal Veterinary Association*, Ames, IA, 1992, Iowa State University Press.
13. Haddad LM, Herman SM: Antibiotics and anthelminthics. In Haddad LM, Shannon MW, Winchester JF, editors: *Clinical management of poisoning and drug overdose*, Philadelphia, 1998, Saunders.
14. Hoitsma AJ, et al: Drug-induced nephrotoxicity aetiology, clinical features, and management, *Drug Safety* 6(2):131, 1991.
15. Plumb DC: *Veterinary drug handbook*, ed 3, Ames, IA, 1999, Iowa State University Press.
16. Bonner BB: Chelonian therapeutics, *Vet Clinics of N Amer Exotic Pract* 3(1):207–232, 2000.
17. Roder JD: Antimicrobials. In Plumlee KH, editor: *Clinical veterinary toxicology*, St Louis, 2004, Mosby.
18. Funk RS: A formulary for lizards, snakes, and crocodilians, *Vet Clinics of N Amer Exotic Pract* 3(1):333–358, 2000.
19. Scott FW, et al: Teratogenesis in cats associated with griseofulvin therapy, *Teratology* 11:79, 1975.
20. Carlton FB, Simpson WM, Haddad LM: The organophosphates and other insecticides. In Haddad LM, Shannon MW, Winchester JF, editors: *Clinical management of poisoning and drug overdose*, Philadelphia, 1998, Saunders.
21. Blodgett DJ: Organophosphate and carbamate insecticides. In Peterson ME, Talcott PA, editors: *Small animal toxicology*, Philadelphia, 2001, Saunders.

22. Jamal GA: Neurological syndromes of organophosphorus compounds, *Adv Drug React Toxicol Rev* 16(3):133–170, 1997.
23. Hansen SR: Pyrethrins and pyrethroids. In Peterson ME, Talcott PA, editors: *Small animal toxicology*, Philadelphia, 2001, Saunders.
24. Denardo D, Wozniak EJ: Understanding the snake mite and current therapies for control, *Proc Assoc of Rept Amph Veterin* 137–147, 1997.
25. Papich MG: Ivermectin. In Papich MG, editor: *Handbook of veterinary drugs*, Philadelphia, 2002, Saunders.
26. Teare JD, Bush M: Toxicity and efficacy of ivermectin in chelonians, *J Am Vet Med Assoc* 183(11):1195, 1983.
27. Wosniak EJ, et al: Ectoparasites, *Jour Herp Med Surg* 10(3):15–21, 2000.
28. Papich M: *Handbook of veterinary drugs*, London, 2002, Saunders.
29. Alvarado TP, et al: Fenbendazole overdose in four Fea's vipers (*Azemiops feae*), *Proc Assoc Rept Amph Vet* 35–36, 1997.
30. Stein G: Reptile and amphibian formulary. In Mader DR, editor: *Reptile medicine and surgery*, Philadelphia, 1996, Saunders.
31. Carpenter JW, Marion CJ: *Exotic animal formulary*, Philadelphia, 2012, Saunders.
32. Dalvi RR: Comparative studies on the effect of fenbendazole on the liver and liver enzymes of goats, quail, and rats, *Vet Res Commun* 13:135–139, 1989.
33. Howard LL, et al: Benzimidazole toxicity in birds, *Proc Annu Conf Am Assoc Zoo Vet* 36, 1999.
34. Papendick RI, et al: Suspected fenbendazole toxicity in birds, *Proc Annu Conf Am Assoc Zoo Vet* 144–146, 1998.
35. Shoda T, et al: Liver tumor promoting effects of fenbendazole in rats, *Toxicol Pathol* 27:553–562, 1999.
36. Stokol T, et al: Development of bone marrow toxicosis after albendazole administration in a dog and a cat, *J Am Vet Med Assoc* 210:1753–1756, 1997.
37. Lloyd ML: Chlorhexidine toxicosis in a pair of red-bellied short-necked turtles, Emydura subglosa, *Bull Assoc Rept Amph Vet* 6(4):6–7, 1996.
38. Mcguigan MA: Bleach, soaps, detergents, and other corrosives. In Haddad EM, Shannon MW, Winchester JF, editors: *Clinical management of poisoning and drug overdose*, ed 3, Philadelphia, 1998, Saunders.
39. Talcott PA: Zinc poisoning. In Peterson ME, Talcott PA, editors: *Small animal toxicology*, Philadelphia, 2001, Saunders.
40. Holstege CP, Kirk MA, et al: Smoke inhalation. In Goldfrank LR, editor: *Toxologic emergencies*, ed 7, New York, 2002, McGraw-Hill.
41. Metts BC, Stewart NJ: Rodenticides. In Haddad LM, Shannon MW, Winchester JF, editors: *Clinical management of poisoning and drug overdose*, Philadelphia, 1998, Saunders.
42. Murphy JM, Talcott PA: Anticoagulant rodenticides. In Peterson ME, Talcott PA, editors: *Small animal toxicology*, Philadelphia, 2001, Saunders.
43. Dorman DL: Bromethalin. In Peterson ME, Talcott PA, editors: *Small animal toxicology*, Saunders, 2001.
44. Rumbeiha WK: Cholecalciferol. In Peterson ME, Talcott PA, editors: *Small animal toxicology*, Philadelphia, 2001, Saunders.
45. Morrow CK, Volmer PA: Cholecalciferol. In Plumlee KH, editor: *Clinical veterinary toxicology*, St Louis, 2004, Mosby.
46. Puschner B, Metaldehyde: In Peterson ME, Talcott PA, editors: *Small animal toxicology*, Philadelphia, 2001, Saunders.
47. Gfeller RW, Messonnier SP: Metaldehyde. In Gfeller RW, Messonnier SP, editors: *Handbook of small animal toxicology and poisonings*, St Louis, 2004, Mosby.
48. Goldfrank LR: Mushrooms. In Goldfrank LR, et al, editors: *Goldfrank's toxicologic emergencies*, ed 7, New York, 2002, McGraw-Hill.
49. Benjamin DR: Mushroom poisoning in infants and children: the Amanita pantherina/muscaria group, *J Toxicol Clin Toxicol* 30:12–22, 1992.
50. Plumlee KH: Plant hazards, *Vet Clin North Amer (Small Animal Pract)* 32(2):383–395, 2002.
51. Puschner B: Grayanotoxins. In Plumlee KH, editor: *Clinical veterinary toxicology*, St Louis, 2004, Mosby.
52. Casteel S: Taxine alkaloids. In Plumlee KH, editor: *Clinical veterinary toxicology*, St Louis, 2004, Mosby.
53. Hall J: Lily. In Plumlee KH, editor: *Clinical veterinary toxicology*, St Louis, 2004, Mosby.
54. Fitzgerald KT: Cyanide. In Peterson ME, Talcott PA, editors: *Small animal toxicology*, Philadelphia, 2001, Saunders.
55. Pickerell JA, Oehme F, Mannala SA: Avocado. In Plumlee KH, editor: *Clinical veterinary toxicology*, St Louis, 2004, Mosby.
56. Albretsen JC: Evaluation of castor bean toxicosis in dogs: 98 cases, *J Am Anim Hosp Assoc* 36(3):229–233, 2000.

57. Albretson JC: Cycasin. In Plumlee KH, editor: *Clinical veterinary toxicology*, St Louis, 2004, Mosby.
58. Kunkel DB, Brailberg G: Poisonous plants. In Haddad LM, Shannon MW, Winchester JF, editors: *Clinical management of poisoning and drug overdose*, Philadelphia, 1998, Saunders.
59. Galey D: Cardiac Glycosides. In Plumlee KH, editor: *Clinical veterinary toxicology*, St Louis, 2004, Mosby.
60. Plumlee KH: Nicotine. In Peterson ME, Talcott PA, editors: *Small animal toxicology*, Philadelphia, 2001, Saunders.
61. Haddad LM: Nicotine. In Haddad LM, Shannon MW, Winchester JF, editors: *Clinical management of poisoning and drug overdose*, Philadelphia, 1998, Saunders.
62. Plumlee KH: Tannic Acid. In Plumlee KH, editor: *Clinical veterinary toxicology*, St Louis, 2004, Mosby.
63. Rotstein DS, et al: Suspected oak Quercus, toxicity in an African Spurred Tortoise, *Geochelone sulcata*, *Jour Herp Med and Surgery* 13(3):20–21, 2003.
64. Martin B, Szara S: Marijuana. In Haddad EM, Shannon MW, Winchester JF, editors: *Clinical management of poisoning and drug overdose*, Philadelphia, 1998, Saunders.
65. Volmer PA: Drugs of abuse. In Peterson M, Talcott PA, editors: *Small animal toxicology*, Philadelphia, 2001, Saunders.
66. Fowler ME: *Veterinary zootoxicology*, Boca Raton, FL, 1993, CRC Press.
67. Peterson ME, Talcott PA: *Small animal toxicology*, Philadelphia, 2001, Saunders.
68. Walter FG, Fernandez MC, Haddad LM: North American venomous snakebites. In Haddad LM, Shannon M, Winchester LF, editors: *Clinical management of poisoning and drug overdose*, Philadelphia, 1998, Saunders.
69. Ovadia M, Kochva E: Neutralization of Viperidae and Elapidae snake venoms by sera of different animals, *Toxicon* 15(6):541, 1977.
70. Philpot VB, Smith RG: Neutralization of pit viper venom by king snake serum, *Proc Soc Exp Biol Med* 74:521, 1950.
71. Peterson ME: Poisonous lizards. In Peterson ME, Talcott PA, editors: *Small animal toxicology*, Philadelphia, 2001, Saunders. 2001.
72. Fowler ME: Venomous lizards. In Fowler ME, editor: *Veterinary zootoxicology*, Boca Raton, FL, 1993, CRC Press.
73. Heradon RA, Tu T: Biochemical characterization of the lizard toxin gilatoxin, *Biochemistry* 20:3517–3522, 1981.
74. Mocha-Morales J, Martin BM, Possani LD: Isolation and characterization of helothermine, a novel toxin from Heloderma horridum horridum (Mexican beaded lizard) venom, *Toxicon* 28:299–309, 1990.
75. Peterson ME: Toad venom toxicity. In Tilley LP, Smith WK, editors: *The five-minute veterinary consult*, Philadelphia, 1997, Williams & Wilkins.
76. Peterson ME: Amphibian toxins. In Peterson ME, Talcott PA, editors: *Small animal toxicology*, Philadelphia, 2001, Saunders.
77. Butler VP, et al: Heterogeneity and liability of endogenous digitalis-like substances in the plasma of the toad *Bufo marinus*, *Am J Physiol* 271:R325–R332, 1996.
78. Tunney FX: Stinging insects. In Haddad LM, Shannon M, Winchester JF, editors: *Clinical management of poisoning and drug overdose*, Philadelphia, 1998, Saunders.
79. Tracy J, et al: The natural history of exposure to the imported fire ant *(Solenopsis invicta)*, *J Allergy Clin Immunol* 95:824, 1995.
80. Eisner T, et al: Lucibufagins: Defensive steroids from the fireflies *Photinus ignitus* and *Photinus marginellus* (Coleoptera:Lampyridae), *Proc Nat Acad Sci* 75:905–908, 1978.
81. Fieser LF, Fieser M: *Natural products related to phenanthrene*, New York, 1999, Reinhold.
82. Glor R, et al: Two cases of firefly toxicosis in bearded dragons, *Pogona vitticeps*, *Proc Assoc Rept Amph Vet*27–30, 1999.
83. Eisner T, et al: Firefly "femme fatales" acquire defensive steroids (lucibufagins) from their firefly prey, *Proc Nat Acad Sci* 94:9723–9728, 1997.
84. Sexton OJ: Differential predation by the lizard Anolis carolinensis on unicoloured and polycoloured insects after an interval of no contact, *Anim Behav* 12:101–110, 1964.
85. Lloyd JE: Firefly parasites and predators, *Coleopt Bull* 27:91–106, 1998.
86. Sydow SL, Lloyd JE: Distasteful fireflies sometimes emetic, but not lethal, *Entomol* 58:312, 1998.
87. Case MT, et al: Acute mouse and chronic dog toxicity studies of danthron, dioctyl sodium sulfosuccinate, poloxalkol and combinations, *Drug Chem Toxicol* 1(1):89–101, 1977-1978.
88. Donowitz M, Binder HJ: Effect of dioctyl sodium sulfosuccinate on colonic fluid and electrolyte movement, *Gastroenterology* 69:941–950, 1975.
89. Da Fox, et al: Surfactants selectively ablate enteric neurons of the rat jejunum, *J Pharmacol Exp Ther* 277(2):539–544, 1983.
90. Karlin DA, et al: Effect on dioctyl sodium sulfasuccinate feeding on rat colorectal 1,2-dimethylhydrazine carcinogenesis, *J Natl Cancer Inst* 64:791–793, 1980.

91. Lish PM: Some pharmacological effects of dioctyl sodium sulfasuccinate on the gastrointestinal tract of the rat, *Toxicol Appl Pharmacol* 41(6):580–584, 1961.
92. Moffat RE, et al: Studies on dioctyl sodium sulfasuccinate toxicity: clinical, gross and microscopic pathology in the horse and guinea pig, *Can J Comp Med* 39:434–441, 1975.
93. Saunders DR, et al: Effect of dioctyl sodium succinate on structure and function of human and rodent intestine, *Gastroenterology* 69(2):380–386, 1975.
94. Paul-Murphy J et al: Necrosis of esophageal and gastric mucosa in snakes given oral dioctyl sodium succinate, *Proceedings of the 1st International Conference of Zoological and Avian Medicine*, Honolulu, HI, 1987.
95. Kirk RW: *Current veterinary therapy in small animal practice*, Philadelphia, 1976, Saunders.
96. Frye FL: *Biomedical and surgical aspects of captive reptile husbandry*, Edwardsville, KY, 1981, Veterinary Medical Publishing.
97. Shumacher J, Kohler G, Maxwell LK, et al: Husbandry and management. In Jacobson ER, editor: *Biology, husbandry, and medicine of the green iguana*, Malabar, FL, 2003, Krieger Publishing.

Small Mammal Toxicology

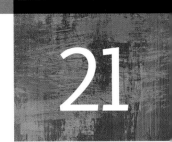

Eric K. Dunayer, MS, VMD, DABT, DABVT

- The poisoned small mammal patient may present a special challenge to the veterinary practitioner although the basic approach should be the same as for dogs and cats.
- Some toxicants are of particular interest in small mammals.
- As with dogs and cats, decontamination is important to limit toxicant absorption.
- Rodents and rabbits do not vomit, so emesis should not be attempted in them.
- Rodenticides are particularly dangerous in rodents as they are target species.
- Rabbits are sensitive to topical flea products containing fipronil; exposure can lead to uncontrollable seizures.
- Ferrets are very sensitive to both ibuprofen and acetaminophen.

Introduction

Many people keep small mammals as pets. These include rodents (rats, mice, hamsters, guinea pigs, gerbils, and chinchillas), rabbits, ferrets, and other small mammals such as sugar gliders and hedgehogs. These animals present challenges from a toxicologic standpoint for several reasons. First, many are curious and easily escape their enclosures and thus can be exposed to toxicants in the environment. Second, their small size means that even small ingestions can lead to very large dosages on a mg/kg or mg/m² basis. Finally, their physiology may present unique challenges in treating a poisoned animal.

Small mammals are exposed to the same toxicants as dogs and cats. In most cases, the approach to treatment is the same. To cover all possible toxicants is beyond the scope of this chapter. Therefore, this chapter mainly covers differences in treatments between small mammals and dog and cats, as well as toxicants of special interest in these species.

Decontamination

The approach to a poisoned small mammal should be the same as for larger animals, with appropriate adjustment for their size and physiology. As with any poisoning, decontamination can be important to lessen exposure and reduce the risk of serious signs developing. Appropriate decontamination is based on species exposed, toxicant, and clinical signs being exhibited.

Although emesis is a standard procedure performed in dogs and cats, it cannot be used in many of these animals. Rodents and rabbits are incapable of vomiting.[1] Ferrets, however, are capable of vomiting. Emesis can be attempted by using 3% hydrogen peroxide (1 mL/lb by mouth [PO], repeated once if no emesis after 15 minutes, not to exceed 10 mL) or apomorphine (0.04 mg/kg intravenous or intramuscular [IM]).[2] As with dogs and cats, emesis should not be attempted in a ferret who is already vomiting or showing signs of central nervous system depression or coma.

Gastric lavage can be used with caution. Normally, gastric lavage should be performed in an anesthetized patient with a cuffed endotracheal tube in place to prevent aspiration of lavage fluid.[1] This may be difficult in the small patients. In addition, aggressive gastric lavage in rabbits, who have thin-walled stomachs,[3] can lead to a gastric rupture.

Some small mammals, such as hamsters, have cheek pouches. These are used to store food and allow the animal to carry food back to their den where it can be eaten in safety. In hamsters, the cheek pouches should be everted and a swab should be used carefully to remove any material from them to prevent later ingestion.[1]

Activated charcoal can be used for toxicants when its use is appropriate. It is most effective against large organic molecules and of limited to no use against small molecules (such as ethanol and ethylene glycol), heavy metals, and inorganic compounds. Careful attention to volume is needed to reduce the risk of aspiration. In general, the dose is 1-3 g/kg or 1-3 mg/g. In many small mammals, the activated charcoal may need to be given by stomach tube because the animal may be reluctant to voluntarily ingest it, or it may be mixed with a tasty food to encourage ingestion.[1,2]

Cathartics, which speed up the movement of the toxicant through the gastrointestinal tract, can be used. Generally, these should not be administered more than once a day if multiple doses of activated charcoal are being given. Additionally, cathartic (especially osmotically active ones like sorbitol) may enhance the loss of free water into the gut and the development of hypernatremia. The patient should be monitored closely for signs of hypernatremia such as depression, tremors, or seizures.[1,2]

For exposure to caustic or corrosive compounds, as well as petroleum distillates, dilution is the treatment of choice. Emesis is contraindicated, as is the use of activated charcoal. In addition, gastric lavage should not be performed. Water, milk, fruit juices, or juicy fruits (e.g., grapes or oranges) can be used as diluents.[1,2] However, the use of acidic fruits and fruit juices should be avoided following an exposure to an alkaline substance as the resulting neutralization reaction can release heat, which may cause further damage to the gastrointestinal tract.[1] The administration of a large volume of diluent, particularly in species that can vomit, can cause emesis and defeat the purpose for their use.

Dermal exposure is another common route of poisoning. Depending on the substance, significant toxicant can be absorbed dermally, leading to system signs. In addition, in species that are active groomers, dermal toxicants can become an oral exposure. As soon as possible after exposure, the animal should be bathed. For water-soluble agents, flushing with large volumes of water may be sufficient. If the substance is oily, a liquid hand dishwashing detergent such as Dawn should be used. Human shampoos, pet shampoos, and flea shampoos should not be used as these don't adequately degrease the fur and may be toxic to the patient. The animal should be bathed and rinsed until there is no toxic residue remaining. The water temperature should be carefully controlled to prevent chilling of small patients. The patient should be stabilized prior to attempting bathing as the stress may worsen clinical signs.[1,2]

In the case of ocular exposure, the eye should be flushed with tepid water or saline solution. Contact lens soaking and cleaning solutions, as well as ocular decongestants, should not be used. In large mammals, a slow stream of water from a tap may be used. In smaller mammals, an eyedropper filled with the appropriate flush can be used to avoid "drowning" the patient under a stream from the faucet. The eye should be flushed for 10-15 minutes but this can be done in short intervals to allow the animal to recover between flushings. After flushing, the eye should be monitored for signs of inflammation or ulceration and treated appropriately.[1,2]

Intravenous fluids, when appropriate, should be administered. Although intravenous catheterization is possible in some species, in smaller animals, intraosseous fluid administration may be required. Careful attention to fluid rates is needed to avoid fluid overload.[1]

Rodents

Ironically, although rodents are commonly used in toxicology testing and in development and regulation of drugs, pesticides, and other consumer products, there is virtually nothing written on clinical toxicology in these species. Although LD_{50} values exist for many chemicals in rats and mice, such data is of limited use clinically. LD_{50} values do not indicate what the minimum toxic or lethal doses are, what signs are expected from an exposure, or what treatments are indicated. Therefore, the use of such results should be used with caution. However, other toxicology data on drugs may be available via a literature search.

A few toxicants are of particular importance in rodents and are discussed.

Rodenticides

Because rodents are the target species for these agents, pet rodents are at particular risk if they are exposed. Again, their curious nature, small size (which allows them to get into small areas where the agents are placed), and low body weight all predispose the animals to increased risk. In addition, baits are formulated to be particularly palatable to rodents; most are grain based and sweetened to attract rodents. Currently there are five rodenticides approved for use in the United States: anticoagulants, bromethalin, cholecalciferol, strychnine, and zinc phosphide. All of these are discussed elsewhere in the book, so I limit discussion here. Many of the comments in this section also apply to rabbits and ferrets.

Anticoagulant rodenticides work by blocking the recycling of vitamin K, which is needed for activation of precoagulation factors to their active form. Most anticoagulant rodenticides sold today are the second-generation or long-acting agents; a single feeding is capable of leading to a fatal bleeding diathesis. Treatment for an exposed rodent is, for the most part, the same as for any other animals. Because emesis is not an option, gastric lavage may be attempted with care. A dose of activated charcoal can be given to reduce absorption of the toxicant. The main treatment is administration of vitamin K_1 (phytonadione) either orally or by injection (injected vitamin K_1 carries an increased risk of anaphylactic reaction regardless of route). The dose for vitamin K_1 in dogs is 2.5-5 mg/kg divided twice a day; length of treatment depends on the compound ingested and ranges from 14-30 days minimum.[4] One source recommends 1-10 mg/kg IM for rodents and rabbits.[5] One of the biggest problems is accurately dosing the vitamin K_1. The smallest tablet available comes as 5 mg, whereas a small rat or mouse may require less than 1 mg for each dose. Although overdose of oral vitamin K_1 is usually well tolerated, there have been reports of hypersensitivity reactions in some animals. To accurately dose the small mammal patient, injectable vitamin K_1 can be given orally. Vitamin K_1 injection is reported to have a foul taste. However, because vitamin K_1 should always be given with a fatty meal to enhance absorption, the liquid can be mixed with peanut butter or other suitable fatty food to mask the taste.[2]

In patients who are actively bleeding, the goal is to restore clotting function and volume as needed. Vitamin K_1 administration is important; however, there may be a lag period of 16-24 hours or more before sufficient levels of active factors can be produced. Therefore exogenous factors, usually through a whole blood or fresh plasma transfusion, need to be given to breach the gap.[5] This involves finding a suitable donor and obtaining blood for administration. Logistically this may be difficult in small mammals. In addition, blood cross matching would need to be done to avoid adverse transfusion reactions, especially if whole blood is used.

Bromethalin is a neurotoxic rodenticide. Guinea pigs are relatively resistant to the toxic effects of bromethalin. Although LD_{50}s in most species are in the 2-10 mg/kg range, it is 1000 mg/kg in guinea pigs. They lack the hepatic enzymes to desmethylate bromethalin to form the much more toxic metabolite desmethylbromethalin.[6]

Unlike anticoagulants, no effective antidotes exist for bromethalin and treatment is often futile once signs begin. Therefore emphasis must be placed on decontamination. Again, because emesis is not an option in rodents and rabbits, administration of activated charcoal is important. Multiple doses of activated charcoal should be given to both prevent absorption of bait in the gastrointestinal tract as well as to interrupt enterohepatic recirculation. In dogs and cats, at least 6 doses of activated charcoal over a 48-hour period are recommended.[6] Once signs begin, treatment is supportive and symptomatic. The use of agents to reduce cerebral edema (such as mannitol, furosemide, and corticosteroids) has not been shown to be useful. One study in rats[7] demonstrated that ginkgo biloba extract administered at 100 mg/kg immediately after an exposure to bromethalin reduced edema formation. However, the study followed rats for only 48 hours postexposure so the long-term efficacy of this treatment is unknown. Apparently no follow-up studies have been performed.

Cholecalciferol (vitamin D_3) rodenticides cause hypercalcemia and hyperphosphatemia leading to mineralization of soft tissue. Death is generally due to acute renal failure. As with bromethalin, aggressive decontamination with multiple doses of activated charcoal is indicated. Standard treatment for cholecalciferol toxicosis includes saline diuresis, furosemide, and corticosteroids to increase renal calcium loss as well decrease gastrointestinal calcium absorption. One of the most effective treatments is the administration of pamidronate, a bisphosphonate, to decrease calcium mobilization from the bone. The drug is expensive and must be administered intravenously, which may limit its use in small patients.[8]

Strychnine ingestion causes rigid paralysis and seizures. Onset of signs can be rapid and death can occur before treatment can be rendered. Generally treatment consists of gastric lavage, administration of activated charcoal (although aspiration is a serious risk), and controlling the neurologic signs. Muscle relaxants (such as methocarbamol), acepromazine, seizure control, and assisted ventilation may be indicated.[9] The prognosis is generally poor.

Zinc phosphide is an inorganic compound. In an acid environment (i.e., the stomach), zinc phosphide is converted to phosphine gas. Signs may be delayed if the stomach is empty and may occur rapidly after a meal. In general, animals who can vomit have a higher tolerance to zinc phosphide because they can self-decontaminate; therefore rodents are more sensitive. Signs include gastrointestinal hemorrhage, seizures, and pulmonary edema; animals who recover may develop renal or hepatic failure up to 2 weeks after the exposure. Treatment is supportive and symptomatic.[10]

Antibiotic Enterocolitis

In certain rodents, particularly guinea pigs and hamsters[11,12] and rabbits,[12] administration of antibiotics can lead to antibiotic-associated enterotoxemia. These animals have a gut flora that is mainly gram-positive bacteria; antibiotics can eradicate these bacteria, leading to an overgrowth of *Clostridium* spp., particularly *C. difficile,* and the release of exotoxin leading to hemorrhagic typhilitis. Antibiotics that cause this condition include β-lactams (ampicillin, penicillin), lincosamides (clindamycin, lincomycin), erythromycin, and chlortetracycline.[13] There may be a dose-related effect, with the animal able to tolerate lower doses of the drugs.

Treatment, which is symptomatic and supportive, includes supporting body temperature and maintaining hydration. Supplemental oral administration of bacteria to reestablish normal flora may speed recovery. The administration of *Lactobacillus* spp. or use of species-appropriate fecal slurries has been recommended. Chloramphenicol (50 mg/kg q8h PO) may suppress the clostridial overgrowth. In rabbits, cholestyramine (an ion-exchange resin) has been shown to absorb bacterial toxin and improve survival; this may be useful in other species.[11]

Prevention includes using the proper antibiotics and at proper dosages. Simultaneous oral administration of *Lactobacillus* spp. or yogurt during antibiotic treatment and for several days beyond may be helpful as well.[11]

Rabbits

A review of toxicology in rabbits has been published in the *Veterinary Clinics of North America—Exotic Practice.*[13]

Fipronil

The use of fipronil-containing flea products such as spot-ons or sprays has been associated with seizures in rabbits.[13] Following exposure, the rabbits develop anorexia and lethargy and then may develop seizures a few days later. Treatment consists of bathing the rabbit in a liquid hand dishwashing detergent (such as Dawn) as soon as possible after the exposure, and symptomatic and supportive care for the anorexia. Some have suggested administering activated charcoal as the rabbit may have ingested the agent. Benzodiazepine anticonvulsants such as diazepam can be used to attempt to control the seizures. However, in my experience, prognosis is guarded once seizures begin.[13]

Avocado

Ingestion of avocado (*Persea americana*) can be toxic to rabbits.[14] Ingestion of the leaves and fruit, which contain the toxin persin, has been associated with toxicity. In lactating does, a sterile mastitis can develop. Although the animals usually recover, they may have a permanent decrease in milk production. At higher dosages of persin, rabbits can develop myocardial necrosis leading to cardiac arrhythmias, submandibular edema, and death. Prognosis for these rabbits is poor.[14]

Household Plants

As grazers, rabbits may ingest household and garden plants. They may be adapted to certain plant toxins and so are more resistant to some plants than carnivores. For instance, rabbits have an atropinase in their blood that makes them resistant to plants that contain tropane alkaloids.[15] Rabbits are also resistant to muscarinic mushrooms because of poor absorption of the toxin. However, ingestion of any plant known to be toxic to other species should be approached with care. The owner should bring the plant in for identification and treatment should be based on general therapies for that plant.

Ferrets

As with rodents, not much information exists about toxic exposures in ferrets. At least one review of exposures reported to the American Society for the Prevention of Cruelty to Animals Animal Poison Control Center has been published.[16] The agents that ferrets were exposed to were very similar to those seen in dogs and cats (Box 21-1). In most cases, signs are similar to those seen in dogs and cats, and treatments are the same. However, some agents of special concern are discussed.

Ibuprofen

Ferrets appear to be particularly sensitive to ibuprofen toxicosis.[17] Signs can develop in as little as 4 hours but may take up to 48 hours to develop. Unlike dogs and cats, in which gastrointestinal and renal signs predominate, ferrets develop neurologic signs, including ataxia, tremors, seizure, and coma. Neurologic signs developed in almost 95% of ferrets in one study.[17] In addition, gastrointestinal and renal signs may develop. Dosages of more than 220 mg/kg can be lethal; this can be as little as one 200-mg tablet in a ferret.

Following ingestion, emesis can be attempted in asymptomatic ferrets. This can be followed with multiple doses of activated charcoal because ibuprofen undergoes enterohepatic recirculation. Ferrets showing neurologic signs are at an increased risk for aspiration if they vomit the activated charcoal. Other treatment should include intravenous diuresis (two times the maintenance dose for at least 48 hours) to protect the kidneys and gastrointestinal protectants such as H_2 blockers and sucralfate (Carafate) to minimize gastric ulcers.[17] Misoprostol, a synthetic prostaglandin, may prevent gastric ulceration. However, because of the ferret's small size, accurately administering the drug is difficult unless it is compounded. Comatose ferrets should be kept warm and closely monitored, particularly in regard to respiration. Seizures should be controlled as needed. The use of naloxone to reverse coma has been suggested but has not been fully evaluated. Generally with early treatment, the ferret can recover. But once neurologic signs develop the prognosis is guarded.

Acetaminophen

Ferrets appear to be particularly sensitive to acetaminophen[18] although not as sensitive as cats. Ferrets given 50 mg/kg of acetaminophen showed signs, whereas approximately half the ferrets given 200 mg/kg died.[19] Acetaminophen overdose can cause hepatic necrosis

---

Box 21-1 **Most Common Exposures Reported to the Animal Poison Control Center for Ferrets**

Miscellaneous medications
Cleaning products (including bleaches)
Insecticides
Flea products
Ibuprofen
Anticoagulant rodenticides
Chocolate
Acetaminophen
Venlafaxine (Effexor)
Bromethalin
Toxic plants
Paint
Soaps and shampoos

Adapted from Dunayer E: Toxicology of ferrets, *Vet Clin Exot Anim* 11:301-314, 2008.

From November 2001-September 2007 (10 or more reports out of 618 cases).

and methemoglobinemia. Treatment consists of aggressive decontamination (emesis and activated charcoal), monitoring hepatic enzymes (especially leakage enzymes such as alanine aminotransferase), monitoring for methemoglobinemia, and *N*-acetylcysteine. *N*-acetylcysteine provides compounds that can conjugate acetaminophen and its toxic metabolite and enhance removal from the body. It is administered as a 5% solution orally; a loading dose of 140-280 mg/kg is given, and then 70 mg/kg is given every 6 hours for an additional 7 doses. The drug can be given intravenously if a sterile solution is available.[20]

Conclusion

Although treating small mammals that have been exposed to poisons may present unique problems, a careful approach, keeping in mind species-specific differences, can lead to a successful therapeutic outcome.

References

1. Lichtenberger M, Richardson JA: Emergency care and managing toxicoses in exotic animal patients, *Vet Clin Exot Anim* 11(2):211–228, 2008.
2. DeClementi C: Prevention and treatment of poisoning. In Gupta RC, editor: *Veterinary toxicology*, St Louis, 2007, Elsevier, pp 1139–1158.
3. Donnelly TM: Rabbits: basic anatomy, physiology, and husbandry. In Hillyer EV, Quesenberry KE, editors: *Ferrets, rabbits, and rodents: clinical medicine and surgery*, Philadelphia, 1997, Saunders, pp 147–168.
4. Means C: Anticoagulant rodenticides. In Plumlee KH, editor: *Clinical veterinary toxicology*, St Louis, 2004, Mosby, pp 444–446.
5. Plumb DC: Phytonadione vitamin K1. *Plumb's veterinary drug handbook*, ed 5, Malden, MA, 2005, Blackwell, pp 635–637.
6. Dunayer E: Bromethalin: the other rodenticide, *Vet Med* 98(9):732–736, 2003.
7. Dorman DC, et al: Effects of an extract of ginkgo biloba on bromethalin-induced cerebral lipid peroxidation and edema in rats, *Am J Vet Res* 53(1):138–142, 1992.
8. Morrow CK, Volmer PA: Cholecalciferol. In Plumlee KH, editor: *Clinical veterinary toxicology*, St Louis, 2004, Mosby, pp 448–451.
9. Talcott PA: Strychnine. In Plumlee KH, editor: *Clinical veterinary toxicology*, St Louis, 2004, Mosby, pp 454–456.
10. Albretsen JC: Zinc phosphide. In Plumlee KH, editor: *Clinical veterinary toxicology*, St Louis, 2004, Mosby, pp 456–458.

11. Schaeffer DO: Gastrointestinal diseases of guinea pigs. In Hillyer EV, Quesenberry KE, editors: *Ferrets, rabbits, and rodents: clinical medicine and surgery*, Philadelphia, 1997, WB Saunders, pp 261–263.
12. Harkness JE, Wagner JE: *The biology and medicine of rabbits and rodents*, ed 3, Philadelphia, 1989, Lea & Febiger, pp 56–57.
13. Johnston MS: Clinical toxicology of domestic rabbits, *Vet Clin Exot Anim* 11:315–326, 2008.
14. Pickrell JA, et al: Avocado. In Plumlee KH, editor: *Clinical veterinary toxicology*, St Louis, 2004, Mosby, pp 424–425.
15. Richardson VCG: *Rabbits: health, husbandry, and disease*, Malden, MA, 2000, Blackwell, p 151.
16. Dunayer E: Toxicology of ferrets, *Vet Clin Exot Anim* 11:301–314, 2008.
17. Richardson JA, Balabuszko RA: Ibuprofen ingestion in ferrets: 43 cases, January 1995-March 2000, *J Vet Emer Crit Care Soc* 11(1):53–59, 2001.
18. Wickstom ML, Eason CT: Literature search for mustelid-specific toxicants, *Sci Conservations* 127E:57–65, 1999.
19. O'Connor CE: *Evaluation of new toxins for mustelid control*. Wellington, New Zealand, 2002, Department of Conservation. From http://www.doc.govt.nz/upload/documents/science-and-technical/DSIS56.pdf. Accessed October 20, 2007.
20. Sellon RK: Acetaminophen. In Peterson ME, Talcott PA, editors: *Small animal toxicology*, ed 2, St Louis, 2006, Elsevier-Saunders, pp 550–558.

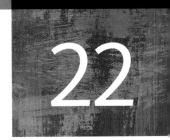

Poisoning in the Avian Patient

22

Jerry J. LaBonde, MS, DVM

Principles of Avian Toxicology

In avian toxicology it is difficult to generalize from mammals to birds because of the uniqueness of the avian physiology. Often, what is considered safe for a human or other mammal may be toxic to a bird. There is considerable variation between avian species in their response to different toxins. In general, the smaller the bird, the more sensitive it is to toxic exposures. Toxins have a more profound effect in very young, very old, or compromised birds (especially with liver disease). The avian respiratory system is extremely sensitive to many different types of gases and smoke. Relatively rapid transit times and gastrointestinal (GI) absorption combined with a high metabolic rate accelerate the effects of an ingested toxin. In aviary or multiple-bird homes, usually many birds are affected. Environmental conditions such as ventilation and temperature affect toxin exposure. Free-ranging wildlife such as raptors, waterfowl, and game fowl can be exposed to numerous toxicants in their environment. Toxicant exposure can result in mortalities, but often morbidity is a more significant factor manifest as decreased reproductive performance and inability to thrive. These exposures can be from primary exposure to a toxicant or a secondary toxicosis from bioaccumulation of toxic substances. Raptors, being at the top of the food chain with a wide range of distribution, play a role as biomonitors or sentinels of ecosystem health.[1]

Toxicoses in avian species are a dose-response relationship. The dose of a toxicant is the most important factor in determining the response in an avian patient. There are many household and environmental substances that may affect a bird's homeostasis. There are also many therapeutic options for birds such as synthetic and natural drugs, nutraceuticals, and alternative therapies for which safe levels have not been established.

The diagnosis of a toxicosis in the avian patient is sometimes a clinical challenge. This diagnosis is based largely on history and clinical signs because specific tests for most toxicants are not available. Most owners are unaware of potential toxic substances and a complete history may be difficult to obtain. Birds readily chew or ingest foreign materials and, as a group, they appear overly sensitive to toxicants. It is difficult to generalize about clinical disease of toxicants and birds because each species may respond in a specific way, there are many classes of poisons, and toxicosis can mimic other diseases. When presented with wildlife cases, toxicosis should always be on the differential diagnosis until proven otherwise.

Diagnosis of Toxicoses

It is not uncommon for birds to be brought to the veterinarian with an acute toxicosis. Toxicity is usually dose dependent. A fundamental diagnostic approach starts with a history, including a review of potential toxicant sources and routes of exposure. However, often the owner is unaware of toxin exposure to the bird. Without a history of toxin exposure, the diagnosis is often made by ruling out infectious, contagious, and metabolic diseases. Occasionally the clinical signs may reveal a fingerprint or toxic syndrome indicative of a specific poison (e.g., hematuria and neurologic signs are a fingerprint for lead toxicosis). Identifying the toxicant is secondary to stabilizing the patient and treating the clinical signs.

Veterinary journals and textbooks provide rapid access to poison information, but may be limited on the vast array of toxicant substances birds may be exposed to. The Veterinary Information Network can provide Internet access to information from board-certified veterinary toxicologists. Poison information centers are helpful and provide rapid access to critical information. The Certified Regional Poison Control Centers, the American Society for the Prevention of Cruelty to Animals Animal Poison Control Center, and Pet Poison HELPLINE may have sketchy amounts of avian-related information, but they do provide information on the physiologic effects of various compounds and chemicals. Knowing the physiologic effects of a toxicant can direct the veterinarian's course of treatment.

Diagnostic laboratories are useful in confirming a toxicosis. One should contact the laboratory to confirm its ability to handle small samples and the amount of sample required before submission. Samples that are submitted include plasma, serum, whole blood, tissue (frozen or fresh), and gastric contents. The submission of paired samples from unaffected birds is helpful in interpreting the results. Gross necropsy and histopathologic examination rarely show a toxicologic cause. Two sets of tissues should be collected at postmortem, one set for histopathologic examination in 10% buffered formalin and one set frozen for toxicologic examination. For toxicologic examinations, brain, spinal cord, and peripheral nerves should be included in both sets of tissues.[2]

Management of Toxicoses

A fundamental six-step approach in the treatment of avian toxicities appears to work best. One must focus on treating the patient, not the toxin.

Step 1: Stabilize the patient. This includes emergency therapy to maintain normal metabolic, respiratory, cardiovascular, and neurologic function.

Step 2: Prevent further exposure. Remove all birds from the affected environment. Ventilate the area. Flush or wash the bird's skin and feathers to remove the toxin. For ingestion of acids (corrosive), internally dilute with milk or water. Externally flush with water and apply sodium bicarbonate paste. For ingestion of alkali compounds (caustic), internally dilute with vinegar (1:4), lemon juice, or diluted egg whites followed by a cathartic. Externally flush with water and apply vinegar.[3]

Step 3: Delay further absorption. Because emetics are contraindicated in birds, absorption of toxins is delayed by crop or proventricular lavage, the use of adsorbents and cathartics, or surgical removal. Intubation of an anesthetized bird is necessary for crop or proventricular lavaging. Activated charcoal is an adsorbent. Prepare a slurry (e.g., 1 g/5-10 mL H_2O) dose 1-4 g/kg.[4,5] Many commercial activated charcoal slurry products contain sorbitol as a cathartic. Dosing is the same as with activated charcoal alone. Pulse dosing every 4-6 hours should be considered with toxins that have enteric coatings or marked hepatic biliary recirculation.[5] Activated charcoal (without sorbitol) is recommended for pulse dosing if the bird is dehydrated. Activated charcoal is not effective for corrosive substances, petroleum distillate, or heavy metals. A second, weak adsorbent is bismuth sulfate at 1-2 mL/kg orally.[4]

Step 4: Institute physiologic antagonist therapy. There are few antidotes for specific toxins.

Step 5: Facilitate removal of absorbed toxicants. Diuresis, heat, and the use of cathartics or bulk diets aid in the removal of toxins. Be careful with cathartics because they can cause dehydration and hypotension. Bulk diet: ½ tsp of psyllium in 60 mL of baby food, gruel, or tube-feeding mixture.[3]

Step 6: Administer supportive therapy. Depending on the condition of the bird, this includes heat, fluids, nutritional supplementation, antibiotics, and other indicated drugs.

Iatrogenic Toxicoses

Any pharmaceutical, supplement, or homeopathic compound is potentially toxic when used in inappropriate doses or routes in birds. There is a wide variety of potential toxic reactions to drug agents used by veterinarians and over-the-counter or prescription drugs used in the home. More notable iatrogenic toxicoses in pet birds are aminoglycosides, fenbendazole and albendazole, and over-supplementation of vitamins D and A.[6,7] If a toxic reaction to an over-the-counter drug is suspected, consulting with poison information centers is advised to learn the potential physiologic effects of the drug. Parrots have been known to chew on owners' medications, but determining how much was ingested can be difficult. Activated charcoal is indicated for suspicious ingestions, and if the bird is presented immediately, gastric lavage should be done prior to administration of activated charcoal. Supportive care is based on clinical signs.

Inhalant Toxins

Inhalant toxicoses are the most common toxicoses observed in pet birds. The efficiency of the avian respiratory system makes birds more susceptible to gases or fumes in the household or aviary and can often result in acute death. The majority of exposures occurring in the home are a result of inappropriate use or proximity near the pet birds. Ventilation, temperature, and humidity can affect the toxic potential of many airborne toxins. Smaller avian species are more susceptible to inhalant toxins. Smoke from cooking or burning material and fumes from aerosols or cleaning agents are frequent causes of inhalant toxicosis. Any strong odor or aerosolized particulates from any household product can be potentially toxic. Many standard vacuum cleaners have a filtered exhaust that can emit microaerosolized particulates into the air. When inhaled, these particulates can cause respiratory compromise. Standard ventilators or stove-top filters do not sufficiently clear the air of toxic particles. When any gases or fumes are present in the home or aviary, the birds should be removed from the house and windows opened for ventilation.

With any toxic inhalant exposure, the veterinarian needs to treat the clinical signs presented. This may include administration of humidified oxygen, bronchodilators, diuretics for pulmonary edema, broad-spectrum antibiotics, antiinflammatories, analgesics, and supportive fluid and heat therapy. The use of antiinflammatory steroids is controversial and in some cases may even worsen the condition.[8] Residues from smoke can be washed off the feathers with diluted dish soap once the bird is stable.

Polytetrafluoroethylene

Polytetrafluoroethylene (PTFE), or polymer fume fever, poisonings are one of the more common airborne toxins reported in birds. Sources of PTFE are nonstick surfaces on products such as cookware, drip pans (which can reach temperatures of 600° F), heat lamp covers, irons, and ironing board covers. The gas is emitted when the surface undergoes pyrolysis at 280° C (536° F) and the PTFE is degraded.[9,10] Acute death resulting from respiratory failure is the most common result, but mild exposures exhibit moist rales, dyspnea, ataxia, depression, or anxious behavior. At necropsy, hemorrhagic and edematous lungs are the most common findings consistent with any irritant gas exposure. Particulates may be noted on histopathologic analysis as well as pulmonary edema, hemorrhage, and necrosis.[11,12]

Smoke Inhalation

The primary cause of death in most smoke inhalation toxicoses is carbon monoxide (CO). There are, however, other irritant (aldehydes, HCl, sulfur dioxide) and nonirritant (CO, CO_2, hydrogen cyanide) gases as well as particulate matter that can cause severe respiratory trauma. Carbon monoxide from incomplete combustion of fires, combustible engines (such as poorly ventilated vehicles, a concern with raptors being transported), and some poorly maintained furnaces can result in acute deaths. Carbon monoxide does not injure the lungs, but it decreases the oxygen-carrying capacity of hemoglobin in the blood resulting in dyspnea, depression, ataxia, nausea, and death. Carbon dioxide buildup will lower available oxygen as well as acting as a respiratory stimulant, resulting in increased inhalation of other toxic constituents of smoke. Hydrogen cyanide causes cellular inability to use oxygen, further complicating smoke inhalation.[13]

The primary concern with irritant gases (aldehydes, HCl, sulfur dioxide) is delayed, complicated pulmonary failure. These clinical problems may not surface for days.[13] Therefore persistent monitoring and treatment should continue for days up to 3 weeks following smoke exposure.[14]

Treatment of smoke inhalation includes access to fresh air immediately, followed by emergency therapy as needed. Oxygen in a dark, stress-free environment is used to stabilize, and, if possible, humidified oxygen or nebulized saline in oxygen will minimize drying of secretions and seeding of bacteria. Bronchodilator therapy can be used to alleviate reflex bronchospasms. Bronchodilator therapy includes terbutaline 0.01 mg/kg intramuscularly (IM) every 6 hours or nebulization of terbutaline at 0.01 mg/kg in 9 mL of 0.9% saline.[4,15] Fluid therapy will aid in cardiac output and enhance oxygen delivery to tissues.

Tobacco smoke via passive inhalation can result in chronic respiratory problems, pulmonary fibrosis, increased susceptibility to bacterial invasion, ocular irritation, and some dermatologic problems, most commonly on the feet or face. Coughing, sneezing, and conjunctivitis are the most common clinical signs. Exposure to second-hand smoke has been shown to increase atherosclerotic plaques in cockerels.[12] The ingestion of nicotine can also cause problems such as vomiting, diarrhea, hyperexcitability, seizures, and death. Therapy for secondary illnesses caused by tobacco exposure will only help if the bird is removed from the chronic exposure to these products.

There are many household products that have been anecdotally reported as toxic to birds. The primary cause of respiratory compromise is due to contact irritation of lungs and air sacs. Any aerosolized product from a spray or aerosolized from wind or vacuuming can be potentially toxic. Many of these products may be considered nontoxic unless airborne and inhaled in a specific concentration.

Inhaled or aspirated particulates or medications can cause severe tracheal inflammation (Box 22-1). Mucoid obstruction can occur in the trachea or at the syrinx. Humidified air, bronchodilators, and placement of an abdominal air sac for breathing should be considered for treatment.

Box 22-1	Inhalant Household Toxins

Air fresheners and scented candles
Ammonia and strong bleach
Automobile exhaust, carbon monoxide
Bug bombs, pesticide strips and sprays
Burning foods and cooking oils
Chemical sprays (i.e., disinfectants, deodorizers, furniture polish, etc.)
Fluoropolymers from spray starch
Glues, paints, nail polish and polish remover
Hair permanents and hair sprays
Hair dryer fumes (primarily from new hair dryers)
Leaded gasoline fumes
Most nonstick cooking surfaces (i.e., pots, pans, woks, drip pans, ovens, baking sheets, irons)
Mothballs (naphthalene, paradichlorobenzene)
Self-cleaning ovens
Smoke (tobacco or any other source)

Miscellaneous Household Toxins

There are numerous household products to which a bird could potentially be exposed. Many products, if used correctly with proper ventilation, can be used safely around birds. When inappropriate use occurs, birds are easily affected, with a clinical history of acute onset with no changes in diet or environment. Pet bird owners should always be questioned if any household products, aerosols, or cleaning agents have been recently used in the home when any bird presents with an unexplained illness. Many owners will be unaware of the sensitivity their birds have to everyday products. For example, an Amazon parrot exhibited severe respiratory distress after an owner applied a spray-on antistain protectant to a nearby sofa.[16] Because of the numerous products used in the home, birds should be treated according to their clinical signs and condition.

Clinical signs and therapy of some common household product exposures are briefly discussed.[17,18]

Alcohol

Exposures can be from ingestion or topical absorption. Clinical signs depend on the amount of exposure and include lethargy, ataxia, regurgitation, and death. Therapy includes fluid therapy and placing the bird in a warm, dark incubator.

Aluminum Chloride

Aluminum chloride is found in deodorants and can cause oral irritation, hemorrhagic gastroenteritis, ataxia, and nephrosis. Treatment includes careful lavage of the crop and proventriculus and administration of GI protectants.

Ammonia

Ammonia is found in cleaning agents. The primary clinical sign is respiratory irritation. Treatment involves fresh air, oxygen, and supportive therapy.

Chlorine

Chlorine is found in bleaches and hot tub and pool chemicals. Clinical signs include epiphora, photophobia, respiratory distress, and GI irritation. Treatment involves flushing the eyes or skin with water or milk, or, in the case of ingestion, milk of magnesia orally or dilution with water.

Cooking Oils

Common problems caused by cooking oils include skin burns and hypothermia with contact exposures. With ingestion (preening feathers), diarrhea, dehydration, regurgitation, and pneumonia may occur. Activated charcoal is helpful, but hypothermia and sepsis from burns are the primary concerns. An absorbent towel or corn starch can be used to soak up excess oil, but a series of warm, mild detergent baths may be needed. Baths should only be given once the bird is warmed and stable.

Disinfectants (Phenolic Compounds)

Phenolic compound products are rapidly absorbed through ingestion, inhalation, or dermal contact. Corrosive burns can occur on the skin, eyes, and respiratory tract. GI burns of the mouth, pharynx, and esophagus may occur. Clinical signs include open-mouth panting, vomiting, ataxia, shock, coma, and death. Treatment is similar to that required by cationic soaps, with special attention to acid base status and renal and hepatic function.

Disinfectants (Pine Oils)

Pine oil products can be mixed with phenols or terpene alcohols. Irritation to mucous membranes can result in conjunctivitis, photophobia, vomiting, and abdominal pain. Respiratory depression, ataxia, and death may also occur. Treatment includes dilution with milk, egg whites, or water, followed by an osmotic cathartic. Supportive care is important.

Nicotine

Sources include tobacco products. Depression, tachycardia, cyanosis, and dyspnea can be observed. Treatments include absorbents, cathartics, and supportive therapy.

Petroleum-Based Products

Petroleum-based products include mineral spirits, nail polish remover, furniture polish, gasoline, and paint removers. Clinical signs include skin irritation, mental depression, and mucosal and respiratory irritation. Hepatorenal damage can occur. For cutaneous exposure, wash with a mild detergent. If ingestion has occurred, sucralfate (25 mg/kg, PO every 8 hours) is indicated if vomiting is not present.[4] Supportive therapy, oxygen, and treatment for potential pneumonia is indicated.

Soaps and Detergents (Anionic)

Anionic soaps and detergents are usually alkaline corrosive products found in laundry detergents, dish washer detergents, and shampoos. Clinical signs include ocular irritation, vomiting, diarrhea, and GI pain. Treat by flushing the eyes with water, or, if ingestion occurs, milk or water should be given to dilute. Activated charcoal may be of benefit. Animals with cutaneous exposures should be thoroughly bathed.

Soaps and Detergents (Cationic)

Cationic soaps and detergents are usually quaternary ammonium compounds found in clearning products, fabric softeners, germicides, and sanitizers. Clinical signs can be severe and include vomiting, corrosive damage, weakness, muscle tremors, seizures, coma, and death. Treatment for oral ingestion is milk, water, or egg whites, followed by activated charcoal and supportive therapy. Patients with ocular exposures should be lavaged with isothermic, isotonic saline for 15-20 minutes.

Food and Plant Toxicoses

Foods

Iron storage liver disease, hemochromatosis, can occur in soft-bill species sensitive to dietary level of iron such as toucans, mynahs, hornbills, birds of paradise, and starlings.[19,20] To a lesser extent, lories show a species predilection to iron storage liver disease, but it is unclear if it is due to high levels of dietary iron or excess of dietary vitamin C or A that facilitate iron absorption.[21] Clinical signs include anorexia, dyspnea, and ascites. Clinical pathologic findings often reveal elevated packed cell volume, liver enzymes, and bile acids. Treatment involves restricted vitamin C and vitamin A and low-iron diets.[22,23] Abdominal centesis of ascetic fluid to aid in respiration can help stabilize a critical patient. Phlebotomies and iron chelators such as deferoxamine mesylate (Desferal) and deferiprone (Ferriprox) should be considered as well.[4,24]

Chocolate toxicosis usually occurs as a result of overindulgent owners or pet psittacines having free range in the home. Toxic doses have not been established in birds, but what may seem a small amount to the owner could be a toxic dose in a small bird. Clinical signs are due to methylxanthines (caffeine and theobromine) and include tachycardia, hypertension, ventricular arrhythmia, diarrhea, polyuria, and seizures. In avian cases, hepatic, renal, pulmonary, and central nervous systems are affected.[12,25]

Onion and *garlic* (*Allium* genus) are human foods that can cause problems when provided in significant amounts related to the size of the bird. Garlic is used by humans as a neutraceutical for parasite control or as an antioxidant that can be dangerous when given to birds.[12,26] A Pionus parrot was presented dead after the owner administered a ¼ clove of garlic orally because the bird was not feeling well. All parts of the plants contain sulfur-containing compound and are considered toxic; they are toxic when fresh, dried, or cooked. Clinical signs are lethargy, weakness, tachycardia, anemia, and death. Pathologic abnormalities include anemia, anisocytosis, intra- and extravascular hemolysis, hemoglobinuria, hemoglobinuric nephrosis, and hemosiderin in the liver.[26]

Avocado (*Persea americana*) ingestion can elicit variable toxic reactions. There may also be variability in toxicity between different types of avocados. Not all species of birds are equally affected, making a dose-response relationship difficult to establish. Studies in budgerigars fed 1-mL doses of a water and avocado mixture led to death within 24 to 48 hours.[27] Larger birds can exhibit agitation, feather pulling, lethargy, and dyspnea. At necropsy, subcutaneous edema, pericardial effusion, and organ congestion are observed. Persin has been identified as the toxin in mammals but has not been established in birds.[12]

Sodium chloride or *salt* toxicities can be observed from ingestion of excessive amounts of salt (salted nuts and crackers) or from contaminated water.[28] Clinical signs include polydipsia, depression, hemoglobinuria, excitement, tremors, torticollis, opisthotonus, ataxia, and death. Neurologic signs are due to cerebral edema. Treatment involves diuretics and fluids such as 5% dextrose in water or 2.5% dextrose in 0.45% saline.[14]

Plants

Plant toxicoses are a common concern among pet bird owners. However, the frequency of clinical toxicoses from exposure is rare. Toxic plant species reported in clinical studies are listed in Table 22-1. There is wide species variation to plant toxins, and adverse effects are often dose dependent. Frequently, the plant is chewed on but not ingested. The most common clinical signs are oral lesions, lethargy, and regurgitation. Treatment includes supportive care, and the use of adsorbents and cathartics may be indicated.

For reported plant toxicities in clinical cases or studies, see Table 22-1.

Heavy-Metal Toxicities

Heavy-metal poisoning is one of the most commonly reported avian toxicoses because of the ubiquitous availability of heavy-metal sources and the tendency of birds to chew on objects in their environment. Lead is the most common toxicity and is followed by zinc, copper, and iron.

Lead

There are numerous sources of lead that birds can chew on and ingest, including toys with lead-based metal, bells with lead clappers, hardware cloth, galvanized wire, stained glass windows, Tiffany lamps, antique or costume jewelry, curtain weights, lead solder, fishing weights, foil from champagne or cognac bottles, improperly glazed ceramics, mirror backs, batteries, and paint applied prior to 1955.[33] For wildlife, the primary concern is ingestion of lead shot or fishing weights. Lead shot has been banned for use on state and federal lands since 1991 in the United States, but can still be used on private land for game bird or rodent hunting. Spent ammunition in these areas can be picked up by waterfowl or game fowl.[34] Exposure can occur in scavenging birds such as crows, ravens, eagles, hawks, vultures, and condors.[35] Ingestion of the metal is most likely needed for a toxicosis. Lead shot or fragments imbedded in tissue does not appear to be a toxic burden to the animal; however, long-term exposure in the tissue can lower the dose needed at ingestion of lead to produce clinical signs.[1,36]

Clinical signs of lead exposure are dose dependent and multisystemic, involving the hematopoietic, neurologic, GI, and renal systems. Renal effects are not observed in raptors.[1] In pet birds, the most common clinical signs, in decreasing order, are depression, weakness, regurgitation, polyuria and polydipsia, seizures, hemoglobinuria, and diarrhea. In waterfowl and raptors, blindness, drooped wings, peripheral neuropathy, GI stasis, bright green diarrhea, and biliverdinuria are additional clinical signs observed.[34,37] Species' tolerance variations are reported in raptors. Turkey vultures (*Cathartes aura*) and red-tailed hawks (*Buteo jamaicensis*) tolerate higher lead levels than other raptors, such as bald eagles (*Haliaeetus leucocephalus*), before showing clinical signs.[1,38] Birds with acute exposures appear in good flesh but may be mildly anemic and hypoproteinemic, with slow labored respirations. They can also present as weak or depressed, have neurologic signs, and have hemoglobinuria or biliverdinuria. Birds suffering from chronic exposures are

Table 22-1 Toxic Plant Species

Plant	Clinical Signs and Pathologic Findings	Toxin and Plant Parts
Avocado (*Persia americana*)	Agitation, feather pulling, anorexia, dyspnea, death; pulmonary and organ congestion, subcutaneous edema, hydropericardium	Persin: All parts of the plant
Bishop's weed (*Ammi majus*)	Photosensitization	Furocoumarins: Seeds and foliage
Black locust (*Robinia pseudoacacia*)	Depression, dyspnea, coughing, sneezing, and regurgitation	Robin: Leaves, seed, and bark
Blue-green algae (*Microcystis, Anabaena, Aphanazomenon, Oscillartoria*)	Acute death, hepatitis, and photosensitization; edema; petechiation and hemorrhage, weakness, depression, seizures	Microcystin, anatoxin-a, anatoxin-a(s)
Castor bean (*Ricinus communis*)	Regurgitation, abdominal pain, bloody diarrhea, seizures, renal failure, and death	Ricin: Seeds (see Color Plate 74-1, C)
Clematis (*Montana rubens*)	Regurgitation	Leaves
Coffee bean (*Sesbania drummondii*)	Restlessness, hyperactivity, tachycardia, polyuria, regurgitation, muscle tremors, and seizures	Caffeine: Bean
Crown vetch (*Coronilla varia*)	Tachypnea and neurologic signs	Nitroglycosides: Leaves
Dieffenbachia (*Dieffenbachia* spp.)	Skin and oral irritation, hypersalivation, and regurgitation	Oxalate raphides
Elephant's ear (*Colocasia* or *Alocasia* spp.)	Skin and oral irritation, hypersalivation, and regurgitation	Oxalate raphides
Ergot (*Claviceps purpurea*)	Vesicular dermatitis, dry gangrenous necrosis of tongue, comb, and wattles	Ergotamine
Lily of the valley (*Convallaria majalis*)	Lethargy, weakness, bradycardia, arrhythmias, diarrhea, and regurgitation	Cardiac glycoside: Leaves
Locoweed (*Astragalus* spp.)	Neurologic signs and hypersalivation	Miserotoxin: All parts of the plant
Maternity plant (*Kalanchoe* spp.)	Regurgitation, diarrhea, ataxia, cardiac failure	Lanceotoxin: Foliage and flowers
Milkweed (*Asclepias* spp.)	Regurgitation, diarrhea, ataxia, respiratory distress, and seizures	Cardenolides: All parts of the plant
Nightshade (*Solanum* spp.) (Color Plate 22-1)	Regurgitation, dyspnea, tachycardia, and weakness	Alkaloids: Berries and leaves
Oak (*Quercus* spp.)	Anorexia, abdominal pain, diarrhea, and regurgitation	Pyrogallol tannins: Acorns, leaves, and buds
Oleander (*Nerium oleander*)	Lethargy, subcutaneous hemorrhage, diarrhea, weakness, tetanic spasms, salivation, and regurgitation	Oleandrin: Leaves (see Color Plate 26-2, C)
Philodendron (*Philodendron* spp.)	Skin and oral irritation, choking, regurgitation, diarrhea	Oxalate raphides
Poinsettia (*Euphorbia pulcherrima*)	Oral irritation, regurgitation, red stained feces, gastroenteritis, and hepatic necrosis	Diterpene ester: Leaves and milky sap
Pokeweed (*Phytolacca americana*)	Gastrointestinal irritation, regurgitation, and diarrhea	Phytolaccatoxin: Roots, berries, leaves
Rhododendron (*Rhododendron* spp.)	Lethargy, weakness, regurgitation, diarrhea, and bradycardia	Grayanotoxins: Leaves
Tobacco (*Nicotiana* spp.)	Regurgitation, tremors, tachycardia, seizures	Nicotine: Leaves
Virginia creeper (*Parthenocissus quinquefloia*)	Lethargy and regurgitation	Leaves
Yew (*Taxus* spp.)	Ataxia, regurgitation, and dyspnea	Taxines: Fruit and leaves

emaciated and have crop stasis or GI signs. Chronic low-grade exposure can be immuno-suppressive. Subclinical lead toxicosis in raptors can be present in birds presented for other causes such as trauma.[1]

The severity of the clinical pathologic condition depends on dose and chronicity of ingestion. Abnormalities include heterophilia, hypochromic regenerative anemia, cytoplasmic vacuolization of red cells, and elevations in lactic dehydrogenase, aspartate transaminase, creatinine phosphokinase, and uric acid.[39,40]

A diagnosis of lead poisoning is based on history of exposure, clinical signs, clinical pathologic findings, blood-lead concentration, and radiographic evidence of metallic densities in the GI tract. The absence of metal particles does not rule out heavy metal toxicosis, especially in raptors. Blood-lead concentration is the definitive test to confirm lead poisoning. When the lead is ingested, it is solubilized in the proventriculus and ventriculus and is absorbed in the small intestine. The lower the pH in the digestive tract (raptors), the more rapid the absorption compared with higher-pH environments (psittacines and granivorous birds).[1] Lead then binds to the red blood cells and is distributed to the body. The blood, parenchymal organs, nervous system, and soft tissues will carry approximately 6% of the total body burden of lead and approximately 94% of the burden will be in bone. Bone has a slower rate of exchange of lead than the soft tissues. Therefore blood-lead values represent only a small amount of the total body burden.[40]

Heparinized whole blood concentrations greater than 20 mcg/dL (0.2 ppm) are suggestive, and concentrations greater than 50 mcg/dL (0.5 ppm) are diagnostic for lead poisoning.[33,41] Prognosis for patients with levels of more than 1 ppm is guarded.[40] Most laboratories need a small sample to assay blood-lead concentrations, but one should check with each individual laboratory before submission. In-house blood-lead levels can be obtained with the Lead Care Analyzer (Lead Care Blood Testing System, ESA Inc.).

Treatment is tailored to the patient's physical condition and the blood-lead concentration. Treatment with chelation therapy forms nontoxic complexes in the blood that are excreted in the bile and urine. The initial chelator of choice is calcium disodium versenate (CaEDTA). CaEDTA appears to have minimal chelation effect in soft tissue but is very effective in bone. CaEDTA injections (35-50 mg/kg IM) are administered every 12 hours for 5 days, then off for 3 days, and then repeat as needed.[4,33] For prolonged therapy CaEDTA can be diluted with saline and administered subcutaneously.[1] Further treatment may be indicated as lead concentrations equilibrate from bone into soft tissue and blood. Treatment ends when the blood-lead concentration is normal, there is no radiographic evidence of metal, and the bird is clinically normal. The blood-lead concentration is rechecked three to four days after CaEDTA treatment has ended. Restarting CaEDTA therapy until results of the blood-lead concentrations are known is recommended. Nephrosis, neurologic toxicity, and incidental chelation of zinc have been reported as side effects of prolonged chelation therapy, but have not been observed clinically in birds.[1] Samour and Naldo reported extended treatment of 23 days in falcons with no deleterious effects.[42]

Alternative chelation therapies include the use of dimercaptosuccinic acid (DMSA). DMSA is the preferred oral chelator (25-35 mg/kg by mouth [PO] q12h) and can be used with CaEDTA if needed.[43] Oral chelators should be used with the same frequency as CaEDTA. Some cases may benefit from oral administration compared with injectable (CaEDTA) for prolonged treatment.[44] DMSA does not chelate lead from bone but is effective in soft tissues. Combination therapy with CaEDTA and DMSA has been shown to be effective and in some cases has shown to increase survivability compared with either chelator used alone.[34] Considering that CaEDTA primarily chelates from the bone and DMSA chelates from soft tissues, combination therapy should be considered in advanced cases.

D-penicillamine (PA) is another chelator that has the advantage of oral administration. PA (30-55 mg/kg PO q12h for 7-14 days) can be used in conjunction with or after CaEDTA injections or by itself. Side effects such as regurgitation are reported, and PA is not recommended if CaEDTA or DMSA are available.

Hastening the removal of particles with the use of bulk diets and cathartics is recommended and may prevent the need for surgical removal. Rat skins with hair can be fed to raptors to stimulate cast formation and egestion of lead particles in the ventriculus.[45] As long as the bird is given chelation therapy and is improving, there is no urgency for surgery. Many of the particles break down and pass on their own. Large burdens of heavy metals in the intestinal tract will need to be removed. Endoscopic removal with or without gastric lavage should be considered before surgery.

Supportive therapy is directed at controlling seizures, anemia, immunosuppression, and anorexia. Antioxidative therapy with vitamin C and vitamin B complex to aid recovery of injury to the nervous system may be helpful.[1]

Zinc

The diagnosis and signs of acute zinc toxicoses are similar to that of lead except hemoglobinuria is rare.[33,45] Frequently, birds simultaneously have lead and zinc poisoning. Zinc plasma concentrations are reported in asymptomatic macaws at 1.3-2 ppm and 1.25-2.29 ppm in clinically normal Hispaniolan Amazon parrots.[41] Clinical signs are observed when concentrations are more than 10 ppm. Zinc concentrations more than 5 ppm are suggestive of toxicosis.[12,46] Plasma is collected in nonrubber-stopper containers or in royal blue–stopper containers to prevent zinc contamination from leaching into the sample. The liver, kidney, and pancreas are the tissues of choice for postmortem zinc analysis.

The more remarkable pathologic lesions of zinc poisoning include ileus and focal mononuclear degeneration of liver, kidney, and the pancreas. In waterfowl, necrotizing ventriculitis and pancreatic lesions are observed.[40]

The treatment of choice is similar to lead therapy employing CaEDTA, DMSA, and PA. A distinct difference between lead and zinc is that zinc is not stored in the bone and therefore equilibrates and chelates faster.[43] Removal of zinc particles can be done by endoscopy, gastric lavage, or surgery if needed.

Sources of zinc include galvanized containers, galvanized mesh, hardware cloth, staples, galvanized nails, fertilizers, some paints, zinc pyrithione shampoos, zinc oxide, zinc undecylenate (Desenex cream), and pennies (post-1982).[33,40,47]

Other Heavy Metals

Other heavy-metal toxicities are rare in pet birds, but poisonings from copper, iron, and mercury can occur. Copper sources include wire and pennies manufactured before 1982. The treatment of choice is PA or DMSA. Iron toxicoses can result from cast-iron feeding bowls with chipped enamel.[3,41] Deferoxamine (Desferol 40 mg/kg PO, subcutaneously [SC], or IM q24hr for 7 days to months) is the treatment of choice in mammals, but safe dosing levels are not established in birds and intestinal absorption is poor when give orally.[3,4] Mercury ingestion is more of a concern in wild birds and DMSA may be effective.[12] Mercury comes in three forms: elemental (fluorescent light bulbs, thermometers, lubricating oils), inorganic (blistering agents, skin creams and soaps, laxatives), and organic or methyl mercury (organomercurial fungicides, industrial contamination of aquatic food chains). Elemental mercury is not absorbed well in the intestinal tract and generally will not cause toxicity except in high amounts.[48] Methyl mercury, the most toxic form for wildlife, is readily absorbed and easily crosses the blood-brain barrier. Clinical signs are neurologic as well as decreased reproductive performance and hatchability.[12,49] Diagnosis is based on history, clinical signs, and kidney tissue residue concentrations exceeding 40 mcg/g wet weight.[46] Gastric lavage and activated charcoal are used for acute oral exposures. DMSA has been used in mammals as an effective chelator.[48]

Pesticides

Pesticide toxicities primarily are the result of inappropriate application or use of insecticides, rodenticides, and herbicides.

Insecticides

Organophosphates (OPs) and *carbamates* (CBMs) are the most common causes of avian insecticide toxicoses. OPs include fenthion, famfur, disulfoton, diazinon, dichlorvos, and malathion. CBMs include carbaryl, carbofuran, and aldicarb. LD_{50} concentrations indicate avian species are up to 20% more susceptible than mammals to the toxic effects of these products.[50] Inhalation is the primary source of exposure in pet birds, but ingestion from contaminated feeds and environment (e.g., ingestion of insects exposed to the pesticides) is a greater concern with confined outdoor birds and wildlife.[51,52]

The mechanism of action of OPs and CBMs is acetylcholinesterase (AChE) inhibition resulting in acetylcholine (ACh) accumulation in cholinergic synapses. Accumulation of ACh causes cholinergic hyperstimulation of end organs such as heart and airways followed by paralysis of skeletal muscles. OP bonds to AChE are essentially irreversible, and the CBM bonds are slowly reversible. Death is usually caused by neurologic and muscular dysfunction. Initial response to OP toxicity is stimulation leading to nerve impulse inhibition.[53] Early clinical signs include anorexia, weakness, diarrhea, crop stasis, ataxia, wing twitching, and prolapsed nictitans. More severe signs are muscular tremors, stiffness, dyspnea with rales, bradycardia, paralysis, and seizures. Death is usually caused by respiratory failure.[16,54]

An organophosphorus ester-induced delayed neuropathy has been observed 2 weeks following exposure to an OP in a white-front Amazon parrot. This bird exhibited ascending progressive paralysis, and death resulted from respiratory failure.[16]

Diagnosis of OP or CBM toxicosis is based on history, clinical signs, and response to treatment. If bradycardia is present and does not reverse with administration of 0.02 mg/kg of atropine intravenously (IV), OP toxicity is considered. Cholinesterase assays from whole blood, plasma, serum, or brain tissue are used to determine toxic exposure. These samples are submitted with paired nonexposed samples to determine whether depressed concentrations of cholinesterase are significant. In acute toxicoses, little or no cholinesterase will be found. Chronic toxicoses show concentrations of less than 50% of the normal sample, and a 20% decrease suggests an exposure. One effect of chronic exposure is decreased egg production and poor hatchability. Depressed AChE concentrations from CBMs may not be found owing to rapid regeneration if the samples are not submitted as soon as possible. Submission of gastric contents and environmental sources aid in diagnostic investigations—these samples, along with liver and kidney postmortem, can be used to test for the specific pesticide.[1,53,54]

Treatment includes atropine (0.2-0.5 mg/kg IM) every 3 to 4 hours as needed. One fourth of the initial dose is administered IV.[4] Atropine, a competitive muscarine receptor antagonist, will interrupt actions of ACh on the heart, GI tract, and airway. Atropine has little or no effect on nicotinic receptors and used alone will not counteract neuromuscular paralysis. Pralidoxime (2-PAM, 10-20 mg/kg IM) is administered every 8 to 12 hours as needed. 2-PAM is only effective if used within the first 24 to 36 hours of exposure.[4,53] A dose of 100 mg/kg given IM within 24 hours of an OP toxicity has been reported as effective in raptors; however, 20 mg/kg has been reported as toxic.[55] 2-PAM is contraindicated or should be used with caution with some CBM toxicities as it has been shown to inhibit AChE activity.[53]

Organochlorine (OC) toxicoses are a concern for free-ranging birds and have been reported in waterfowl ingesting treated grains or germinating seedlings. Sources can persist in the environment for long periods and include chlordane, dieldrin, aldrin, toxaphene, heptachlor, and dichlorodiphenyltrichloroethane (DDT) analogues.[34] Clinical signs include weight loss, muscle fasciculations, clonic convulsions, disorientation, ataxia, and death. Chronic low level exposures result in decreased fertility, egg shell thinning, and decreased hatchability.[56] During periods of stress or malnutrition OC compounds are released from fat stores, resulting in clinical signs. Treatment is supportive care and pathologically there are no gross lesions. High levels of OCs in brain and liver tissues may be helpful in confirming a diagnosis.[46]

Naphthalene and *paradichlorobenzene* (mothballs and mite protectors) toxicities result from contaminated foods or inappropriate ingestion. Clinical signs include diarrhea, weight loss, immunosuppression, hepatitis, tremors, and seizures. Treatment is supportive therapy. Paradichlorobenzene can be radiopaque on radiographs.

Inappropriate *pyrethrin* exposure can occur in birds. Pyrethrins work by alteration of sodium, calcium, and chloride channels.[12] Clinical signs are similar to those seen in mammals and include tremors, hyperthermia, seizures, and death. Treatment includes diazepam, methocarbamol, supportive care, and bathing with diluted dish soap once the bird is stable.

Rodenticides

Anticoagulant rodenticide toxicity occurs through direct exposure and through secondary ingestion of affected rodents.[57] First-generation rodenticides (i.e., warfarin) have short biologic half-lives and may require chronic exposure to produce clinical signs. Second-generation compounds (i.e., brodifacoum) are more toxic and only require a single exposure. This necessitates long-term therapy because of their long half-life.[58]

Interference with vitamin K epoxide reductase cycle results in decreased vitamin K and is the primary mechanism of action of anticoagulant rodenticides.[58] Birds rely more on the intrinsic clotting pathway than the extrinsic (vitamin K dependent), which may explain their decreased sensitivity to anticoagulant rodenticides.[12] However, toxicoses do occur, but species sensitivity has been documented at doses less than 1 mg/kg and up to 20 mg/kg.[12] Clinical signs include depression, anorexia, subcutaneous hemorrhage, bleeding from the nares, bloody droppings, and oral petechia.[33,57] Diagnosis is based on history and clinical signs. Clotting profiles on avian blood have not yet proven effective in diagnosis of these toxicoses.

Treatment includes vitamin K_1 (Veda-K1, 0.2 to 2.2 mg/kg IM or PO) every 4 to 8 hours until stable.[4] Daily oral administration of vitamin K is used until the toxin is metabolized. Treatment length for brodifacoum toxicities is as long as 3 to 4 weeks. Gastric lavage followed by administration of activated charcoal is helpful in acute exposures.

Other rodenticides include *cholecalciferol* analogs that produce a hypercalcemia and hyperphosphatemia. The increase in calcium can cause regurgitation, diarrhea, depression, polyuria and polydipsia, cardiac conduction disturbances, renal failure, and metastatic calcification.[58] Treatment is directed to lowering blood calcium concentrations by diuresis, glucocorticoids, and an antihypercalcemic.[59] Once calcium levels are normal for 96 hours, treatment can be discontinued.[15] Doses of antihypercalcemics have not been established in birds.

Zinc phosphide and *crimidine* toxicants are used as grain-based rodent baits. Grain-eating birds such as waterfowl, wild turkeys, doves, pigeons, quail, and pheasants are most likely to be exposed.[12] Clinical signs are regurgitation, cyanosis, and decreased blood pressure. Treatment is supportive care and reducing acidosis.

Oil Toxicoses

Oil toxicoses are primarily observed in wild avian species. Topical exposure decreases the feathers' ability for water proofing, insulation, and flight. Ingestion or aspiration causes pneumonia, GI irritation, ulceration, and hemolytic anemia.[12,34] Numerous accidental exposures have occurred in pet birds. Cooking oils, household petroleum-based products, and inappropriate use of oil-based pharmaceutical ointments are common sources of toxicoses. Clinical signs include burns and hypothermia from external contact and diarrhea, regurgitation, and dehydration from ingestion (i.e., preening feathers).[18] Pneumonia and tracheitis are also concerns that results from aspiration of oil-based products. Treatment includes heat; supportive care; nutritional support; and warm, mild detergent baths with frequent rinses after the bird is stabilized. A "dry" way to treat oil exposures in birds too stressed for detergent baths involves a dusting with corn starch to absorb the oils. The use of iron powder and magnetic removal of oil from feathers has been studied, but risk of toxicity from ingestion should be considered.[12] Silver sulfadiazine cream is very effective for burn therapy.

Mycotoxins

Mycotoxins are fungal metabolites most commonly found in grains and feeds stored in humid conditions.[46] Hundreds of mycotoxins have been identified, but mycotoxicosis is often a difficult diagnosis to confirm. There are numerous potential toxins, and the specific toxin may not be in the feed at the time of testing. Therefore what is tested may not be the same as what was ingested. Presence of the fungus does not guarantee presence of the toxin. Toxicities are usually dose dependent, and acute overt intoxications are rare. Avian species appear to be more sensitive than other species to *aflatoxicosis*.[12] Cases can be insidious and chronic, resulting in nonspecific signs such as poor production, unthriftiness, diphtheritic lesions in the oral cavity and esophagus, ataxia, and blindness. Immunosuppression, chronic hepatitis, poor reproductive performance, and renal disease are some of the more common conditions caused by mycotoxins.[12,46]

Prevention includes proper handling and storage of feed material. The shells from mycotoxin-contaminated peanuts have been the most common source of mycotoxin-induced hepatitis in parrots. There is no specific treatment; however, birds may benefit from glucomannans and organic selenium to decrease the hepatotoxic and neurologic changes associated with exposure.[12]

References

1. Redig PT, Arent LR: Raptor toxicology, *Vet Clin North Am Exot Anim Pract* 11(2):261–282, 2008.
2. Poppenga RH: Diagnostic sampling and establishing a minimum data base in exotic animal toxicology, *Vet Clin North Am Exot Anim Pract* 11(2):195–210, 2008.
3. LaBonde JJ: Toxic disorders. In Rosskopf WJ, Woerpel RW, editors: *Diseases of caged and aviary birds*, ed 3, Philadelphia, 1996, Williams and Wilkins, pp 511–522.
4. Carpenter JW: *Exotic animal formulary*, ed 3, St Louis, 2005, Elsevier Saunders, pp 226–229.
5. Peterson ME: Toxicological decontamination. In Peterson ME, Talcott PA, editors: *Small animal toxicology*, ed 2, St Louis, 2006, Elsevier Saunders, pp 127–140.
6. Howard LL, Papendick R, Stalis IH, et al: Fenbendazole and albendazole toxicity in pigeons and doves, *J Avian Med Surg* 16(3):203–210, 2002.
7. Lightfoot T: Warning: fenbendazole in cockatiels, *Exot DVM Vet Mag* 1(4):39, 1999.
8. Verstappen FALM, Dorrestein GM: Aspergillosis in amazon parrots after corticosteroid therapy for smoke-inhalation injury, *J Avian Med Surg* 19(2):138–141, 2005.
9. Forbes NA, Jones D: PTFE toxicity in birds, *Vet Rec* 140(19):512, 1997.
10. Lyman R: Polytetrafluoroethylene toxicity. In Harrison G, Harrison L, editors: *Clinical avian medicine and surgery*, Philadelphia, 1986, Saunders, p 487.
11. Wells RE, Slocombe RF: Acute toxicosis of budgerigars (*Melopsittacus undulates*) caused by pyrolysis products from heated Polytetrafluoroethylene: microscopic study, *Am J Vet Res* 43(7):1243–1248, 1982.
12. Lightfoot TL, Yeager MY: Pet bird toxicity and related environmental concerns, *Vet Clin North Am Exot Anim Pract* 11(2):229–260, 2008.
13. Beasley VR: Smoke inhalation, *Vet Clin North Am Small Animal Pract* 20(2):545–556, 1990.
14. LaBonde JJ: Toxicity in pet avian patients, *Sem Avian Exot Pet Med* 4(1):23–31, 1995.
15. Lichtenebrger M, Richardson JA: Emergency care and managing toxicoses in the exotic animal patient, *Vet Clin North Am Exot Anim Pract* 11(2):211–228, 2008.
16. LaBonde JJ: Two clinical cases of exposure to household use of organophosphate and carbamate insecticides, *Assoc Avian Vet Conference*, New Orleans, 113–118, 1992.
17. Kore AM, Kiesche-Nesselrodt A: Toxicology of household cleaning products and disinfectants, *Vet Clin North Am Small Animal Pract* 20(2):529–538, 1990.
18. LaBonde JJ: Household poisonings in caged birds. In Bonagura JD, Kirk RW, editors: *Kirk's current veterinary therapy XII small animal practice*, Philadelphia, 1995, W.B. Saunders, pp 1299–1302.
19. Sheppard C, Dierenfeld E: Iron storage disease in birds: speculation on etiology and implications for captive husbandry, *J Avian Med Surg* 16(3):192–197, 2002.
20. Crissy SD, Ward AM, Block SE, et al: Hepatic iron accumulation over time in starlings (*Sturnus vulgaris*) fed two levels of iron, *J Zoo Wildl Med* 31(4):491–496, 2003.

21. West GD, Garner MM, Talcott PA: Hemochromatosis in several species of lories with high dietary iron, *J Avian Med Surg* 15(4):297–301, 2000.
22. Otten BA, Orosz SE, Auge S, et al: Mineral content of food items commonly ingested by toucans (*Ramphastos sulfuratus*), *J Avian Med Surg* 15(3):194–196, 2001.
23. Drews AV, Redrobe SP, Patterson-Kane JC: Successful reduction of hepatocellular hemosiderin content by dietary modification in toco toucans (*Ramphastos toco*) with iron storage disease, *J Avian Med Surg* 18(2):101–105, 2004.
24. LaBonde JJ: Medicine and surgery of mynahs. In Rosskopf WJ, Woerpel RW, editors: *Diseases of caged and aviary birds*, ed 3, Philadelphia, 1996, Williams and Wilkins, pp 928–932.
25. Cole G, Murray M: Suspected chocolate toxicosis in an African Grey parrot (*Psittacus erithacus*), *Assoc Avian Vet Conference and Expo*, Monterey, CA, 8–12, 2005.
26. Wade LL, Newman SJ: Hemoglobinuric nephrosis and hepatosplenic erythrophagocytosis in a dusky-headed conure (*Aratinga weddelli*) after ingestion of garlic (*Allium sativum*), *J Avian Med Surg* 18(3): 155–161, 2004.
27. Hargis AM, Stauber E, Casteel S, et al: Avocado (*Persea americana*) intoxication in caged birds, *J Am Vet Med Assoc* 194:64–66, 1989.
28. Wilson H, Brown CA, Greenacre CB, et al: Suspected sodium hypochlorite toxicosis in a group of psittacine birds, *J Avian Med Surg* 15(3):209–215, 2001.
29. Barr AC: Household and garden plants. In Peterson ME, Talcott PA, editors: *Small animal toxicology*, ed 2, St Louis, 2006, Elsevier Saunders, pp 345–409.
30. Shropshire C, Stauber E, Arai M: A screening study of potential toxic plants in budgerigars, Unpublished paper, Pullman, 1989, Washington State University. 1989.
31. Oehme FW, Davis J: Plants poisonous to free living or caged birds. In Hoff G, Davis J, editors: *Noninfectious diseases of wildlife*, 1982, Ames, Iowa State University Press, pp 8–23.
32. Cambell TW: Crown vetch (*Cornilla varia*) poisoning in a budgerigar (*Melopsittacus undulates*), *J Avian Med Surg* 20(2):97–100, 2006.
33. LaBonde JJ: Avian toxicology, *Vet Clin North Am Exot Anim Pract* 21(6):1329–1343, 1991.
34. Degerness L: Waterfowl toxicology: a review, *Vet Clin North AM Exot Animal Pract* 11(2):283–299, 2008.
35. Church ME, Gwiazda R, Risebrough RW, et al: Ammunition is the principle source of lead accumulated by California Condors re-introduced to the wild, *Environ Sci Technol* 40(19):6143–6150, 2006.
36. Sanderson GC, Anderson WL, Foley GL, et al: Effects of lead, iron, and bismuth alloy shot embedded in the breast muscles of game-farm mallards, *J Wildl Dis* 34:688–697, 1998.
37. Platt SR, Helmick KE, Graham J, et al: Peripheral neuropathy in a turkey vulture with lead toxicosis, *J Am Vet Med Assoc* 214:1218–1220, 1999.
38. Carpenter JW, Pattee OH, Fritts SH, et al: Experimental lead poisoning in turkey vultures (*Cathartes aura*), *J Wildl Dis* 39:95–104, 2003.
39. Hoffman DL, Patee OH, Wiemeyer SN, et al: Effects of lead shot ingestion on delta-aminolevulinic acid dehydratase activity, hemoglobin concentration, and serum chemistry in bald eagles, *J Wildl Dis* 17(3):423–431, 1981.
40. Mautino M: Lead and zinc intoxication in zoological medicine: a review, *J Zoo Wildl Med* 28:28–35, 1997.
41. Osofsky A, Jowett P, Hosgood G, et al: Determination of normal blood concentrations of lead, zinc, copper and iron in Hispaniolan Amazon (*Amazona vetralis*), *J Avian Med Surg* 15(1):31–36, 2001.
42. Samour J, Naldo JL: Lead toxicosis in falcons: a method for lead retrieval, *Sem Avian Exot Pet Med* 14(2):143–148, 2005.
43. Denver MC, Tell LA, Galey FD, et al: Comparison of two heavy metal chelators for treatment of lead toxicosis in cockatiels, *Am J Vet Res* 61(8):935–940, 2000.
44. Hoogesteijn AL, Raphael BL, Calle P, et al: Oral treatment of avian lead intoxication with meso-2,3-dimercaptosuccinic acid, *J Zoo Wildl Med* 34(1):82–87, 2003.
45. Holz P, Phelan J, Slocombe R, et al: Suspected zinc toxicosis as a cause of sudden death in orange bellied parrots (*Neophema chrysogaster*), *J Avian Med Surg* 15(3):209–215, 2000.
46. Degerness L: Avian toxicology: common problems, *Proc Ann Meeting Assoc Avian Vet*, San Diego, CA, 193–205, 2010.
47. Reece R: Zinc toxicity (new wire disease) in aviary birds, *Aust Vet J* 63:199, 1986.
48. Tegzes JH: Mercury. In Peterson ME, Talcott PA, editors: *Small animal toxicology*, ed 2, St Louis, 2006, Elsevier Saunders, pp 822–829.
49. Richardson J: Implications of toxic substances in clinical disorders. In Harrison GJ, Lightfoot T, editors: *Clinical Avian Medicine*, Palm Beach, 1999, HBD International Inc, pp 1030–1049.
50. Humphreys DJ: *Veterinary toxicology*, ed 3, London, 1998, Baillere Tindall. 179–182.
51. Reece RL, Handson P: Observations on the accidental poisonings of birds by organophosphate insecticides and other toxic substances, *Vet Rec* 111:453–455, 1982.

52. Kwan Y: Pesticide poisoning events in wild birds in Korea from 1998-2002, *J Wildl Dis* 40(4):737–740, 2004.

53. Meerdink GL: Organophosphorous and carbamate insecticide poisoning. In Kirk RW, editor: *Current veterinary therapy*, vol. 10, Philadelphia, 1989, WB Saunders, pp 135–137.

54. Hill EF, Fleming WJ: Anticholinesterase poisoning of birds: field monitoring and diagnosis of acute poisonings, *Environ Toxicol Chem* 1:27–38, 1982.

55. Shlosberg A: Treatment of monocrotophos-poisoned birds of prey with pralidoxamine iodide, *J Am Vet Assoc* 169(9):989–990, 1976.

56. Lightfoot T: Organochlorine disaster in Florida—2 years later, *J Avian Med Surg* 15(2):138–140, 2001.

57. Kenny D, Kinsey M: Brodifacoum toxicity in avian species at the Denver Zoologic Gardens, *Regional Proc AM Assoc Zoological Parks and Aquariums*, 1987.

58. Dorman DC: Anticoagulant, cholecalciferol, and bromethaline-based rodenticides, *Vet Clin North Am Small Animal Pract* 20(2):339–352, 1990.

59. Mellema MS, Haskins SC: Supportive care of the poisoned patient. In Peterson ME, Talcott PA, editors: *Small animal toxicology*, ed 2, St Louis, 2006, Elsevier Saunders, pp 116–118.

Adverse Drug Reactions*

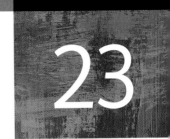

23

Alastair E. Cribb, DVM, PhD, FCAHS
Mathieu Peyrou, DVM, MSc

An adverse drug reaction (ADR) is any noxious or unintended response to a drug that occurs at appropriate doses used for prophylaxis, diagnosis, or therapy. They may vary from minor annoyances to severe, life-threatening events. Because ADRs are an ever-present threat when drugs are used in clinical practice, communication with owners about risk and response to ADRs are an important part of client education. The frequency with which ADRs occur in the average clinical veterinary practice or in teaching hospitals is not known, but it is generally accepted that an ADR is a significant contributor to patient morbidity and mortality.

Drug toxicity includes all toxicity associated with a drug, including that observed in overdose situations (e.g., poisonings with drugs). *Side effects,* on the other hand, generally refers to relatively minor adverse effects that occur during therapy, such as polydipsia or polyuria in dogs on corticosteroids. Lack of therapeutic efficacy may also be an ADR. However, lack of response may also be caused by an incorrect diagnosis or inappropriate treatment and so is not necessarily an ADR.

When using a drug, the veterinarian has an obligation to minimize the likelihood of an ADR occurring, to be aware of the potential clinical signs of an ADR so that a prompt diagnosis can be made, and to know the appropriate clinical care to administer should an ADR occur. The veterinarian should educate clients as to the risk of ADRs associated with the drug so that they can rationally balance this risk against the expected therapeutic benefit of the drug for their animal. The owners must also be informed of the clinical signs expected should an ADR occur and what steps they should take on observing these signs (e.g., stop the drug, transport the patient to the clinic).

Assessment of Risk

The decision to use a drug is based on a risk-benefit analysis for the individual patient. No drug is without some risk; however, the willingness of the owner and the veterinarian to accept the risk associated with a therapy depends on the relative risks and benefits of the drug compared with the risk of no treatment or the risk associated with alternative treatments, such as surgery. A drug should not be used without a specific therapeutic goal, so that efficacy and toxicity can be balanced appropriately.

When assessing risk, the veterinarian needs to look at the population risk (how frequent and severe is the ADR?) and the individual risk (does this patient have any characteristics that increase or decrease risk?). Assessing the risks of an ADR may be frustrating because the information necessary to truly assess risk is not available. Veterinarians are often using

---

*FDA Adverse Event Reporting System; +1 888 463-6332; +1 301 796-3400; druginfo@fda.hhs.gov
FDA Adverse Event Reporting System website: http://www.fda.gov/Drugs/GuidanceComplianceRegulatoryInformation/Surveillance/AdverseDrugEffects/default.htm

drugs with limited published clinical data in veterinary species and what information is available on ADRs is often vague. Finding information on the actual frequency and severity of ADRs is often difficult. Therefore, an understanding of the mechanism or pathogenesis of ADRs is often helpful, as discussed in detail in this chapter.

Although mechanisms are in place for reviewing and recording ADRs of licensed products, information for drugs used off-label is less readily available. Many standard veterinary textbooks list adverse reactions that have been reported to drugs without incorporating information on species differences or indeed noting if the adverse reactions have been reported in veterinary species. Furthermore, information on the frequency and severity of ADRs is often lacking. For licensed animal products, the company marketing the product is a good source of information, either through information on the package insert or through direct contact with the company. The Center for Veterinary Medicine, U.S. Food and Drug Administration (FDA) and the Veterinary Drugs Directorate, Health Canada, maintain a record of adverse events that have been reported and use this information to recommend changes in drug labels when appropriate. The FDA's database is available through its website (see the "Animal and Veterinary" section of the FDA website) and is a good source of up-to-date information on potential ADRs that have been reported.

Once an animal is receiving treatment, the identification and response to an ADR becomes important. The same caveats for prospectively assessing risk for the patient apply to deciding if a clinical event represents an ADR. That is, we often rely on cross-species extrapolation and a rather limited database to decide if an ADR has occurred. We must often rely on our knowledge of the pharmacologic and toxicologic characteristics of the drug in making a rational decision as to whether a clinical event is potentially drug-related and in deciding appropriate therapy. The diagnosis and response to ADRs is discussed in the following sections.

In summary, to make the most use of the information available, to tailor our decisions to the individual patient, and to make rational clinical decisions, an understanding of the basic principles of ADRs is invaluable. Therefore this chapter first presents general principles that can be applied in many clinical situations to guide therapeutic decisions. This is followed by a brief overview of hepatic and renal ADRs.

Classification of Adverse Drug Reactions

Several different systems for classifying ADRs exist, based on either clinical presentation or mechanism of toxicity. The clinical presentations of ADRs depend on the pharmacologic and chemical properties of the drug and the target organ damaged. In many cases, the exact mechanism of toxicity is not known or understood. This can make classification of drug toxicities difficult but does not prevent us from employing a broad mechanistic classification that will assist in making clinical decisions.

Dose-Dependent Adverse Drug Reactions

Most ADRs are dose-dependent. That is, the larger the dose, the greater the number of patients affected and the more severe the reaction. These types of ADRs or toxicities are generally predictable and can be reproduced in experimental models. The majority of patients experience a dose-dependent ADR if the drug is given at a sufficient dose or for a sufficient time period. In a clinical setting, the frequency of these reactions depends largely on the care with which the products are used and knowledge of specific dose adjustment that may be required. They can occur at therapeutic doses or plasma concentrations in some individuals, but they are commonly associated with elevated drug plasma concentrations resulting from altered pharmacokinetics in the patient caused by concurrent disease, pregnancy, age, or a drug interaction. This is particularly true for drugs with a narrow therapeutic index, in which changes in pharmacokinetics result in a functional overdose despite use of a normally safe therapeutic dosage regimen. The majority of dose-dependent toxicities can be avoided by careful and appropriate selection of the dose, taking into consideration patient characteristics and concurrent drug use.

> **Box 23-1**   Examples of Pharmacologic Toxicities
>
> Digoxin-induced cardiac arrhythmias
> Ulcers associated with inhibition of cyclooxygenase activity by nonsteroidal antiin-
>   flammatory drugs
> Pancytopenia from estrogens in dogs
> Hypotension from acepromazine (α-1 antagonism)
> Iatrogenic Cushing's from excessive corticosteroid use
> Ivermectin neurotoxicity

> **Box 23-2**   Examples of Intrinsic Toxicities
>
> Aminoglycoside nephrotoxicity and
>   ototoxicity
> Acetaminophen methemoglobinemia
>   and hemolytic anemia
> Acetaminophen hepatotoxicity
> Sulfonamide-induced hypothyroidism
> Doxorubicin cardiotoxicity

Patients may be hypersusceptible to a dose-dependent ADR, so that they have a reaction at doses (or plasma concentrations) lower than typically observed. Hypersusceptibility may result from altered pharmacokinetics, either through disease, genetic variation, or a drug interaction, that leads to higher than expected drug concentrations in the circulation or at specific sites for a given drug dose. Alternatively, there may be a receptor or target organ sensitivity that results in an adverse reaction at a lower concentration.

The occurrence of a dose-dependent toxicity in a patient is not necessarily an absolute contraindication to future use of the drug. If possible, the reason for the occurrence of the ADR should be ascertained. For example, was a dosing error made or was the ADR the result of a drug interaction?

Dose-dependent ADRs can be further subdivided into pharmacologic toxicity or intrinsic toxicity. The general principles of dose-dependent ADRs apply, but the diagnosis and treatment of these two different classes of ADRs may differ.

Pharmacologic Toxicity

Pharmacologic toxicity (also referred to as *mechanism-based, receptor-mediated, augmented,* or *Type A adverse reactions*) is a form of dose-dependent ADR that arises through exaggerated or undesirable pharmacologic effects of a drug (Box 23-1). Pharmacologic toxicity depends on an interaction of the parent drug or a pharmacologically active metabolite with a specific target or receptor. These effects may be related to the intended therapeutic target or to additional, inseparable secondary pharmacologic actions. In the latter instance, the ADRs are often called "side effects." For example, a minor side effect is mydriasis associated with the use of atropine as a preanesthetic agent.

Intrinsic Toxicity

Intrinsic toxicity is determined by the chemical properties of the drug, not its pharmacologic properties. That is, the toxicity depends on the intrinsic chemical properties of the drug—hence the term *intrinsic toxicity.* The drug or its metabolites do not bind to specific receptors to cause these toxicities, but instead bind nonspecifically to a variety of proteins or nucleic acids or disrupt membranes or organelle function (Box 23-2). Intrinsic toxicity may have a short course (e.g., acetaminophen toxicity) or a longer course (e.g., bone marrow suppression with chemotherapy). It is also referred to as *Type A (augmented)* or *Type C (chronic)* adverse reactions, depending on the nature and course of the reaction.

Intrinsic toxicity frequently depends on the metabolism of the parent drug to toxic metabolites, a process referred to as *bioactivation.* The site of toxicity therefore depends on the sites of accumulation of the toxin, the localization of enzymes necessary for metabolism of the compound, and the susceptibility of specific cells to the toxic effects. A typical intrinsic toxin is acetaminophen. Acetaminophen is metabolized to reactive metabolites that cause methemoglobinemia, hemolytic anemia, or liver damage, the primary clinical manifestations depending on the species of animal affected. Drugs or chemicals with carcinogenic properties, which bind to deoxyribonucleic acid (DNA) or damage DNA through other mechanisms, would be included in this category.

Clinical Pharmacologic Characteristics of Dose-Dependent Adverse Drug Reactions

Dose-dependent ADRs have the potential to occur in all patients, but they may be avoided in many instances by careful selection of the dose, taking into account the patient characteristics. Patient evaluation becomes very important in deciding whether an adjustment in the recommended standard dose is required or if it is safe to use the drug. In some cases, sex and age (e.g., fluoroquinolone-induced cartilage changes) are important characteristics that must be considered. Susceptibility to dose-dependent ADRs can be enhanced through factors that lead to greater drug exposure (i.e., decreased clearance and increased absorption) or that enhance the pharmacologic effect (e.g., concurrent medications; presence of epileptic foci in the brain). This hypersusceptibility may also be referred to as *patient idiosyncrasy*. For example, hypersusceptibility of collie dogs to ivermectin neurotoxicosis is related to an increased penetration of ivermectin into the central nervous system resulting from a genetic variation in P-glycoprotein responsible for pumping ivermectin out of the central nervous system.[1,2] Inhibition of metabolism or clearance of a drug can lead to accumulation to toxic levels. Glucocorticoids and nonsteroidal antiinflammatory drugs (NSAIDs) have synergistic effects on the occurrence of gastropathy. In the case of intrinsic toxicities that depend on bioactivation to toxic metabolites, factors that alter metabolism of the drug or affect cell defense mechanisms (e.g., deplete cellular glutathione) also enhance susceptibility.

The target organ and clinical signs depend on a number of factors. For pharmacologic toxicity, the observed signs depend on the pharmacologic effects. For intrinsic toxicities, the clinical manifestations depend on the affected organ. The target organ depends on accumulation of the drug, the cell defense mechanisms present in those organs, and the presence of the enzymes required for bioactivation of the drug. For example, the nephrotoxicity of aminoglycosides depends in part on their accumulation in renal tubular cells. If this accumulation is prevented by appropriate dosing regimens, then the risk of nephrotoxicity is decreased.

Treatment in dose-dependent toxicities should involve discontinuation of the drug and, if clinically indicated, removal of the drug from the body through appropriate measures. When appropriate, therapy can be directed at the specific pharmacologic target to either treat or prevent the ADR. Targeting to the appropriate pharmacologic target is critical. For example, misoprostol is the best and most effective therapy to prevent NSAID-induced gastropathy.[3] Once ulcers or erosions have occurred, discontinuation of the NSAID followed by appropriate therapy with sucralfate or an acid inhibitor such as omeprazole is appropriate. On the other hand, because loss of prostaglandin is not the primary mechanism behind steroid-induced gastric bleeding, misoprostol is not effective in preventing steroid-induced gastropathy.[4,5]

For intrinsic toxicities, drug withdrawal and supportive care are the most important steps. In certain cases, treatment directed at supporting specific cell-defense mechanisms may be appropriate. N-acetylcysteine can function both as an antioxidant to alleviate methemoglobinemia associated with acetaminophen toxicity and as a precursor for glutathione to scavenge reactive metabolites associated with hepatotoxicity.[6] Other antioxidants can also be employed to minimize the hematologic toxicity associated with acetaminophen.

In summary, dose-dependent ADRs are the most common class of ADRs encountered clinically. They can be minimized by careful and judicious use of the drug, taking into account the individual patient. The clinical manifestation and treatment is directed by the pharmacologic properties of the drug or the mechanism of the chemically based toxicity and the target organ. The previous occurrence of a dose-dependent ADR in an animal is a clear indication for modification of the therapeutic regimen but does not necessarily contraindicate the use of the causative or a related drug in the patient.

Idiosyncratic Adverse Drug Reactions

Idiosyncratic ADRs are the second major class of ADRs. They are also referred to as *host-dependent, dose-independent, Type B (bizarre), Type II*, or *patient-related* ADR. These terms are often used interchangeably (Box 23-3). Unfortunately, because of our lack of understanding of the pathogenesis of many idiosyncratic ADRs, considerable confusion remains. Many clinicians use the term *idiosyncratic* to denote "unknown mechanism." This, however, is an inappropriate use of the term, particularly as the mechanisms of some idiosyncratic ADRs become elucidated. The defining characteristic of idiosyncratic ADRs is that they occur in patients at serum concentrations within the therapeutic range and will not occur in the majority of patients despite increasing the dose to otherwise toxic levels. That is, a specific interaction must occur between the patient and the drug to result in the adverse reaction. They are not classically dose-dependent and are highly dependent on the characteristics of the individual patient (host-dependent or patient-related). They usually cannot be reliably reproduced in an experimental setting. Thus both experimentally and in the clinical setting, their occurrence is unpredictable. The incidence of idiosyncratic ADRs is usually much lower than dose-dependent ADRs, but in certain populations they may be relatively frequent. Idiosyncratic ADRs depend on the chemical properties, not the pharmacologic properties, of the drug. They are distinguished from hypersusceptibility to pharmacologic or intrinsic toxicities in that they cannot be produced simply by elevating the dose or increasing the exposure in the target population or in experimental animals.

The clinical presentation of idiosyncratic drug reactions is variable and depends on the exact mechanism underlying the reaction. For example, malignant hyperthermia from halothane exposure in pigs and hepatotoxicity from sulfonamide antimicrobials are both idiosyncratic ADRs. They have a distinct pathogenesis and distinct clinical signs. However, the majority of idiosyncratic ADRs have characteristics associated with an immunologic pathogenesis and many people are referring to these types of reactions (hypersensitivity reactions, "drug allergies," immune-mediated drug reactions) when they use the term *idiosyncratic reactions*.

Drug hypersensitivity syndrome reactions, drug-induced hemolytic anemia or *thrombocytopenia, drug-induced lupus, drug fever,* and *drug-induced immune-mediated hepatitis* are all terms used to describe idiosyncratic reactions that are thought to have an immunologic basis. The clinical manifestations of *idiosyncratic hypersensitivity syndrome reactions* include such pathologic states as fever, lymphadenopathy, dermatopathies, hepatitis, nephritis, leukopenia, agranulocytosis, eosinophilia, thrombocytopenia, and aplastic anemia. This type of idiosyncratic reaction is relatively rare (frequency estimated to be <1/1000) and has a delayed onset, with clinical signs generally manifesting 7 to 14 days or longer after the start of therapy.[7] They are distinct from the typical drug allergy characterized by anaphylaxis or urticaria occurring immediately after drug administration, which is

Box 23-3	Examples of Idiosyncratic Adverse Drug Reactions in Veterinary Species

Propylthiouracil and methimazole toxicity in cats
Sulfonamide polyarthritis, thrombocytopenia, hepatotoxicity in dogs
Diazepam hepatotoxicity in cats
Mebendazole hepatotoxicity in dogs
Malignant hyperthermia triggered by halothane in pigs and dogs
Carprofen hepatitis

an immunoglobulin (Ig) E–mediated immediate hypersensitivity reaction directed against the drug.

Idiosyncratic reactions are important in veterinary medicine from a patient treatment standpoint, but they also have an influence on veterinary practice from another perspective. Fear of idiosyncratic toxicity in humans may be the reason for the banning of products for use in food animals (e.g., chloramphenicol causes aplastic anemia in rare individuals) or may lead to the withdrawal of a drug from the market. Some practitioners are reluctant to prescribe drugs that have been associated with idiosyncratic ADR in humans for fear of precipitating an event in the owner. In general, owners should be warned about the potential for drugs employed in veterinary practice to cause idiosyncratic reactions in humans (Box 23-4) and be instructed to wash their hands immediately after administering the drug to their animals. It is wise to inquire if the client or any immediate family members have drug allergies before dispensing a drug so that they can take appropriate precautions, such as wearing gloves and washing hands.

Pathogenesis of Idiosyncratic Adverse Drug Reactions

The pathogenesis of idiosyncratic ADRs is complex and depends on the reaction under consideration. For example, malignant hyperthermia is related primarily to mutations in the ryanodine receptor in the muscle sarcoplasmic reticulum[8] so that muscle calcium homeostasis cannot be maintained in the face of challenge with certain muscle relaxants, caffeine, and halothane. It is an idiosyncratic reaction because it requires a specific patient genotype and, although a mutated receptor is responsible for susceptibility, interaction of halothane with a specific receptor is not required to trigger the clinical event. The most common types of idiosyncratic reactions, however, involve cellular damage, leading to organ-specific damage, such as nephropathies, hepatopathies, blood dyscrasias, and dermatopathies. These reactions commonly depend on bioactivation to a reactive intermediate that can either directly cause cellular damage or trigger a pathologic immune response.

Clinical signs consistent with an immunologic pathogenesis for many idiosyncratic reactions include a delayed onset, typically 7 to 14 days after the start of therapy, fever, skin rash, and occasionally eosinophilia. The clinical signs are highly variable, depending on the patient and other clinical factors. Patients may display a clearly systemic disease with multiple organs affected, or may have a single abnormality, such as thrombocytopenia, neutropenia, skin rash, or hepatitis. A previous exposure to the drug may have occurred, but is not necessary. If an animal has tolerated a drug for more than 6 to 8 weeks, the likelihood of experiencing an idiosyncratic reaction drops. Despite the variable clinical presentation, it appears that common pathogenic events underlie the clinical disease.

The immunologic responses that have been identified in cases of idiosyncratic reactions in humans and animals have been directed against either drug-modified proteins or autoantigens. Drugs are themselves generally too small to trigger an immunologic response; however, if they are metabolized to reactive metabolites, they may form drug-protein conjugates (Figure 23-1) that are capable of triggering an immunologic response.[3,9] The immune response may be directed against the drug-protein conjugate or against the protein itself (autoantigen) that was altered by the drug. The factors that determine which animals will

---

Box 23-4 Some Drugs Associated with Idiosyncratic Reactions in Humans

Penicillins
Cephalosporins
Erythromycin
Sulfonamides
Trimethoprim
Chloramphenicol
Aromatic anticonvulsants, including phenobarbital, phenytoin, carbamazepine, and felbamate
Phenylbutazone
Dipyrone
Phenothiazine derivatives (chlorpromazine)
Halothane, isoflurane
Methimazole, propylthiouracil
Captopril
Procainamide

experience an idiosyncratic reaction remain obscure, although genetic and environmental differences in metabolic capacity and immunologic responsiveness appear to play roles.

The general scheme of Gell and Coombs for the classification of immunologic reactions is frequently applied to drug-induced immune reactions but is of limited usefulness in classifying idiosyncratic reactions. True drug allergies are typical type I (IgE-mediated) immediate hypersensitivity–type reactions, but idiosyncratic hypersensitivity syndrome reactions can have manifestations of type II (antibody-directed cell cytotoxicity), type III (immune-complex disease), and type IV (delayed hypersensitivity—cell-mediated) reactions to varying degrees within an individual patient. The basis of the target-organ specificity of idiosyncratic adverse reactions and the variable clinical presentations are not fully understood but appear to depend on the sites of bioactivation of the drug, the stability of the reactive metabolites formed, and the sites of covalent binding of the reactive metabolites, and the nature of the immune response in individual animals.

Clinical Pharmacology of Idiosyncratic Adverse Drug Reactions

From a clinical perspective, the major difficulty with idiosyncratic ADRs is their unpredictability. They are not dose-dependent and so cannot be avoided by careful dose selection. Although they are usually rare, they are potentially fatal. Although their delayed onset means that a previous short-term exposure does not guarantee safety, if an idiosyncratic reaction has not occurred during or after a prolonged exposure (e.g., 4-8 weeks), it is unlikely to occur on subsequent exposures. If a reaction is a true drug allergy (e.g., IgE mediated), a previous exposure is required and reexposure may precipitate an acute anaphylactic response. The temporal relationships for immediate hypersensitivity reactions are thus very different from the delayed-onset hypersensitivity reaction described previously.

A major dilemma with idiosyncratic reactions is diagnosis. Often the clinical signs may not be clearly distinguishable from those associated with the primary disease process. The clinician should consider idiosyncratic reactions on their differential diagnosis list when unexpected changes in clinical progress occur.

Owners should be warned of the possibility of idiosyncratic ADRs. Drug withdrawal is the most important step and owners should be told to stop the drug immediately should any untoward events occur. Clinical manifestations depend on the target cell or organ, but they are usually systemic reactions. Often the first signs noted by the owner are lethargy, depression, and anorexia. The treatment should be directed at the clinical manifestation of the ADR. The effectiveness of corticosteroids in treating idiosyncratic hypersensitivity ADRs is poorly documented. However, anecdotal experience in humans and the documentation of an immunologic component to the reactions suggests that animals not responding to supportive care should be treated with high-dose corticosteroids (e.g., immunosuppressive doses, not antiinflammatory doses). Animals that manifest neutropenia as a clinical sign

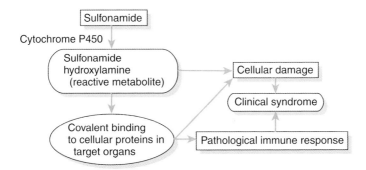

Figure 23-1 Simplified scheme of the pathogenesis of sulfonamide hypersensitivity reactions.

should be treated with an appropriate broad-spectrum prophylactic antibiotic to protect against secondary bacterial infections.

If an animal has experienced an idiosyncratic ADR, use of the suspected or a chemically related drug should be considered contraindicated unless no other alternative exists for a life-threatening illness. In that case, a desensitization protocol should be considered as part of the reinitiation of therapy. Unfortunately, there is essentially no published experience with these protocols in veterinary patients.

Incidence of Adverse Drug Reactions

The incidence of many ADRs in veterinary medicine is often unknown because of the difficulties in attributing clinical events to drug administration and the dependence on spontaneous reporting of ADRs. Many ADRs are not apparent until the drug has been used in a large number of genetically variant animals. The newest drug available is not necessarily the best or safest choice for therapy, particularly when considering drugs developed for use in humans. A drug relatively safe for use in humans is not necessarily safe in dogs and cats. Clinical studies demonstrating safety of drugs should also be evaluated carefully to determine if the patient population studied is representative of the population in which you wish to use the drug.

Small experimental studies at higher-than-normal clinical doses may indicate what dose-dependent toxicities to be aware of and give an indication of the therapeutic index, but they do not determine the incidence of dose-dependent or idiosyncratic reactions to expect at typical clinical doses in the general patient population. In general, the large clinical trials and postmarketing surveillance necessary to determine the incidence of ADRs are not available in veterinary medicine. Many times the impression of the incidence or importance of an ADR is colored by personal experience. Although this may be useful experience, it can often be misleading. In general, dose-dependent ADRs tend to be more common but less serious, whereas idiosyncratic ADRs tend to be relatively rare but more serious (e.g., the incidence of sulfonamide hypersensitivity reactions in dogs is probably less than 1/1000). The unpredictability and potential severity of idiosyncratic toxicities gives them an effect disproportionate with their incidence.

It is always important to remember that the likelihood of an ADR in the patient being treated is more important than the frequency of occurrence in the general population and the decision to use the drug should be based on an assessment of risk in the individual patient. Particular vigilance for adverse reactions in neonates, older animals, animals with a previous history of an ADR, and animals receiving multidrug therapy is required. Many factors contribute to the occurrence of an ADR in a given patient. Drug factors include dose, duration, vehicle, and drug interactions from concomitant therapy. Patient factors include species or breed, genetic and environmental variation in drug metabolism, age, sex, body composition (fat vs. lean weight), pregnancy status (teratogenicity), concurrent disease states, immunologic status, and concurrent drug or chemical exposures. How these factors contribute to the development of an ADR depends on the drug and the type of toxicity.

Diagnosis of an Adverse Drug Reaction

Attribution of a clinical event to a drug can be difficult. Perhaps the most important clues to link a clinical event with drug treatment are an appropriate temporal relationship, a previous report of a similar ADR associated with the drug, and a lack of another clinical explanation of the event. There are many algorithms or probability methods that have been developed for diagnosing potential ADRs. However, essentially they simplify down to the following questions, which reflect a rational approach to attributing a clinical event to an ADR:

1. Is the temporal association of the event with drug treatment appropriate for the type of ADR? If signs were present before drug administration or occur long (generally 1 month, but could be longer in some situations) after drug discontinuation, they are

unlikely to be related to the drug. The temporal association should be appropriate for the suspected ADR and not incompatible with the pathogenesis of the suspected reaction. For example, an anaphylactic reaction would not occur 7 days after drug administration.

2. Has the suspected ADR been previously reported? If the signs are consistent with a previously reported ADR, the probability is much higher that the signs are the result of an ADR. If the ADR has not been previously reported, the probability is lower but this does not necessarily eliminate the possibility of an ADR. The drug company, the drug insert (particularly the safety section), the FDA's Adverse Event Reporting System website and drug handbooks are good places to find drug-specific information.

3. Are there other possible explanations for the clinical signs? It is important to differentiate clinical signs attributable to the disease from those that may be related to the drug. Other drugs that the animal may have been receiving should also be considered.

4. Has the drug been administered previously to the patient and what was the outcome? This needs to be interpreted in a manner consistent with the suspected ADR. If a previous exposure produced a similar response, it is more likely to be drug related. On the other hand, a previous uneventful exposure, although decreasing the likelihood, does not rule out an ADR.

5. Do the signs disappear with drug withdrawal and recur with reexposure? It is generally not ethical to reexpose an animal to a drug suspected of causing an ADR, but this may occur inadvertently or in clinical situations in which alternative therapies are limited.

6. Is there evidence of dosing error or elevated plasma concentrations? When in doubt, the dose should always be recalculated. If available, therapeutic drug monitoring (TDM) can be a useful tool in deciding if toxic drug concentrations exist.

7. Are predisposing factors present in the patient? Is the animal receiving other drugs likely to have pharmacodynamic or pharmacokinetic interactions with the drug in question? For example, use of an NSAID and an aminoglycoside may increase the risk of nephrotoxicity, whereas concurrent use of an NSAID and a glucocorticoid will increase the likelihood of gastric ulceration. Does the animal have a concurrent disease, which may increase susceptibility to an adverse event (i.e., underlying hepatic or renal disease or diabetes)?

Drug Interactions

Drug interactions refer to in vivo interactions between drugs. Drug interactions may be relative or absolute contraindications to the concurrent use of drugs. Drug interactions may lead to a diminished or an enhanced effect of a drug or may lead to the occurrence of toxicity. In general, drug interactions have either a pharmacodynamic or a pharmacokinetic basis.

Pharmacodynamic interactions are the pharmacologic effects of two drugs that may be opposite to each other (e.g., metoclopramide and dopamine have opposite effects on renal blood flow), work at the same site (e.g., two NSAIDs), or enhance the effects through sequential or complementary effects (e.g., effects of glucocorticoids on β_2-receptors and use of a β_2-agonist, such as terbutaline; effects of corticosteroids and NSAIDs on gastric integrity). Drug combinations should be assessed carefully for drug interactions before their use. There are many possible pharmacodynamic interactions, some of which are listed in Table 23-1.

Pharmacokinetic interactions occur when drugs inhibit or enhance each other's metabolism or renal excretion (Table 23-2). One drug may also displace another from protein binding sites, leading to greater free drug concentrations and hence pharmacologic effect. Drug interactions can lead to the occurrence of ADRs at doses or plasma concentrations lower than typically expected, depending on the mechanism of the interaction.

Knowledge of pharmacokinetic drug interactions in small animals remains limited. Probably the most common mechanism for pharmacokinetic interactions is metabolic

Table 23-1	Some Pharmacodynamic Drug Interactions	
Drugs	**Interaction**	**Mechanism**
Glucocorticoids and NSAIDs	Increased gastrointestinal toxicity	NSAIDs primarily inhibit prostaglandin production, whereas corticosteroids increase gastric acid secretion and decrease mucosal defenses.
Furosemide and ACE inhibitors	Increased diuretic effect	ACE inhibitors decrease aldosterone secretion, which subsequently increases the diuretic effect of furosemide.
Furosemide and thiazide diuretics	Increased diuretic effect	Work at different sites in diuretics the renal tubule, leading to a synergistic diuretic effect.
Glucocorticoids and β-2 agonists	Increased bronchodilatory effect	Glucocorticoids upregulate and increase the responsiveness of β-receptors.
Sucralfate and gastric acid secretion inhibitors	Decreased efficacy of sucralfate	Sucralfate requires an acid pH for maximal efficacy; if gastric acid secretion inhibitors (e.g., cimetidine, ranitidine, omeprazole) increase gastric pH, efficacy of sucralfate may be decreased.
NSAIDs and anticoagulants	Increased bleeding	Combination of inhibition of platelet aggregation (NSAIDs) with inhibition of other coagulation pathways (heparin, warfarin) will lead to increased bleeding tendency.
Opioids and general anesthetics	Enhanced respiratory depression by opioids	General anesthetics generally enhance the respiratory depressant effects of opioids.

ACE, Angiotensin-converting enzyme; *NSAID,* nonsteroidal antiinflammatory drug.

interaction at the level of cytochrome P450 in the liver. The cytochrome P450 family of drug-metabolizing enzymes is a unique system. It is composed of more than 20 different enzymes, of which 4 or 5 are likely responsible for the majority of drug metabolism. There are significant species differences in the regulation and substrate specificity of these enzymes. Thus although there are many similarities between species, cytochrome P450-based drug interactions in dogs or cats are not necessarily the same as those in humans. Hence, although we rely heavily on extrapolation of potential drug interactions in humans to drug interactions in dogs and cats, this may not always be reliable. Further work is required in companion animals to fully elucidate the extent of clinically significant metabolic drug interactions. Nevertheless, a reasonable rule of thumb is to avoid when possible combining drugs with a clearance that depends on metabolism and when interactions have been reported in other species unless they have been shown not to occur in veterinary species. Table 23-2 summarizes some of the possible drug interactions and their mechanisms in small animals, primarily dogs.

Drug Incompatibilities

Drug incompatibilities are chemical interactions that occur between drugs in vitro. Drugs that are incompatible should not be mixed together in a syringe or fluid bag. As a general rule, do not mix drugs unless necessary and then only if you know they are compatible.

Table 23-2	Some Pharmacokinetic Drug Interactions in Dogs	
Drug	Interaction	Mechanism
PB	Propranolol—decreased efficacy Lidocaine—increased clearance Chloramphenicol—decreased efficacy	PB induces several cytochrome P450 enzymes, increasing the metabolism of several drugs. The increased hepatotoxicity when combinations of anticonvulsants are used is likely because of increased bioactivation.
Cimetidine	Theophylline—increased toxicity Metronidazole—increased toxicity Midazolam—increased effects Propranolol—increased effects	Cimetidine is a moderate inhibitor of several different P450 enzymes and so decreases metabolism of several drugs.
Chloramphenicol	Phenobarbital—pharmacologic toxicity	Chloramphenicol inhibits phenobarbital metabolism.
Enrofloxacin	Theophylline—pharmacologic toxicity	Enrofloxacin inhibits theophylline clearance.
Digoxin	Quinidine, verapamil, keto-conazole, itraconazole—decrease digoxin clearance leading to toxicity	These drugs inhibit P-glycoprotein–dependent renal clearance of digoxin.

PB, Phenobarbital.

Most standard drug handbooks contain information on drug incompatibilities and should be consulted before mixing drugs.

Drug-Induced Hepatotoxicity

Drug-induced liver damage remains one of the most important ADRs. Because of its strategic location between the intestine and the systemic circulation, the liver can be exposed to relatively high drug concentrations. When coupled with its high metabolic capacity, particularly through the cytochrome P450 enzymes, the liver has the greatest exposure to reactive metabolites. Intrinsic hepatotoxicity is often related to bioactivation to reactive metabolites that damage liver cells and cause hepatic necrosis (e.g., acetaminophen hepatotoxicity; see Chapter 30). It may also occur subsequent to disruption of mitochondrial function or disruption of bile transport, leading to cholestatic injury. Idiosyncratic hepatotoxicity is nearly always related to bioactivation to reactive intermediates. Dose-dependent hepatopathies are usually identified during the drug development process but may still contribute to clinically important drug-induced toxicity. However, the majority of serious cases of hepatotoxicity are idiosyncratic in nature.

Box 23-5 provides a list of the most clinically important hepatotoxic drugs in small animals. This is not a complete list of potential hepatotoxins but rather a list of drugs that have been associated with hepatotoxicity in dogs and cats. There are other drugs that have been shown to be hepatotoxic in other species (humans and rodents) but that have not been reported or observed to cause clinically significant hepatotoxicity in veterinary species. For example, many complementary or alternative health products (e.g., certain kava products and germander) have been reported to cause hepatotoxicity in humans and conceivably may do so in animals, but no specific reports exist.

Phenobarbital

One of the most commonly used hepatotoxins that remains a clinical challenge for veterinarians is phenobarbital. A small percentage of dogs on chronic phenobarbital administration will develop hepatopathy and eventually hepatic cirrhosis.[10,11] Phenobarbital is known to cause elevations in serum liver enzyme activities that are not directly correlated to the occurrence or degree of hepatotoxicity.[12,13] Although elevations in serum liver enzyme activities have been attributed to enzyme induction, this is far from clear.[12,13] Minor elevations in serum alanine aminotransferase (ALT) and alkaline phosphatase (AP) activities are generally not a cause for concern, but elevations in ALT that are three to five times the upper limit of normal should be monitored carefully. It should also be noted that dogs with significant hepatic cirrhosis may not have marked elevations in serum liver enzyme activities despite extensive liver damage. If elevations in AP and ALT activities are accompanied by decreases in albumin concentration or serum urea nitrogen, they should be considered more seriously. Additional diagnostic work-up, including a bile acid test, is indicated. Although hepatic biopsy may help to document actual liver damage, no histopathologic changes that are hallmarks of early phenobarbital hepatotoxicity have been identified.[12]

Dogs with high serum concentrations of phenobarbital (>30 to 40 mcg/mL) are thought to be at increased risk of phenobarbital-associated liver damage. Although elevated serum phenobarbital concentrations are often observed in dogs that have developed hepatopathy,[11] it has been difficult to separate cause and effect. That is, loss of liver function may lead to decreased clearance of phenobarbital and elevated serum concentrations. Dogs with low serum concentrations of phenobarbital may still develop liver disease (Cribb, unpublished observations). Yearly evaluation of serum enzyme activities is often recommended but has not been clearly shown to prospectively identify dogs at risk of developing hepatotoxicity. Unexpected increases in serum phenobarbital concentrations may also be an indication of hepatic dysfunction. If dogs are removed from phenobarbital early in the course of hepatic damage, recovery can occur. However, once the hepatic damage has proceeded to the stage of significant cirrhosis, recovery appears less likely. Dogs should be carefully weaned from phenobarbital and therapy with an alternative anticonvulsant, such as potassium bromide or levetiracetam, instituted if hepatopathy is demonstrated or highly suspected.

Box 23-5   Clinically Important Hepatotoxins

Intrinsic Hepatotoxins
Acetaminophen (dogs)
Phenobarbital, primidone, phenytoin
Glucocorticoids
Mitotane
Tetracycline
Cyclosporine
Griseofulvin
Thiacetarsamide
Ketoconazole

Idiosyncratic Hepatotoxins
Diazepam in cats
Propylthiouracil and methimazole in cats
Trimethoprim and sulfonamide antimicrobials in dogs
Mebendazole
Carprofen
Diethylcarbamazine and oxibendazole

Idiosyncratic Hepatotoxicity

Idiosyncratic hepatitis clearly occurs with sulfonamides, carprofen, methimazole, diethylcarbamazine-oxibendazole, mebendazole, and diazepam in companion animals. In all cases, the incidence is rare (probably less than 1/1000). The most common signs of idiosyncratic hepatotoxicity are acute onset of anorexia and malaise within the first 2 to 8 weeks of therapy. However, hepatotoxicity can develop sooner or may have a delayed onset. Although periodic screening for elevations in serum liver enzyme activities is sometimes recommended for idiosyncratic hepatotoxins, there is no evidence that this is effective in predicting or preventing hepatotoxicity. The onset of liver damage is quick once it occurs so that dogs or cats can go from normal serum activities to clinical liver damage in a few days' time. When commencing drugs that are associated with idiosyncratic hepatotoxicity, it is useful to establish a baseline for serum activities before the start of therapy. It is also important to remember that fluctuations of serum enzyme activities out of the normal range are not uncommon and simple elevation is not necessarily an indication to stop the medication, although it is a clear indication for enhanced clinical and biochemical monitoring of the patient.

The most important treatment for idiosyncratic hepatotoxicity is immediate cessation of therapy and diagnosis. The owners should be instructed to immediately stop the drug and bring the animal in for evaluation should it become anorexic or depressed. Serum liver enzyme activities should be determined and, if elevated, a presumptive diagnosis of idiosyncratic hepatotoxicity is made. Clinical experience suggests that continued treatment once the reaction has started is more likely to lead to a fatal outcome. Although hepatic biopsy may serve to confirm the hepatic damage, this is rarely indicated and is probably not helpful in differentiating idiosyncratic hepatotoxicity from other causes. There is no specific therapy for idiosyncratic hepatotoxicity. In severe cases that continue to deteriorate, treatment with corticosteroids, on the assumption that there is an underlying immune-mediated pathogenesis, can be tried, but there are no good clinical studies to support this approach in human or veterinary medicine.

Drug-Induced Nephrotoxicity

Because of their large perfusion (approximately 25% of the cardiac output), their ability to concentrate and accumulate toxicants, and their high metabolic activity, kidneys are highly vulnerable to drug-induced toxic injury. The most common drugs associated with nephrotoxicity in small animals are presented in Box 23-6. It is important to note that Box 23-6 and this section describe toxic events associated with drugs that are intrinsically nephrotoxic and do not address drugs, such as furosemide, that can cause renal dysfunction through their pharmacologic properties. As a general principle, two potentially nephrotoxic drugs should not be used together and nephrotoxic drugs should be avoided in animals with known or suspected renal dysfunction. To minimize the risk of nephrotoxicity, it is important to maintain the hydration status of the animal and ensure adequate urine output.

Aminoglycosides

Nephrotoxicity is a major limiting factor for aminoglycoside administration. Aminoglycoside toxicity results in renal failure with hypoosmotic polyuria, enzymuria, glucosuria, and proteinuria. Serum creatinine can be increased after a few days of administration. Renal failure is usually reversible but can become irreversible if administration is prolonged. Toxic mechanisms are not fully understood but probably involve active uptake of the drug by tubular cells and accumulation in lysosomes, Golgi apparatus, and endoplasmic reticulum. Histopathologically, aminoglycoside tubular cell toxicity is associated with formation of myeloid bodies that result from the accumulation of phospholipids in a concentric lamellar disposition within enlarged and dysfunctional lysosomes. Rupture of overwhelmed lysosomes is believed to be a major trigger for tubular cell death. Impaired synthesis of protective prostaglandins and inhibition of mitochondrial respiration and of protein synthesis have also been proposed as additional toxic mechanisms.

As low trough levels of aminoglycosides have been associated with decreased nephrotoxicity in multiple human trials, single daily administration is currently used in humans and horses.[14,15] However, multiple once-daily intramuscular administrations of gentamicin have been associated with signs of renal damage in dogs (increased serum creatinine and blood urea nitrogen, renal tubular casts, and decreased specific urine gravity) and so care must still be exercised.[16]

Box 23-6	Drugs Associated with Nephrotoxicity

Aminoglycosides
Amphotericin B
Cyclosporin A
Nonsteroidal antiinflammatory drugs
Sulfonamides
Tetracyclines
Radiocontrast agents
Methoxyflurane

To minimize the risks associated with aminoglycoside-induced nephrotoxicity, patient hydration should be maintained, co-administration with other nephrotoxic or diuretic drugs (antiinflammatory drugs, furosemide) should be avoided, and TDM should be used. TDM dose adjustment is related to the patient's pharmacokinetic parameters and minimal inhibitory concentration (MIC) of the causative bacteria. The goal is to provide a dosage regimen that produces a peak concentration 8 to 10 times more than the MIC and a trough concentration of less than 2 mcg/mL, and preferably less than 1 mcg/mL. Prostaglandin analogue supplementation (misoprostol) does not seem to be effective for the prevention or treatment of gentamicin-induced renal injury.

β-Lactams

Cephalosporins have been commonly cited as being potentially nephrotoxic drugs. The early cephalosporins (i.e., cephaloridine) had clear nephrotoxic properties and a number of analogues were also shown to cause renal damage. The damage related to cephalosporins was selective to the S2 segment of the proximal tubule as a result of active uptake through the organic anion transport system. However, none of the currently used cephalosporins appears to be associated with a significant risk of nephrotoxicity.

Among other β-lactams, only imipenem is significantly nephrotoxic. Therefore it is administered in combination with cilastatin to inhibit its metabolism by dehydropeptidase I on the brush borders of renal tubular cells to minimize its uptake into renal tubular cells and subsequent nephrotoxicity.

Amphotericin B

In its conventional colloidal dispersion form (Fungizone), amphotericin B is associated with high risks of renal toxicity in humans and in veterinary species. It induces an intense renal arteriolar vasoconstriction and is directly cytotoxic in relation with its ability to bind cholesterol and form membrane pores, leading to tubular necrosis. Several protocols have been developed for the administration of amphotericin B to minimize nephrotoxicity. New lipid-based formulations have lowered the toxic events related to amphotericin B administration in human medicine.[17] Clinical trials have not been performed in veterinary medicine to date and therefore use of safer azole antifungals is preferred to amphotericin B wherever possible.

Cisplatin

Nephrotoxicity is the major limiting factor of cisplatin administration in humans and is associated with acute renal failure and chronic renal failure. Although not fully documented in veterinary clinical settings, renal toxicity of cisplatin should be carefully monitored. Toxicity results from bioactivation of cisplatin to more toxic metabolites in the renal tubular cells, oxidative stress, and direct cytotoxicity of cisplatin through the inhibition of DNA and protein synthesis.

Cyclosporine A

As cyclosporine A renal toxicity is a common problem in human medicine, its increased use in veterinary medicine, especially for dermatologic diseases, has raised the question of nephrotoxic risks in veterinary species. In contrast to humans, dog and cat kidneys do not seem to be a major target of cyclosporine toxicity. Very few cases of renal impairment have been reported in the literature.[18]

Nonsteroidal Antiinflammatory Drugs

Renal synthesis of prostaglandins by cyclooxygenase constitutes a regulatory mechanism to cope with diminished renal perfusion that may occur in volume-contracted states (i.e., dehydration, diuretics) or reduced cardiac output (i.e., congestive heart failure).[19] Because NSAIDs can inhibit prostaglandin synthesis, they may impair renal function in high-risk patients, culminating with acute renal failure. The nephrotoxic potential of selective COX-2 inhibitors is unclear in human medicine[20] and has not been addressed thoroughly in veterinary species. It is clear, however, that relatively selective COX-2 inhibitors can cause nephrotoxicity under the right circumstances. NSAIDs can also damage the kidney by direct toxicity, usually after massive administration. Both mechanisms may be involved in acute renal papillary necrosis, which has been reported in dogs and cats.[21,22]

Radiocontrast Agents

Hyperosmolar radiocontrast agents have been associated with renal damage and decreased renal clearance, especially in dogs with heart failure. Transient renal ischemia, direct tubular toxicity, and changes in glomerular capillary permeability have been proposed to explain these alterations.[23] New nonionic agents with lower osmolarity (i.e., iopamidol) have decreased risks of toxicity.

Sulfonamides

Idiosyncratic toxicity of sulfonamides in dogs has been associated with proteinuria, which may result from drug-induced glomerulonephritis.[24,25] However, renal toxicity is less common than some other signs (i.e., fever, arthropathy, and blood dyscrasias). Sulfonamides may also cause crystalluria if high doses are administered to animals or if they are dehydrated.

Tetracyclines

In dogs, high doses of oxytetracycline (25 mg/kg intravenously) have been associated with tubular nephropathy. Clinical signs include vomiting, diarrhea, dehydration, and isosthenuria with azotemia, hypercreatininemia, and hyperphosphatemia.[26] Renal damage has also been described with the use of outdated or degraded tetracycline.

Conclusion

By taking a rational approach to ADRs based on an understanding of the general principles of mechanisms of toxicity, the veterinary clinician can go beyond the consultation of a list of adverse reactions to a thoughtful assessment of risk and causality in our patients. This will lead to the safer, more appropriate use of drugs and better patient care. Although all veterinarians will experience the occurrence of ADRs in their patients, careful use of drugs will minimize the frequency and consequences.

References

1. Mealey KL, Bentjen SA, Gay JM, et al: Ivermectin sensitivity in collies is associated with a deletion mutation of the mdr1 gene, *Pharmacogenetics* 11:727–733, 2001.
2. Paul AJ, Tranquilli WJ, Seward RL, et al: Clinical observations in collies given ivermectin orally, *Am J Vet Res* 48:684–685, 1987.
3. Cribb AE: Adverse effects of non-steroidal anti-inflammatory drugs. In Ka W, editor: *Clinical pharmacology: principles and practice*, Las Vegas, 1998, Western Veterinary Conference.
4. Hanson SM, Bostwick DR, Twedt DC, et al: Clinical evaluation of cimetidine, sucralfate, and misoprostol for prevention of gastrointestinal tract bleeding in dogs undergoing spinal surgery, *Am J Vet Res* 58:1320–1323, 1997.
5. Rohrer CR, Hill RC, Fischer A, et al: Efficacy of misoprostol in prevention of gastric hemorrhage in dogs treated with high doses of methylprednisolone sodium succinate, *Am J Vet Res* 60:982–985, 1999.
6. St Omer VV, McKnight ED III: Acetylcysteine for treatment of acetaminophen toxicosis in the cat, *J Am Vet Med Assoc* 176:911–913, 1980.
7. Cribb AE, Lee BL, Trepanier LA, et al: Adverse reactions to sulphonamide and sulphonamide-trimethoprim antimicrobials: clinical syndromes and pathogenesis, *Adverse Drug React Toxicol Rev* 15:9–50, 1996.
8. Fujii J, Otsu K, Zorzato F, et al: Identification of a mutation in porcine ryanodine receptor associated with malignant hyperthermia, *Science* 253:448–451, 1991.
9. Park BK, Coleman JW, Kitteringham NR, et al: Drug disposition and drug hypersensitivity, *Biochem Pharmacol* 36:581–589, 1987.
10. Bunch SE: Hepatotoxicity associated with pharmacologic agents in dogs and cats, *Vet Clin North Am Small Anim Pract* 23:659–670, 1993.

11. Dayrell-Hart B, Steinberg SA, VanWinkle TJ, et al: Hepatotoxicity of phenobarbital in dogs: 18 cases (1985-1989), *J Am Vet Med Assoc* 199:1060–1066, 1991.
12. Gaskill C, Miller LM, Mattoon JS, et al: Liver histopathology and serum alanine aminotransferase and alkaline phosphatase activities in epileptic dogs receiving phenobarbital, *Vet Pathol* 42:147–160, 2005.
13. Muller PB, Taboada J, Hosgood G, et al: Effects of long-term phenobarbital treatment on the liver in dogs, *J Vet Intern Med* 14:165–171, 2000.
14. Godber LM, Walker RD, Stein GE, et al: Pharmacokinetics, nephrotoxicosis, and in vitro antibacterial activity associated with single versus multiple (three times) daily gentamicin treatments in horses, *Am J Vet Res* 56:613–618, 1995.
15. Tudor RA, Papich MG, Redding WR, et al: Drug disposition and dosage determination of once daily administration of gentamicin sulfate in horses after abdominal surgery, *J Am Vet Med Assoc* 215:503–506, 1999.
16. Albarellos G, Montoya L, Ambros L, et al: Multiple once-daily dose pharmacokinetics and renal safety of gentamicin in dogs, *J Vet Pharmacol Ther* 27:21–25, 2004.
17. Fukui H, Koike T, Saheki A, et al: Evaluation of the efficacy and toxicity of amphotericin B incorporated in lipid nano-sphere (LNS), *Int J Pharm* 263:51–60, 2003.
18. Robson D: Review of the pharmacokinetics, interactions and adverse reactions of cyclosporine in people, dogs and cats, *Vet Rec* 152:739–748, 2003.
19. Whelton A: Nephrotoxicity of nonsteroidal anti-inflammatory drugs: physiologic foundations and clinical implications, *Am J Med* 106:13S–24S, 1999.
20. Sandhu GK, Heyneman CA: Nephrotoxic potential of selective cyclooxygenase-2 inhibitors, *Ann Pharmacother* 38:700–704, 2004.
21. Silverman LR, Khan KN: "Have you seen this?" Nonsteroidal anti-inflammatory drug-induced renal papillary necrosis in a dog, *Toxicol Pathol* 27:244–245, 1999.
22. Wolf DC, Lenz SD, Carlton WW, et al: Renal papillary necrosis in two domestic cats and a tiger, *Vet Pathol* 28:84–87, 1991.
23. Margulies K, Schirger J, Burnett J Jr: Radiocontrast-induced nephropathy: current status and future prospects, *Int Angiol* 11:20–25, 1992.
24. Giger U, Werner LL, Millichamp NJ, et al: Sulfadiazine-induced allergy in six Doberman pinschers, *J Am Vet Med Assoc* 186:479–484, 1985.
25. Trepanier LA, Danhof R, Toll J, et al: Clinical findings in 40 dogs with hypersensitivity associated with administration of potentiated sulfonamides, *J Vet Intern Med* 17:647–652, 2003.
26. Moalli MR, Dysko RC, Rush HG, et al: Oxytetracycline-induced nephrotoxicosis in dogs after intravenous administration for experimental bone labeling, *Lab Anim Sci* 46:497–502, 1996.

Miscellaneous Indoor Toxicants

24

Sharon M. Gwaltney-Brant, DVM, PhD, DABVT, DABT

Hundreds of household and commercial products are available in homes and businesses. Although many household products are not highly toxic, cleaning substances, cosmetics, and personal care products are a common source of exposure for pets.

Household products are often complex chemical mixtures of organic and inorganic compounds designed for specific applications. When an animal has been exposed to a household product, it is important for the veterinarian to obtain the following information if possible: full trade name of the product, ingredients in the product (both active and inert) and their concentrations, amount and dilution of the product the animal came in contact with, clinical signs and their progression in relation to the time of exposure, and any treatments given by the owner before coming in with the animal. It is helpful to instruct the owner to bring in the original container of the product in question.

Even when this information is obtained, it may still be difficult for the clinician to assess the situation because the toxicity of many household products is not always predictable on the basis of the chemical and physical properties of the individual ingredients. Interactions among ingredients within a single product and among different products when present in combination further complicate the toxicologic risk assessment. This predicament may be alleviated in part by appropriate consultations. Information on the ingredients and clinical toxicology of a particular product may be obtained from human and animal poison control centers, emergency medical centers, and manufacturers' product safety and information hotlines. Many commercial products have specific manufacturer's information and telephone numbers as part of their labels, and poison control center numbers are available in local telephone directories.

This chapter updates an earlier review of the clinical toxicology of common indoor toxicants, such as cleaning agents, corrosive and caustic agents, disinfectants, alcohols, and other miscellaneous products.[1] Described also is general management of companion animals with oral, dermal, and ocular exposures to these classes of compounds.

Soaps, Detergents, and Cleaning Agents

Soaps and detergents are among the most frequently encountered household products. This class of compounds includes hand soaps, shampoos, spray cleaners, dishwashing liquids and powders, and laundry products. Soaps and detergents are surfactants (i.e., agents that lower the surface tension of water to enable it to wet surfaces more efficiently). Surfactants also help to remove dirt, disperse soil, and emulsify fat or grease.

Soaps and detergents are classified according to their chemical structure. True soaps are salts of fatty acids, usually made by the reaction of alkali with natural fats and oils or with the fatty acids obtained from animal or vegetable sources. Detergents are surfactants that contain inorganic ingredients, such as phosphates, silicates, or carbonates. Detergents are further classified as nonionic surfactants, anionic surfactants, or cationic surfactants based on their ionic charge when in solution.

Soaps

Soaps are generally low in oral toxicity. However, some soaps, such as homemade soaps and laundry soaps, have an appreciable content of free alkali, thus presenting a possible corrosive hazard.[2,3] Commercial bar soaps generally have a low order of toxicity, but may cause emesis and diarrhea because of gastrointestinal irritation. This irritation may result in part from the essential oils used as fragrances in bar soaps.[2] Treatment involves the use of demulcents and diluents, such as milk or water. Induction of emesis may be considered if the ingested quantity exceeds 20 g of soap/kg body weight (BW), and the soap is nonalkaline (noncorrosive), or if spontaneous emesis has not occurred within 30 minutes of ingestion. If diarrhea or excessive vomiting occurs, symptomatic treatment and efforts should be started to maintain fluid and electrolyte balance.

Nonionic Detergents

Many products contain nonionic synthetic detergents formulated into hand dishwashing detergents, shampoos, and some laundry detergents. Nonionic surfactants are uncharged in aqueous solutions at neutral pH. Examples of nonionic detergents are alkyl ethoxylate, alkyl phenoxy polyethoxy ethanols, and polyethylene glycol stearate.[4]

The majority of nonionic detergents have a low order of irritation and thus low toxicity. Ingestion of nonionic detergents usually results in only vomiting and diarrhea, and ocular exposures to nonionic detergents generally do not produce extensive liquefaction of the corneal epithelium.[2] Depending on the exposure route, treatments for nonionic detergent exposures should include diluting ingestions with milk or water, rinsing exposed eyes with copious amounts of water, or thorough rinsing of detergents from skin and hair coats. If protracted vomiting occurs, treatments to reverse the effects and measures should be performed to maintain fluid and electrolyte balance.

Anionic Detergents

Anionic surfactants are primarily sulfonated or phosphorylated straight-chain hydrocarbons. These compounds are used commonly in laundry detergents, electric dishwashing detergents, and in some shampoos. Among the more common anionic detergents are alkyl sodium sulfates, alkyl sodium sulfonates, dioctyl sodium sulfosuccinate, sodium lauryl sulfate, tetrapropylene benzene sulfonate, and linear alkyl benzene sulfonates.[4] Many of these materials contain alkali builders, such as sodium phosphate, sodium carbonate, sodium metasilicate, or sodium silicate, to increase their effectiveness in hard water.

Most anionic detergents are slightly to moderately toxic. Electric or automatic dishwashing detergent products are considered most toxic because of their high alkalinity. The caustic potential of automatic dishwashing detergents has recently been evaluated and remains the topic of great controversy. The pH of 1% solutions of automatic dishwashing detergents is less than the supposedly critical pH traditionally associated with corrosive injury to the esophagus[5]; however, large ingestions of automatic dishwasher detergents are still practical risks to cause corrosive damage, depending on the composition, concentration, physical form, duration of exposure, and viscosity of the product. In general nonphosphate-containing electric dishwashing detergents induce greater tissue irritation and injury than phosphate-containing automatic dish detergents.[6]

Ingested anionic detergents are well absorbed from the intestinal tract. Healthy skin appears to be a good barrier to anionic surfactants, but such surfactants can be absorbed through irritated or broken skin. Anionic detergents are metabolized by the liver, and the metabolites are excreted in the urine.[2] Intravascular hemolysis may occur with anionic detergent exposure in patients with impaired liver function; the liver dysfunction is thought to be related to the detergent concentrations in the blood.[2] Prolonged or repeated cutaneous exposure to anionic detergents may result in irritation. Ocular exposure to automatic dish detergents has been reported to cause corneal erosion and opacity.[5] Ingestions of anionic detergents often result in vomiting, nausea, diarrhea, and gastrointestinal discomfort. Most exposures cause illness but are not fatal.

Oral administration of milk or water to dilute the detergent is advised. Activated charcoal should be given if large quantities of detergent have been ingested and if corrosive injury has not occurred to the gastrointestinal tract. With ocular exposure, the eyes should be rinsed with copious amounts of water. Thorough bathing and rinsing is recommended for dermal exposures. If protracted vomiting occurs, symptomatic treatment and measures should be instituted to maintain systemic fluid and electrolyte balance. The patient should be monitored for the development of hemolysis. If hemolysis does occur, intravascular fluids are recommended to prevent renal tubular damage from the precipitation of hemoglobin in renal tubules or the resultant hypoxia, and renal function should be monitored. In patients that have ingested automatic dishwashing detergent, evaluation may be warranted of the mouth, oropharynx, and esophagus for corrosive injury. Treatment for corrosive injuries should be started as described later in this chapter in the section "Corrosives."

Cationic Detergents and Potpourris

Cationic detergents are used as fabric softeners, liquid potpourris, germicides, and sanitizers and are considered highly or extremely toxic. The American Society for the Prevention of Cruelty to Animals Animal Poison Control Center (ASPCA-APCC) reports that exposures to liquid potpourri are the sixth most common toxicosis reported in cats.[7] In addition to the cationic detergents, potpourris contain essential oils that are well absorbed dermally and through mucous membranes and can cause mucous membrane and GI irritation, along with central nervous system depression and dermal hypersensitivity and irritation. The cationic surfactants are quaternary ammonium compounds with aryl or alkyl substituent groups, one of which is often a long hydrophobic carbon chain. Generally a halogen, such as bromide, iodide, or chloride, is also attached. These agents include benzethonium chloride, benzalkonium chloride, alkyl dimethyl 3,4-dichlorobenzene, and cetyl pyridinium chloride.[4]

Toxicoses in animals and humans have been reported from quaternary ammonium compounds.[8-10] The observed toxicity of cationic detergents can be divided into local effects, depending on concentration and systemic effects, which are dose related.[10] Cationic detergent concentrations as low as 1% are damaging to mucous membranes, and solutions containing more than 7.5% of cationic detergents may cause corrosive burns of the mouth, pharynx, and esophagus.

Quaternary ammonium compounds are absorbed from the gastrointestinal tract, but several factors modify this systemic absorption. Ethanol and isopropanol, which are often found in cationic detergent preparations, significantly enhance gastrointestinal absorption. In contrast, food and chyme in the stomach reduce absorption by forming unabsorbable complexes.[2-11] Percutaneous absorption through intact skin is not a major route of absorption for these compounds, although quaternary ammonium compounds may be absorbed through damaged skin.[2] Ingestion of these detergents from licking or grooming irritated skin surfaces and paws is also a significant exposure pathway for dogs and cats.

A mechanism explaining the systemic effects of cationic detergent toxicity has not been established. There are conflicting reports of cholinesterase inhibition caused by quaternary ammonium compounds.[3] These compounds also possess ganglionic blocking potential and a curare-like action that causes paralysis of the neuromuscular junctions of striated muscles.[2,3,10] This hypothesis is supported by the structural similarities between quaternary ammonium compounds and decamethonium, a neuromuscular blocking agent, and hexamethonium, a ganglionic blocking agent.[3]

The principal clinical signs of these poisonings are profuse salivation, vomiting with possible hematemesis, muscle weakness, fasciculations, central nervous system (CNS) and respiratory depression, fever, seizures, collapse, and coma. These effects are very similar to, and must be differentiated from, those of pesticide poisonings. In cats, exposures to liquid potpourri products resulted in hypersalivation, hyperthermia, vomiting or retching, depression, dyspnea and abnormal respiratory sounds, and oral ulcers.[12] Cationic detergent ingestions usually result in corrosive damage to the mucous membranes of the mouth, tongue, pharynx, and esophagus. Shock may develop early or as the toxicosis progresses.

Hair loss and skin ulcerations are frequently seen in cats,[9] and inflammatory lesions of the paws are reported in dogs after exposure to quaternary ammonium compounds.[8] Ocular exposure may result in clinical effects of mild discomfort to very serious corneal damage, depending on the concentration of the detergent.

Treatment of ingestions requires the giving of milk, water, or egg whites. Vomiting should not be induced when the concentration of cationic detergent in the product consumed is greater than 7.5%. Oral dilution may be followed by the administration of activated charcoal and a saline cathartic. Esophagoscopy for evaluation of the degree of corrosive damage is appropriate if stridor, dysphagia, or prolonged hypersalivation is present. General supportive care should include maintenance of respiration, adequate caloric intake (e.g., placement of a percutaneous esophageal gastric [PEG] tube), GI protectants (e.g., sucralfate), antibiotics, analgesics (e.g., butorphanol tartrate, fentanyl), corticosteroids, intravenous (IV) fluid therapy (monitor blood gas and acid-base status, and serum electrolytes), and treatment of any seizures that may occur. Patients should be monitored closely for shock. Any exposed skin should be gently but thoroughly washed with soap and water. The eyes should be thoroughly evaluated, and if ocular exposure has occurred, the eyes should be lavaged with isothermic isotonic saline for 20 to 30 minutes. Corneal ulcers should be promptly and persistently treated if present.[2]

Corrosives

A number of household products are capable of causing corrosive injury to contacting membranes. Most corrosives are classified as acids or alkalis, depending on their pH in solutions. Strongly alkaline or basic compounds tend to produce more severe injury than acidic materials.[13,14]

Acidic household products typically contain hydrochloric (muriatic), sulfuric, nitric, or phosphoric acid, or sodium bisulfite, which forms sulfuric acid in water. In addition, aqueous solutions of free halogens (e.g., chlorine, bromine, or iodine) can also be corrosive. Common acidic products include antirust compounds, toilet bowl cleaners, gun barrel cleaning fluid, automobile batteries, and swimming pool cleaning agents. Acids typically produce a localized coagulative necrotic lesion. Because of the rapid surface protein coagulation, acidic burns rarely penetrate the entire thickness of the mucosal membrane. Contact with strong acids induces immediate intense pain, so most animals become alerted to the danger and do not ingest significant quantities.[3]

Alkaline agents are also found in a variety of household products, such as drain cleaners, washing products, liquid cleansers, and toilet bowl products. Common ingredients are lye formulations (e.g., sodium and potassium hydroxide or potash, sodium and potassium carbonate), ammonium hydroxide, and potassium permanganate.[2] These alkaline products cause immediate liquefactive necrosis on contact. The lesions tend to be deeper and more penetrating than those caused by acidic materials. Because alkaline agents produce little immediate pain on contact, unlike acids, there is less potential for animals to be repelled by discomfort, making more extensive exposure possible. Full-thickness esophageal burns may occur. The strength of pH has an important effect on the degree of injury.[2,13,15] Most cases of severe esophageal injury and resulting secondary stricture have occurred from contact with substances with a pH greater than 10.

Concentrated ammonia solution ingested by a cat was shown to cause obliteration of the esophageal wall, seizures, and death within 5 minutes. The increased viscosity of alkalis may contribute to faster and deeper penetration of the esophageal mucosa.[15]

In general, corrosive burns of mucosal membranes first appear milky white or gray. Soon, however, the area turns black and may look wrinkled because of eschar formation. The animal may vocalize or become depressed; some animals manifest pain by panting. Hypersalivation and inability to swallow may be noted. Other effects are hematemesis, abdominal pain, polydipsia, epiglottic edema with secondary respiratory distress, and possible shock. Secondary pneumonitis may result from aspiration or exposure to acid vapors.[2,13]

Esophageal involvement is less common with acid exposures than with alkali ingestions. The character of the commercial formulation also affects the resulting toxicity—solid or granular substances tend to be more painful initially, and burns are more common in the perioral area.[14] Liquids may be less painful initially and thus tend to be swallowed, leading to esophageal and gastric injuries. One cannot assume that the absence of oral lesions indicates that the esophagus and gastric mucosa are not damaged—0% to 30% of patients with esophageal burns have no oral lesions; the reverse can also be true.[13,15]

Once a corrosive substance comes into contact with mucosal membranes, blood vessel thrombosis, cellular necrosis, bacterial infiltration, and lipid saponification occur and are followed by mucosal sloughing. There is an increase in fibroblastic activity. Strictures may form several weeks after the initial injury. It is believed that strictures are most likely to occur after circumferential burns.[13]

Food and fluid tend to buffer alkaline substances in the stomach; however, corrosive substances tend to induce pylorospasm. The most severe gastric injuries thus occur around the pylorus, and pyloric stenosis or perforations with secondary peritonitis are possible sequelae.[3,13] In addition to strictures and perforation, other clinical complications are gastrointestinal bleeding, edema, aspiration, fistulae, and gastric outlet obstruction.

If ocular or dermal exposure occurs, serious burns can result. Ocular exposures to either alkaline or acidic solutions are extremely painful and can lead to corneal and conjunctival necrosis. The extent of corneal damage may not be immediately evident. When the stroma of the cornea is injured, perforation or opaque scarring may result. Acids tend to penetrate the eye more slowly than do bases.[2,3,13]

Treatment consists of immediate dilution of the exposure with milk or water. Dilution with milk in vitro causes the lowest peak temperature, whereas water produces the quickest return to physiologic normalcy. Attempts to neutralize the burn chemically (e.g., acids added to basic exposures and basic solutions added to acid exposures) are contraindicated because exothermic reactions will result, producing elevated local heat and causing thermal burns. Unfortunately, the action of corrosives is so rapid that dilution is sometimes of little apparent benefit. Controversially, excessive dilution may lead to vomiting, thus increasing esophageal contact time and the opportunity for secondary aspiration. In general, however, dilution is recommended and should be appropriately performed.[13]

Gastric lavage is contraindicated in caustic ingestions, and charcoal is ineffective in binding caustics. After administration of a diluent, the animal should be given supportive care. IV fluids are often indicated. If severe pharyngeal edema is present, an endotracheal or tracheostomy tube may be placed to ensure unobstructed respirations. Careful endoscopy with a flexible scope is valuable the first 12 to 24 hours after ingestion, because outward clinical signs do not always correlate with the severity of injury. The procedure should be halted at the first sign of esophageal mucosal injury. Radiographic evaluation is another alternative. Surgical resection of damaged tissue is sometimes advised; however, it is not always possible to easily identify the damaged area, and after-resection leaking of esophageal contents may occur at sites of anastomoses. Corticosteroids, because they decrease fibroblastic activity and inflammation, have been recommended to reduce stricture from circumferential alkali burns. Steroid treatment should be started within the first 48 hours and be accompanied by prophylactic antibiotic therapy. Analgesics are often indicated for pain control. Antibiotics are specifically indicated in animals with perforations. Severely affected patients may require placement of a PEG tube for alimentary nutritional support. It is useful to monitor blood gas and acid-base status and concentrations of serum electrolytes. Therapy for shock may also be required; uncorrected circulatory collapse can lead to renal failure, ischemic lesions of vital organs, and acute death. Affected skin should be aggressively flushed with copious amounts of water, and exposed eyes must be flushed with sterile saline for at least 30 minutes. Topical anesthetics are helpful in patient manipulations and comfort.[2,3,13-15]

Disinfectants

Disinfectants are applied to inanimate objects to destroy microorganisms or inhibit their growth. Such cleaners are often formulated as combinations of one or more disinfectant compounds and detergents.

Disinfectant cleaners are more toxic than soap and plain detergent compounds. Disinfectants found in cleaning products include quaternary ammonium compounds, phenols, pine oils, bleaches, and alcohols. Quaternary ammonium compounds were reviewed earlier in the section on cationic detergents; the alcohols are discussed in "Solvents and Alcohols" later in this chapter.

Phenols

Phenol is an aromatic alcohol derived from coal tar that is a highly reactive and corrosive contact poison. Phenolic disinfectants are generally formulated with chlorophenols (3% to 8%), phenylphenol (2% to 10%), soaps and detergents (10% to 20%), glycerin (1% to 2%), and alcohols and glycols (1% to 20%). Some concentrated phenolic disinfectants contain pure phenol at concentrations from 20% to 50%.

The oral LD_{50} of phenol in dogs is approximately 0.5 g/kg BW. Cats are more sensitive than dogs to phenol and phenolic products because of their limited detoxifying glucuronide transferase activity. Phenol and phenolic compounds are rapidly absorbed through ingestion, inhalation, or dermal contact. The degree of dermal absorption depends more on the magnitude of exposed skin area than on the concentration of the solution.[3] Phenols are detoxified by the liver and excreted in urine as glucuronide and sulfate conjugates.

Phenol denatures and precipitates cellular proteins and thus directly poisons all contacting cells. Phenol at concentrations greater than 5% has resulted in oral burns, and concentrations of more than 1% have produced dermal burns. Phenol derivatives are considered less corrosive than phenol. Ocular and cutaneous exposure to phenols is often accompanied by a short interval of intense pain followed by local anesthesia.[2] Animals tend to be more sensitive to the formation of coagulative necrotic skin lesions from phenols because their hair coat serves to retain the phenol-containing solution, thus providing longer contact time with the skin.[16] Affected areas tend to turn white and then develop dry eschars over the next several days. Ocular exposure to phenolic compounds results in severe burns and penetrating corneal lesions.

Oral exposure to phenolic compounds produces corrosive burns of the mouth, oropharynx, and esophagus. Initial clinical signs are vomiting, hypersalivation, apprehension, hyperactivity, ataxia, and panting. As the clinical syndrome progresses, fasciculations, shock, cardiac arrhythmias, methemoglobinemia, and coma may develop.[2] Hepatic and renal damage may occur within the next 12 to 24 hours. Respiratory alkalosis develops secondary to centrally mediated respiratory stimulation.[17] Histologic examination of the liver shows severe centrilobular hyperemia, fatty degeneration, and necrosis, and the kidneys display renal tubular degeneration and necrosis.

Toxicoses from exposure to phenolic disinfectants are medical emergencies. Dilution of phenol exposures with water is controversial because such dilution may enhance systemic absorption. It is advantageous that gastrointestinal demulcents (milk or eggs) be given at home before the owner brings the exposed animal to the veterinary clinic. Severity of mucosal damage to the oropharynx must be assessed before attempting gastric lavage. If severe mucosal damage is present, gastric lavage and emesis are contraindicated. Activated charcoal and a saline cathartic may be administered if no or minimal mucosal damage is present. For dermal exposure, the preferred agent for the dilution and removal of phenolic compounds is polyethylene glycol or glycerol, followed by washing with a mild liquid dish detergent and thorough rinsing with water. Humans who contact the exposed areas should wear heavy rubber gloves and protective clothing to protect themselves from contamination. After the final rinsing, dressings soaked in 0.5% sodium bicarbonate may be applied to injured areas. Oily dermatologic dressings should be avoided because they enhance absorption of phenol. For ocular exposures, the eyes should be flushed with isothermic isotonic saline for 20 to 30 minutes. Corneal erosions are managed by appropriate medical procedures.[2]

Aggressive supportive care is necessary to manage phenol toxicoses. Acid-base status, cardiovascular function, renal function, and hepatic function must all be closely monitored. Shock and respiratory depression are complicating concerns and require fluids and supporting respiratory efforts. *N*-acetylcysteine (140 mg/kg loading dose IV and, then 70 mg/kg four times daily orally for 3 days) may limit hepatic and renal toxicity.[2]

Pine Oils and Turpentine

Pine oils, derived by steam distillation of wood from pines, consist of a mixture of terpene alcohols. Pine oil–based compounds may contain small amounts of phenol derivatives. The concentration of pine oil in disinfectant cleaners varies from 0.3% to 60%.[18] Many "pine oil" cleaners marketed in the United States are pine scented but contain little or no actual pine oil, so it is important to check the label on pine-scented cleaners. Pine Sol, one of the most widely used pine oil cleaners, contains 8% to 12% pine oil, 3% to 7% alkyl alcohol ethoxylates, 1% to 5% isopropanol, and 1% to 5% sodium petroleum sulfonate in its "Original" formulation[19]; other cleaners branded as Pine Sol contain no pine oil. Turpentine is a hydrocarbon mixture of terpenes derived from pine oil rather than petroleum and is often applied as a paint thinner.

The oral LD_{50} of pine oil ranges from 1 to 2.7 mL/kg BW. A substantially lower dose results in severe toxicosis.[2] Pine oil is readily absorbed from the gastrointestinal tract and is metabolized by the liver to be excreted in urine as glucuronide conjugates. High concentrations of ingested pine oil are demonstrable in lung tissue, lending a characteristic pine or turpentine odor to the breath.[18] As is true for phenolic compounds, cats are more susceptible than other species to pine oil toxicoses.[20]

Pine oils are directly irritating to mucous membranes, producing erythema of the oropharynx, mouth, and skin. Ocular exposure causes marked blepharospasm, epiphora, photosensitivity, and erythema of the conjunctiva and sclera.[2] Ingestion results in nausea, hypersalivation, bloody vomiting, and abdominal pain. Systemic effects include weakness and CNS depression, ataxia, hypotension, and respiratory depression. Pulmonary toxicity is due to aspiration during ingestion or from emesis or may be due to chemical pneumonitis from absorption of the pine oil through the gastrointestinal tract with subsequent deposition in the lung.[18] Myoglobinuria and acute renal failure may develop following massive ingestions. A cat that ingested 100 mL of undiluted Pine Sol had severe depression, ataxia, unresponsive pupils, and shock, and died within 12 hours.[20] Pulmonary edema, acute centrilobular hepatic necrosis, and total renal cortical necrosis were present at necropsy examination.[20]

Prompt dilution with milk, egg white, or water should occur following ingestion of pine oil disinfectants. Because of rapid onset of depression and the danger of aspiration pneumonia, emesis is often contraindicated, and even gastric lavage with placement of a cuffed endotracheal tube poses risk. Dilution should be followed by the administration of activated charcoal and a saline or osmotic cathartic. Symptomatic and supportive care, consisting of maintenance of renal perfusion and acid-base and electrolyte balance, is crucial. Animals that have their dermis exposed should be bathed with soap and then rinsed with copious amounts of water as soon as feasible after the exposure.

Bleaches

Most common household bleach preparations contain sodium hypochlorite at concentrations between 3% and 6%. Hypochlorite salts are widely used as disinfectants, deodorizers, and water purifiers. Industrial strength bleaching solutions and swimming pool chlorine products may contain up to 50% hypochlorite. Powdered chlorine laundry bleaches have calcium hypochlorite, trichloroisocyanuric acid, or dichlorodimethylhydantoin compounds that slowly form hypochlorite in aqueous solutions.[3] Nonchlorine bleach preparations, known as *colorfast bleaches,* may contain sodium peroxide, sodium perborate, or enzymatic detergents.[4]

Chlorine bleaches are hazardous when mixed with strong acids or ammonia solutions because such mixtures produce chlorine or chloramine gas, respectively, which are severe respiratory and eye irritants.

Hypochlorite toxicosis results from its corrosive effect on skin and mucous membranes. This action is due to the oxidizing potency of the hypochlorite ion, which is measured as "available chlorine" and approximates that of similar concentrations of sodium hydroxide solutions. The clinical effects of ingested hypochlorite depend on the product's hypochlorite ion concentration and resulting pH rather than the ingested dose (quantity). In the acidic environment of the stomach, hypochlorite forms hypochlorous acid, which penetrates mucous membranes, is reduced by proteins, and causes local protein coagulation.[21]

Household chlorine bleaches are mild to moderate irritants and generally are not associated with significant tissue destruction. Oropharyngeal, esophageal, and gastric burns have been reported from some chlorine bleach ingestions, but the clinical incidence of effects is extremely low. The more concentrated hypochlorite solutions and bleaching powders can produce corrosive burns if the physical form of the product favors significant membrane exposure, and the duration of exposure is prolonged. The common toxic effects from household chlorine bleaches are irritation of the oropharynx, salivation, vomiting, and abdominal pain. The exposed animal may smell of chlorine, and bleaching of the hair may be seen.[2] Systemic reactions to chlorine bleaches are rare, and if present often are secondary to local membrane and tissue injury. Inhalation of fumes or powders from chlorine bleach products initiates pulmonary irritation and coughing, retching, and dyspnea.

Nonchlorine bleach products are of low toxicity. Sodium peroxide dissociates in the gastrointestinal tract to release oxygen and may cause mild gastritis and emesis. Sodium perborate–containing bleaches decompose to peroxide and borate; these bleaches are more alkaline and thus irritating. They may also produce systemic effects from boric acid.[4]

Ingestions of bleaching solutions are best treated by the administration of milk or water to dilute the ingested solution and to serve as demulcents. Acidic antidote medications should not be used because they enhance tissue penetration and injury by forming hypochlorous acid. Areas of dermal contact should be washed with soap and rinsed with abundant amounts of water. Because of the low incidence of esophageal damage likely from household chlorine bleach ingestions, the decision to perform endoscopy should be made based on the patient's clinical signs and prognostic necessity. Animals with dysphagia, dyspnea, or significant oropharyngeal burns should undergo careful evaluative endoscopy and be treated appropriately for any corrosive injuries present.[21]

Solvents and Alcohols

Acetone

Acetone is common in nail polish removers, varnishes, glues, and rubber cements as a clear, colorless, volatile, highly flammable liquid with a characteristic aromatic fruity odor and pungent, sweetish taste. It may be absorbed orally, by inhalation, and through dermal application. Although acetone is relatively low in toxicity (lowest oral canine lethal dose, LD_{LO}, is approximately 8 mL/kg), ingestions greater than 2 to 3 mL/kg may be toxic.

Signs of exposure roughly simulate those of ethanol intoxication, although the CNS depressant action of acetone is greater. The characteristic odor of acetone on the breath and elevated urinary ketones are sensitive indicators of exposure. CNS depression, ataxia, and vomiting occur following mild exposure; stupor and coma are present in severe intoxications. Hyperglycemia and ketonemia with acidosis may be present and require differentiation from acute diabetic coma.

Effective treatment is largely symptomatic and appropriate supportive care. Patients with signs of recent ingestions (i.e., within 2 hours with an intact gag reflex) may benefit from emesis followed by oral administration of activated charcoal and a cathartic. Giving IV fluids containing sodium bicarbonate will help manage the associated acidosis. The plasma half-life of acetone is relatively long (28 hours); hence clinical improvement may be relatively slow.

Isopropanol

Isopropyl alcohol is a common household disinfectant and solvent. It is also common in perfumes, colognes, and other grooming products. Ingestion causes CNS depression similar to the effects of ethanol, but more severe. Isopropanol is metabolized by alcohol dehydrogenase more slowly than ethanol to produce acetone, itself a CNS depressant, as the major metabolite. The reported toxic dose of 70% isopropanol (rubbing alcohol) is 1 mL/kg, but as little as 0.5 mL/kg may cause adverse effects. Signs of toxicosis develop within 30 to 60 minutes; ataxia, vomiting, and hematemesis can develop, which may progress to CNS and respiratory depression, severe hypotension, mild acidosis, coma, and loss of deep tendon reflexes.

Treatment of isopropanol toxicoses involves induction of emesis if ingestion occurred within 1 hour and the animal is relatively asymptomatic at the time of presentation. Activated charcoal administration is of little value because it is relatively ineffective in binding alcohols. IV fluids should be administered, and electrolyte and acid-base status must be monitored. Hemodialysis is effective in reversing severe hypotension and coma from isopropanol.

Methanol

Methyl alcohol, or wood alcohol, is often found in automotive windshield cleaner fluids and lock antifreeze products (see Chapter 59). It is metabolized by alcohol dehydrogenase to formaldehyde as its major metabolite; the formaldehyde is further metabolized to formic acid by aldehyde dehydrogenase. Although formic acid accumulation is associated with severe acidosis and blindness in humans exposed to methanol, blindness and acidosis do not occur in dogs or cats ingesting methanol. This clinical difference is due to differences in the rate of methanol metabolism between humans and animals and the greater availability of tetrahydrofolate in the livers of nonprimate species.[22] The lethal dose of oral methanol in dogs is 4 to 8 mL/kg.

Clinical signs of methanol intoxication in dogs are CNS depression, ataxia, hypothermia, respiratory depression, and coma. Treatment of such poisonings is similar to that for isopropanol toxicosis.

Miscellaneous Household Hazards

Batteries

The small disc or button batteries used to power calculators, hearing aids, cameras, and watches pose significant ingestion hazards for pets. Dry-cell batteries of varying size found in toys, flashlights, and so on can be a risk as well. Fortunately, most disc batteries pass through the digestive system intact without producing any clinical signs. The disc batteries that may require intervention are the larger manganese (21 to 23 mm) and mercury batteries (sales of mercury batteries were discontinued in the United States in 1996).

Dry-cell batteries can contain sodium or potassium hydroxide (alkaline dry cell) or ammonium chloride and manganese dioxide (acidic dry cell), along with varying amounts of heavy metals (e.g., lithium, nickel, zinc, silver, cadmium). Mercury button batteries contain 15% to 50% mercuric oxide or, on average, 1 to 5 g of mercury.[23] The main hazard from batteries is corrosive damage to the esophagus from batteries impacted in the esophagus. This tissue damage is caused by leakage of the battery alkalis, the electrical current generated by the battery's contact with the cells of the esophageal wall and within the electrolyte-rich fluids of the gastrointestinal tract, and various degrees of pressure necroses to the esophageal wall from the impacted batteries.

Most ingested disc batteries pass through the digestive tract spontaneously within 24 to 36 hours without producing any adverse effects. The presence of gastrointestinal distress or related signs suggests possible battery retention and impaction with resulting obstruction, tissue necrosis, and potential pending perforation. Clinical signs that may develop include fever, dysphagia, vomiting, tachypnea, abdominal tenderness, anorexia, and black nonmelanotic stools.[23] The location of an ingested battery may be determined by radiography. If an initial radiograph is taken shortly after ingestion, the radiopaque object may be followed through the gastrointestinal tract and delayed passage identified. Batteries retained for more than 36 hours should be given priority for removal.

Batteries lodged in the esophagus and stomach should be removed by endoscopy. Patients with batteries passing through the stomach should be monitored for the development of clinical effects; however, if the battery has been chewed or split apart, more aggressive actions may be necessary to ensure rapid passage through the intestines. This may require the use of fiber bulk laxatives, saline cathartics, and enemas in asymptomatic patients. Timely surgical retrieval of impacted or chewed pieces of batteries is necessary in patients with evidence of mucosal hemorrhage or bowel perforation. Following ingestion of damaged mercury-containing disc batteries, monitoring of urinary mercury levels is especially important when the battery has been split or chewed into pieces. Chelation therapy with dimercaptosuccinic acid or d-penicillamine, as for lead poisoning, may be required for patients with elevated urine mercury levels or those having signs of mercury toxicity: weight loss, anorexia, ataxia, and CNS stimulation and dysfunction.

Birth Control Pills

Although there are a variety of birth control pills on the market, they all have very similar compositions: estrogen and progesterone in very low concentration. "Mini-pill" birth control pills have only progesterone in them. Some birth control pills also contain supplemental iron. Birth control pills are dispensed in containers of 21, 28, 81, or 84 tablets; 28-count containers generally have 4-7 inert pills. Most of the active tablets contain 0.035 mg or less of estrogen and varying amounts of progesterone.[24] Birth control pills are quite different from hormone replacement pills, which some women refer to as "birth control pills" but which contain much higher levels of estrogen. It is always safest to verify the product involved when birth control pills have been ingested by pets. In general, it is the estrogen content of the tablets that is of concern, as estrogen doses of more than 1 mg/kg may result in bone marrow suppression; given the low level of estrogen in birth control pills, it is very difficult to get near this dose even if all the tablets of a month's supply are ingested. Single high doses of the progesterone content of the tablets are unlikely to cause more than mild gastrointestinal upset. For iron-containing tablets, calculate the dosage of iron; doses of more than 20 mg/kg merit decontamination (see Chapter 51). Decontamination is rarely needed even when patients have ingested an entire month's worth of tablets, unless there is a foreign body concern resulting from package ingestion.

Cold Packs and Ice Packs

Cold packs and ice packs are commonly used as first aid to reduce swelling and inflammation and to help refrigerate foods, drugs, and other perishables during transit in coolers. Some are designed for cold use only, whereas others can be heated and used as hot packs, primarily as first aid. "Instant" cold packs contain water surrounding a tube or bag of ammonium nitrate; the pack is activated by crushing the interior container, which releases ammonium nitrate and precipitates an endothermic reaction that can cool the pack to approximately 35° F for 10-15 minutes. Large amounts of ingested ammonium nitrate can cause gastritis, acidosis, and nitrite toxicity manifesting as methemoglobinemia, but severe toxicosis is not expected from the amounts present in most cold packs.[25] Mild gastrointestinal upset may occur and should be treated symptomatically.

Gel-based cold packs are refrigerated or frozen to the desired temperature and retain that temperature for a prolonged period. Gel-based packs are composed of approximately 60% to 75% water combined with a variety of compounds including hydroxyethyl cellulose, carboxyl methyl cellulose, glycerin, vinyl-coated silica gel, and polyacrylamites. These products have relatively low oral toxicity and are unlikely to cause more than mild gastrointestinal upset if ingested by pets. However, some cold packs may contain more toxic components, such as diethylene glycol or ethylene glycol. In January 2012, the U.S. Consumer Product Safety Commission issued a recall on gel cold packs included in some lunch boxes and food carriers after receiving reports of two dogs becoming ill following ingestion of the cold pack contents.[26] One dog was reported to have died, although the other recovered with treatment. The cold packs were determined to contain both ethylene glycol and diethylene glycol.

Cough Drops (with Menthol)

There are many different formulations of cough drops, consisting mostly of menthol and sugars. Menthol has a wide margin of safety, with an oral LD_{50} in dogs of 3-4 g/kg BW. Exposures to extremely large amounts of cough drops can cause gastrointestinal distress (e.g., abdominal pain, diarrhea) due to the sugar and sugar alcohols. In extreme cases, the menthol can lead to renal, lung, and heart dysfunction along with central nervous system depression. Menthol can also be found in candy, cigarettes, creams, gum, mouthwash, and many ointments.

Cyanoacrylate Adhesives (Superglue)

Cured cyanoacrylate adhesives are nontoxic if ingested; however, uncured cyanoacrylate adhesives form an almost instantaneous bond when applied to the hair or skin, resulting in an annoyed animal and a frustrated owner presenting the animal to a veterinarian. Adhered skin may be manipulated by soaking the affected areas with warm, soapy water as quickly as possible, one hopes before a full adhesive cure occurs. After irrigation the surfaces may be peeled apart gently or the surfaces may be rolled apart using a blunt object. Do not pull the surfaces apart with direct opposing actions. Clipping the hair may be required to reduce tension on skin or eyelids. If small areas of skin away from the face and eyes are affected, the area may be soaked with acetone for several minutes and repeated attempts made to separate the hair or skin. In the case of eyelid or eyeball adhesions, wash the area thoroughly with warm water and apply a gauze patch and an Elizabethan collar to prevent self-trauma by the animal; do not attempt opening the eye with forceful manipulation or the use of solvents. The eye should be able to be opened within a few hours to a few days with no residual tissue damage.

Expanding Wood Glues (Gorilla Glue, Elmer's ProBond Wood Glue, etc.)

Woodworking adhesives and expanding insulations that contain polymeric diphenylmethane diisocyanate react with hydrogen ions in acids, alcohols, and water to form urethane and related compounds. These products typically expand, foam, and cure within 15 minutes and are technically "nontoxic."[27] However, when ingested, a relatively rapid increase of the material volume within the confined space of the stomach produces acute gastric or gastrointestinal blockage. An in vitro study documented a greater than eightfold increase in material volume over a 2-hour period.[28] Vomiting, lethargy, and a painful abdomen may be apparent within hours of ingestion. Emesis to remove the material is contraindicated; it is recommended that the animal take nothing by mouth and that radiographs be taken to localize the mass. Abdominal surgery is often required to remove the digestive tract obstruction.

Glow Jewelry (Dibutyl Phthalate, Zinc Sulfide, Strontium Aluminate)

Dibutyl phthalate is present in many of the glow-in-the-dark products, and its toxicity potential is considered to be quite low. However, indoor pets chewing on these products and releasing the liquid contents may experience salivation, along with hyperactivity and aggressive behavior. The chemical is considered to be unpleasant, thereby limiting excessive exposures. Rinsing the mouth is generally all that is required to potentially dilute the dibutyl phthalate, and generally all signs resolve within a few hours.

Some glow-in-the-dark products contain a combination of zinc sulfide and strontium aluminate. These compounds are also known to have irritating properties, along with causing ataxia, confusion, cardiac irregularities, and acute respiratory arrest. Treatment aims are symptomatic and supportive in nature.

Glucosamine-Based Joint Supplements

Glucosamine-based joint supplements have been used in veterinary patients with osteoarthritis for over two decades. Although there is some debate on the efficacy of these supplements in limiting pain and improving mobility, recent studies and reviews have concluded that some patients do appear to have positive responses to these products.[29] Although no prescription products exist, a myriad of differing products are available over the counter and through veterinarians. Most products contain glucosamine in combination with other ingredients, including chondroitin sulfate, dimethyl sulfone, creatine monohydrate, docosahexanoic acid, eicosapentaenoic acid, ascorbic acid, vitamin E, and thioctic acid, along with a variety of other trace elements, flavors, and fillers. Although safety studies on these products are not readily available, they tend to be well tolerated by most animals at the recommended doses. These products tend to be formulated to be highly palatable and chewable, which increases the risk for excessive ingestion if animals obtain access to the product containers.

In most cases, overdoses are not expected to cause more than mild gastrointestinal upset.[30] However, the ASPCA APCC has reported on 21 dogs that developed liver injury following ingestion of large amounts of glucosamine-based joint supplements.[31] Amounts ingested ranged from 20 to 240 chewable tablets, resulting in doses of 183-6667 mg/kg glucosamine, 418-2667 mg/kg creatine, and 45-4000 mg/kg dimethyl sulfone. Signs included vomiting, diarrhea, and lethargy, which developed anywhere from 30 minutes to 2 days following ingestion. Increases in serum alanine aminotransferase (ALT) activity were detected as early as 5 hours following ingestion, although the majority of increases in ALT were noted between 24 and 48 hours following exposure; in two thirds of the dogs, ALT values exceeded 1000 U/L. Of nine dogs with follow-up information, four dogs recovered with veterinary care, two were euthanized because of poor response to treatment, and three remained on hepatoprotectants at the time of follow-up. Postmortem lesions on one dog euthanized 11 days after exposure revealed severe centrilobular necrosis, acute renal tubular necrosis, pancreatic necrosis, and myocardial necrosis. The cause of liver injury in these cases was not known; possibilities include some type of contaminant in the supplement, interaction between active ingredients or other medications, or preexisting health issues. Based on these cases, toxicologists at APCC recommend aggressive decontamination, monitoring, and symptomatic and supportive care in dogs that present with overdose of glucosamine-based joint supplements.

Homemade and Commercial Play Dough

Ingestion of homemade and commercial play dough has been associated with severe hypernatremia in dogs.[32] The lowest toxic dose for dogs is 2 g NaCl/kg BW and the lowest lethal dose is 4 g NaCl/kg BW. A typical recipe found on an Internet search for homemade play dough consists of 2 cups of flour, 1 cup of salt, and ½ to 1 cup of water; this is roughly equivalent to 8.4 g of sodium chloride per tablespoon of play dough.[32] A commercial playdough was found to contain 4.3% sodium. Clinical signs have been observed in dogs following ingestion of as little as 1.9 g of play dough/kg BW; they include vomiting, polydipsia, polyuria, tremors, hyperthermia, and seizures.[32] Treatment procedures for potentially toxic exposures should include basic decontamination procedures in the asymptomatic patient, followed by monitoring serum sodium levels. Seizures were commonly reported in those dogs in which sodium concentrations exceeded 180 mEq/L.[32] Correcting the acute hypernatremia is a necessity and involves the use of IV fluids and warm water enemas to help dilute the serum sodium level.[33] In cases in which hypernatremia has persisted for more than 18-24 hours, the formation of idiogenic osmoles in the CNS make treatment more challenging, as rapid rehydration may result in cerebral edema caused by the osmotic effect in the brain.[34] In these more chronic hypernatremia cases, slowly lowering the sodium concentrations over a 48- to 72-hour period with isotonic or hypertonic fluids is necessary. It has been recommended not to lower the sodium concentrations faster than 0.5 to 1 mEq/L/h.[32] Additional treatment options are based on the signs that the animal is exhibiting at the time.

Hops

Hops (*Humulus lupulus*) are cultivated for their use in beer making; the flowers of the female plant are used to impart the bitter flavor and pungent aroma to beer. Ingestion of both fresh and spent hops has been associated with the development of malignant hyperthermia in dogs.[35] Breeds that may appear to be particularly susceptible to this problem include greyhounds and golden retrievers. Treatment is directed toward basic decontamination of the gastrointestinal tract if the exposure is recent, and controlling the high temperatures in clinically affected animals (e.g., IV fluids, various cooling measures). If available, dantrolene, a skeletal muscle relaxant that has been used in humans to manage malignant hyperthermia, may be used at an initial dose of 2-3 mg/kg IV or 3.5 mg/kg PO followed by 3.5 mg/kg every 12 hours as needed.[36]

Ice Melts

Ice melts can cause mild to moderate risk to pets, depending on the active ingredient present. Most of the ingredients present act as gastric irritants, and vomiting and diarrhea are the most commonly observed clinical signs immediately following oral exposures. These include products that contain urea, calcium carbonate, and calcium magnesium acetate. Ice melts that contain sodium chloride also can lead to serious hypernatremia and an osmotic diuresis if the exposure dose is high enough, which can ultimately lead to muscle tremors, acidosis, and seizure activity. Muscle weakness and cardiac abnormalities can result from ingestion of ice melts that contain potassium chloride. Products that contain magnesium chloride can additionally cause muscle weakness, cardiac abnormalities, and hypotension. Treatment of exposures is symptomatic and supportive in nature.

Iron-Based Hand Warmers

Air-activated hand warmers contain reduced iron, activated charcoal, water, water reservoirs (e.g., vermiculite), cellulose (e.g., wood powder), and salt.[37,38] Similar formulations are also used as "oxygen absorbers" that are included in packaged dehydrated foods to prolong shelf life. On contact with oxygen, the iron is converted to iron oxide (rust), releasing heat in the process. Depending on the individual formulation, temperatures generated by hand warmers can range from 100° F to 180° F for a duration of 1 to 20 hours.[39] Rats dosed with hand warmer contents (2 g/kg) developed no evidence of toxicosis.[40] A case series of four older adult humans who had ingested hand warmer contents revealed no or mild clinical effects, although two had transient elevations in serum iron levels.[40] Significant esophageal and gastric corrosive injury was reported in an older adult woman who ingested the contents of multiple hand warmers.[38] A dog that ingested one or two oxygen absorber packets developed vomiting, melena, elevated serum iron levels, and elevated ALT.[37] In most cases, few clinical effects are expected following ingestion of hand warmers, but a few patients may develop mild to moderate gastrointestinal signs. Gastrointestinal protectants (e.g., sucralfate, acid reducer) and, as needed, antiemetics should be initiated in animals with signs of gastrointestinal upset. Animals with gastrointestinal irritation or corrosive injury from iron ingestion are at increased risk for systemic absorption of iron across the damaged gastrointestinal mucosa.[41] For this reason, animals showing more than mild gastrointestinal upset following hand warmer ingestion should have serum iron levels evaluated. Chelation with deferoxamine is rarely warranted and is contraindicated if iron is still present in the gastrointestinal tract, as the chelator can increase gastrointestinal absorption of iron.[42] For patients with iron remaining in the gut that are in need of chelation therapy, the use of the oral iron chelator deferasirox should be considered. Deferasirox (20 mg/kg by mouth [PO] single ingestion) has been shown to significantly reduce serum iron levels in humans following ingestion of supratherapeutic levels of iron.[43]

Matches, Fireworks, and Flares

Matches are generally considered nontoxic when ingested, but they do contain 40% to 60% potassium chlorate in the match heads. Potassium chlorate is a moderately effective oxidizing agent that can cause methemoglobinemia. The oral LD_{LO} of potassium chlorate in dogs is 1200 mg/kg (75 sticks/kg BW); a box of 20 wooden matches (16 mg/stick) has 320 mg of potassium chlorate, whereas a book of paper matches contains 110 mg of potassium chlorate. The development of clinical signs from the ingestion of several books or boxes of matches would not be expected, but in the occasional animal that ingests a large number of matches, vomiting, CNS depression, hypotension, cyanosis, and hemolysis can occur. The affected animal may be successfully treated symptomatically unless clinically significant methemoglobinemia develops. The methemoglobinemia may be treated intravenously with 1% methylene blue at 4 mg/kg in dogs or once at 1.5 mg/kg in cats. The oral use of 20 mg/kg ascorbic acid is often recommended in cats, but its effectiveness is usually too slow for practical use.

Most household fireworks are relatively harmless if swallowed. The toxic ingredients are typically oxidizing agents that may include potassium nitrate, potassium chloride, sodium nitrate, and potassium perchlorate. Flares typically contain sodium nitrate, sulfur, and various hydrocarbons. The most common problems associated with ingestion include gastrointestinal irritation and ulceration (e.g., vomiting, salivation, abdominal pain). Severe ingestions can lead to the formation of methemoglobin, hemolysis, and seizure activity (rare). Ingestion of "snake" fireworks has been associated with barium toxicosis in a human.[44] Severe obtundation, cardiac dysrhythmia, and respiratory failure were associated with profound hypokalemia and serum barium levels of more than 20,000 mcg/L (normal <200 mcg/L). Large fireworks for commercial or municipal use can contain potentially toxic compounds such as arsenic, antimony, bismuth, barium, concentrated chlorates and perchlorates, lead, thallium, and white and red phosphorus.

Methionine-Based Lawn "Savers" (Urine Scald Preventers)

There is a wide range of products available on the market purported to help prevent scalding of lawns by dog urine through alteration of urine chemistry. One of the more popular ingredients used in these products is DL-methionine, a sulfur-containing amino acid that aids in acidifying urine. At the levels in the individual chewable tablet or chews (usually 100-150 mg per item), DL-methionine poses no hazard to dogs, but because of the palatability of these products, accidental overdoses can occur when dogs obtain access to entire packages of product.[45] At DL-methionine doses of less than 200 mg/kg, mild, self-limiting gastrointestinal upset may occur, whereas doses of more than 200 mg/kg may result in ataxia and doses of more than 400 mg/kg may result in signs resembling hepatic encephalopathy, including ataxia, disorientation, tachypnea, hyperesthesia, seizures, and coma (ASPCA APCC, unpublished data, 2011). Doses of 2 g/kg of methionine in cats has been associated with anorexia, methemoglobinemia, Heinz body formation, ataxia, cyanosis, and hemolysis.[46] Patients should be managed by early decontamination (emesis and activated charcoal within 2 hours of exposure), and, if symptomatic, IV fluid diuresis and oral or rectal lactulose can aid in reducing the signs. Symptomatic care should be given for acid or base, hematologic, or CNS signs. Most animals make full recoveries within 24-48 hours when provided with appropriate veterinary care.

Mothballs

The major types of mothballs available commercially for home use contain naphthalene or paradichlorobenzene (i.e., 1,4-dichlorobenzene). Naphthalene mothballs are present in "old-fashioned" preparations, whereas paradichlorobenzene mothballs are used as cake deodorizers in garbage and diaper pails and in bathrooms.

The LD_{LO} of naphthalene is approximately 400 mg/kg, but cats are more sensitive to the chemical than dogs. A naphthalene mothball can weigh between 2.7 and 4 g; therefore ingestion of a single mothball is a potential toxic risk for a companion animal. Clinical signs associated with the ingestion of naphthalene mothballs are vomiting, naphthalene-scented breath, methemoglobinemia, hemolytic Heinz body anemia, hemoglobinuria, hepatic injury, and possible nephrosis from the hemoglobinuria or hypoxia. Appropriate treatment following naphthalene mothball ingestion is induction of emesis followed by oral administration of activated charcoal and a saline cathartic, 4 mg of 1% methylene blue/kg IV in dogs or one dose of 1.5 mg 1% methylene blue/kg in cats for methemoglobinemia (20 mg ascorbic acid/kg orally in cats is usually inefficient therapy), and IV bicarbonate-containing fluids to reduce hemoglobin precipitation in the kidneys from the red blood cell hemolysis.

Paradichlorobenzene is an organochlorine insecticide with an LD_{50} of approximately 500 mg/kg. Clinical signs associated with ingestion are vomiting, abdominal pain, tremors, seizures, and liver and kidney damage. Treatment for paradichlorobenzene ingestions should include prompt gastrointestinal decontamination, fluid administration to induce diuresis, symptomatic response to adverse signs, supportive care of vital functions, and seizure control with parenteral benzodiazepines.

Paintballs

Potential ingredients in paintballs include polyethylene glycol, glycerin, gelatin, sorbitol, dipropylene glycol, mineral oil, dye, ground pigskin, and water.[33] Ingestions in dogs have led to vomiting, ataxia, diarrhea, and tremors; less commonly observed signs include tachycardia, weakness, hyperactivity, hyperthermia, blindness, and seizures.[33] Clinical pathologic changes reported include hypernatremia, hyperchloremia, acidosis, and hypokalemia.[33] The exact toxic dose is yet to be well defined. Treatment in asymptomatic patients includes basic traditional decontamination procedures, such as emesis and gastric lavage. The use of activated charcoal and a cathartic should be considered carefully; their use may provide little benefit and some of the ingredients of paintballs may act as osmotic cathartics themselves. One should also carefully monitor the patient for potential problems in acid-base status, along with various electrolyte changes. Hypernatremic patients should benefit from IV fluid, 5% dextrose in water or 2.5% dextrose in 0.45% saline, at 1.5 to 2 times maintenance.[33] IV potassium should be instituted to those hypokalemic patients at a rate not to exceed 0.5 mEq/kg/h.[46] Other treatment modalities are based on the clinical needs of the patient. Most cases resolve within a 24-hour period after basic supportive measures are instituted.

Silica Gel Containing Desiccant Packs

These moisture absorbents are commonly found in shoe boxes, lamps, medication bottles, electronic equipment and food items (e.g., jerky). The packs can be paper or plastic packets or plastic cylinders with powder, granular or liquid contents. The main active ingredient is silica gel, though some can contain iron. Silica gel has a low degree of toxicity and mild gastrointestinal upset is generally the most one would expect to see following oral exposures. However, there is a recent report of a dog that ingested one or two oxygen absorber packets that developed vomiting, melena, elevated serum iron levels, and elevated ALT.[37]

Xylitol

As a sweetener in sugar-free products, xylitol induces hypoglycemia by stimulating insulin secretion from the pancreas of dogs[27,47] (see Chapter 83). Its increased marketing and use have resulted in canine intoxications associated with products containing this sweetener, including sugar-free gums, candies, and baked goods. Xylitol can also be found in some sugar-free medicinal syrups or elixirs and in some veterinary dental products (e.g., mouthwash, toothpaste); in the latter, toxicosis would be of concern only if a dog was to ingest the concentrated product. Some of the dental products contain a high concentration of xylitol. A recent case of a dog ingesting a children's tooth gel revealed that the product contained 35% xylitol. Current literature reports that xylitol doses of more than 100 mg/kg have caused hypoglycemia in dogs, although the APCC reports at least one case of hypoglycemia in a dog ingesting as little as 75 mg/kg (ASPCA APCC, unpublished data, 2011). Clinical signs may develop in as little as 30 to 60 minutes following ingestion of xylitol, or signs may be delayed up to 12 hours.[48] Weakness, ataxia, collapse, and seizures may persist as long as 12 to 24 hours, perhaps caused by the slow release and absorption of xylitol from the ingested formulations.[49] Serum chemistry abnormalities in affected dogs include hypoglycemia, hyperglycemia (Somogyi-like phenomenon), hypokalemia, and hypophosphatemia. Additionally, some dogs ingesting xylitol have subsequently developed acute liver failure.[48] Six of eight dogs that developed liver failure subsequent to ingestion of xylitol did not have initial signs of hypoglycemia, but instead developed vomiting and lethargy 9-72 hours following exposure to xylitol. Dogs with xylitol-associated liver failure developed coagulopathy, severely elevated ALT activity, hyperbilirubinemia, thrombocytopenia, mildly elevated alkaline phosphatase activity, moderate hypoglycemia (attributed to liver failure rather than direct xylitol effect), and mild to moderate hyperphosphatemia. Development of hyperphosphatemia was considered a poor prognostic indicator. The lowest estimated xylitol dose associated with liver injury was 500 mg/kg, but it is not known whether liver injury is dose-related or idiosyncratic in nature.[48] Twelve Pekingese dogs experimentally dosed with 1 or 4 g/kg of xylitol did not develop liver failure, although all developed hypoglycemia that resolved within 3-4 hours, and all dogs developed mild and transient elevations in ALT and aspartate aminotransferase.[47] Other clinicopathologic abnormalities reported in these dogs included hypophosphatemia, hypokalemia, and hypercalcemia.

Because signs can begin within 30-60 minutes of xylitol ingestion, induction of vomiting should be done soon after ingestion and only in dogs that are clinically normal. Activated charcoal binds poorly to xylitol and is not likely to be beneficial.[48,50] Dogs that have ingested between 75 mg/kg and 500 mg/kg of xylitol should be hospitalized and blood glucose measurements taken every 1-2 hours for at least 12 hours.[46] If hypoglycemia develops, manage with IV dextrose and monitor for hypokalemia (supplement as needed). If more than 500 mg/kg has been ingested, the recommendation is to start IV dextrose immediately, as well as hepatoprotectants and antioxidants. If hospitalization of dogs ingesting low doses of xylitol is not possible, oral feeding of several small amounts of sugar or sugar-containing meals is reasonable, with clients instructed to present the dog should signs of hypoglycemia develop.[49] Response from hypoglycemia is usually rapid, with most dogs recovering within 12 to 24 hours. Mild elevations in liver enzyme activities generally resolve within a few days, although a recheck at 72 hours is recommended. Dogs experiencing significant liver injury have a more guarded prognosis, although many have survived with aggressive and appropriate treatment for liver failure. A Staffordshire terrier developed vomiting 3 hours after ingesting eight home-baked muffins containing 250 g of xylitol (10.5 g/kg).[51] The dog presented to the veterinarian 48 hours later with persistent vomiting, reluctance to walk, dehydration, and marked icterus. Clinicopathologic findings included hyperbilirubinemia, hypoglycemia, and ALT too high to measure, as well as elevated hematocrit, blood urea nitrogen and albumin consistent with dehydration. The dog subsequently developed coagulopathy and thrombocytopenia and had a documented ALT of 25,050 IU/L (reference: 16-90 IU/L). The dog was treated with IV fluids, glucose, hepatoprotectants, vitamin K_1, gastrointestinal protectants, and antibiotics, and fully recovered over the course of 10 days.

Conclusions

Hundreds of different household products along with over-the-counter and prescription medications are available in homes, presenting potential hazards to pets as complex mixtures of chemicals that vary widely in their toxic potential. Prevention of toxicoses in companion animals follows the same guidelines as those recommended for children: Hazardous cleaning and other chemical products should be kept out of the reach of pets, they should not be left in open containers, solutions of cleaning products should not be unattended where animals may get into them, the product containers should be tightly sealed and properly labeled, and cleaning or other chemical household solutions intended for waste should be promptly discarded. Medications should always be kept out of reach of all companion animals.

If a companion animal has ingested or spilled a cleaning product or disinfectant on itself, it is important to promptly assess the risk to the animal. Most product labels contain warnings about the corrosive, irritating, or toxic potential of the product together with instructions for preliminary action in the event of accidental oral, dermal, or ocular exposures. These instructions offer initial guidance until further information about the product can be obtained or until specific advice can be received from the emergency hotline of the product's manufacturer (frequently part of the label information), from available animal poison control contacts, or through the nationwide 24-hour toll-free telephone number (800-222-1222) of human poison control information centers. Clinicians seeking more direct "in clinic" information on the numerous possible household chemical hazards are referred to the many written resources available.[52,53]

Acknowledgment

The editors wish to acknowledge the exceptional contribution of Drs. Anita Kore and Fred Oehme, who authored this chapter for the previous editions of the book. Their contribution served as the foundation for the material appearing in this edition.

References

1. Oehme FW, Kore AM: Common indoor toxicants. In Peterson ME, Talcott PA, editors: *Small animal toxicology*, ed 2, Philadelphia, 2006, WB Saunders.
2. Coppock RW, Mostrom MS, Lillie LE: The toxicology of detergents, bleaches, antiseptics and disinfectants in small animals, *Vet Hum Toxicol* 30:463–473, 1988.
3. Gosselin RE, Smith RP, Hodge HC: *Clinical toxicology of commercial products*, ed 5, section III, Baltimore, 1984, Williams & Wilkins.
4. McGuigan MA: Bleach, soaps, detergents, and other corrosives. In Haddad LM, Shannon MW, Winchester JF, editors: *Clinical management of poison and drug overdose*, ed 3, Philadelphia, 1998, WB Saunders, pp 830–835.
5. Krenzelok EP: Liquid automatic dishwashing detergents: a profile of toxicity, *Ann Emerg Med* 18:60–63, 1989.
6. Lee JF, Simonowitz D, Block GE: Corrosive injury of the stomach and esophagus by nonphosphate detergents, *Am J Surg* 123:652–656, 1972.
7. Merola VM, Dunayer EK: The 10 most common toxicoses in cats, *Vet Med* 101:339–342, 2006.
8. Grier RL: Quaternary ammonium compound toxicosis in the dog, *J Am Vet Med Assoc* 150:984–987, 1967.
9. Trapani M, Brooks DL, Tillman PC: Quaternary ammonium toxicosis in cats, *Lab Anim Sci* 32:520–522, 1982.
10. VanBerkel M, DeWolff FA: Survival after acute benzalkonium chloride poisoning, *Hum Toxicol* 7:191–193, 1988.
11. Arena JM: Poisonings and other health hazards associated with use of detergents, *JAMA* 190:56–58, 1964.
12. Richardson JA: Potpourri hazards in cats, *Vet Med* 94(12):1010–1012, 1999.
13. Howell JM: Alkaline ingestions, *Ann Emerg Med* 15:820–825, 1986.
14. Muhlendahl KEV, Oberdisse U, Krienke EG: Local injuries by accidental ingestion of corrosive substances by children, *Arch Toxicol* 139:299–314, 1978.
15. Vancura EM, Clinton JE, Ruiz E, et al: Toxicity of alkaline solutions, *Ann Emerg Med* 9:118–122, 1980.
16. Abdullahi SU: Phenol toxicity in a dog, *Vet Hum Toxicol* 25:407, 1983.
17. Dreisbach RH: *Handbook of poisoning: prevention, diagnosis and treatment*, Los Altos, CA, 1980, Lange Medical Publications.
18. Brook MP, McCarron MM, Mueller JA: Pine oil cleaner ingestion, *Ann Emerg Med* 18:391–395, 1989.
19. The Clorox Company: *Pine Sol material safety data sheet*, Oakland, 2005. Retrieved January 2012 from http://www.thecloroxcompany.com/downloads/msds/pinesol/originalpine-solbrandcleaner1.pdf.
20. Rousseaux CG, Smith RA, Nicholson S: Acute Pine Sol toxicity in a domestic cat, *Vet Hum Toxicol* 28:316–317, 1986.
21. Bryson PD: Other chemicals that burn. In Bryson PD, editor: *Comprehensive review in toxicology*, ed 2, Rockville, MD, 1989, Aspen Publishers.
22. Koestner A, Norton S: Nervous system. In Haschek WM, Rousseaux CG, editors: *Handbook of toxicologic pathology*, New York, 1991, Academic Press.
23. Ellenhorn MJ, Barceloux DG: *Medical toxicology: diagnosis and treatment of human poisoning*, New York, 1988, Elsevier.
24. Gwaltney-Brant SM: *Toxicology of common household hazards*, Baltimore, MD, 2010, Proceedings of the CVC.
25. Challoner KR, McCarron MM: Ammonium nitrate cold pack ingestion, *J Emerg Med* 6(4):289–293, 1988.
26. US Consumer Product Safety Commission: *Expandable lunch boxes recalled by California Innovations due to freezer gel pack ingestion hazard*. Release #12–089, January 23, 2012. Retrieved February 2012 from http://www.cpsc.gov/cpscpub/prerel/prhtml12/12089.html?tab=recalls.
27. Cope RB: Four new small animal toxicoses, *Aust Vet Practit* 34:121–123, 2004.
28. Lubich C, Mrvos R, Krenzelok: Beware of canine Gorilla Glue ingestions, *Vet Hum Toxicol* 46:153–154, 2004.

29. Aragon CL, Hofmeister EH, Budsberg SC: Systematic review of clinical trials of treatments for osteoarthritis in dogs, *J Am Vet Med Assoc* 230(4):514–521, 2007.
30. American Society for the Prevention of Cruelty to Animals Animal Poison Control Center database (unpublished data), 2009.
31. Khan SA, McLean MK, Gwaltney-Brant S: Accidental overdosage of joint supplements in dogs, *J Am Vet Med Assoc* 236(5):509–510, 2010.
32. Barr JM, Khan SA, McCullough SM, et al: Hypernatremia secondary to homemade play dough ingestion in dogs: a review of 14 cases from 1998-2001, *J Vet Emer Critical Care* 14(3):196–202, 2004.
33. Donaldson CW: Paintball toxicosis in dogs, *Vet Med* 98:995–997, 2003.
34. Thompson LJ: Sodium chloride (salt). *Veterinary toxicology: basic and clinical principles*, New York, 2007, Academic Press.
35. Duncan KL, Hare WR, Buck WB: Malignant hyperthermia-like reaction secondary to ingestion of hops in five dogs, *J Am Vet Med Assoc* 210(1):51–54, 1997.
36. Talcott PA: *Foods, medications and other household hazards your pet should avoid*, Las Vegas, 2008, Proceedings of the Western Veterinary Conference.
37. Brutlag AG, Flint CTC, Puschner B: Iron intoxication in a dog consequent to the ingestion of oxygen absorber sachets in pet treat packaging, *J Med Toxicol* 8(1):76–79, 2012.
38. Tseng YJ, Chen CH, Chen WK, Dong-Zong H: Hand warmer related corrosive injury, *Clin Toxicol* 39(9):870–871, 2011.
39. Cassel CA: *HeatMax product information material safety data sheet*. Myers Custom Supply, retrieved January 2012 from http//www.heatmax.info.
40. Tam AY, Chan YC, Lau FL: A case series of accidental ingestion of hand warmer, *Clin Toxicol* 46(9):900–904, 2008.
41. Hooser SB: Iron. *Veterinary toxicology: basic and clinical principles*, New York, 2007, Academic Press.
42. Gwaltney-Brant SM, Rumbeiha WK: Newer antidotal therapies, *Vet Clin North Am Small Anim Pract* 32(2):323–339, 2002.
43. Griffith EA, Fallgatter KC, Tantama SS, Tanen DA, Matteucci MJ: Effect of deferasirox on iron absorption in a randomized, placebo-controlled, crossover study in a human model of acute supratherapeutic iron ingestion, *Ann Emerg Med* 58(1):69–73, 2011.
44. Rhyee SH, Heard K: Acute barium toxicity from ingestion of "snake" fireworks, *J Med Toxicol* 5(4):209–213, 2009.
45. Villar D, Carson TL, Osweiler G, Bryan R: Overingestion of methionine tablets by a dog, *Vet Hum Toxicol* 45(6):311–312, 2003.
46. Plumb DC: *Veterinary drug handbook*, Ames, Iowa, 2002, Iowa State University Press.
47. Xia Z, He Y, Yu J: Experimental acute toxicity of xylitol in dogs, *J Vet Pharmacol Ther* 32(5):465–469, 2009.
48. Dunayer EK: New findings on the effects of xylitol ingestion in dogs, *Vet Med* 101:791–796, 2006.
49. Dunayer EK: Hypoglycemia following canine ingestion of xylitol-containing gum, *Vet Hum Toxicol* 46:87–88, 2004.
50. Cope RB: A screening study of xylitol binding in vitro to activated charcoal, *Vet Hum Toxicol* 46:336–337, 2004.
51. Fawcett A, Phillips A, Malik R: Hypoglycaemia and acute hepatic failure associated with accidental xylitol ingestion in a dog, *Aust Vet Pract* 40(4):142–147, 2010.
52. Kore AM, Kiesche-Nesselrodt A: Toxicology of household cleaning products and disinfectants, *Vet Clin North Am Small Anim Pract* 20:525–537, 1990.
53. Owens JG, Dorman DC: Common household hazards for small animals, *Vet Med* 92:140–148, 1997.

"Recreational" Drugs

Petra A. Volmer, DVM, MS, DABVT, DABT

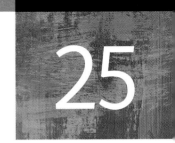

25

- Many illicit drug preparations contain impurities that can confuse the clinical picture.
- **Amphetamines** are commonly prescribed for the treatment of obesity, narcolepsy, and attention deficit disorder in humans.
  - They are highly toxic, rapidly absorbed, and eliminated in the urine.
  - Treatment is aimed at controlling seizures and cardiac arrhythmias and promoting elimination.
- **Barbiturates** are used therapeutically as sedatives and anticonvulsants and for the induction of anesthesia.
  - They tend to be lipophilic drugs that readily enter the central nervous system (CNS) to produce sedation.
  - Treatment is aimed at maintaining respiratory function and enhancing elimination with repeated doses of activated charcoal.
- The **benzodiazepines** are used as sedatives, antianxiety agents, and anticonvulsants.
  - They are well absorbed orally, are metabolized in the liver, and can produce active metabolites.
  - Most exposures can be treated with good supportive care. Flumazenil is a specific benzodiazepine antagonist that is effective in cases of extreme CNS depression.
- **Cocaine** has very restrictive medical uses, and most exposures are due to access to illicit supplies.
  - It is highly toxic, well absorbed orally, and excreted in the urine.
  - Treatment is aimed at stabilizing the neurologic and cardiac systems and at maintaining acid-base status.
- **Lysergic acid diethylamide** (LSD) is rapidly absorbed, metabolized in the liver, and excreted in the bile.
  - Treatment is symptomatic. Most exposures are self-limiting, requiring no medical intervention.
- The active ingredient in **marijuana** is delta-9-tetrahydrocannabinol, which has a wide safety margin.
  - Exposures are rarely fatal, and treatment is symptomatic and supportive. IV lipid therapy might be tried.
- **Phencyclidine** can be easily and cheaply synthesized.
  - It is well absorbed from the alkaline intestinal environment and undergoes extensive enterohepatic recirculation, prolonging its half-life.

- Phencyclidine can produce unpredictable clinical effects, and treatment is symptomatic. Activated charcoal is effective in decreasing the half-life and enhancing elimination.
- **Opioids** cause CNS and respiratory depression in dogs; they can have a stimulatory effect in cats.
  - Individual agents can act as agonists, partial agonists, or antagonists at opioid receptors.
  - Treatment is aimed at preventing CNS and respiratory depression. Naloxone is a specific opioid antagonist that has no agonistic activity and can be used to reverse opioid-induced respiratory and CNS depression.
- The **tricyclic antidepressants** can be lethal at doses of 15 mg/kg or more.
  - They are rapidly absorbed and metabolized in the liver and undergo enterohepatic recirculation. Their half-lives can be quite variable and long.
  - Treatment is aimed at preventing seizures and cardiac toxicity. Activated charcoal interrupts enterohepatic recirculation, and intravenous (IV) sodium bicarbonate has been shown to reduce cardiac toxicity.

Although animal exposures to human "drugs of abuse" do not occur frequently in veterinary medicine, most such exposures are emergency situations. Owners are often reluctant to admit the possibility of illicit drug exposure until the animal is in severe distress. The veterinary clinician should be familiar with the most common drugs of abuse, clinical courses, and treatments. It is important to remember that most "street" drugs are not pure and may contain combinations of drugs, thereby confusing the clinical picture. Because of the surge of recreational drug use and the addictive properties of many of these agents in humans, most of these compounds have been closely regulated. A thorough history of federal drug regulation can be found on the United States Drug Enforcement Agency (DEA) website at http://www.usdoj.gov/dea/pubs/history/.[1] A brief synopsis follows.

In response to America's increasing drug problem, in 1968 the Bureau of Narcotic and Dangerous Drugs (BNDD) was formed by merging the Bureau of Narcotics (under the Treasury Department) with the Bureau of Drug Abuse Control (under the Department of Health, Education, and Welfare). The new agency, BNDD, was placed under the Department of Justice and became the primary drug law enforcement agency overseeing international and interstate drug activities.

In 1970 the Controlled Substances Act (CSA) was passed by Congress. It went into effect in 1971, was enforced by the BNDD, and ultimately replaced more than 50 pieces of drug legislation. This law established a single system of control for narcotic and psychotropic drugs for the first time in U.S. history. It also established five schedules classifying controlled substances according to how dangerous they are, their potential for abuse and addiction, and whether they possess legitimate medical value. The CSA, although amended on several occasions, has remained the legal framework from which the DEA has derived its authority.

A lack of coordination, communication, and cooperation among the various entities involved in drug control (including the BNDD, U.S. Customs Service, Office for Drug Abuse Law Enforcement, and the Office of National Narcotics Intelligence) prompted President Richard Nixon in 1973 to declare "an all-out global war on the drug menace." Reorganization Plan No. 2 was sent to Congress and resulted in the establishment of the DEA within the Department of Justice. This move consolidated drug enforcement operations and placed a single administrator in charge of federal drug enforcement.

The DEA specifies schedules for each controlled substance and assigns them to a schedule depending on their abuse potential. A summary of the regulatory aspects of addictive and abused drugs follows.[2]

Schedule I (C-I) drugs have a high abuse potential and are not currently accepted in the United States for use in any practice situation, although they may be obtained for research or instructional use. Examples include heroin, lysergic acid diethylamide (LSD), mescaline, dihydromorphine, and morphine methyl sulfonate.

Schedule II (C-II) drugs have a high abuse potential. Their use can produce severe psychic or physical dependence in humans, and they apparently have similar effects in animals. Examples include opium, morphine, codeine, methadone, meperidine (Demerol), cocaine, phenmetrazine (Preludin), methylphenidate (Ritalin), methaqualone (Quaalude), amobarbital (Amytal), pentobarbital (Nembutal), and secobarbital (Seconal).

Schedule III (C-III) drugs have less abuse potential than those in the previous two schedules. These drugs produce moderate or low physical dependence but often induce high psychologic dependence in humans. They include nalorphine, benzphetamine, paregoric, and some barbiturates.

Schedule IV (C-IV) drugs have a low abuse potential that can lead to limited physical or psychological dependence in humans. Examples include barbital, phenobarbital, methyl phenobarbital, chloral hydrate, ethinamate, meprobamate, chlordiazepoxide (Librium), and diazepam (Valium).

Schedule V (C-V) drugs have the lowest abuse potential.

Amphetamines

Sources

The amphetamine class of drugs consists of a number of derivative molecules that are structurally related to the parent compound amphetamine. Amphetamine is the common name for alpha-methylphenylethylamine, and is a member of the family of phenylethylamines. Numerous substitutions are possible, resulting in a number of amphetamine analogues. They are subject to close regulation under the federal CSA of 1970. Amphetamine itself is no longer used in veterinary medicine. Before the CSA was passed, amphetamine was used as a central nervous system (CNS) and respiratory stimulant in dogs to overcome the depressant effects of barbiturates.[2]

There are a large number of legitimate amphetamine pharmaceuticals that contain various amphetamine analogues. They are indicated for the treatment of obesity, attention deficit disorder, and narcolepsy in humans. By far, most small animal exposures occur as accidental ingestions of these prescribed medications. Table 25-1 lists the most commonly prescribed amphetamines, their trade names, and therapeutic uses. Illegal amphetamine production also occurs in clandestine laboratories. Some street names include "speed," "uppers," "dex," "dexies," and "bennies" for amphetamine,[4] "ice" and "glass" for the clear, translucent crystals of methamphetamine, and "crystal," "crank," and "meth" for the white or yellow powder form of methamphetamine.[4] Designer amphetamines include 4-methylaminorex ("ice," "U4EUh"), 3,4-methylenedioxymethamphetamine ("ecstasy," "XTC," "Adam," "MDA"), 3,4-methylenedioxy-N-ethylamphetamine ("Eve"), and methcathinone ("cat").[5] Methylphenidate (Ritalin) has become an increasingly popular stimulant in college students studying for exams. The U.S. DEA reports methylphenidate as one of the most frequently stolen medications.[6] Psychoactive "bath salts" have become popular in recent years. The ingredients in these synthetic designer drugs are not chemically related to any detergent or soap, but are stimulant compounds claiming to produce an amphetamine-like high. These products can contain 3,4-methylenedioxypyrovalerone or 4-methylmethcathinone (mephedrone) under the street names "White Rush," "Cloud Nine," "Ivory Wave," or "Vanilla Sky."[7,8]

Table 25-1   Some Prescription Amphetamine Products, Their Trade Names, and Therapeutic Uses

Compound	Trade Name	Therapeutic Uses
Amphetamine (C-II)	Benzedrine	CNS stimulant
Benzphetamine (C-III)	Didrex	Anorexiant
Dextroamphetamine (C-II)	Dexedrine	Narcolepsy, ADD, anorexiant
Diethylpropion (C-IV)	Tenuate, Tenuate Dospan (long acting)	Anorexiant
Fenfluramine (C-IV)	Pondimin	Anorexiant
Mazindol (C-IV)	Mazanor, Sanorex	Anorexiant
Methamphetamine (C-II)	Desoxyn, Methampex, Desoxyn Gradumets (long acting)	ADD, anorexiant
Methylphenidate (C-II)	Ritalin, Ritalin SR	ADD, narcolepsy
Pemoline (C-IV)	Cylert	ADD
Phendimetrazine (C-III)	Bontril-PDM, Wehless, Metra Phenzine, Plegine, Statobex Prelu-2, Adipost, PT-105, Melfiat-105 Unicelles, Timecells (long acting)	Anorexiant
Phenmetrazine (C-II)	Preludin	Anorexiant
Phentermine (C-IV)	Fastin, Adipex-P, Ionamin, Termene, Phentrol, Obermine Phentride, Obestin-30 Obephen, T-Diet, Dapex, Obenix	Anorexiant
Dextroamphetamine and amphetamine	Adderall	ADD, anorexiant
Fenfluramine and phentermine	"Fen-Phen"*	Anorexiant

ADD, Attention deficit disorder; CNS, central nervous system.

*Marketing was discontinued in 1997 because of the associated incidence of cardiac valvulopathy.[3]

Toxic Dose

The oral median lethal dose (LD_{50}) for amphetamine sulfate in the dog is 20 to 27 mg/kg, and for methamphetamine hydrochloride it is 9 to 11 mg/kg.[9] The IV LD_{50} for amphetamine in the dog is 5.85 mg/kg.[10] Death from methamphetamine has been reported in humans at a dose of 1.5 mg/kg.[11]

Toxicokinetics

In general, amphetamines are well absorbed orally with peak plasma levels occurring by 1 to 3 hours. Sustained-release preparations have a slower rate of absorption, and peak levels are delayed. Amphetamines are highly lipophilic, readily crossing the blood-brain barrier.[4] They undergo hepatic metabolism, and both unchanged amphetamine and its metabolites are excreted in the urine. Some metabolites may be pharmacologically active.[4] Renal excretion of unchanged amphetamine is pH dependent, with an acidic urine greatly enhancing elimination.[4,12] The half-life in humans with a urine pH of less than 6.6 is 7 to 14 hours, whereas it is 18 to 34 hours in those with a urine pH of greater than 6.7.[13] A study in dogs demonstrated a half-life of 6.13 hours at a urine pH of 7.5 and 3.67 hours at a urine pH of 5.96.[14]

Mechanism of Toxicity

The exact mechanism for the CNS effects of the amphetamines is unknown, but they have a stimulant effect on the cerebral cortex, on the reticular-activating system,[12] and on the medullary respiratory center.[15] Peripherally, amphetamines cause release of norepinephrine from adrenergic nerve terminals and have a direct stimulant effect on α-adrenergic and β-adrenergic receptors.[12] They are also inhibitors of monoamine oxidase, thus depressing catecholamine metabolism.[15] Amphetamine is a dopamine excitatory receptor agonist and can be blocked centrally by phenothiazine derivatives that have dopamine excitatory receptor antagonism.[16]

Clinical Signs

Signs expected following exposure to an amphetamine include hyperactivity, restlessness, mydriasis, hypersalivation, vocalization, tachypnea, tremors, hyperthermia, ataxia, seizures, and tachycardia. Some animals exhibit depression, weakness, and bradycardia.

Minimum Database

The minimum database should include a serum chemistry profile and blood gas analysis in symptomatic animals to determine acid-base status, electrolyte abnormalities, and the extent of hypoglycemia. The cardiac rate and rhythm should be monitored for tachyarrhythmias. Animals should also be observed for signs of CNS stimulation and hyperthermia.

Confirmatory Tests

Amphetamines can be detected in blood, urine, and saliva. Consultation with a diagnostic toxicologist is recommended before sample collection and submission.

Treatment and Prognosis

For recent exposures (less than 30 minutes) emesis can be induced and activated charcoal administered. The animal should then be monitored closely for signs of amphetamine toxicosis. For extremely large ingestions or for animals exhibiting clinical signs, gastric lavage followed by activated charcoal is indicated. Sustained-release preparations may require repeated doses of activated charcoal.

Seizures have been successfully controlled with diazepam, pentobarbital, or propofol. However, benzodiazepines may paradoxically exacerbate the neurologic effects from amphetamines and are generally not recommended. Chlorpromazine given IV at 10 to 18 mg/kg prevented lethal effects of amphetamine in experimentally dosed dogs[17] and has also been recommended for controlling CNS excitation and seizures because of its dopamine excitatory receptor antagonist properties.[16] Phenothiazines should be used with the knowledge that they may lower the seizure threshold. Hyperthermia should be corrected using cool IV fluids, ice packs, fans, or cool-water baths. Animals should be closely monitored to prevent subsequent hypothermia.

Tachyarrhythmias can be controlled with a beta blocker, such as propranolol or metoprolol. Ventricular dysrhythmias can be treated with lidocaine.

IV fluids are necessary to maintain renal function and promote elimination of amphetamines. Urinary acidification using ascorbic acid or ammonium chloride has been shown to enhance the elimination of amphetamine,[13] but this procedure is contraindicated if the patient's acid-base status cannot be closely monitored or if myoglobinuria is present. Intense muscle activity caused by tremors or seizures can result in a metabolic acidosis and rhabdomyolysis. Fluid diuresis will help to prevent acute renal failure from myoglobinuria secondary to rhabdomyolysis, which is very rare but can occur. IV lipid therapy can possibly be considered with the more lipophilic compounds.

Prognosis depends on the severity and duration of clinical signs at presentation. Trauma, hypoxia, hyperthermia, or cerebral edema can result from uncontrolled seizure activity. Renal failure can result from myoglobinuria (rare) and acidosis.

Differential Diagnoses

Other agents that can cause CNS stimulation should be included in the differential diagnosis list. These include methylxanthines, metaldehyde, tremorgenic mycotoxins, pseudoephedrine, strychnine, tricyclic antidepressants, permethrin (cats), 5-fluorouracil, organochlorine insecticides, organophosphorus and carbamate insecticides, 4-aminopyridine, sodium ion toxicosis, lead, and herbal preparations containing ma huang, guarana root, or ephedra.

Barbiturates

Sources

The barbiturates as a class are barbituric acid derivatives. Barbituric acid itself has no CNS activity. Various side chain substitutions on barbituric acid influence the particular barbiturate's lipophilicity, potency, and rate of elimination. The barbiturates are used therapeutically as sedatives and anticonvulsants and to induce anesthesia. Barbiturate use has declined in favor of safer alternatives, such as the benzodiazepines.[18] The barbiturates have been classified as ultrashort-, short-, intermediate-, or long-acting based on their duration of action (0.3, 3, 3 to 6, and 6 to 12 hours, respectively).[19] Table 25-2 lists the most common barbiturate preparations, trade names, and classifications based on duration of action. Primidone is a phenobarbital congener that is metabolized to produce phenobarbital and phenylethylmalonamide. The parent compound and its metabolites have anticonvulsant activity.

Most small-animal exposures occur as a result of accidental ingestion of human or veterinary prescription preparations. However, toxicoses have also resulted from iatrogenic overdose, ingestion of illicit preparations (known as "downers," "reds," "Christmas trees," and "dolls"),[10] accidental administration of euthanasia solutions, and ingestion of tissue of euthanized animals.[20,21] Barbiturates can persist in euthanized carcasses for months and even years depending on environmental conditions. The barbiturate found in most euthanasia solutions is pentobarbital. Table 25-3 lists some commonly used euthanasia solutions and their active ingredients. Recently the Food and Drug Administration's Center for Veterinary Medicine added an environmental warning to labels of pentobarbital-containing euthanasia solutions.[22] Veterinarians and animal owners are responsible for proper disposal of euthanized carcasses. Accidental poisoning of wildlife that scavenge euthanized carcasses may result in criminal penalties for the animal owner and veterinarian.[23,24]

Table 25-2 Some Pharmaceutical Barbiturates Classified According to Duration of Action

Barbiturate	Trade Names	Classification
Thiamylal (C-III)	Surital, Bio-Tal	Ultrashort
Thiopental (C-III)	Pentothal	Ultrashort
Methohexital (C-IV)	Brevital	Ultrashort
Pentobarbital (C-II)	Nembutal	Short
Secobarbital (C-II)	Seconal	Short
Butabarbital (C-III)	Buticaps, Butisol, Barbased, Butalan, Sarisol	Intermediate
Amobarbital (C-II)	Amytal	Intermediate
Mephobarbital (C-IV)	Mebaral	Long
Phenobarbital (C-IV)	Luminal, Solfoton, Barbital	Long
Amobarbital and secobarbital (C-II for combination)	Tuinal	Short

Toxic Dose

The oral LD_{50} for phenobarbital in the dog is 150 mg/kg; the minimum published oral lethal dose (LD_{LO}) for phenobarbital in the cat is 125 mg/kg.[10]

Toxicokinetics

The barbiturates are well absorbed orally or following intramuscular (IM) injection. The sodium salts are more rapidly absorbed than the free acids. Lipid solubility of the drug determines distribution of the barbiturate in the body and thus the duration of action. Short-acting barbiturate anesthetics (e.g., thiamylal) are highly lipid soluble, are distributed into all body tissues (including the brain) very rapidly, and then are redistributed very rapidly into fat and total body water. The anesthetic effect is terminated when the drug exits the brain. Less lipophilic barbiturates enter and leave the brain more slowly, resulting in a more gradual onset and longer duration of action (e.g., phenobarbital). Because of the rapid distribution phase of the highly lipophilic anesthetic barbiturates, it is difficult to correlate true half-life with duration of action for these compounds.[19]

The barbiturates are metabolized in the liver by hepatic microsomal enzymes and both unchanged compound and metabolites are excreted in the urine. Acutely the barbiturates may bind to P450 enzymes and interfere with the metabolism of other compounds. Chronic use of barbiturates increases hepatic microsomal enzyme activity (e.g., enzyme induction) and can accelerate biotransformation of exogenous and some endogenous substances (e.g., steroids). In very young or very old animals or those with hepatic disease, metabolism of barbiturates may be slow, resulting in a prolonged half-life. Approximately 25% of phenobarbital is excreted unchanged in the urine. Urine alkalinization enhances phenobarbital excretion by ion trapping.[19] For phenobarbital, urinary alkalinization can increase excretion fivefold to tenfold. Urine alkalinization is ineffective for the short-acting barbiturates because they are more highly protein bound, have higher pKa values, and are primarily metabolized by the liver with very little urinary excretion.[25]

Table 25-3 Trade Names of Some Euthanasia Solutions and Their Active Ingredients

Trade Name	Active Ingredients (mg/mL)
Beuthanasia-D Special (C-III)	Pentobarbital sodium (390)
	Phenytoin sodium (50)
Euthanasia-6 (C-II)	Pentobarbital sodium (390)
Euthanasia solution (C-II)	Pentobarbital sodium (324)
Euthasol (C-III)	Pentobarbital sodium (390)
	Phenytoin sodium (50)
FP-3 (C-III)	Pentobarbital sodium (390)
	Lidocaine (20)
Pentobarbital sodium injection (C-II)	Pentobarbital sodium (390)
Repose (C-III)	Secobarbital (400)
	Dibucaine (25)
Sleepaway (C-II)	Pentobarbital sodium (260)
Socumb-6 Gr (C-II)	Pentobarbital (360)
Somlethol (C-II)	Pentobarbital sodium (389)
T-61*	Embutramide (200)
	Mebezonium (50)
	Tetracaine (5)
Uthol (C-II)	Pentobarbital sodium (324)

*T-61 was a widely used euthanasia solution and was not subject to the Controlled Substances Act of 1970. It contains no barbiturate but a narcotic analgesic (embutramide), a neuromuscular blocker to cause skeletal muscle relaxation (mebezonium), and a local anesthetic (tetracaine).

Mechanism of Toxicity

The barbiturates activate inhibitory γ-aminobutyric acid-a (GABA$_a$) receptors and inhibit excitatory glutamate receptors.[18] They can also inhibit the release of norepinephrine and acetylcholine.[26] They are considered CNS depressants, but in some patients they can produce excitement. High doses of barbiturates suppress the hypoxic drive and the chemoreceptor drive, resulting in respiratory depression. Anesthetic concentrations of barbiturates can depress sodium and potassium channels in the heart, and direct depression of cardiac contractility occurs at extremely high doses.[18] Severe oliguria or anuria may occur because of extreme hypotension in patients with acute barbiturate intoxication.

Clinical Signs

Clinical signs include depression, ataxia, incoordination, weakness, disorientation, recumbency, coma, hypothermia, tachycardia or bradycardia, and death.

Minimum Database

A complete blood count and chemistry profile should be performed, and acid-base status should be evaluated in patients exhibiting severe clinical signs. Cardiac and respiratory function should be evaluated.

Confirmatory Tests

Barbiturates can be detected in stomach contents, blood, urine, and feces. Consultation with a veterinary diagnostic toxicologist is recommended before sample collection and submission.

Treatment and Prognosis

For recent ingestions, emesis followed by repeated doses of activated charcoal and a cathartic should be administered. For animals exhibiting severe depression, emesis is contraindicated because of the risk of aspiration. In these cases, gastric lavage should be performed, followed by repeated doses of activated charcoal and a cathartic. Magnesium-containing cathartics (Epsom salts) should be avoided because magnesium may exacerbate CNS depression.[27] It has been shown that repeated doses of activated charcoal greatly reduce the plasma half-life of phenobarbital.[28-32] Activated charcoal acts as a "sink" to enhance diffusion of barbiturates from the circulation into the gastrointestinal tract, even for compounds given parenterally.[26]

Respiratory depression is the major cause of death, so initial treatment should include assessment of respiratory function. Intubation, administration of oxygen, and assisted ventilation may be required. Hypothermia is a common sequela in severely depressed animals and should be monitored and corrected. Cardiac monitoring is required because some barbiturates (e.g., thiopental sodium and thiamylal sodium) are arrhythmogenic.[27] Also, profound hypothermia resulting from barbiturate intoxication can cause ventricular fibrillation and cardiac arrest.[19]

Some barbiturates undergo hepatic metabolism with renal excretion, so increased renal blood flow with IV fluids may enhance elimination. Forced alkaline diuresis may promote removal of some barbiturates, especially phenobarbital, which is subject to ion trapping in the urine.[19] Intravenous lipid therapy might be considered in severely affected patients.

Differential Diagnoses

Other causes of CNS and respiratory depression should be included in the differential diagnosis. These include benzodiazepines, xylitol, macrolide antiparasiticides (e.g., ivermectin), encephalopathies, amitraz, ethanol, ethylene glycol, propylene glycol, diethylene glycol, methanol, isopropanol, acetone, phenothiazines, opioids, and hypoglycemia.

Benzodiazepines

Sources

The benzodiazepines are used as sedatives, antianxiety agents, and anticonvulsants. The first benzodiazepine, chlordiazepoxide, was synthesized by accident in 1961 by the laboratories

Table 25-4	Some Common Benzodiazepines and Their Trade Names
Compound	**Trade Name**
Alprazolam (C-IV)	Xanax
Chlordiazepoxide (C-IV)	Libritabs, Librium, Sereen
Clobazam (C-IV)	Frisium
Clonazepam (C-IV)	Klonopin
Clorazepate (C-IV)	Cloraze Caps, Cloraze Tabs, GenENE, Tranxene
Diazepam (C-IV)	Valium, Valrelease (sustained release)
Estazolam (C-IV)	ProSom
Flurazepam (C-IV)	Dalmane
Halazepam (C-IV)	Paxipam
Lorazepam (C-IV)	Ativan
Midazolam (C-IV)	Versed
Oxazepam (C-IV)	Serax
Quazepam (C-IV)	Doral
Temazepam (C-IV)	Restoril
Triazolam (C-IV)	Halcion
Zolazepam	Telazole (zolazepam in combination with tiletamine is Telazol)

of Hoffman La Roche.[33] The term *benzodiazepine* refers to the chemical structure of the compound: a benzene ring bound to a seven-member diazepine ring. Modifications in this structure have led to the development of a number of benzodiazepine derivatives that vary in therapeutic use and half-life. Table 25-4 lists some of the commonly used benzodiazepines and their trade names. All of the benzodiazepines are schedule C-IV drugs according to the CSA of 1970. Most small-animal exposures result from ingestion of prescription formulations. A very potent benzodiazepine, flunitrazepam (Rohypnol), has made its way into illicit use as a "date rape" drug. It produces sedation in humans within 20 to 30 minutes that may last for hours.[34]

Toxic Dose

The oral LD_{50} for diazepam in the rat is 249 mg/kg and for the mouse, 48 mg/kg. The IV LD_{50} in the rat and mouse is 32 and 25 mg/kg, respectively.[10] The oral LD_{50} of alprazolam in the rat and mouse is 1220 and 770 mg/kg, respectively.[10]

Toxicokinetics

The benzodiazepines are well absorbed from the gastrointestinal tract. They are highly lipid soluble and highly protein bound. The benzodiazepines are widely and rapidly distributed in brain, liver, and spleen and are then more slowly redistributed to more poorly perfused sites, such as adipose tissue and muscle.[35] Biotransformation occurs in the liver, and some benzodiazepines produce active metabolites with half-lives that exceed those of the parent compound. Conjugation with glucuronide occurs with elimination in the urine.[36] Benzodiazepines without major active metabolites include alprazolam, clonazepam, oxazepam, temazepam, and triazolam.[34,37]

The major metabolite of diazepam in the dog is nordiazepam. It is just as pharmacologically active on the CNS as diazepam.[38] The plasma half-life of diazepam following IV injection in the dog is 2.4 hours; the half-life of nordiazepam is 2.85 hours. In the cat, the mean elimination half-life of diazepam is 5.46 hours, and of nordiazepam it is 21.3 hours following IV administration.[38]

Mechanism of Toxicity

The benzodiazepines interact with benzodiazepine receptors that modulate GABA, an inhibitory neurotransmitter. Benzodiazepine receptors are widely distributed in the CNS but are also present in kidney, liver, heart, and lung.[38] The function of peripheral benzodiazepine receptors is unknown.[33] Of the GABA receptor subunits, $GABA_a$ appears to contain the benzodiazepine receptor, which is distinct from the GABA binding site. When benzodiazepines bind, gating for chloride channels is triggered, resulting in hyperpolarization of the cell and a decrease in neuronal excitation.[38] The effect on GABA appears to be the main mechanism by which benzodiazepines act, but a number of other neurotransmitters, including acetylcholine, catecholamines, serotonin, and glycine may be involved in benzodiazepine activity as well.[38]

Clinical Signs

The respiratory and cardiac effects of the benzodiazepines are minor in normal healthy individuals.[39] Clinical presentations can include ataxia, depression, disorientation, and incoordination. Severely depressed animals may become hypothermic. Extremely high doses can produce coma and even seizures. In some normal animals therapeutic doses of diazepam can produce excitation.[38] There have been reports of cats developing liver failure following exposure to oral formulations of diazepam.

Minimum Database

In animals exhibiting severe signs, body temperature and cardiac rate and rhythm should be monitored.

Confirmatory Tests

Benzodiazepines and their metabolites can be detected in blood and urine.[40] Consultation with a diagnostic toxicologist is recommended before sample collection and submission.

Treatment and Prognosis

Most benzodiazepine exposures can be treated with appropriate supportive care. In patients with recent ingestions, emesis should be induced, and activated charcoal with a cathartic should then be administered. If the animal is severely depressed, emesis is contraindicated because of the risk of aspiration. Most patients require no further treatment beyond gastric emptying, activated charcoal, and monitoring.[35] For patients exhibiting extreme CNS depression, the specific benzodiazepine antagonist flumazenil (Romazicon) can be administered at a dose of 0.1 mg/kg IV.[41] Flumazenil is a competitive benzodiazepine blocker with an average half-life in humans of approximately 1 hour.[35] Because of the short half-life of flumazenil compared with those of most of the benzodiazepines or their active metabolites, animals should be closely monitored and flumazenil repeated if clinical signs recur. Body temperature should be monitored and corrected. For the highly fat-soluble compounds, IV lipid therapy might be considered in severely affected patients.

Differential Diagnoses

Barbiturates, opioids, ethanol, ethylene glycol, propylene glycol, diethylene glycol, methanol, macrolide parasiticides (e.g., ivermectin), amitraz, phenothiazines, isopropanol, acetone, xylitol, hypoglycemia, and encephalopathies should be included in the differential diagnosis.

Cocaine

Sources

Cocaine is a natural alkaloid that is derived from the leaves of *Erythroxylon coca*. This shrub grows predominantly in Mexico, South America, the West Indies, and Indonesia.[42] Colombia produces approximately 75% of the world's cocaine from cocaine base that is imported from Peru and Bolivia or produced locally in Colombia.[6] Cocaine is a schedule II drug and, as such, is under very strict control according to the CSA of 1970. Medical uses are restricted to topical administration as a local anesthetic on the mucous membranes of the oral, laryngeal, and nasal cavities. It can also be used diagnostically to ascertain the cause of a miotic pupil (i.e., Horner's syndrome). Most exposures in small animals are due to ingestions of illicit cocaine supplies.

Cocaine is often adulterated with inert substances used to dilute it (e.g., lactose, inositol, mannitol, cornstarch, or sugar) or with active drugs, such as procaine, lidocaine, amphetamines, caffeine, heroin, phencyclidine, ergot, or strychnine.[6,42] There are two main forms of cocaine: the hydrochloride salt and "free base." The hydrochloride salt is the powdered form of cocaine and readily dissolves in water. It can be taken intravenously or intranasally. Free base is the conversion of the hydrochloride form to the pure cocaine alkaloid resulting in flakes, crystals, or a rock form that makes a popping or cracking sound when heated (i.e., "crack," "rock," or "flake").[6,42] It readily vaporizes rather than burns and so can be smoked. It can also be taken orally. It is lipophilic and crosses alveolar-capillary and blood-brain barriers.[42] Street names for cocaine powder include "bernies," "coke," "girl," "gold dust," "star dust,"[43] "snow," "C," "white girl," "leaf," "blow," "nose candy," "her," and "white lady."[6,44]

Toxic Dose

The LD_{50} for pure cocaine in the dog is 13 mg/kg IV, and orally in the mouse it is 99 mg/kg.[10] The lowest published lethal dose in the dog is 3.5 mg/kg subcutaneously (SC); in the cat it is 7.5 mg/kg IV and 16 mg/kg SC.[10]

Toxicokinetics

Cocaine is well absorbed from all mucosal surfaces. Peak plasma concentrations in humans can occur 15 to 120 minutes following nasal mucosal application, but peak concentrations can occur sooner following administration by the oral route.[45] Inflamed or irritated surfaces enhance absorption. Cocaine is hydrolyzed by serum esterases and undergoes demethylation in the liver. Cocaine and its metabolites are excreted in the urine. Less than 10% to 20% is excreted unchanged in the urine.

Mechanism of Toxicity

Cocaine is a strong CNS stimulant because of its sympathomimetic effects. It blocks the reuptake of norepinephrine and serotonin at adrenergic nerve terminals, resulting in an excess of neurotransmitters at receptor sites. In addition it sensitizes sympathetic effector cells to give an exaggerated response to catecholamines (i.e., tachycardia).[43] IV injection of cocaine in dogs causes significant increases in mean arterial pressure, heart rate, cardiac output, and body temperature, and a significant decrease in arterial pH.[46] Conduction disturbances, coronary vasospasm and hypoxia, and a direct toxic effect on the myocardium may all be involved to produce cardiac arrest.[47-49]

Clinical Signs

Signs expected following cocaine ingestion in animals include hyperactivity, ataxia, mydriasis, vomiting, hypersalivation, tremors, seizures, tachycardia, and tachypnea.

Minimum Database

A serum chemistry profile and blood gas analysis should be performed immediately to determine the patient's electrolyte and acid-base status. Monitoring of cardiac rate and rhythm and body temperature is required.

Confirmatory Tests

Cocaine can be detected in serum and plasma, stomach contents, and urine.[49,50] Consultation with the diagnostic laboratory is recommended before sample collection and submission.

Treatment and Prognosis

Treatment is aimed at decontamination, stabilizing the neurologic and cardiac systems, and maintaining acid-base status.

Acute ingestions in animals not exhibiting clinical signs should be managed by inducing vomiting immediately. Because cocaine is rapidly absorbed, and clinical signs can become severe in a short time, induction of emesis should be undertaken with caution. The stimulation of inducing emesis in a symptomatic animal may precipitate a seizure, resulting in aspiration. Sedation and gastric lavage followed by administration of activated charcoal may be a better alternative.

The initial drug of choice for tremors and seizures is diazepam. For refractory seizures a barbiturate may be required. Chlorpromazine given before treatment (12 mg/kg IV) effectively antagonized the effects of cocaine in experimentally dosed dogs.[46] It reduced the severity of the seizures and maintained arterial pH and body temperature at predrug control levels. Because chlorpromazine is a phenothiazine tranquilizer, consideration must be given to the possibility of lowering the seizure threshold.

Life-threatening tachyarrhythmias should be treated with a beta blocker, such as propranolol. IV fluids maintain renal blood flow and promote diuresis. Acidosis should be monitored and treated with sodium bicarbonate. Hyperthermia can be corrected with cool IV fluids, cool water baths, and fans. Close monitoring is necessary to prevent the occurrence of hypothermia once excess muscle activity has been controlled.

Differential Diagnoses

Amphetamines, pseudoephedrine, caffeine, chocolate, metaldehyde, permethrin (in cats), organophosphorus and carbamate insecticides, chlorinated hydrocarbons, epilepsy, strychnine, lead, tremorgenic mycotoxins, and herbal preparations containing ma huang, ephedra, or guarana root should be on the differential diagnosis list.

Lysergic Acid Diethylamide (LSD)

Sources

The synthesis of LSD was the result of research with the ergot alkaloids derived from *Claviceps purpurea*.[51] The Swiss chemist Albert Hofmann accidentally discovered its hallucinogenic properties when he unintentionally was exposed via the topical route.[51] LSD was marketed by Sandoz under the trade name Delysid in 1947. In the 1950s LSD was used experimentally as a model for schizophrenia and as an aid in analytical psychotherapy. It was thought that LSD could aid the patient in releasing repressed information. The Central Intelligence Agency experimented with the use of LSD as a mind-control agent and as a tool for interrogating suspected criminals.[51] In the 1960s LSD became popular as a recreational drug and was banned by federal law in 1966. LSD is classified as a schedule I agent with high abuse potential. There is a lack of established safety data for LSD, even under medical supervision, and there is no known use of LSD in medical treatment.[51]

LSD is a mixture of four stereoisomers: D-, L-, D-iso, and L-iso LSD. Only the D-LSD isomer has hallucinogenic activity. It is a water-soluble, colorless, tasteless, and odorless powder. LSD is taken orally in capsules or applied to a variety of ingestible substances.[52] It is typically sold as liquid-impregnated blotter paper, microdots, tiny tablets, and "window-pane" gelatin squares.[6,51] Street names for LSD include "acid," "blotter acid," "cubes," "dots," "heavenly blue," "microdot," "pearly gates," "royal blue," "sugar cubes," "trip," "pane," "window-pane," "window glass," and "wedding bells."[6,10] Lysergic acid hydroxyethylamide can be found in morning glory seeds and has one-tenth the potency of LSD.[51] The estimated human hallucinogenic dose is 200 to 300 seeds.[52] The intact seed coat prevents absorption, and so the seeds must be pulverized to release the toxin.[51] Animal exposures to LSD are uncommon.

Toxic Dose

The minimum oral toxic dose of LSD in humans ranges from 700 ng/kg to 2800 ng/kg.[10] The IV LD_{50} in the rat is 16 mg/kg.[10]

Toxicokinetics

LSD is rapidly absorbed following oral administration, and peak plasma levels occur within 30 minutes to 5 hours.[53] Plasma protein binding is more than 80%.[51] Effects in humans begin at 40 to 60 minutes, peak at 2 to 4 hours, and gradually return to baseline over 6 to 8 hours.[54] LSD is metabolized in the liver via hydroxylation and glucuronidation, and 80% is excreted in the bile to be eliminated in the feces.[53] The excreted metabolites are pharmacologically inactive.[51] The elimination half-life is between 2 and 5 hours.

Mechanism of Toxicity

The actual mechanism of action of LSD has not been clearly defined, and it appears to act at multiple sites in the CNS. However, research supports a common site of action at the central serotonin (5-hydroxytryptamine [5-HT]) receptors.[51] The 5-HT$_{2A}$ receptor is thought to modulate hallucinogens.[51] Other neurotransmitters may also be involved in hallucinations, in particular, glutamate and dopamine.[51] The effects can be either inhibitory or stimulatory. Consequently the clinical course of LSD exposure can be difficult to predict.

Clinical Signs

In humans LSD alters visual and sensory perception and can produce states of euphoria. During "bad trips," however, psychotic attacks and panic reactions can occur. It is not known if animals experience similar effects. Signs in animals may include disorientation, mydriasis, depression, excitation, and vocalization.

Confirmatory Tests

LSD can be detected in urine, serum,[55] and feces.[52] Testing only confirms exposure and is often quite difficult because LSD undergoes rapid metabolism. Most veterinary diagnostic laboratories are not prepared to analyze for LSD. The practitioner is encouraged to contact the laboratory's diagnostic toxicologist before sample collection and submission. Analysis at a human laboratory may be required.

Treatment and Prognosis

Treatment is symptomatic and supportive. Most cases of LSD ingestions are self-limiting and require no medical intervention.[52] Decontamination with activated charcoal is recommended before the onset of signs, but may worsen signs if already present. In humans gastric lavage is ineffective and may exacerbate psychotic reactions.[55] Diazepam can be used for extreme agitation, and the animal should be monitored for tachycardia and hyperthermia. Placing the animal in a dark, quiet environment is recommended. Excessive restraint should be avoided because of concerns for hyperthermia and rhabdomyolysis (rare, but may occur).[51]

Differential Diagnoses

Differential diagnoses include phencyclidine, marijuana, hallucinogenic mushrooms, stimulants, and depressants.

Marijuana

Sources

Crude marijuana consists of the dried and chopped stems, leaves, seeds, and flowers of the plant *Cannabis sativa* (Color Plate 25-1). The major active constituent in marijuana is delta-9-tetrahydrocannabinol (THC), although as many as 66 cannabinoids have been identified.[56] The concentration of THC found in plants depends on environmental conditions, including amounts of light, moisture, soil type, pH, nutrients, and trace elements. The amount of THC in a sample decreases with time.[57] In humans the most common routes of exposure are inhalation ("marijuana cigarettes," "joints," "reefers," and "bongs") and oral ("hash brownies").

Marijuana is often used in conjunction with other drugs, such as opium, alcohol, cocaine, heroin, phencyclidine, ketamine, and formaldehyde.[57] Most animal exposures occur as a result of ingestion of the owner's illicit supply, although secondhand smoke exposures can occur. It is becoming much more popular for pets to ingest "marijuana butter." Since the THC is fat soluble, it is becoming common practice to sautee the plant in butter so that the THC will leach into the butter (the plant material is ultimately strained out of the mixture). The butter can then be used in baking where food items can be ingested for the THC effect without experiencing the bitter/crunchy taste of the plant. In most areas of the country, possession of marijuana is illegal, but some states, such as California and Arizona, have allowed the medicinal use of crude marijuana under certain circumstances. However, in 1997 Arizona passed a law nullifying a physician's right to prescribe schedule I substances without federal approval.[56] Purified THC analogues are now available by prescription (dronabinol [Marinol]—schedule III, nabilone [Cesamet]—schedule II) for the treatment of nausea associated with cancer chemotherapy, appetite stimulation for acquired immune deficiency syndrome patients, glaucoma, and multiple sclerosis.[56,58] THC and crude marijuana are schedule I drugs under the CSA.[59] Attempts have been made to reclassify crude marijuana as a schedule II drug, but these have failed.[56,58]

Marijuana refers to any part of the plant. Some street names include "pot," "Mary Jane," "MJ," "weed," "grass," "puff," and "hemp."[58] Hashish is the dried resin from flower tops and can contain up to 10% or more THC. Hashish oil can contain up to 20% THC.[58] Sinsemilla is seedless marijuana with a THC content of around 5%. This form accounts for 85% of domestic production.[58]

In 2010 the popularity of synthetic marijuana surged. Marketed as designer marijuana and herbal incense, these combinations of potent synthetic cannabinoids were sold in gas stations and head shops under names such as "Spice," "K2," "Skunk," "Wild Greens," "Head Trip," "Purple Haze," and "Zombie Matter." Although labeled as "not for human consumption," smoking produced more severe effects than that of marijuana alone, including seizures, hallucinations, tremors, and paranoia, with resulting injury and death in users, prompting the passage of the Synthetic Drug Control Act of 2011.[60]

Toxic Dose

The minimum lethal oral dose in the dog for THC is greater than 3 g/kg.[61] This dose is 1000 times the behaviorally effective dose in the dog, indicating a wide safety margin for THC.[62]

Toxicokinetics

Oral absorption of THC, the most common route in animals, is increased with fatty foods, and the onset of effects begins within 30 to 60 minutes. In humans THC is 97% to 99% protein bound, and peak plasma levels occur within 2 to 3 hours. THC is highly lipid soluble and is distributed into body fat, liver, brain, and kidney. It is rapidly metabolized in the liver; 11-hydroxy-delta-9-THC is the primary metabolite. It is more potent than THC and readily crosses the blood-brain barrier.[63] Ten percent to 15% of THC or its metabolites is excreted in the urine, and the remainder is eliminated in the feces through biliary excretion. It is enterohepatically recirculated.[57] Because of its high lipid solubility, THC has a very short initial plasma half-life. Adipose storage produces a biological half-life of 25 to 30 hours.[64] Nabilone, a THC analogue, has a half-life of 2 hours for the parent compound and 35 hours for its metabolites.[64]

Mechanism of Toxicity

Two cannabinoid receptors have been identified: CB1 and CB2. CB1's wide distribution in the brain correlates well with the cannabinoid effects on memory, perception, and control of movement.[63] CB2 has not been detected in the CNS and is restricted to the periphery. This distribution suggests a potential analgesic effect for THC.[57] Both CB1 and CB2 receptors have been identified in immune cells and modulate the effect of THC on the immune response.[57]

Clinical Signs

The most common signs reported in dogs include depression, ataxia or incoordination, hypermetria, urinary incontinence, vomiting, tremor, mydriasis, hypothermia, weakness, bradycardia, disorientation, and hypersalivation.[65] Other possible signs include stupor, nystagmus, tachycardia, hyperexcitability, apprehension, tachypnea, hyperthermia, and vocalization.

Minimum Database

Body temperature and cardiac rate and rhythm are usually the only signs that must be monitored.

Confirmatory Tests

Stomach contents and urine can be tested for cannabinoids. Because of their lipophilicity and enterohepatic recirculation, urine levels can remain detectable for several days following acute exposure.[66] Consultation with the diagnostic laboratory before sample collection and submission is recommended. It is common to see false negatives with store-bought drug kits that test for marijuana in human urine.

Treatment and Prognosis

Treatment is primarily symptomatic and supportive. Because of the wide margin of safety of the cannabinoids, toxicosis is rarely fatal. Emesis should be induced following an acute ingestion. Repeated doses of activated charcoal and a cathartic may reduce the half-life of THC by interrupting enterohepatic recirculation. If signs of CNS stimulation occur, treat with a benzodiazepine. Body temperature must be closely monitored and corrected if abnormal. Recovery may take 24 to 72 hours, or longer (up to 5 days), depending on the dose ingested. IV lipid therapy might be considered in severely affected patients.

Differential Diagnoses

Opioids, LSD, phencyclidine hydrochloride (PCP), ethanol, tranquilizers, ethylene glycol, propylene glycol, diethylene glycol, methanol, isopropanol, acetone, macrolide parasiticides (e.g., ivermectin), xylitol, depressants, muscle relaxants, and hallucinogenic mushrooms can cause similar clinical signs.

Opioids

Sources

Opium is the dried milky exudate derived from the unripe seed capsules of the poppy plant, *Papaver somniferum*.[67] Opium contains 24 alkaloids including morphine, codeine, and thebaine (dimethylmorphine).[67] Raw opium consists of at least 10% morphine, but variability exists by growing region.[68] Laudanum is the deodorized tincture of opium, and paregoric is the camphorated tincture of opium.[68] The opioids have found great use medicinally for their analgesic properties and recreationally for their psychoactive effects. In 1914 because of concerns regarding addiction and toxicity, the Harrison Narcotic Act was enacted to make the nonmedical use of opioids illegal. The opioids are classified as agonists, partial agonists, or antagonists based on their ability to bind and exert pharmacologic effects at the various opioid receptors (Table 25-5). Most animal exposures occur as a result of oral exposures to pharmaceutical preparations; however, malicious exposures sometimes occur (i.e., a case involving a suicidal heroin addict who injected her dog before herself).

Toxic Dose

The minimum lethal subcutaneous dose in the dog for morphine is 210 mg/kg, and in the cat, 40 mg/kg.[10] The IV LD_{50} for morphine in the dog is 133 mg/kg.[10] The oral LD_{50} for morphine in the rat is 335 mg/kg, and in the mouse, 524 mg/kg.[10] The minimum lethal dose

Table 25-5	Some Opioid Agonists, Partial Agonists, and Antagonists and Their Classification According to the Controlled Substance Act*
Agonists	**Schedule Classification**
Opioid Agonists	
Alfentanil	C-II
Codeine	C-II
Diphenoxylate	C-V in combination
Etorphine	C-I
Fentanyl	C-II
Heroin	C-I
Hydrocodone	C-II alone or C-III in combination
Hydromorphone	C-II
Levomethadyl acetate	C-II
Levorphanol	C-II
Loperamide	Not scheduled
Meperidine	C-II
Methadone	C-II
Morphine	C-II alone or C-III in combination
Opium	C-II alone or C-III or C-V in combination
Oxycodone	C-II
Oxymorphone	C-II
Propoxyphene	C-IV
Sufentanil	C-II
Partial Agonists	
Buprenorphine	C-V
Butorphanol	Not scheduled
Nalbuphine	Not scheduled
Pentazocine	C-IV
Antagonists	
Diprenorphine	C-II
Nalorphine	C-III
Naloxone	Not scheduled
Naltrexone	Not scheduled
Nalmefene	Not scheduled

*Some drugs have received alternate scheduling status based on their use alone or in combination with other drugs (i.e., cold and flu preparations). Etorphine and its antagonist, diprenorphine, are approved in the United States for use in wild or exotic species.[67]

for heroin in the dog is 25 mg/kg SC, and in the cat, is 20 mg/kg orally.[10] The IV LD$_{50}$ for codeine in the dog is 69 mg/kg; the oral LD$_{50}$ for codeine in the rat is 427 mg/kg, and in the mouse, 250 mg/kg.[10]

Toxicokinetics

The opioids are well absorbed from the gastrointestinal tract and are rapidly metabolized in the liver. Most morphine-like drugs undergo significant first-pass metabolism and are markedly less potent when administered orally versus parenterally.[69] Morphine is approximately 33% protein bound. Morphine is conjugated with glucuronic acid to produce morphine-6-glucuronide, the major pharmacologically active metabolite.[70] Morphine-6-glucuronide is more active as an analgesic than morphine itself.[69] Codeine is metabolized to morphine, which accounts for its pharmacologic activity. Most morphine-6-glucuronide is excreted by the kidney; very little morphine is excreted unchanged. Some of the glucuronides are excreted in the bile and are hydrolyzed in the gut.[69] Enterohepatic recirculation of morphine and its glucuronide occurs.[70] Cats are deficient in glucuronyl-S-transferase, and this may account for their sensitivity to opioid compounds.

Mechanism of Toxicity

Four major opioid receptors have been identified (μ [mu], κ [kappa], δ [delta], and σ [sigma]) as well as other minor opioid receptor subtypes (ε- [epsilon], ζ [zeta]). Opioid receptors have been found in the central and autonomic nervous systems, gastrointestinal tract, heart, kidney, vas deferens, pancreas, fat cells, lymphocytes, and adrenal glands.[67] Opioids differ in their specificity and efficacy at different types of receptors. Some agents act as agonists at one type of receptor and as partial agonists or antagonists at another.[69] Most of the clinically useful opioids bind to μ receptors. The analgesic effects of morphine-like drugs are a result of binding to the μ_1 subtype, whereas the μ_2 subtype mediates respiratory depression.[67] Partial agonists have agonistic activity at one or more types of opioid receptors and antagonistic effects at others. Naloxone is the most commonly used antagonist. It is a pure competitive antagonist with no agonist activity and has a high affinity for the μ receptor.

Apomorphine is a morphine analogue. It is a rapidly acting emetic, which exerts its clinical effects through dopamine-2 receptor subtype agonism within the chemoreceptor trigger zone of the medulla.[68] Excessive doses may result in respiratory, cardiac, or CNS depression, and protracted vomiting. Naloxone may reverse the CNS and respiratory effects of the drug but is not expected to stop the vomiting.[71] Apomorphine is not scheduled.

Clinical Signs

Signs in dogs can include vomiting, defecation, salivation, CNS depression, miosis, and ataxia. In severe cases, respiratory depression, constipation, hypothermia, coma, seizures, and cyanosis can occur. Pulmonary edema is recognized as a possible sequela of opioid overdose in humans. Patients awakening from an opioid coma, either spontaneously or following administration of a reversal agent, may develop hypoxemia and pulmonary rales. It is not clear whether the pulmonary edema is a result of naloxone administration or if the administration of the reversal agent uncovered an acute lung injury.[68] Cats often exhibit excitatory behavior.[72]

Minimum Database

At a minimum, one should evaluate the respiratory function, body temperature, and blood gases of an exposed patient.

Confirmatory Tests

Morphine may be detected in urine or serum. Consultation with the diagnostic laboratory before submission is recommended.

Treatment and Prognosis

For recent ingestions with no clinical signs, vomiting should be induced and activated charcoal administered with a cathartic. The animal should be monitored for signs of CNS depression. Respiratory depression with resultant hypoxia is the most common cause of death in cases of opioid overdose. Establishment of a patent airway, assisted ventilation, and oxygen may be required. In animals exhibiting CNS or respiratory depression, naloxone at a dose of 0.01 to 0.04 mg/kg IV, IM, or SC is indicated.[73] Naloxone may have to be repeated because of its short half-life in relation to that of the opioids. It will reverse respiratory depression but may not restore full consciousness.[70] Naloxone has a high affinity for the μ receptor, but less for the other receptors. Larger doses are required to reverse the effects of pentazocine, propoxyphene, and buprenorphine, which also bind to κ and σ receptors.[74,75] Gastric lavage, activated charcoal, and a cathartic may be effective even several hours after exposure because pylorospasm is produced by the opioid, causing much of the drug to remain in the stomach.[76]

Differential Diagnoses

Barbiturates, ethanol, ethylene glycol, propylene glycol, diethylene glycol, methanol, iso-propanol, acetone, marijuana, amitraz, encephalopathies, macrolide parasiticides (e.g., ivermectin), benzodiazepines, xylitol, and phenothiazines should be included on the differential diagnosis list.

Phencyclidine and Ketamine

Sources

In the 1950s PCP (1-[1-phenylcyclohexyl] piperidine) was originally marketed for human anesthesia under the trade name Sernyl, but it was discontinued in 1965 because of a high incidence of postoperative psychoses and dysphoria. It was briefly reintroduced for veterinary anesthesia in 1967 as Sernylan but was quickly removed because of its emergence as a drug of abuse.[77] PCP is known for inducing violent rages, seizures, coma, and death.[6] It has been classified as a schedule II drug under the CSA. Phencyclidine can be easily and cheaply synthesized in clandestine laboratories and is available as a powder, tablet, crystal, or liquid. In its original state, PCP is a white crystalline powder. Its most popular form is a liquid mixture of PCP dissolved in formaldehyde and methanol ("embalming fluid").[6] Tobacco or marijuana cigarettes are dipped into the liquid and smoked. Some street names include "angel dust," "angel hair," "boat," "love boat," "dummy dust," "CJ," "embalming fluid," "hog," "hog dust," "jet fuel," "PCP," "PeaCe Pill," "rocket fuel," "super grass," "stardust," "whack," and "zombie dust."[6,77]

PCP has more than 60 analogues, including ketamine, a chloroketone analogue. Ketamine has approximately one-tenth to one-twentieth the potency of PCP. It has a much shorter duration of action and produces fewer seizures than PCP.[78] Like PCP, individuals anesthetized with ketamine feel detached or disconnected from their pain and environment. PCP and ketamine are therefore known as *dissociative anesthetics,* not *hallucinogens.* In addition, ketamine has both analgesic and amnesic properties.[6] Because of the greater control it provides in clinical use compared with PCP, ketamine is regularly used in human operating rooms, emergency departments, and veterinary clinics.[78] The pharmacologic properties that have made ketamine clinically popular account for its nonmedical popularity as a drug of abuse. Ketamine is not produced in clandestine laboratories as is PCP but is obtained illicitly from medical, dental, and veterinary sources and has been sold over the Internet as a "date-rape" drug.[78] Because of its abuse potential, ketamine was classified as a schedule III drug in 1999. Ketamine can be ingested, injected IM or IV, smoked, or snorted.[6] On the street ketamine is sold as "green,"[6,77] "K," "Super K," "Special K," "Vitamin K," "Super Acid," "Super C," "Purple," "Jet," and "Cat Valium."[6]

Toxic Dose

The oral LD_{50} for phencyclidine in mice is 75 mg/kg.[10] Marked clinical signs of intoxication in the dog can occur at oral doses of 2.5 to 10 mg/kg and in the cat at 1.1 to 12 mg/kg.[79] IV, signs can occur at exposures as low as 1 mg/kg in dogs.[80,81]

Toxicokinetics

Phencyclidine is poorly absorbed from the stomach. It is a weak base with a pKa of between 8.6 and 9.4 and has a high lipid-to-water partition coefficient.[78] Thus it tends to be ionized in the gastric environment. It is, however, well absorbed from the comparatively alkaline intestinal environment and the respiratory tract. Extensive recirculation occurs as phencyclidine is secreted into the stomach and then is reabsorbed from the intestinal lumen, prolonging its half-life. In humans the onset of effect occurs within 30 to 60 minutes following oral exposure, and the effects can last up to 24 to 48 hours.[77]

Phencyclidine is well distributed and because of its lipophilicity and pKa, it is found in high concentrations in the CNS and in adipose tissue. In dogs 68% of a single dose is metabolized in the liver, and only 32% is excreted unchanged by the kidneys. In cats 88% of the parent compound is renally excreted.[79] Phencyclidine can be ion trapped in the nephron when the urine pH is less than 5.5.[79]

Ketamine is primarily metabolized in the liver by demethylation and hydroxylation. Ketamine and its metabolites are eliminated in the urine. Following IM injection in the cat, peak plasma levels occur in approximately 10 minutes. Elimination half-life in the cat, calf, and horse is approximately 1 hour.[82]

Mechanism of Toxicity

PCP and ketamine functionally and electrophysiologically "dissociate" the somatosensory cortex from higher centers. The precise mechanism by which this is achieved is not fully understood.[78] PCP, ketamine, and their analogues bind with high affinity to the cortex and limbic structures of the brain, blocking the N-methyl-D-aspartate (NMDA) receptors. The NMDA receptor is normally activated by glutamate, an excitatory amino acid. Dissociative agents, such as PCP and ketamine, bind to the NMDA receptor at a site independent of glutamate and thus block the receptor noncompetitively.[78] PCP and ketamine also bind to the biogenic amine reuptake complex (i.e., norepinephrine and dopamine) but with less affinity than to the NMDA receptor. This may account for the sympathomimetic and psychomotor effects seen clinically. Both PCP and ketamine affect heart rate, blood pressure, and cardiac output but PCP more inconsistently so.[78] NDMA antagonists affect behavior, sensation, and cognition to produce a clinical condition resembling schizophrenia. They also produce negative effects on concentration, recall, learning, and retention of new information.[78] Other effects that may be involved in the action of dissociative agents are inhibition of GABA and stimulation of alpha and opiate receptors.[77]

Clinical Signs

Effects on muscle tone are variable, but generally ketamine either causes no change in muscle tone or increased muscle tone.[82] It does not abolish the pinnal and pedal reflexes, nor the photic, corneal, laryngeal, or pharyngeal reflexes.[82] Ketamine increases cardiac output, heart rate, mean aortic pressure, pulmonary artery pressure, and central venous pressure.[82]

In humans, phencyclidine overdose can cause coma, seizures, hypotension or hypertension, and muscular rigidity accompanied by hyperthermia and rhabdomyolysis.[83] Signs may last for days. Lower doses can cause ataxia, slurred speech, hyperesthesia, blank staring, or hostility.[77] Dogs dosed with phencyclidine exhibit grimacing, jaw snapping, muscular rigidity, salivation, seizures, and blank staring.[81,84]

Minimum Database

Animals exhibiting severe signs should be evaluated for acidosis, hypoglycemia, electrolyte abnormalities, hypothermia or hyperthermia, and myoglobinuria.

Confirmatory Tests

Most veterinary diagnostic laboratories are not prepared to analyze for PCP, ketamine, or their analogues. The practitioner is urged to check with the laboratory or diagnostic toxicologist before sample collection and submission. Submission to a human laboratory for identification may be required. Urine is most commonly analyzed, although PCP may be detected in serum and possibly gastric contents.[78]

Because of the distribution of phencyclidine, blood levels do not correlate well with clinical findings.[85] Phencyclidine may be detected in urine for 2 weeks or longer after exposure.[77] PCP, ketamine, and their analogues and metabolites may cross-react in immunoassay kits, although the extent to which this occurs may be variable.[78]

Treatment and Prognosis

Phencyclidine produces unpredictable effects, so treatment is symptomatic. In mild cases the patient should be maintained in a dark, quiet, nonstimulating environment. For animals exhibiting severe hyperactivity, rigidity, aggression, or seizures, diazepam can be administered. Phenothiazine tranquilizers are contraindicated because they may lower the seizure threshold, exacerbate anticholinergic effects of PCP, and produce hypotension.[77] In patients with severe seizures, barbiturates or general anesthesia may be required.

Activated charcoal has been shown to decrease the toxicity and increase the LD_{50} of phencyclidine in dogs and rats, respectively.[84] Activated charcoal prevents the recirculation of phencyclidine in the gut and enhances elimination. Charcoal should be administered with a cathartic to promote passage of the drug.

Forced diuresis, mannitol, and furosemide can increase the rate of urinary clearance of phencyclidine. Urinary acidification can greatly enhance elimination of phencyclidine, but this should not be attempted unless the patient's acid-base status can be closely monitored. Acidification may exacerbate a metabolic acidosis and increases the risk of myoglobinuric renal failure (rare). Dextrose may be required for hypoglycemic patients. Body temperature should be closely monitored.

Prognosis depends on the clinical condition of the animal at the time of presentation. Patients with a large degree of self-inflicted trauma or rhabdomyolysis (rare, but may occur) have a poorer prognosis. Those that undergo immediate decontamination, monitoring, and supportive care have a good prognosis.

Differential Diagnoses

Some differential diagnoses include LSD, hallucinogenic mushrooms, hops, and marijuana.

Tricyclic Antidepressants

Sources

Tricyclic antidepressants were developed in the 1950s and are still commonly prescribed today. They are named for their three-ringed chemical structure, which is common to most agents in this class (exception: the tetracyclic drug maprotiline and the dibenzoxazepine drug amoxapine).[86] Imipramine was the first tricyclic antidepressant used for depression. Newer cyclic antidepressants have been developed in an attempt to decrease the cardiovascular and CNS toxicity of older members of the class. Although other antidepressants, such as the monoamine oxidase inhibitors (MAOIs) (e.g., phenelzine sulfate, tranylcypromine sulfate), selective serotonin reuptake inhibitors (SSRIs) (e.g., fluoxetine, paroxetine, and nefazodone), and novel antidepressants like bupropion have been introduced, the tricyclics are still widely prescribed in human medicine. They have also been used in veterinary medicine for the treatment of certain behavior disorders. Table 25-6 lists some tricyclic antidepressants and their trade names.

Table 25-6   Some Commonly Prescribed Tricyclic Antidepressants and Their Trade Names

Tricyclic Antidepressant	Trade Name
Amitriptyline	Elavil, Amitid, Endep, Amitril
Amoxapine	Asendin
Clomipramine	Anafranil, Clomicalm
Desipramine	Norpramin, Pertofrane
Doxepin	Adapin, Sinequan
Imipramine	Tofranil, Presamine, SK-Pramine, Janimine
Maprotiline	Ludiomil
Nortriptyline	Aventyl, Pamelor
Protriptyline	Vivactil
Trimipramine	Surmontil

Toxic Dose

Tricyclic antidepressants have a low margin of safety because even small overdoses may produce toxicity. Exposures of more than 15 mg/kg should be considered potentially lethal doses.[87]

A review of the ASPCA APCC database indicates that dogs have exhibited tremors with oral doses as low as 5.5 mg/kg and 2.2 mg/kg of the MAOIs phenelzine and tranylcypromine, respectively.[88] The toxicity of the SSRIs varies greatly with the individual compound. Sertraline at 10 mg/kg in dogs was shown to cause mydriasis and anorexia, with the minimum oral lethal dose of 80 mg/kg.[89,90] Fluvoxamine is another SSRI, and oral exposures of 10 mg/kg were shown to cause depression and tremors.[88] Doses of nefazodone hydrochloride of 100 mg/kg given orally twice a day in dogs did not lead to fatalities.[91] Trazodone hydrochloride, another popular SSRI, has a reported LD_{50} in dogs of 500 mg/kg, and clinical signs can occur (ataxia, tremors, seizures) at 6-8 mg/kg dosages.[92] Venlafaxine hydrochloride, another SSRI, can cause mild depression at oral doses of 1 mg/kg, and tremors are observed at 10 mg/kg.[88] Bupropion hydrochloride, a novel antidepressant, has a very short half-life of 1.73 hours in dogs and depression can be seen with dosages of 10 mg/kg orally.[88,93]

Toxicokinetics

The tricyclic antidepressants are readily absorbed from the gastrointestinal tract, although absorption may be prolonged, especially in overdose situations, because of the anticholinergic effects of the drugs. Peak plasma levels generally occur within 2 to 8 hours but can be delayed for more than 12 hours.[94] Clinical signs can occur within 1 hour of ingestion. Oral bioavailability is low and variable because of extensive first-pass metabolism.[86] The tricyclic antidepressants are highly lipophilic and distribute widely to the brain, heart, lungs, and liver. There appears to be selective accumulation of tricyclic antidepressants in the heart. Imipramine in rabbits and amitriptyline in mice and rats are more highly concentrated in heart than in skeletal muscle. The concentrations of several tricyclic antidepressants administered to rabbits were found to be 40 to 200 times greater in cardiac tissue than in plasma.[95] The tricyclic antidepressants are highly protein bound, readily cross the placenta, and are distributed into the milk.[96] A low blood pH may make the drug more available by decreasing protein binding.[86] Metabolism occurs in the liver, and enterohepatic recirculation may occur as lipophilic metabolites are reabsorbed. Half-lives of the tricyclic antidepressants are quite variable but tend to be long, ranging from 9 to 84 hours.[97] The major route of excretion is urinary, although some compounds may be excreted in the feces through bile.[96]

MAOIs are rapidly absorbed and signs are generally seen within 1 to 2 hours of ingestion, but can be delayed for up to 24 hours.[88] The SSRIs are all well absorbed and highly protein bound. In general, half-lives for the SSRIs are less than 20 to 30 hours.

Mechanism of Toxicity

The major organ systems involved in tricyclic antidepressant toxicosis (as well as the other classes of antidepressants) are the cardiovascular and neurologic systems. Tricyclic antidepressants inhibit the fast sodium channels in the ventricular myocardium, slowing ventricular depolarization and resulting in a prolongation of the QRS interval. In this respect they act similarly to class I antiarrhythmic drugs, such as quinidine. Slowed conduction may contribute to the development of electrical reentry impulses, resulting in ventricular tachycardia or fibrillation. Electrocardiographic changes can include increased PR intervals, QT intervals, and QRS duration.[87] Clinically, bradycardia, cardiac arrhythmias, and severe hypotension may be noted. Elevation of blood pH has had a beneficial effect in animal models of tricyclic antidepressant toxicosis.[98] Studies in dogs have shown a correlation between an elevated blood pH and reversal of tricyclic antidepressant-induced cardiac toxicity.[99,100]

The CNS toxicity of tricyclic antidepressants is complex and has not been fully elucidated. A combination of factors, including increased concentrations of monoamines, such as norepinephrine, antidopaminergic effects, anticholinergic properties, inhibition of sodium channels, and interactions with GABA receptors, are all likely involved.[86]

Clinical Signs

The onset of signs and the progression of the clinical course may be rapid. Initial signs can include vomiting, hyperexcitability, hyperthermia, tremors, tachycardia, mydriasis, vocalization, and seizures. As the toxic syndrome progresses, lethargy, ataxia, bradycardia, coma, hypotension, and cardiac arrhythmias can develop. The major cause of death in tricyclic antidepressant exposures is cardiac failure. With MAOI exposures, signs can include hyper(hypo)tension, ataxia, restlessness, tachycardia, arrhythmias, respiratory depression, shock, coma, and seizures.[88] Clinical signs associated with SSRI overdose include lethargy or agitation, vomiting, ataxia, tremors, seizures, hypertension and tachycardia.[88] Clinical signs of bupropion overdose include vomiting, dypnea, salivation, ataxia, arrhythmias, tremors, hypotension, and seizures.[88]

Minimum Database

The minimum database should include an evaluation of neurologic status, cardiac rate and rhythm, and acid-base status.

Confirmatory Tests

Tricyclic antidepressants, along with the other antidepressants, can potentially be detected in plasma, serum, whole blood, and urine.[98,101] Consultation with a diagnostic toxicologist is suggested before submission of samples.

Treatment and Prognosis

Clinical signs of tricyclic antidepressant overdose can develop rapidly, and induction of vomiting in recently exposed animals should be undertaken with caution. Emesis can trigger seizure activity in tricyclic antidepressant–poisoned animals, causing risk of aspiration. Sedation with an ultrashort-acting barbiturate and gastric lavage followed by activated charcoal may be a better alternative.[87] Atropine should be avoided because of the anticholinergic properties of the tricyclic antidepressants. A cathartic should be administered with the charcoal, but magnesium sulfate (Epsom salts) should not be used; tricyclic antidepressants decrease gastrointestinal motility, and large amounts of magnesium could be absorbed. Alternative cathartics are sorbitol or sodium sulfate (Glauber's salts). Repeated doses of activated charcoal are recommended to interrupt enterohepatic recirculation of the tricyclic antidepressants.

Animals should be closely monitored because of the possibility of rapid deterioration. Sodium bicarbonate should be administered for acidosis or signs of cardiac toxicity. Tricyclic antidepressant-induced cardiac toxicity can be reversed by elevating the blood pH.[99,100] Maintaining blood pH at more than 7.5 prevented death in experimentally poisoned dogs.[87,102] In the absence of acid-base monitoring, sodium bicarbonate at a dose of 2 to 3 mEq/kg IV during a period of 15 to 30 minutes is recommended.[87] Cardiac monitoring should continue, and sodium bicarbonate should be repeated as clinical signs recur.

Seizures can be treated with diazepam or phenobarbital.[87] Good supportive care including fluid therapy and thermoregulation is indicated. The animal may require hospitalization in excess of 24 hours because of the often long and variable half-lives of individual tricyclic antidepressant agents.

Treatment options for MAOI- and SSRI-exposed patients are similar and should include consideration of decontamination procedures (emesis, activated charcoal, cathartic), along with symptomatic and supportive care. Patients exhibiting the serotonin syndrome may be treated with cyproheptadine hydrochloride at a dose of 1.1 mg/kg orally.[88]

Differential Diagnoses

Some agents that should be considered in the differential diagnosis include amphetamines, cocaine, methylxanthines, pseudoephedrine, herbal preparations containing ma huang or guarana root, quinidine, propranolol, and albuterol.

References

1. United States Drug Enforcement Administration: *A tradition of excellence*, http://www.usdoj.gov/dea/pubs/history/.
2. Adams HR: Drugs acting on the autonomic and somatic nervous systems. In Adams HR, editor: *Veterinary pharmacology and therapeutics*, ed 7, Ames, 1995, Iowa State University Press. 1995.
3. Connolly HM, Crary JL, McGoon MD, et al: Valvular heart disease associated with fenfluramine-phentermine, *N Engl J Med* 337(9):581, 1997.
4. Albertson TE, Van Hoozen BE, Allen RP: Amphetamines. In Haddad LM, Shannon MW, Winchester JF, editors: *Clinical management of poisoning and drug overdose*, ed 3, Philadelphia, 1998, WB Saunders.
5. Amphetamines and designer drugs. In Ellenhorn MJ, editor: *Ellenhorn's medical toxicology*, ed 2, Baltimore, 1997, Williams & Wilkins. 1997.
6. *Street drugs: a drug identification guide*, Plymouth, MN, 2003, Publishers Group LLC, www.streetdrugs.org.
7. Benzie F, Hekman K, Cameron L, et al: Emergency department visits after use of a drug sold as "bath salts"—Michigan, November 12, 2010–March 31, 2011, *MMWR* 60(19):624–627, 2011.
8. Ross EA, Watson M, Goldberger B: "Bath salts" intoxication, *N Engl J Med* 365:967–968, 2011.
9. Zalis EG, Kaplan G, Lundberg GD, et al: Acute lethality of the amphetamines in dogs and its antagonism by curare, *Proc Soc Exp Biol Med* 118(2):557, 1965.
10. RTECS: Registry of toxic effects of chemical substances. From MDL Information Systems Inc. (electronic version). *Thomson MICROMEDEX*, Greenwood Village, CO, Vol. 61, expires August 31, 2004.
11. Zalis EG, Parmley LF: Fatal amphetamine poisoning, *Arch Intern Med* 101:822–826, 1963.
12. Amphetamines general statement. In McEvoy GK, editor: *AHFS drug information*, Bethesda, MD, 2003, American Society of Health-System Pharmacists Inc.
13. Anggard E, Jonsson LR, Hogmark AL, et al: Amphetamine metabolism in amphetamine psychosis, *Clin Pharmacol Ther* 14(5):870, 1973.
14. Baggot JD, Davis LW: Pharmacokinetic study of amphetamine elimination in dogs and swine, *Biochem Pharmacol* 21:1967, 1972.
15. Editorial Staff: Amphetamines (pharmacology/toxicology). In Klasco RK, editor: *POISINDEX System*, *Thomson MICROMEDEX*, Greenwood Village, CO, Vol. 121, expires September 2004.
16. Gross ME, Booth NH: Tranquilizers, α_2-adrenergic agonists, and related agents. In Adams HR, editor: *Veterinary pharmacology and therapeutics*, ed 7, Ames, 1995, Iowa State University Press.
17. Catravas JD, Waters IW, Hickenbottom JP, et al: The effects of haloperidol, chlorpromazine and propranolol on acute amphetamine poisoning in the conscious dog, *J Pharmacol Exp Ther* 202(1):230, 1977.
18. Hobbs WR, Rall TW, Verdoorn TA: Hypnotics and sedatives; ethanol. In Hardman JG, Limbird LE, editors: *Goodman and Gilman's the pharmacological basis of therapeutics*, New York, 1996, McGraw-Hill.
19. Haddad LM, Winchester JF: Barbiturates. In Haddad LM, Shannon MW, Winchester JF, editors: *Clinical management of poisoning and drug overdose*, ed 3, Philadelphia, 1998, WB Saunders.
20. Reid TC: Barbiturate poisoning in dogs, *NZ Vet J* 6(7):190, 1978.
21. Humphreys DJ, Longstaffe JA, Stodulski JBJ, et al: Barbiturate poisoning from pet shop meat: possible association with perivascular injection, *Vet Rec* 107(22):517, 1980.
22. Warning added to euthanasia products, *J Am Vet Med Assoc* 223(6):773, 2003.
23. Euthanatized animals can poison wildlife: veterinarians receive fines, *J Am Vet Med Assoc* 220(2):146–147, 2002.
24. Secondary pentobarbital poisoning of wildlife. US Fish Wildlife Service fact sheet. December 2003. http://cpharm.vetmed.vt.edu/USFWS/USFWSFPentobarbFactSheet.pdf.
25. Lee DC: Sedative-hypnotics agents. In Goldfrank LR, Flomenbaum NE, Lewin NA, et al. *Goldfrank's toxicologic emergencies*, ed 7, New York, 2002, McGraw-Hill.
26. Barbiturate pharmacology. In Plumb DC, editor: *Veterinary drug handbook*, ed 4, Ames, 2002, Iowa State University Press.
27. Kisseberth WC, Trammel HL: Illicit and abused drugs, *Vet Clin North Am Small Anim Pract* 20(2):413, 1990.
28. Boldy DAR, Vale JA, Prescott LF: Treatment of phenobarbitone poisoning with repeated oral administration of activated charcoal, *Q J Med* 61(235):997, 1986.
29. Vale JA, Ruddock FS, Boldy DAR: Multiple doses of activated charcoal in the treatment of phenobarbitone and carbamazepine poisoning, *Vet Hum Toxicol* 29(2):152, 1987.
30. Amitai Y, Degani Y: Treatment of phenobarbital poisoning with multiple dose activated charcoal in an infant, *J Emerg Med* 8(4):449, 1990.
31. Veerman M, Espejo MG, Christopher MA, et al: Use of activated charcoal to reduce elevated serum phenobarbital concentration in a neonate, *Clin Toxicol* 29(1):53, 1991.

32. Lindberg MC, Cunningham JA, Lindberg NH: Acute phenobarbital intoxication, *South Med J* 85(8):803, 1992.
33. Anxiolytic and hypnotic drugs. In Rang HP, Dale MM, Ritter JM, et al: *Pharmacology*, ed 5, Philadelphia, 2003, Churchill Livingstone.
34. Editorial Staff: Benzodiazepines (Overview). In Klasco RK, editor: *POISINDEX System. Thomson MICROMEDEX*, Greenwood Village, CO, Vol. 121, expires 9/2004.
35. Farrell SE, Roberts JR: Benzodiazepines. In Haddad LM, Shannon MW, Winchester JF, editors: *Clinical management of poisoning and drug overdose*, ed 3, Philadelphia, 1998, WB Saunders.
36. Diazepam. In Plumb DC, editor: *Veterinary drug handbook*, ed 4, Ames, 2002, Iowa State University Press.
37. Benzodiazepines general statement. In McEvoy GK, editor: *AHFS drug information*, Bethesda, MD, 2003, American Society of Health-System Pharmacists Inc.
38. Gross ME, Booth NH: Tranquilizers, α_2-adrenergic agonists, and related agents. In Adams HR, editor: *Veterinary pharmacology and therapeutics*, ed 7, Ames, 1995, Iowa State University Press.
39. Hobbs WR, Rall TW, Verdoorn TA: Hypnotics and sedatives: ethanol. In Hardman JG, Limbird LE, editors: *Goodman and Gilman's the pharmacological basis of therapeutics*, New York, 1996, McGraw-Hill.
40. Benzodiazepines. In Ellenhorn MJ, editor: *Ellenhorn's medical toxicology*, ed 2, Baltimore, 1997, Williams & Wilkins.
41. Flumazenil. In Plumb DC, editor: *Veterinary drug handbook*, ed 4, Ames, 2002, Iowa State University Press.
42. Hollander JE, Hoffman RS: Cocaine. In Goldfrank LR, Flomenbaum NE, Lewin NA, et al: *Goldfrank's toxicologic emergencies*, ed 7, New York, 2002, McGraw-Hill.
43. Steffey EP, Booth NH: Local anesthetics. In Adams HR, editor: *Veterinary pharmacology and therapeutics*, ed 7, Ames, 1995, Iowa State University Press.
44. Albertson TE, Marelich GP, Tharratt RS: Cocaine. In Haddad LM, Shannon MW, Winchester JF, editors: *Clinical management of poisoning and drug overdose*, ed 3, Philadelphia, 1998, WB Saunders.
45. Cocaine hydrochloride. In McEvoy GK, editor: *AHFS drug information*, Bethesda, MD, 2003, American Society of Health-System Pharmacists Inc.
46. Catravas JD, Waters IW: Acute cocaine intoxication in the conscious dog: studies on the mechanism of lethality, *J Pharmacol Exp Ther* 217(2):350–356, 1981.
47. Kabas JS, Blanchard SM, Matsuyama Y, et al: Cocaine-mediated impairment of cardiac conduction in the dog: a potential mechanism for sudden death after cocaine, *J Pharmacol Exp Ther* 252(1):185, 1990.
48. Williams RG, Kavanagh KM, Teo KK: Pathophysiology and treatment of cocaine toxicity: implications for the heart and cardiovascular system, *Can J Cardiol* 12(12):1295, 1996.
49. Frazier K, Colvin B, Hullinger G: Postmortem diagnosis of accidental cocaine intoxication in a dog, *Vet Hum Toxicol* 40(3):154–155, 1998.
50. Lindgren JE: Guide to the analysis of cocaine and its metabolites in biological material, *J Ethnopharmacol* 3:337, 1981.
51. Tucker JR, Ferm RP: Lysergic acid and diethylamide and other hallucinogens. In Goldfrank LR, Flomengbaum NE, Lewin NA, et al: *Goldfrank's toxicologic emergencies*, ed 7, New York, 2002, McGraw-Hill.
52. Haddad LM: LSD, natural hallucinogens, and miscellany. In Haddad LM, Shannon MW, Winchester JF, editors: *Clinical management of poisoning and drug overdose*, ed 3, Philadelphia, 1998, WB Saunders.
53. Editorial Staff: LSD (Kinetics). In Klasco RK, editor: *POISINDEX System, Thomson MICROMEDEX*, Greenwood Village, CO, Vol. 121, expires September 2004.
54. O'Brien CP: Drug addiction and drug abuse. In Hardman JG, Limbird LE, editors: *Goodman and Gilman's the pharmacological basis of therapeutics*, New York, 1996, McGraw-Hill.
55. Hallucinogenic drugs. In Ellenhorn MJ, editor: *Ellenhorn's medical toxicology*, ed 2, Baltimore, 1997, Williams & Wilkins. 1997.
56. Voth EA, Schwartz RH: Medicinal applications of delta-9-tetrahydrocannabinol and marijuana, *Ann Intern Med* 126(10):791, 1997.
57. Otten EJ: Marijuana. In Goldfrank LR, Flomengbaum NE, Lewin NA, et al: *Goldfrank's toxicologic emergencies*, ed 7, New York, 2002, McGraw-Hill.
58. Marijuana and other cannabinoids. In Ellenhorn MJ, editor: *Ellenhorn's medical toxicology*, ed 2, Baltimore, 1997, Williams & Wilkins.
59. *U.S. Department of Justice Drug Enforcement Administration: Controlled substance schedules*, http://www.deadiversion.usdoj.gov/schedules/index.html.
60. Synthetic drug control act of 2011, H.R. 1254: http://www.gpo.gov/fdsys/pkg/BILLS-112hr1254rh.pdf.
61. Thompson GR, Rosenkrantz H, Schaeppi UH, et al: Comparison of acute oral toxicity of cannabinoids in rats, dogs, and monkeys, *Toxicol Appl Pharmacol* 25(3):363, 1973.

62. Waller CW: Chemistry, toxicology and psychic effects of cannabis. In Keeler RF, Tu AT, editors: *Handbook of natural toxins, Vol. I, Plant and fungal toxins*, New York, 1983, Marcel Dekker.

63. Ameri A: The effects of cannabinoids on the brain, *Prog Neurobio* 58:315–348, 1999.

64. Editorial Staff: Marijuana (kinetics). In Klasco RK, editor: *POISINDEX System, Thomson MICROMEDEX*, Greenwood Village, CO, Vol. 121, expires September 2004.

65. Janczyk P, Donaldson CW, Gwaltney S: Two hundred and thirteen cases of marijuana toxicoses in dogs, *Vet Human Toxicol* 46(1):19–21, 2004.

66. Hallucinogenic drugs. In Ellenhorn MJ, editor: *Ellenhorn's medical toxicology*, ed 2, Baltimore, 1997, Williams & Wilkins.

67. Branson KR, Gross ME, Booth NH: Opioid agonists and antagonists. In Adams HR, editor: *Veterinary pharmacology and therapeutics*, ed 7, Ames, 1995, Iowa State University Press.

68. Nelson LS: Opioids. In Goldfrank LR, Flomenbaum NE, Lewin NA, et al: *Goldfrank's toxicologic emergencies*, ed 7, New York, 2002, McGraw-Hill.

69. Analgesic drugs. In Rang HP, Dale MM, Ritter JM, editors: *Pharmacology*, ed 5, Philadelphia, 2003, Churchill Livingstone.

70. Reisine T, Pasternak G: Opioid analgesics and antagonists. In Hardman JG, Limbird LE, editors: *Goodman and Gilman's the pharmacological basis of therapeutics*, New York, 1996, McGraw-Hill.

71. Apomorphine. In Plumb DC, editor: *Veterinary drug handbook*, ed 4, Ames, 2002, Iowa State University Press.

72. Davis LE, Donnelly EJ: Analgesic drugs in the cat, *J Am Vet Med Assoc* 53(9):161, 1968.

73. Kisseberth WC, Trammel HL: Illicit and abused drugs, *Vet Clin North Am Small Anim Pract* 20(2):413, 1990.

74. Acute reactions to drugs of abuse, *Med Lett Drugs Ther* 38(974):45, 1996.

75. Schwartz M: Opiates and narcotics. In Haddad LM, Shannon MW, Winchester JF, editors: *Clinical management of poisoning and drug overdose*, ed 3, Philadelphia, 1998, WB Saunders.

76. Opiate agonists general statement. In McEvoy GK, editor: *AHFS drug information*, Bethesda, MD, 2003, American Society of Health-System Pharmacists Inc.

77. Wright RO, Woolf AD: Phencyclidine. In Haddad LM, Shannon MW, Winchester JF, editors: *Clinical management of poisoning and drug overdose*, ed 3, Philadelphia, 1998, WB Saunders. 1998.

78. Olmedo R: Phencyclidine and ketamine. In Goldfrank LR, Flomenbaum NE, Lewin NA, et al: *Goldfrank's toxicologic emergencies*, ed 7, New York, 2002, McGraw-Hill.

79. Coppock RW, Mostrom MS, Lillie LE: Ethanol and illicit drugs of abuse. In Kirk RW, editor: *Current veterinary therapy X: small animal practice*, Philadelphia, 1989, WB Saunders.

80. Vaupel DB, Jasinski DR: Acute single dose effects of phencyclidine (PCP) in dogs, *Fed Proc* 38(3,1):435, 1979.

81. Boren JL, Consroe PF: Behavioral effects of phencyclidine (PCP) in the dog: a possible animal model of PCP toxicity in humans, *Life Sci* 28(11):1245, 1981.

82. Ketamine. In Plumb DC, editor: *Veterinary drug handbook*, ed 4, Ames, 2002, Iowa State University Press.

83. Acute reactions to drugs of abuse, *Med Lett Drugs Ther* 38(974):45, 1996.

84. Picchioni AL, Consroe PF: Activated charcoal-a phencyclidine antidote, or hog in dogs, *N Engl J Med* 300(4):202, 1979.

85. Phencyclidine. In Ellenhorn MJ, editor: *Ellenhorn's medical toxicology*, ed 2, Baltimore, 1997, Williams & Wilkins.

86. Liebelt EL, Francis PD: Cyclic antidepressants. In Goldfrank LR, Flomenbaum NE, Lewin NA, et al: *Goldfrank's toxicologic emergencies*, ed 7, New York, 2002, McGraw-Hill.

87. Johnson LR: Tricyclic antidepressant toxicosis, *Vet Clin North Am Small Anim Pract* 20(2):393, 1990.

88. Wismer TA: Antidepressant drug overdoses in dogs, *Vet Med* 95(7):520, 2000.

89. Koe BK, Weissman A, Welch WM, Browne RG: Sertraline, 1S,4S-N-methyl-4-(3,4-dichlorophenyl)-1,2,3,4-tetrahydro-1-naphthylamine, a new uptake inhibitor with selectivity for serotonin, *J Pharmacol Exp Ther* 226(3):686, 1983.

90. RTECS: Registry of Toxic Effects of Chemical Substances., National Institute for Occupational Safety and Health, Cincinnati, OH, Micromedex, Englewood, CO.

91. Shukla UA, Kaul S, Marathe PH, Pittman KA, Barbhaiya RH: Pharmacokinetics of nefazodone following multiple escalating oral doses in the dog, *Eur J Drug Metab Pharmacokinet* 17(4):309, 1992.

92. Antidepressants. *American Hospital Formulary Service*, Bethesda, MD, 1999, American Society of Health-System Pharmacists 1894.

93. Butz RF, Schroeder DH, Welch RM, Mehta NB, Phillips AP, Findlay JW: Radioimmunoassay and pharmacokinetic profile of bupropion in the dog, *J Pharmacol Exp Ther* 217(3):602–610, 1981.

94. Baldessarini RJ: Drugs and the treatment of psychiatric disorders: depression and mania. In Hardman JG, Limbird LE, editors: *Goodman and Gilman's the pharmacological basis of therapeutics,* New York, 1996, McGraw-Hill.

95. Jandhyala BS, Steenberg ML, Perel JM, et al: Effects of several tricyclic antidepressants on the hemodynamics and myocardial contractility of the anesthetized dogs, *Eur J Pharmacol* 42:403–410, 1977.

96. Tricyclic antidepressants general statement. In McEvoy GK, editor: *AHFS drug information,* Bethesda, MD, 2003, American Society of Health-System Pharmacists Inc.

97. Editorial Staff: Tricyclic antidepressants (kinetics). In Klasco RK, editor: *POISINDEX System, Thomson MICROMEDEX,* Greenwood Village, CO, Vol. 121, expires 9/2004.

98. Pentel PR, Keyler DE, Haddad LM: Tricyclic antidepressants and selective serotonin reuptake inhibitors. In Haddad LM, Shannon MW, Winchester JF, editors: *Clinical management of poisoning and drug overdose,* ed 3, Philadelphia, 1998, WB Saunders.

99. Sasyniuk BI, Jhamandas V, Valois M: Experimental amitriptyline intoxication: treatment of cardiac toxicity with sodium bicarbonate, *Ann Emerg Med* 15(9):1052, 1986.

100. Stone CK, Kraemer CM, Carroll R, et al: Does a sodium-free buffer affect QRS width in experimental amitriptyline overdose? *Ann Emerg Med* 26(1):58, 1995.

101. Cyclic antidepressants. In Ellenhorn MJ, editor: *Ellenhorn's medical toxicology,* ed 2, Baltimore, 1997, Williams & Wilkins.

102. Callaham M, Schumaker H, Pentel P: Phenytoin prophylaxis of cardiotoxicity in experimental amitriptyline poisoning, *J Pharmacol Exp Ther* 245(1):216, 1988.

Hazards Associated with the Use of Herbal and Other Natural Products*

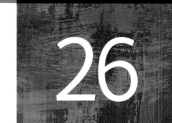

Elizabeth A. Hausner, DVM, PhD, DABVT, DABT

Robert H. Poppenga, DVM, PhD, DABVT

- The use of herbal remedies for the prevention and treatment of a variety of illnesses in small animals has increased tremendously in recent years.
- Although most herbal remedies, when used as directed and under the supervision of knowledgeable individuals, are safe, the potential for adverse effects or intoxications certainly exists.
- Because of inherent toxicity, some herbal remedies should not be used under any circumstances.
- Because nearly all herbal remedies contain multiple biologically active constituents, interaction with conventional drugs is a concern. It is incumbent on clinicians to be aware of those herbs that can cause intoxication and to be cognizant of potential herb-drug interactions.
- There are a number of evidence-based resources available to assist clinicians in the safe use of herbal remedies.

Broadly defined, *herbs* are plants used for medicinal purposes or for their olfactory or flavoring properties. There is increasing interest in the use of herbs and other "natural" products by both veterinarians and animal owners to treat medical problems (herbal medicine). The reasons underlying the increased use of herbal and other "alternative" medical modalities in human health have been investigated extensively and are multifactorial.[1-3] Social, economic, and philosophical reasons often underlie the decision by an individual to turn to alternative modalities, such as herbal medicine. Unfortunately, similar investigations into the motivation of pet owners to employ such modalities for the treatment of their pets have not been conducted. However, it is likely that the same motivations apply.

Plants have been used for medicinal purposes by people since the beginning of recorded history and undoubtedly well before. In the West, many modern medicines, either in the form of a "parent" compound or as a synthetic derivative, originated from plants. Examples of parent compounds include salicylates (from *Salix* spp. or willow bark), digitoxin and

---

*The views and opinions expressed are those of the authors and do not represent the Food and Drug Administration.

digoxin (from *Digitalis* spp. or foxglove), quinine (from *Cinchona* spp. or cinchona bark), and morphine (*Papaver* spp. or opium poppy). The pharmaceutical industry continues to search for new and effective plant-derived compounds. Herbs are important components of traditional Chinese medicine, ayurvedic medicine, and the medical practices of many indigenous cultures. Herbs were important components of both human and veterinary medicine in Europe and North America before the advent of purified natural and synthetic drugs.

Herbal medicine and conventional pharmacology differ in three fundamental ways.[4] First, herbalists use unpurified plant extracts containing several different constituents in the belief that the various constituents work synergistically (the effect of the whole herb is greater than the summed effects of its individual components). In addition, herbalists believe that toxicity is reduced when the whole herb is used instead of its purified active constituents; this is termed *buffering*. Secondly, several herbs are often used together. The theories of synergism and buffering are believed to be applicable when herb combinations are employed. In conventional medicine, polypharmacy is generally not considered to be desirable because of increased risks of adverse drug reactions (ADRs) or interactions. Lastly, herbalists and many other alternative medical practitioners approach patients in a more "holistic" way than do many conventional medical practitioners who tend to focus more narrowly on the disease and exclude consideration of the patient as an individual.

Regulations

In 1994 Congress passed the Dietary Supplement Health and Education Act (DSHEA), which limits government oversight of products categorized as dietary supplements. Dietary supplements include minerals, vitamins, amino acids, herbs and any product sold as a "dietary supplement" before October 15, 1994. Thus, in the United States, dietary supplements are regulated as food. The Dietary Supplement and Nonprescription Drug Consumer Protection Act became effective in December 2007. The law requires collection of adverse event reports by the manufacturers, distributors, and retailers of dietary supplements. The labels of these products are also required to provide information to facilitate such reporting. Under the Food, Drug, and Cosmetic Act and the Public Service Health Act, the Food and Drug Administration (FDA) has also implemented requirements for the safety and quality of dietary supplements. Part of this entails good manufacturing practices. Another part is the establishment of adulteration standards specific to supplements. The burden of proof is on the government to demonstrate that adulteration of a product presents "significant and unreasonable risk of illness or injury." It should be noted that supplements are also adulterated if they are prepared, packed, or held under conditions that do not meet current good manufacturing practice regulations.[5] A complication to these safeguards comes from the Internet. Pet owners have the opportunity to purchase products from vendors who may or may not adhere to these regulations.

Active Herbal Constituents

There are five broad classes of active chemical constituents in plants: volatile oils, resins, alkaloids, glycosides, and fixed oils.[6] Volatile oils are odorous plant ingredients. Examples of plants that contain volatile oils include catnip, garlic, and citrus. Ingestion or dermal exposure to volatile oils can result in intoxication. Resins are complex chemical mixtures that can be strong gastrointestinal irritants. Alkaloids are a heterogeneous group of alkaline, organic, and nitrogenous compounds. Often these compounds are the most pharmacologically active plant constituents. Glycosides are sugar esters containing a sugar (glycol) and a nonsugar (aglycon). Glycosides are not typically toxic. However, hydrolysis of the glycosides after ingestion can release toxic aglycones. Fixed oils are esters of long-chain fatty acids and alcohols. Herbs containing fixed oils are often used as emollients, demulcents, and bases for other agents; in general these are the least toxic of the plant constituents.

Many of these plant-derived chemicals are biologically active and potentially toxic. There are numerous case reports in the medical literature documenting serious and potentially life-threatening adverse effects following human and animal exposure to herbal preparations. It is worth noting that in several instances the incidence of animal intoxication from an herb, herbal preparation, or dietary supplement seems to parallel its popularity.[7,8] However, it is important to point out that, considered as a whole, the use of herbal products does not appear to be associated with a higher incidence of serious adverse effects than ingestion of conventional prescription or over-the-counter (OTC) pharmaceuticals. Serious ADRs to conventional pharmaceuticals in hospitalized patients have been estimated to be approximately 7%.[9] An approximately equal incidence of hospital admissions caused by ADRs has been reported.[10] A recent study estimated that approximately 25% of all herbal remedy– and dietary supplement–related calls to a regional human poison control center could be classified as ADRs.[11] The most common ADRs were associated with zinc (38.2%), echinacea (7.7%), chromium picolinate (6.4%), and witch hazel (6%). Only 3 out of 233 ADRs were considered serious enough to warrant hospitalization. It is likely that ADRs are underreported for both conventional drugs and herbal remedies. Unfortunately, there is almost no information regarding the overall incidence of ADRs to conventional drugs or herbal remedies in veterinary medicine.

There are various ways in which poisoning of an animal might occur. Use of a correctly identified herbal that contains a known toxin is one possibility. For example, chronic use of an herbal remedy containing hepatotoxic pyrrolizidine alkaloids (PAs) may result in liver failure. Pennyroyal oil containing the putative hepatotoxin, pulegone, was responsible for the death of a dog after it was applied dermally to control fleas.[12] Alternatively, administration of a misidentified plant may result in poisoning. Contamination of commercially prepared herbal remedies with toxic plants has been documented in the medical literature.[13,14] Seeds of poison hemlock (*Conium maculatum*) have been found in anise seed. Recently, plantain sold as a dietary supplement was found to contain cardiac glycosides from *Digitalis* spp. Just as with traditional prescription medications, pet intoxication following accidental ingestion of an improperly stored remedy may occur. This is particularly true with dogs because of their indiscriminate eating habits. Dr. Poppenga was involved in a case in which a miniature poodle ingested several tablets of its owner's medication containing rauwolfia alkaloids and developed clinical signs within 2 hours of ingestion. Reserpine was detected in the medication and the urine of the dog.

Some herbal remedies, particularly Chinese patent medicines, may contain heavy metals, such as arsenic, lead, or mercury, which were added intentionally as part of the formula or unintentionally, along with contaminant pesticide residues. Intentionally added pharmaceuticals, such as nonsteroidal antiinflammatory drugs (NSAIDs), corticosteroids, caffeine, or sedatives, have also been reported.[15,16] Natural toxins commonly found in Chinese patent medicines include borneol, aconite, toad secretions (*Bufo* spp., *Ch' an Su*), mylabris, scorpion, borax, acorus, and strychnine (*Strychnos nux-vomica*).[15]

Because herbal preparations contain numerous biologically active compounds, the potential exists for ADRs when they are used in conjunction with conventional pharmaceuticals. In addition, many naturally occurring chemicals found in herbal remedies cause induction of one or more liver cytochrome P450 metabolizing enzymes or share other metabolic pathways with conventional pharmaceuticals. For example, eucalyptus oil induces liver enzyme activity.[17] This can result in altered metabolism of other drugs or chemicals resulting in either enhanced or diminished drug efficacy or toxicity. Coexisting liver or renal disease can alter the metabolism and elimination of herbal constituents, thus predisposing to adverse reactions. Apparent idiosyncratic reactions to herbal remedies have been documented in people. Such reactions might be due to individual differences in drug metabolizing capacity.[18,19]

Of particular concern to veterinarians is the possibility of species differences in susceptibility to the toxic effects of herbal constituents. For example, cat hemoglobin is quite susceptible to oxidative damage. The volatile oil in garlic contains oxidants, such as allicin.

Thus one can hypothesize that oxidant-induced Heinz body anemia would be more likely to occur in cats given garlic than in other species. However, there is no information to substantiate or refute such a hypothesis. Unfortunately, little evidence-based information exists on which informed judgments may be made about potential hazards of specific herbs to different animal species.

According to annual surveys of herbs sold in the United States, the most commonly used herbs include coneflower (*Echinacea* spp., Color Plate 26-1), garlic (*Allium sativa*), ginseng (*Panax* spp.), ginkgo (*Ginkgo biloba*), St. John's-wort (*Hypericum perforatum*), saw palmetto (*Serenoa repens*), sweetleaf (*Stevia rebaudiana*), aloe (*Aloe* spp.), resveratrol (*Vitis vinifera*), cayenne (*Capsicum* spp.), bilberry (*Vaccinium myrtillus*), and cat's claw (*Uncaria tomentosa*). Presumably, these are the herbs to which pets are most likely to be exposed. According to the *Botanical Safety Handbook*,[20] coneflower, saw palmetto, aloe (gel used internally), and cayenne (used internally) should be considered safe when used appropriately. Garlic, ginseng, ginkgo, St. John's-wort, goldenseal, aloe (gel used externally, dried juice used internally), and cayenne (used externally) have some restrictions for use.[20] For example, in humans garlic should not be used by nursing mothers, and cayenne should not be applied to injured skin or near eyes. Both ginkgo and St. John's-wort are contraindicated in individuals taking monoamine oxidase inhibitors because of potential herb-drug interactions. There is little data available for bilberry, sweetleaf, resveratrol, or cat's claw to make a determination regarding their safety across species. However, no observed adverse effect level for resveratrol of 600 mg/kg/day was determined in a subchronic oral toxicity study using beagles.[21]

The overall incidence of human dietary supplement adverse events (DSAE) appears to be relatively low, although inadequate and poor-quality reporting of DSAE are major limitations of dietary supplement safety monitoring in the United States.[22] Of interest are studies listing the most common herb-related calls to a regional human poison control center.[23,24] The most frequent calls, in descending order of frequency, involved St. John's wort, ma huang, echinacea, guarana, ginkgo, ginseng, valerian, tea tree oil, goldenseal, arnica, yohimbe, and kava kava. Not all of the calls could be categorized as ADRs.

Summaries of the Safety of Common Herbs

Not all of the following herbs, essential oils, and dietary supplements are used in herbal medicine because of well-recognized risks of intoxication. However, they are included in the following discussion precisely because of their inherent toxicity. Unless otherwise specified, the following information is taken from three primary sources: *Botanical Safety Handbook*,[20] *The Complete German Commission E Monographs: Therapeutic Guide to Herbal Medicines*,[25] and *Review of Natural Products*.[26] Other herbs of toxicologic concern are listed in Table 26-1.

5-Hydroxytryptophan

5-Hydroxytryptophan (5-HTP), also known as *Griffonia seed extract,* is a popular dietary supplement that is available OTC for a variety of conditions including depression, chronic headaches, obesity, and insomnia in humans. A retrospective study by the American Society for the Prevention of Cruelty to Animals Animal Poison Control Center (ASPCA-APCC) reported 21 cases of accidental ingestion of products containing 5-HTP by dogs between 1989 and 1999.[8] Clinical signs of intoxication developed in 19 of the 21 dogs and consisted primarily of seizures, depression, tremors, hyperesthesia, ataxia, and hyperthermia. Vomiting and diarrhea were also frequently reported. The pharmacologic and toxicologic action of 5-HTP is believed to be due to increased concentrations of serotonin in the central nervous system (CNS).[27] The estimated minimum toxic oral dose from the APCC study was 23.6 mg/kg, and the minimum lethal oral dose was estimated to be 128 mg/kg. Of the 19 symptomatic dogs, 3 died, and 16 of 17 dogs receiving symptomatic and supportive care recovered.

Table 26-1   Additional Herbs of Toxicologic Concern

Scientific Name	Common Names	Active Constituents	Target Organs
Acorus calamus	Acorus, calamus, sweet flag, sweet root, sweet cane, sweet cinnamon	β-Asarone (procarcinogen)	Liver—potent hepatocarcinogen
Aesculus hippocastanum	Horse chestnut, buckeye	Esculin, nicotine, quercetin, rutin, saponins, shikimic acid	Gastrointestinal, nervous
Arnica montana and A. latifolia	Arnica, wolf's bane, leopard's bane	Sesquiterpene lactones	Skin—dermatitis
Atropa belladonna	Belladonna, deadly nightshade	Atropine	Nervous—anticholinergic syndrome
Conium maculatum	Poison hemlock	Coniine, other similar alkaloids	Nervous—nicotine-like toxicosis
Convallaria majalis	Lily-of-the-valley, mayflower, conval lily	Cardiac glycosides	Cardiovascular
Cytisus scoparius	Scotch broom, broom, broom tops	L-Sparteine	Nervous—nicotinic-like toxicosis
Datura stramonium (Color Plate 26-3)	Jimsonweed, thorn apple	Atropine, scopolamine, hyoscyamine	Nervous—anticholinergic syndrome
Dipteryx odorata	Tonka bean	Coumarin	Hematologic—anticoagulant
Euonymus europaeus; E. atropurpureus	European spindle tree; wahoo, eastern burning bush	Cardiac glycosides	Cardiovascular
Eupatorium perfoliatum; E. purpureum	Boneset, thoroughwort; joe pye weed, gravel root, queen-of-the meadow	Pyrrolizidine alkaloids	Liver
Heliotropium europaeum	Heliotrope	Pyrrolizidine alkaloids	Liver
Hyoscyamus niger	Henbane, fetid nightshade, poison tobacco, insane root, stinky nightshade	Hyoscyamine, hyoscine	Nervous—anticholinergic syndrome
Ipomoea purga	Jalap	Convolvulin	Gastrointestinal
Mandragora officinarum	Mandrake	Scopolamine, hyoscyamine	Nervous—anticholinergic syndrome
Podophyllum peltatum	Mayapple, mandrake	Podophyllin	Gastrointestinal—gastroenteritis
Sanguinaria canadensis	Bloodroot, red puccoon, red root	Berberine	Gastrointestinal
Solanum dulcamara, other Solanum spp. (Color Plate 22-1)	Woody, bittersweet, or climbing nightshade	Numerous glycoalkaloids including solanine and chaconine	Gastrointestinal, nervous, cardiovascular
Tussilago farfara	Coltsfoot	PA alkaloid, senkirkine	Liver
Vinca major and V. minor	Common periwinkle, periwinkle	Vincamine	Immune system

Absinthe (Wormwood)

The name *wormwood* is derived from the ancient use of the plant (*Artemesia absinthium*) and its extracts as an intestinal anthelmintic. Wormwood was the main ingredient in absinthe, a largely banned, toxic liqueur, the chronic consumption of which was associated with absinthism. Absinthism was characterized by mental enfeeblement, hallucinations, psychosis, delirium, vertigo, trembling of the limbs, digestive disorders, thirst, paralysis, and death. The toxins found in wormwood are α- and β-thujone. In rats, intravenous (IV) injection of thujone at 40 mg/kg and 120 mg/kg induces convulsions and death, respectively. According to the German Commission E, indications for the use of wormwood include loss of appetite, dyspepsia, and biliary dyskinesia. Thujone-free plant extract is used as a flavoring agent in alcoholic beverages, such as vermouth. The FDA classifies the plant as an unsafe herb. The American Herbal Products Association (AHPA) indicates that the herb should not be used during pregnancy or lactation or for long-term use.

Aconite

Traditionally, aconite (*Aconitum* spp.) root was used for topical analgesia, neuralgia, asthma, and heart disease. It contains several cardioactive alkaloids including aconitine, aconine, picraconitine, and napelline. These act on the heart by increasing sodium flux through sodium channels. Acute toxicosis can be induced following the ingestion of 5 mL of aconite tincture, 2 mg of pure aconitine, or approximately 1 g of the plant. Clinical signs include burning sensation of the lips, tongue, and throat, and gastrointestinal upset characterized by salivation, nausea, and emesis. Cardiac arrhythmias with unusual electrical characteristics have been observed following intoxication. Death can occur from minutes to days following ingestion. Although little used in the United States, it continues to be used in traditional medicine in Asia and Europe. The most common herb-related adverse reaction in China involves aconite root.[15] The AHPA suggests that the herb be taken only under the advice of an expert qualified in its appropriate use.

Aloe

Mucilaginous leaf gel (aloe gel) from parenchymatous leaf cells of *Aloe* spp. is used as an emollient and for wound healing. Dried juice or latex (aloe) from cells below the leaf skin has been used as a laxative. The gel is the product most frequently used by the cosmetic and health food industries. The gel is not intended for internal use. External use of the gel on intact skin is generally considered safe and is not associated with adverse reactions. The latex contains a number of chemicals of which the anthraquinone, barbaloin (a glucoside of aloe-emodin), is the most abundant. Aloe-emodin and other anthraquinones are gastrointestinal irritants that exert a strong purgative effect and cause severe cramping.

Aristolochia

Traditionally, aristolochia (*Aristolochia* spp.) has been used as an antiinflammatory agent and for the treatment of snakebites. More recently, it was found to be a contaminant of a weight loss preparation.[14] The active ingredient in aristolochia is aristolochic acid, which is carcinogenic, mutagenic, and nephrotoxic. The rodent IV LD_{50} is 38 to 203 mg/kg. In rats doses as low as 5 mg/kg for 3 weeks have been associated with various neoplasias. This herb is not recommended for use.

Blue-Green Algae (Cyanobacteria)

Blue-green (BG) algae are single-celled organisms that have been promoted for their nutritional properties and used to enhance plumage color in birds. Several BG algal species produce potent toxins. *Microcystis aeruginosa* produces the hepatotoxic microcystins. *Anabaena flos-aquae* produce the neurotoxins anatoxin-a and anatoxin-a$_s$. *Aphanizomenon flos-aquae* can also produce the neurotoxins saxitoxin and neosaxitoxin. Efforts are underway to better define the risks associated with ingestion of potentially toxigenic BG algae and to establish safe concentrations of total microcystins in marketed products. *Spirulina* has also been promoted as a nutritional supplement and is not considered a toxigenic BG algae genus. However, some products have been found to be contaminated with mercury, and microbial contamination could possibly be a concern if harvested algae grow in water contaminated with human or animal wastes.

Chaparral

Traditionally, a tea made from chaparral (*Larrea tridentate*) has been used to treat acne, abdominal cramps, bronchitis, common colds, chickenpox, and snakebites. Additionally, the plant was believed to have analgesic, anticarcinogenic, and antiaging properties. Currently, this plant is not recommended for use because of its hepatotoxic properties, carcinogenicity, and ability to cause contact dermatitis, and it was removed from the generally recognized as safe category by the FDA in 1970. Nordihydroguaiaretic acid is believed to be responsible for most of the biological activity of the plant. Several human case reports associated the ingestion of chaparral tablets or capsules for 6 to 12 weeks with reversible hepatotoxicity.

Comfrey

Chronic consumption of *Symphytum* spp. has been associated with hepatotoxicity caused by the presence of pyrrolizidine alkaloids (PAs) in the plant. PA metabolites form adducts with proteins, deoxyribonucleic acid, and ribonucleic acid in hepatocytes resulting in cell damage and death. In addition, several PAs in comfrey are carcinogenic to rats. Traditionally, the plant has been used externally to promote wound healing and treat hemorrhoids and internally to treat gastric ulcers and as a blood purifier. Even when applied externally to rat skin, PAs have been detected in urine. Comfrey is unsafe for use in any form.

Digitalis

Digitalis spp. contain several cardiac glycosides including digitoxin, gitoxin, and lanatosides that inhibit sodium-potassium adenosine triphosphatase (ATPase) activity. All parts of the plant are toxic. Toxic doses of fresh leaves are reported to be approximately 6 to 7 oz for a cow, approximately 4 to 5 oz for a horse, and less than 1 oz for a pig. Sucking on the flowers or ingesting seeds and leaves of the plant have intoxicated children. Ornamental varieties of foxglove contain notably lower concentrations of the glycosides. Clinical signs of intoxication include gastrointestinal upset, dizziness, weakness, muscle tremors, miosis, and potentially fatal cardiac arrhythmias. *Digitalis* glycosides have a relatively long half-life and may accumulate, leading to intoxication. Poisoning by foxglove is one of the few plant intoxications for which there is a specific antidote. Digoxin-specific Fab antibodies are effective in treating acute intoxications.[28] A number of other plants contain cardiac glycosides including *Nerium oleander, Thevetia peruviana, Convallaria majalis, Taxus* spp., *Strophanthus* spp., *Acocanthera* spp., and *Urginea maritima.*

Ephedra (Ma Huang)

The dried young branches of ephedra (*Ephedra* spp.) have been used for their stimulating and vasoactive effects. In addition, ephedra has been used in several products promoted for weight loss. The plant constituents responsible for biologic activity are the alkaloids ephedrine and pseudoephedrine. In commercial use, dried ephedra should contain no less than 1.25% ephedrine. Ephedrine and pseudoephedrine are sympathomimetics, and acute intoxication is associated with insomnia, restlessness, tachycardia, and cardiac arrhythmias. Nausea and emesis are also reported to occur. A case series involving intoxication of dogs following ingestion of a weight loss product containing guarana (caffeine) and ma huang (ephedrine) was reported.[7] Estimated doses of the respective plants associated with adverse effects were 4.4 to 296.2 mg/kg and 1.3 to 88.9 mg/kg, respectively. Clinical signs included hyperactivity, tremors, seizures, behavioral changes, emesis, tachycardia, and hyperthermia. Ingestion was associated with mortality in 17% of the cases. North American species of ephedra (also called "Mormon tea") have not been shown to contain any pharmacologically active alkaloids.

The use of ephedra in humans has been associated with a greatly increased risk for adverse effects compared with other commonly used herbs. One study reported that products containing ephedra accounted for 64% of all reported adverse effects from herbs, although they accounted for only 1% of herbal product sales.[24-29] The actual frequency of adverse effects in patients using ephedra could not be determined because the study was based on calls received by human poison control centers. However, based on such studies the FDA initiated a ban on ephedra-containing products in April of 2004. This marked the first time that the FDA banned the sale of a dietary supplement since the passage of the DSHEA in 1994.

Garlic

Allium sativum is a member of the onion family. The plant contains 0.1% to 0.3% of a strong-smelling, volatile oil containing allyl disulfides, such as allicin. Extracts from garlic are reported to have a number of biocidal activities, to decrease lipid and cholesterol levels, to prolong clotting times, to inhibit platelet aggregation, and to increase fibrinolytic activity.[30,31] Acute toxicity of allicin for dogs and cats is unknown; its LD_{50} for mice following subcutaneous or IV administration is 120 mg/kg and 60 mg/kg, respectively. The oral LD_{50} for garlic extracts given to rats and mice ranges from 0.5 mL/kg to 30 mL/kg. In chronic toxicity studies with garlic oil or garlic extracts, anemia has been observed in dogs. A single 25-mL dose of fresh garlic extract has caused burning of the mouth, esophagus and stomach, nausea, sweating, and lightheadedness.[31] Topical application of garlic oil causes local irritation, which can be quite severe. The sensitivity of cat hemoglobin to oxidative damage may make cats more sensitive to adverse effects.

Germander

Germander (*Teucrium chamaedrys*) contains polyphenol derivatives, diterpenes, flavonoids, and tannins. Plant constituents are hepatotoxic, perhaps requiring metabolism to toxic metabolites. The toxicity of germander is not well defined. It is categorized as a class 3 herb by the AHPA, which indicates that it should not be administered except under the advice of an individual qualified in its appropriate use.

Guarana

Guarana is the dried paste made from the crushed seeds of *Paullinia cupana* or *P. sorbilis,* a fast-growing shrub native to South America. Currently, the most common forms of guarana include syrups, extracts, and distillates used as flavoring agents and as a source of caffeine for the soft drink industry. More recently, it has been added to weight loss formulations in combination with ephedra. Caffeine concentrations in the plant range from 3% to 5%, which compares with 1% to 2% for coffee beans. Oral lethal doses of caffeine in dogs and cats range from 110 to 200 mg/kg body weight and 80 to 150 mg/kg body weight, respectively.[32] See "Ephedra" earlier in this chapter for a discussion of a case series involving dogs ingesting a product containing guarana and ephedra.[33]

Kava Kava

The German Commission E has recommended the root and rhizome of *Piper methysticum* for the treatment of nervous anxiety, stress, and restlessness. The plant contains at least 18 kava pyrones, which are possible dopaminergic receptor antagonists. The toxicity of kava kava is not well defined, although chronic use in humans is associated with dry, flaking, discolored skin, and reddened eyes (kavaism). More recently, kava kava has received increased scrutiny because of potential hepatotoxicity, and kava extracts have, in fact, been banned by the European Union and Canada.[34] A total of 78 cases of possible hepatotoxicity following use of the herb are available from a variety of databases. Only a few of these cases can be reliably linked to kava kava use, and hepatotoxicity appears to be idiosyncratic.

Postulated mechanisms of hepatotoxicity include inhibition of cytochrome P450 enzymes, reduced liver glutathione concentrations, and inhibition of cyclooxygenase enzyme activity.[34,35] Overall the safety of kava kava extracts is good and compares favorably with the safety of conventional anxiolytics.[34] Kava kava does have the potential to interact with a number of other drugs and exacerbate the toxicity of other hepatotoxic agents. Where kava kava extracts are still available they should not be used during pregnancy, lactation, or clinical depression. In humans the duration of use should be limited to 3 months to prevent habituation.

Khat

Severe adverse effects in humans, including migraine, cerebral hemorrhage, myocardial infarction, and pulmonary edema have been associated with khat (*Catha edulis*) use. Khat contains tannins that are potentially hepatotoxic. The active constituents in khat include cathine and cathinone; both have stimulant properties with the potency of stimulation between that of caffeine and amphetamine. Animal studies indicate that cathinone can depress testosterone levels, cause testicular tissue degeneration, and decrease sperm numbers and motility. Khat use by pregnant women has been associated with notably lower birth rates. It may also be teratogenic and mutagenic.

Kratom

Kratom usually refers to the leaves of *Mitragyna speciosa,* a plant indigenous to Southeast Asia. Kratom, or Krypton, has been used traditionally for pain, depression, and anxiety. There is some recent use for opiate withdrawal. The leaves contain several active components, including mitragynine and 7-hydroxymitragynine.[36] Despite structural similarity to yohimbine, mitragynine acts as a μ-opioid receptor partial agonist. The relatively minor component, the indole alkaloid 7-hydroxymitragynine, is reported to be more potent than morphine. Kratom is a controlled substance in some countries but not in the United States.[37] There are some published case reports of adverse events in humans, but as yet little clinical information for animals exists.[38]

Lobelia

Traditionally, *Lobelia inflata* has been used as an antispasmodic, respiratory stimulant, relaxant, emetic, and euphoriant. The plant contains pyridine alkaloids, such as lobeline, lobelanine, and lobelanidine. Lobeline has nicotinic agonist properties (~5% to 20% of the potency of nicotine). Toxicity has been associated with ingestion of 50 mg of dried herb, 1 mL of a tincture, and 8 mg of pure lobeline. Clinical signs of intoxication include hypothermia, hypertension, respiratory depression, paralysis, seizures, euphoria, nausea, emesis, abdominal pain, salivation, tachycardia, and coma. The German Commission E does not recommend it for use, but the AHPA suggests that there is no substantiated evidence of severe signs or death following use of the plant. The AHPA does suggest that the plant not be used during pregnancy or taken in large doses.

Mistletoe

Mistletoes are grouped into two broad categories: the European mistletoe (*Viscum album*) and the American mistletoe (*Phoradendron serotinum*) (see Chapters 27 and 39). The European mistletoe is suggested for use in degenerative joint disease and as a palliative for malignant tumors. Plant constituents include β-phenylethylamine, tyramine, and structurally related compounds. In addition, European and American mistletoes contain proteins called *viscotoxins* and *phoratoxins,* respectively, with similar toxicity to abrin and ricin (found in *Abrus precatorius* and *Ricinus communis,* respectively). These compounds produce dose-dependent hypertension or hypotension, bradycardia, and increased uterine and gastrointestinal motility. All parts of the plant are considered toxic, and prompt gastrointestinal decontamination and symptomatic and supportive care should be instituted following ingestion. However, a review of the human toxicity of mistletoe indicated that the majority of patients ingesting the plant remained asymptomatic with no reported

344 SECTION 3 Miscellaneous Toxicant Groups

deaths.[39] Ingestion of up to three berries or two leaves is unlikely to produce serious human toxicity.

Noni Juice

Noni juice is derived from *Morinda citrifolia*, sometimes called "starvation fruit" or "vomit fruit" because of a taste unappealing to humans. Traditionally, noni juice, also called *Bq Ji'Tian, Indian Mulberry*, or *Wild Pine*, has been used for conditions ranging from asthma to smallpox, premenstrual syndrome, and leprosy, but is not well studied for any one of those conditions. The herbal has a high potassium content, which may predispose to interactions with potassium-sparing diuretics and certain antihypertensive medications. Xeronine and proxeronine are components mentioned in advertising but at this time have not been chemically identified or studied medically. Although there are several reports of hepatic damage in humans, there is insufficient data at this time to assess safety and efficacy in animals.[40-42]

Nutmeg and Mace

Nutmeg is derived from the seed of *Myristica fragrans*, and the spice, mace, is derived from the seed coat. Current uses of the plant include the treatment of gastrointestinal disturbances, such as cramps, flatulence, and diarrhea. It has been investigated as an antidiarrheal medication in calves.[33] It has potential anticancer and biocidal activities. The toxicity of nutmeg is uncertain, although case reports suggest that if ingested doses are sufficient, acute toxicity can occur. Two tablespoons of ground nutmeg, one to three whole nutmegs, or 5 g of powdered nutmeg may cause clinical signs of hallucinations, nausea, and severe emesis. The German Commission E lists the plant as an unapproved herb, and the AHPA suggests that it only be used under the supervision of an individual knowledgeable about its potential effects.

Oleander

Despite its toxicity, oleander (*Nerium oleander*) has been used for its medicinal properties for centuries (Color Plate 26-2). The plant contains a number of cardiac glycosides with activities similar to those of digitalis. In birds ingestion of as little as 0.12 to 0.7 g of the plant can be fatal. Ingestion of as little as 0.005% of an animal's body weight in dry oleander leaves can be fatal (~10 to 20 leaves for an adult horse).[44] Ingestion of oleander should be considered serious and prompt medical attention sought. The editor is aware of a fatal exposure of oleander leaves in a dog. An emergency gastrotomy was performed to remove the compacted oleander leaves that could not be removed via gastric lavage. The dog exhibited severe cardiac arrhythmias and ultimately died from seizures and cardiac arrest. Digoxin-specific Fab fragments are antidotal. The extreme toxicity of the plant precludes its use in any form.

Pleurisy Root

Asclepias tuberosa root traditionally has been used to ease the pain and facilitate breathing in patients with pleurisy. The toxicity of the plant is not well defined; cardiac glycosides and neurotoxic resinoids are found in many *Asclepias* spp.. The glycosides inhibit sodium-potassium ATPase. Clinical signs of intoxication include fatigue, anorexia, emesis, cardiac arrhythmias, bradycardia, and hypokalemia. This plant is best avoided.

Pokeweed

Phytolacca spp. are ubiquitous in the United States and have a long history of use in folk remedies for rheumatism and arthritis and as an emetic and purgative. Active plant constituents include triterpene saponins, a tannin, a resin, and a protein called pokeweed mitogen. All parts of the plant are toxic except the above ground leaves that grow in the early spring, which can be eaten after proper preparation. Toxic components are highest in the rootstock, less in the mature leaves and stems, and least in the fruit. Ingestion of poisonous plant parts causes severe stomach cramping, nausea, emesis, persistent diarrhea, dyspnea, weakness, spasms, hypotension, seizures, and death. Severe poisonings have been reported in adult humans who ingested mature pokeweed leaves and as little as one cup of tea brewed with ½ tsp of powdered pokeroot. There is unlikely to be a valid medical indication for the use of this plant.

Senna

Cassia spp. have been used for their laxative effects caused by anthraquinone glycosides (sennosides) present in the plant. These compounds increase gastrointestinal motility, induce fluid movement in the lumen, and have direct irritant effects. Catharsis can result from ingestion of teas containing 1 to 2 tsp of dried senna leaves. Chronic use of laxatives, including senna, can cause a laxative dependency syndrome, which is characterized by poor gastrointestinal motility in the absence of their use. Appropriate use of senna may be associated with mild abdominal cramping. More prolonged use can cause electrolyte disturbances, especially hypokalemia.

St. John's wort

A number of chemical constituents have been isolated from St. John's wort (*Hypericum perforatum*), including anthraquinone derivatives (hypericin and pseudohypericin), the phloroglucinols hyperforin and adhyperforin, flavonoids, phenols, tannins, and a volatile oil. External indications for use include acute injuries or contusions, myalgia, and first-degree burns. Taken internally, it is used to treat depression, anxiety, or nervous unrest. Assessment of possible antiviral properties is ongoing. Hyperforin is the most neuroactive component of the plant and is believed to be responsible for its CNS effects. It modulates neuronal ionic conductance and inhibits serotonin reuptake. Hypericin is a photodynamic agent, and when ingested it can induce photosensitization. Most reports of photosensitization in humans are associated with excessive intake of the plant. Other side effects are usually mild. As an aside, considerable variations in active constituent concentrations have been documented in different brands of St. John's wort. In humans, the use of St. John's wort can interfere with the safety and efficacy of numerous other drugs, including carbamazepine, citalopram, cyclosporine, digoxin, fluoxetine, fluvoxamine, naratriptan, oral contraceptives, paroxetine, phenobarbital, phenytoin, rizatriptan, sertraline, sumatriptan, theophylline, warfarin, and zolmitriptan.

White Willow

Active constituents in willow (*Salix* spp.) include salicylates (primarily in the form of glycosides salicortin and salicin) and tannins. Current indications for plant use include fever, rheumatism, and as an antiinflammatory. Therapeutic and adverse effects occur through inhibition of prostaglandin synthesis. In addition, salicylates inhibit oxidative phosphorylation and Krebs cycle enzymes. In cats acetylsalicylic (AS) acid is toxic at 80 to 120 mg/kg given orally for 10 to 12 days. In dogs AS at 50 mg/kg given orally twice a day is associated with emesis; higher doses can cause depression and metabolic acidosis. A dose of 100 to 300 mg/kg orally once daily for 1 to 4 weeks is associated with gastric ulceration; more prolonged dosing is potentially fatal.[45] Cats are particularly vulnerable to overdose because of an inability to rapidly metabolize salicylates. Presumably, salicylates in willow have approximately equivalent toxicity. Most standards for medicinal willow bark require salicylates to be present at greater than 1% dry weight, although this is difficult to achieve with many source species. There are a number of other plants that contain salicylates, including *Betula* spp. (birch), *Filipendula ulmaria* (meadowsweet), and *Populus* spp.

Yohimbine

Pausinystalia yohimbe bark contains the alkaloid yohimbine at a concentration of ~6%. Yohimbine is an α_2-adrenergic receptor blocker and has purported aphrodisiac and hallucinogenic properties. Yohimbine causes peripheral vasodilatation and CNS stimulation. In intoxications, yohimbine causes severe hypotension, abdominal distress, and weakness. CNS stimulation and paralysis have been reported. An acute IV toxic dose for dogs is 0.55 mg/kg.

The drug or crude product should never be given without adequate medical supervision. Human formulations have been combined with other purported sexual stimulants.

Essential Oils

Essential oils are the volatile, organic constituents of fragrant plant matter and contribute to plant fragrance and taste. They are extracted from plant material by distillation or cold pressing. There are a number of essential oils that are not recommended for use because of their toxicity or potential for toxicity.[46] They are listed in Table 26-2. These oils have unknown or oral LD_{50} values in animals of 1 g/kg or less. Most toxicity information has been derived using laboratory rodents or mice; such data should only be used as a rough guide because it cannot always be extrapolated to other species. They are best avoided for aromatherapy or for dermal or oral use. Essential oils that are more difficult to assess for safety, but which are best avoided, are given in Tables 26-2 and 26-3, along with their oral LD_{50} values (between 1 and 2 g/kg). *Essential Oil Safety: A Guide for Health Care Professionals*[46] is an excellent reference for in-depth discussions of general and specific essential oil toxicity. The following essential oils are of particular concern.

Camphor

Camphor is an aromatic, volatile, terpene ketone derived from the wood of *Cinnamomum camphora* or synthesized from turpentine. Camphor oil is separated into four distinct fractions: white, brown, yellow, and blue camphor.[46] White camphor is the form used in aromatherapy and in OTC products (brown and yellow fractions contain the carcinogen safrole, and are not normally available). OTC products vary in form and camphor content; external products contain 10% to 20% in semisolid forms or 1% to 10% in camphor spirits. It is used as a topical rubefacient and antipruritic agent. Camphor is rapidly absorbed from

Table 26-2	Toxic Essential Oils[34]		
Oil	**Genus, Species**	**Oral LD$_{50}$ (g/kg)**	**Toxic Component**
Boldo leaf	*Peumus boldus*	0.13	Ascaridole 16%
Wormseed	*Chenopodium ambrosioides*	0.25	Ascaridole 60%-80%
Mustard	*Brassica nigra*	0.34	Allyl isothiocyanate 99%
Armoise	*Artemisia herba-alba*	0.37	Thujone 35%
Pennyroyal (Eur.)	*Mentha pulegium*	0.40	Pulegone 55%-95%
Tansy	*Tanacetum vulgare*	0.73	Thujone 66%-81%
Thuja	*Thuja occidentalis*	0.83	Thujone 30%-80%
Calamus	*Acorus calamus* var. *angustatus*	0.84	Asarone 45%-80%
Wormwood	*Artemisia absinthium*	0.96	Thujone 34%-71%
Bitter almond	*Prunus amygdalus* var. *amara*	0.96	Prussic acid 3%
Tree wormwood, large wormwood	*Artemisia arborescens*	Not established	Iso-thujone 30%-45%
Buchu	*Barosma betulina;* *B. crenulata*	Not established	Pulegone 50%
Horseradish	*Cochlearia armoracia*	Not established	Allyl isocyanate 50%
Lanyana	*Artemisia afra*	Not established	Thujone 4%-66%
Pennyroyal (N. Am.)	*Hedeoma pulegioides*	Not established	Pulegone 60%-80%
Southernwood	*Artemisia abrotanum*	Not established	Thujone
Western red cedar	*Thuja plicata*	Not established	Thujone 85%

the skin and gastrointestinal tract, and toxic effects can occur within minutes of exposure. In humans signs of intoxication include emesis, abdominal distress, excitement, tremors, and seizures followed by CNS depression characterized by apnea and coma. Fatalities have occurred in humans ingesting 1 to 2 g of camphor-containing products, although the adult human lethal dose has been reported to be 5 to 20 g.[46,47] One teaspoon of camphorated oil (~1 mL of camphor) was lethal to 16-month-old and 19-month-old children. Chronic ingestion in children can result in hepatotoxicity and neurotoxicity.

Citrus Oil

Citrus oil and citrus oil constituents, such as D-limonene and linalool, have been shown to have insecticidal activity. Although D-limonene has been used safely as an insecticide on dogs and cats, some citrus oil formulations or use of pure citrus oil may pose a poisoning hazard.[48] Fatal adverse reactions have been reported in cats following the use of an "organic" citrus oil dip.[49] Hypersalivation, muscle tremors, ataxia, lateral recumbency, coma, and death were noted experimentally in three cats following use of the dip according to label directions.

Table 26-3	Potentially Toxic Essential Oils[34]		
Oil	Genus, Species	Oral LD$_{50}$ (g/kg)	Toxic Component
Wintergreen	*Gaultheria procumbens*	1.20	Methyl salicylate 98%
Cornmint	*Mentha arvensis* var. *piperascens*	1.25	L-menthol 35%-50% Menthone 15%-30% Pulegone 0.2%-5%
Savory (summer)	*Satureia hortensis; S. montana*	1.37	Carvacol 3%-67%; Thymol 1%-49% Para-cymene 7%-26%
Clove leaf	*Syzygium aromaticum*	1.37	Eugenol 70%-95% Isoeugenol 0.14%-0.23%
Basil	*Ocimum basilicum*	1.40	Estragole 40%-87% Methyleugenol 0.3%-4.2% Linalool 0.5%-6.3%
Hyssop	*Hyssopus officinalis*	1.40	Pinocamphone 40%; Iso-pinocamphone 30%
Sassafras (Brazilian)	*Ocotea pretiosa*	1.58	Safrole 85%-90%
Myrrh	*Commiphora* spp	1.65	Not established
Birch (sweet)	*Betula lenta*	1.70	Methyl salicylate 98%
Bay leaf (W. Indian)	*Pimenta racemosa*	1.80	Eugenol 38%-75%
Oregano	*Origanum vulgare; Coridothymus capitatus* and others	1.85	Thymol-varies Carvacrol-varies
Sassafras	*Sassafras albidum*	1.90	Safrole 85%-90%
Tarragon	*Artemisia dracunculus*	1.90	Estragole 70%-87% Methyleugenol 0.1%-1.5%
Tea tree	*Melaleuca alternifolia*	1.90	Terpenes 50%-60% Cineole 6%-8%
Savin	*Juniperus sabina*	Not established	Sabinyl acetate 20%-53% Sabinene 20%-42%

Melaleuca Oil

Derived from the leaves of the Australia tea tree (*Melaleuca alternifolia*), melaleuca oil is often referred to as *tea tree oil*. The oil contains terpenes, sesquiterpenes, and hydrocarbons. A variety of commercially available products contain the oil (e.g., shampoos), and the pure oil has been sold for use on dogs, cats, ferrets, and horses. Tea tree oil toxicosis has been reported in dogs and cats.[50,51] A case report describes the illness of three cats exposed dermally to pure melaleuca oil for flea control.[51] Clinical signs in one or more of the cats included hypothermia, ataxia, dehydration, nervousness, trembling, and coma. There were moderate increases in serum alanine transaminase and aspartate transaminase concentrations. Two cats recovered within 48 hours following decontamination and supportive care. However, one cat died approximately 3 days following exposure. The primary constituent of the oil, terpinen-4-ol, was detected in the urine of the cats. Another case involved the dermal application of seven to eight drops of oil along the backs of two dogs as a flea repellent.[52] Within approximately 12 hours, partial paralysis of the hind limbs developed in one dog, along with ataxia and depression. The other dog only displayed depression. Decontamination (bathing) and symptomatic and supportive care resulted in rapid recovery within 24 hours.

Pennyroyal Oil

A volatile oil derived from *Mentha pulegium* and *Hedeoma pulegiodes,* pennyroyal oil has a long history of use as a flea repellent and has been used to induce menstruation and abortions in humans. There is one case report of pennyroyal oil toxicosis in the veterinary literature in which a dog was dermally exposed to pennyroyal oil at approximately 2 g/kg.[12] Within 1 hour of application, the dog became listless and within 2 hours began vomiting. Thirty hours after exposure, the dog exhibited diarrhea, hemoptysis, and epistaxis. Soon thereafter, the dog had seizures and died. Histopathologic examination of liver tissue showed massive hepatocellular necrosis. The toxin in pennyroyal oil is thought to be pulegone, which is bioactivated to a hepatotoxic metabolite called menthofuran.

Oil of Wintergreen

Derived from *Gaultheria procumbens,* this oil contains a glycoside that, when hydrolyzed, releases methyl salicylate. The oil is readily absorbed through skin and is used to treat muscle aches and pains. Salicylates are toxic to dogs and cats. Because cats metabolize salicylates much more slowly than other species, they are more likely to be overdosed. Intoxicated cats may present with depression, anorexia, emesis, gastric hemorrhage, toxic hepatitis, anemia, bone marrow hypoplasia, hyperpnea, and hyperpyrexia.

Sassafras Oil

Sassafras is the name applied to two trees native to eastern Asia and one native to eastern North America (*Sassafras albidum*). All parts of the tree are aromatic, and the oil is obtained from the peeled root. The main constituent of the oil is safrole (up to 80%). Sassafras has been used as a sudorific and flavoring agent and for the treatment of eye inflammations. The oil has been used externally for relief of insect bites and stings and for removing lice. Because safrole is carcinogenic, the FDA has banned the use of the oil as a food additive. A dose of safrole of 0.66 mg/kg is considered hazardous for humans. Tea samples, prepared as recommended in commonly used herbal medicine information sources or on product labels, contain between 0.09 mg and 4.66 mg per cup.[53] One product, containing 2.5 g of sassafras bark per tea bag, was estimated to provide up to a 200-mg dose of safrole.[54] The actual amount of safrole ingested depends on the safrole content, the duration of the infusion, and the amount of tea consumed. Oil of sassafras is toxic in doses as small as 5 mL to adult humans.[55] Because of toxicity, carcinogenicity, and lack of therapeutic benefit, the use of this plant cannot be recommended under any circumstance.

Product Adulteration

There is a long history of Chinese patent medicines, especially those originating from Hong Kong, being adulterated with metals, conventional pharmaceuticals, or natural toxins.[15,56-58]

Sedatives, stimulants, and NSAIDs are common conventional pharmaceuticals added to patent medicines without labels indicating their presence. Commonly found natural toxins in Chinese patent medicines include borneol, aconite, toad secretions (*Bufo* spp., *Ch' an Su*), mylabris, scorpion, borax, acorus, and strychnine (*Strychnos nux-vomica*).[15]

The motivation for adulterating patent medicines is unclear. Perhaps there is a belief that the conventional pharmaceuticals are necessary to provide immediate relief to the patient while waiting for the herbs, with a slower onset of action, to have their desired effect. It is also possible that without the addition of potent conventional drugs, the herbal preparations would not be efficacious.

Chinese patent medicines often contain cinnabar (mercuric sulfide), realgar (arsenic sulfide), or litharge (lead oxide) as part of the traditional formula. Recently, dietary supplements, purchased largely from retail stores, were tested for arsenic, cadmium, lead, and mercury.[58] Of the 95 products tested, 84 contained botanicals as a major component of the formulation. Of those 95 products, 11 contained lead at concentrations that would have caused lead intake to exceed recommended maximum levels for children and pregnant women had the products been used according to label directions.

Serious adverse health effects have been documented in humans using adulterated Chinese herbal medicines.[57] There are no published cases in the veterinary literature, although Dr. Poppenga is aware of one case in which a small dog ingested a number of herbal tea "balls," which were prescribed to its owner for arthritis. The dog came to a veterinary clinic in acute renal failure several days after the ingestion. Analysis of the formulation revealed low-level heavy metal contamination (mercury and lead) and rather large concentrations of caffeine and the NSAID indomethacin. The acute renal failure was most likely caused by NSAID-induced renal damage.

Herb-Drug Interactions

Herb-drug interactions refer to the possibility that an herbal constituent may alter the pharmacologic effects of a conventional drug given concurrently or vice versa. The result may be either enhanced or diminished drug or herb effects or the appearance of a new effect that is not anticipated from the use of the drug or herb alone. Although there are several proposed ways to categorize herb-drug interactions, the most logical characterizes interactions from either a pharmacokinetic or a pharmacodynamic perspective.[59] Possible pharmacokinetic interactions include those that alter the absorption, metabolism, distribution, or elimination of a drug or herbal constituent and result in an increase or decrease in the concentration of active agent at the site of action. For example, herbs that contain dietary fiber, mucilages, or tannins might alter the absorption of another drug or herbal constituent. Herbs containing constituents that induce liver enzymes might be expected to affect drug metabolism or elimination. Induction of liver-metabolizing enzymes can increase the toxicity of drugs and other chemicals via increased production of reactive metabolites. The production of more toxic reactive metabolites is termed *bioactivation*.[19] Alternatively, enhanced detoxification of drugs and other chemicals can decrease their toxicity. Long-term use of herbs and other dietary supplements can induce enzymes associated with procarcinogen activation, thus increasing the risk of some cancers.[19,60] The displacement of one drug from protein binding sites by another agent increases the concentration of unbound drug available to target tissue. Pharmacodynamic interactions or interactions at receptor sites can occur; these can be agonistic or antagonistic in nature.

The quality of evidence documenting various herb-drug interactions varies. Some interactions are documented in clinical trials and some are inferred from in vitro experiments, whereas others are only suspected based on theoretical grounds. In one study evaluating the reliability of published reports of herb-drug interactions, only 13% of the reports were considered to be well documented, whereas 68% could not be evaluated because of poor or incomplete information.[61]

Table 26-4 lists potential herb-drug interactions based on conventional drug therapeutic class. Obviously, some therapeutic classes of drugs are not used in veterinary medicine, such as antiparkinsonism drugs, but they are included to provide as complete an overview

Table 26-4   Potential Herb-Drug Interactions Based on Drug Therapeutic Class[53]

Therapeutic Class	Potential Herb Interactions	Possible Adverse Effects
Analgesics	Herbs with diuretic activity (e.g., corn silk, dandelion, juniper, uva ursi)	Increased risk of toxicity with antiinflammatory analgesics
	Herbs with corticosteroid activity (e.g., licorice, bayberry)	Potential reduction of plasma salicylate concentration
	Herbs with sedative effects (e.g., calamus, nettle, ground ivy, sage, borage)	Possible enhancement of sedative effect
Anticonvulsants	Herbs with sedative effects (e.g., calamus, nettle, ground ivy, sage, borage)	Possible increase in sedative side effects
	Herbs containing salicylates (e.g., poplar willow)	Increased risk of seizure
	Ayurvedic Shankapuspi	Potentiation of phenytoin action
		Decreased phenytoin half-life
Antidepressants	Herbs with sympathomimetic amines (e.g., agnus castus, calamus, cola broom, licorice)	Increased risk of hypertension with MAOIs
	Ginkgo biloba	Potential sedative side effects
		Use with tricyclic antidepressants or other medications that ↓ seizure threshold not advised
Antiemetic and antivertigo drugs	Herbs with sedative effects (e.g., calamus, nettle, ground ivy, sage, borage)	Potential increased sedative effect
	Herbs with anticholinergic effect	Antagonism
Antiparkinsonism drugs	Herbs with anticholinergic effect	Potentiation of effects
	Herbs with cholinergic effect	Antagonism
Antipsychotics	Herbs with diuretic activity (e.g., corn silk, dandelion, juniper, uva ursi)	Potentiation of lithium action; increased risk of intoxication
	Herbs with anticholinergic effect	Reduction of phenothiazine concentrations; increased risk of seizures
	Ginseng, yohimbine, and ephedra	Concomitant use with phenelzine and monoamine oxidase inhibitors may result in increased side effects
Anxiolytics/hypnotics	Herbs with sedative effects (e.g., calamus, nettle, ground ivy, sage, borage)	Potentiation
Phenobarbital	Thujone-containing herbs (e.g., wormwood, sage, or gamolenic)	May lower seizure threshold
	Acid-containing herbs (e.g., evening primrose oil borage)	
NSAIDs	Feverfew	Reduced effectiveness of feverfew
	Herbs with antiplatelet activity (e.g., ginkgo biloba, ginger, ginseng, garlic)	May increase risk of bleeding caused by gastric irritation by NSAIDs

Stimulants	Ginseng	Increased risk of side effects
Antiarrhythmics	Herbs with cardioactive effects	Antagonism
	Herbs with diuretic activity (e.g., corn silk, dandelion, juniper, uva ursi)	Antagonism if hypokalemia occurs
Anticoagulants	Herbs with coagulant or anticoagulant activity (e.g., alfalfa, red clover, chamomile, ginkgo)	Antagonism or potentiation
	Garlic	Decreased platelet activity
	Ginger	Inhibition of thromboxane synthetase activity, thus increasing bleeding time
	Herbs containing salicylates (e.g., poplar, willow)	Potentiation
Antihyperlipid-emic drugs	Herbs with hypolipidemic activity (e.g., black cohosh, fenugreek, garlic, plantain)	Additive effect
Antihypertensives	Herbs containing hypertensive (blue cohosh, cola, ginger) or mineralocorticoid (e.g., licorice, bayberry) action	Potentiation
	Herbs with hypotensive action (e.g., agrimony, celery, ginger, hawthorn)	Antagonism
	Herbs with high levels of amines or sympathomimetic action (e.g., agnus castus black cohosh, cola, mate, St. John's-wort)	Potentiation
	Herbs with diuretic activity (e.g., corn silk, dandelion, juniper, uva ursi)	Antagonism
β-Blockers	Herbs containing cardioactive constituents	Antagonism
	Herbs with high levels amines or sympathomimetic action (e.g., agnus castus, black cohosh, cola, mate, St. John's wort)	Risk of severe hypertension
Cardiac glycosides	Herbs with cardioactive constituents (e.g., broom, squill, mistletoe, cola nut, figwort)	Antagonism or potentiation
	Hawthorn, Siberian ginseng, Kyushin, uzara root	Increased risk of bleeding
Diuretics	Herbs with diuretic activity (e.g., corn silk, dandelion, juniper, uva ursi)	Increased risk of hypokalemia
	Herbs with hypotensive action (e.g., agrimony, celery, ginger, hawthorn)	Difficulty controlling diuresis
Nitrates and cal-cium channel blockers	Herbs with cardioactive constituents (e.g., broom, squill)	Antagonism
	Herbs with hypertensive action (e.g., bayberry, broom, blue cohosh, licorice)	Antagonism
	Herbs with anticholinergic effects (e.g., corkwood tree)	Reduced buccal absorption of nitroglycerin
Sympathomimetics	Herbs containing sympathomimetic amines (e.g., aniseed, capsicum, parsley, vervain)	Increased risk of hypertension
	Herbs with hypertensive action (e.g., bayberry, broom, blue cohosh, licorice)	Increased risk of hypertension
	Herbs with hypotensive action (e.g., agrimony, celery, ginger, hawthorn)	Antagonism

Continued

Table 26-4 Potential Herb-Drug Interactions Based on Drug Therapeutic Class[53]—cont'd

Therapeutic Class	Potential Herb Interactions	Possible Adverse Effects
Antifungals (ketoconazole)	Herbs with anticholinergic effects (e.g., corkwood tree)	Decreased absorption of ketoconazole
Antidiabetic agents	Herbs with hypoglycemic or hyperglycemic principles (e.g., alfalfa, fenugreek, ginseng)	Antagonism or potentiation
	Herbs with diuretic activity (e.g., corn silk, dandelion, juniper, uva ursi)	Antagonism
	Chromium, karela	Effect on blood glucose levels altering drug requirements
Corticosteroids	Herbs with diuretic activity (e.g., corn silk, dandelion, juniper, uva ursi)	Risk of increased potassium loss
	Herbs with corticosteroid activity (e.g., licorice, bayberry)	Increased risk of side effects, such as sodium retention
	Herbs with immunostimulant effects	Antagonism of immunosuppressive effect
Sex hormones	Herbs with hormonal activity (e.g., alfalfa, bayberry, black cohosh, licorice)	Potential antagonism or potentiation
Estrogens	Herbs containing phytoestrogens (e.g., dong quai, red clover, alfalfa, licorice, black cohosh, soybeans)	Hyperestrogenism
Drugs for hyper-thyroidism or hypothyroidism	Herbs with high concentrations of iodine Horseradish and kelp	Interference with therapy
Oral contraceptives	Herbs with hormonal activity (e.g., black cohosh, licorice)	May reduce oral contraceptive effectiveness
Methotrexate	Herbs with salicylates (e.g., meadowsweet, poplar, willow)	Potential for toxicity
Drugs with immu-nostimulant or immunosup-pressive action	Herbs with immunostimulant effects (e.g., boneset, *Echinacea*, mistletoe)	Antagonism or potentiation
Probenecid	Herbs with salicylates (e.g., meadowsweet, poplar, willow)	Inhibition of uricosuric effect of probenecid
Acetazolamide	Herbs with salicylates (e.g., meadowsweet, poplar, willow)	Potential for toxicity
General anesthetics	Herbs with hypotensive constituents (e.g., black cohosh, goldenseal, hawthorn)	Potentiation of hypotension
Muscle relaxants	Herbs with diuretic action (e.g., broom, buchu, corn silk)	Possible potentiation if hypokalemia
Depolarizing mus-cle relaxants	Herbs with cardioactive constituents (e.g., cola, figwort, hawthorn)	Risk of arrhythmias

MAOI, Monoamine oxidase inhibitor; *NSAID,* nonsteroidal antiinflammatory drug.

as possible. If an interaction is listed, the reader should consult more detailed sources of information to determine its clinical relevance. It is important to point out that information regarding herb-drug interactions is expanding rapidly. There are several references that can be consulted to obtain in-depth information about specific herb-drug interactions.[17,20,59,62,63]

Diagnosis of Intoxication

Without a history of exposure to an herbal remedy, the diagnosis of intoxication is difficult. Clinical signs are often nonspecific, and the animal may have concurrent signs caused by an underlying disease condition. Vomitus or gastric lavage material should be examined for the presence of plants or other possible herbal formulations. Essential oil exposure might be suspected based on the odor of stomach contents or skin. In some instances, a constituent of an herbal remedy may be detected in a biological specimen. For example, pulegone was found in liver tissue from a dog intoxicated by pennyroyal oil.[12] Some laboratories have the capability to detect potential patent medicine adulterants. However, many veterinary diagnostic laboratories do not have such broad capabilities to detect natural products, and laboratory confirmation of exposure or intoxication is often impossible. In suspected herbal poisonings, a veterinary toxicologist should be consulted about available laboratory procedures and appropriate tissue samples for submission.

Treatment of Intoxication

Treatment is directed toward undertaking appropriate decontamination procedures, such as inducing emesis and administering activated charcoal with or without a cathartic.[64] Indications and contraindications for decontamination procedures should be followed. In general, other treatment is symptomatic and supportive. In rare cases, an antidote might be available (i.e., digoxin Fab fragments for cardiac glycosides). The adage "treat the symptoms and not the patient" is appropriate in most suspected poisonings caused by herbal preparations.

Sources of Information

Because of the increased interest in natural products, there is an explosion of information regarding their use and potential hazards of use. It is important to have access to objective, science-based information to make rational decisions regarding the safety and efficacy of plant-derived chemicals. Three excellent resources are the *Botanical Safety Handbook*,[20] prepared for the standards committee of the AHPA; the German Commission E monographs,[25] which have become available in English; and, more recently, the *Review of Natural Products*.[26] An excellent lay-oriented reference is entitled *The Honest Herbal: A Sensible Guide to the Use of Herbs and Related Remedies*.[33] In addition, there are excellent chapters regarding risks associated with the use of natural products in several human-oriented toxicology textbooks.[6,15,65] Essential oil toxicology is extensively covered in a text by Tisserand and Balacs and a chapter by Vassallo.[46,66]

A relatively recent study suggested that six commonly used herbal references contained insufficient information for the assessment and management of suspected ADRs of herbal remedies.[24] We considered the Natural Medicines Comprehensive Database (www.natural database.com) to be the most complete and useful reference source.

Finally, several other websites provide herb-related information and links to other herb information resources. These include the American Botanical Council (www.herbalgram.org), the Herb Research Foundation (www.herbs.org) and the American Society of Pharmacognosy (www.phcog.org) websites. Unfortunately, membership or a subscription is required to fully access the information on the sites. The FDA (www.fda.gov) and the National Institute of Health's National Center for Complementary and Alternative Medicine (NCCAM) (nccam.nih.gov) are two government-sponsored sites that provide free information. The FDA site provides consumer alerts and advisories about herbs and dietary supplements and mechanisms for reporting possible adverse effects related to herb and dietary supplement use. The NCCAM site, in addition to providing alerts and advisories, provides suggestions for evaluating medical resources on the web for objectivity and accuracy. HerbMed (www.herbmed.org) is an interactive, electronic herbal database sponsored by the Alternative Medicine Foundation that provides hyperlinked access to evidence-based data on the use of herbs for health. A subscription is required to obtain all of the information from the site. For access to the scientific literature, PubMed (http://www.ncbi.nlm.nih.gov/entrez/query.fcgi), sponsored by the National Library of Medicine, contains more than 14 million citations from the biomedical literature dating back to the 1950s.

References

1. Astin JA: Why patients use alternative medicine: results of a national study, *JAMA* 279:1548–1553, 1998.
2. Blais R, Maïga A, Aboubacar A: How different are users and non-users of alternative medicine? *Can J Pub Health* 88:159–162, 1997.
3. Elder NC, Gillcrist A, Minz R: Use of alternative health care by family practice patients, *Arch Fam Med* 6:181–184, 1997.
4. Vickers A, Zollman C: ABC of complementary medicine: herbal medicine, *BMJ* 319:1050–1053, 1999.
5. Abdel-Rahman A, Anyangwe N, Carlacci L, et al: The safety and regulation of natural products used as foods and food ingredients, *Toxicol Sci* 123(2):333–348, 2011.
6. Hung OL, Lewin NA: Howland MA: Herbal preparations. In Goldrank LR, Flomenbaum NE, Lewin NA, et al: *Goldfrank's toxicologic emergencies*, ed 6, Stamford, CT, 1998, Appleton and Lange.
7. Ooms TG, Khan SA, Means C: Suspected caffeine and ephedrine toxicosis resulting from ingestion of an herbal supplement containing quarana and ma huang in dogs: 47 cases (1997-1999), *J Am Vet Med Assoc* 218:225–229, 2001.
8. Gwaltney-Brant SM, Albretsen JC, Khan SA: 5-Hydroxytryptophan toxicosis in dogs: 21 cases (1989-1999), *J Am Vet Med Assoc* 216:1937–1940, 2000.
9. Lazarou J, Pomeranz BH, Corey PN: Incidence of adverse drug reactions in hospitalized patients. A meta-analysis of prospective studies, *JAMA* 279:1200–1205, 1998.
10. Pirmohamed M, James S, Meakin S, et al: Adverse drug reactions as a cause of admission to hospital: prospective analysis of 18,820 patients, *BMJ* 329:15–19, 2004.
11. Yang S, Dennehy CE, Tsourournis C: Characterizing adverse events reported to the California poison control system on herbal remedies and dietary supplements: a pilot study, *J Herb Pharmacother* 2:1–11, 2003.
12. Sudekum M, Poppenga RH, Raju N, et al: Pennyroyal oil toxicosis in a dog, *J Am Vet Med Assoc* 200: 817–818, 1992.
13. DeSmet PAGM: Toxicological outlook on the quality assurance of herbal remedies. In De Smet PAGM, Keller K, Hansel R, et al: *Adverse effects of herbal drugs 1*, Berlin, 1991, Springer-Verlag.
14. Vanherweghem LJ: Misuse of herbal remedies: the case of an outbreak of terminal renal failure in Belgium (Chinese herbs nephropathy), *J Altern Complement Med* 4:9–13, 1998.
15. Ko RJ: Herbal products information. In Leikin JB, Paloucek FP, editors: *Poisoning and toxicology compendium*, Cleveland, OH, 1998, Lexi-Comp.
16. Harris ES, Cao S, Littlefield BA, et al: Heavy metal and pesticide content in commonly prescribed individual raw Chinese herbal medicines, *Sci Total Environ* 409(20):4297–4305, 2011.
17. Blumenthal M: Perspectives on the safety of herbal medicines. In Leikin JB, Paloucek FP, editors: *Poisoning and toxicology compendium*, Cleveland, OH, 1998, Lexi-Comp.
18. Stedman C: Herbal hepatotoxicity, *Sem Liv Dis* 22:195–206, 2002.
19. Zhou S, Koh H, Gao Y, et al: Herbal bioactivation: the good, the bad and the ugly, *Life Sci* 74:935–968, 2004.
20. McGuffin M, Hobbs C, Upton R, et al: *Botanical safety handbook*, Boca Raton, FL, 1997, CRC Press.
21. Johnson WD, Morrissey RL, Usborne AL, et al: Subchronic oral toxicity and cardiovascular safety pharmacology studies of resveratrol, a naturally occurring polyphenol with cancer preventive activity, *Food Chem Toxicol* 49:3319–3327, 2011.
22. Gardiner P, Sarma DN, Dog TL, et al: The state of dietary supplement adverse event reporting in the United States, *Pharmacoepidem Dr S* 17:962–970, 2008.
23. Haller C, Kearney T, Bent S, et al: Dietary supplement adverse events: report of a one-year poison center surveillance project, *J Med Toxicol* 4:84–92, 2008.
24. Haller CA, Anderson IB, Kim SY: An evaluation of selected herbal reference texts and comparison to published reports of adverse herbal events, *Adverse Drug React Toxicol Rev* 21:143–150, 2002.

25. Blumenthal M, Busse WR, Goldberg A, et al: *The complete German Commission E monographs*, Boston, 1998, Integrative Medicine Communications.
26. DerMarderosian A, editor: *Review of natural products*, St Louis, 2001, Facts and Comparisons.
27. Birdsall TC: 5-Hydroxytryptophan: a clinically effective serotonin precursor, *Altern Med Rev* 3:271–280, 1998.
28. Roberts DJ: Plants: cardiovascular toxicity. In Ford MD, Delaney KA, Ling LJ, et al: *Clinical toxicology*, Philadelphia, 2001, WB Saunders Co.
29. Bent S, Tiedt TN, Odden MC, et al: The relative safety of ephedra compared to other herbal products, *Ann Intern Med* 138, 468–447, 2003.
30. Siegers CP: *Allium sativum.* In DeSmet PAGM, Keller K, Hänsel R, et al: *Adverse effects of herbal drugs 1*, Berlin, 1991, Springer-Verlag.
31. DerMarderosian A, editor: *Review of natural products*, St Louis, 2001, Facts and Comparisons.
32. Carson TL: Methylxanthines. In Peterson ME, Talcott PA, editors: *Small animal toxicology*, Philadelphia, 2001, WB Saunders Co.
33. Tyler VE: *The honest herbal: a sensible guide to the use of herbs and related remedies*, ed 3, New York, 1993, Pharmaceutical Products Press.
34. Clouatre DL: Kava kava: Examining new reports of toxicity, *Toxicol Lett* 150:85–96, 2004.
35. Anke J, Ramzan I: Kava hepatotoxicity: are we any closer to the truth? *Planta Med* 70:193–196, 2004.
36. Horie S, Koyama F, Takayama H, et al: Indole alkaloids of a Thai medicinal herb, *Mitragyna speciosa*, that has opioid agonistic effect in guinea pig ileum, *Planta Med* 71(3):231–236, 2005.
37. Babu KM, McCurdy CR, Boyer EW: Opioid receptors and legal highs: *Salvia divinorum* and kratom, *Clin Toxicol* 46(2):146–152, 2008.
38. Kapp FG, Maurer HH, Auwarter V, Winkelmann M, Heimanns-Claussen M: Intra-hepatic cholestasis following abuse of powdered kratom (*M. speciosa*), *J Med Toxicol* 3:227–231, 2011.
39. Hall AH, Spoerke DG, Rumack BH: Assessing mistletoe toxicity, *Ann Emer Med* 15:1320–1323, 1986.
40. Yu EL, Sivagnamam M, Ellis L, Huang JS: Acute hepatotoxicity after ingestion of *Morinda citrifolia* (noni juice) in a 14-year-old boy, *J Pediatr Gastroenterology Nutr* 52:222, 2011.
41. Millonig G, Stadmann S, Vogel W: Herbal hepatotoxicity: acute hepatitis caused by a noni preparation (*Morinda citrifolia*), *Eur J Gastroenterol Hepatol* 17:445, 2005.
42. Stadlbauer V, et al: Hepatotoxicity of noni juice: report of 2 cases, *World J Gastroenterol* 11(30):4758–4760, 2008.
43. Stamford IF, Bennett A: Treatment of diarrhea in calves with nutmeg, *Vet Rec* 106:389, 1980.
44. Kingsbury JM: *Poisonous plants of the United States and Canada*, Engelwood Cliffs, NJ, 1964, Prentice-Hall.
45. Osweiler GD: Over-the-counter drugs and illicit drugs of abuse. *The national veterinary medical series: toxicology*, Philadelphia, 1996, Williams and Wilkins.
46. Tisserand R, Balacs T: *Essential oil safety: a guide for health care professionals*, Edinburgh, 1999, Churchill Livingstone.
47. Emery DP, Corban JG: Camphor toxicity, *J Paediatr Child Health* 35:105–106, 1999.
48. Powers KA, Hooser SB, Sundberg JP, et al: An evaluation of the acute toxicity of an insecticidal spray containing linalool, D-limonene, and piperonyl butoxide applied topically to domestic cats, *Vet Human Toxicol* 30:206–210, 1988.
49. Hooser SB, Beasley VR, Everitt JI: Effects of an insecticidal dip containing D-limonene in the cat, *J Am Vet Med Assoc* 189:905–908, 1986.
50. Villar D, Knight MJ, Hansen SR, et al: Toxicity of melaleuca oil and related essential oils applied topically on dogs and cats, *Vet Hum Toxicol* 36:139–142, 1994.
51. Bischoff K, Guale F: Australian tea tree (*Melaleuca alternifolia*) oil poisoning in three purebred cats, *J Vet Diagn Invest* 10:208–210, 1998.
52. Kaluzienski M: Partial paralysis and altered behavior in dogs treated with melaleuca oil, *J Toxicol Clin Toxicol* 38:518, 2000.
53. Carlson M, Thompson RD: Liquid chromatographic determination of safrole in sassafras-derived herbal products, *JAOAC* 80:1023–1028, 1997.
54. Segelman AB, Segelman FP, Karliner J, et al: Sassafras and herb tea. Potential health hazards, *JAMA* 236:477, 1976.
55. Grande GA, Dannewitz SR: Symptomatic sassafras oil ingestion, *Vet Human Toxicol* 29:447, 1987.
56. Au AM, Ko R, Boo FO, et al: Screening methods for drugs and heavy metals in Chinese patent medicines, *Bull Environ Contam Toxicol* 65:112–119, 2000.
57. Ernst E: Adulteration of Chinese herbal medicines with synthetic drugs: a systematic review, *J Intern Med* 252:107–113, 2002.
58. Dolan SP, Nortrup DA, Bolger M, et al: Analysis of dietary supplements for arsenic, cadmium, mercury, and lead using inductively coupled plasma mass spectrometry, *J Agr Food Chem* 51:1307–1312, 2003.

59. Blumenthal M: Interactions between herbs and conventional drugs: introductory considerations, *HerbalGram* 49:52–63, 2000.
60. Ryu S, Chung W: Induction of the procarcinogen-activating CYP1A2 by a herbal dietary supplement in rats and humans, *Food Cosmet Toxicol* 41:861–866, 2003.
61. Fugh-Berman A, Ernst E: Herb-drug interactions: a review and assessment of report reliability, *J Clin Pharmacol* 52:587–595, 2001.
62. American Botanical Council: *Herb reference guide (pamphlet)*, 1998.
63. Herr SM: *Herb-drug interaction handbook*, ed 2, Nassau, NY, 2002, Church Street Books.
64. Poppenga R: Treatment. In Plumlee KH, editor: *Clinical veterinary toxicology*, St Louis, 2004, Mosby.
65. Palmer ME, Howland MA: Herbals and other dietary supplements. In Ford MD, Delaney KA, Ling LJ, et al: *Clinical toxicology*, Philadelphia, 2001, WB Saunders.
66. Vassallo S: Essential oils. In Ford MD, Delaney KA, Ling LJ, et al: *Clinical toxicology*, Philadelphia, 2001, WB Saunders.

Household and Garden Plants

27

A. Catherine Barr, PhD, DABT

- An excellent website for a listing of toxic and non-toxic plants to cats and dogs: http://www.aspca.org/pet-care/poison-control/plants/

This chapter is designed to support small animal veterinarians in cases of potential toxic plant ingestion. With the client's help, the veterinarian should refer to Box 27-1 to determine whether any of the plants listed have been available to the patient. Note that plants have been listed in multiple categories when associated with multiple clinical signs. Veterinarians should be aware that common names of plants can differ in different locations of the United States. Accurate physical identification of the plants is essential, and this may necessitate gaining access to other resources (e.g., garden nurseries, horticulturists, college, university, or extension support staff, botanists, books, and the Internet). For the plants listed, one can then refer to Table 27-1 to determine the potential scope of the toxic syndrome and its prognosis. The patient is then treated as indicated. Information about the plant or plants involved is shared with the client, and isolation of the patient from the plants is recommended in the future. When possible, alternative plants from Table 27-2 should be suggested.

Treatment of Plant Intoxications

In most cases the primary treatments for toxic plant ingestion include decontamination and symptomatic supportive care. A large proportion of toxic plants cause vomiting, which in many cases alleviates the necessity for further decontamination. However, with some plants vomiting is delayed, and decontamination procedures should include induced emesis or gastric lavage (depending on patient condition). Stomach content or vomitus is reserved for later examination because plant material may be helpful in identifying causative agents and guiding clients toward preventing future incidents. Emesis is followed with activated charcoal and saline cathartic to extend decontamination. The patient is monitored during catharsis, and fluids are administered as necessary. There are very few specific treatments for plant intoxications; when they exist, they have been listed in Table 27-1. Only treatments that are consistently helpful have been noted. For the remainder, the patient is treated symptomatically and given supportive care. Veterinarians who have questions should call a diagnostic toxicologist, generally located at their nearest full-service veterinary diagnostic facility (see Chapter 12).

Box 27-1	Toxic Plant Quick Reference Based on Clinical Signs

Gastrointestinal System

African milk bush (*Synadenium grantii*)

Ageratum, floss-flower (*Ageratum* spp.)

Alder buckthorn (*Rhamnus* spp.)

Amaryllis (*Amaryllis* spp.)

Anemone, Pasque flower, windflower, meadow anemone, crowfoot (*Anemone* spp.)

Apple (*Malus* spp.)

Apricot, peach, plum, bitter almond, cherry, choke cherry (*Prunus* spp.)

Arnica (*Arnica montana*)

Arum (*Aram italicum*)

Aucuba, Japanese aucuba, Japanese laurel, spotted laurel (*Aucuba japonica*)

Azalea (*Rhododendron* spp.)

Baby's breath (*Gypsophlia paniculata*)

Bagpod sesbane (*Sesbania vesicaria*)

Barberry, pipperidge (*Berberis* spp.)

Bird of paradise (*Caesalpinia* spp.)

Bittersweet, woody nightshade, wild nightshade (*Solanum dulcamara*)

Black bryony (*Tamus communis*)

Black laurel, mountain laurel (*Leucothoe davisiae*)

Black locust (*Robinia pseudoacacia*)

Black nightshade (*Solanum nigrum*)

Bleeding heart, Dutchman's breeches, squirrel corn, staggerweed (*Dicentra* spp.)

Blood lily, powderpuff lily (*Haemanthus multiflorus*)

Bluebell (*Hyacinthoides non-scripta*)

Blue cohosh (*Caulophyllum thalictroides*)

Blue tannia, blue taro, caladium, elephant's ear, malanga, tannia, yautia (*Xanthosoma* spp.)

Box, common box, boxwood (*Buxus sempervirens*)

Broom (*Cytisus* spp.)

Buttercup, meadow buttercup, crowfoot, lesser spearwort (*Ranunculus* spp.)

Caladium, elephant's ear (*Caladium* spp.)

Calla lily (*Zantedeschia* spp.)

Candelabra aloe, octopus plant, torch plant, Barbados aloe, medicinal aloe (*Aloe* spp.)

Candelabra cactus, false cactus, mottled spurge, dragon bones (*Euphorbia lactea*)

Castor bean (*Ricinus communis*)

Century plant, maguey, American aloe (*Agave americanum*)

Ceriman, Swiss cheese plant, fruit-salad plant, split-leaf philodendron, Mexican breadfruit (*Monstera* spp.)

Chenille plant, red-hot cattail (*Acalypha hispida*)

Cherry laurel (*Prunus laurocerasus*)

Chinaberry tree (*Melia azederach*)

Chinese evergreen (*Aglaonema* spp.)

Chinese lantern, winter cherry, Cape gooseberry (*Physalis alkekengi*)

Chinese yam, cinnamon vine (*Dioscorea batatas*)

Christmas rose, black hellebore (*Helleborus* spp.)

Cohosh, baneberry, doll's eyes (*Actaea* spp.)

Common bean (*Phaseolus vulgaris*)

Coontie, cardboard palm, camptie, yugulla (*Zamia* spp.)

Coral bean, coral tree (*Erythrina* spp.)

Crinum lily, spider lily, swamp lily (*Crinum* spp.)

Croton (*Codiaeum variegatum* or *Croton tiglium*)

Crown of thorns (*Euphorbia milii*)

Box 27–1	Toxic Plant Quick Reference Based on Clinical Signs—cont'd

Daffodil, trumpet narcissus, jonquil (*Narcissus* spp.)
Death camas (*Zigadenus* spp.)
Devil's ivy, ivy arum, pothos, hunter's robe, taro vine (*Epipremnum aureum*)
Dieffenbachia, dumb cane (*Dieffenbachia* spp.)
Dogbane, Indian hemp (*Apocynum cannabinum*)
Easter lily, star-gazer lily, tiger lily (*Lilium* spp.)
Elder, dwarf elder, Danewort (*Sambucus ebulus*)
Elephant's ear (*Alocasia* spp.)
English ivy, Irish ivy, common ivy (*Hedera helix*)
Ephedra, ma huang, Mormon tea (*Ephedra* spp.)
Eucalyptus, blue gum, cider gum, silver dollar, Australian fever tree (*Eucalyptus* spp.)
Euonymus, spindle (*Euonymus* spp.)
Euphorbium (*Euphorbia resinifera*)
European mistletoe (*Viscum album*)
False hellebore, white hellebore (*Veratrum* spp.)
Fetter bush, stagger bush (*Lyonia* spp.)
Firethorn (*Pyracantha* spp.)
Fishtail palm (*Caryota mitis*)
Flamingo flower (*Anthurium* spp.)
Foxglove, common foxglove, long purples, dead men's fingers
  (*Digitalis* spp., (Color Plate 27-1))
Gloriosa lily, glory lily, climbing lily (*Gloriosa superba*)
Golden chain tree (*Laburnum anagyroides*)
Golden corydalis, bulbous corydalis, scrambled eggs, fitweed, fumitory (*Corydalis* spp.)
Golden dewdrop (*Duranta repens*)
Goldenseal (*Hydrastis canadensis*)
Golden spider lily, red spider lily, magic lily (*Lycoris* spp.)
Goosefoot, nephthytis, African evergreen, arrowhead vine (*Syngonium* spp.)
Greater celandine (*Chelidonium majus*)
Green earth star (*Cryptanthus acaulis*)
Guelder-rose, high-bush cranberry (*Viburnum* spp.)
Herb-Paris (*Paris quadrifolia*)
Holly, yaupon, possum-haw (*Ilex* spp.)
Horse chestnut, buckeye (*Aesculus* spp.)
Horseradish, red cole (*Armoracia rusticana*)
Hyacinth, garden hyacinth, Dutch hyacinth (*Hyacinthus orientalis*)
Hydrangea, hills of snow, French hydrangea, hortensia (*Hydrangea macrophylla*)
India rubber vine, purple allemande (*Cryptostegia* spp.)
Iris, crested iris, dwarf iris, fleur-de-lis, blue flag, butterfly iris, poison flag, yellow iris
  (*Iris* spp.)
Jack-in-the-pulpit (*Arisaema triphyllum*)
Jerusalem cherry, Christmas cherry, winter cherry, Natal cherry (*Solanum pseudocapsicum*)
Kaffir lily (*Clivia miniata*)
Kalanchoe, Palm-Beach-bells, feltbush, velvet elephant ear, devil's backbone, lavender-scallops (*Kalanchoe* spp.)
Kingcup, marsh marigold (*Caltha palustris*)
Lantana, shrub verbena, yellow sage, bunchberry (*Lantana camara*)
Larkspur (*Delphinium* spp.)
Laurel, bay laurel, sweet bay (*Laurus nobilis*)
Lily of the palace, naked lady, amaryllis (*Hippeastrum* spp.)
Lily of the valley (*Convallaria majalis*)

Continued

Box 27–1	Toxic Plant Quick Reference Based on Clinical Signs—cont'd

Liriope (*Liriope* spp.)

Lobelia, cardinal flower, blue lobelia (*Lobelia* spp.)

Loquat, Japanese plum (*Eriobotrya japonica*)

Lords-and-ladies, cuckoo pint, Adam and Eve (*Arum maculatum*)

Lupin, lupine, bluebonnet (*Lupinus* spp.)

Male fern (*Dryopteris filix-mas*)

Manchineel tree, manzanillo (*Hippomane mancinella*)

Marigold, African marigold, French marigold, bog marigold, Aztec marigold (*Tagetes* spp.)

Marsh marigold, kingcup (*Caltha palustris*)

May apple, mandrake (*Podophyllum* spp.)

May lily (*Maianthemum bifolium*)

Meadow saffron, autumn crocus (*Colchicum autumnale*)

Mescal bean, mountain laurel, frijolito, Eve's necklace (*Sophora* spp.)

Mezereon, spurge olive (*Daphne* spp.)

Milkweed, butterfly weed (*Asclepias* spp.)

Mock azalea, rusty-leaf (*Menziesia ferruginea*)

Monkshood (*Aconitum* spp.)

Mountain laurel, dwarf laurel (*Kalmia* spp.)

Netted vriesea (*Vriesea fenestralis*)

Nettle, stinging nettle, noseburn (*Urtica* spp., *Cnidoscolus* spp., *Tragia* spp.)

Ngaio tree (*Myoporum laetum*)

Night-blooming jessamine, Chinese inkberry (*Cestrum nocturnum*)

Nightshade (*Solanum* spp.)

Oak (*Quercus* spp.)

Old man's beard, traveler's joy, virgin's bower (*Clematis* spp.)

Oleander (*Nerium oleander*)

Oregon grape, trailing mahonia (*Mahonia* spp.)

Ornamental pepper (*Capsicum annuum*)

Oyster plant, boat lily, Moses in a boat (*Rhoeo spathacea*)

Peace lily, white sails, white anthurium, spathe flower, Mauna Loa (*Spathiphyllum* spp.)—very low toxicity

Pencil tree, milkbush, Indian tree, rubber euphorbia, finger tree, naked lady (*Euphorbia tirucalli*)

Periwinkle (*Vinca* spp.)

Persian violet, alpine violet, sowbread (*Cyclamen* spp.)

Peyote, mescal, mescal buttons (*Lophophora williamsii*)

Pheasant's eye (*Adonis* spp.)

Philodendron, sweetheart plant, panda plant, parlor ivy (*Philodendron* spp.)

Physic nut, Berlander nettlespurge (*Jatropha* spp.)

Pieris (*Pieris japonica*)

Pineapple, pineapple tree (*Ananas comosus*)

Pink quill (*Tillandsia cyanea*)

Plumbago, Cape plumbago, Cape leadwort, Ceylon leadwort (*Plumbago* spp.)

Poinsettia, Christmas star (*Euphorbia pulcherrima*)—very low toxicity

Pokeweed, pokeberry, pokesalad (*Phytolacca americana*)

Potato (*Solanum tuberosum*)

Primrose, German primrose, poison primrose (*Primula* spp.)

Privet, wax-leaf ligustrum (*Ligustrum* spp.)

Pulsatilla (*Pulsatilla* spp.)

Red bryony, white bryony (*Bryonia* spp.)

Rhododendron (*Rhododendron* spp.)

Box 27–1	Toxic Plant Quick Reference Based on Clinical Signs—cont'd

Rhubarb, garden rhubarb, pie plant, water plant, wine plant (*Rheum rhabarbarum*)
Rosary pea, prayer bean, jequirity, precatory bean (*Abrus precatorius*)
Rouge plant, pigeon berry (*Rivina humilis*)
Rowan, mountain ash, service tree, whitebeam (*Sorbus* spp.)
Sago palm, leatherleaf palm, Japanese fern palm (*Cycas revoluta, Cycas* spp.)
Sandbox tree, monkey pistol (*Hura crepitans*)
Savin (*Juniperus sabina*)
Schefflera, umbrella tree, rubber tree, starleaf (*Schefflera* spp.)
Sea onion (*Urginea maritima*)
Sensitive plant, shame plant, touch-me-not, action plant, humble plant (*Mimosa pudica*)
Skunk cabbage (*Symplocarpus foetidus*), yellow skunk cabbage (*Lysichiton americanum*)
Snowberry, wolfberry, Indian currant (*Symphoricarpus* spp.)
Snowdrop (*Galanthus nivalis*)
Solomon's seal (*Polygonatum* spp.)
Sorrel, wood sorrel (*Oxalis* spp.)
Spider lily, crown-beauty, sea daffodil, basket flower, alligator lily (*Hymenocallis* spp.)
Spurge, creeping spurge, donkey tail (*Euphorbia myrsinites*)
Squill, starry hyacinth, autumn scilla, hyacinth scilla, Cuban lily, Peruvian jacinth, hyacinth of Peru, bluebell (*Scilla* spp.)
Star of Bethlehem, summer snowflake, dove's dung, nap-at-noon (*Ornithogalum* spp.)
Sweet-flag (*Acorus calamus*)
Taro, dasheen cocoyam (*Colocasia esculenta*)
Tobacco, tree tobacco (*Nicotiana* spp.)
Tomato (*Lycopersicon lycopersicum*)
Tuberous begonia (*Begonia tuberhybrida*)
Tulip (*Tulipa* spp., hyb)
Tung oil tree (*Aleurites* spp.)
Urn plant (*Aechmea fasciata*)
Water hemlock, cowbane (*Cicuta* spp.)
Water lettuce, shellflower (*Pistia stratiotes*)
Wax begonia (*Begonia sempervirens-cultorum*)
Weeping fig, Java willow, Benjamin tree, small-leaved rubber plant (*Ficus benjamina*)
White cedar (*Thuja occidentalis*)
White mustard, charlock (*Sinapis* spp.)
White snakeroot (*Eupatorium rugosum*)
Wild calla, wild arum (*Calla palustris*)
Wild radish (*Raphanus rhaphinistrum*)
Wild rosemary (*Ledum palustre*)
Wisteria, Chinese kidney bean (*Wisteria sinensis*)
Wormwood, sagewort, sagebrush (*Artemisia* spp.)
Yellow allamanda, Nani Ali'i, flor de barbero (*Allamanda cathartica*)
Yellow oleander (*Thevetia peruviana*)
Yesterday today and tomorrow (*Brunfelsia* spp.)
Yew, Japanese yew (*Taxus* spp.)
Zamia (*Macrozamia* spp.)
Zephyr lily, rain lily, fairy lily, fire lily (*Zephyranthes* spp.)
Zulu potato, climbing onion (*Bowiea volubilis*)

Central or Peripheral Nervous System
Pinpoint Pupils
Azalea (*Rhododendron* spp.)
Black laurel, mountain laurel (*Leucothoe davisiae*)

Continued

Box 27–1	Toxic Plant Quick Reference Based on Clinical Signs—cont'd

California poppy (*Eschscholzia californica*)
Herb-Paris (*Paris quadrifolia*)
Kaffir lily (*Clivia miniata*)
Mountain laurel, dwarf laurel (*Kalmia* spp.)
Opium poppy (*Papaver somniferum*)
Pieris (*Pieris japonica*)
Poppy (*Papaver* spp.)
Rhododendron (*Rhododendron* spp.)
Wild rosemary (*Ledum palustre*)

Dilated Pupils (Mydriasis)
Angel's trumpet (*Brugmansia* spp.)
Aralia, Balfour aralia, dinner plate aralia, Ming aralia, geranium-leaf aralia, wild
    coffee, coffee tree (*Polyscias* spp.)
Bittersweet, woody nightshade, wild nightshade (*Solanum dulcamara*)
Black nightshade (*Solanum nigrum*)
Candelabra cactus, false cactus, mottled spurge, dragon bones (*Euphorbia lactea*)
Christmas rose, black hellebore (*Helleborus* spp.)
Croton (*Croton tiglium*)
Deadly nightshade (*Atropa belladonna*)
English ivy, Irish ivy, common ivy (*Hedera helix*)
Euphorbium (*Euphorbia resinifera*)
Golden dewdrop (*Duranta repens*)
Hemlock (*Conium maculatum*)
Henbane (*Hyoscyamus niger*)
Jerusalem cherry, Christmas cherry, winter cherry, Natal cherry (*Solanum
    pseudocapsicum*)
Jimsonweed, thorn-apple, moonflower (*Datura stramonium*)
Kentucky coffee tree (*Gymnocladus dioicus*)
Milkweed, butterfly weed (*Asclepias* spp.)
Morning glory, bindweed, pearly gates (*Ipomoea* spp.)
Pencil tree, milkbush, Indian tree, rubber euphorbia, finger tree, naked lady
    (*Euphorbia tirucalli*)
Peyote, mescal, mescal button (*Lophophora williamsii*)
Potato (*Solanum tuberosum*)
Sandbox tree, monkey pistol (*Hura crepitans*)
Schefflera, umbrella tree, rubber tree, starleaf (*Schefflera* spp.)
Tomato (*Lycopersicon lycopersicum*)
Tung oil tree (*Aleurites* spp.)
Yew, Japanese yew (*Taxus* spp.)

Hyperexcitability, Muscle Twitches
Azalea (*Rhododendron* spp.)
Black laurel, mountain laurel (*Leucothoe davisiae*)
Coffee (*Coffee arabica*)
Day-blooming jessamine (*Cestrum diurnum*)
Deadly nightshade (*Atropa belladonna*)
Golden chain tree (*Laburnum anagyroides*)
Golden corydalis, bulbous corydalis, scrambled eggs, fitweed, fumitory (*Corydalis*
    spp.)
Henbane (*Hyoscyamus niger*)
Horse chestnut, buckeye (*Aesculus* spp.)
Jimsonweed, thorn-apple, moonflower (*Datura stramonium*)
Karaka nut (*Corynocarpus laevigatus*)

Box 27–1	Toxic Plant Quick Reference Based on Clinical Signs—cont'd

Kentucky coffee tree (*Gymnocladus dioicus*)
Marijuana (*Cannabis sativa*)
Mezereon, spurge olive (*Daphne mezereum*)
Mock azalea, rusty-leaf (*Menziesia ferruginea*)
Moonseed, sarsparilla (*Menispermum canadense*)
Mountain laurel, dwarf laurel (*Kalmia* spp.)
Pieris (*Pieris japonica*)
Pinkroot, West Indian pinkroot (*Spigelia* spp.)
Rhododendron (*Rhododendron* spp.)
Wild rosemary (*Ledum palustre*)
Yesterday today and tomorrow (*Brunfelsia calycina*)

Delirium, Hallucinations, Behavioral Changes
Angel's trumpet (*Brugmansia* spp.)
Christmas rose, black hellebore (*Helleborus* spp.)
Deadly nightshade (*Atropa belladonna*)
Golden chain tree (*Laburnum anagyroides*)
Henbane (*Hyoscyamus niger*)
Jimsonweed, thorn-apple, moonflower (*Datura stramonium*)
Madagascar periwinkle (*Catharanthus roseus*)
Male fern (*Dryopteris filix-mas*)
Marijuana (*Cannabis sativa*)
Mescal bean, mountain laurel, frijolito, Eve's necklace (*Sophora* spp.)
Morning glory, bindweed, pearly gates (*Ipomoea* spp.)
Nutmeg (*Myristica fragrans*)
Peyote, mescal, mescal buttons (*Lophophora williamsii*)

Trembling, Ataxia, Weakness, Depression
Ageratum, floss-flower (*Ageratum* spp.)
Amaryllis (*Amaryllis* spp.)
Aralia, Balfour aralia, dinner plate aralia, Ming aralia, geranium-leaf aralia, wild coffee, coffee tree (*Polyscias* spp.)
Azalea (*Rhododendron* spp.)
Bittersweet, woody nightshade, wild nightshade (*Solanum dulcamara*)
Black nightshade (*Solanum nigrum*)
Bleeding heart, Dutchman's breeches, squirrel corn, staggerweed (*Dicentra* spp.)
Bluebell (*Hyacinthoides non-scripta*)
Blue cohosh (*Caulophyllum thalictroides*)
Box, common box, boxwood (*Buxus sempervirens*)
Chinaberry tree (*Melia azederach*)
Coral bean, coral tree (*Erythrina* spp.)
Daffodil, trumpet narcissus, jonquil (*Narcissus* spp.)
Easter lily, star-gazer lily, tiger lily (*Lilium* spp.)
Ephedra, ma huang, Mormon tea (*Ephedra* spp.)
Foxglove, common foxglove, long purples, dead men's fingers (*Digitalis purpurea*)
Gloriosa lily, glory lily, climbing lily (*Gloriosa superba*)
Golden corydalis, bulbous corydalis, scrambled eggs, fitweed, fumitory (*Corydalis* spp.)
Hemlock (*Conium maculatum*)
Horse chestnut, buckeye (*Aesculus* spp.)
Horsetail (*Equisetum* spp.)
Hound's-tongue (*Cynoglossum officinale*)
Jerusalem cherry, Christmas cherry, winter cherry, Natal cherry (*Solanum pseudocapsicum*)

Continued

| Box 27–1 | Toxic Plant Quick Reference Based on Clinical Signs—cont'd |

Kalanchoe, Palm-Beach-bells, feltbush, velvet elephant ear, devil's backbone, lavender-scallops (*Kalanchoe* spp.)
Kentucky coffee tree (*Gymnocladus dioicus*)
Lantana, shrub verbena, yellow sage, bunchberry (*Lantana camara*)
Larkspur (*Delphinium* spp.)
Lobelia, cardinal flower, blue lobelia (*Lobelia* spp.)
Lupin, lupine, bluebonnet (*Lupinus* spp.)
Mescal bean, mountain laurel, frijolito, Eve's necklace (*Sophora* spp.)
Mezereon, spurge olive (*Daphne mezereum*)
Milkweed, butterfly weed (*Asclepias* spp.)
Mimosa, silk tree (*Albizia julibrissin*)
Monkshood (*Aconitum* spp.)
Mountain laurel, dwarf laurel (*Kalmia* spp.)
Nettle, stinging nettle, noseburn (*Urtica* spp., *Cnidoscolus* spp., *Tragia* spp.)
Opium poppy (*Papaver somniferum*)
Pieris (*Pieris japonica*)
Poppy (*Papaver* spp.)
Red bryony, white bryony (*Bryonia* spp.)
Rhododendron (*Rhododendron* spp.)
Sago palm, leatherleaf palm, Japanese fern palm (*Cycas revoluta, Cycas* spp.)
Schefflera, umbrella tree, rubber tree, starleaf (*Schefflera* spp.)
Tobacco, tree tobacco (*Nicotiana* spp.)
Water hemlock, cowbane (*Cicuta* spp.)
White snakeroot (*Eupatorium rugosum*)
Wild rosemary (*Ledum palustre*)
Yesterday today and tomorrow (*Brunfelsia calycina*)
Zamia (*Macrozamia* spp.)
Zephyr lily, rain lily, fairy lily, fire lily (*Zephyranthes* spp.)

Paralysis
Angel's trumpet (*Brugmansia* spp.)
Azalea (*Rhododendron* spp.)
Black laurel, mountain laurel (*Leucothoe davisiae*)
Blood lily, powderpuff lily (*Haemanthus multiflorus*)
Broom (*Cytisus* spp.)
Coral bean, coral tree (*Erythrina* spp.)
Coyotilla, tullidora (*Karwinskia humboldtiana*)
Day-blooming jessamine (*Cestrum diurnum*)
Death camas (*Zigadenus* spp.)
False hellebore, black hellebore (*Veratrum* spp.)
Hemlock (*Conium maculatum*)
Kaffir lily (*Clivia miniata*)
Kentucky coffee tree (*Gymnocladus dioicus*)
Larkspur (*Delphinium* spp.)
Lily of the palace, naked lady, amaryllis (*Hippeastrum* spp.)
Meadow saffron, autumn crocus (*Colchicum autumnale*)
Monkshood (*Aconitum* spp.)
Mountain laurel, dwarf laurel (*Kalmia* spp.)
Persian violet, alpine violet, sowbread (*Cyclamen* spp.)
Pieris (*Pieris* spp.)
Rhododendron (*Rhododendron* spp.)
Wild rosemary (*Ledum palustre*)

| Box 27–1 | Toxic Plant Quick Reference Based on Clinical Signs—cont'd |

Convulsions

Amaryllis (*Amaryllis* spp.)

Angel's trumpet (*Brugmansia* spp.)

Aralia, Balfour aralia, dinner plate aralia, Ming aralia, geranium-leaf aralia, wild coffee, coffee tree (*Polyscias* spp.)

Black locust (*Robinia pseudoacacia*)

Bleeding heart, Dutchman's breeches, squirrel corn, staggerweed (*Dicentra* spp.)

Box, common box, boxwood (*Buxus sempervirens*)

Broom (*Cytisus* spp.)

Candelabra cactus, false cactus, mottled spurge, dragon bones (*Euphorbia lactea*)

Castor bean (*Ricinus communis*)

Chinaberry tree (*Melia azederach*)

Croton (*Croton tiglium*)

English ivy, Irish ivy, common ivy (*Hedera helix*)

Euphorbium (*Euphorbia resinifera*)

Fetter bush, stagger bush (*Lyonia* spp.)

Golden chain tree (*Laburnum anagyroides*)

Golden corydalis, bulbous corydalis, scrambled eggs, fitweed, fumitory (*Corydalis* spp.)

Golden dewdrop (*Duranta repens*)

Karaka nut (*Corynocarpus laevigatus*)

Loquat (*Eriobotrya japonica*)

Meadow saffron, autumn crocus (*Colchicum autumnale*)

Mediterranean thistle (*Atractylis gummifera*)

Milkweed, butterfly weed (*Asclepias* spp.)

Mimosa, silk tree (*Albizia julibrissin*)

Moonseed, sarsaparilla (*Menispermum canadense*)

Ngiao tree (*Myoporum laetum*)

Pencil tree, milkbush, Indian tree, rubber euphorbia, finger tree, naked lady (*Euphorbia tirucalli*)

Persian violet, alpine violet, sowbread (*Cyclamen* spp.)

Sago palm, leatherleaf palm, Japanese fern palm (*Cycas revoluta, Cycas* spp.)

Sandbox tree, monkey pistol (*Hura crepitans*)

Schefflera, umbrella tree, rubber tree, starleaf (*Schefflera* spp.)

Sea onion (*Urginea maritima*)

Spurge, creeping spurge, donkey tail (*Euphorbia myrisinites*)

Squill, starry hyacinth, autumn scilla, hyacinth scilla, Cuban lily, Peruvian jacinth, hyacinth of Peru, bluebell (*Scilla* spp.)

Snowdrop (*Galanthus nivalis*)

Tobacco, tree tobacco (*Nicotiana* spp.)

Tung oil tree (*Aleurites* spp.)

Water hemlock, cowbane (*Cicuta* spp.)

White cedar (*Thuja occidentalis*)

Yellow jessamine, Carolina jessamine (*Gelsemium sempervirens*)

Yesterday today and tomorrow (*Brunfelsia* spp.)

Zamia (*Macrozamia* spp.)

Zulu potato, climbing onion (*Bowiea volubilis*)

Hepatoencephalopathy

Comfrey (*Symphytum officinale*)

Common ragwort, tansy ragwort (*Senecio jacobaea*)

Crotalaria (*Crotalaria* spp.)

Continued

Box 27–1	Toxic Plant Quick Reference Based on Clinical Signs—cont'd

Dusty miller, cineraria, butterweed, Cape ivy, German ivy, Natal ivy, parlor ivy, water ivy, wax vine (*Senecio* spp.)
Fiddleneck, tarweed (*Amsinckia* spp.)
Hound's-tongue (*Cynoglossum officinale*, Color Plate 27-14)
Lantana, shrub verbena, yellow sage, bunchberry (*Lantana camara*)
Purple viper's-bugloss, Calamity Jane, Patterson's curse (*Echium lycopsis*)
Sago palm, leatherleaf palm, Japanese fern palm (*Cycas revoluta, Cycas* spp.)
Zamia (*Macrozamia* spp.)

Unconsciousness, Coma
Ageratum, floss-flower (*Ageratum* spp.)
Amaryllis (*Amaryllis* spp.)
Apple (*Malus* spp.)
Azalea (*Rhododendron* spp.)
Black laurel, mountain laurel (*Leucothoe davisiae*)
California poppy (*Eschscholzia californica*)
Calla lily (*Zantedeschia* spp.)
Cherry laurel (*Prunus laurocerasus*)
Chinaberry tree (*Melia azederach*)
Coontie, cardboard palm, camptie, yugulla (*Zamia* spp.)
Deadly nightshade (*Atropa belladonna*)
English ivy, Irish ivy, common ivy (*Hedera helix*)
Fetter bush, stagger bush (*Lyonia* spp.)
Hemlock (*Conium maculatum*)
Henbane (*Hyoscyamus niger*)
Horseradish, red cole (*Armoracia rusticana*)
Jimsonweed, thorn-apple, moonflower (*Datura stramonium*)
Kentucky coffee tree (*Gymnocladus dioicus*)
Lobelia, cardinal flower, blue lobelia (*Lobelia* spp.)
Loquat, Japanese plum (*Eriobotrya japonica*)
Mescal bean, mountain laurel, frijolito, Eve's necklace (*Sophora* spp.)
Mezereon, spurge olive (*Daphne mezereum*)
Mountain laurel, dwarf laurel (*Kalmia* spp.)
Opium poppy (*Papaver somniferum*)
Poppy (*Papaver* spp.)
Potato (*Solanum tuberosum*)
Sago palm, leatherleaf palm, Japanese fern palm (*Cycas revoluta, Cycas* spp.)
Sandbox tree, monkey pistol (*Hura crepitans*)
Sorrel, wood sorrel (*Oxalis* spp.)
Spurge (*Euphorbia* spp.)
Sweet-flag (*Acorus calamus*)
Tobacco, tree tobacco (*Nicotiana* spp.)
Water hemlock, cowbane (*Cicuta* spp.)
White snakeroot (*Eupatorium rugosum*)
Wild rosemary (*Ledum palustre*)
Zamia (*Macrozamia* spp.)

Cardiovascular System
Amaryllis (*Amaryllis* spp.)
Angel's trumpet (*Brugmansia* spp.)
Aralia, Balfour aralia, dinner plate aralia, Ming aralia, geranium-leaf aralia, wild coffee, coffee tree (*Polyscias* spp.)
Arnica (*Arnica montana*)

Box 27–1	Toxic Plant Quick Reference Based on Clinical Signs—cont'd

Avocado (*Persea americana*)
Azalea (*Rhododendron* spp.)
Black laurel, mountain laurel (*Leucothoe davisiae*)
Black locust (*Robinia pseudoacacia*)
Broom (*Cytisus* spp.)
Castor bean (*Ricinus communis*)
Christmas rose, black hellebore (*Helleborus* spp.)
Common bean (*Phaseolus vulgaris*)
Croton (*Croton tiglium*)
Daffodil, trumpet narcissus, jonquil (*Narcissus* spp.)
Day-blooming jessamine (*Cestrum diurnum*)
Deadly nightshade (*Atropa belladonna*)
Death camas (*Zigadenus* spp.)
Desert rose, mock azalea (*Adenium* spp.)
Dogbane, Indian hemp (*Apocynum cannabium*)
English ivy, Irish ivy, common ivy (*Hedera helix*)
Ephedra, ma huang, Mormon tea (*Ephedra* spp.)
Euonymus, spindle (*Euonymus* spp.)
False hellebore, white hellebore (*Veratrum* spp.)
Fetter bush, stagger bush (*Lyonia* spp.)
Foxglove, common foxglove, long purples, dead men's fingers (*Digitalis purpurea*)
Golden dewdrop (*Duranta repens*)
Hemlock (*Conium maculatum*)
Henbane (*Hyoscyamus niger*)
Horseradish, red cole (*Armoracia rusticana*)
India rubber vine, purple allamanda (*Cryptostegia* spp.)
Jimsonweed, thorn-apple, moonflower (*Datura stramonium*)
Kalanchoe, feltbush, velvet elephant ear, devil's backbone, lavender-scallops
   (*Kalanchoe* spp.)
Licorice (*Glycyrrhiza glabra*)
Lily of the palace, naked lady, amaryllis (*Hippeastrum* spp.)
Lily-of-the-valley (*Convallaria majalis*)
Lobelia, cardinal flower, blue lobelia (*Lobelia* spp.)
Lupin, lupine, bluebonnet (*Lupinus* spp.)
Monkshood (*Aconitum* spp.)
Moonseed, sarsaparilla (*Menispermum canadense*)
Morning glory, bindweed, pearly gates (*Ipomoea* spp.)
Mountain laurel, dwarf laurel (*Kalmia* spp.)
Nettle, stinging nettle, noseburn (*Urtica* spp., *Cnidoscolus* spp., *Tragia* spp.)
Night-blooming jessamine (*Cestrum nocturnum*)
Oleander (*Nerium oleander*)
Periwinkle (*Vinca* spp.)
Pheasant's eye (*Adonis* spp.)—very low toxicity
Pieris (*Pieris japonica*)
Potato (*Solanum tuberosum*)
Privet, wax-leaf ligustrum (*Ligustrum* spp.)
Rhododendron (*Rhododendron* spp.)
Saffron crocus, meadow saffron (*Crocus sativus*)
Schefflera, umbrella tree, rubber tree, starleaf (*Schefflera* spp.)
Sea onion (*Urginea maritima*)
Silk vine (*Periploca graeca*)
Snowdrop (*Galanthus nivalis*)

Continued

Box 27–1	Toxic Plant Quick Reference Based on Clinical Signs—cont'd

Squill, starry hyacinth, autumn scilla, hyacinth scilla, Cuban lily, Peruvian jacinth, hyacinth of Peru, bluebell (*Scilla* spp.)

Star of Bethlehem, summer snowflake, dove's dung, nap-at-noon (*Ornithogalum* spp.)

Tobacco, tree tobacco (*Nicotiana* spp.)

Tulip (*Tulipa* spp., hyb.)

Wild rosemary (*Ledum palustre*)

Wintersweet, Bushman's poison, poison bush (*Acokanthera* spp.)

Yellow oleander (*Thevetia peruviana*)

Yew, Japanese yew (*Taxus* spp.)

Zephyr lily, rain lily, fair lily, fire lily (*Zephyranthes* spp.)

Zulu potato, climbing onion (*Bowiea volubilis*)

Respiratory System

Dyspnea, Cyanosis

Apple (*Malus* spp.)

Apricot, peach, plum, bitter almond, cherry, choke cherry (*Prunus* spp.)

Arnica (*Arnica montana*)

Bleeding heart, Dutchman's breeches, squirrel corn, staggerweed (*Dicentra* spp.)

Box, common box, boxwood (*Buxus sempervirens*)

Caladium (*Caladium* spp.)

California poppy (*Eschscholzia californica*)

Calla lily (*Zantedeschia* spp.)

Ceriman, Swiss cheese plant, fruit-salad plant, split-leaf philodendron, Mexican breadfruit (*Monstera* spp.)

Cherry laurel (*Prunus laurocerasus*)

Day-blooming jessamine (*Cestrum diurnum*)

Devil's ivy, ivy arum, pothos, hunter's robe, taro vine (*Epipremnum aureum*)

Dieffenbachia, dumb cane (*Dieffenbachia* spp.)

Elephant's ear (*Alocasia* spp.)

False hellebore, white hellebore (*Veratrum* spp.)

Flamingo flower (*Anthurium* spp.)

Golden corydalis, bulbous corydalis, scrambled eggs, fitweed, fumitory (*Corydalis* spp.)

Goosefoot, nephthytis, African evergreen, arrowhead vine (*Syngonium* spp.)

Lords-and-ladies, cuckoo pint, Adam and Eve (*Arum maculatum*)

Marijuana (*Cannabis sativa*)

Nettle, stinging nettle, noseburn (*Urtica* spp., *Cnidoscolus* spp., *Tragia* spp.)

Philodendron, sweetheart plant (*Philodendron* spp.)

Potato (*Solanum tuberosum*)

Tulip (*Tulipa* spp., hyb.)

Respiratory Depression or Paralysis

Angel's trumpet (*Brugmansia* spp.)

Barberry, pipperidge (*Berberis* spp.)

Bittersweet, woody nightshade, wild nightshade (*Solanum dulcamara*)

Box, common box, boxwood (*Buxus sempervirens*)

Broom (*Cytisus* spp.)

Coral bean, coral tree (*Erythrina* spp.)

Deadly nightshade (*Atropa belladonna*)

False hellebore, white hellebore (*Veratrum* spp.)

Gloriosa lily, glory lily, climbing lily (*Gloriosa superba*)

Golden chain tree (*Laburnum anagyroides*)

Hemlock (*Conium maculatum*)

Box 27–1	Toxic Plant Quick Reference Based on Clinical Signs—cont'd

Henbane (*Hyoscyamus niger*)
Jimsonweed, thorn-apple, moonflower (*Datura stramonium*)
Kentucky coffee tree (*Gymnocladus dioicus*)
Larkspur (*Delphinium* spp.)
Lupin, lupine, bluebonnet (*Lupinus* spp.)
Meadow saffron, autumn crocus (*Colchicum autumnale*)
Milkweed, butterfly weed (*Asclepias* spp.)
Monkshood (*Aconitum* spp.)
Opium poppy (*Papaver somniferum*)
Oregon grape, trailing mahonia (*Mahonia* spp.)
Red bryony, white bryony (*Bryonia* spp.)
Rhododendron (*Rhododendron* spp.)
Tobacco, tree tobacco (*Nicotiana* spp.)
Yew, Japanese yew (*Taxus* spp.)

Renal System
Barberry, pipperidge (*Berberis* spp.)
Black locust (*Robinia pseudoacacia*)
Castor bean (*Ricinus communis*)
Day-blooming jessamine (*Cestrum diurnum*)
Easter lily, star-gazer lily, tiger lily (*Lilium* spp.)
Gloriosa lily, glory lily, climbing lily (*Gloriosa superba*)
Licorice (*Glycyrrhiza glabra*)
Oregon grape, trailing mahonia (*Mahonia* spp.)
Red bryony, white bryony (*Bryonia* spp.)
Saffron crocus, meadow saffron (*Crocus sativus*)
White cedar (*Thuja occidentalis*)
Wild radish (*Raphanus rhaphinistrum*)

Calcium Oxalate Crystalluria
Dock, curly dock (*Rumex* spp.)
Rhubarb (*Rheum rhabarbarum*)
Sorrel, wood sorrel (*Oxalis* spp.)

Hematuria, Azotemia
Barberry, pipperidge (*Berberis* spp.)
Black locust (*Robinia pseudoacacia*)
Castor bean (*Ricinus communis*)
Garlic (*Allium* spp.)
Onion (*Allium* spp.)
Oregon grape, trailing mahonia (*Mahonia* spp.)
Rosary pea, prayer bean, jequirity, precatory bean (*Abrus precatorius*)

Liver Damage
Amaryllis (*Amaryllis* spp.)
Borage (*Borago officinalis*)
Comfrey (*Symphytum officinale*)
Common ragwort, tansy ragwort (*Senecio jacobaea*)
Coontie, cardboard palm, camptie, yugulla (*Zamia* spp.)
Crotalaria (*Crotalaria* spp.)
Daffodil, trumpet narcissus, jonquil (*Narcissus* spp.)
Day-blooming jessamine (*Cestrum diurnum*)
Dusty miller, cineraria, butterweed, Cape ivy, German ivy, Natal ivy, parlor ivy, water ivy, wax vine (*Senecio* spp.)

Continued

Box 27–1	Toxic Plant Quick Reference Based on Clinical Signs—cont'd

Fiddleneck, tarweed (*Amsinckia* spp.)
Heliotrope (*Heliotropium* spp.)
Hound's-tongue (*Cynoglossum officinale*)
Lantana, shrub verbena, yellow sage, bunchberry (*Lantana camara*)
Oak (*Quercus* spp.)
Purple viper's-bugloss, Calamity Jane, Patterson's curse (*Echium lycopsis*)
Rhubarb, garden rhubarb, pie plant, water plant, wine plant (*Rheum rhabarbarum*)
Sago palm, leatherleaf palm, Japanese fern palm (*Cycas revoluta, Cycas* spp.)
Snowdrop (*Galanthus nivalis*)
White cedar (*Thuja occidentalis*)
Wild radish (*Raphanus rhaphinistrum*)
Zamia (*Macrozamia* spp.)

Jaundice, Icterus
Borage (*Borago officinalis*)
Comfrey (*Symphytum officinale*)
Coontie, cardboard palm, camptie, yugulla (*Zamia* spp.)
Crotalaria (*Crotalaria* spp.)
Fiddleneck, tarweed (*Amsinckia* spp.)
Heliotrope (*Heliotropium* spp.)
Hound's-tongue (*Cynoglossum officinale*)
Lantana, shrub verbena, yellow sage, bunchberry (*Lantana camara*)
Purple viper's-bugloss, Patterson's curse, Calamity Jane (*Echium lycopsis*)

Primary Photosensitization
Bishop's weed, Queen Anne's lace (*Ammi majus*)
Dutchman's breeches (*Thamnosma texana*)
Hogweed, giant hogweed, common parsnip (*Heracleum* spp.)
Marigold, African marigold, French marigold, bog marigold, Aztec marigold (*Tagetes* spp.)
St. John's wort (*Hypericum perforatum*)

Emaciation, Ascites, Edema of Dependent Extremities
Borage (*Borago officinalis*)
Comfrey (*Symphytum officinalis*)
Common ragwort, tansy ragwort (*Senecio jacobaea*)
Crotalaria (*Crotalaria* spp.)
Dusty miller, cineraria, butterweed, Cape ivy, German ivy, Natal ivy, parlor ivy, water ivy, wax vine (*Senecio* spp.)
Fiddleneck, tarweed (*Amsinckia* spp.)
Heliotrope (*Heliotropium* spp.)
Hound's-tongue (*Cynoglossum officinale*)
Purple viper's-bugloss, Calamity Jane, Patterson's curse (*Echium lycopsis*)

Sudden Death
Bagpod sesbane (*Sesbania vesicaria*)
Foxglove (*Digitalis purpurea*)
Kalanchoë, feltbush, velvet elephant ear, devil's backbone, lavender-scallops (*Kalanchoe* spp.)
Oleander (*Nerium oleander*)
Yellow oleander (*Thevetia peruviana*)
Yew, Japanese yew (*Taxus* spp.)

Table 27-1 Toxic Plant Information Summary

Latin Name	Common Names	Clinical Signs, Prognosis, Additional Treatment	Toxins, Plant Parts, Lethal Doses
Abrus precatorius	Rosary pea, prayer bean, jequirity, precatory bean—broken seeds only	Delayed 3 hours to 2 days; severe gastroenteritis, vomiting, serious hemorrhagic enteropathy, fluid loss; bleeding from retina and serous membranes is characteristic	Abrin (toxalbumin/lectin, 2 chain) stops protein synthesis
LD: adults 0.5-2 seeds, children 1-2 seeds
Acalypha hispida	Chenille plant, red-hot cattail	Gastroenteritis, gastrointestinal inflammation; eye irritant	Euphorb latex, diterpene esters
Aconitum spp.	Monkshood	Burning and tingling of mouth, fingers, and toes within 10-20 minutes; distal paresthesia gradually extending centrally, followed later by vomiting, diarrhea, paralysis, intense pain, respiratory paralysis, cardiac failure, and death while conscious	Aconitine and others (diterpene or norditerpene alkaloids with ethylated or methylated amine); aconitine 0.3%-2% in tubers, 0.2%-1.2% in leaves; LD adult human 3-6 mg/kg (=few grams plant material); also well absorbed percutaneously
Acokanthera spp.	Wintersweet, Bushman's poison, poison bush	Arrhythmias, bradycardia; potentially hyperkalemia	Cardiotoxic cardenolides
Acorus calamus	Sweet-flag	Rapid respirations, stupor, vomiting, bloody diarrhea, coma, hypocalcemic tetany	Soluble oxalates
Actaea spp.	Cohosh, baneberry, dolls' eyes	Hypersalivation, vomiting, abdominal pain, possible diarrhea; blistering, ulceration of mucosae	Fruits and roots only; contact irritant, vesicant toxin not identified
Adenium spp.	Desert rose, mock azalea	Arrhythmias, bradycardia; potentially hyperkalemia	Entire plant; cardiac glycosides
Adonis spp.	Pheasant's eye	Vomiting, hyperkalemia, bradycardia, arrhythmias; subepidermal vesicant essentially nontoxic	Adonitoxin, 20 other cardenolides 0.25% in plant; poorly absorbed protoanemonin (vesicant irritant)
Aechmea fasciata	Urn plant	Severe irritation of skin and mucous membranes, itching, burning, inflammation, possible blistering hoarseness, salivation, vomiting	Insoluble calcium oxalate, proteolytic enzymes

Continued

Table 27-1   Toxic Plant Information Summary—cont'd

Latin Name	Common Names	Clinical Signs, Prognosis, Additional Treatment	Toxins, Plant Parts, Lethal Doses
Aesculus spp.	Horse chestnut, buckeye	Vomiting, diarrhea; ataxia, muscle twitches, sluggishness or excitation	Aescin (saponin complex) in seeds and twigs; unknown additional neurotoxin; poorly absorbed
Agapanthus orientalis	African blue lily; blue African lily	Conjunctivitis; irritation and mouth ulceration, vomiting	Unknown; not likely to be fatal because of immediate oral discomfort
Agave americanum	Century plant, maguey, American aloe	Local mucosal irritation	Insoluble calcium oxalate
Ageratum spp.	Ageratum, floss-flower	Vomiting, ataxia, unconsciousness	Precocenes I and II, hepatotoxic chromenes
Aglaonema spp.	Chinese evergreen	Irritation of skin and mucous membranes, inflammation, hoarseness, salivation, vomiting; rarely oxaluria	Insoluble calcium oxalate; also soluble oxalates
Albizia julibrissin	Mimosa, silk tree	Tremors, convulsions appear abruptly	5-Acetoxymethyl-3-hydroxy-4-methoxymethyl-2-methylpyridine (alkaloid) in the legumes; seizures prevented by pyridoxine; mechanism may be impaired GABA synthesis
Aleurites spp.	Tung oil tree	Vomiting, abdominal pain, diarrhea	Tigliane-type phorbol esters in seed oil/sap
Allamanda catharctica	Yellow allamanda, Nani Ali'i; flor de barbero	Conjunctivitis; irritation of lips, tongue, and mouth; vomiting, diarrhea	Plumericin, bioactive iridoid irritant; seeds, fruit, leaves, bark, sap; herbal cathartic
Allium spp.	Garlic, onion	Contact allergens; Heinz body anemia (hemolytic)	Tulipalins; n-propyl disulfide
Alocasia spp.	Elephant's ear	Severe irritation of skin and mucous membranes, inflammation, possible blistering, hoarseness, salivation, vomiting; if large amounts, dysphagia, respiratory compromise; severe pain in mouth, lips, throat, stomach	Calcium oxalate raphides and idioblasts; also some unknown proteinaceous toxin Small amounts of root or leaf may be fatal because of restricted airway in very small animals
Aloe spp.	Candelabra aloe, octopus plant, torch plant, Barbados aloe, medicinal aloe	Inhibits stomach acid secretion; inhibits water and electrolyte absorption from colon; potent cathartic—causes abdominal cramping and diarrhea	Barbaloin (0.1%-1.2% dry weight in leaf), other anthraquinone glycosides; small amount of leaf = purgative dose

Scientific name	Common name	Clinical signs	Toxic principle
Alpinia spp.	Shell ginger, shell flower, ginger-lily, pink porcelain lily	Eye irritation; not much else	One species, mild cardioactive compound (Yakuchinone-A) (herbal)
Alstroemeria aurantiaca, hyb.	Peruvian lily, lily of the Incas	Allergic dermatitis	Tulipalin A (1%-2% throughout plant)
Amaryllis spp.	Amaryllis	Hypersalivation, vomiting, abdominal pain, diarrhea, hypotension, dehydration, electrolyte imbalance	Amaryllidaceae alkaloids, lycorine, mostly in the outer layers of the bulb
Ammi majus	Bishop's weed, Queen Anne's lace	Primary photosensitization	Furocoumarins, highest in seeds, also in foliage
Amsinckia sp. (Color Plate 27-2)	Fiddleneck, tarweed	Much delayed (weeks to months) anorexia, depression, rough pelage, diarrhea, emaciation, constipation icterus, hepatoencephalopathy, death	Pyrrolizidine alkaloids; probably requires chronic consumption
Ananas comosus	Pineapple, pineapple tree	Irritation of lips, tongue, and mucosal surfaces, vomiting; allergen	Bromelin (digestive enzyme), calcium oxalate raphides, ethyl acrylate (skin sensitizer)
Anemone spp.	Anemone, Pasque flower, windflower, meadow anemone, crowfoot	Mucosal blistering and ulceration, profuse salivation, intense gastrointestinal irritation, abdominal pain, vomiting with blood, diarrhea; ataxia, seizures	Protoanemonin (related to cantharidin), subepidermal vesicant; also saponins
Anthurium spp.	Flamingo flower	Severe mucosal irritation and inflammation, possible blistering, dysphagia, salivation, vomiting	Calcium oxalate raphides and idioblasts; also soluble oxalates
Apocynum cannabium	Dogbane, Indian hemp	Vomiting, diarrhea, cardiovascular collapse	Apocynamarin (cardioactive glycoside)
Arisaema triphyllum	Jack-in-the-pulpit, green dragon	Oral, pharyngeal, and esophageal irritation, salivation, edema, vomiting	Insoluble calcium oxalates
Armoracia rusticana	Horseradish, red cole	Potent skin and eye irritant, vomiting; horseradish syncope occurs in some individuals—vasodepressor mechanism initiated by direct irritation of the gastric or upper respiratory tract	Sinigrin (allyl glucosinolate)

Continued

Table 27-1   Toxic Plant Information Summary—cont'd

Latin Name	Common Names	Clinical Signs, Prognosis, Additional Treatment	Toxins, Plant Parts, Lethal Doses
Arnica montana	Arnica	Vomiting, diarrhea, bleeding, edema, respiratory stimulation, brief tachycardia dyspnea, followed by cardiac paralysis, death; allergic contact dermatitis	Helenalin ester (sesquiterpene lactone with strong SH crosslinking ability)
Artemisia absinthium	Wormwood, sagewort, sagebrush	Mucosal irritation and erythema, vomiting, diarrhea	Thujone (monoterpene) in essential oil
Arum maculatum, *Arum italicum*	Lords-and-ladies, cuckoo pint, Adam and Eve, arum	Mucosal irritation, possible ulceration, hypersalivation, vomiting, abdominal pain, diarrhea; possible dehydration	Insoluble calcium oxalates; toxicity varies with ripeness of berries and locality of plants
Asclepias sp. (Color Plate 27-3)	Milkweed, butterfly weed	Vomiting, diarrhea, ataxia, weakness, dilated pupils, convulsions, respiratory paralysis, death	Cardenolides; 0.05%-2% of animal's body weight in plant material can be fatal
Asparagus spp.	Asparagus	Contact allergen; slight "indisposition"	Sitosterol, stigmasterol, and their glucosides (steroidal saponins); highest levels found in berries
Atractylis gummifera	Mediterranean thistle	Strychnine-like convulsions	Atractyligenin, atractyloside, and carboxyatractyloside; blocks oxidative phosphorylation
Atropa belladonna	Deadly nightshade	Tachycardia, dryness of mucous membranes, mydriasis, excitation, confusion, frenzy, hyperthermia, coma; occasional hypersensitive individuals	Atropine, scopolamine, L-hyoscyamine; all plant parts toxic, 0.4%-0.85% dry weight; seeds, unripe fruits almost all hyoscyamine; ripe fruits have racemate atropine (approximately half the CNS activity); birds are immune, mammals are not; yellow varieties and those in heavier soils and higher altitudes contain alkaloids up to 30% dry weight; may be glycosidase inhibitors (long-term neurologic deficits)
Aucuba japonica	Aucuba, Japanese aucuba, Japanese laurel spotted laurel	Vomiting, occasionally fever	Aucubin (triterpenoid saponin of the β-amyrin group); berries

Scientific name	Common name	Clinical signs	Toxic principle
Begonia semperflorens-cultorum	Wax begonia	Mucosal irritation and inflammation, hypersalivation, vomiting; no cases reported	Insoluble calcium oxalates, soluble oxalates; underground parts only
Begonia tuberhybrida	Tuberous begonia	Mucosal irritation and inflammation, hypersalivation, vomiting	Insoluble calcium oxalates, soluble oxalates, cucurbitacin B; tubers only
Berberis spp.	Barberry, pipperidge	Confusion, epistaxis, vomiting, diarrhea, renal irritation; high doses cause primary respiratory arrest, hemorrhagic nephritis	Berberine (isoquinoline alkaloid); root and stem bark, at 5.3%-15.3% dry weight; berries harmless
Borago officinalis	Borage	Much delayed (weeks to months) anorexia, depression, rough pelage, diarrhea, emaciation, constipation, icterus, hepatoencephalopathy, death	Pyrrolizidine alkaloids; probably requires chronic consumption
Bowiea volubilis	Zulu potato, climbing onion	Vomiting, diarrhea, bradycardia, arrhythmias, conduction defects, Ca^{2+}-binding hyperkalemia, seizure agents reduce lethality	Bufadienolide cardiotoxins: bovicide A, B, C, and D, hellebrin; entire plant and bulb
Brassaia actinophylla (*Schefflera actinophylla*)	Schefflera, umbrella tree, rubber tree, starleaf	Vomiting, copious diarrhea, ataxia, anorexia, leukopenia, tachycardia, stupor, mydriasis, seizures	Soluble oxalates (0.9%-15%) wet weight leaves; falcarinol (alkylating agent, irritant)
Brunfelsia spp. (Color Plate 27-4)	Yesterday-today-and-tomorrow	Anxiety, excitation, persistent sneezing, vomiting, muscle tremors worsening to ataxia, seizures, death within a few hours	Unknown
Bryonia spp.	Red bryony, white bryony	Drastic purgative, abdominal pain, bloody diarrhea, ataxia, renal inflammation, respiratory paralysis; dermal irritant, progressing to inflammation and blistering	Cucurbitacins (9) (tetracyclic triterpenes); 6-8 berries
Buxus sempervirens	Box, boxwood, common box	Vomiting, diarrhea, awkward gait, dyspnea, vocalizing, ataxia, convulsions, respiratory failure death	Buxine (cyclobuxine, pregnane alkaloids); leaves up to 1% dry weight; 0.1 g/kg fatal to dogs; 750-g leaves fatal to horse; tannins

Continued

Table 27-1 Toxic Plant Information Summary—cont'd

Latin Name	Common Names	Clinical Signs, Prognosis, Additional Treatment	Toxins, Plant Parts, Lethal Doses
Caesalpinia spp.	Bird-of-paradise, pride of Barbados, poinciana	Delay of ½ to several hours; profuse, persistent vomiting; later diarrhea, possible dehydration; recovery within 24 hours	Seeds and pods contain tannins; child hospitalized after ingesting 5 pods
Caladium spp.	Caladium	Severe mucosal irritation, inflammation, possible blistering, hypersalivation, vomiting; if large amounts, dysphagia, airway obstruction, respiratory compromise	Calcium oxalate raphides and idioblasts; leaves and bulbs
Calla palustris	Wild calla, wild arum	Severe mucosal irritation, inflammation, possible blistering, hypersalivation, vomiting; if large amounts, dysphagia, airway obstruction, respiratory compromise	Insoluble calcium oxalates
Caltha spp.	Marsh marigold, cowslip, kingcup	Mucosal irritation and inflammation, profuse salivation, bloody vomiting and diarrhea, severe abdominal pain, ataxia, seizures	Alkaloids and saponins, protoanemonin
Cannabis sativa	Marijuana	Depression, excitation, dyspnea, muscle tremors, hallucination, aberrant behavior, subnormal temperature, sweating	Tetrahydrocannabinol
Capsicum annuum	Ornamental and cultivated peppers	Mucosal irritation, inflammation, abdominal pain, vomiting, diarrhea	Capsaicin, 0.2%-1%; less dihydro-, nordihydro-, homo-, and homodihydro-capsaicin; capsaicin accounts for 70% of irritant capacity, release of substance P from sensory nerves, pain response and inflammation
Caryota mitis	Fishtail palm	Mucosal irritation and inflammation, blistering, hypersalivation, vomiting, airway constriction	Calcium oxalate raphides; berry contains 0.05%
Catharanthus roseus	Madagascar periwinkle	Severe abdominal pain and profuse diarrhea, dehydration, electrolyte imbalance; later peripheral neuropathy, bone marrow suppression, cardiovascular collapse	Vinca alkaloids (cytotoxic, inhibit microtubule formation); all parts of plant

Species	Common name	Clinical signs	Toxin
Caulophyllum thalictroides	Blue cohosh	Vomiting, abdominal pain, diarrhea, dehydration, hypertension, muscular weakness, coma, respiratory paralysis, death	Lupin alkaloids (quinolizidine alkaloids), N-methylcytosine (nicotinic alkaloid), saponins
Cestrum diurnum	Day-blooming jessamine	Hypercalcemia, hypophosphatemia, bone weakness, calcinosis of heart, liver, kidneys, and lungs	1,25-Dihydroxy-cholecalciferol
Cestrum nocturnum	Night-blooming jessamine, Chinese inkberry	Dry mucosa, tachycardia, hyperthermia, mydriasis, excitation	Anticholinergic alkaloids; green berries most toxic; ripe berries not very toxic; also present in foliage
Chelidonium majus	Greater celandine (bright yellow sap)	Vomiting, abdominal pain, severe bloody diarrhea, dehydration	21 alkaloids (benzo-phenanthridine and protoberberine) with chelidonic acid; herb 0.3%-1.0%, root up to 2%, fruits approximately 0.15%; seasonally variable; benzyltetrahydro-isoquinoline alkaloids (10 groups) and triterpenoid saponins (weak)
Cicuta spp.	Water hemlock, cowbane	Within an hour of ingestion, vomiting, salivation, abdominal pain, dizziness, vomiting, unconsciousness, tonic-clonic convulsions, death	Cicutoxin (GABA receptor antagonist or potassium channel blocker); one bite of chambered rootstock can kill a child; even bitten and spit out, artificial respiration and muscle relaxant therapy required
Clematis spp.	Old man's beard, traveler's joy, virgin's bower	Subepidermal vesicant; mucosal inflammation and blistering, profuse salivation, intense abdominal pain, bloody vomiting and diarrhea; ataxia, seizures	Protoanemonin (related to cantharidin)
Clivia miniata	Kaffir lily	Delayed severe vomiting, hypersalivation, diarrhea, dehydration, electrolyte imbalance	Lycorine (0.43% dry weight) and galanthamine; few grams of bulb may be fatal to a child
Cnidoscolus spp.	Nettle, stinging nettle, noseburn	Salivation, vomiting, arrhythmias, dyspnea, weakness, collapse	Acetylcholine, histamine in plant hairs
Coffea arabica	Coffee	Central stimulation; allergic reactions	Methylxanthines, 1%-2%; allergen

Continued

Table 27-1	Toxic Plant Information Summary—cont'd		
Latin Name	Common Names	Clinical Signs, Prognosis, Additional Treatment	Toxins, Plant Parts, Lethal Doses
Colchicum autumnale	Meadow saffron, autumn crocus	Within 2-12 hours, abdominal pain, vomiting, profuse diarrhea, fatal shock caused by dehydration; in 4-5 days, bone marrow suppression, peripheral neuropathy, cardiovascular collapse	Colchicine (antimitotic, inhibits microtubule formation) in all parts; flowers (0.1%), seeds (0.8%), corm (0.6%); 1.5-2 g plant material, 2-3 seeds, or ½ flower fatal
Colocasia esculenta	Taro, dasheen, cocoyam	Mucosal irritation and inflammation, possible blistering, hypersalivation; if large amounts, dysphagia, airway obstruction, respiratory compromise	Insoluble calcium oxalates
Conium maculatum (Color Plate 27-5)	Hemlock, poison hemlock	Beginning approximately 12 minutes after ingestion, pupillary dilatation, hypertension, trembling, ataxia, muscle weakness, paralysis, coma, respiratory paralysis, death	Coniine (piperidine alkaloid); nicotinic alkaloid; content seasonally variable in plant; 0.25%-4% of body weight in green material can be fatal
Convallaria majalis	Lily-of-the-valley	Vomiting, abdominal pain, diarrhea, bradycardia, cardiac arrhythmias; hyperkalemia Ipecac emetic contraindicated as cardiac glycosides affect the vagus	Cardenolide cardiotoxins (primarily convallotoxin, convallamarin) highest in seeds (0.45%), flowers (0.4%), leaves (0.13%-0.2% dry weight); poorly absorbed; fruit skin, flowers contain steroidal saponins
Corynocarpus laevigatus	Karaka nut	Convulsions, cardiovascular collapse	Prototoxin karakin is hydrolyzed to beta-nitropropionic acid; inhibits succinate dehydrogenase (Krebs cycle); seeds are toxic; ripe fruit (excluding seeds) is edible
Crinum spp.	Crinum lily, spider lily, swamp lily	Vomiting, abdominal pain, diarrhea, potential electrolyte imbalance	Lycorine, crinidine, bulbispermine, crinine, powelline, hippadine, and other phenanthridine alkaloids; all plant parts are toxic, bulbs contain highest levels; like *Narcissus*
Crocus sativus	Saffron crocus, autumn crocus	Extensive bleeding from skin, severe collapse, nephrotoxicity	Safranal (from protocrocin precursor, a tetraterpene glycoside); 5-10 g powdered stigmas (saffron) deadly

Scientific name	Common name	Clinical signs	Toxic principle/comments
Crotalaria spp.	Crotalaria, rattle box	Much delayed (weeks to months) anorexia, depression, rough pelage, diarrhea, emaciation, constipation, icterus, hepatoencephalopathy, death	Monocrotaline and other pyrrolizidine alkaloids; rarely, acute hepatic failure
Croton tiglium	Croton	Vomiting, diarrhea; pupillary dilatation, giddiness, delirium, convulsions	Crotin (toxalbumin) in seeds; tigliane phorbol esters in seed oil and sap; few drops of sap can cause a reaction
Cryptanthus acaulis	Green earth star	Severe mucosal irritation and inflammation, possible blistering, salivation, vomiting	Insoluble calcium oxalates, proteolytic enzymes
Cryptostegia spp.	India rubber vine, purple allamanda	Vomiting, abdominal pain, diarrhea, bradycardia, cardiac arrhythmias; hyperkalemia	Cardioactive glycosides
Cycas spp.	Sago palm, leatherleaf palm, Japanese fern palm	Violent emesis, diarrhea, ataxia, seizures, coma, death; few bites cause massive hepatic necrosis in dogs; hepatoencephalopathy; lower doses carcinogenic and teratogenic	Cycasin, neocycasin A and B, macrozamin; BMAA; MAM; 0.2%-0.3% dry weight in seeds; also high levels in root, less in foliage
Cyclamen persicum	Persian violet, alpine violet, sowbread	Nausea, vomiting, diarrhea; if absorbed, convulsions and paralysis	Cyclamin (triterpenoid saponin); mostly in roots, little in leaves; small pieces of tuber may cause convulsions
Cytisus spp.	Broom	Vomiting, abdominal pain, circulatory collapse, cardiac arrhythmias, gradual paralysis, convulsions, respiratory paralysis, death	Sparteine (quinolizidine alkaloid)
Daphne mezereum	Daphne, mezereon, spurge olive	Severe mucosal irritation and inflammation, hypersalivation, dysphagia, severe abdominal pain, vomiting, bloody diarrhea, narcosis, muscle twitching	Mezerein (daphnane diterpene ester); LD_{50} mouse: 0.275 mg/kg; vesicant found in all parts; 2-3 fruits fatal to child
Datura spp. (Color Plate 26-3, *Brugmansia* spp.)	Jimsonweed, thorn-apple, moonflower, devil's trumpet	Classically described: "Red as a beet, dry as a bone, blind as a bat, and mad as a hatter!" Excitation, tachycardia, hyperthermia, confusion, mydriasis, dry mouth, constipation, hallucinations, frenzy, coma	Atropine, scopolamine, L-hyoscyamine; alkaloid in leaves 0.38%, flowers 0.61%, shoots 0.16%, fruits 0.66%, pericarp 0.05%, seeds 0.58%, roots 0.23% dry weight; scopolamine up to 65% of alkaloid content in some flowers

Continued

Table 27-1 Toxic Plant Information Summary—cont'd

Latin Name	Common Names	Clinical Signs, Prognosis, Additional Treatment	Toxins, Plant Parts, Lethal Doses
Delphinium spp	Larkspur	Uneasiness, vomiting, weakness, ataxia, paralysis, respiratory paralysis, death Neostigmine or physostigmine is of limited use	MLA, other reversible nicotinic ACh receptor binders; highest levels found in seeds and immature plant, decrease as flowers bud
Dicentra spp. (Color Plate 27-6)	Bleeding heart, squirrel corn, Dutchman's breeches, staggerweed	Trembling and staggering; convulsions; frothing at the mouth; vomiting; dyspnea; diarrhea; glassy-eyed, pain-filled expressions	Aporphine, bulbocapnine, protoberberine, protopine (isoquinoline alkaloids); all parts toxic; foliage 0.17%, root 0.76% dry weight alkaloids *D. spectabilis*
Dieffenbachia sp. (Color Plate 27-7)	Dieffenbachia, dumb cane	Severe mucosal irritation and inflammation, possible blistering, hypersalivation, vomiting; if large amounts, dysphagia, airway obstruction, respiratory compromise	Calcium oxalate raphides and idioblasts; also soluble oxalates and dumbcain, a proteolytic enzyme
Digitalis purpurea	Foxglove, common foxglove, long purples, dead men's fingers	Vomiting, abdominal pain, diarrhea, lethargy, bradycardia, ventricular arrhythmias; hyperkalemia Ipecac emesis contraindicated because of effect of cardiac glycosides on the vagus	Cardenolide cardiotoxins: up to 1% dry weight in leaves: desacetyldigilanid A, desacetyldigilanid B, glucogitaloxin; 10%-20% hydrolyzed to digitoxin, gitoxin, gitaloxin; seeds more toxic than leaves; also saponins digitonin, gitonin, tigonin
Duranta repens	Golden dewdrop	Hyperthermia, mydriasis, tachycardia, convulsions; gastrointestinal irritation, vomiting, diarrhea, electrolyte imbalance	Saponins
Echium spp.	Purple viper's-bugloss, Paterson's curse, Calamity Jane	Much delayed (weeks to months) signs: anorexia, depression, rough pelage, diarrhea, emaciation, constipation, icterus, hepatoencephalopathy, death	Pyrrolizidine alkaloids; probably requires chronic consumption
Ephedra spp.	Ephedra, ma huang, Mormon tea	Vomiting, tachycardia, hypertension, ataxia, weakness, potential myocardial infarction	Ephedrine, pseudo- and norpseudoephedrine; sympathomimetic amines
Epipremnum aureum (Color Plate 27-8)	Devil's ivy, ivy arum, pothos, hunter's robe, taro vine	Mucosal irritation and inflammation, vomiting, hypersalivation; if large amounts, dysphagia, airway obstruction, respiratory compromise	Insoluble calcium oxalate raphides

Eriobotrya japonica	Loquat, Japanese plum	Delayed abdominal pain, vomiting, lethargy, coma, convulsions, cardiovascular collapse	Seed pits contain amygdalin (cyanogenic glycoside)
Erythrina spp.	Coral bean, coral tree	Uneasiness, vomiting, weakness, ataxia, paralysis, respiratory paralysis, death	Isoquinoline alkaloids, reversible nicotinic ACh receptor binders
Eschscholzia californica	California poppy	Narcosis, muscular relaxation, depression of the central respiratory center; pinpoint pupils, cyanosis, respiratory failure, death	Rhoeadine-type alkaloids: thebaine, papaverrubines, papaverine; small amounts compared with opium poppy
Eucalyptus spp.	Eucalyptus, blue gum, cider gum, silver dollar, Australian fever tree	Mucosal irritation and erythema, vomiting, diarrhea	Essential oils 4.8%-6.6% of leaf dry weight, largely cineole
Euonymus europaeus	Euonymus, European spindle tree	Delayed vomiting, abdominal pain, severe diarrhea, bradycardia, arrhythmias Emesis contraindicated because of cardiac glycoside effect on vagus	Evonoside, evobioside, evomonoside (cardiac glycosides) in berries and seeds, evonine, neoevonine, 4-deoxyevonine (alkaloids)
Eupatorium rugosum	White snakeroot	Delayed 3-11 days: trembling, ataxia, weakness, severe repeated vomiting, constipation and thirst, acetone breath, prostration, delirium, coma, death	Tremetol and tremetone; 0.5%-1.5% of body weight is fatal; recovery rare, slow, can be incomplete
Euphorbia lactea	Candelabra cactus, false cactus, mottled spurge, dragon bones	Vomiting, abdominal pain, diarrhea	Diterpene esters in milky sap (type not specified)
Euphorbia milii	Crown of thorns	Vomiting, abdominal pain, diarrhea; thorns tend to limit consumption and access	Hydroxyphorbol diterpene esters in milky sap (milliamines A through I); also triterpenes, flavonoids
Euphorbia myrisinites	Spurge, creeping spurge, donkey tail	Dermal blistering can take a week to heal; no mention of oral route	Ingenane diterpene esters in milky sap
Euphorbia pulcherrima	Poinsettia, Christmas star	Hothouse varieties: at most mouth irritation and some vomiting	Very little diterpene ester; considerable natural variability in milky sap

Continued

Table 27-1 Toxic Plant Information Summary—cont'd

Latin Name	Common Names	Clinical Signs, Prognosis, Additional Treatment	Toxins, Plant Parts, Lethal Doses
Euphorbia resinifera	Euphorbium	Vomiting, abdominal pain, diarrhea; one of the most irritating euphorbs	Daphnane diterpene esters (resiniferatoxin) in milky sap
Euphorbia tirucalli	Pencil tree, milkbush, Indian tree, rubber euphorbia, finger tree, naked lady	Vomiting, abdominal pain, diarrhea	Phorbol diterpene esters in milky sap
Euphorbia spp.	Spurges	Mucosal inflammation, gastroenteritis, vomiting, abdominal pain, diarrhea	Phorbol, daphnane, and ingenane diterpene esters in milky sap; toxicity varies with season, species exposed, amount of latex and time exposed
Galanthus nivalis	Snowdrop	Persistent vomiting, diarrhea, sedation, hypotension, seizures, electrolyte imbalance	Lycorine; galanthamine (centrally acting anticholinesterase); bulb
Gelsemium sempervirens	Yellow jessamine, Carolina jasmine	Dry mouth, ataxia, dysphagia, strychninelike muscular contractions	Indolizidine alkaloids, gelsemine, gelsemicine
Ginkgo biloba	Ginkgo	Large amounts of seeds, possible delayed, recurrent seizures, preceded by vomiting and diarrhea	4-o-methylpyridoxine (suppresses GABA production); urushiol-like compounds in the seed coat
Gloriosa superba	Gloriosa lily, glory lily, climbing lily	Within 2-12 hours: abdominal pain, profuse vomiting, diarrhea, dysphagia, oliguria or anuria; fatal hypovolemic shock; if lower dose, bone marrow depression in 4-5 days; alopecia at 12 days; respiratory failure	Gloriosine and colchicine, both antimitotic; 3 mg/g tuber; 7-11 mg colchicine is fatal to adult humans
Glycyrrhiza glabra	Licorice	Water retention, hypertension, congestive heart failure	Glycyrrhizin (triterpenoid saponin)
Gymnocladus dioicus	Kentucky coffee tree	Hypertension, mydriasis, seizures; weakness, paralysis, coma, respiratory paralysis	Cytisine (nicotinic alkaloid)
Gypsophila paniculata	Baby's breath	Dermal irritant and allergen; vomiting, diarrhea	Unknown

Haemanthus multiflorus (Color Plate 27-9)	Blood lily, powderpuff lily	Salivation, vomiting, diarrhea, paralysis, collapse	Lycorine, chidanthine, hippeastrine, haemanthidine, haemultine; bulb
Hedera helix	English ivy, common ivy, Irish ivy	Hypersalivation, vomiting, abdominal pain, diarrhea, electrolyte imbalance tachycardia, stupor, mydriasis, convulsions	Hederasaponins B and C, rutin, caffeic acid, chlorogenic acid, alpha-hederin, emetine, berries; falcarinol, falcarinone, didehydrofalcarinol (alkylating agents, irritants)
Heliotropium spp.	Heliotrope, scorpion's tail	Much delayed (weeks to months): anorexia, depression, rough pelage, diarrhea, emaciation, constipation, icterus, hepatoencephalopathy, death	Pyrrolizidine alkaloids; effect probably requires chronic consumption
Helleborus spp.	Christmas rose, black hellebore	Intense vomiting, abdominal pain, diarrhea, mydriasis, bradycardia, arrhythmia, idioventricular rhythm, ventricular fibrillation, hyperkalemia, hallucination Lidocaine has been effective to control arrhythmias	Hellebrin, other bufadienolide cardiotoxins; protoanemonin, ranunculin in foliage; helleborin (steroidal saponin)
Heracleum spp.	Hogweed, giant hogweed, common parsnip	Primary photosensitization	6,7-Furanocoumarins
Hippeastrum aulicum	Lily of the palace, naked lady: amaryllis	Nausea, vomiting, salivation, some diarrhea, paralysis, and central collapse	Lycorine (phenanthridine alkaloid) in bulb
Hippomane mancinella	Manchineel tree, manzanillo	Mucosal irritation and damage, vomiting, severe abdominal pain, diarrhea	White latex includes hippomane A (same as huratoxin) and B, daphnane diterpene esters
Hura crepitans	Sandbox tree, monkey pistol	Mucosal irritation and damage, vomiting, severe abdominal pain, diarrhea	Hurin (toxalbumin), huratoxin in seeds; daphnane diterpene esters in seed oil/sap
Hyacinthoides nonscripta	Bluebell	Choking, central depression, attempted vomiting, weak, slow pulse, hypothermia, bloody diarrhea	Glucosidase inhibitors; leaves, fruits, and bulbs: DMDP (up to 1% dry weight); in leaves: D-AB1

Continued

Table 27-1   Toxic Plant Information Summary—cont'd

Latin Name	Common Names	Clinical Signs, Prognosis, Additional Treatment	Toxins, Plant Parts, Lethal Doses
Hyacinthus orientalis	Hyacinth, Dutch hyacinth	Vomiting, hypersalivation, diarrhea	Lycorine (phenanthridine alkaloids) in bulb; less toxic than *Narcissus*
Hydrangea macrophylla	Hydrangea, hills of snow, French hydrangea, hortensia	Abdominal pain, vomiting, lethargy; in high doses, coma, convulsions, cardiovascular collapse	Hydrangin (cyanogenic glycoside): highest levels in flower buds
Hydrastis canadensis	Goldenseal	Vomiting, abdominal pain, diarrhea	Berberine
Hymenocallis spp.	Spider lily, crown-beauty, sea daffodil, basket flower, alligator lily	Very persistent vomiting, abdominal pain, diarrhea, dehydration, electrolyte imbalance	Lycorine (emetic) and tazettine (hypotensive) (phenanthridine alkaloids) in bulb
Hyoscyamus niger	Henbane	Dry mouth, dysphagia, tachycardia, mydriasis, confusion, frenzy, coma	Atropine, L-hyoscyamine, scopolamine up to 40% of total alkaloid; roots 0.08%, leaves 0.17%, seeds 0.3% dry weight
Hypericum perforatum	St. John's wort, Klamath weed	Primary photosensitization	Hypericin and hyperforin
Ilex spp.	Holly; yaupon, possumhaw	Abdominal pain, vomiting, diarrhea with more than two berries	Foliage: tannins, caffeine, theobromine; berries: triterpene compounds, saponins, low level cardiotonic activity
Ipomoea spp.	Morning glory, bindweed, pearly gates	Depression, mydriasis, muscle tremors, ataxia, increased deep tendon reflexes, diarrhea, hypotension, hallucinations	Indole alkaloids; D-lysergic acid amide, D-isolysergic acid amide, and elymoclavine; seeds only; 200-300 seeds necessary to produce hallucinations
Iris spp.	Iris, crested iris, dwarf iris, flag, fleur-de-lis, blue flag	Vomiting, abdominal pain, bloody diarrhea	Iridin (irritant phenolic glycoside), myristic acid, irisoquin (benzoquinone); highest in rhizomes

Species	Common Names	Clinical Signs	Toxins
Jatropha spp.	Physic nut, jicamilla, peregrine, bellyache bush	Vomiting; profuse, sometimes bloody diarrhea; ataxia; dehydration; electrolyte imbalance	Curcin (toxalbumin); phorbol esters; seeds approximately 60% oil
Juniperus sabina	Savin	Profuse vomiting, diarrhea	Podophyllotoxins: sabinene, sabinyl acetate (terpene derivatives); has been used to control warts
Kalanchoe spp. (Color Plate 39-5)	Kalanchoe, feltbush, velvet elephant ear, devil's backbone, lavender-scallops	Vomiting, diarrhea, ataxia, trembling, sudden death by cardiac failure	Lanceotoxin A (cumulative bufadienolide cardiotoxins)
Kalmia spp.	Mountain laurel, dwarf laurel	Copious salivation, excitation, vomiting, miosis, diarrhea, bradycardia, severe hypotension, conduction disturbances, weakness, ataxia, paralysis, coma, occasional seizures. Emetic contraindicated owing to vagal effects	Grayanotoxins (cardioactive diterpenoid), sodium channel activators
Karwinskia humboldtiana	Coyotilla, buckthorn, tullidora	Long (weeks) latency; ascending posterior paresis by demyelination; terminal respiratory paralysis	Karwinol A (neurotoxic polycyclic polyphenol) in berries (also called buckthorn toxins T-496, T-514, T-544)
Laburnum anagyroides	Golden chain tree, laburnum	Vomiting, hypersalivation; hypertension, excitation, seizures; higher doses: weakness, paralysis, coma, respiratory paralysis, death	Cytisine (nicotinic quinolizidine alkaloid); entire plant is toxic, especially seeds; laburnine, laburnamine
Lantana camara	Lantana, shrub verbena, yellow sage, buncberry	Vomiting, abdominal pain, diarrhea, ataxia, depression, cholestasis, bilirubinemia, hepatic damage, lethargy, coma, death	Unripe berries most toxic; pentacyclic triterpenes lantadene A and B, 0.5%-2.2% dry weight, in leaves
Ledum palustre	Wild rosemary	Delayed approximately 1 hour: copious salivation, excitation, vomiting, miosis, diarrhea, bradycardia, severe hypotension, conduction disturbances, weakness, ataxia, paralysis, coma, seizures. Induced emesis contraindicated owing to vagal effects	Grayanotoxin I (cardioactive diterpenoid); ledol, palustrol (sesquiterpene alcohols) found in essential oil

Continued

Table 27-1 Toxic Plant Information Summary—cont'd

Latin Name	Common Names	Clinical Signs, Prognosis, Additional Treatment	Toxins, Plant Parts, Lethal Doses
Leucothoe spp.	Black laurel, mountain laurel	Delayed approximately 1 hour: copious salivation, excitation, vomiting, perspiration, miosis, diarrhea, bradycardia, severe hypotension, conduction disturbances, weakness, ataxia, paralysis, coma, occasional seizures Induced emesis contraindicated owing to vagal effects	Grayanotoxins (cardioactive diterpenoid); ledol, palustrol (sesquiterpene alcohols) found in essential oil
Lilium spp., hybrids	Easter lily, star-gazer lily, tiger lily (Color Plate 20-3)	Vomiting, depression; renal failure in cats	Unknown: small amounts of flower, stem, and leaves
Ligustrum spp.	Privet, wax-leaf ligustrum	Abdominal pains, vomiting, watery diarrhea, rapid pulse	Syringin (ligustrin), irritant glycoside; whole plant, especially berries
Lobelia spp.	Lobelia, cardinal flower, blue lobelia, Indian tobacco	Salivation, vomiting, tachycardia, hypertension, mydriasis, seizures; in larger amounts, weakness, ataxia, depression, coma, death	Lobeline, nicotinic alkaloids
Lonicera spp.	Honeysuckle	No clinical signs, to vomiting, abdominal pain, diarrhea	Saponins in berries; at least 30 berries for clinical signs (adult human)
Lophophora williamsii	Peyote, mescal, mescal button	Mydriasis, vomiting, diarrhea, ataxia, hallucinations	Mescaline; all parts toxic
Lupinus spp.	Lupin, lupine, bluebonnet (not Texas bluebonnet)	Dry mucous membranes, hyperthermia, mydriasis, confusion	Sparteine, lupinine, lupanine (quinolizidine alkaloids); entire plant; anticholinergic
Lycopersicon lycopersicum	Tomato	Delayed 4-9 hours: vomiting, severe diarrhea, possible dehydration and electrolyte imbalance	Solanines in foliage; cholinesterase inhibition; ripened fruits are nontoxic
Lycoris spp.	Golden spider lily, red spider lily, magic lily	Vomiting, abdominal pain, diarrhea, dehydration, electrolyte imbalance	Lycorine, phenanthridine alkaloids
Lyonia spp.	Fetter bush, stagger bush	Hypersalivation, vomiting, abdominal pain, diarrhea, bradycardia, dysrhythmias, coma, convulsions	Lyoniol A, similar to grayanotoxins, sodium channel activator

Lysichiton americanum	Yellow skunk cabbage	Irritation to the GIT; if large amounts ingested, airway obstruction, respiratory compromise	Insoluble calcium oxalates
Macrozamia spp.	Zamia	Violent emesis, diarrhea, ataxia, seizures, coma, death; massive hepatic necrosis in dogs; lower doses carcinogenic and teratogenic	Macrozamin, cycasin, neocycasin A and B; amino acid MAA; MAM
Mahonia spp.	Oregon grape, trailing mahonia	Confusion, epistaxis, vomiting, diarrhea, renal irritation; high doses: primary respiratory arrest and hemorrhagic nephritis	Berberine (isoquinoline alkaloid); root and stem bark contain 0.06% dry weight; berries harmless
Maianthemum bifolium	May lily	Gastrointestinal irritation, vomiting	Saponins
Malus spp.	Apple	Hypersalivation, vomiting, lethargy, coma, convulsions, cardiovascular collapse	Amygdalin (cyanogenic glycoside) in seeds only; 1 cup seeds fatal to adult human
Melia azederach	Chinaberry, chinaberry tree	Vomiting, diarrhea, weakness, ataxia, depression, convulsions, coma	Meliatoxins A1, A2, B1 (limonoid tetranorterpenes) in fruits and bark; 5-6 fruits fatal to young dog within 48 hours
Menispermum canadense	Moonseed, sarsaparilla	Cardiac dysrhythmias, neurologic excitation, seizures	Dauricine, potassium channel inhibitor, in fruits
Menziesia ferruginea	Mock azalea, rusty leaf	Hypersalivation, excitation, vomiting, miosis, diarrhea, bradycardia, severe hypotension, conduction disturbances, weakness, ataxia, paralysis, coma, occasional seizures Induced emesis contraindicated because of vagal effects	Grayanotoxin I (cardioactive diterpenoid); ledol, palustrol (sesquiterpene alcohols) found in essential oil
Monstera spp.	Split-leaf philodendron, ceriman, Swiss cheese plant, fruit-salad plant, Mexican breadfruit	Mucosal irritation and inflammation, possible blistering, hypersalivation, vomiting; if large amounts: dysphagia, airway obstruction, respiratory compromise	Calcium oxalate raphides and idioblasts; found throughout the plant
Myoporum laetum	Ngaio tree	Vomiting, abdominal pain, diarrhea, dehydration, electrolyte imbalance; seizures	Ngaione (essential oil) furanoid sesquiterpene ketone in leaves and fruit
Myristica fragrans	Nutmeg	Depression, aggression, disturbed vision	Myristicin

Continued

Table 27-1 Toxic Plant Information Summary—cont'd

Latin Name	Common Names	Clinical Signs, Prognosis, Additional Treatment	Toxins, Plant Parts, Lethal Doses
Nandina domestica	Heavenly bamboo	Incoordination, weakness, seizures, respiratory failure	Cyanogenic glycosides: all parts potentially problematic
Narcissus spp.	Daffodil, jonquil, narcissus	Vomiting, hypersalivation, diarrhea, dehydration, sedation, hypotension, electrolyte imbalance	Lycorine, other phenanthridine alkaloids, highest levels in bulb, also found in stem and leaves
Nerium oleander	Oleander	Vomiting, diarrhea, bradycardia, arrhythmias, hyperkalemia, sudden death. Induced emesis contraindicated because of vagal effects	Oleandrin (cardenolide cardiac glycoside), as little as 0.005% of animal's body weight in plant material can be fatal
Nicotiana spp.	Tobacco, tree tobacco	Vomiting, diarrhea, tremors, hypertension, mydriasis, seizures; in larger doses, weakness, paralysis, coma, respiratory failure	Nicotine; leaves 0.5%–9.0% dry weight; all parts toxic; also anabasine in some spp.; rapidly absorbed through skin, mucous membranes
Ornithogalum spp.	Star of Bethlehem, wonder flower, dove's dung, nap-at-noon	Vomiting, diarrhea, hyperkalemia, bradycardia, heart block, arrhythmias. Induced emesis contraindicated because of effect on the vagus	Convallotoxin (0.04%), convalloside, and other cardioactive glycosides found mostly in bulb
Oxalis spp.	Sorrel, wood sorrel	Rapid respirations, stupor, vomiting, bloody diarrhea, coma, hypocalcemic tetany; renal oxalosis can occur if large amounts consumed	Soluble sodium and potassium oxalates throughout entire plant
Papaver spp.	Poppies	Narcosis, muscular relaxation, central respiratory depression, miosis, cyanosis, respiratory failure, death	Rhoeadine-type alkaloids, papaverrubines, thebaine, papaverine; very small amounts compared with opium poppy
Paris quadrifolia	Herb Paris	Vomiting, diarrhea, miosis	Steroidal saponins (old names: paristyphin, paridin); whole plant toxic
Periploca graeca	Silk vine	Vomiting, diarrhea, bradycardia, arrhythmias, collapse, death	Cardioactive glycosides
Philodendron sp. (Color Plate 27-10)	Philodendron, sweetheart plant, parlor ivy	Mucosal irritation and inflammation, hypersalivation, vomiting, diarrhea	Calcium oxalate (up to 0.7% dry weight) found throughout the plant

Physalis spp.	Chinese lantern, ground cherry, Cape gooseberry	Vomiting, diarrhea	Solanine glycosides in unripe fruits
Phytolacca americana	Pokeweed, pokeberry, poke salad, ink plant	Gastrointestinal irritation, delayed vomiting, abdominal pain, diarrhea	Phytolaccatoxin and other triterpenoid saponins; levels much higher in roots than in leaves; least in berries
Pieris spp.	Pieris, fetterbush, lily-of-the-valley bush	Delayed hypersalivation, excitation, vomiting, diarrhea, bradycardia, arrhythmias, hypotension, weakness, ataxia, paralysis, coma, occasional seizures. Induced emesis contraindicated because of vagal effects	Grayanotoxin (cardioactive diterpenoid sodium channel activator); as little as 1 g of fresh leaves/kg fatal to goats
Pista stratiotes	Water lettuce, shellflower	Mucosal irritation and inflammation, possible blistering, hypersalivation, vomiting	Insoluble calcium oxalates
Plumbago spp.	Cape plumbago, cape leadwort, Ceylon leadwort	Vomiting, gastritis, diarrhea	Plumbagin (quinone) found in root; vesicant irritant
Podophyllum spp.	May apple, mandrake	Oropharyngeal pain, delayed intense abdominal pain, profuse watery diarrhea, dehydration, electrolyte imbalance, peripheral neuropathy, bone marrow suppression, cardiovascular collapse	Podophyllatoxins (lignan beta-glycosides); cytotoxic, inhibiting microtubule formation; fruit least toxic
Polyscias spp.	Balfour aralia, dinner plate aralia, Ming aralia, geranium-leaf aralia, wild coffee, coffee tree	Tachycardia, stupor, mydriasis, seizures	Falcarinone (alkylating agent, irritant); saponins
Polygonatum spp.	Solomon's seal	Vomiting, diarrhea	Steroidal saponins, especially fruits, seeds; aglycone is diosgenin

Continued

Table 27-1 Toxic Plant Information Summary—cont'd

Latin Name	Common Names	Clinical Signs, Prognosis, Additional Treatment	Toxins, Plant Parts, Lethal Doses
Prunus spp.	Apricot, Damson plum, bitter almond, bird cherry, choke cherry, peach, wild black cherry	Sublethal HCN acid poisoning: dizziness, local irritation, vomiting (may smell of bitter almonds), pink mucous membranes, dyspnea	Kernel within the pit contains varying concentrations of amygdalin (up to 8%); cyanide blocks cellular respiration at cytochrome oxidase
Prunus laurocerasus	Cherry laurel	Sublethal HCN poisoning: see *P. armeniaca*	Prunasin: in leaves 1%-1.5%, very low levels in fruit pulp; amygdalin very high in seeds
Pulsatilla spp.	Pulsatilla	Intense oropharyngeal pain and inflammation, mucosal blistering, hypersalivation, bloody vomiting and diarrhea; ataxia, seizures	Protoanemonin (lactone of γ-hydroxyvinyl-acrylic acid); subepidermal vesicant
Quercus spp.	Oak	Marked lack of appetite, diarrhea, hepatic injury, colic	Pyrogallol, tannins in acorns
Ranunculus spp.	Buttercup, blister wort, crowfoot	Intense oropharyngeal pain and inflammation, mucosal blistering, hypersalivation, bloody vomiting and diarrhea; ataxia, seizures	Protoanemonin and ranunculin in sap (subepidermal vesicant); 0.27%-2.5% dry weight in foliage of various species
Raphanus raphinistrum	Wild radish	Gastroenteritis, liver and kidney disorders	Glucosinolates
Rhamnus spp.	Alder buckthorn, bear-berry, coffeeberry, cascara sagrada	Vomiting, abdominal pain, diarrhea	Glucofrangulin (anthracene glycoside) in fruits, bark, seeds; bark and fruits used as a purgative and laxative
Rheum spp., hyb.	Rhubarb, pie plant, wine plant	Vomiting, abdominal pain, diarrhea; with large amounts, hypocalcemia, renal damage	Anthraquinone glycoside cathartics in leaves; soluble oxalate (0.28% dry weight of leaf material)
Rhododendron spp.	Azaleas, rhododendrons	Delayed hypersalivation, excitation, vomiting, miosis, diarrhea, bradycardia, arrhythmias, hypotension, weakness, ataxia, paralysis, coma, occasional seizures Induced emesis contraindicated because of vagal effects	Grayanotoxins I, II, III (cardioactive diterpenoids); in flowers, leaves, nectar, honey; not all species and hybrids toxic, great variability; sodium channel activator

Rhoeo spathacea	Oyster plant, Moses in a boat	Mucosal irritation, vomiting, abdominal pain	Unidentified irritant
Ricinus communis (Color Plate 74-1)	Castor bean plant	Delayed 2-72 hours, dose dependent: vomiting, abdominal pain, bloody diarrhea, dehydration circulatory collapse, death	Ricin (toxalbumin, two chains) stops protein synthesis; one chewed seed can be fatal; 1 mg ricin/g seed; LD mouse (rat, dog) = 1 mcg/kg; rabbit = 0.1 mcg/kg
Rivina humilis	Rouge plant, pigeon berry	Vomiting, abdominal pain, diarrhea	Unknown toxin similar to phytolaccatoxin
Robinia pseudoacacia	Black locust	Vomiting, abdominal pain, bloody diarrhea, dehydration	Robin (toxalbumin/lectin, two chains, not linked) found in seeds, bark, leaves; less toxic than abrin or ricin
Sambucus spp. (Color Plate 27-12)	Elderberry, elder, dwarf elder	Vomiting, abdominal pain, diarrhea, coma, convulsions	Cyanogenic glycosides, or a toxalbumin, entire plant, especially root
Schefflera spp.	Schefflera, umbrella tree, rubber tree, starleaf	Vomiting, copious diarrhea, ataxia, anorexia, leukopenia, tachycardia, stupor, mydriasis, seizures	Falcarinol (alkylating agent, irritant); soluble oxalates, 0.9%-1.5% wet weight in leaves
Scilla spp.	Squill; star hyacinth, Cuban lily, Peruvian jacinth, hyacinth of Peru	Vomiting, diarrhea, bradycardia, arrhythmias	Proscillaridin A (bufadienolide cardiotoxin); inhibits glycosidases
Senecio spp.	Ragwort, cineraria, butterweed, groundsel	Acute hepatitis if large amount; chronic or low level: much delayed anorexia, depression, rough coat, diarrhea or constipation, emaciation, icterus, hepatoencephalopathy, death	Pyrrolizidine alkaloids: 0.3%-0.4% dry weight; not all species proved to contain alkaloids
Sinapis spp.	White mustard, charlock	Acute gastroenteritis, pain, diarrhea	Glucosinolates
Solanum spp. (Color Plate 27-13)	Nightshade, bittersweet, love apple, Carolina horsenettle, nipple-fruit, potato vine	Vomiting, abdominal pain, diarrhea, tachycardia, weakness, ataxia, respiratory failure, death	Variable major alkaloids: solanine, tomatine, solamarine, solasodine; green berries often contain highest concentrations, followed by leaves, shoots, and ripe berries

Continued

Table 27-1 Toxic Plant Information Summary—cont'd

Latin Name	Common Names	Clinical Signs, Prognosis, Additional Treatment	Toxins, Plant Parts, Lethal Doses
Solanum pseudocapsicum (Color Plate 22-1)	Jerusalem cherry, Christmas cherry, Natal cherry, winter cherry, ornamental pepper	Vomiting, mydriasis, drowsiness	Solanocapsine, solanocapsidine, solanine found in all plant parts; ripe and unripe berries similarly toxic; cholinesterase inhibition
Sophora spp.	Mescal bean, mountain laurel, frijolito, Eve's necklace	Hypersalivation, vomiting, diarrhea; hypertension, mydriasis, trembling, weakness, paralysis, death due to respiratory failure	Cytisine, nicotinic alkaloids (lupine-type); one seed, masticated, is lethal; foliage at 1% body weight is toxic, 2% is fatal
Sorbus spp.	Rowan, mountain ash, service tree, whitebeam	Minor gastroenteritis	Low levels amygdalin in seeds; parasorbic acid (local irritant)
Spathiphyllum sp. (Color Plate 27-11)	Peace lily, white anthurium, spathe flower, Mauna Loa	Mucosal irritation and inflammation	Insoluble calcium oxalate raphides; possible proteinaceous toxin
Spigelia spp.	Pinkroot, West Indian pinkroot	Muscle spasms to severe seizures; possible rhabdomyolysis and resultant renal effects	Spigeline (strychnine-like alkaloid)
Symphoricarpus spp.	Snowberry, wolfberry, Indian currant	Vomiting, abdominal pain, diarrhea	Saponin, and some chelidonine (isoquinoline alkaloid) in berries
Symphytum officinale	Comfrey	Much delayed (weeks to months): anorexia, depression, rough pelage, diarrhea, emaciation, constipation, icterus, hepatoencephalopathy, death	Pyrrolizidine alkaloids; toxicity probably requires chronic consumption
Symplocarpus foetidus	Skunk cabbage	Mucosal irritation and inflammation, possible blistering, hypersalivation, vomiting; if large amounts, dysphagia, airway obstruction, respiratory compromise	Insoluble calcium oxalate raphides and possible proteinaceous toxin
Synadenium grantii	African milkbush	Mucosal irritation and inflammation, potential blistering; vomiting, diarrhea	Tigliane-type diterpene esters (primary irritants, cocarcinogens)

Species	Common name	Clinical effects	Toxin/mechanism
Syngonium spp.	Goosefoot, nephthytis, African evergreen, arrowhead vine	Mucosal irritation and inflammation, possible blistering, hypersalivation, vomiting; if large amounts: dysphagia, airway obstruction, respiratory compromise; rapid respiration, stupor; rarely hypocalcemic tetany	Calcium oxalate raphides and idioblasts; also soluble oxalates
Tamus communis	Black bryony	Mucosal irritation and inflammation, possible blistering, hypersalivation, vomiting, diarrhea	Calcium oxalate raphides and idioblasts; traces of alkaloids; saponins (20 mg diosgenin/kg); photosensitive phenanthrene derivative
Taxus spp.	Yew; Japanese, English, western, Canadian, and Florida yew	Ataxia, mydriasis; abdominal pain, hypersalivation, vomiting, bradycardia, hypotension, hyperkalemia, death. Induced emesis contraindicated because of effects on the vagus	Taxines (cardioactive glycoalkaloids); various bioflavonoids with CNS-depressant, analgesic, or antipyretic activity; cyanogenic glycosides (not significant); fleshy red aril around seeds not toxic
Thevetia peruviana	Yellow oleander	Vomiting, diarrhea, bradycardia, arrhythmias, hyperkalemia, collapse, death. Induced emesis contraindicated because of effects on the vagus	Peruvoside, thevetins, thevetoxin (cardiac glycosides); entire plant is toxic, 8-10 seeds necessary to kill an adult human
Thuja occidentalis	White cedar	Gastric bleeding, hepatic degeneration, renal damage, tetanic convulsions	Thujone (monoterpene, strong local irritant)
Tillandsia cyanea	Pink quill	Severe mucosal irritation and inflammation, possible blistering, hypersalivation, vomiting	Insoluble calcium oxalates, proteolytic enzymes
Tragia spp.	Nettle, stinging nettle, noseburn	Salivation, vomiting, arrhythmias, dyspnea, weakness, collapse	Acetylcholine, histamine in plant hairs
Tulipa spp.	Tulip, garden tulip	Vomiting, hypersalivation, arrhythmias, dyspnea	Tuliposides A, B (convert to tulipalins A, B, lactone allergens); a lectin that inhibits DNA synthesis; mostly in bulb
Urginea maritima	Red squill, sea onion	Vomiting, diarrhea, bradycardia, arrhythmias, hyperkalemia, seizures; Ca^{2+}-binding agents decrease lethality	Proscillaridin A (bufadienolide cardiotoxins), noncumulative

Continued

Table 27-1 Toxic Plant Information Summary—cont'd

Latin Name	Common Names	Clinical Signs, Prognosis, Additional Treatment	Toxins, Plant Parts, Lethal Doses
Urtica spp.	Nettle, stinging nettle, noseburn	Salivation, vomiting, arrhythmias, dyspnea, weakness, collapse	Acetylcholine, histamine in plant hairs
Veratrum spp.	False hellebore, white hellebore	Distal paresthesia gradually extending centrally, followed by vomiting, diarrhea, paralysis, intense pain, hypothermia, dyspnea, arrhythmias, hypotension, collapse, respiratory paralysis, cardiac failure	Protoveratrines A and B (tetraesters), jerveratrum (furanopiperidines); steroidal alkaloids; sodium channel activators
Viburnum spp.	Guelder rose, highbush cranberry	Mild smooth muscle stimulant, vomiting, diarrhea	Bark, leaves only; berries edible in moderation
Vinca spp.	Periwinkle	Vomiting, collapse	Vincamine, vinblastine, vincristine (indole alkaloids)
Viscum album	European mistletoe	Local irritant, vomiting, diarrhea, hypotension	Viscotoxins; viscumin (toxalbumin) in leaves, stems, berries
Vriesea fenestralis	Netted vriesea	Severe mucosal irritation and inflammation, possible blistering, hypersalivation, vomiting	Insoluble calcium oxalate, proteolytic enzymes
Wisteria sinensis	Wisteria, Chinese kidney bean	Vomiting, abdominal pain, diarrhea	Wisterin "sapotoxin"; bark and roots; lectins in all parts
Xanthosoma spp.	Malanga, blue taro, tannia, yautia	Mucosal irritation and inflammation, possible blistering, hypersalivation, vomiting; if large amounts, dysphagia, airway obstruction, respiratory compromise	Insoluble calcium oxalate raphides, possible proteinaceous toxin

Zamia spp.	Coontie, cardboard palm, camptie, yugulla	Violent emesis, diarrhea, ataxia, seizures, coma, death; hepatoencephalopathy; lower doses carcinogenic and teratogenic	Cycasin (hydrolyzes to MAM)
Zantedeschia spp.	Calla lily, arum lily	Mucosal irritation and inflammation, possible blistering, hypersalivation, vomiting; if large amounts: dysphagia, airway obstruction, respiratory compromise	Calcium oxalate raphides and idioblasts; all plant parts are toxic; one spadix put a child in a 12-hour coma; recovered at 24 hours; can be fatal
Zephyranthes spp.	Zephyr lily, rain lily, fairy lily, fire lily	Vomiting, abdominal pain, diarrhea (may be bloody), dehydration, electrolyte imbalance	Lycorine, haemanthamine; bulbs and leaves are toxic, bulbs more so
Zigadenus spp.	Death camas	Distal paresthesia gradually extending centrally followed by hypersalivation, vomiting, diarrhea, hypothermia, muscle tremors, dyspnea, bradycardia, hypotension, paralysis, respiratory paralysis, cardiac failure	Zygadenine, zygacine, isogermidine, neogermidine, protoveratridine (steroidal alkaloids like those of Veratrum); sodium channel activators

ACh, Acetylcholine; *BMAA*, beta-methyl amino-L-alanine; *Ca²⁺*, calcium; *CNS*, central nervous system; *D-ABI*, 1,4-dideoxy-1,4-imino-D-arabinitol; *DMDP*, 2,5-dihydroxymethyl-3,4-dihydroxypyrrolidine; *GABA*, γ-aminobutyric acid; *HCN*, hydrocyanic acid; *LD*, lethal dose; *MAA*, methylazoxymethanol; *MAM*, metabolite methylazoxymethanol; *MLA*, methlycaconitine.

Table 27-2 Listing of Common Household and Garden Plants for Which No Incriminating Information Has Been Discovered—Possible Pet-Friendly Alternatives

Latin Name	Common Name(s)
*Abutilon hybridum**	Chinese bellflower, flowering maple, parlor maple
Acanthus spinosus	Bear's bush, bear's breech, spiny bear's breech
*Achillea millefolium**	Yarrow, fernleaf yarrow, sneezewort
Achimenes hyb.	Hot-water plant
Aeschynanthus spp.	Basket plant, lipstick plant
Ajuga spp.	Ajuga, bugleweed
Alcea rosea	Hollyhock
Alchemilla spp.	Lady's mantle, mountain lady's mantle
Alyssum saxatilia	Basket-of-gold
Amelanchier spp.*	Juneberry
Anaphalis spp.	Pearly everlasting
Anthemis tinctoria	Marguerite, golden marguerite, chamomile
Aphelandra hyb.	Zebra plant
Arabis spp.	Rock cress
Araucaria heterophylla	Norfolk Island pine
Arenaria spp.	Mountain sandwort, moss sandwort
Aruncus spp.	Goat's beard
Aster spp.	Alpine aster, Michaelmas daisy
Aubrieta deltoidea	Rock cress
Beloperone guttata	Shrimp plant
Bletia hyb.	Orchids
Bougainvillea glabra hyb.	Bougainvillea, paper flower
Bouvardia hyb.	Bouvardia
Brassia hyb.	Orchids
Buddleia davidii	Buddleia, butterfly bush
Cactaceae family	Rattail cactus, Peruvian torch, Christmas and Easter cacti
Calathea spp.	Peacock plant
Callisia elegans	Striped inch plant
Callistephus chinensis	China aster
Canna indica	Canna, canna lily (not a true lily), Indian-shot
Catalpa speciosa	Western catalpa tree
Cerastrium spp.	Snow-in-summer
Chaenomeles spp.*	Ornamental quince
Chrysanthemum spp., hyb.	Chrysanthemum, marguerite, painted daisy (human contact allergen)
Chrysopsis spp.	Golden asters
*Cichorium endivia**	Endive
Citrofortunella mitis hyb.	Calamondin
Citrus limon "Meyer"	Meyer's lemon
Clarkia grandiflora	Godetia, satinflower
Coleus spp.*	Painted nettle, Spanish thyme, Indian borage
Coreopsis grandiflora	Coreopsis, tickseed
Cornus spp.*	Dogwood, dogberry, Cornelian cherry, pink flowering dogwood
Cosmos bipinnatus	Cosmos
Cotoneaster spp.*	Cotoneaster, service berry
Crassula spp.	Silver jade plant, silver dollar, happiness tree, sickle plant
Crataegus spp.*	Hawthorne
Crossandra infundibuliformis	Firecracker flower

Table 27-2 Listing of Common Household and Garden Plants for Which No Incriminating Information Has Been Discovered—Possible Pet-Friendly Alternatives—cont'd

Latin Name	Common Name(s)
Cryptotaenia japonica*	Mitsuba
Cuphea spp.*	Firecracker plant, cigar flower, red-white-and-blue flower
Cydonia spp.*	Quince
Cymbidium hyb.	Orchids
Cyperus spp.	Egyptian paper plant, papyrus, umbrella plant
Cyrtomium falcatum	Japanese holly ferns
Dahlia pinnata hyb.*	Dahlia, dwarf dahlia
Dendrobium hyb.	Orchids
Deutzia scabra	Deutzia
Dianthus spp.*	Carnations, pinks, sweet William
Dioscorea batatas*	Chinese yam, cinnamon vine
Dryopteris filix-mas*	Male fern
Echeveria spp.	Baby echeveria, painted-lady, red echeveria
Echinacea spp.	Coneflowers, purple coneflower
Echinops spp.	Globe thistles
Epimedium spp., hyb.	Epimedium (evergreen flowering mat)
Eryngium spp.	Eryngo, sea holly, rattlesnake master
Erythronium spp.*	Dog-tooth violet, trout lily, avalanche lily
Ficus benjamina*	Weeping fig, Java willow, Benjamin tree, small-leaved rubber plant
Fittonia verschaffeltii	Mosaic plant
Forsythia spp.	Forsythia, golden bell, border forsythia
Fraxinus ornus	Flowering ash, manna ash
Fuchsia spp., hyb.*	Fuchsia, lady's eardrops
Gaillardia spp.	Gaillardia, blanketflower
Ganzania spp.	Ganzania, treasure flower
Gardenia jasminoides	Gardenia, Cape jasmine
Gaultheria procumbens*	Checkerberry, creeping wintergreen
Gaura spp.	Gaura, white gaura
Geranium spp., hyb.	Cranesbill, geranium, filaree
Gerbera jamesonii	Gerber daisy, Barberton, Transvaal daisy
Geum spp.	Scarlet avens, Chilean avens, prairie smoke
Grevillea spp.*	Silky oak, grevillea, kahili flower, silver oak, he-oak
Helianthus spp.	Sunflowers
Heliopsis helianthoides	Oxeye, sunflower, heliopsis
Hypoestes phyllostachya	Freckle-face, polka-dot plant
Iberis spp.	Candytuft, perennial candytuft
Impatiens spp.*	Impatiens, garden balsam, busy Lizzie, jewelweed
Justicia carnea	Brazilian plume, king's crown, flamingo plant
Lactuca spp.*	Great lettuce, garden lettuce
Laeliocattleya hyb.	Orchids
Lagerstroemia indica	Crape myrtle
Laurus nobilis*	Laurel, bay laurel, sweet bay
Leontopodium alpinum	Edelweiss
Liatris spicata	Gayfeather, blazing star
Linum spp.	Flax, blue flax, golden flax
Magnolia spp.	Magnolias: laurel, Oyama, saucer, southern, star

Continued

Table 27-2 Listing of Common Household and Garden Plants for Which No Incriminating Information Has Been Discovered—Possible Pet-Friendly Alternatives—cont'd

Latin Name	Common Name(s)
Malva spp.	Hollyhock, mallow, musk mallow
*Matricaria chamomilla**	Wild chamomile
Mespilus spp.*	Medlar
*Mimosa pudica**	Sensitive plant, shame plant, touch-me-not plant, action plant
Nephrolepis spp.*	Boston fern, dwarf Boston fern, ladder fern, sword fern
Odontoglossum hyb.	Orchids
Oenethera spp.	Primroses: beach, evening, Ozark, white evening; fluttermills
Oncidium hyb.	Orchids
Palmae family	Palms: Areca, butterfly, coconut, date, fan, Weddell (not Cycads or Caryota)
Pelargonium spp., hyb.*	Geraniums: horseshoe, ivy-leaved, zonal
Peperomia spp.*	American rubber plant, pepper face, emerald-ripple
Phalaenopsis hyb.	Orchids
Philadelphus coronarius	Mock orange, syringe
Phlox spp.	Phlox, creeping phlox, moss pink, ground pink, moss phlox
Photinia spp.	Photinia, red-tip photinia
Phyllitis scolopendrium	Hart's-tongue fern
*Pilea cadierei**	Watermelon plant
Polemonium spp.	Jacob's ladder, creeping Jacob's ladder
Portulaca spp.	Portulaca, purslane, rose moss
Potentilla spp.	Cinquefoils: bush, Himalayan, shrubby
Primulus spp.*	Primrose, German primrose, poison primrose
Pyrus spp.*	Pear, ornamental pear
Rudbeckia spp.	Coneflower, rudbeckia
Saintpaulia ionantha hyb.	African violets
Salvia spp.	Sages: silver, azure, mealycup, velvet, meadow
*Sansevieria trifasciata**	Mother-in-law's tongue, snake plant
Schlumbergera bridgesii	Christmas cactus, Easter cactus
Sedum spp.*	Sedum, gold moss, stonecrop, wall pepper, October plant
Sempervivum spp.*	Hens-and-chickens, houseleek, stonecrop
Setcreasea pallida var. *purpurea*	Purple heart
Sinningia speciosa hyb.	Gloxinia
*Sparmannia africana**	African hemp, indoor linden
Targetes spp.*	Marigold
*Tolmiea menziesii**	Piggyback plant, pickaback plant, thousand mothers, youth-on-age
Toxicodendron spp.*	Poison ivy, poison oak, poison sumac
Tradescantia spp.*	Wandering Jew, flowering inch plant, spiderwort, widow's tears
Zebrina pendula	Wandering Jew
Zinnia elegans	Zinnia, youth-and-old-age

*May produce hypersensitivity reactions in some humans.

References

1. Bianchini F, Pantano AC: *Simon and Schuster's guide to plants and flowers*, New York, 1974, Simon and Schuster.
2. Botha CJ, van der Lugt JJ, Erasmus GL, et al: Krimpsiekte, a paretic condition of small stock poisoned by bufadienolide-containing plants of the Crassulaceae in South Africa. In Garland T, Barr AC, editors: *Toxic plants and other natural toxicants*, Wallingford, Oxon, UK, 1998, CAB International.
3. Burrows GE, Tyrl RJ: *Toxic plants of North America*, Ames, 2001, Iowa State University Press.
4. Calanasan CA, Capon RJ, Gaul KL, et al: Toxic analogues of wedeloside and carboxyatractyloside from Australian plant species. In Colegate SM, Dorling PR, editors: *Plant-associated toxins: agricultural, phytochemical and agricultural aspects*, Wallingford, Oxon, UK, 1994, CAB International.
5. Carson TL, Sanderson TP, Halbur PG: *Acute nephrotoxicosis in cats following ingestion of lily (*Lilium *sp)*. Abstracts of the 37th Annual American Association of Veterinary Laboratory Diagnosticians, Grand Rapids, 1994, Mich.
6. Chiusoli A, Boriani ML: *Simon and Schuster's guide to house plants*, New York, 1986, Simon and Schuster/Fireside Books.
7. De Balogh KKIM, Dimande AP, van der Lugt JJ, et al: *Ipomoea carnea*: the cause of lysosomal storage disease in goats in Mozambique. In Garland T, Barr AC, editors: *Toxic plants and other natural toxicants*, Wallingford, Oxon, UK, 1998, CAB International.
8. Fowler M, editor: *Poisonous plants: a veterinary guide to toxic syndromes (CD-ROM)*, Davis, CA, 1998, School of Veterinary Medicine, University of California–Davis.
9. Frohne D, Pfander HJ: *A colour atlas of poisonous plants (English translation)*, London, 1984, Wolfe Publishing Ltd.
10. Hare WR: Chinaberry (*Melia azederach*) poisoning in animals. In Garland T, Barr AC, editors: *Toxic plants and other natural toxicant*, Wallingford, Oxon, UK, 1998, CAB International.
11. Ivie GW: Toxicological significance of plant furocoumarins. In Keeler RF, Van Kampen KR, James LF, editors: *Effects of poisonous plants on livestock*, London, 1978, Academic Press.
12. Kim HL, Stipanovic RD: Isolation of karwinol A from coyotillo (*Karwinskia humboldtiana*) fruits. In Garland T, Barr AC, editors: *Toxic plants and other natural toxicants*, Wallingford, Oxon, UK, 1998, CAB International.
13. Kingsbury JM: *Poisonous plants of the United States and Canada*, Englewood Cliffs, NJ, 1964, Prentice-Hall.
14. Nash RJ, Watson AA, Winters AL, et al: Glycosidase inhibitors in British plants as causes of livestock disorders. In Garland T, Barr AC, editors: *Toxic plants and other natural toxicants*, Wallingford, Oxon, UK, 1998, CAB International. 1998.
15. Nelson LS, Shih RD, Balick MJ: *Handbook of poisonous and injurious plants*, New York, 2007, The New York Botanical Garden, Springer Science and Business Media.
16. Norton S: Toxic effects of plants. In Klaassen CD, editor: *Casarett & Doull's toxicology: the basic science of poisons*, ed 5, New York, 1996, McGraw-Hill.
17. Oelrichs PB, Kratzmann S, MacLeod JK, et al: A study of persin, the mammary cell necrosis agent from avocado (*Persea americana*), and its furan derivative in lactating mice. In Garland T, Barr AC, editors: *Toxic plants and other natural toxicants*, Wallingford, Oxon, UK, 1998, CAB International.
18. Osweiler GD, Carson TL: Toxic plants and zootoxins. In Morgan RV, editor: *Handbook of small animal medicine*, ed 3, Philadelphia, 1997, WB Saunders.
19. Riet-Correa F, Pfister J, Schild AL, et al: *Poisoning by plants, mycotoxins and related toxins*, Wallingford, Oxon, UK, 2011, CAB International.
19a. Robinson GH, Burrows GE, Holt EM, et al: Evaluation of the toxic effects of the legumes of mimosa (*Albizia julibrissin*) and identification of the toxicant. In Garland T, Barr AC, editors: *Toxic plants and other natural toxicants*, Wallingford, Oxon, UK, 1998, CAB International.
20. Rumbeiha WK, Francis JA, Fitzgerald SD, et al: A comprehensive study of Easter lily poisoning in cats, *J Vet Diagn Invest* 16:527–541, 2004.
21. Seiber JN, Lee SM, McChesney MM, et al: New cardiac glycosides (cardenolides) from *Asclepias* species. In Seawright AA, Hegarty MP, James LF, et al: *Plant toxicology, Yeerongpilly, Queensland Poisonous Plant Committee, Queensland Department of Primary Industries*, 1985, Animal Research Institute.
22. Sharma OP: Plant toxicoses in northwestern India. In Colegate SM, Dorling PR, editors: *Plant-associated toxins: agricultural, phytochemical and agricultural aspects*, Wallingford, Oxon, UK, 1994, CAB International.
23. Shlosberg A, Ohad DG, Bellaiche M, et al: Monitoring of physiological and pathological changes in turkey poults fed leaves of potentially cardiomyotoxic *Nerium oleander* and *Persea americana*. In Garland T, Barr AC, editors: *Toxic plants and other natural toxicants*, Wallingford, Oxon, UK, 1998, CAB International.

24. Spainhour CB, Flory W, Reagor JC: The intoxication of a canine by the fruit of the garden shrub *Brunfelsia calycina* var, *floribunda, Texas Vet Med J* 51:22–23, 1989.
25. Spoerke DG Jr, Smolinske SC: *Toxicity of houseplants*, Boca Raton, FL, 1990, CRC Press.
26. Stegelmeier BL, Panter KE, Pfister JA, et al: Experimental modification of larkspur (*Delphinium* spp) toxicity. In Garland T, Barr AC, editors: *Toxic plants and other natural toxicants*, Wallingford, Oxon, UK, 1998, CAB International.

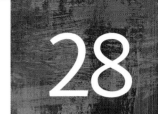

Miscellaneous Herbicides, Fungicides, and Nematocides

28

Patricia A. Talcott, MS, DVM, PhD, DABVT

- Suspected pet poisonings with herbicides, fungicides, and nematocides are proportional to the frequency of use by the general population.
- Vomiting is a nonspecific commonly observed clinical sign.
- There are no specific antidotes for most herbicide, fungicide, or nematocide poisonings.
- Exposure to pesticide-treated plants is unlikely to result in intoxication in companion animals. Misapplication of herbicides at some point produces visible signs of phytotoxicity.
- Acute exposures to these pesticides rarely produce altered clinical chemical data, which are commonly seen in long-term animal feeding trials.
- The EXtension TOXicology NETwork is an excellent resource for toxicologic information of many pesticides: http://extoxnet.orst.edu/.

Public perception of risk is greatly influenced by the voluntary nature of the risk. Thus consumers who purchase pesticide products for their own use often have a different perception of risk from these products compared with products used by others, such as veterinarians, farmers, or pest control or lawn care service operators. With the exception of the anticoagulant rodenticides, inquiries about possible pesticide poisoning in pet animals are more directly proportional to the frequency of use of the pesticide than to the toxicity ranking of the pesticide. The Environmental Protection Agency reports that U.S. pesticide expenditures totaled $11.8 billion in 2006 and $12.5 billion in 2007.[1] Herbicides are the largest group of pesticides purchased, followed by insecticides and miticides, fungicides, and others.[1] U.S. pesticide amount used in both 2006 and 2007 exceeded 1.1 billion pounds.[1] The most commonly used pesticides around the home and garden are shown in Table 28-1. Cancellations of the residential uses of chlorpyrifos and diazinon have resulted in a significant decrease in the use of organophosphate insecticides in the home and garden sector.

Most often a pet owner suspects a pesticide poisoning when the pet shows clinical signs within a short time following a known environmental pesticide application. In virtually all incidents of illness, the pet owner wants a diagnosis of causation. If exposure to a toxic substance is suspected, an effort should be made to identify the substance, the date of application and exposure, and the method of pesticide use and exposure.

The clinical signs should be biologically consistent with the toxicology of the suspected toxicant. Seizures, for example, will not occur from exposure to urea fertilizer at any dose. The Internet is an excellent resource for information on pesticides. The Extoxnet site contains summaries of many pesticides.[2] Material safety data sheets (MSDSs) are available from suppliers and manufacturer home pages. And of course, "the dose makes the poison." Therefore, because the MSDS for a product lists the potential toxic effects, it is important to determine if the exposure was to the undiluted product or to some end-use dilution before concluding that there was a cause-and-effect relationship. For example, many liquid formulations of herbicides that must be diluted before use are severe eye irritants and may even be corrosive to the eye in the undiluted form. Yet when diluted for use (e.g., 1 tsp/gal of water), the end-use dilution can be less irritating to the eye than ordinary hair shampoo.

Vomiting is a common complaint in dogs and cats and is so nonspecific that the sign itself is not sufficient to establish a cause-and-effect relationship to a known pesticide exposure. It is generally well known that dogs and cats vomit after eating grass, whether or not it has been treated with an herbicide. The time course of onset of signs following pesticide exposure is also important. Both environmental degradation and low application rates make it most unlikely that exposure to pesticide application residues several days after the application would be toxicologically significant. Errors that result in overapplication of herbicides to plants most often produce visible damage to the plant. A twofold to threefold error in application of herbicide-fertilizer combinations to lawns produces obvious signs of phytotoxicity.

Phenoxy Herbicides

2,4-D

Chemically, 2,4-D is 2-chloro-4-phenoxyacetic acid. It is usually formulated as salts, esters, or amine derivatives.[2] 2,4-D is used for control of broadleaf weeds on residential and commercial properties and in some areas on roadside rights-of-way. Residues on treated turf are in the range of 35 to 75 ppm and dissipate rapidly in the first several days following the application. A residue tolerance of 300 ppm has been established on pasture grasses.

Poisoning is almost always caused by accidental ingestion of concentrates or sprays. Technical-grade phenoxy herbicides are irritating to the eye and mucous membranes and somewhat less irritating to skin, and are also phytotoxic to most plants. Dogs appear to be somewhat more sensitive to phenoxy herbicides than other species of domestic animals. The approximate oral median lethal dose (LD_{50}) for 2,4-D in the dog has been reported to be 100 mg/kg.[3] However, Beasley and colleagues[4] orally dosed English pointers with 8.8, 43.7, 86.7, 175, and 200 mg/kg 2,4-D, and all survived. Doses of 175 or 220 mg/kg of body weight produced overt signs of toxicosis characterized by myotonia, vomiting, and weakness. The lower doses did not produce overt clinical signs, but electromyographic abnormalities were detectable at exposures of 8.8 mg/kg. Multiple dosages of 20 mg/kg daily for approximately 3 weeks or 25 mg/kg for 6 days were lethal for dogs.[3,5]

Even at an exposure of 20 mg/kg of body weight, it is not likely that dogs will be significantly poisoned by exposure to properly treated lawns. The greatest hazard to dogs is ingestion of undiluted product, discarded or excess spray that had been previously mixed, or pools of spray that have collected in low spots or in containers. Arnold and colleagues[6] attempted to produce 2,4-D toxicosis by placing English pointers on enclosed turf plots to confine

Table 28-1	Quantities of Pesticides Most Commonly Used in Nonagricultural Sectors of the U.S. Home and Garden Market	
Pesticide	**Millions of Pounds**
1. 2,4-D	8-11
2. Glyphosate	5-8
3. Carbaryl	4-6
4. MCPP	4-6
5. Pendimethalin	3-5
6. Pyrethroids	2-4
7. Malathion	2-4
8. Dicamba	1-3
9. Trifluralin	1-3
10. Pelarganoc acid	<1

Approximate quantities, 2005 and 2007.

the animals for controlled periods of continuous exposure. One enclosure was sprayed with 2,4-D at a rate of 168 mg/square meter, which is the maximum recommended rate for lawns, and another enclosure was sprayed at four times the maximum recommended rate. The dogs were placed in the enclosures within 30 minutes of spraying and were observed five times each day for a period of 7 days. Detailed clinical examinations included electromyograms, which were performed on days 1 and 7 after exposure. No adverse effects were detected in any of the clinical, hematologic, biochemical, electrophysiologic, or postmortem examinations. A 2,4-D concentration of 500 ppm (25 mg/kg of body weight) in the diet caused no ill effects in dogs during a 2-year study. The level of 2,4-D at which no observable effects were noted in chronic toxicity in dogs was determined to be 1 mg/kg/day.[7]

Orally administered 2,4-D is rapidly and extensively absorbed by the gastrointestinal tract. The extent of dermal absorption varies according to the chemical form of the product and the species of animal, varying from approximately 5% for the acid in humans to 85% for the ester in rats. Absorbed 2,4-D salts and esters are rapidly converted to 2,4-D acid and excreted by the renal anion transport system. The renal anion transport system is saturable and appears to account for the longer half-life and greater sensitivity to toxicity in the dog. 2,4-D concentrations of 718 mcg/mL and 1075 mcg/mL were present in the serum of dogs dosed with 175 or 220 mg 2,4-D/kg of body weight, respectively. The peak serum concentration was 121 mcg/mL following an oral exposure of 8.8 mg/kg of body weight.

2,4-D is widely distributed in tissues with little accumulation in fat. Plasma or serum appears to be the best specimen to use for laboratory confirmations of 2,4-D (as well as other phenoxy herbicides) poisoning. Kidney tissue and urine are alternative samples that can be used. Pharmacokinetic data suggest that kidney to plasma ratios approach unity as the renal organic anion system becomes saturated. Data also suggest that plasma and kidney concentrations of up to 100 ppm may be present in animals that do not show signs of intoxication.

The clinical signs in dogs are characteristic and include vomiting and an initial disinclination to move and a passivity that gradually becomes worse as a pattern of myotonia develops.[8] This rigidity of skeletal muscles is combined with ataxia, progressive apathy, depression, and muscular weakness, particularly of the posterior limbs. Myotonia has been produced by exposure to 2,4-D and 2,4,5-T in dogs. At high doses, the condition can be induced in less than 1 hour after administration. Spontaneous movement ceases, and when startled, animals make sudden spastic movements and sometimes lose the ability to stand or rise. Opisthotonos may also occur. A potential biochemical lesion associated with myotonia is an increase in basic paranitrophenyl phosphatase related to increased passive flux of potassium. This may lead to myotonia through a compensatory decrease in chloride conductance. Periodic clonic spasms and finally coma are the typical sequelae of phenoxy herbicide poisoning in dogs. During the clinical course of poisoning there is marked anorexia; there may be vomiting and occasionally passage of blood-tinged feces. Postmortem examination often reveals necrotic ulcers of the oral mucosa, signs of irritation in the gastrointestinal tract, and sometimes necrosis of the small intestine, and focal necrosis in the liver and degeneration of renal tubules. However, there are no reports of renal failure in dogs from any exposure to 2,4-D.

There are no specific antidotes. Because 2,4-D is excreted almost quantitatively in urine as the free acid, forced alkaline diuresis should enhance excretion. Unless there is severe central nervous system (CNS) depression (rare), recovery should be rapid.

An association between 2,4-D and canine malignant lymphoma in dogs was reported in the Journal of the National Cancer Institute (NCI) in 1991.[9] This report not only raised concern by homeowners and veterinarians, but also in some instances was used to indict lawn care in a generic sense. The NCI reported a twofold increase in risk of canine malignant lymphoma associated with four or more yearly homeowner applications of 2,4-D. It is unusual for any homeowner (or commercial lawn care companies) to apply 2,4-D four or more times per year; thus the validity of pet owners' responses to the NCI questionnaire or interviews concerning the application of lawn care products is questionable.

Two critiques of the NCI report have been published. A panel of experts concluded that because of numerous limitations in the design of the study, an association was not established between 2,4-D and canine malignant lymphoma.[10,11]

Kaneene and Miller did not confirm a dose-response relationship between 2,4-D use and canine malignant lymphoma and concluded that the occurrence of canine malignant lymphoma was not significantly associated with the use of 2,4-D.[11]

An increased risk of transitional cell carcinoma of the urinary bladder of Scottish Terriers exposed to lawns or gardens treated with phenoxy herbicides was reported by Glickman and colleagues.[12] The authors proposed a gene-environment interaction to the development of the bladder tumors. The cause-effect relationship was based on information obtained by questionnaires completed by owners of dogs in the case and control groups. Additional studies are needed to replicate the results and to more specifically confirm exposures.

MCPA

4-Chloro-2-methylphenoxyacetic acid (MCPA) has been used in the United States, but has been the more widely used phenoxy herbicide in Europe, where it has been extensively used in forest management. MCPA is used for control of broadleaf weeds on residential lawns.

The rat oral LD_{50} for MCPA ranges from 600 mg/kg to 1470 mg/kg of body weight. Dogs given single oral doses of MCPA at 25 mg/kg of body weight exhibited no clinical signs during a 48-hour observation period. Oral administration of MCPA to male and female beagles at doses of up to 48 mg/kg of body weight for 13 weeks resulted in increases in hepatic enzymes and blood urea nitrogen, with severe signs of toxicity observed at the highest dosage tested. The dogs had pustules, dead skin spots, persistent mouth lesions, diarrhea, loss of appetite, decreased food consumption, loss of body weight, pus-forming conjunctivitis, jaundice, anemia, and lethargy. The no observable effect dosage was 1 mg/kg of body weight/day. In a 1-year dietary feeding study in dogs fed 6, 30, or 150 ppm of MCPA, there were no deaths, but dose-related increases in creatinine and blood urea nitrogen were observed. The effects were minor at the 30 ppm level, and none were observed at the 6 ppm exposure level.

The toxicokinetics, clinical signs, and treatment are similar to those described for 2,4-D exposures. At necropsy, jaundice, an enlarged gallbladder, discolored liver, and hemorrhages of the lungs, stomach, and intestines were observed in dogs receiving MCPA by gelatin capsule for 13 weeks.[13]

MCPP

2-Methyl-4-chlorophenoxypropanoic acid (MCPP) has the generic name *mecoprop*. MCPP is used exclusively for nonagricultural purposes, primarily for broadleaf weed control on lawns. The toxicology of MCPP is very similar to that of 2,4-D and MCPA. The rat oral LD_{50} ranges from 650 to 1200 mg/kg of body weight.

Glyphosate

Glyphosate is N-(phosphonomethyl)glycine. It is a systemic herbicide with agricultural, industrial right-of-way, and urban domestic applications. Glyphosate is the second most widely used herbicide in the home and garden market and is a nonselective herbicide (i.e., it will kill all plants). It is used to kill all unwanted vegetation along fences, edges of grassed areas, mulched ornamental beds, and perimeters near trees, parking lots, and driveways. Residues on grass following normal application range from 0.2 ppm to 100 ppm.

The rat oral LD_{50} is 4320 mg/kg of body weight, and the rabbit dermal LD_{50} is greater than 794 mg/kg of body weight for females and greater than 5000 mg/kg of body weight for males. Technical glyphosate is not an irritant, but the formulated products contain approximately 15% surfactant, which may be irritating. Dogs receiving glyphosate by gelatin capsule at dosages of 100 and 500 mg/kg/day for 1 year exhibited a decrease in pituitary weights. No detectable toxic effects were observed when rats were fed glyphosate for 2 years at dietary concentrations of 0, 30, 100, and 300 ppm. In a subsequent study, rats were fed levels of 0, 1000, 5000, and 30,000 ppm glyphosate for 2 years. There was a slight increase in the incidence of renal tumors that was not statistically significant from the control animals.

The metabolism of glyphosate in the dog or cat has not been reported. In the rat, glyphosate does not undergo biotransformation. Approximately 36% and 51% of an oral glyphosate dose of 10 mg/kg of body weight was eliminated in the urine and feces within 7 days.

Intoxication of pet animals by glyphosate is an extremely rare event because of the low toxicity of the compound. Human ingestion of the formulated product Roundup has produced massive fluid and electrolyte loss attributed to the surfactant, which composes 15% of the formulated product. The fluid and electrolyte loss triggered acute renal tubular necrosis.[14] Activated charcoal should adsorb glyphosate in the gastrointestinal tract. Fluid therapy should be implemented to maintain urine flow and replace diminished electrolytes.

Dicamba

Dicamba is a benzoic acid herbicide (3,6-dichloro-2-methoxybenzoic acid). It is widely used as a postemergent broadleaf herbicide on lawns or grasslands and on numerous crops. Dicamba has low toxicity, with oral LD_{50} values in rats, mice, guinea pigs, and rabbits that range from 566 to 3000 mg/kg of body weight.[15] Dogs fed dicamba for 2 years at a dietary concentration of 50 ppm exhibited no observable effects. When dicamba was fed at a dose of 250 ppm, the only adverse finding was mild hepatic discoloration.

Dicamba is rapidly absorbed from the gastrointestinal tract and is readily excreted in urine, with about 80% to 90% of the dose excreted within the first 24 hours. The major excretory product is unchanged dicamba and a glucuronide conjugate.

Signs of acute dicamba toxicosis in animals are muscle spasms, urinary incontinence, shortness of breath, cyanosis, and collapse. Poisoning by dicamba is not commonly reported in dogs or cats, nor is there data on gross or histologic lesions. The relatively rapid rate of excretion suggests that conservative supportive therapy, if any, should lead to a satisfactory outcome. Exposure to dicamba can be confirmed through plasma serum and urine testing.

Pendimethalin

Pendimethalin is a dinitroaniline compound (N-[1-ethylpropyl]-3,4-dimethyl-2,6-dinitrobenzenamine). It is an orange-yellow dye and stains hair and vinyl floor coverings. White hair stains green. Pendimethalin is the most widely used preemergent herbicide in the urban residential environment. It is used in the spring and has increasingly replaced bensulide and dacthal. Pendimethalin is also used to control grasses and weeds in field crops.

The rat oral LD_{50} is 1250 mg/kg of body weight, and the rabbit dermal LD_{50} is greater than 5000 mg/kg of body weight. Pendimethalin was given to beagles by gelatin capsule for 2 years at doses of 12.5, 50, and 200 mg/kg of body weight. The no observable effect level was determined to be 12.5 mg/kg. Although there was no effect on body weight or food intake, there was a dose-related increase in serum alkaline phosphatase concentrations, and microscopic liver lesions were seen at the higher doses of 50 and 200 mg/kg.

Pendimethalin is poorly absorbed from the gastrointestinal tract and is largely excreted unchanged in feces. Poisoning by pendimethalin in dogs and cats is not common. Pendimethalin is unlikely to cause significant hepatotoxicity at any level of exposure. The pendimethalin stain may be removed by application of a waterless hand cleaner such as GOJO or D&L Hand Cleaner followed by a shampoo and thorough rinsing. To be effective, the waterless cleaner should be applied to dry hair and blotted off, and the hair then shampooed and rinsed.

Prodiamine

Prodiamine is another dinitroaniline herbicide, which has fewer staining properties than pendimethalin, yet has similar properties as a preemergent herbicide. The rat oral LD_{50} is greater than 5000 mg/kg of body weight and the dermal LD_{50} is greater than 2000 mg/kg of body weight. Because of its high degree of safety, prodiamine represents minimal risk to pets.

Fungicides

Fungicides that are used to control diseases of plants are generally low in mammalian toxicity. A major use of fungicides is in the preservation of wood. Pentachlorophenol-treated lumber is used primarily for barns, fence posts, railroad ties, and wooden bridges. In residential settings, chromated copper arsenate (CCA)-treated lumber was historically the choice, but its purchase and use for residential purposes has been largely discontinued. CCA-treated lumber can still be used in agricultural and industrial settings. This is often called *Wolmanized lumber*. The safer alkaline copper quaternary (types B and D) and copper azole (CBA-A, CA-B) compounds are largely replacing the CCA-containing products. The organic tins, triphenyltin and tributyltin, have been used in antifouling paints on ships and to prevent mold growth on carpeting that has become wet from flooding. Organic tin compounds leach into water, resulting in unacceptable toxicity to lower forms of aquatic life, and their use has been restricted.

Pentachlorophenol

The toxicity of pentachlorophenol has been clouded by the poor characterization of the technical material and the presence of dioxin contaminants. The oral LD_{50} for pentachlorophenol ranges from 27 to 211 mg/kg of body weight in rats. Pentachlorophenol is volatile and is toxic by inhalation. This can be significant in cases of exposure in confined spaces with little ventilation. For example, plants rarely survive in log cabins built from pentachlorophenol-treated logs. Pentachlorophenol is also toxic via the dermal route, with dermal LD_{50} values ranging from 96 to 330 mg/kg of body weight. Dermal exposure is the most toxic route of exposure and is particularly hazardous for newborn animals.

Pentachlorophenol is readily absorbed from all routes of exposure and is excreted unchanged or as a glucuronide conjugate. The half-life in blood ranges from 15 to 78 hours. Pentachlorophenol is an uncoupler of oxidative phosphorylation and therefore produces pyrexia in poisoned animals. It is an irritant and may produce eye and skin irritation, hair loss, throat or respiratory irritation, and abdominal pain. High exposure conditions can lead to CNS effects, such as excitation or seizures. Chronic exposures cause decreases in body weight.

Except for signs of irritation, gross lesions are not remarkable. The liver, kidneys, and CNS are the major target organs. Removal of the patient from the site of exposure and supportive treatment should result in a favorable prognosis. Decontamination of skin is advisable following exposure to recently treated surfaces.

Chromated Copper Arsenate–Treated Lumber

The safety of CCA-treated lumber has been reviewed extensively in consideration of cancer risks to children using treated playground equipment. The arsenic is highly bound to wood, and the dislodgeable residues are negligible in relation to background levels of arsenic from soil. Therefore risks to pets are also negligible. CCA-treated lumber is no longer being commercially made as of December 2003 for residential use. But stores can continue to sell remaining stock after production ceases. Toxicities have been seen in livestock that ingest ash of burned treated lumber; arsenic appears to be the element responsible for the problems observed.

Thiram

Thiram is tetramethylthiuram disulfide. Although it is a crop protection fungicide, the use of thiram as an animal repellent is the most likely source of exposure to pet animals. Thiram has a low acute toxicity, with oral LD_{50} values ranging from 620 to 1900 mg/kg of body weight in rats and dermal LD_{50} values greater than 5000 mg/kg of body weight. Thiram is irritating to the eyes, skin, and respiratory tract and is also a potent sensitizer. A dietary level of 200 ppm fed for 1 year (4 mg/kg) had no effect in dogs.

It is logical to assume that the sulfur odor contributes to the repellent properties of thiram. Carbon disulfide is formed during the metabolism of thiram. Thiram inhibits a variety of enzymes, including cytochrome P450 and alcohol dehydrogenase. Worker exposures have shown an interaction with alcohol but not with drugs metabolized by the cytochrome P450 system.

In rats and mice, thiram produces incoordination, hyperactivity, loss of muscle tone, dyspnea, and seizures. In humans, allergic hypersensitivity to thiram is common. Repeated and daily oral doses of 49 mg/kg/day in laboratory animals produced weakness, muscle incoordination, and limb paralysis. There are no diagnostic lesions.

Nematocides

Several classes of chemicals are used as nematocides. The organophosphate and carbamate classes are discussed elsewhere (Chapter 67).

Imidacloprid

Imidacloprid is a member of a newer class of insecticides, the chloronicotinyl class. The mode of action of imidacloprid is to block neurotransmission by postsynaptic antagonism of nicotinic acetylcholine receptors. It is used to control grubs in lawns and as a termiticide in residential environments.

The acute toxicity of imidacloprid is low, with the oral LD_{50} ranging from 511 to 1084 mg/kg of body weight in rats. The dermal LD_{50} is greater than 5000 mg/kg of body weight. Rabbits were administered imidacloprid by the dermal route for 3 weeks at a dose of 1000 mg/kg for 6 hours a day, 5 days a week. Local or systemic effects were not observed. Dogs were administered imidacloprid for 1 year at dietary concentrations of 200, 500, or 1250 ppm. Because of the absence of significant effects, the high dose was increased to 2500 ppm at 17 weeks for the remainder of the study. Effects observed at the high dose included decreased food consumption, increased liver weights, and elevated serum cholesterol levels. The no observable effect level was determined to be 500 ppm (12.5 mg/kg of body weight).

Imidacloprid is rapidly absorbed from the gastrointestinal tract and excreted via urine and feces. Approximately 96% of the dose is recovered within 48 hours. Poisoning by imidacloprid has not been reported in dogs and cats. Insects become disoriented at sublethal doses and stop foraging for food. The limited data reported on dogs suggest that mild hepatotoxicity might occur with prolonged exposure, but neurologic effects have not been reported at doses up to 2500 ppm.

Acknowledgments

The author would like to recognize the previous contributions of an esteemed colleague Dr. Roger A. Yeary to this chapter.

References

1. Environmental Protection Agency: *Pesticide industry sales and usage, 2006 and 2007 market estimates*. February 2011. http://www.epa.gov/opp00001/pestsales/07pestsales/market_estimates2007.pdf.
2. Extoxnet: the extension toxicology network, http://ace.orst.edu/info/extoxnet. (Although not specifically cited, the Extoxnet pesticide information files were reviewed for each of the pesticides in this chapter.)
3. Drill VA, Hiratzka T: Toxicity of 2,4-dichlorophenoxyacetic acid and 2,4,5-trichlorophenoxyacetic acid: a report on their acute and chronic toxicity of dogs, *Arch Ind Hyg Occup Med* 7:61–67, 1953.
4. Beasley VR, Arnold EK, Lovell RA: 2,4-D toxicosis I: a pilot study of 2, 4-dichlorophenoxyacetic acid and dicamba-induced myotonia in experimental dogs, *Vet Hum Toxicol* 33:435–440, 1991.

5. Hill EV, Carlisle H: Toxicity of 2,4-dichlorophenoxyacetic acid in experimental animals, *Ind Hyg Toxicol* 29:85–95, 1947.
6. Arnold EK, Lovell RA, Beasley VR: 2,4-D toxicosis III: an attempt to produce 2,4-D toxicosis in dogs on treated grass plots, *Vet Hum Toxicol* 33:457–461, 1991.
7. Charles JM, Dulgard DW, Army HC, et al: Comparative subchronic dietary toxicity studies on 2,4-dichlorophenoxyacetic acid, amine, and ester in the dog, *Fund Appl Toxicol* 29:78–85, 1996.
8. Chen AV, Bagley RS, Talcott PA: Confirmed 2,4-dichlorophenoxyacetic acid toxicosis in a dog, JAAHA 46:1–5.
9. Hayes HM, Tarone RE, Cantor KP, et al: A case control study of canine malignant lymphoma: positive association with dog owners' use of 2,4-dicholorphenoxyacetic acid herbicides, *J Natl Cancer Inst* 83:1226–1231, 1991.
10. Carlo GL, Cole P, Miller AB, et al: Review of a study reporting an association between 2,4-dichlororphenoxyacetic acid and canine malignant lymphoma: report of an expert panel, *Reg Toxicol Pharmacol* 16:245–252, 1992.
11. Kaneene JB, Miller R: Re-analysis of 2,4-D use and the occurrence of canine malignant lymphoma, *Vet Human Toxicol* 41:164–170, 1999.
12. Glickman LT, Raghavan M, Knapp DW, et al: Herbicide exposure and the risk of transitional carcinoma of the urinary bladder in Scottish Terriers, *J Am Vet Med Assoc* 224:1290–1297, 2004.
13. European Commission, Health & Consumer Protection Directorate-General, MCPA, July 2008, http://ec.europa.eu/food/plant/protection/evaluation/existactive/list_mcpa.pdf.
14. Menkes DB, Temple WA, Edwards JR: Intentional poisoning with glyphosate-containing herbicides, *Hum Exp Toxicol* 10:103–107, 1991.
15. Hayes WJ, editor: *Herbicides and pesticides studied in man*, Baltimore, 1982, Williams & Wilkins.

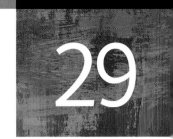

Smoke Inhalation

Kevin T. Fitzgerald, PhD, DVM, DABVP

29

- Smoke inhalation is the leading cause of death from fire.
- Temperature, oxygen concentration, and the chemical composition of the material burning determine the combustion products.
- The astonishing array of different materials in an animal's environment and their wide variety of toxic combustion products guarantee that there is no "typical" smoke.
- Toxic combustion products are grouped as simple asphyxiants, irritant toxins, and chemical asphyxiants.
- Water solubility of toxins is the most important chemical characteristic in determining level of the respiratory tract injury.
- Smoke is a complex mixture of heated air, suspended solid and liquid particles, gases, fumes, aerosols, and vapors.
- The most common clinical sign of smoke inhalation is respiratory compromise.
- The most valuable diagnostic tools in evaluation of a suspected smoke inhalation victim are arterial blood gas analysis, carboxyhemoglobin levels, methemoglobin concentration, and thoracic radiographs.
- Smoke inhalation treatment includes maintenance of airway patency, ventilation and oxygenation, countering pulmonary debris, and stabilization of hemodynamic imbalances.
- Differential diagnoses for smoke inhalation include any syndrome that manifests itself as respiratory compromise.

Sources

Smoke inhalation is the leading cause of death from fires for both humans and animals. More than 80% of fire-related deaths are the result of smoke inhalation and not from surface burns.[1] Smoke itself is the complex mixture of vapors, gases, fumes, heated air and particulate matter, and liquid and solid aerosols produced by thermal decomposition. Thermal decomposition can result from flaming combustion or from pyrolysis, which is the application of intense heat. These thermal decompositions can result in the rapid oxidation of a substance by heat. Pyrolysis occurring with high heat and relatively low oxygen concentration is known as smoldering. Although flaming combustion generates light (flame), heat, and smoke; smoke can be produced in the absence of flames. Thus flames are not a prerequisite for smoke production, and furthermore the gaseous product of combustion (smoke) is not always visible.

Table 29-1	Combustion Products of Frequently Encountered Material
Source	Combustion Product
Wood, paper, cotton	Carbon monoxide, acetaldehyde, formaldehyde, acetic acid, formic acid, methane
Silk	Ammonia, cyanide, hydrogen sulfide, sulfur dioxide
Wool	Phosgene, cyanide, hydrogen chloride, chlorine
Nylon	Ammonia, cyanide
Rubber	Hydrogen sulfide, sulfur dioxide
Plastics	Ammonia, aldehydes, cyanide, phosgene, chlorine, hydrogen chloride
Polyvinyl chloride	Carbon monoxide, phosgene, chlorine, hydrogen chloride
Polyurethane	Cyanide, isocyanates
Fluorinated resin	Hydrogen fluoride
Sulfur-containing material	Sulfur dioxide
Nitrogen-containing material	Cyanide, isocyanates
Fire-retardants	Hydrogen bromide, hydrogen chloride
Petroleum products	Carbon monoxide, acetic acid, formic acid
Polystyrene	Styrene
Acrylic	Carbon monoxide, hydrogen chloride, acrolein

Combustion products are difficult to predict in fires. Even within the same fire, the concentration of the smoke may vary.[2] Temperature, oxygen concentration, and the chemical composition of the burning material determine the combustion products.

In recent years, the use of newer synthetic building materials and furnishings has led to an increase in inhalational injuries caused by fires.[3] Although more rigorous building codes make new structures less likely to burn, the materials used to make them have become more dangerous when they do catch fire through their production of more toxic smoke. At about the time of World War II, differences were noted between natural materials and synthetics in terms of their combustion products and relative toxicity when burning. It is now recognized that, compared with natural materials (e.g., cotton, wood, wool), plastics generate more heat more swiftly, spread flames faster, generate larger amounts of denser visible smoke, and release more toxic and greater concentrations of invisible products of thermal decomposition. Despite testimonials to the contrary, plastics are neither nonburning nor self-extinguishing and, like many other synthetic substances, burn hotter and smokier than wood or other natural substances. Some of the more common and more toxic combustion products are listed in Tables 29-1 and 29-2 and Box 29-1.

Every 12 seconds a fire department responds to a fire alarm in the United States.[4] When compared with other countries, the United States has one of the highest numbers of fire-related deaths in the world. The majority of fires in the United States (more than 70%) occur in residential homes. Carelessness with cigarettes, heating devices, matches, flammable liquids, and malfunctioning electrical appliances is overwhelmingly the most common initiatory cause of fires. Every year there are nearly 3600 human deaths in the United States related to fires. More than half of smoke inhalation cases (53%) occur between November and February.[5] This may be explained by the greater number of house fires in the colder months resulting from space heater malfunctions, increased use of potentially faulty heating pads and electric blankets, malfunctioning heaters, and the increased use of candles and Christmas tree lights during this time. Deaths in companion animals as a consequence of fire are harder to quantify, but certainly thousands of animals suffer fire-related injuries and smoke inhalation each year. Although smoke inhalation is infrequently presented to veterinary hospitals in companion animals, when it does appear victims must be dealt with swiftly and efficiently. Practicing clinicians must recognize the

Table 29-2	Common Toxic Products of Thermal Decomposition	
Agent	**Toxic Products**	**Effects**
Physical Agent		
Heat and flame	Flaming combustion	Burns, laryngotracheitis
Soot	Organic material	Airway obstruction
Steam	Water heated to boiling	Laryngotracheitis, bronchitis, alveolitis
Oxygen depletion	Combustion, pyrolysis	Burns, laryngotracheitis
Trauma	Explosions, collapsing structures	Burns
Chemical Agent		
Acrolein	Cotton, paper, wood, acrylics, polystyrene	Respiratory tract irritation
Aldehydes	ABS, polyester (alkyds) phenolics	Respiratory tract irritation
Carbon monoxide	Incomplete combustion of organic material	Functional anemia, cellular asphyxia
Carbon dioxide	Complete combustion of organic material	Simple asphyxia, narcosis
Halogen acids, such as hydrochloric, hydrobromic, and hydrofluoric acid	Acrylics, vinyl (polyvinyl chloride), film, resins, fire retardants	Respiratory tract irritation
Cyanide	Paper, silk, wool, urethane acrylonitriles	Cellular asphyxia
Isocyanates	Urethane (foam)	Respiratory tract irritation
Organic acids	Cotton, paper, wool, wood	Respiratory tract irritation
Nitrogen oxide	Paper, petroleum products, wood	Respiratory tract irritation
Phosgene	Fire retardants, vinyls, polyvinyl chloride	Respiratory tract irritation
Styrene	ABS, polystyrene	Respiratory tract irritation
Sulfur oxides	Rubber, fur, hair, hide, wool, petroleum	Respiratory tract irritation

ABS, Acrylonitrile butadiene styrene.

clinical signs of smoke inhalation, its pathophysiologic characteristics, and the proper treatment protocol. It has been documented that younger animals (younger than 3 years of age) are most likely to present suffering from smoke inhalation. It has been suggested that younger animals are not more at risk but rather more likely to survive smoke exposure. Studies have documented that older dogs fare worse than younger ones following such experiences.[6]

Toxic Dose

There is no standard toxic or lethal dose for smoke inhalation in animals. The composition of smoke can vary tremendously even from the same fire. Combustion products and their concentrations are difficult to predict, and the relative toxicity of smoke produced depends on the composition of the substance burning, amount of oxygen available, the temperature of the fire, the length of exposure, and the size of the animal involved. In addition, the incredible variety of materials currently used in an animal's

Box 29-1	Toxic Combustion Products

Simple Asphyxiants
Carbon dioxide
Methane
Oxygen-deprived environment

Chemical Asphyxiants
Carbon monoxide
Hydrogen cyanide
Hydrogen sulfide
Oxides of nitrogen

Irritants
High water solubility (upper airway injury)
Acrolein
Sulfur dioxide
Ammonia
Hydrogen chloride
Intermediate water solubility (upper and lower airway injury)
Chlorine
Isocyanates
Poor water solubility (pulmonary parenchymal injury)
Phosgene
Oxides of nitrogen

environment and their wide spectrum of toxic combustion products ensure that there is no such thing as "typical" smoke.

If burns are present and respiratory tract tissue displays burn edema, the episode becomes much more serious and much more likely to be life threatening. Increased vascular permeability of burned, edematous respiratory tissue greatly enhances the toxic effects of smoke inhalation. In one study in humans, mortality as a result of smoke inhalation alone was 12%; in cases in which smoke inhalation was also associated with burns, 61% were fatal.[7] Thus mortality from smoke inhalation is dramatically increased in animals with concomitant thermal burns.

Toxicokinetics and Mechanism of Toxicity

The pathophysiologic characteristics of smoke inhalation can be traced to the mechanism of action of the individual toxins involved, their subsequent physiologic effects, and the cause of clinical toxicity after exposure. Toxic combustion products are classified as *simple asphyxiants, irritant toxins,* and *chemical asphyxiants.* These categories and their production products are included in Box 29-1.

Simple asphyxiants are space occupying and fill enclosed spaces at the expense of oxygen. In addition to this effect, combustion uses oxygen and creates an oxygen-deprived environment. The net effect is less oxygen available to the animal.

Irritant toxins are chemically reactive substances. They produce local effects on the tissue or the respiratory tract. Ammonia is produced by burning wool, silk, nylon, and synthetic resins.[8] Ammonia has high water solubility and dissolves in moist membranes of the upper respiratory tract, resulting in nasopharyngeal, laryngeal, and tracheal inflammation. Acrolein is lipid soluble and penetrates cell membranes. It denatures nucleic acid and intracellular proteins and results in cell death. Acrolein is a very common irritant gas generated by combustion. Sulfur dioxide is found in more than 50% of smoke from fires.[9] Sulfur dioxide reacts with the moist respiratory membrane mucosa, producing the potent caustic, sulfurous acid. Polyvinyl chloride is ubiquitous in floor coverings, office and home furniture, electrical insulation, and clothing. The resultant combustion products phosgene, chlorine, and hydrogen chloride are produced in many residential fires.[10] Together with water in the mucosa, chlorine produces hydrogen chloride free oxygen radicals and is very damaging to tissue. Phosgene descends and produces more delayed alveolar injuries. Isocyanates are produced from burning and smoldering upholstery, and intense irritation of both upper and lower respiratory tissue results.

Organic material produces finely divided carbonaceous particulate matter on combustion. This particulate matter or soot is suspended in the gases and hot air of smoke. Soot has not only carbon, but also aldehydes, acids, and reactive radicals that adhere to its surface.[8] The inhalation of soot and associated aerosols heightens the effect of other irritant toxins. Soot binds with respiratory mucosal surfaces, allowing other irritant chemicals to adhere and react with adjacent tissue. The penetrance and deposition of these particles within the respiratory tract depend on size. Small particles (1 to 3 μm) reach the alveoli. In various animals, lung injury decreases when smoke is filtered to remove particulate matter. Sulfur dioxide shows a high propensity to adhere to soot. In addition, polyvinyl chloride combustion produces a large amount of soot-containing smoke coated with its particular combustion products phosgene, chloride, and hydrogen chloride. In addition to soot and related particles, irritant gases, acids, and other combustion products can also adhere to aerosol droplets.

The most important determining factor in predicting the level of respiratory injury is the water solubility of the toxin. Water-soluble chemicals injure the mucosa of upper respiratory airways by releasing the mediators of inflammation and deleterious free radicals. This type of inflammation increases microvascular membrane permeability and results in a net influx of fluid from intravascular spaces into the upper respiratory tissue. The underlying tissue of the supraglottic larynx may become terrifically swollen and edematous. This edematous reaction can result in minutes to hours postexposure, continue to progress, and close off upper airways completely.

Low water-soluble molecules react with the lung parenchyma. They react more slowly and produce delayed toxic effects. Concentration of the toxic element inhaled, particle size, duration of exposure, respiratory rate, absence of protective reflexes, preexisting disease, and size and age of the animal also contribute to the level and degree of respiratory injury in addition to the water solubility of toxic products.

An intense inflammatory reaction develops secondary to the initial injury to respiratory mucosal cells by toxic combustion products.[11] Inhaled soot and toxic gases generate increased airway resistance caused by inspissated secretions, increased mucosal airway edema, and associated bronchospasm. Damaged mucosal cells stimulate copious exudates rich in protein, inflammatory cells, and necrotic debris. If this reaction continues, mucosal sloughing ensues. The degenerative exudates, bronchorrhea, and extensive sloughing produce casts of the airways. In animal victims of smoke inhalation, these casts increase airway resistance by blocking major airways and prevent oxygen passage to the alveoli. In addition, increased vascular permeability of respiratory tissue contributes to airway blockage. Bronchoconstriction and reflexive wheezing follow in response to inflammation and the toxic mucosal injury.

Chemical asphyxiants produce toxic systemic effects at tissue distant from the lung. Carbon monoxide is generated during incomplete combustion and is regarded as the most serious systemic agent to smoke inhalation victims. Carbon monoxide prevents oxygen binding to hemoglobin, thereby producing a functional anemia.[12] Furthermore, carbon monoxide inhibits release of oxygen, thereby shifting the oxyhemoglobin dissociation curve to the left. Carbon monoxide itself has other toxic effects that cause lipid peroxidation and directly damage cellular membranes. Carbon monoxide is invariably present in smoke from fires and is thought to be the cause of most immediate deaths from smoke inhalation.[13] Nitrogen-containing products, such as wool, silk, nylon, plastics, paper, rubber, pyroxylin, polyurethanes, and polyacrylonitriles, all produce cyanide at combustion.

Cyanide has been detected in samples from many other types of fires as well. Together with carbon monoxide, cyanide has at least an additive and perhaps synergistic toxic effect in victims of smoke inhalation. Nitrogen-containing compounds produce oxides of nitrogen on their burning, which are potent respiratory irritants. Other combustion products can cause systemic and local toxicity. Metal oxides, hydrogen fluoride, hydrogen bromide, and various hydrocarbons can all be retrieved from toxic smoke. Benzene can be detected in the smoke of plastic and petroleum fires.[14] Antimony, cadmium, chromium, cobalt, gold, iron, lead, and zinc have all been recovered from smoke samples during fires. Natural disasters, accidents at illegal drug labs, transportation accidents, industrial fires, and acts of terrorism are situations in which unusual types of toxic smoke combustion products may be encountered. In fact the entire spectrum of potentially toxic combustion products from fires is endless, and we must remain vigilant.

Super-heated air and steam in smoke result in thermal burns to tissue of the respiratory tract. In animals, the higher the air temperature and humidity, the greater is the mortality in affected individuals. Exposure to dry air heated to 200° C for 5 minutes or to 125° C for 15 minutes is potentially lethal in mammals.[15] Shorter exposure to dry air at temperatures of 350° C to 500° C results in tracheitis in dogs. Exposure to steam alone results in tracheitis, bronchitis, and pulmonary parenchymal damage. Respiratory tract injury secondary to steam or heat alone is relatively uncommon in animals.

Combustion progressively consumes oxygen. This decrease in oxygen concentration produces hypoxic asphyxia. The normal oxygen fraction at sea level is roughly 21%. Acute reductions in ambient oxygen fractions to 15% result in dyspnea. A reduction to 10% produces dyspnea and altered mentation, and fractions from 8% to 6% cause loss of consciousness followed by death in less than 8 minutes.

It is noteworthy to examine the dynamics of smoke dispersal from fires. Spreading smoke initially accumulates and forms a hot layer mainly at the ceiling, which gradually descends to the floor. The main toxic combustion agent threats (e.g., heat, irritants, asphyxiants, noxious gases, and particulate material) are found in this ceiling layer.[16] Depending on the size of the enclosed room, the amount of smoke produced, and duration of time, the toxic products will eventually disperse to the floor. Thus, at least initially, animals at the floor are breathing cooler and much less contaminated air and are receiving less radiant heat. Because of this pattern of dispersal, the chance for survival exists for limited periods.

Carcinogens are also some of the toxic products of thermal decomposition. All fires produce benzopyrene, the classic initiator of carcinogenesis. Plastic fires, particularly those involving polyvinyl chloride, produce arsenic, benzene, chromium, and acrylonitrile, all of which are suspected human and animal carcinogens. Smoke from wood and plastic produces the potent carcinogen, formaldehyde. Soot, so long known to cause cancer in chimney sweeps and tobacco smokers, is a principal product of most fires. The exact association of smoke inhalation and the development of cancer are unknown for animals at present.

Smoke inhalation causes progressive physiologic dysfunction and ultimately can lead to death. Irrespective of cause, asphyxia is the underlying mechanism. This asphyxia may be due to inhibition of cellular respiration, impaired oxygen transport and delivery, central respiratory depression, direct or indirect occlusion of airways, or a decreased supply of oxygen. For smoke inhalation, there is a direct correlation between the duration of exposure and the severity of effects. Finally, the greater the exposure the more rapid and pronounced are the effects observed.

Clinical Signs

Smoke inhalation victims generally have signs of respiratory compromise, systemic toxicity, or a combination of both.[17,18] Concomitant surface burns may be noted and cutaneous burns of more than 15% body surface area, a history of exposure in an enclosed space, altered mentation and carbonaceous sputum or saliva production are all associated with a high incidence of bronchopulmonary injury.[19] The presence of extensive body burns indicates greater exposure and a potentially larger, hotter fire, and is typically associated with a higher incidence of both upper and lower respiratory tract injury and a worse prognosis. A respiratory abnormality may worsen with time after presentation, and signs of systemic toxicity are maximal at the time of exposure.

Signs of smoke inhalation may be notoriously nonspecific and include cough, dyspnea, tachycardia, tachypnea, and hypoxemia. Almost always, signs of lacrimation, conjunctivitis, pharyngitis, and rhinitis are present. Erythema, edema, and soot may be evident on examination of the nose, mouth, and throat. Corneal abrasions are common, and exposure to fire or prolonged heat can produce corneal burns. Mucosal ulcerations and hemorrhagic areas may be present.

Drooling, dysphagia, hoarseness, and stridor are all signs of laryngotracheal involvement and injury. In severe cases, copious exudates combined with severe laryngeal edema can result in complete upper airway obstruction. Blistering, erythema, ulcerations, mucosal sloughing, mucosal edema, hemorrhage, and laryngospasm may all be evident with the aid of a laryngoscope.[20] The increased secretions may contain soot and carbonaceous particulate matter. Laryngeal edema and tracheal narrowing may be visible on radiographs.

Auscultation of the lungs may reveal rales, rhonchi, and wheezing. In bronchospasm breath sounds can be virtually inaudible. Rales or crackles may be localized (atelectasis) or diffuse (pneumonitis). Fever and leukocytosis may accompany atelectasis and pneumonitis. Radiographs obtained soon after fire exposure may be normal. After progression, chest radiographs can reveal peribronchial cuffing (caused by airway edema) and diffuse infiltrates (caused by atelectasis, pneumonitis, or pulmonary edema).[21] Crusts, casts of debris and exudates, and plugs of mucus and soot may develop and block airways.

Central nervous system (CNS) signs and cardiovascular dysfunction signs reveal systemic toxicity caused by hypoxia and hypercapnia. Further CNS effects can include agitation, confusion, ataxia, abnormal posturing, transient loss of consciousness, and seizures. Cardiovascular signs include hypotension, dysrhythmias, and cardiac arrest.

Ocular injuries are not uncommon in animals involved in fires or subsequently exposed to smoke. Pawing at the eyes, blepharitis, epiphora, conjunctivitis, corneal ulceration, and edema may all occur as the result of exposure. Therefore a thorough ophthalmic examination of the lids, conjunctiva, cornea, and sclera must be performed on all potential smoke victims.

As with any severe shock or prolonged period of tissue hypoxia, elevated plasma lactate concentration (0.1 mEq/L) may be present. However, this finding is by no means specific to smoke inhalation. The methemoglobin fractions are elevated in virtually all animals with significant signs of either smoke inhalation or systemic toxicity. Notable methemoglobinemia appears to be a rare finding. Signs indicating increased risk of smoke inhalation injury are summarized in Box 29-2.

Minimum Database and Confirmatory Tests

Details of fire and smoke exposure, current medications, past medical treatment, and any therapy before hospital arrival should all be obtained in a good history from family members of the victim. Of particular importance is what substance generated the smoke (e.g., wood, plastic, polyvinyl chloride), a description of the smoke (odor, intensity, and color), the duration of the exposure, and whether the exposure took place indoors or in the open.

The nature and types of signs displayed by the animal at the time of the exposure and at the time of hospital arrival are helpful in determining the severity of the exposure. Altered mentation, ataxia, collapse, and syncope at the time of exposure all suggest carbon monoxide or cyanide intoxication. These substances can be easily missed if delayed presentation has allowed clinical improvement by the time of hospital presentation or if oxygen was administered in the field.

Vital signs cannot be overlooked. Physical examination should first focus on determining the patency and condition of airways, adequacy of respirations, and assessment of ventilation. The respiratory rate of the animal involved is critical. The heart rate, mucous membrane color, CNS function, body temperature, and skin turgor should all be closely

Box 29-2	Signs Indicating Increased Risk of Smoke Inhalation Injury

Being confined to a small, closed space
Loss of consciousness
Respiratory compromise
Central nervous signs
Carbonaceous sputum
Edema of larynx-pharynx
Presence of burns
Singed hairs
Stridor
Ocular manifestations (blepharitis, conjunctivitis, epiphora, corneal ulcer, etc.)

monitored. Animals showing respiratory signs must be assessed for hypoxia, hypercapnia, and upper airway obstruction. All fire victims should receive a thorough ophthalmic evaluation, including retinal examination, checking for particulate matter under the lids, and fluorescein stain evaluation of the cornea for ulcerations.

In addition to the heart rate, respiratory rate, body temperature, and central nervous function, pulse oximetry (SpO_2) should be obtained in all smoke-inhalation animals. Oxygen saturation obtained through this method may be falsely elevated and near normal when methemoglobinemia and carboxyhemoglobinemia are present. Cyanosis that is unresponsive to oxygen in an animal without respiratory distress is suggestive of methemoglobinemia. Any animal with cyanosis with normal vital signs and an SpO_2 greater than 90% should have a methemoglobin fraction measured.

Animals with altered mental status, respiratory distress, and atypical chest auscultations should be assessed for hypercapnia and acid-base imbalances by formal blood gas analysis. Decreased oxygen saturation measured by cooximetry in conjunction with a normal PO_2 (and hence normal calculated oxygen) suggests a diagnosis of either carbon monoxide poisoning or methemoglobinemia. The difference between calculated and measured oxygen saturation can be used to estimate either the fraction of carbon monoxide or methemoglobin. If a metabolic lactic acidosis is present, and carboxyhemoglobin and methemoglobin and PO_2 are all normal, then cyanide poisoning should be suspected. Unresponsive hypotension and coma are likewise suggestive of cyanide poisoning.

Diagnostic tests must focus on the animal's oxygenation and ventilation. Thus, for the suspected smoke inhalation victim, arterial blood gas analysis, carboxyhemoglobin concentration, methemoglobin levels, and chest radiographs are the most valuable diagnostic tools to be used. Establishing whether a metabolic acidosis is present can help in diagnosing underlying tissue hypoxia.

The presence of elevated carboxyhemoglobin concentrations in smoke victims indicates substantial exposure to toxic combustion products has occurred, and the potential for ongoing, developing smoke-related pathologic conditions exists. However, carboxyhemoglobin concentrations alone are poor predictors of severity of exposure because low or nondetectable concentrations do not rule out the possibility of significant underlying tissue damage and potential for progressive pathologic conditions. Admission carboxyhemoglobin levels do not reflect peak blood concentrations and are usually significantly decreased by the time the animal reaches the veterinary hospital. Furthermore, it is important to note that transcutaneous measurement of oxygen saturation (pulse oximetry) is unreliable in smoke inhalation patients because it overestimates actual oxygen saturation in the presence of methemoglobin.

Lactic acidosis seen in animals suffering from smoke inhalation is a result of tissue hypoperfusion, carbon monoxide poisoning, and cyanide poisoning resulting in pulmonary dysfunction. Nevertheless, lactic acidosis also is an insensitive indicator of smoke inhalation because hypoxia from any cause impedes aerobic metabolism and generates lactic acid.

Chest radiographs are most commonly normal at the time of and for the first few hours following smoke inhalation. Thus early radiographs are another inaccurate predictor of pulmonary injury. Within 24 to 36 hours of exposure, radiographic changes ranging from patchy atelectasis to diffuse interstitial and alveolar involvement may be evident. Subtle radiographic findings within the first 24 hours of exposure can include perivascular haziness, peribronchial cuffing, bronchial wall thickening, and subglottic edema.[22] For radiographic studies to be helpful in diagnosis of smoke inhalation, serial chest radiographs must be obtained over time. The hallmark pulmonary injuries secondary to smoke inhalation usually develop more than 24 hours after smoke inhalation and can include acute lung tissue injury, aspiration, infection, volume overload, respiratory distress, and cardiogenic pulmonary edema.

Animals demonstrating abnormal cardiac rhythms and hypertension and those suffering from underlying cardiovascular disease should receive an electrocardiogram after episodes of smoke inhalation. Sedation and bronchoscopy can be performed in larger animals, but is rarely done in veterinary medicine for diagnosis alone.

Finally, effective, aggressive therapy for smoke inhalation victims should never be postponed while awaiting blood results. Blood results (e.g., carboxyhemoglobin levels, methemoglobin concentrations, confirmation of blood cyanide levels) may take hours or longer to obtain. Initiation of treatment for acutely smoke-poisoned animals must never await results of laboratory analysis.

Treatment

Successful management of smoke inhalation begins with prompt and safe removal of the animal from the smoke-filled environment. Care must be taken, and unless rescuers possess skin, respiratory, and eye protection, removing animals from fires is best left to professional firefighters. Never enter smoky environments without adequate protection. Basic emergency support measures can be instituted as necessary at the scene of the exposure. Decontamination measures, such as irrigation of eyes and skin, can be initiated immediately.

The cornerstones of smoke inhalation therapy are maintenance of airway patency, adequate ventilation and oxygenation, aggressive measures for countering pulmonary debris, and stabilization of hemodynamic imbalances. A major concern in managing smoke inhalation patients is failing to appreciate their potential for rapid deterioration. Critical airway compromise can develop suddenly and insidiously in these animals. The patency of upper airways must be rapidly ascertained and established if compromised. Upper airway injury is always almost certain if obvious oropharyngeal burns are present. If telltale burns are not present, it is very easy to underestimate the degree of injury after episodes of smoke inhalation. If evidence of upper airway injury is present, endotracheal intubation should be undertaken rather than waiting for the injured animal to decompensate and deteriorate. Animals displaying coma, visible burns, full-thickness neck burns, edema of the oropharynx, and stridor should all be swiftly intubated. Fluid administration to burn victims contributes to the formation of upper airway edema. As a result, burned animals receiving aggressive fluid therapy also require intubation.

Inhalant β_2-adrenergic agonists are the first line of defense for acute reversible bronchoconstriction (e.g., asthma and chronic obstructive pulmonary disease). Although effective for these conditions, their efficacy has not been established in smoke inhalation victims.[23] Because pathophysiologic changes induced by irritant toxins in smoke are partially reversible, β_2-adrenergic agonists should have some beneficial effects on airway obstruction. Corticosteroids are effective in treatment of refractory acute asthma, but mortality and infection rates are increased in animals with smoke inhalation that receive steroids. Furthermore, benefits of corticosteroid treatment of smoke injury have not been demonstrated in clinical animal studies.[24,25,26] Both cough suppressants and pain-relieving opioids should be avoided because they suppress the cough reflex necessary for the expectoration of inhaled smoke particles.

Mammalian lungs may show progressive pathophysiologic changes over time (hours to days) after exposure to smoke. Counters for progressive respiratory compromise and failure include mechanical ventilation techniques, continuous positive airway pressure, positive end-expiratory pressure, and vigorous clearing of pulmonary secretions and debris. Frequent airway suctioning may be necessary to clear plugs, casts, inspissated secretions, and necrotic debris.

Toxic combustion products damage the respiratory tract but also potentially the skin, eyes, and other mucous membranes. The extent of chemical injury to eyes, skin, and other membranes is largely determined by the duration of contact between the irritant or toxin and the animal's tissue. The eyes of all animals suffering from smoke inhalation must be thoroughly examined for corneal burns caused by thermal, chemical, or irritant injury. Animals with signs of ocular injury should have the eyes irrigated copiously with artificial tears or normal saline. Dermal decontamination should be initiated if necessary to prevent ongoing dermal burns from toxin-laden soot adherent to the skin. Rapid removal of soot and smoke debris from skin may prevent continued injury and burns.

Candidates for immediate endotracheal intubation include animals with respiratory distress and signs of upper airway obstructions and animals that are cyanotic or hypoxic (SpO_2 <90%) despite aggressive maximum oxygen therapy with a nonrebreathing mask. Animals with respiratory depression (<10 to 12/min or PCO_2 >50 mm Hg), pulmonary edema, depressed mentation, and full-thickness neck or face burns also should be intubated. Any animal should be considered for intubation that does not improve with oxygen delivered by mask. Intubation should be done with the largest possible endotracheal tube so that suction can be employed, or bronchoscopy can be performed if required. The use of nasal catheters for oxygen delivery may be necessary in animals with excessive airway edema, if extensive perioral burns and constricting neck burns are present, or if direct visualization of the larynx for intubation is impossible. Be certain to evaluate the whole animal for other injuries (e.g., neck trauma and cervical spine injury) by performing a thorough physical examination. Do not focus only on the smoke inhalation. The potential for other injuries occurring during fires should never be overlooked.

Once intubated, the airway should be suctioned regularly to remove secretions, inhaled debris, and necrotic material. Supplemental oxygen must be humidified to prevent drying of respiratory tissue and secretions. Positive and expiratory pressure should be routinely administered to prevent and to treat atelectasis and for those who remain hypoxic despite administration of 100% oxygen. Bronchoscopy can be employed to help direct effective removal of bronchial secretions. Repeated suctioning may be necessary to help break up inspissated mucous plugs, casts, and accumulated debris.

Tracheostomy is reserved only for animals with complete airway obstruction, either caused by constriction, edema, or trauma, or for those that may require prolonged intubation. Performing a tracheostomy must be carefully considered because it requires upkeep, can be associated with significant complications, and is usually reserved for animals that are tremendously compromised.

Animals that do not require intubation nonetheless may benefit from inhalant, aerosolized, and racemic epinephrine. However, they still must be carefully monitored for sudden deterioration and may still need to be intubated.

Experimental evidence exists for a variety of smoke-inhalation therapies, ranging from nonsteroidal antiinflammatory drug administration, antioxidants, and free radical scavengers to inhaled nitric oxide. Hyperbaric oxygen may be of benefit in the treatment of pulmonary edema and pneumonitis. Hyperbaric oxygen can also be effective in treating carbon monoxide poisoning, cyanide poisoning, cerebral edema, and thermal burns associated with fires and smoke inhalation. It can also be considered in animals with refractory hypoxemia. Nevertheless, the availability of hyperbaric oxygen is still limited for veterinary medical applications.

The treatment of carbon monoxide poisoning in animals associated with smoke inhalation is supplemental oxygen therapy administered through a tight-fitting mask or endotracheal tube. The amount of cyanide exposure in animal victims of smoke inhalation is not predictable. However, cyanide poisoning should be suspected in animals with serious episodes of smoke exposure. Because hydroxocobalamin therapy has become available in the United States, cyanide poisoning is treated according to the usual guidelines. Methemoglobinemia can result from inhalation of certain toxic products of combustion. Oxygen therapy alone is effective for most instances. Methylene blue should be reserved for only those cases in which methemoglobin concentration is greater than 20% to 30%.

Treatment with antibiotics should only be initiated in patients with a documented infection. The prophylactic use of antibiotic therapy begun immediately in cases of smoke inhalation is of no benefit and in fact may help implement the development of infection with antibiotic-resistant organisms. Selection of antibiotics should be directed by the results from the Gram stain and culture and sensitivity of the sputum and secretions collected. Animals with fever and persistent leukocytosis more than 2 days postexposure should be treated with antibiotics. Empirical therapy with agents effective against *Staphylococcus aureus* (such as cefazolin) and gram-negative organisms like *Pseudomonas* (gentamicin) can be started in the absence of culture results.

Intravenous fluid therapy may be indicated for animals displaying hypotension and to prevent drying of normal airway secretions. Nevertheless, fluid therapy must be administered prudently because smoke damage to pulmonary endothelial cells can result in increased pulmonary vascularity and overhydration may result in accumulations of pulmonary fluids, compounding respiratory distress.

Because of the high incidence of sudden deterioration and decompensation in cases of smoke inhalation, it is recommended that exposed animals be observed closely for 6 to 8 hours postexposure before they are released. No smoke inhalation victims should be discharged until they are asymptomatic, normal on physical examination and ancillary tests, and otherwise stable. All discharged animals should be seen again within 72 hours to ensure that underlying pulmonary injuries are not progressing.

Definite therapy and treatment is available for animals suffering from smoke inhalation. Early intervention and respiratory support are essential in these cases. Establishing and maintaining patent airways and the delivery of high-flow oxygen is the basis for successful treatment of smoke inhalation. The use of hyperbaric oxygen and other therapeutic regimens is being explored in the hope of more effective therapy for smoke-intoxicated animals.

Prevention and Prognosis

Prevention of smoke inhalation injuries begins with the prompt and safe removal of animals from environments filling with smoke. However, no rescues can be attempted unless rescuers have adequate skin, eye, and respiratory protection. In many instances removing animals from fires and contact with toxic smoke is best left to professional firefighters. Common sense must outweigh emotion and hazardous heroics.

The simple use of smoke alarms and sprinkler systems cannot be underestimated in reducing the hazardous effects of fires. The mere presence of a smoke alarm is a tremendous deterrent to fire-related injury simply through its early-warning merits. If sprinkler systems are in place and activated, its response to a fire is swift and unmistakable. Sprinkler systems require no action from occupants, do not depend on their presence or location, and immediately quench the toxic potential of fire and smoke.[27] In the absence of smoke detectors and sprinkler systems, fires can progress to their most dangerous potential. Both smoke detectors and sprinkler systems are widely available, fairly inexpensive, and relatively easy to install.

Commercial fire extinguishers using a variety of retardants are also easily and inexpensively obtainable at home improvement outlets. Family members should all be well versed in where smoke alarms and fire extinguishers are located in the home and be instructed in their function. Stickers for doors are available informing rescuers how many and what types of animals live in that residence. These should be prominently placed and currently updated.

Following smoke inhalation, a whole spectrum of related injuries is possible, ranging from asymptomatic, unaffected animals to rapid upper airway occlusion, to a few to several days later the appearance of delayed pulmonary edema and progressive pathologic changes. Prognosis depends on several factors, such as duration of exposure, the concentration of the inhaled smoke, the toxic combustion products of the smoke involved, and the presence of preexisting underlying disease. Animals suffering from smoke inhalation may have a variety of complications caused by a number of pulmonary sequelae. Wheezing and chronic cough may reflect underlying chronic hyperreactive airways. Chronic bronchitis, bronchiectasis, bronchial stenosis, pulmonary fibrosis, bronchiolitis obliterans, and atelectasis may result after exposure to smoke and subsequent inflammation and scarring. Tracheal stenosis has been seen as a complication of long-term endotracheal intubation.[28] The precise outcome of smoke inhalation exposure may not be evident for some time. As a result, these cases often require extensive follow-up, serial radiographs, bronchoscopy, and other diagnostics to document the extent and the nature of pulmonary injuries and how much normal function will be maintained. Studies have revealed that, for both dogs and cats displaying respiratory signs on presentation following smoke inhalation, the best prognostic indicator may be close monitoring for progression of clinical signs the day following admission.[29,30] Because of the potential deterioration of patients in the days following admission, smoke victims should be hospitalized for at least 48 hours for observation, monitoring, and to perform diagnostic tests. Early intervention certainly is beneficial in the prognosis and outcome of smoke inhalation cases. Finally, we must continue to strive to identify safer, less toxic construction and furnishing materials that do not release poisonous combustion products when burned.

Gross and Histologic Lesions

The effects of smoke inhalation can be characterized with regard to the mechanism of action of the individual toxicants, their physiologic effects, or their course of toxicity after exposure. Thermal burns are caused by hot air and steam, and chemical and thermal burns are produced by irritant gases. Target tissue for smoke are skin, mucosal surfaces (eyes and respiratory tract), and any mucous membranes. The effects of smoke irritation are mediated by polymorphonuclear leukocytes, arachidonic acid metabolites (leukotrienes, thromboxanes, and prostacyclins), cytokines (platelet activity factors), and free radicals (such as superoxides, peroxides, and hydroxyl).[31] Minimal exposure results only in inflammation, but prolonged exposure to smoke can cause ulceration and cellular necrosis. Smoke causes inflammation of the larynx, trachea, bronchi, bronchioles, and alveoli, which then produces local edema, bronchospasm, cessation of ciliary function, loss of surfactant, and increased permeability of microvasculature membranes, upper and lower airway obstruction, atelectasis, loss of lung compliance, and ventilation-perfusion mismatch may develop.[32]

From the perspective of time, smoke inhalation produces a progressive pulmonary dysfunction that can ultimately be fatal. Asphyxia is the end result, no matter what the predisposing causes or smoke sources. Asphyxia can be due to a number of causes: inhibition of cellular respiration (carbon monoxide and cyanide), impaired oxygen transport and delivery (carboxyhemoglobin and methemoglobin), central respiratory depression (carbon monoxide, cyanide, and carbon dioxide), direct or indirect occlusion of airways (effects of irritant gases, heat, soot, and humidity), or a decreased supply of oxygen (air robbed of oxygen by combustion or containing toxic gases that lower the partial pressure of oxygen). There is a strong correlation between duration of exposure and severity of pathologic injuries.

Following smoke inhalation the clinical sequence of events can be divided into early, intermediate, and late phases. In the initial 24 to 36 hours, the systemic effects of carbon monoxide, cyanide, and methemoglobin and the airway effects of heat, humidity, irritant gases, and soot predominate. From 6 hours to 5 days following exposure, pulmonary edema becomes the most significant problem.[33] It can develop swiftly, progress to severe respiratory distress, and a high mortality rate. Cerebral edema is present in animals with severe or prolonged hypoxia. Lesions attributed to carbon monoxide toxicity associated with smoke inhalation have been identified in the brains of exposed dogs.[34] These lesions were detected primarily in the caudate nucleus, the globus pallidus, and substantia nigra but were also found in the cerebellum, cerebral cortex, and dorsal thalamus.

In days to weeks after exposure, late manifestations include permanent CNS damage secondary to anoxia, bronchiectasis, and subglottic stenosis as a result of airway injury and prolonged endotracheal intubation, and sepsis and pneumonia secondary to edema, debris, impaired defense mechanisms, and opportunistic bacteria. Pneumonia is the most common late complication, and it can have a mortality rate approaching 50%. Early pneumonia (within 3 to days of exposure) is usually due to *S. aureus*, and *Escherichia coli* is usually the culprit when pneumonia occurs later in the progression of pathologic events. Chronic sequelae, such as asthma, pulmonary fibrosis, chronic obstructive pulmonary disease, bronchiolitis obliterans, and neoplasia, can develop months to years after the original exposure injury.

Nuclear imaging, pulmonary function tests, and bronchoscopy can all be used to document chronic pulmonary lesions following smoke inhalation. These types of studies are often more sensitive than changes detectable by radiographs.

The morbidity and mortality of smoke inhalation increase greatly when associated with thermal burns. Burned animals demonstrate increased vascular permeability that leads to a large fluid flux from the circulatory plasma to the interstitial spaces.[13,33] The more extensive the cutaneous burns, the more severe is the resultant lung edema formation. Animals with combined burn and smoke inhalation injuries show an increase in transpulmonary fluid flux (lung lymph flow), an increase in lung water content, and a significant drop in the partial pressure of inspired oxygen as a result of the edema. This constriction also produces significant airway obstruction. The major cause of progressively worsening pulmonary gas exchange is the development of airway obstruction. By 48 to 72 hours postexposure, there is a progressive reduction in bronchi and bronchiolar luminal cross section. This reduction in cross section is due to the progressive development of obstructive casts and exudative material that occludes the lumen of the airway. This poor oxygenation of blood leads to hypoxemic events in tissue distant to the respiratory tract. Therapy targeting these pathologic mechanisms, removing obstructive materials and cellular debris, and preventing the development of permanent pathologic pulmonary changes might be a more effective way of successful airway management and smoke inhalation treatments in the future.

Differential Diagnoses

The manifestations of smoke inhalation can be unfortunately nonspecific. Most of the time, smoke inhalation causes injuries that preponderantly involve the lower respiratory tract. Look-alikes of smoke inhalation include any situation leading to respiratory compromise. A list of potential differential diagnoses for smoke inhalation is shown in Box 29-3.

Box 29-3	Differential Diagnoses for Smoke Inhalation

Asthma
Heart disease
Allergic bronchitis
Inhalation of other toxic solvents
Pneumonia
Metabolic disease
Neoplasia
Trauma
Chronic obstructive pulmonary disease
Pneumothorax

References

1. Gad SC, Anderson RC: *Combustion toxicology*, Boca Raton, FL, 1990, CRC Press.
2. Orzel RA: Toxicologic aspects of fire smoke: polymer pyrolysis and combustion, *Occup Med* 8:414–429, 1993.
3. Bowes PC: Casualties attributed to toxic gas and smoke at fires: a survey of statistics, *Med Sci Law* 16: 104–110, 1976.
4. Karter M: *Fire loss in the United States during 1999*, Quincy, MA, 2000, National Fire Protection Association.
5. Drobatz KJ: Smoke inhalation. In King KG, editor: *Textbook of respiratory disease in dogs and cats*, St Louis, 2004, Saunders, pp 480–486.
6. Nieman G, Clark WR, Wax S, et al: The effect of smoke inhalation on pulmonary surfactant, *Ann Surg* 191:171–181, 1980.
7. Clark WR, Nieman GF: Smoke inhalation, *Burns* 14:473–494, 1988.
8. Holstege CP: Smoke inhalation. In Goldfrank LR, et al, editors: *Goldfrank's toxicologic emergencies*, ed 7, New York, 2002, McGraw-Hill.
9. Charan NB, et al: Pulmonary injuries associated with acute sulfur dioxide intoxication, *Am Resp Dis* 119:555–560, 1979.
10. Dyer RF, Esch VH: Polyvinyl chloride toxicity in fires: hydrogen chloride toxicity in firefighters, *JAMA* 235:393–397, 1976.
11. Thurning DR, et al: Pulmonary responses to smoke inhalation: morphological changes in rabbits exposed to pine wood smoke, *Hum Pathol* 13:355–364, 1982.
12. Bizovi KE, Leikin JD: Smoke inhalation among firefighters, *Occup Med* 10:721–733, 1995.
13. Anderson RA, Watson AA: Fire deaths in the Glasgow area: the role of carbon monoxide, *Med Sci Law* 21:288, 1981.
14. Treitman RD, Burgess WA, Gold A: Air contaminants encountered by firefighters, *Am Ind Hyg Assoc J* 41:796–802, 1980.
15. Terril JB, Montgomery RR, Reinhardt CF: Toxic gases from fires, *Science* 200:1343, 1978.
16. Enkhbaatar P, Traber DL: Pathophysiology of acute lung injury in combined burn and smoke inhalation injury, *Clin Sci* 107:137–143, 2004.
17. Jasani S, Hughes D: Smoke inhalation. In Silverstein DC, Hupper K, editors: *Small animal critical care medicine*, St Louis, 2009, Saunders.
18. Clarke DL, Drobutz KJ: Smoke inhalation. In Osweiler GD, Hovda LR, Brutlag AG, Lee JA, editors: *Small animal toxicology*, Ames, IA, 2011, Wiley and Sons.
19. Mosley S: Inhalation injury: a review of the literature, *Heart Lung* 17:3, 1988.
20. Linden CH: Smoke inhalation. In Haddad LM, Hannon MW, Winchester JF, editors: *Clinical management of poisoning and drug overdose*, Philadelphia, 1988, WB Saunders, pp 876–885.
21. Peitzman AB, et al: Smoke inhalation: evaluation of radiographic manifestations and pulmonary dysfunction, *J Trauma* 29:1232, 1989.
22. Lee MJ, O'Connell DJ: The plain chest radiograph after acute smoke inhalation, *Clin Radiol* 39:33–37, 1988.
23. McFadden ER: Therapy for acute asthma, *J Allergy Clin Immunol* 84:151–158, 1989.
24. Nieman GF, Clark WR, Hakim T: Methylprednisolone does not protect the lung from inhalation injury, *Burns* 17:384–390, 1991.
25. Dressler DP, Skornik WA, Kupersmith S: Corticosteroid treatment of experimental smoke inhalation, *Ann Surg* 183:46–52, 1976.
26. Robinson NB, Hudson LD, Reim M, et al: Steroid therapy following isolated smoke inhalation injury, *J Trauma* 22:876–879, 1982.
27. Alarie Y: Toxicity of fire smoke, *Crit Rev Toxicol* 32(4):259–289, 2002.
28. Lee-Chiong TL: Smoke inhalation injury, *Postgrad Med* 105(2):55–62, 1999.
29. Drobatz KJ, Walker LM, Hendricks JC: Smoke exposure in dogs: 27 cases (1988-1997), *J Am Vet Med Assoc* 215(9):1306–1311, 1999.
30. Drobbatz KJ, Walker LM, Hendricks JC: Smoke exposure in cats: 22 cases (1988-1997), *J Am Vet Med Assoc* 215(9):1312–1316, 1999.
31. Traber DI, Linares HA, Herndon DN: The pathophysiology of smoke inhalation—a review, *Burns* 14:357, 1988.
32. Parrish JS, Bradshaw DA: Toxic inhalation injury: gas, vapor, and vesicant exposure, *Respir Care Clin* 10:43–58, 2004.
33. Marsh PS: Fire and smoke inhalation injury in horses, *Vet Clin North Am Equine Pract* 23(1):19–30, 2007.
34. Kent M, Creevy KE, Delahunta A: Clinical and neuropathological findings of acute carbon monoxide toxicity in Chihuahuas following smoke inhalation, *J Am Anim Hosp Assoc* 46(4):259–264, 2010.

CHAPTER

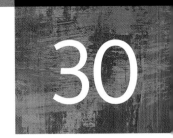

Acetaminophen

Rance K. Sellon, DVM, PhD, DACVIM

- Expected single toxic doses of acetaminophen range from 50 to 100 mg/kg (cats) to 600 mg/kg (dogs). Toxicity may be observed with lower doses, particularly with chronic exposure.
- Clinical signs of toxicity usually reflect hepatic injury or failure (dogs) and hemolytic anemia from methemoglobinemia (cats).
- Diagnosis is typically made from a history of exposure coupled with compatible clinical and laboratory findings.
- The mainstay of therapy is administration of N-acetylcysteine at a loading dose of 140 mg/kg intravenously (IV) or orally (PO) every 6 hours, followed by 70 mg/kg IV or PO every 6 hours for five to seven or more doses. Accompanying treatment options include cimetidine and ascorbic acid. S-adenosylmethionine (SAMe) may also be therapeutic for intoxicated animals.
- Supportive treatment measures, such as IV fluids and blood, are necessary in many cases.

Sources

Acetaminophen is a widely available analgesic and antipyretic (weak anti-inflammatory properties) contained in many over-the-counter and prescription preparations intended for human use. Exposure to dogs and cats occurs through administration of one of these preparations by an uninformed but well-meaning owner intending to treat fever or pain perceived in the pet or by accidental ingestion of a toxic dose. Accidental ingestion of a toxic dose has been the most common cause of toxicosis in dogs.[1] The editor is also aware of acetaminophen being used to maliciously poison companion animals. Acetaminophen may also be generated from the metabolism of phenacetin, an ingredient of some analgesic mixtures. In Australia and Great Britain, paracetamol is the equivalent of acetaminophen.

Toxic Dose

Dogs

The recommended therapeutic dosage of acetaminophen in dogs is 15 mg/kg given orally (PO) every 8 hours. The reported dosage required to produce signs of toxicity in dogs is approximately 600 mg/kg, although clinical signs of toxicity have been seen in dogs at dosages much less than this.[2] One should be concerned when exposure doses exceed 50 mg/kg, and signs are commonly observed when exposures exceed 100 mg/kg. Higher exposure doses (>200 mg/kg) are generally required to cause methemoglobinemia in dogs.

423

In one published report, a dog with hematologic evidence of acetaminophen toxicosis was administered roughly 46 mg/kg daily for 6 weeks.[3] The author is aware of cases of clinical toxicosis in dogs following chronic administration of therapeutic doses. Acetaminophen exposures lower than reported toxic doses can lead to keratoconjunctivitis sicca (KCS), particularly in small breed dogs.

Cats

Compared with dogs, cats are extremely sensitive to the toxic effects of acetaminophen and can have clinical signs of toxicity with dosages in the range of 50 to 100 mg/kg. Toxicosis has been occasionally observed with dosages as low as 10 mg/kg.[4] In cats that have received subtoxic doses of acetaminophen, subsequent doses can prove rapidly fatal.

Toxicokinetics

Because of product formulations, most acetaminophen poisonings that develop in dogs and cats follow oral ingestion. After ingestion, the drug is rapidly absorbed into the portal circulation and metabolized in the liver by glucuronidation, sulfation, and cytochrome P450-mediated pathways. In dogs, as in many other species, low doses of acetaminophen are metabolized primarily through the glucuronidation and sulfation pathways, with the resulting nontoxic conjugates excreted in bile and urine.[5] Although the amount of acetaminophen metabolized through the cytochrome P450 pathway is usually small, the product of this metabolic pathway, N-acetyl-p-benzoquinone imine (NAPQI), is toxic. The toxic effects of NAPQI are normally limited by its conjugation with glutathione, a compound essential for cellular protection against oxidative injury, to form nontoxic cysteine and mercapturic acid conjugates. Because the metabolism of acetaminophen by glucuronidation and sulfation pathways is capacity limited, increasing doses of acetaminophen lead to an increased proportion of the drug that is metabolized by the cytochrome P450 system and an increase in the production of the toxic NAPQI. Cellular stores of glutathione become depleted during conjugation of the increased amounts of NAPQI. In addition, synthesis of glutathione is suppressed in the face of high concentrations of acetaminophen. The end result is increased concentrations of unconjugated NAPQI. In dogs the biotransformation of acetaminophen is also a dose-dependent event: The higher the dose, the longer it takes for the biotransformation process to occur.[2]

Cats, like dogs, also exhibit dose-dependent toxicokinetics, albeit with some important differences.[2] Relative to a number of other species, cats have low hepatic levels of high-affinity acetaminophen uridine diphosphate–glucuronosyltransferase.[6] Therefore, compared with dogs, cats have a diminished capacity to metabolize acetaminophen through the glucuronidation pathway, and more of the drug is transformed through the sulfation pathway. As in dogs, the sulfation pathway of cats is also capacity limited. Additionally, the dose dependency of biotransformation in cats occurs at doses approximately one-tenth those observed for dogs. A capacity-limited sulfation pathway, poor glucuronidation capacity, and lower threshold for dose-dependent biotransformation explain the sensitivity of cats to acetaminophen toxicity, which occurs at much lower doses than in dogs.

Mechanism of Toxicity

Central to the mechanism of acetaminophen poisoning in dogs and cats is depletion of cellular glutathione. In the absence of glutathione conjugation, increased concentrations of NAPQI accumulate. Because of its electrophilic properties, NAPQI covalently binds to cellular proteins (e.g., enzymes, structural and regulatory proteins), thereby disrupting protein function and damaging cellular membranes through lipid peroxidation. Additionally, glutathione depletion renders cells susceptible to oxidative injury that contributes to loss of mitochondrial function, depletion of adenosine triphosphate, and cell necrosis. In dogs the liver is more susceptible to the toxicity of acetaminophen (it is estimated that 70% of hepatic glutathione must be depleted before hepatotoxicity occurs), whereas in cats the red blood cell is most susceptible to oxidative injury following glutathione depletion. Historically, the reasons for the differences in tissue affected have been attributed to the comparative susceptibility of red blood cells to oxidative injury. Feline hemoglobin contains eight sulfhydryl groups, compared with four sulfhydryl groups in other species. Feline erythrocytes are thus much more prone to oxidative injury, making the development of methemoglobinemia a much earlier and more prominent feature of toxicosis in cats than in dogs.

A recent study has suggested that another metabolite, para-aminophenol, contributes to the development of acetaminophen toxicity, specifically methemoglobinemia.[7] The generation of para-aminophenol in dogs and cats is fostered by an absolute or relative deficiency of the enzyme *N*-acetyltransferase as compared with other species and may be the more likely cause of methemoglobinemia than NAPQI.

In addition to the direct effects of toxic metabolites, consequences of cell death induced by acetaminophen toxicity have gained attention as contributors to the clinical consequences of intoxication—in particular, hepatic injury. Numerous lines of evidence, primarily from rodent models of acetaminophen-induced hepatic injury, are demonstrating that sterile inflammatory cascades initiated by hepatocellular necrosis provoke further hepatocellular injury and necrosis.[8,9]

Clinical Signs

Dogs

In dogs the clinical signs of acetaminophen toxicosis most commonly reflect hepatocellular injury and necrosis. At higher toxic doses, clinical signs of methemoglobinemia may become apparent. It is possible for an occasional dog to exhibit signs more referable to methemoglobinemia than to hepatotoxicity.[10,11] Vomiting, lethargy, trembling, chemosis, anorexia, tachycardia, and tachypnea are most often described. There may be abdominal pain and icterus. If methemoglobinemia is present, cyanosis, hemoglobinuria, and hematuria may also be observed. Facial and paw edema are commonly reported (Color Plate 30-1).

Cats

Clinical signs of acetaminophen toxicosis in cats are similar to those for dogs except that cats do not develop hepatotoxicosis as readily. The most common clinical signs reported include cyanosis (Color Plate 30-2) or muddy mucous membranes, methemoglobinemia, lethargy, anorexia, respiratory distress, edema of the face and paws, hypothermia, and vomiting. Icterus may also develop, most commonly as a consequence of hemolysis. Signs associated with hepatotoxicosis in cats are more commonly seen in high-dose exposures and in males.

Minimum Database

Abnormalities seen in a laboratory database in both dogs and cats may include methemoglobinemia, which may impart a brown tinge to whole blood, possibly followed by hemolysis depending on the extent of the oxidative damage. Hemolytic changes include anemia, hemoglobinemia, and hemoglobinuria. Increased activity of serum alanine transaminase (ALT) may be seen in both species, in dogs because of direct hepatotoxicity, and in dogs and cats secondary to hypoxic hepatocellular injury. The temporal changes that occur in serum transaminase activity following acetaminophen toxicity have been described in dogs.[12] In the first 24 hours, ALT and aspartate transaminase increase, with extreme (more than 1500 times higher than normal) increases possible by 48 hours. Progressive decreases in blood urea nitrogen, cholesterol, and albumin and increases in serum bilirubin are considered indicative of impaired hepatic function. On urinalysis there may be evidence of hemoglobinuria or hematuria.

In animals with chronic liver injury, hyperbilirubinemia may be found. In cats hyperbilirubinemia occurs early in the course of toxicity (within 48 hours) secondary to hemolysis, with increases in liver enzymes possible 3 to 6 days following ingestion. In animals with severe liver injury, there may be evidence of marked hepatic failure accompanied by prolongation of prothrombin time and activated partial thromboplastin time.

People, like dogs, are more susceptible to hepatotoxicity induced by acetaminophen. However, in a small proportion of people intoxicated with acetaminophen, the laboratory database suggests acute renal failure in the absence of evidence of hepatocellular injury. In one study, acute renal failure developed 2 to 5 days after ingestion of toxic doses of acetaminophen.[13] Although acute renal failure has not been reported in dogs or cats with acetaminophen toxicity, the similarities to people in the clinical picture of toxicity, especially in dogs, suggest the possibility that such could occur in rare instances.

Confirmatory Tests

When confirmation of a diagnosis of acetaminophen poisoning is necessary, plasma, serum, or urine concentrations of acetaminophen may be measured by many methods (e.g., immunoassay, gas-liquid chromatography, thin-layer chromatography, high-performance liquid chromatography). However, assays are not widely available in veterinary diagnostic laboratories, and documentation of toxic concentrations of acetaminophen is rarely accomplished in clinical practice. Human hospitals or diagnostic facilities can offer assays with relatively short turnaround times (less than 24 hours). In dogs and cats, a diagnosis of acetaminophen poisoning is typically established following correlation of clinical signs and laboratory abnormalities with documentation of exposure to the drug obtained through the history.

Treatment

The treatment of acetaminophen toxicosis is directed at preventing additional absorption of the drug, providing supportive measures, and administering drugs that more directly counteract the toxic mechanisms (e.g., replenish glutathione stores, convert methemoglobin to hemoglobin, prevent or treat hepatic necrosis). Induction of emesis or gastric lavage, followed by administration of activated charcoal (2 g/kg PO) within the first 4 to 6 hours, may help prevent absorption of acetaminophen remaining in the gastrointestinal tract. Supportive therapy often includes administration of oxygen and intravenous (IV) fluids to maintain hydration and electrolyte balance, especially in the presence of vomiting. Although the best fluid to administer to dogs or cats with acetaminophen toxicity has not been established, one study in mice reported a benefit in hepatic recovery with administration of lactated Ringer's solution (LRS).[14] Compared with saline-treated mice, mice administered LRS had more rapid reductions in ALT and less hepatocellular necrosis 72 hours after induction of toxicity. If anemia is severe enough (as judged by the hematocrit or packed cell volume and clinical signs of anemia), administration of packed red blood cells or whole blood may be required to preserve oxygen-carrying capacity. Blood substitutes, such as purified bovine hemoglobin, can support tissue oxygenation in the absence of traditional blood products. However, clinical studies of the treatment of acetaminophen poisoning using blood substitutes in veterinary patients have not been reported, and use of such products in this situation represents an extra-label use.

The specific "antidote" for acetaminophen poisoning provides a source of glutathione precursors for repletion of cellular glutathione stores. N-acetylcysteine, available as a 10% or 20% sterile solution, has been the historical standard and is administered at a dose of 140 mg/kg initially either IV or PO in animals that are not vomiting; it is then repeated at a dosage of 70 mg/kg IV or PO every 6 hours for an additional five to seven treatments. N-acetylcysteine may be administered IV either undiluted or diluted in a 5% dextrose solution. A human study suggests that administration of activated charcoal before N-acetylcysteine treatment does not reduce the effectiveness of orally administered N-acetylcysteine,[15] but comparable studies have not been done in dogs or cats.

Other sources of sulfur donors may be of benefit if N-acetylcysteine is not available. SAMe serves as an important intermediary in pathways that generate phospholipids, important for cell membrane function, and glutathione. SAMe has proven beneficial in the treatment of a dog with acetaminophen toxicity, and in cats it has shown protective effects against the development of acetaminophen-induced erythrocyte oxidative injury.[16,17] The suggested dosage of SAMe for dogs is 40 mg/kg PO once followed by 20 mg/kg PO every 24 hours for 9 days.[16] Optimum dosages for cats with clinical toxicity have not been established, but protective benefits were demonstrated in an experimental model of feline toxicity when SAMe was administered at 180 mg PO every 12 hours for 3 days, then 90 mg PO every 12 hours for 14 days.[17] It has not been determined whether administration of activated charcoal around the time of SAMe administration impairs absorption of SAMe. Sodium sulfate (50 mg/kg of a 1.6% solution IV every 4 hours for six treatments) is another alternative that has proven beneficial effects.[18] Treatment of acetaminophen toxicity is encouraged even if not initiated until late (more than 18 hours) in the course of intoxication because positive clinical outcomes can still be obtained with administration of antidotes and appropriate supportive care.

Ascorbic acid (30 mg/kg PO every 6 hours for 6 treatments) and methylene blue (1 mg/kg IV of a 1 solution given every 2 to 3 hours for two to three treatments) can be administered to reduce methemoglobin to hemoglobin. In a study of limited numbers of experimentally intoxicated cats, combination therapy with methylene blue and *N*-acetylcysteine offered little advantage over *N*-acetylcysteine alone.[19] Methylene blue was shown not to be toxic to cats when used at therapeutic doses for a limited number of treatments.[20] Methylene blue offers the advantage over ascorbic acid in that it has a more rapid onset of action.

Cimetidine has been advocated as a component of the treatment protocol for dogs and cats with acetaminophen toxicity.[12,20] The rationale behind its inclusion is that, as an inhibitor of the cytochrome P450 system, it will inhibit metabolism of acetaminophen into toxic compounds. Experimental evidence in rodent models of toxicity supports its use,[21] but its administration to people with acetaminophen toxicosis has not been consistently recommended.[13,22,23] Some have suggested that the concentrations of cimetidine required to achieve adequate inhibition of cytochrome P450 enzymes are more than tenfold higher than is typically achieved with routine human therapeutic doses.[24] Controlled prospective clinical studies addressing the use of cimetidine or other cytochrome P450 antagonists in the treatment of acetaminophen toxicosis have not, to my knowledge, been conducted in dogs or cats. The few studies that have addressed the use of H_2 antagonists as cytochrome P450 inhibitors in the setting of acetaminophen toxicosis have been performed in experimentally intoxicated dogs treated with the antagonist before acetaminophen was administered.[25,26]

Prognosis

The prognosis of animals with acetaminophen poisoning is a function of the dose received and the amount of time that passes before treatment is instituted. In a study of 17 cats with acetaminophen poisoning, fatalities were observed with doses as low as 10 mg/kg, but cats that had received higher doses survived.[4] Survivors were generally treated within 14 hours, whereas cats that died were not treated until 17 hours or more after exposure. Dogs may die within the first 72 hours if left untreated.[12] As with many toxicoses, the sooner therapy is implemented, the better the prognosis. Elevations in serum liver enzymes have been suggested as being a useful prognostic indicator.

Gross and Histologic Lesions

Dogs and cats that die or are euthanized from acetaminophen poisoning may exhibit evidence of methemoglobinemia and pulmonary edema. Icterus may also be seen secondary to hemolytic disease or to cholestasis with chronic toxicity or repeated acute insults. Other changes that have been described, typically in animals with more chronic toxicity, include proliferation of bile ducts, cholangitis, and infiltrates of mononuclear cells. Hepatocytes may be necrotic, have vacuolar changes, or show lipid accumulation.[27]

In dogs, and in occasional cats, that die from acute toxicity, centrilobular necrosis and congestion of the liver is observed. Renal tubular edema and degeneration and proteinaceous tubular casts have also been described in dogs with experimentally induced toxicosis.[27]

Differential Diagnoses

Several other substances are known to cause methemoglobinemia in dogs and cats. These include nitrites, phenacetin, nitrobenzene, naphthalene, phenol and cresol, sulfites, and some topically applied anesthetics, such as benzocaine.[28] Questions that address the drug exposure of a patient with methemoglobinemia are critical in differentiating the different toxicoses. The list of substances capable of causing acute hepatic injury is long, and the reader is referred to other sources for this information.[12] Some of the more common hepatotoxins in companion animals include cyanobacteria (blue-green algae), copper, zinc, iron, xylitol, mushrooms, aflatoxin, and sago palm. Some of the more common differential diagnoses for the clinical signs seen in dogs include pancreatitis, infectious hepatitis (particularly leptospirosis and Rocky Mountain spotted fever), and toxicoses induced by many drugs.

References

1. Jones RD, Baynes RE, Nimitz CT: Nonsteroidal anti-inflammatory drug toxicosis in dogs and cats: 240 cases (1989-1990), *J Am Vet Med Assoc* 201:475–477, 1992.
2. Hjelle JJ, Grauer GF: Acetaminophen-induced toxicosis in dogs and cats, *J Am Vet Med Assoc* 188: 742–746, 1986.
3. Harvey JW, French TW, Senior DF: Hematologic abnormalities associated with chronic acetaminophen administration in a dog, *J Am Vet Med Assoc* 189:1334–1335, 1986.
4. Aronson LR, Drobatz K: Acetaminophen toxicosis in 17 cats, *J Vet Emerg Crit Care* 6:65–69, 1996.
5. Center SA: Pathophysiology of liver disease: Normal and abnormal function. In Guilford WG, Center SA, Strombeck DR, et al, editors: *Strombeck's small animal gastroenterology*, ed 3, Philadelphia, 1996, WB Saunders.
6. Court MH, Greenblatt DJ: Molecular basis for deficient acetaminophen glucuronidation in cats. An interspecies comparison of enzyme kinetics in liver microsomes, *Biochem Pharmacol* 53:1041–1047, 1997.
7. McConkey SE, Grant DM, Cribb AE: The role of para-aminophenol in acetaminophen-induced methemoglobinemia in dogs and cats, *J Vet Pharmacol Therap* 32:585–595, 2009.
8. Hinson JA, Roberts DW, James LP: Mechanisms of acetaminophen-induced liver necrosis, *Handb Exp Pharmacol* 196:369–405, 2010.
9. Imaeda AB, Watanabe A, Sohail MA, et al: Acetaminophen-induced hepatotoxicity in mice is dependent on Tlr9 and the Nalp3 inflammasome, *J Clin Invest* 119:305–314, 2009.
10. Schlesinger DP: Methemoglobinemia and anemia in a dog with acetaminophen toxicity, *Can Vet J* 36:515–517, 1995.
11. MacNaughton SM: Acetaminophen toxicosis in a Dalmatian, *Can Vet J* 44:142–144, 2003.
12. Center SA: Acute hepatic injury: hepatic necrosis and fulminant hepatic failure. In Guilford WG, Center SA, Strombeck DR, et al, editors: *Strombeck's small animal gastroenterology*, ed 3, Philadelphia, 1996, WB Saunders.
13. Eguia L, Materson BJ: Acetaminophen-related acute renal failure without fulminant liver failure, *Pharmacotherapy* 17:363–370, 1997.
14. Yang R, Zhang S, Kajander H, et al: Ringer's lactate improves liver recovery in a murine model of acetaminophen toxicity, *BMC Gastroenterol* 11:125–134, 2011.
15. Spiller HA, Krenzelok EP, Grande GA, et al: A prospective evaluation of the effect of activated charcoal before oral N-acetylcysteine in acetaminophen overdose, *Ann Emerg Med* 23:519–523, 1994.
16. Wallace KP, Center SA, Hickford FH, et al: S-adenosyl-L-methionine (SAMe) for the treatment of acetaminophen toxicity in a dog, *J Am Anim Hosp Assoc* 38:246–254, 2002.
17. Webb CB, Twedt DC, Fettman MJ, et al: S-adenosylmethionine (SAMe) in a feline acetaminophen model of oxidative injury, *J Feline Med Surg* 5:69–75, 2003.
18. Savides MC, Oehme FW, Leipold HW: Effects of various antidotal treatments on acetaminophen toxicosis and biotransformation in cats, *Am J Vet Res* 46:1485–1489, 1985.
19. Rumbeiha WK, Lin Y-S, Oehme FW: Comparison of N-acetylcysteine and methylene blue, alone or in combination, for treatment of acetaminophen toxicosis in cats, *Am J Vet Res* 56:1529–1533, 1995.

20. Rumbeiha WK, Oehme FW: Methylene blue can be used to treat methemoglobinemia in cats without inducing Heinz body hemolytic anemia, *Vet Hum Toxicol* 34:120–122, 1992.
21. Al-Mustafa ZH, Al-Ali AK, Qaw FS, et al: Cimetidine enhances the hepatoprotective action of *N*-acetylcysteine in mice treated with toxic doses of paracetamol, *Toxicology* 121:223–228, 1997.
22. Burkhart KK, Janco N, Kulig KW, et al: Cimetidine as adjunctive treatment for acetaminophen overdose, *Hum Exp Toxicol* 14:299–304, 1995.
23. Zed PJ, Krenzelok EP: Treatment of acetaminophen overdose, *Am J Health Syst Pharm* 56:1081–1091, 1999.
24. Slattery JT, McRorie TI, Reynolds R, et al: Lack of effect of cimetidine on acetaminophen disposition in humans, *Clin Pharmacol Ther* 46:591–597, 1989.
25. Francavilla A, Makowka L, Polimeno L, et al: A dog model for acetaminophen-induced fulminant hepatic failure, *Gastroenterology* 96:470–478, 1989.
26. Panella C, Makowka L, Barone M, et al: Effect of ranitidine on acetaminophen-induced hepatotoxicity in dogs, *Dig Dis Sci* 35:385–391, 1990.
27. Savides MC, Oehme FW, Nash SL, et al: The toxicity and biotransformation of single doses of acetaminophen in dogs and cats, *Toxicol Appl Pharmacol* 74:26–34, 1984.
28. Houston DM, Myers SL: A review of Heinz-body anemia in the dog induced by toxins, *Vet Hum Toxicol* 35:158–161, 1993.

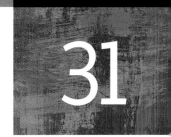

Amitraz

Jill A. Richardson, DVM

31

- Amitraz is primarily used to treat demodicosis in dogs but is also used for external parasites in several species.
- The most common signs of amitraz toxicity include sedation, bradycardia, and ataxia.
- *Yohimbine* and *atipamezole* have been used successfully to treat amitraz toxicity.

Sources

Amitraz is a formamidine antiparasitic agent. Amitraz dips are primarily used to treat demodicosis in dogs, but are also used for external parasites in several species, including cattle, rabbits, goats, and cats.[1] Mitaban® is available as a 19.9% topical solution for dilution in 10.6 mL bottles; this product is approved in dogs only. Amitraz is also found in tick control collars for dogs and contains 9.0% amitraz. Collars weigh 27.5 g, are 25" long, and there are 2500 mg of amitraz per collar (Preventic® package label insert). These collars are labeled for dogs 12 weeks and older. ProMeris® for Dogs is a topical spot-on 150 mg/mL solution approved for dogs and puppies 8 weeks of age or older.

Toxic Dose

The oral median lethal dose (LD_{50}) of amitraz in dogs is 250 mg/kg [Registry of Toxic Effects of Chemical Substances (RTECS)]. According to a study, beagles receiving 4 mg/kg PO daily for 90 days exhibited signs of transient ataxia, CNS depression, hyperglycemia, decreased pulse rates, and lowered body temperature.[1] In another study, dogs that were given 100 mg of amitraz/kg body weight at three dose rates showed clinical signs of sedation, bradycardia, polyuria, hypothermia, and hyperglycemia.[3] It is recommended to use amitraz cautiously in cats, rabbits, and diabetic patients.

Toxicokinetics

Amitraz is rapidly absorbed orally. Following doses of 100 mg/kg in dogs, peak plasma concentrations were observed after 5 hours with an elimination half-life of approximately 24 hours.[3]

Mechanism of Toxicity

The exact pharmacologic action of amitraz is not completely known; however, it does possess α_2-adrenergic activity.[1] Amitraz can cause a notable increase in plasma glucose levels, possibly from inhibiting insulin release through α_2-adrenergic activity.[1,4]

Clinical Signs

Clinical signs of amitraz toxicosis include hypersalivation, lethargy, ataxia, bradycardia, vomiting, dyspnea, hypothermia, tremors, and seizures.[1,5] The most commonly reported adverse effect after amitraz topical administration in dogs is transient sedation, which may persist for 24 to 72 hours.[1] Adverse effects are more likely to be seen in debilitated, geriatric, or toy breed dogs. Because of the drug's effects on plasma glucose, use amitraz with caution in diabetic patients.[1,4] Severe effects can be expected with ingestion of amitraz-containing insecticide collars.

Minimum Database and Confirmatory Tests

Assessment of the hydration status and urinary function are necessary because the kidneys are the primary sites of elimination of amitraz. Evaluation of heart rate, serum glucose, and blood pressure are also recommended. Some laboratories can test for amitraz in plasma, urine, skin, blood, or stomach contents.[6,7] However, these results can only confirm the exposure and absorption of amitraz because toxic levels have not been determined for tissue. There are no specific gross or histologic lesions on postmortem examination.

Treatment

If the exposure is dermal, treatment would include initial stabilization and bathing with a mild dishwashing detergent.

Treatment of animals ingesting amitraz-containing collars should consist of emesis in asymptomatic animals, retrieval of the collar using endoscopy, if possible, and administration of activated charcoal and a cathartic to remove any remaining collar fragments.

Yohimbine at a dose of 0.11 to 0.2 mg/kg IV (start with low dose) may be of benefit for overdose effects.[1,8,9] Because yohimbine has a short half-life, it may need to be repeated, particularly if the animal has ingested an amitraz-containing collar that has not been retrieved from the gastrointestinal (GI) tract. Atipamezole, at a dose of 50 mcg/kg IM, has also been used to treat amitraz toxicity and is thought to have fewer cardiorespiratory effects than yohimbine.[1,10]

Supportive hydration and close monitoring of the cardiovascular system is also recommended.

Prognosis

In most situations, exposed animals usually recover in 24 to 72 hours with prompt veterinary care and use of α_2-adrenoreceptor agonists.

Differential Diagnoses

Other toxicants causing CNS depression, along with possible ataxia, bradycardia, and sedation include ethanol, methanol, isopropanol, macrolide antiparasitics, marijuana, ethylene glycol, propylene glycol, 2-butoxyethanol, barbiturates, benzodiazepines, xylitol, antidepressants, CNS trauma, and primary CNS disease.

References

1. Plumb DC: *Veterinary drug handbook*, ed 4, Ames, IA, 2002, Iowa State University Press.
2. RTECS®: *Registry of toxic effects of chemical substances*. National Institute for Occupational Safety and Health, Cincinnati, CD ROM, Englewood, CO, 2000, MICROMEDEX.
3. Hugnet C, Buronrosee F, Pineau X, et al: Toxicity and kinetics of amitraz in dogs, *Am J Vet Res* 57(10):1506–1510, 1996.
4. Hsu WH, Schaffer DD: Effects of topical application of amitraz on plasma glucose and insulin concentrations in dogs, *Am J Vet Res* 49(1):130–131, 1988.

5. Cullen LK, Reynoldson JA: Cardiovascular and respiratory effects of the acaricide amitraz, *J Vet Pharmacol Ther* 10(2):134–143, 1987.

6. Queiroz ME, Valadao CA, Farias A, et al: Determination of amitraz in canine plasma by solid-phase microextraction-gas chromatography with thermionic specific detection, *J Chromatogr B Analyt Technol Biomed Life Sci* 794(2):337–342, 2003.

7. Ameno K, Fuke C, Ameno S, et al: A rapid and sensitive quantitation of amitraz in plasma by gas chromatography with nitrogen-phosphorus detection and its application for pharmacokinetics, *J Anal Toxicol* 15(3):116–118, 1991.

8. Hsu WH, Lu ZX, Hembrough FB: Effect of amitraz on heart rate and aortic blood pressure in conscious dogs: influence of atropine, prazosin, tolazoline, and yohimbine, *Toxicol Appl Pharmacol* 84(2):418–422, 1986.

9. Hsu WH, Hopper DL: Effect of yohimbine on amitraz-induced CNS depression and bradycardia in dogs, *J Toxicol Environ Health* 18(3):423–429, 1986.

10. Andrade SF, Sakate M: The comparative efficacy of yohimbine and atipamezole to treat amitraz intoxication in dogs, *Vet Hum Toxicol* 45(3):124, 2003.

Anticoagulant Rodenticides

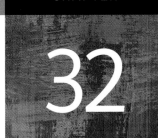

32

Michael J. Murphy, DVM, PhD, JD, DABVT

Patricia A. Talcott, MS, DVM, PhD, DABVT

- Anticoagulant rodenticides available in the United States may include brodifacoum, bromadiolone, chlorophacinone, coumafuryl, difenacoum, difethialone, diphenadione (diphacinone), pindone, valone, and warfarin.
- Dogs are intoxicated more commonly than cats or other domestic animals. Anticoagulant rodenticides act by inhibiting the "recycling" of vitamin K_1 to induce a coagulopathy. Animals with an anticoagulant rodenticide–induced coagulopathy may spontaneously bleed from any site.
- The site, volume, and rate of hemorrhage determine the clinical signs observed. The clinical signs observed in more than half of anticoagulant rodenticide-intoxicated animals are anorexia, weakness, coughing, epistaxis, or dyspnea caused by hemorrhage within the lung. However, hemorrhage can occur anywhere; ranging from petechiation and ecchymoses all the way to hematuria, hemoabdomen and even subdural hemorrhages of the central nervous system.
- Abnormalities observed in clinical laboratory tests may include a regenerative or nonregenerative anemia, hypoproteinemia, thrombocytopenia, slight elevation in alkaline phosphatase activity, hyperfibrinogenemia, elevated FDPs, low CO_2, low Po_2, and most important—elevated coagulation times (ACT, OSPT, and APTT). Although all these abnormalities are not present at all times in a given case, elevated coagulation times distinguish exposure from toxicity in all cases.
- Exposure can be confirmed by analysis of serum or whole blood or liver (postmortem) for the specific anticoagulant.
- Treatment options include blood or plasma transfusions, oral or SC vitamin K_1 (4-week duration), oxygen, antibiotics, thoracentesis or abdominal paracentesis, cage rest, and attention to caloric intake as indicated by the status of the animal.
- The prognosis is guarded to good, depending on the severity and location of the hemorrhage.

Pesticides are involved in more animal exposures and deaths than any other category of toxins. The term *pesticide* includes rodenticides, insecticides, herbicides, fungicides, avicides, and other miscellaneous compounds. Common rodenticide toxicoses involve anticoagulant rodenticides, bromethalin, cholecalciferol, strychnine, and zinc phosphide. This chapter is devoted to anticoagulant rodenticide toxicosis. It has been estimated that greater than 90% of all rodenticides used commercially are of the anticoagulant type.

Sources

The anticoagulant rodenticides were developed following investigations of moldy sweet clover poisoning in cattle. In this historical, well-known syndrome, the naturally occurring coumarin in the clover is converted by fungi to dicumarol, the toxic agent.[1] Warfarin was initially synthesized during these investigations of moldy sweet clover poisoning and was subsequently marketed as a rodenticide. Rodent species, however, have since developed resistance to it,[2] so compounds effective against warfarin-resistant rodents have been developed. The first-generation rodenticides, like warfarin and pindone, generally have shorter elimination half-lives and require higher concentrations and consecutive intake over days in order to deliver a lethal dose. Second-generation anticoagulant rodenticides were developed and are far more toxic than the first-generation anticoagulant compounds. Second-generation compounds are now more commonly encountered in veterinary exposures. They include brodifacoum, bromadiolone, chlorophacinone, coumafuryl, difenacoum, difethialone, and diphacinone. Coumachlor, coumatetralyl, and flocoumafen have not been marketed in the United States, and valone distribution in the United States was discontinued in 1993. The greater efficacy of these products against rodents is associated with a greater potential toxicity to nontarget species.

Domestic animals are sometimes inadvertently, and occasionally maliciously, exposed to anticoagulant rodenticide baits. In fact, anticoagulant rodenticides are second only to cholinesterase inhibitors as a cause of death in dogs and cats. Dogs are more commonly poisoned than cats. Some reports have indicated no seasonal predilection; however, in the Pacific Northwest, the majority of confirmed anticoagulant cases occurs in the late fall and early spring when rodent activity is high. This apparent discrepancy may be associated with the source of the samples received—such as urban versus rural and national versus regional. Nevertheless, brodifacoum is the active ingredient most commonly identified in cases of anticoagulant rodenticide–induced coagulopathies diagnosed in the Washington State University (WSU) Veterinary Teaching Hospital. Diphacinone (diphenadione), bromadiolone, and chlorophacinone come in as distant second, third, and fourth. Warfarin and other compounds account for less than 5% of diagnoses. A partial list of the many anticoagulant rodenticide products on the market is presented in Table 32-1. Anticoagulant rodenticide products come in grain-based pellets, minipellets, wax-paraffin blocks, meal baits, dry concentrates, water bait, tracking powder, ground spray, whole and broken grains, nylon pouches, coated talc, and dust. Concentrations of the active ingredient vary from 0.05% to 0.25% between products, but are generally consistent for a given product. To decrease the incidence of exposure of these compounds to children, pets, and wildlife, the U.S. Environmental Protection Agency has instituted measures that require over-the-counter sales of some products for residential use be available in tamper-resistant bait stations and that some compounds be classified for restricted use.

Toxic Dose

At least 10 anticoagulant rodenticide active ingredients are distributed in the United States. They may be obtained over the counter or through pest control operators. They are categorized as first- or second-generation anticoagulant rodenticides on the basis of their efficacy against warfarin-resistant rats. Anticoagulant rodenticide compounds that are effective against warfarin-resistant rats are termed second-generation anticoagulant rodenticides by definition.

The second-generation anticoagulant rodenticides are more potent, longer acting, or both when compared with first-generation compounds. The dose is higher, and the length of vitamin K_1 treatment is longer when treating nontarget species with toxicoses from second-generation compounds compared with the first-generation compounds (Table 32-2).

The likelihood of secondary toxicity occurring in a rodent-eating pet is of interest when anticoagulant rodenticides are used. Although secondary poisoning is theoretically more likely with the second-generation compounds, it is extremely uncommon to confirm field

Table 32-1   Trade Names and Names of the Active Ingredient for Some Anticoagulant Rodenticide Products*

Trade Name	Chemical Name
Acilone	Bromadiolone
Actosin C	Chlorophacinone
Banarat	Bromadiolone
Bar Bait	Warfarin
Boot Hill	Bromadiolone
Bromacal	Bromadiolone
Bromalone	Bromadiolone
Bromapoint	Bromadiolone
Bromone	Bromadiolone
Caid	Chlorophacinone
Castrix D	Difenacoum
Cekurat	Bromadiolone
Chlorocal	Chlorophacinone
Contracts	Bromadiolone
Contrax-W	Warfarin
Contrax-D	Diphenadione
Co-Rax	Warfarin
Coumafene	Warfarin
Cov-R-Tox	Warfarin
D-Cease	Difethialone
D-Con	Brodifacoum
D-Con Mouse-Prufe II	Brodifacoum
Denkarin	Warfarin
Dethmor	Warfarin
Dicusat M	Chlorophacinone
Dicusat E	Warfarin
Diphacin	Diphenadione
Ditrac	Diphenadione
Drat	Chlorophacinone
Enforcer Mouse Kill	Brodifacoum
Famarin	Coumachlor
Final	Warfarin
Forwarat	Brodifacoum
Frunax-DS	Difenacoum
Fumarin	Coumafuryl
Havoc	Brodifacoum
Hawk	Bromadiolone
Jaquar 50 Rodenticide Place Pac	Brodifacoum
Just One Bite	Bromadiolone
Killrat	Bromadiolone
Kill-Ko Rat and Mouse Blues	Coumafuryl
Kill-Ko Rat Killer	Diphenadione
Klerat	Brodifacoum
Kukbo Rat KO	Bromadiolone
Kukbo Stunt	Coumatetralyl
Kukbo Yaong	Brodifacoum
Kypfarin	Warfarin
Lafar	Bromadiolone
Lepit	Chlorophacinone
Lightning	Bromadiolone

Continued

Table 32-1 Trade Names and Names of the Active Ingredient for Some Anticoagulant Rodenticide Products*—*cont'd*

Trade Name	Chemical Name
Lim-N8	Brodifacoum
Liphadione	Chlorophacinone
Kill-Ko Rat and Mouse Blues	Difenacoum/Brodifacoum
LM 91	Chlorophacinone
Luxarin	Warfarin
Maki	Bromadiolone
Matikus	Brodifacoum
Matrak	Difenacoum
Microzul	Chlorophacinone
Mole Patrol	Chlorophacinone
Mouse Maze	Diphenadione
Mouse Out	Chlorophacinone
Neosorexa	Brodifacoum/Difenacoum
Nofar	Brodifacoum
Parakakes	Diphenadione
PCQ	Diphenadione
Pivacin	Pindone
Pival	Pindone
Pivaldione	Pindone
Pival Parakakes	Pindone
Pivalyn	Pindone
Place-Pax	Warfarin
PMP tracking powder	Valone
Prolin	Warfarin
Promar	Diphenadione
Prozap	Diphenadione
Racumin	Coumatetralyl
Ramik	Diphenadione
Ramik Mouse Pack	Diphenadione
Ramik Mouser	Diphenadione
Ramorin	Warfarin
Ramucide	Chlorophacinone
Ratak	Difenacoum
Ratak Plus	Brodifacoum
Rat & Mouse Blues II	Diphenadione
Rat and Mouse Killer	Warfarin
Raterex	Bromadiolone
Ratilan	Coumachlor
Ratimus	Bromadiolone
Ratomet	Chlorophacinone
Ratox	Bromadiolone
Ratoxin	Warfarin
Ratimus	Bromadiolone
Rat Zap rodent bar	Diphenadione
Raviac	Chlorophacinone
RAX	Warfarin
Redentin	Chlorophacinone
Rodent Cake	Diphenadione
Rodex	Warfarin
Rodex Blox	Warfarin

Table 32-1 Trade Names and Names of the Active Ingredient for Some Anticoagulant Rodenticide Products*—*cont'd*

Trade Name	Chemical Name
Ropax	Brodifacoum
Rosex	Bromadiolone
Rozol	Chlorophacinone
Salsbury Ropax Bars	Warfarin
Sorexa	Difenacoum/Brodifacoum
Storm	Flocoumafen
Stratagem	Flocoumafen
Super Caid	Bromadiolone
Talon	Brodifacoum
Tomcat	Bromadiolone
Tomorin	Coumachlor
Topitox	Chlorophacinone
Tox-Hid	Warfarin
Trap-NA-Sak	Diphenadione
Tri-ban	Pindone
Trokat Bait	Chlorophacinone
Volid	Brodifacoum
Warf 42	Bromadiolone
Warfarin Concentrate	Warfarin
Warfarin Plus	Warfarin
Warfarin Q	Warfarin
Warficide	Bromadiolone
Warfotox	Warfarin
WeatherBlok	Brodifacoum
Woprodenticide	Warfarin
Zoocoumarin	Warfarin

*Some products may be discontinued and unavailable for purchase.

cases of toxicosis in domestic species caused by secondary poisoning. This may be related to the "dilution effect" of the rodent species ingesting the bait. For example, a brodifacoum-poisoned rodent may have a liver concentration of brodifacoum of 2 to 5 ppm, whereas the bait is typically 50 ppm. Secondary poisonings are commonly seen in raptors or any animals whose diet consists mostly of rodents and who stay in areas where there is high use of the anticoagulant rodenticide baits.

Toxicokinetics

Plasma, liver, milk, and fetus are the tissues of most interest in a veterinary setting, although anticoagulant rodenticides may travel to a number of other tissues. Peak plasma concentrations of anticoagulant rodenticides occur within minutes to hours of oral exposure. However, the onset of clinical signs (accompanied with abnormal clotting times) is normally at least 36 hours after exposure for the reasons discussed in the mechanism section below. Plasma elimination half-lives in the dog are about 14 hours for warfarin, 4½ days for diphenadione, and about 6 days for brodifacoum. Consequently, whole blood is the specimen of choice by some laboratories for anticoagulant rodenticide analysis in a live animal.

Liver is the tissue of choice for analysis in a dead animal because it has the highest concentration of most anticoagulant rodenticides. Conclusive studies on the passage of the anticoagulant rodenticides into milk or into the fetus have not been reported in dogs or cats. Warfarin is known to pass in the milk of lactating humans. A few field cases indicate

Table 32-2	Toxicity of Some Anticoagulant Rodenticides			
		Acute oral LD$_{50}$		
		Compound (mg/kg BW)		Bait* (oz/# BW)
Active Ingredient	Bait Concentration (ppm or mg/kg bait)	Dog	Cat	Dog
Short Acting				
Warfarin	250	20-50	5-30	1.3
Fumarin	250	NA	NA	NA
Pindone	250	5-75	NA	0.3
Valone	250	NA	NA	NA
Long Acting				
Chlorophacinone	50 (0.005%)	50-100	NA	NA
Brodifacoum	50 (0.005%)	0.2-4	25[†]	0.06
Bromadiolone	50 (0.005%)	11-15	>25[‡]	3.5
Difethialone	25 (0.0025%)	4	>16	2.6
Diphacinone	50 (0.005%)	3-7.5	14.7	1

*Ounces of finished bait per pound of body weight required to achieve the lowest LD$_{50}$ value reported in the dog.
[†]Animals should be closely observed and reexamined at the end of therapy.
[‡]Limited data.
NA, Data not available.

that intramammary and transplacental distribution of anticoagulant rodenticides should be considered in lactating or pregnant pets exposed to these products.

Mechanism of Toxicity

The clinically relevant toxic event in anticoagulant rodenticide poisoning is a coagulopathy. The coagulopathy occurs because of reduction in activatable forms of clotting factors II, VII, IX, and X. The reduction in activatable forms of these clotting factors occurs because of insufficient amounts of vitamin K$_1$ at the site of posttranslational modification of these clotting factors.

Vitamin K$_1$ is required for synthesis of the forms of clotting factors II, VII, IX, and X that are active in fibrin formation. To be active in fibrin formation, these factors need to be able to bind calcium. To bind calcium, there need to be dicarboxylic acid groups on several locations on each clotting factor. Initial synthesis of each of these clotting factors provides only a single carboxylic acid on these locations. Vitamin K$_1$ is required for the addition of the second carboxylic acid group—this is termed a posttranslational modification of the clotting factor protein. Vitamin K$_1$ becomes oxidized to vitamin K$_1$-epoxide during the process of adding the second carboxylic acid group. Vitamin K$_1$-epoxide is normally reduced back to vitamin K$_1$ by one or more enzymes. This reduction is sometimes referred to as the *recycling* of vitamin K$_1$. The activity of recycling enzymes is inhibited by the anticoagulant rodenticide compounds. This inhibition results in a decrease in vitamin K$_1$ and an increase in vitamin K$_1$-epoxide concentrations in hepatocytes and plasma.[3]

Synthesis of activatable clotting factors II, VII, IX, and X is subsequently impaired. Factors VII, IX, and X have plasma half-lives of 6.2, 13.9, and 16.5 hours, respectively, in the dog, so they become somewhat reduced in circulation 24 to 64 hours after exposure of the animal to the anticoagulant rodenticide. Clinical coagulopathy occurs after depletion of vitamin K$_1$ in the liver and then depletion of activatable factors VII, IX, and X in plasma. This indirect mechanism of action is responsible for the lag time commonly observed between the ingestion of bait and the onset of clinical signs. This lag time is normally 3 to 5 days. These proteins are ineffective in clot formation because they do not have sufficient dicarboxylic acid groups to bind calcium. The vitamin K_1–dependent clotting factors are involved in both the intrinsic and extrinsic clotting cascades, so one-stage prothrombin time (OSPT), activated partial thromboplastin time (APTT), and activated clotting time (ACT) become prolonged.

Clinical Signs

Following depletion of active clotting factors, animals may hemorrhage from virtually any site. It is the authors' experience that approximately half of anticoagulant exposed companion animals will hemorrhage into their lungs; therefore, bilateral epistaxis, hemoptysis, weakness, lethargy, pallor, exercise intolerance, and dyspnea are commonly reported clinical signs.[4] Unfortunately, since the other half of exposed animals can bleed anywhere, presenting signs are quite varied: melena, hematochezia, hematuria, lameness (joint hemorrhage), paresis or paralysis (epidural or subdural hemorrhage), ecchymoses, gingival bleeding, acute collapse (hemorrhage into a major body cavity), seizures (cerebral hemorrhage), acute upper airway obstruction (laryngeal or thymic hemorrhage), abdominal distention and pain, and shaking.[5] Extensive bruising of the skin can occur, depending on how the patient was handled at the time the coagulopathy was present. Occasionally a diagnosis of anticoagulant rodenticide poisoning is made after surgical procedures have been performed on patients when uncontrolled hemorrhage occurs at the incision site after surgery. Checking an ACT time before surgery is wise if there is a suspicion of a rodenticide being consumed.

Minimum Database

The minimum database should include collection of blood before treatment for a complete blood count, serum chemistry panel, hemostasis screen, and major and minor cross matches. Red cell counts, total protein, platelet count, and prothrombin time (PT)/partial thromboplastin time (PTT) are parameters that should be frequently monitored throughout the progression of the disease. Mild to severe anemia, thrombocytopenia (rarely do they fall to <35,000/μL), and hypoproteinemia are observed in most patients. These abnormalities are not seen all the time and depend on the site and severity of hemorrhage. Lack of these abnormalities should not rule out the possibility that problems might occur in the future, particularly when exposure is well documented. Depending on how soon the patient is examined, the anemia may or may not be regenerative. A mild elevation in alkaline phosphatase level is considered nonspecific and is most likely related to the degree of hypoxia present. Notable elevations in liver enzymes are probably an indicator of severe liver damage from other causes and should be considered an important predisposing factor for the development of clinical illness. We are aware of a case of a dog suffering from both brodifacoum poisoning and liver failure secondary to metastasis of a mammary adenocarcinoma. This dog did not respond to vitamin K_1 therapy, most likely because of the liver's inability to produce the necessary coagulation proteins.

Evaluation of clotting times is crucial in confirming a coagulopathy. An ACT can be rapidly performed in house while awaiting OSPT or APTT results. The OSPT is prolonged first in poisoned patients, but prolongation of both OSPT and APTT is normally present before the onset of clinical signs. Fibrin degradation products and hyperfibrinogenemia have also been documented in approximately 50% of anticoagulant-poisoned patients.[5] A reduction in elevated coagulation parameters 12 to 24 hours after adequate vitamin K_1 treatment supports a diagnosis of vitamin K_1–responsive coagulopathy, which is virtually always an anticoagulant rodenticide–induced coagulopathy.

Blood gas analysis can be useful in guiding supportive treatment if it is readily available. A mild acidosis with low CO_2 levels, PO_2 values of less than 50 mm Hg, and an anion gap that is normal to slightly elevated are common observations.

Thoracic or abdominal radiographs or ultrasound can be very useful in identifying the site of hemorrhage—such as a pericardial, thoracic, or pulmonary hemorrhage. The most commonly reported abnormalities include pleural effusion with increases in lung opacification, hemothorax, air bronchogram signs, interlobar fissure lines, extraluminal compression of the trachea, and loss of abdominal or retroperitoneal detail.[5] Thoracentesis or abdominal paracentesis may yield a bloody effusion with a high packed-cell volume that does not clot in a serum tube.[6]

Confirmatory Tests

Identifying the specific compound involved may influence the dose or duration of vitamin K_1 treatment. It is reasonable to assume that an exposure would be to a long-acting, anti-coagulant compound until proved otherwise, given how easily available these products are to pets.

Analytical methods are available to identify specific anticoagulant rodenticides in blood, serum, plasma, liver, gastrointestinal contents, and suspect bait. High-performance liquid chromatography and gas chromatography–mass spectrometry methods are available in several veterinary diagnostic laboratories in the United States. These methods are most commonly used when the specific agent must be identified. However, analytical results are often not available for several days, and clinicians should not delay initiating treatment waiting on confirmation of the specific chemical involved. The concentration of the specific anticoagulant rodenticide detected in blood or liver is not related to the severity of the disease because of the toxicokinetics of the various compounds and the fact that the exposure dose is rarely known with certainty in field cases. Detecting the presence of an anticoagulant rodenticide chemical in an animal with a coagulopathy supports a diagnosis of an anticoagulant rodenticide–induced coagulopathy. In a clinical setting, the main reason for needing to know the specific anticoagulant rodenticide is to help establish the dose and duration of vitamin K_1 therapy. The easiest way to make this decision is to evaluate the ingredient listing on the box of bait used at the home if available.

Treatment

Treatment regimens vary depending on when the exposed patient is presented to the clinic and whether there is evidence of a coagulopathy. Traditional decontamination procedures of inducing emesis, then administering activated charcoal, followed by a cathartic may be performed in patients that come in within a few hours of exposure. These procedures are not generally indicated if coagulation abnormalities are already present. The dilemma that most clinicians face at this point is whether or not to initiate vitamin K_1 therapy or have the patient return 36 hours later to check PT and PTT times. This decision should be based on an estimate of the exposure dose, the success of decontamination procedures, and the time interval between exposure and presentation of the patient.

Determining the risk to the patient can be done by either estimating the exposure dose and then comparing with a known toxic dose (if amount consumed and percentage of active ingredient of the anticoagulant in the bait are both known), or determining how much of the bait the patient would have had to ingest in order to receive a toxic/lethal dose and determining whether this scenario is feasible or not, based on history. Regardless of how the risk assessment is done, one must use available toxicity data for the known compounds (see Table 32-2). It is important to note that most toxicity data for the anticoagulants are reported as LD_{50}s—the dose that will induce lethality in 50% of the exposed patients. It is the authors' suggestion that when using the data to assess risk, you should reduce the LD_{50} by a factor of 10 when performing your mathematical computations for risk. This will provide a margin of safety in an attempt to make a safer prediction of risk.

When vitamin K_1 therapy is not initiated, a clotting parameter, such as OSPT, PTT, and ACT, can be checked at 36 hours and perhaps again at 96 hours after exposure. Additional treatment is not warranted if the clotting times are not prolonged at this time. If the clotting times are prolonged, aggressive vitamin K_1 treatment and plasma transfusion are warranted.

Primary treatment aims for the bleeding patient are to replace the inactive clotting factors by transfusion(s) and vitamin K_1, to maintain adequate cardiovascular support, and to administer basic appropriate supportive care and exercise restriction. All patients in this category that are admitted to the WSU Veterinary Teaching Hospital are transferred immediately to the intensive care unit where they can be continuously monitored for at least the first 24 hours. The length of stay can range from 24 hours to several days. Clotting factors can be immediately restored with one or more transfusions of either plasma or whole blood once blood samples have been collected for clinical evaluation. The choice of fluid therapy depends on the degree of anemia present. Plasma should be administered at 6 to 10 mL/kg or whole blood at 12 to 20 mL/kg depending on whether clotting factors or red cells, respectively, are indicated. An estimate of the total volume of whole blood transfused should be based on the packed-cell volume. Autotransfusion with thoracentesis or abdominal paracentesis fluid may be used in emergency situations to replace red cells and plasma fluid volume, but not clotting factors. Consultation with a clinical pathologist may be necessary in some cases.

Vitamin K_1—but not vitamin K_3—should always be administered to patients with an anticoagulant rodenticide coagulopathy or to patients where the risk is high of developing a coagulopathy. This form of the vitamin is immediately available for synthesis of new clotting factors. Other chemical forms of vitamin K are not. In fact, vitamin K_3 is ineffective in the treatment of warfarin[7] or dicoumarol toxicosis, so it is contraindicated for the treatment of anticoagulant rodenticide toxicosis. Dogs dosed with 25 mg/kg of vitamin K_3 may develop Heinz body anemias, hemoglobinuria, urobilinuria and urobilinogenuria, methemoglobinemia, cyanosis, and hepatic damage.[7] Production and marketing of injectable vitamin K_3 was suspended in 1985 for safety and efficacy reasons by the Center for Veterinary Medicine of the Food and Drug Administration.

However, vitamin K_1 has no direct effect on coagulation, and clinically significant synthesis of new clotting factors commonly requires approximately 6 to 12 hours. Thus, emergency need for replacement of circulating clotting factors can only be met with a transfusion.

Oral or subcutaneous are the most commonly used routes of administering vitamin K_1. Vitamin K_1 may be administered by the intravenous (IV), intramuscular (IM), subcutaneous (SC), or oral routes. Differences of minutes in the absorption of vitamin K_1 are not clinically significant between the administration routes, so patient factors determine the preferred route of administration. The IV route is not recommended for reasons of safety—the potential for anaphylaxis is always present with IV vitamin K_1 administration.[8] Similarly the IM route is not recommended for reasons of safety because of the pain and hemorrhage that may result. In general, the clinician is often faced with deciding whether to use the oral or SQ route; the oral route should be chosen unless the patient parameters indicate otherwise. Animals with severe hypovolemia may have poorly perfused peripheral tissue, thus reducing vitamin K_1 absorption from a SC site. Oral administration of vitamin K_1 should be reconsidered in animals known to have a fat malabsorption problem, those that are vomiting, or those that were given oral activated charcoal.

Nevertheless, the two most commonly recommended routes of vitamin K_1 administration are oral and SC. The bioavailability of oral vitamin K_1 is increased four to five times when given with canned food.[9] Feeding is likely to stimulate the availability of bile salts and formation of chylomicrons necessary for vitamin K_1 absorption.[10]

Daily dosage recommendations of vitamin K_1 range from 0.25 to 2.5 mg/kg in animals exposed to warfarin; however, these warfarin compounds are rarely encountered by pets because of limited use. A commonly utilized dosage recommendation for most exposures in pets is 1.25 to 2.5 mg/kg every 12 hours (twice daily). The author recommends twice daily dosing; however, there are others who advocate one-time daily dosages of 2.5 to 5 mg/kg. Loading doses are sometimes given at the same dose recommended for daily treatment. The exact dose chosen depends on an estimate of the amount of the exposure and the severity of the coagulopathy. Be aggressive! Adverse effects from proper administration of vitamin K_1 are not known to occur.

Vitamin K_1 treatment must be maintained until toxic amounts of the compound are no longer present in the animal, because vitamin K_1 does not appear to affect the metabolism or elimination of the rodenticide. The length of vitamin K_1 treatment depends on the dose and kinetics of the specific anticoagulant rodenticide. Abnormal coagulation may last for 7 days after warfarin exposure or 4 weeks after exposure to second-generation anticoagulant rodenticides (see Table 32-2). The times necessary for therapy in this table are based on dogs that were experimentally dosed with an oral LD_{50} dose of the respective rodenticide. In a given case, the length of therapy required is directly related to the amount of anticoagulant ingested. Most field cases of anticoagulant rodenticide toxicosis receive a 3- to 4-week treatment protocol with good success.

In clinical situations the exposure dose and the specific anticoagulant may not be known, so some practitioners elect to evaluate patients periodically. In this approach patients should receive vitamin K_1 therapy for 3 to 4 weeks. Then OSPT or ACT evaluations are performed 36 to 48 hours after cessation of vitamin K_1 treatment. If the clotting time is prolonged, therapy is continued for another week. If the clotting time is normal, the rodenticide may be adequately eliminated and treatment can be discontinued. Remember that even though clotting times are normal, individual clotting factors may still be greatly reduced.[11]

Animals recovering from second-generation anticoagulant rodenticide toxicosis appear to be more sensitive to reexposure to anticoagulant rodenticides. The fact that the clotting times have returned to normal does not mean that the animal has completely eliminated the second-generation anticoagulant rodenticide compound. Animals may develop a coagulopathy after exposure to a dose of a second-generation compound that is less than that listed in Table 32-2. Owners should be strongly urged to remove all bait before reintroducing their pet to the environment.

Additional nonspecific supportive care measures include cage rest to prevent self-induced trauma, oxygen therapy (e.g., nasal catheter, oxygen cage, and tracheotomy), IV fluid therapy to maintain cardiovascular support, and broad-spectrum antibiotics (e.g., enrofloxacin, ciprofloxacin, and cephalosporins), particularly in patients with pleural effusions. Thoracentesis may be necessary to alleviate severe dyspnea, and pericardiocentesis may be necessary to alleviate cardiac tamponade. Approximately 50% of blood in the thorax or abdomen will be reabsorbed in 48 hours, so many patients will undergo some degree of auto-transfusion. A multitude of drugs has been either documented or theorized to interact with anticoagulant rodenticides; clinicians should refer to hospital formularies or veterinary drug handbooks for a comprehensive list. Paretic patients require intensive care to prevent pressure sores. Because most patients may remain anorexic for a few days, attention should be paid to meeting their nutritional needs.

Lactating and pregnant animals present a special problem. The most conservative approach to treating exposed lactating animals is to wean the pups or kittens early and provide them with oral vitamin K_1 for 2 to 3 weeks. The bitch or queen can also be treated with vitamin K_1 depending on the evaluation of exposure dose and evidence of coagulopathy. Another option is not to wean the pups or kittens but treat the bitch or queen directly while monitoring the coagulation status of the pups or kittens and/or treating the pups and kittens. Bitches and queens exposed to anticoagulant rodenticides while pregnant should be treated with vitamin K_1 until whelping or queening occurs.

Prognosis

The prognosis in patients with anticoagulant rodenticide poisoning is generally guarded to good, depending on the site and severity of hemorrhage. Predisposing liver disease or other complications may of course interfere with the animal's ability to respond to therapy or to control life-threatening hemorrhage.

Gross and Histologic Lesions

It is important to emphasize that anticoagulant rodenticide–poisoned animals may hemorrhage at any site. Approximately 50% of anticoagulant rodenticide–poisoned patients coming to either the WSU Veterinary Teaching Hospital or presenting to the Washington Animal Disease Diagnostic Laboratory experience pulmonary hemorrhage. Other reported sites include cerebral, thymic, laryngeal, intramedullary, renal, perirenal, thoracic, abdominal, hepatic, pericardial, gastrointestinal, and mediastinal hemorrhages. Petechiation and ecchymosis are sometimes seen on the skin and within the mesentery and gastrointestinal tract. The author is aware of a case involving a pregnant dog that died from an anticoagulant rodenticide. The bitch was necropsied, and the pups showed gross evidence of internal bleeding. This provides further evidence that anticoagulants can pose a risk to developing pups and kittens in utero.

Differential Diagnoses

Anticoagulant rodenticide poisoning (prolonged ACT, PT, PTT) in the dog and cat must be differentiated clinically from other causes of coagulopathy, such as disseminated intravascular coagulopathy, congenital factor deficiencies (e.g., von Willebrand's disease), liver disease, chronic gastrointestinal malabsorption, and exposure to sulfaquinoxaline. Response to appropriate vitamin K_1 treatment distinguishes the anticoagulant rodenticides from many of these differentials.

References

1. Smith WK: Relation of bitterness to the toxic principle in sweetclover, *J Agr Res* 56:145, 1938.
2. Jackson WB, Brooks JE, Bowerman AM, et al: Anticoagulant resistance in Norway rats, *Pest Control* 5:14, 1975.
3. Suttie JW: *Current advances in vitamin K research*, Proceedings of the Seventeenth Steenbock Symposium, June 21-25, 1987.
4. DuVall MD, Murphy MJ, Ray AC, et al: Case studies of second-generation anticoagulant rodenticide toxicities in non-target species, *J Vet Diagn Invest* 1(1):66, 1989.
5. Sheafor SE, Couto CG: Anticoagulant rodenticide toxicity in 21 dogs, *J Am Anim Hosp Assoc* 35:38, 1999.
6. Sheafor SE, Couto CG: Clinical approach to a dog with anticoagulant rodenticide poisoning, *Vet Med* 94(5):466–471, 1999.
7. Nangeroni LL: Injectable vitamin K_3, *J Am Vet Med Assoc* 189:850, 1986.
8. Clark WT, Halliwell REW: The treatment with vitamin K preparations of warfarin poisoning in dogs, *Vet Rec* 75(46):1210–1213, 1963.
9. Gerken DF: Unpublished data, 1987.
10. Mandel HG, Cohn VH: Fat soluble vitamins. In Gilman AG, Goodman LS, Rall TW, et al: *The pharmacological basis of therapeutics*, New York, 1985, Macmillan.
11. Mount ME, Feldman BF: Mechanism of diphenadione rodenticide toxicosis in the dog and its therapeutic implication, *Am J Vet Res* 44:2009–2017, 1983.

Anticonvulsants

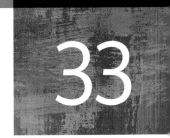

Rodney S. Bagley, DVM, DACVIM
Annie V. Chen, DVM, MS, DACVIM

- There are numerous anticonvulsant medications on the market today for companion animals, each with its own unique side effects and toxic effects.
- Poisoning may result from acute oral exposures, or more commonly, poisonings can be the result of chronic, long-term use.
- Detailed history taking, complete clinical diagnostic workup, and determination of serum concentrations of the drug are necessary for an accurate diagnosis of an anticonvulsant problem.

Anticonvulsants are used for the treatment of tremor and seizure disorders in animals.[1-8] Tremors are defined as involuntary, rhythmic, oscillating movements of a body part. Tremors can result from toxins affecting the cerebellum or from toxins directly stimulating muscles and nerves. Seizures are defined as involuntary, paroxysmal brain disturbances that are a non-specific response to insults to the cerebral cortex. Seizures are considered reactive when the insult arises from outside the brain, like with toxins. Most reactive seizures are generalized in nature and are typically manifested by uncontrollable muscular activity (paddling), autonomic dysfunction (urination, defecation, salivation), loss of consciousness and altered behavior during the immediate post-ictal phase. Cluster seizures are defined as two or more seizures in a 12 to 24 hour period, with the patient regaining consciousness between seizures. Status epilepticus is defined as continuous seizure activity that lasts for more than 5 minutes or as 2 or more discrete seizures with incomplete recovery of consciousness between seizures. Numerous anticonvulsants have been used for treatment of seizures in animals, with some being more commonly used in the modern era, and others having been used historically and are less commonly used today. Additionally, newer anticonvulsants are constantly being identified for use in human seizure disorders.[9] These newer anticonvulsants invariably are administered to animals, usually when standard anticonvulsants are ineffective or are associated with side effects. Although these newer anticonvulsants often have theoretical benefits, much less toxicologic data exist for these drugs in the clinical setting. In rare instances, animals may ingest anticonvulsants that are intended for the owner or another family member.

Therapeutic anticonvulsants are primarily administered either to acutely terminate seizures, such as in an emergency setting, or are administered more chronically as a maintenance medication to reduce or eliminate overall seizure frequency or severity. For rapid termination of seizure activity, such as in the emergency setting, diazepam is most commonly administered. The two most commonly used maintenance anticonvulsants in animals in the current era are phenobarbital and potassium bromide. Historically, anticonvulsants, such as primidone and phenytoin, were used in some dogs, but are infrequently administered in the modern era. Newer maintenance anticonvulsants include drugs such as gabapentin (Neurontin), lamotrigine (Lamictal), zonisamide (Zonegran), and levetiracetam (Keppra).

Phenobarbital

Sources

Phenobarbital is a barbiturate that has been used for a number of years as a monotherapy for seizures in dogs and cats. Phenobarbital is available through a number of human pharmaceutical distributors. Phenobarbital is available by prescription only because this is a class II scheduled drug. Phenobarbital is most often administered orally, intravenously, or rarely, intramuscularly.[1-8]

Toxicokinetics

Bioavailability of oral phenobarbital is between 88% and 95%. The serum half-life ($T_{1/2}$) is approximately 47 to 74 hours in most mongrel dogs. The $T_{1/2}$ in beagles is 25 to 38 hours. The $T_{1/2}$ is approximately 34 to 43 hours in cats.[10] When phenobarbital is administered chronically, such as a maintenance anticonvulsant, half-lives will decline as a result of autoinduction of the drug's own metabolism. Maximum concentrations are observed 4 to 8 hours after oral administration, although food may delay peak concentrations by an additional 2 to 4 hours.[1-8,11]

Phenobarbital is primarily metabolized via hepatic microsomal enzymes, although up to 25% of the unchanged drug is eliminated by pH-dependent renal excretion.[1-8] Glucuronidation is not an important mechanism of elimination, and therefore cats do not appear to metabolize this drug differently from dogs. Metabolism increases with use because of hepatic enzyme induction.

Mechanism of Toxicity and Clinical Signs

Doses of phenobarbital that are associated with both efficacy and toxicity may vary between individual animals. Serum concentrations have been more closely correlated with therapeutic benefit than the administered dose. Therapeutic levels of 20 to 40 mcg/mL have been suggested to maximize seizure control while minimizing side effects.[1-8,11] The risk of hepatotoxicity is greater when the level is above 35 mcg/mL. Trough levels historically correlate better with therapeutic outcome than with peak levels; however, this may not be as significant as initially thought.

Side effects associated with phenobarbital administration include sedation, ataxia, polyuria, polydipsia, polyphagia, nystagmus, restlessness or hyperexcitability, drug rash, hyperprothrombinemia, blood dyscrasias, and osteomalacia.[1-8] Polyuria is thought to be caused by central inhibition of aldosterone release, whereas polyphagia is believed to result from suppression of the satiety center in the ventromedial hypothalamus. Phenobarbital has been shown to induce coagulation defects in cats by reducing vitamin K–dependent clotting factors (II, VII, IX, and X). Phenobarbital, displaced by sulfonamides and salicylates, may lead to an increase in the metabolism of other co-administered drugs. Phenobarbital may decrease measured serum T4 levels caused by increased biliary excretion and possibly an increase in deiodination of T4.[1-8,12-14] Importantly, phenobarbital administration may induce the production of some commonly measured serum indicators of liver dysfunction, such as alkaline phosphatase (AP) and alanine transaminase (ALT).[1-8,15-17] Liver enzyme elevations may take anywhere from 5 weeks up to 7 months to return to normal after discontinuing the drug. Elevation of liver enzymes, with alkaline phosphatase higher than alanine aminotransferase, is common and does not necessarily indicate clinical liver disease.

Toxicity with phenobarbital administration includes those clinical signs associated with acute barbiturate overdose, but may also result in liver failure and cirrhosis. Common clinical signs of acute phenobarbital overdose include sedation (which may progress to coma), respiratory depression, ataxia, paresis, and possibly death. Co-administered drugs, such as chloramphenicol, decrease the metabolism of phenobarbital, and this can cause severe depression, sedation, and coma.[1-8]

Clinical signs of phenobarbital-associated liver disease are similar to signs of liver disease in general. General ill thrift, polyuria, gastrointestinal abnormalities (vomiting and diarrhea), abdominal enlargement, and icterus are possible. Increases in liver-associated enzymes (ALT, AP) and liver function tests (bile acids) and decreases in albumin, glucose, and cholesterol may be observed.[1-8,15-18]

Diagnosis

The diagnosis of phenobarbital toxicity is supported by the appropriate clinical signs in association with serum phenobarbital concentrations increased above the commonly recognized therapeutic range (i.e., greater than 35 mcg/mL). The diagnosis of liver disease is often aided by liver biopsy.

Treatment

Treatment for phenobarbital toxicity is directed toward maintaining respiratory function, basic supportive care for life, and elimination of additional phenobarbital administration. Drugs that may potentiate phenobarbital's effects or decrease phenobarbital metabolism should similarly be discontinued. Adminstration of multiple dose activated charcoal and alteration of urine pH to 7.5 to 8.0 may increase the elmination of parent compound. If liver failure accompanies phenobarbital toxicity, therapy for liver disease should be employed. The prognosis for recovery from phenobarbital toxicity varies with severity of clinical signs before recognition of this toxicity. Phenobarbital should only be used if the patient has no underlying liver disease as assessed by blood work and post-prandial bile acids.

Potassium Bromide

Sources

Potassium bromide (KBr) is actually a chemical product, not a drug formulation.[1-3,5-8,19-23] Potassium bromide has reasonable efficacy for treatment of seizures in dogs and may be used as a monotherapy or in combination with other anticonvulsants. This chemical was historically difficult to obtain in formulations for administration to dogs, but this is less of a problem currently because there are a number of veterinary compounding laboratories that provide therapeutic distribution of the drug.

Toxicokinetics

Potassium bromide has a relatively long serum half-life (~24 days in dogs and 11 days in cats) and therefore requires a significant amount of time to reach a steady state (up to 4 months in dogs and 6 weeks in cats).[1-3,5-8,19-23] In an effort to increase the therapeutic drug level of potassium bromide sooner, a loading dose of potassium bromide can be given at the initiation of treatment. Potassium bromide is often loaded orally and then maintained at 20 and 35 mg/kg/day. Therapeutic blood level of potassium bromide is 1 to 3 mg/mL. If sodium bromide is used, the dosage is slightly reduced to 17 to 30 mg/kg/day. If more rapid seizure control is necessary, an initial dose of 400 to 600 mg/kg, usually divided over a 2 to 3 day period, can be administered. Potassium bromide, when administered in increased concentrations in a single dosing period, is often irritating to the stomach and results in vomiting. To prevent this problem, the loading dose is administered in multiple, smaller doses over the 2- to 3-day period. It often helps when using the loading dose to first calculate the maintenance dose expected. This will most likely be the capsule size that can be formulated by a compounding laboratory. During the loading period, the total loading dose is given over 48 to 72 hours by giving multiple doses of the maintenance dose of the medication.

Clinical Signs

Potassium bromide is reasonably safe but has some side effects. The bromide component is toxic to humans, who can exhibit headaches, skin rashes, tremors, and gastrointestinal disturbances following administration of the chemical.[1-3,5-8,19-22,24] Owners should be careful therefore in handling the medication and not expose themselves to the chemical. This may require placing the medication in the food, wearing gloves when pilling, and washing hands after touching the capsule. Diets with relatively high chloride (sodium chloride) content may increase bromide elimination because bromide competes with chloride for elimination. Renal disease may decrease elimination of bromide, requiring decreases in the dose of bromide up to 50% of normal levels to prevent toxicity.[19-24]

The most common side effects of potassium bromide administration in dogs include sedation and ataxia. Pancreatitis is associated with the use of this drug, but the actual cause and effect relationship is not clear.[26] With some doses, vomiting may occur because of the local irritant effects on the stomach. Diet, alterations in fluid intake, or dehydration may alter the therapeutic KBr levels in the blood. Rarely, skin irritation, itchiness, or rashes may be noted. Other reported side effects include polydipsia, polyuria, polyphagia, and hyperactivity. Importantly in cats, KBr can result in pneumonitis or a fatal asthmatic condition.[5] Caution should be exercised when using this drug in cats, and if any respiratory signs are noted, the drug should be stopped immediately. Rarely, dogs may become aggressive while receiving bromide therapy. When performing routine serum chemistry evaluations, measured serum chloride concentrations will appear to be increased because some analytical methods may measure the serum bromide as chloride.

Diagnosis

Similar to phenobarbital, serum concentrations of KBr can be measured to provide a more objective measure of circulating KBr concentrations. Therapeutic levels should range from 1 to 3 mg/mL. This range, however, is not correlated with efficacy or toxicity as reliably as serum phenobarbital concentrations. With KBr, toxic effects are usually evident clinically (primarily sedation and ataxia).

Treatment

If toxic levels of bromide are present, diuresis is used to eliminate the drug from the body in addition to discontinuation of the drug. Intravenous administration of NaCl-containing fluids is used for diuresis over a 12- to 24-hour period. Clinical signs of ataxia and sedation will usually resolve within 1 to 4 days following discontinuation of the drug and diuresis. Obviously, if KBr is providing some antiseizure effect, decreasing the KBr serum concentrations may result in increases in seizure activity. The risk of increasing seizure activity is often weighed against the toxicity risks. Because KBr has a relatively long serum half-life, the drug may be discontinued for 1 to 3 days, but then reinstituted at a lower dose.

Diazepam

Sources

Diazepam is a benzodiazepine that has been used for a number of years to more rapidly terminate seizures in dogs and cats.[1-8] Diazepam is available through a number of human pharmaceutical distributors. Diazepam is a class II drug and is thus available by prescription only. Because of the short half-life of diazepam in dogs (2-4 hours) and the development of tolerance, diazepam should only be used for emergency management of seizures. Diazepam can be given IV, intranasally, and rectally as boluses, and can be repeated as needed to control seizures. Diazepam can also be given as a constant rate infusion (CRI), titrated to effect. The CRI is usually discontinued slowly after the patient has been seizure free for 8 to 12 hours. The CRI is decreased by 50% every 4 to 6 hours for two decreases. Diazepam has a tendency to precipitate when mixed with other products so it is the safest to give the drug straight through a syringe pump and in a designated diazepam-only catheter. Diazepam is also light sensitive, so all exposed lines and syringe will need to be covered by dark-colored Vet Wrap or towel. Diazepam binds to plastic, so minimizing the amount of line to the patient is best.

Toxicokinetics and Mechanism of Action

Diazepam is metabolized via the liver primarily by demethylation to nordiazepam (desmethyldiazepam) and oxazepam. Metabolites have 25% to 33% of diazepam's anticonvulsant activity. Because of an extensive first pass effect, oral systemic availability is only 1%

to 3%. Drugs, such as cimetidine, that inhibit hepatic microsomal enzyme activity will prolong the serum half-lives of diazepam and nordiazepam. Tachyphylaxis is noted with repeated doses of benzodiazepines, probably caused by a feedback-regulated increase in benzodiazepine receptors or a decreased production of γ-aminobutyric acid (GABA).

Diazepam appears to bind to benzodiazepine receptors, causing allosteric changes that facilitate binding of GABA to its receptor. This binding opens Cl⁻ channels, allowing for Cl⁻ influx and enhanced inhibition of the postsynaptic neuron.

Doses of diazepam necessary for termination of acute seizure activity vary in individual animals. Initial doses range from 1 to 2 mg/kg IV or rectally for acute seizures.[1-8,27,28] In status epilepticus or severe, recurrent seizure activity, diazepam can be administered as a continuous intravenous infusion at dosages between 5 and 20 mg/h and is administered for at least 4 hours beyond the last seizure episode.

Clinical Signs and Treatment

Signs associated with acute toxicity include sedation, drowsiness, lethargy, and malaise. In animals with hepatic portovascular anomalies or liver functional abnormalities, even relatively small doses of diazepam can result in stupor, coma, and death. In cats diazepam administration has been associated with idiosyncratic liver failure.[29,30] This side effect may not be dose- or administration rate-dependent and may occur with either oral or intravenous administration.

Treatment of diazepam toxicity includes discontinuation of the drug and general supportive care. In cats with liver failure, general treatment of animals with liver disease should be considered.

Historical Anticonvulsants

Primidone

Primidone is rapidly oxidized to phenobarbital and phenylethylmalonamide (PEMA) by hepatic microsomal enzymes.[1-8,31] The phenobarbital metabolite contributes 85% of the anticonvulsant activity, and the effectiveness of primidone correlates best with serum phenobarbital concentrations. The $T_{1/2}$ of PEMA and primidone is 10 to 14 hours. Primidone was usually administered at dosages of between 10 and 55 mg/kg/day divided every 8 hours.

This drug was not approved for use in cats and has been suggested to be toxic in cats.[1-8] This may be because cats metabolize the drug differently from dogs. Acute toxicity with primidone includes sedation, ataxia, polyuria and polydipsia, nystagmus, profound tachycardia, episodic hyperventilation, and anorexia. Hepatotoxicity may be associated with the duration of treatment rather than daily dose.[1-8,32] Histopathologic changes in the liver after 6 months of therapy in dogs include hepatocellular hypertrophy and necrosis, lipidosis, and extramedullary hematopoiesis. If medication is discontinued after this time, these changes will result in hepatic fibrosis with some permanent loss of function. Dermatitis associated with the use of primidone in a dog included excessive licking of paws, alopecia, pruritus, scaling, pigmentation, and ulceration over the back, elbows, hocks, face, and ears. Biopsy of these skin lesions showed severe diffuse parakeratotic hyperkeratosis of the epidermis and hair follicles, frequently associated with epidermal hyperplasia, dyskeratosis, and intra-cellular vacuolation.

Phenytoin

Phenytoin is a more common anticonvulsant in human beings. It is degraded to parahydroxy metabolites, which have a $T_{1/2}$ of approximately 22 hours.[1-8] In dogs phenytoin is metabolized primarily to a metahydroxy metabolite that has a $T_{1/2}$ of 4 hours. Biotransformation of this drug occurs via hepatic microsomal enzymes. A smaller volume of distribution and shorter elimination half-life in puppies as compared with adult dogs appears to result in higher peak serum concentrations of this drug in puppies. Conversely, phenytoin is eliminated very slowly in cats. The elimination half-life is approximately 41 hours in adult cats and kittens following intravenous administration and between 24 and 108 hours after oral administration.

Phenytoin appears to interfere with sodium ion conductance, thereby stabilizing neuronal membranes and restricting the spread of electrical discharges. Dosages up to 35 to 50 mg/kg orally every 8 hours or more often may be required to maintain serum therapeutic concentrations.

Acute toxicity results in sedation, ataxia, and anorexia in dogs. A hepatopathy has been associated with chronic administration of this drug in dogs.[32] This hepatopathy results in hepatocellular hypertrophy and necrosis, lipidosis, and extramedullary hematopoiesis. This drug may also result in vitamin K–dependent coagulation defects. A reversible dermal atrophy in cats and gingival hyperplasia in dogs has also been associated with the use of this drug. Similar to phenobarbital, concurrent chloramphenicol administration increases phenytoin toxicity and may decrease measured serum thyroid hormone (T4) concentrations. Phenytoin appears toxic to cats because of an inability to hydroxylate phenolic compounds, and its use can result in sialosis, frequent vomiting, and weight loss. Because of poor efficacy and associated side effects, phenytoin is not used as a maintenance anticonvulsant in animals in the modern era.

Clonazepam (Klonopin)

Clonazepam is an extremely potent benzodiazepine that is occasionally used for treatment of seizures in dogs.[1-8] The hepatic clearance is apparently much greater in dogs compared with human beings, which may result in relatively short (1.6 to 2.9 hours) elimination half-lives. Elimination of clonazepam is further enhanced by phenobarbital; this is an effect caused by hepatic enzyme induction rather than an alteration in hepatic blood flow. Clonazepam is suggested to be administered at a dosage of 0.5 mg/kg orally every 8 to 12 hours to achieve peak serum concentrations of 130 to 179 ng/mL and trough concentrations of 22 to 77 ng/mL. These serum concentrations are near the therapeutic range in human beings. Side effects and toxicity of this drug primarily include sedation progressing to stupor and coma. After prolonged treatment with this drug, abrupt cessation of therapy may result in acute withdrawal signs including "wet dog shakes," listlessness, weight loss, increased body temperature, and dorsal recumbency. Signs are most severe 2 days after cessation of the drug and usually subside within 1 week of withdrawal.

Clorazepate (Tranxene)

Clorazepate is a less potent benzodiazepine product compared with clonazepam.[33-35] This drug is rapidly and completely hydrolyzed in the stomach to nordiazepam, but less information exists for clinical use of this drug in dogs. Preliminary evidence indicates that the dosage of 2 mg/kg every 12 hours produces peak nordiazepam concentrations near 1 mcg/mL, with maximum concentrations occurring between 1 and 2 hours after oral administration. Additional dosage recommendations for this drug in dogs include 0.5 to 1 mg/kg orally every 8 hours.

Little information also exists regarding side effects and toxicity with this drug. It is assumed to have similar side effects to other benzodiazepines with regard to sedation.

Carbamazepine

Carbamazepine is an iminostilbene derivative used as an anticonvulsant and also for relief of pain in trigeminal neuralgia in human beings.[1-8] This drug appears structurally related to tricyclic antidepressants. Published reports regarding clinical use, side effects, and toxicity in dogs are unavailable. In humans this drug may have sedative, anticholinergic, antidepressant, muscle relaxant, antiarrhythmic, antidiuretic, and neuromuscular transmission-inhibitory actions.

Vigabatrin (gamma-vinyl-gamma-aminobutyric acid)[36]

This drug is a structural analogue of GABA and is a selective and irreversible inhibitor of GABA-aminotransferase (GABA-T). One clinical report exists of the use of this drug as an anticonvulsant in dogs. An optimum dose is not known. Clinically, dogs have been given between 35 and 125 mg/kg/day (divided every 8 to 12 hours) therapeutically; the drug was often given concurrently with phenobarbital.[36]

Side effects and toxicity with this drug are poorly established in dogs. In the single report of use in dogs, immune-mediated anemia developed in one treated dog. Intramyelinic edema was present in dogs experimentally administered this drug. Sedation, dizziness, and headache may be noted in humans in association with this drug's use.

Newer Anticonvulsants

Felbamate (Felbatol) (2-phenyl-1,3-propanediol dicarbamate)

Felbamate has been used in some instances of medically refractory seizures in dogs.[37-40] This drug is extensively metabolized by the liver via hydroxylation and conjugation, with an approximate half-life in dogs of 5 to 6 hours. This drug appears to be well absorbed after oral administration. The precise mechanism of action is not known; however, this drug appears to work on the N-methyl-D-aspartate (NMDA) receptor. The optimum dose of the drug is not known. Some dosing protocols have been described for dogs; for dogs less than 10 kg, it is 200 mg orally every 8 hours with a 200-mg/wk increase up to a maximum dose of 600 mg orally every 8 hours or until seizure control is obtained. For dogs greater than 10 kg, it is 400 mg orally every 8 hours with a 400-mg/wk increase up to a maximum dose of 1200 mg orally every 8 hours or until seizures are controlled. Another dosing recommendation describes an initial dose of 15 mg/kg every 8 to 12 hours orally and increasing in 15-mg/kg increments every 2 weeks until seizures are controlled. Doses of 60 to 70 mg/kg were not shown to be toxic to dogs. A reported toxic dose of felbamate appears to be approximately 300 mg/kg.

Felbamate has been associated with aplastic anemia and hepatic failure in humans, which has resulted in its limited use. In dogs severe hepatic disease has been described when this drug was used as a monotherapy or in combination therapy with phenobarbital. Other reported side effects associated with felbamate in humans include anorexia, insomnia, weight loss, nausea, dizziness, fatigue, ataxia, and lethargy.

Gabapentin (Neurontin)

This drug was developed to be structurally similar to GABA; however, it does not appear to work at the GABA receptor.[9,41-43] The mechanism of action and optimum drug dose is not known for dogs. Some dosage protocols have been described for dogs. One suggests beginning at 100 mg orally every 8 hours with a gradual increase up to 900 mg orally every 8 hours over the next 4 weeks or until seizures are controlled. Other recommendations include beginning at 100 to 300 mg/dog every 8 hours orally, with increases in the dose upward every 1 to 2 weeks until seizures are controlled or the maximum dosage of 1200 mg/dog orally every 8 hours is obtained. An additional recommendation is 25 to 60 mg/kg/day divided every 6 to 8 hours. Another recommended anticonvulsant dose in dogs is 2.5 to 10 mg/kg every 8 to 12 hours, orally; 5 to 10 mg/kg every 12 hours, orally, is a recommended dosage in cats.

Drowsiness, tiredness, fatigue, somnolence, dizziness, ataxia, nystagmus, headache, tremors, nausea, and vomiting may be seen in association with administration of this drug in human beings. Side effects in dogs at higher doses include sedation and gastrointestinal upset. Side effects and toxicity associated with this drug in pets are currently unknown. The oral solution contains xylitol, which can be toxic to dogs at doses exceeding 0.1 g/kg. With standard gabapentin doses, it is unlikely that a toxic dose of xylitol will be achieved, but one should use caution.

Management of overdose is generally supportive. There is no evidence that forced diuresis increases urinary elimination.

Lamotrigine (Lamictal) (3,5-diamino-6-[2,3-dichlorophenyl]-1,2,4-triazine)

This drug is believed to stabilize presynaptic neuronal membranes by blocking voltage-dependent sodium channels, thereby preventing the release of excitatory neurotransmitters, such as glutamate and aspartate.[9] An optimum dose is not known for dogs and cats. Skin rashes, anorexia, ataxia, insomnia, headache, ataxia, diplopia, nausea, dizziness, vomiting, somnolence, and weight loss have been associated with administration of this drug in human beings.

Zonisamide (Zonegran)

This drug is a sulfonamide-based anticonvulsant. Its mechanism of action is unknown, but may include blockage of T-type calcium and voltage-gated sodium channels in the brain, modulation of CNS dopaminergic metabolism, scavenging free radicals, enhancing CNS GABA release, or inhibiting carbonic anhydrase.[9,41,44,45] An efficacy dose is not known for dogs or cats. One suggested dosage is 10 mg/kg orally every 12 hours, and another dosage is 4 to 8 mg/kg/day. Serum therapeutic levels in humans are suggested to be 10 to 40 mg/L, whereas in dogs, it may be 18 to 24 mcg/mL. Minimal side effects were noted in beagles treated with 75/mg/kg/day. Ataxia, drowsiness, and gastrointestinal dysfunction may be associated with this drug's use.

Levetiracetam (Keppra)

This drug is a pyrrolidine-based anticonvulsant.[41,46-50] Levetiracetam works by binding to synaptic vesicle protein 2A in the brain. Levetiracetam is not metabolized by the liver, so it is especially advantageous for use for liver patients exhibiting seizure activity. The elimination half-life is 4 hours in the dog and 3 hours in the cat. An efficacious dose of this drug is not known for dogs or cats. Suggested dosages are 20 mg/kg orally every 8 hours or 500 to 4000 mg/day. Levetiracetam can also be given as a 30 mg/kg single IV bolus for the treatment of cluster seizures and status epilepticus. Minimal side effects occurred in beagles treated with less than 400 mg/kg/day. Salivation, restlessness, vomiting, and ataxia are possible, with signs resolving within 24 hours of discontinuation of the drug.

References

1. Boothe DM: Anticonvulsant therapy in small animals, *Vet Clin N Amer Sm Anim Pract* 28:411, 1998.
2. Boothe DM: Anticonvulsants and other neurologic therapies. In Boothe DM, editor: *Small animal clinical pharmacology and therapeutics*, Philadelphia, 2001, WB Saunders Co.
3. Knowles K: Idiopathic epilepsy, *Clin Tech Small Anim Pract* 13:144, 1998.
4. LeCouteur RA, Child G: Clinical management of epilepsy in dogs and cats, *Prob Vet Med* 1:578, 1989.
5. Podell M: Antiepileptic drug therapy, *Clin Tech Small Anim Pract* 13:185, 1998.
6. Podell M: Seizures in dogs, *Vet Clin N Am Small Animal Pract* 26:779, 1996.
7. Thomas WB: Idiopathic epilepsy in dogs, *Vet Clin N Amer Sm Anim Pract* 30(1):183, 2000.
8. Thomas WB: Seizures and narcolepsy. In Dewey CW, editor: *A practical guide to canine and feline neurology*, Ames, 2003, Iowa State Press.
9. Dichter MA, Brodie MJ: New antiepileptic drugs, *N Engl J Med* 334(24):1583, 1996.
10. Cochrane SM, Parent JM, Black WD, et al: Pharmacokinetics of phenobarbital in the cat following multiple oral administration, *Can J Vet Res* 54:309–312, 1990.
11. Levitski RE, Trepanier LA: Effects of timing of blood collection on serum phenobarbital concentrations in dogs with epilepsy, *J Am Vet Med Assoc* 217(2):200, 2000.
12. Kantrowitz LB, Peterson ME, Trepanier LA, et al: Serum total thyroxine, total triiodothyronine, free thyroxine, and thyrotropin concentrations in epileptic dogs treated with anticonvulsants, *J Am Vet Med Assoc* 214:1804, 1999.
13. Müller PB, Wolfsheimer KJ, Taboada J, et al: Effects of long-term phenobarbital treatment on the thyroid and adrenal axis and adrenal function tests in dogs, *J Vet Intern Med* 14:157, 2000.
14. Gaskill CL, Burton SA, Gelens HCJ, et al: Effects of phenobarbital treatment on serum thyroxine and thyroid-stimulated hormone ceoncentration in epileptic dogs, *J Am Vet Med Assoc* 215:489, 1999.
15. Chauvet AE, Feldman EC, Kass PH: Effects of phenobarbital administration on results of serum biochemical analyses and adrenocortical function tests in epileptic dogs, *J Am Vet Med Assoc* 207:1305, 1995.
16. Dayrell-Hart B, Steinberg SA, Van Winkle TJ, et al: Hepatoxicity of phenobarbital in dogs: 18 cases (1985-1989), *J Am Vet Med Assoc* 199:1060, 1991.
17. Müller PB, Taboada J, Hosgood G, et al: Effects of long-term phenobarbital treatment on the liver in dogs, *J Vet Intern Med* 14:165, 2000.
18. Bunch SE, Baldwin BH, Hornbuckle WE, et al: Compromised hepatic function in dogs treated with anticonvulsant drugs, *J Am Vet Med Assoc* 184:444, 1984.
19. Podell M, Fenner WR: Bromide therapy in refractory canine idiopathic epilepsy, *J Vet Intern Med* 7:318, 1993.

20. Podell M, Fenner WR: Use of bromide as an antiepileptic drug in dogs, *Compend Contin Educ Pract Vet* 16:767, 1994.
21. Trepanier LA, Schoick A, Schwark WS, et al: Therapeutic serum drug concentrations in epileptic dogs treated with potassium bromide alone or in combination with other anticonvulsants: 122 cases (1992-1996), *J Am Vet Med Assoc* 213:1449, 1998.
22. Trepanier LA: *Pharmokinetics and clinical use of bromide*, Proceedings of 11th ACVIM Forum 878–880, 1993.
23. Boothe DM, George K, Couch P, et al: Disposition and clinical use of bromide in cats, *J Am Vet Med Assoc* 221(8):1131, 2002.
24. Yohn SE, Morrison WB, Sharp PE: Bromide toxicosis (bromism) in a dog treated with potassium bromide for refractory seizures, *J Am Vet Med Assoc* 201:468, 1992.
25. Nichols ES, Trepanier LA, Linn K: Bromide toxicosis secondary to renal insufficiency in an epileptic dog, *J Am Vet Med Assoc* 208:231, 1996.
26. Gaskill CL, Cribb AE: Pancreatitis associated with potassium bromide/phenobarbital combination therapy in epileptic dogs, *Can Vet J* 41:555, 2000.
27. Papich MG, Alcorn J: Absorption of diazepam after its rectal administration in dogs, *Am J Vet Res* 56:1629, 1995.
28. Podell M: The use of diazepam per rectum at home for the acute management of cluster seizures in dogs, *J Vet Intern Med* 9:68, 1995.
29. Center SA, Elston TH, Rowland PH, et al: Fulminant hepatic failure associated with oral administration of diazepam in 11 cats, *J Am Vet Med Assoc* 209:618, 1996.
30. Hughes D, Moreau RE, Overall KL, et al: Acute hepatic necrosis and liver failure associated with benzodiazepine therapy in six cats, 1986-1995, *J Vet Emerg Crit Care* 6(1):13, 1996.
31. Schwartz-Porsche D, Loscher W, Frey HH: Therapeutic efficacy of phenobarbital and primidone in canine epilepsy: a comparison, *J Vet Pharmacol Therap* 8:113, 1985.
32. Bunch SE, Cascleman WL, Baldwin BH, et al: Effects of long-term primidone and phenytoin administration on canine hepatic function and morphology, *Am J Vet Res* 46:105, 1985.
33. Brown SA, Forrester SD: Serum disposition of oral clorazepate from regular-release and sustained-delivery tablets in dogs, *J Vet Pharmacol Theurap* 14:126, 1991.
34. Forrester SD, Wilcke JR, Jacobson JD, et al: Effects of a 44-day administration of phenobarbital on disposition of clorazepate in dogs, *Am J Vet Res* 54:1136, 1993.
35. Scherkl R, Kurudi D, Frey HH: Clorazepate in dogs: tolerance to the anticonvulsant effect and signs of physical dependence, *Epilepsy Res* 3:144, 1989.
36. Speciale J, Dayrell-Hart B, Steinberg SA: Clinical evaluation of gamma-vinyl-gamma-aminobutyric acid for control of seizures in dogs, *J Am Vet Med Assoc* 198:995, 1991.
37. Adusumalli YE, Gilchrist JR, Wichmann JK, et al: Pharmacokinetics of felbamate in pediatric and adult beagle dogs, *Epilepsia* 33:955, 1992.
38. Adusumalli YE, Yang JT, Wong KK, et al: Felbamate pharmacokinetics in the rat, rabbit, and dog, *Drug Met Disp* 19:1116, 1991.
39. Dayrell-Hart B, Tiches D, Vite C, et al: Efficacy and safety of felbamate as an anticonvulsant in dogs with refractory seizures, *J Vet Int Med* 10:174, 1996.
40. Ruehlmann D, Podell M, March P: Treatment of partial seizures and seizure-like activity with felbamate in six dogs, *J Small Anim Pract* 42:403, 2001.
41. Podell M: Strategies of antiepileptic drug therapy, In proceedings of 19th ACVIM Forum, Denver, 430, 2001.
42. Radulovic LL, Turck D, von Hodenberg A, et al: Disposition of gabapentin (neurontin) in mice, rats, dogs, and monkeys, *Drug Metab Disposition* 23(4):441, 1995.
43. Vollmer KG, von Hodenberg A, Kolle EU: Pharmacokinetics and metabolism of gabapentin in rat, dog and man, *Drug Res* 36(1):830, 1986.
44. Matsumoto K, Miyazaki H, Fujii T, et al: Absorption, distribution and excretion of 3-(sulfamoyl [^{14}C] methyl)-1,2,benzisoxazole (AD-810) in rats, dogs and monkeys and of AD-810 in men, *Drug Res* 33:961, 1983.
45. Walker RM, DiFonzo CJ, Barsoum NJ, et al: Chronic toxicity of the anticonvulsant zonisamide in Beagle dogs, *Fundammt Appl Toxicology* 11:333, 1988.
46. Harden C: Safety profile of levetiracetam, *Epilepsia* 42(Suppl 4):36, 2001.
47. Hovinga CA: Levetiracetam: a novel antiepileptic drug, *Pharmacotherapy* 21(11):1375–1388, 2001.
48. Krakow K, Walker M, Otoul C, et al: Long-term continuation of levetiracetam in patients with refractory epilepsy, *Neurology* 56:1772, 2001.
49. Leppik IE: The place of levetiracetam in the treatment of epilepsy, *Epilepsia* 42(Suppl4):44, 2001.
50. Shorvon SD, van Rijkevorsel K: A new antiepileptic drug: Levetiracetam, a pyrrolidone recently licensed as an epileptic drug, (Editorial), *J Neurol Neurosurg Psychiatry* 72:426, 2002.

Arsenic

Camille DeClementi, VMD, DABT, DABVT

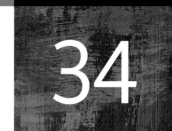

34

- Arsenic is a ubiquitous element.
- Ingestion of arsenic-containing ant and roach baits is the most common exposure scenario in dogs and cats.
- Average oral lethal dose of sodium arsenite in most species is 1 to 25 mg/kg of body weight.
- Clinical signs of acute poisoning include severe gastrointestinal distress along with signs associated with dehydration.
- Treatment aims include aggressive intravenous fluid therapy and chelation with dimercaprol.
- Confirmation of poisoning is best done antemortem by assessing urine arsenic levels, and it is best done postmortem by assessing liver and kidney levels.
- Prognosis is grave once clinical signs become severe.

Sources

Arsenic (As) is actually a metalloid but is often referred to as arsenic metal. It is ubiquitous and can be found naturally in rocks, soil, water, and living organisms in concentrations of parts per million (ppm) or parts per billion (ppb).[1] It is rare to find elemental arsenic free in the natural environment. Instead arsenic combines with oxygen and hydrogen and many other elements including sulfur, nickel, cobalt, copper, iron, aluminum, barium, bismuth, calcium, lead, magnesium, manganese, uranium, and zinc. Arsenic can be found in both organic and inorganic forms and it occurs in both the pentavalent (+5) and trivalent (+3) forms. Human activities concentrate and redistribute arsenic in the environment.[2]

It is impossible for animals, including humans, to avoid exposure to natural sources of arsenic. Complete avoidance may not be a good thing even if it were possible because animal studies show that trace amounts of dietary arsenic are beneficial.[3] Because of arsenic's pervasive nature, all food sources contain some arsenic.

Arsenic is present in all natural water supplies, but the concentrations vary greatly. Arsenic in water usually comes from natural sources. Naturally high arsenic concentrations occur in water from hot springs, ground water in areas of thermal activity, ground water in areas with high arsenic content in rocks, and water with a high dissolved salt content. High arsenic levels in rivers and lakes are usually caused by human sources (e.g., mining).

Commercial use of arsenic has been declining since the 1960s. A large percentage of commercial arsenic is still used in wood preservation; however, the EPA banned the use of chromated copper arsenate (CCA)–treated lumber for residential use as of January 2004. This ban targets areas around the home, including decks and playsets. According to the U.S. Department of Health and Human Services, potential sources of arsenic exposure include the following:[4]

Natural sources: volcanoes (as released into air), arsenic-containing mineral ores, and ground water (especially near geothermal activity).

Commercial products: wood preservatives, pesticides, herbicides (weed killers, defoliants), fungicides, cotton desiccants, cattle and sheep dips, paints and pigments, antifouling paints, leaded gasoline, and fire salts.

Food: wine (grapes sprayed with arsenic-containing pesticides), tobacco (plants sprayed with arsenic-containing pesticides), seafood (especially bivalves, certain cold water and bottom-feeding finfish, and seaweed).

Industrial processes: smelting, purifying industrial gases (removal of sulfur), burning fossil fuels, burning wood treated with arsenic preservatives, electronics manufacturing, hardening metal alloys, preserving animal hides, bronze plating, and clarifying glass and ceramics.

Medicinals: feed additives for domestic animals, Fowler's solution, antiparasitic drugs, Donovan's solution, folk remedies, kelp-containing health foods, and some naturopathic remedies.

In the past, roach and ant baits were common sources of arsenic poisoning in small animals. However, in 1989 the Environmental Protection Agency instituted a phase-out of certain arsenic-containing ant poisons in an attempt to reduce the risk of children ingesting arsenic.[4] The ASPCA Animal Poison Control Center (APCC) receives fewer calls about arsenic than it did 15 to 20 years ago. However, most current calls about arsenic exposure pertain to ingestion of ant baits still on the market. In the past, the organic arsenic thiacetarsamide (Caparsolate®) was used for the treatment of heartworm disease and could cause systemic poisoning in apparently healthy dogs.[5] Currently the only drug approved to treat heartworm disease in dogs is another organic arsenical called melarsomine (Immiticide®).

Toxic Dose

I am an evil, poisonous smoke . . .
But when from poison I am freed,
Through art and sleight of hand
Then can I cure both man and beast,
From dire disease ofttimes direct them;
But prepare me correctly, and take great care
That you faithfully keep watchful guard over me;
For else I am poison, and poison remain,
That pierces the heart of many a one.

Valentini, 1694

This poem exposes the double-edged nature of arsenic. By 2000 BC arsenic trioxide, produced as a byproduct of copper smelting, was used as a medicine and a poison. Professional poisoners used arsenic extensively in the Middle Ages. In fact, in the nineteenth century, one third of the criminal poisonings in France were blamed on arsenic.[6]

In the 1700s and 1800s, a 1% solution of arsenic trioxide called Fowler's solution was used extensively as medicine to such diseases as psoriasis and bronchial asthma. The mild toxic side effects of gastrointestinal discomfort and pain were ignored. If the oral dose could not be tolerated, per rectum administration was used. If the treatment caused severe signs of vomiting and diarrhea, the dose was lowered.[6]

Factors affecting the toxicity of inorganic arsenic include purity, solubility, particle size, valence, the species exposed, and physical condition of the animal exposed. The toxicity increases as the purity and solubility increase, and the particle size decreases. Trivalent arsenicals are 4 to 10 times more toxic than pentavalent arsenicals. Susceptibility to inorganic arsenic varies among domestic species and is highest in cats (lethal dose <5 mg/kg of sodium arsenate) followed by horses, cattle, sheep, swine, and birds.[7] Humans are also very susceptibile to poisoning by inorganic arsenic.[8] As expected, weak, debilitated, and dehydrated animals are more susceptible to arsenic toxicosis than are normal healthy animals.[9] The lethal dose, because of the aforementioned factors, varies greatly; however, the single lethal oral dose of inorganic trivalent arsenic in most species falls within a range of 1 to 25 mg/kg of body weight. In swine, exposure to 500 ppm arsanilic acid in the feed for 7–10 days caused feed additive toxicosis.[7] In a dog, 7.3 mg/kg of thiacetarsemide (three times overdosage) resulted in death caused by severe respiratory depression and pulmonary edema, and melarsomine at 7.5 mg/kg (three times overdosage) in healthy dogs caused death.[10]

Toxicokinetics

The gastrointestinal tract and skin readily absorb soluble arsenicals.[7] If the arsenical is relatively insoluble, it will have limited contact with the gastrointestinal mucosa and will not be extensively absorbed. Limited gastrointestinal absorption also occurs if the particle size of a powdered arsenical is too large. Lack of absorption is why insoluble arsenical compounds or arsenicals consisting of coarse particles are less toxic than are highly soluble arsenicals. Topically applied inorganic arsenicals not only cause local skin damage, but also can cause systemic poisoning. Respiratory absorption depends on the chemical form of the inorganic arsenical inhaled.

After absorption, arsenic is transported in the blood to all organs of the body. Clearance of arsenic from the blood of most species follows a two- or three-phase exponential curve. The first phase is the largest (>90%). Arsenic is eliminated rapidly with a half-life of 1 to 2 hours. The second and third phases have estimated half-lives of 30 and 200 hours, respectively.

From the blood, arsenic accumulates to the greatest extent in the liver, spleen, kidney, lungs, and gastrointestinal tract. Clearance from these organs is rapid. Chronic residues are found in tissues that contain keratin, such as skin, hair, and nails.[4] Placental transfer of arsenic has been shown in hamsters, mice, and monkeys.[11,12] Two to 3 days after a one-time exposure to inorganic arsenic, the concentration of arsenic in most organs falls off rapidly.

In most species, 40% to 70% of an absorbed dose of inorganic arsenic is excreted in the urine within 48 hours.[13] Urinary excretion rates of arsenic are affected by valence, degree of methylation, dose, route of exposure, and animal species.[13] Urinary arsenic is present as inorganic arsenic, methylarsonic acid, or cacodylic acid.

The proposed detoxification of inorganic arsenic goes as follows: The pentavalent form is reduced to the trivalent form, then a methyl group is added to form methylarsonic acid, and a second methyl group is added to form dimethylarsinic acid. The more efficient the methylation process is, the more efficient the urinary excretion. Sweat, hair, milk, skin desquamation, and exhalation are arsenic elimination routes of low significance relative to urinary excretion. Limited amounts of systemic arsenic are eliminated in the feces.

Mechanism of Toxicity

Trivalent arsenicals are 4 to 10 times more toxic than pentavalent arsenicals. Trivalent arsenicals interact with sulfhydryl groups of compounds in biologic systems. In many cases this alters the activity of vital pathways and causes toxicosis. Although most documentation involves inactivation of enzymes, coenzymes and substrates also can be affected.[14] Long lists have been compiled of enzymes susceptible to disruption by trivalent arsenic.[14,15]

Pentavalent arsenicals are reduced to more toxic trivalent forms in vivo. However, pentavalent arsenic ion (arsenate) can also cause direct toxic effects. Squibb and Fowler[14] have summarized the literature that shows that arsenate ion is isosteric and isoelectric with the phosphate ion. Therefore arsenate can substitute for phosphate in many important metabolic reactions. The arsenate esters formed undergo instantaneous spontaneous hydrolysis that is termed *arsenolysis*. This process interrupts metabolic pathways by spontaneous breakdown of crucial intermediates, such as glucose-6-arsenate. Also, cell energy stores can be depleted by the production of adenosine diphosphate arsenate instead of adenosine triphosphate, which spontaneously hydrolyzes, thereby producing no energy.[14,16]

Many acute toxic effects of inorganic arsenicals are attributed to effects on the vascular system.[4,17,18] Congestion, edema, and hemorrhage are commonly found in the visceral organs of animals with acute poisoning. This effect appears to be due to the relaxation and increased permeability of capillaries. Research in dogs with thiacetarsemide, a trivalent organic arsenical, shows a direct effect on arteries and the coagulation system.[19,20] Because trivalent organoarsenicals and inorganic arsenicals are considered to have the same mechanism of action, this finding supports the previous conclusion that inorganic arsenic is a "vascular poison." It is clear that splanchnic capillary networks are affected by arsenic.[18]

Even though arsenic has been associated with multiple types of cancer in humans, attempts to produce cancer in experimental animals have been inconclusive.[4,21]

Clinical Signs

Inorganic and organic trivalent arsenicals cause similar clinical signs. Peracute to acute oral poisonings induce dramatic signs, with resulting high morbidity and mortality. Signs may occur within minutes and death within hours if a high dose of dissolved arsenic is ingested. Signs develop as follows: intense abdominal pain, salivation, vomiting, staggering gait and weakness, diarrhea, rapid weak pulse, prostration, subnormal temperature, collapse, and death. The course of subacute oral poisoning is basically the same as the acute course but is slightly prolonged. Death occurs in several days. This is long enough for anorexia and oliguria to develop and be assessed. Urine may contain protein, red blood cells, and casts.[1,9]

If acute toxicosis occurs by skin contact, systemic signs may occur. However, skin lesions are prominent with blistering, edema, cracking, bleeding, and secondary infection.[1,22]

There is little documentation of spontaneous chronic arsenic poisoning in animals. However, the human medical literature is filled with descriptions of human populations that have been chronically exposed to arsenic. The descriptions vary considerably and may even conflict, reflecting the variation in exposure scenarios. Pershagen[6] reviewed numerous epidemiological studies of chronic human exposure to arsenic. The major changes cited were hyperpigmentation, palmoplantar hyperkeratosis, basal cell carcinoma, and squamous cell carcinoma of the skin; rhinopharyngolaryngitis; nasal septum perforation; bronchitis; emphysema; lung cancer; portal hypertension, cirrhosis, and angiosarcoma in the liver; cardiovascular disease; anemia; granulocytopenia; lymphocyte chromosome abnormalities; neoplasia of the hematopoietic and lymphatic systems; peripheral neuropathy; encephalopathy; congenital defects; and spontaneous abortion.

Subchronic to chronic experimental oral exposure of dogs to inorganic arsenic causes a dose-dependent weight loss or reduced weight gain.[23,24] Weight loss in dogs was shown to be an effect of feed rejection, not a direct effect of arsenic.[24]

Although the liver and the kidneys are considered major target organs, only subtle changes occur consistently in chronic studies. After 6 months of exposure to dietary arsenic, dogs exhibited mild increases in serum aspartate transaminase (AST) and serum alanine transaminase (ALT). Other notable changes in the cell blood counts, urinalyses, and serum chemistries were not present.[24] Anemia has been reported in cases of chronic arsenic intoxication in dogs.[23]

Organic pentavalent arsenical feed additives cause different clinical signs than those caused by inorganic arsenic. These arsenicals cause incoordination and paralysis as a result of peripheral neuropathy.[1] Adverse effects associated with therapeutic use of thiacetarsamide sodium in treating heartworm disease in dogs include vomiting, nephrotoxicity, hepatotoxity, thrombocytopenia, and pulmonary artery emboli. If the product leaks from the vein during injection, swelling and pain and skin sloughing may occur at the injection site. Overdosage may cause respiratory depression, pulmonary edema, and death. Adverse effects associated with therapeutic use of melarsomine in treating heartworm disease in dogs may include injection site reactions, coughing, lethargy, anorexia, hypersalivation, hyperthermia, lung congestion, vomiting, and pulmonary thromboembolism. An overdosage of melarsomine can cause respiratory distress, hypersalivation, restlessness, panting, vomiting, diarrhea, tremors, ataxia, cyanosis, and death.[10]

Minimum Database

A serum chemistry panel and complete blood count are indicated in cases of poisonings, but the results are generally nonspecific. Evidence of dehydration with hemoconcentration, along with mild elevations in liver enzymes, are consistently observed changes. An urinalysis should be performed to determine the extent of renal damage and assess the animal's ability to excrete the arsenic.

Confirmatory Tests

If an animal has a history and clinical signs that are consistent with arsenic toxicosis, chemical analysis should be performed to confirm the presence of arsenic. Specimens that can be used for analysis include urine, liver, kidney, gastrointestinal contents, and the suspected source of contamination. Results of the analysis must be interpreted in light of the specific circumstances of the case, such as clinical signs, species of animal, type of specimen, time since exposure, exposure route, and type of arsenical.

Urine may be the best specimen for the determination of current exposure to arsenic. Normal background levels of arsenic in urine from dogs and cats should be less than 1 ppm. Depending on the factors listed earlier, urine arsenic levels in confirmed cases can vary from 2 to 100 ppm.[9,24] Urine concentrations drop dramatically within days once the exposure to arsenic has ceased. The kidney and liver are the next best specimens for arsenic analysis. Kidney and liver concentrations also drop rapidly after arsenic exposure has stopped. Normal liver and kidney arsenic values are 0.5 ppm or less. Concentrations of elemental arsenic greater than 10 ppm on a wet weight basis in the liver and kidney confirm arsenic poisoning.[9,25] Hair is a good dose-dependent indicator of chronic arsenic exposure in humans. However, confirmation of arsenic toxicosis using hair concentrations is not well documented in dogs and cats. In a 6-month dietary arsenic study, the control dogs had hair concentrations of 0.4 ppm of elemental arsenic.[24] With exposures of up to 4 mg of dietary sodium arsenite per kilogram of body weight per day for 6 months, hair concentrations averaged around 25 ppm of elemental arsenic. However, all dogs in the study were asymptomatic. Blood is generally not a useful specimen for the confirmation of arsenic exposure in domestic species, due to its short half-life. However, this test is offered by most laboratories and can be useful in some exposure circumstances.

Treatment

Critical patients should be stabilized before performing decontamination procedures. Patients that are exhibiting hypovolemic shock should be started on oxygen therapy and intravenous access obtained. Appropriate fluid therapy may include crystalloids, blood products, or colloids.[26] Once the patient is stabilized, decontamination measures can be instituted if the clinician feels the benefits of doing them outweigh the risks.

Decontamination for asymptomatic patients may include induction of emesis. For patients that can safely vomit, emesis may be effective if performed within 4 hours of ingestion.[27] If the patient is unable to safely vomit (e.g., is a species that cannot vomit or is symptomatic), gastric lavage using warm water or a 1% sodium bicarbonate solution can be considered.[9] Lavage should be performed with care since arsenic causes significant damage to the gastrointestinal (GI) tract. Activated charcoal is not recommended in arsenic exposures because it does not bind well to metals[28] and may complicate the course of treatment in the case of a GI perforation.

Depending on the solubility and concentration of the arsenical ingested, the time before onset of clinical signs of vomiting and GI distress can range from several minutes to several hours. The rapid onset of vomiting may protect dogs from severe toxicosis, depending on the amount of arsenic absorbed before the animal vomits. In other cases, especially in cats, if the arsenical ingested is highly concentrated and water soluble, a lethal dose can be absorbed even if vomiting starts within minutes of ingestion.

Chelation should be considered in arsenic exposures. Dimercaprol (British anti-lewisite, BAL) is a sulfhydryl-containing compound that chelates arsenic. British anti-lewisite is not very effective in advanced cases, so it should be given early after exposure. The drug itself is toxic, and therapy should be administered with care and clinical judgment. Signs of BAL toxicosis are vomiting, tremors, convulsions, and coma, culminating in death. However, toxic effects of BAL at therapeutic levels are not severe and are reversible as the drug is excreted. British anti-lewisite is excreted rapidly over a period of 3 to 4 hours. Therefore it is best to administer BAL at recommended (frequent) intervals to maximize its therapeutic effects and minimize its toxic effects.[29] Arsenic stored in tissue may be mobilized by chelator treatment, causing increased circulating arsenic levels and exacerbation of clinical signs of arsenic toxicosis. If this happens, a little extra BAL might be given. If therapy makes the animal worse over 2 to 3 days, the BAL dose may be too large for that animal.[29] When BAL binds to arsenic, the resulting relatively nontoxic complex is water soluble and is readily excreted in the urine.

In small animals, the dose of BAL is 2.5 to 5 mg/kg of body weight given intramuscularly as a 10% solution in oil. The dose of 5 mg/kg of body weight should be used only in acute cases and only on the first day of treatment. Injections should be repeated every 4 hours for the first 2 days, every 8 hours on the third day, and twice a day for the next 10 days until full recovery occurs.[30]

Meso-2,3-dimercaptosuccinic acid (DMSA or succimer) is a metal chelating agent that is less toxic than BAL. Because DMSA is hydrophilic, it may not remove arsenic that has escaped from the extracellular space as rapidly or completely as BAL. Therefore in cases of severe acute intoxication, especially with lipophilic organoarsenicals, BAL is preferred.[31] Meso-2,3-dimercaptosuccinic acid has been shown to be an effective antidote in dogs exposed to methylmercury and lead[32,33] and in mice, rats, and rabbits exposed to arsenic.[34,35,36] DMSA has been used successfully to chelate arsenic in humans, often following initial treatment with BAL once gastrointestinal injury has resolved and gut motility has returned in acutely ill patients.[37] At this time there are no arsenic studies in dogs to show the effectiveness or appropriate dose of this compound. However, the dose that is effective in dogs exposed to lead is 10 mg/kg of body weight per os every 8 hours for 10 days.[33] Experimentally hemodialysis facilitates an increased removal rate of arsenic from dogs.[38]

Intensive supportive care is crucial to a successful outcome in an arsenic exposure. Aggressive fluid therapy may be necessary to reverse dehydration caused by vomiting and diarrhea, and enhance arsenic excretion through the kidneys. Renal failure, liver damage, and electrolyte abnormalities should be monitored and appropriate therapy administered as indicated. The animal should be kept warm and comfortable and given symptomatic care.[39] Parenteral antibiotics are recommended to prevent secondary bacterial infections in the gut.[9] Antiemetic medications may be needed and other symptomatic and supportive care to control diarrhea. A high-quality diet should be fed in small portions, and the amounts given increased as the patient's GI tract can tolerate the food.[40]

Treatment of chronic poisoning starts with the removal of the source of the arsenic. Chelation therapy is usually not necessary because of the rapid excretion rate of arsenic.[36]

Prognosis

Prognosis for animals with acute poisoning is grave unless the diagnosis is made and treatment is started before clinical signs are advanced.[9,40]

Gross and Histologic Lesions

Peracute poisoning causes death so rapidly that no gross or microscopic lesions may be present. Gross lesions of acute and subacute poisoning consist of multifocal to diffuse reddening of the mucosa of the stomach and proximal small intestine; variable amounts of watery fluid in the gastrointestinal tract; a soft, yellow liver; and wet, red lungs. If the animal lives longer than a few hours, edema, hemorrhage, and necrosis of the gastrointestinal tract can lead to the presence of blood and shreds of mucosa in the stool. Perforation of the stomach or intestine may occur. There is splanchnic organ congestion with petechial hemorrhage of serous membranes. Hemorrhages are especially prominent in the heart.[1,16] Gastrointestinal lesions are the most consistent and prominent of those listed; the others may not be present.

Histologic lesions may include gastrointestinal mucosal and submucosal congestion, edema, and variable hemorrhage; gastrointestinal mucosal epithelial necrosis and sloughing; mild fatty degeneration and necrosis of the liver; renal tubular degeneration; and, if the animal lives 3 to 4 days following exposure, cerebral edema and petechiation.[1,9,16] Frank liver necrosis is not common, but has been reported in rabbits exposed to inorganic arsenicals and dogs exposed to arsphenamine (an aromatic organic arsenical).[41,42]

Renal tubular degeneration is reported by many authors as a common lesion produced by inorganic arsenicals. Tsukamoto and colleagues[43] reported renal tubular degeneration and necrosis in dogs exposed to intravenous sodium arsenate.

If the poisoning occurs by skin contact, many of the same systemic signs described previously occur. However, in these cases skin lesions are also prominent with blistering, edema, cracking, bleeding, and secondary infection.[1,21] Jubb and colleagues describe arsenic-induced dermatitis as intense erythema, necrosis, and sloughing. The residual ulcerative lesions are indolent.[17]

Differential Diagnoses

Because of the severe gastrointestinal signs, the differential diagnoses include viral or bacterial gastroenteritis (e.g., canine parvovirus), pancreatitis, paraquat, zinc phosphide poisoning, and ingestion of caustic agents or irritating plants. Other heavy metal toxicoses may cause similar signs (e.g., copper, zinc, inorganic mercury, thallium).

References

1. National Academy of Science: *Arsenic (NAS)*, Washington, DC, 1977, National Academy of Science.
2. Liu J, Goyer RA, Waalkes MP: Metals. In Klaassen CD, editor: *Casarett and Doull's toxicology*, ed 7, New York, 2008, McGraw-Hill Medical.
3. World Health Organization: *Arsenic: trace elements in human nutrition and health*, Geneva, 1996, World Health Organization.
4. Agency for Toxic Substances and Disease Registry: *Arsenic toxicity, case studies in environmental medicine*, Washington, DC, 1990, US Department of Health and Human Services.
5. Hoskins JD: Thiacetarsamide and its adverse effects. In Kirk RW, editor: *Current veterinary therapy X, small animal practice*, Philadelphia, 1989, WB Saunders.
6. Pershagen G: The epidemiology of human arsenic exposure. In Fowler BA, editor: *Biological and environmental effects of arsenic*, New York, 1983, Elsevier.
7. Osweiler GD: *Toxicology*, Philadelphia, 1996, Lippincott Williams & Wilkins.
8. Hayes WJ: *Pesticides studied in man*, Baltimore, 1982, Williams & Wilkins.
9. Osweiler GD, Carson TL, Buck WB, et al: *Clinical and diagnostic veterinary toxicology*, Dubuque, IA, 1985, Kendall/Hunt.
10. Plumb DC: *Plumb's veterinary drug handbook*, ed 5, Ames, IA, 2005, Blackwell Publishing.
11. Hanlon DP, Ferm VH: Placental permeability of arsenate ion during early embryogenesis in the hamster, *Experientia* 33:1221–1222, 1977.
12. Lindgren A, Vahter M, Dencker L: Autoradiographic studies on the distribution of arsenic in mice and hamsters administered (74)As-arsenite or -arsenate, *Acta Pharmacol Toxicol* 51:253–265, 1982.
13. Vahter M: Metabolism of arsenic. In Fowler BA, editor: *Biological and environmental effects of arsenic*, New York, 1983, Elsevier.
14. Squibb KS, Fowler BA: The toxicity of arsenic and its compounds. In Fowler BA, editor: *Biological and environmental effects of arsenic*, New York, 1983, Elsevier.
15. Webb JL: *Enzyme and metabolic inhibitors*, vol 3, New York, 1966, Academic Press.
16. Moore SA, Moennich DMC, Gresser MJ: Synthesis and hydrolysis of ADP-arsenate by beef heart submitochondrial particles, *J Biol Chem* 258:6266–6271, 1983.

17. Jubb KVF, Huxtable CR: The nervous system. In Jubb KVF, Kennedy PC, Palmer N, editors: *Pathology of domestic animals*, ed 4, vol 1, New York, 1993, Academic Press.
18. Hanna C, McHugo PB: Studies on the capillary and cardiovascular actions of intravenous sodium arsenate and arsenite, *Toxicol Appl Pharmacol* 2:674–682, 1960.
19. Boudreaux MK, Dillon AR: Platelet function, antithrombin-III activity, and fibrinogen concentration in heartworm-infected and heartworm-negative dogs treated with thiacetarsamide, *Am J Vet Res* 52(12):1986–1991, 1991.
20. Maksimowich DS, Bell TG, Williams J, et al: Effect of arsenical drugs on in vitro vascular responses of pulmonary artery from heartworm-infected dogs, *Am J Vet Res* 58(4):389–393, 1997.
21. Chan PC, Huff J: Arsenic carcinogenesis in animals and in humans: mechanistic, experimental, and epidemiological evidence, *Environ Carcino and Ecotox Rev* 15(2):83–122, 1997.
22. Evinger JV, Blakemaore JC: Dermatitis in a dog associated with exposure to an arsenic compound, *J Am Vet Med Assoc* 184:1281–1282, 1984.
23. Byron WR, Bierbower GW, Brouwer JB, et al: Pathological changes in rats and dogs from two-year feeding of sodium arsenite or sodium arsenate, *Toxicol Appl Pharmacol* 10:132–147, 1967.
24. Neiger RD, Osweiler GD: Effect of subacute low level dietary sodium arsenite on dogs, *Fund Appl Toxicol* 13:439–451, 1989.
25. Neiger RD, Osweiler GD: Arsenic concentrations in tissues and body fluids of dogs on chronic low-level dietary sodium arsenite, *J Vet Diagn Invest* 4:334–337, 1992.
26. Matthews KA: *Veterinary emergency and critical care manual*, Guelph, 2006, Lifelearn.
27. Garland T: Arsenic. In Gupta RC, editor: *Veterinary toxicology basic and clinical principles*, New York, 2007, Academic Press.
28. Rosedale ME: Decontamination strategies, *Vet Clin Small Anim* 32:311–321, 2002.
29. Hatch RC: Poisons causing abdominal distress or liver or kidney damage. In Booth NH, McDonald LE, editors: *Veterinary pharmacology and therapeutics*, ed 6, Ames, IA, 1988, Iowa State University Press.
30. Szabuniewiez M, Bailey EM, Wiersig DO: Treatment of some common poisonings in animals, *Vet Med Small Anim Clin* 66:1197, 1971.
31. Muckter H, Leibl B, Reichl FX, et al: Are we ready to replace dimercaprol (BAL) as an arsenic antidote? *Hum Exp Toxicol* 16(8):460–465, 1997.
32. Kostyniak PJ: Methylmercury removal in the dog during infusion of 2,3-dimercaptosuccinic acid (DMSA), *J Toxicol Environ Health* 11(4-6):947–957, 1983.
33. Ramsey DT, Casteel SW, Faggella AM, et al: Use of orally administered succimer (meso-2,3-dimercaptosuccinic acid) for treatment of lead poisoning in dogs, *J Am Vet Med Assoc* 208(3):371–375, 1996.
34. Tripathi N, Flora SJ: Effects of some thiol chelators on enzymatic activities in blood, liver and kidneys of acute arsenic (III) exposed mice, *Biomed Environ Sci* 11(1):38–45, 1998.
35. Flora SJ, Dube SN, Arora U, et al: Therapeutic potential of meso 2,3-dimercaptosuccinic acid or 2,3-dimercaptopropane 1-sulfonate in chronic arsenic intoxication in rats, *Biometals* 8(2):111–116, 1995.
36. Inns RH, Rice P, Bright JE, et al: Evaluation of the efficacy of dimercapto chelating agents for the treatment of systemic organic arsenic poisoning in rabbits, *Hum Exp Toxicol* 9(4):215–220, 1990.
37. Lenz K, Hruby K, Druml W, et al: 2,3-dimercaptosuccinic acid in human arsenic poisoning, *Arch Toxicl* 47:241–243, 1981.
38. Sheabar FZ, Yannai S, Taitelman U: Efficiency of arsenic clearance from human blood in vitro and from dogs in vivo by extracorporeal complexing haemodialysis, *Pharmacol Toxicol* 64(4):329–333, 1989.
39. Gossel TA, Bricker JD: *Principles of clinical toxicology*, New York, 1984, Raven Press.
40. Furr AL: Arsenic poisoning. In Kirk RW, editor: *Current veterinary therapy VI: small animal practice*, Philadelphia, 1977, WB Saunders.
41. Soffer LJ, Dantes DA, Sobotka H: Electrolytes of blood and urine of dogs with acute hepatic injury produced by arsphenamine, *Arch Intern Med* 60:509–521, 1937.
42. Von Glahn WC, Flinn FB, Keim WF: Effect of certain arsenates on the liver, *Arch Pathol* 25:488–505, 1938.
43. Tsukamoto H, Parker HR, Gribble DH, et al: Nephrotoxicity of sodium arsenate in dogs, *Am J Vet Res* 4:2324–2330, 1983.

Botulism

E. Murl Bailey Jr., DVM, PhD, DABVT

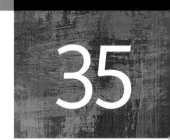

- Botulinum toxins are the most toxic substances known.
- Animals are susceptible to at least three of the seven known types of botulism toxins.
- Exposures may be either oral or inhalation.
- The disease is characterized by a progressive, ascending paralysis. Cranial nerve involvement also occurs.
- Death results from skeletal muscle paralysis and ventilatory failure.
- Identification of the toxin is difficult in cases of inhalation exposure, but can be identified from intestinal contents following oral exposures.
- An antitoxin is available but not effective after the toxin has entered the nerves.
- Treatment includes respiratory support and good nursing care.

Botulism is a disease caused by one or more of the seven toxins that may be produced by various strains of *Clostridium botulinum,* a spore-forming, obligate anaerobic bacillus, commonly found in the soil and very easily isolated.[1] The clostridial neurotoxins are the most toxic substances known, and only tetanus toxin from *C. tetani* and *Shigella* neurotoxins appear to have potencies of the same order of magnitude.[2,3,4]

In the 1930s the Japanese biological warfare group (Unit 731) fed *C. botulinum* cultures to prisoners in Manchuria, and the United States' biological weapons program, which was ended in 1970, produced botulism toxin and botulism toxoid in the 1940s in response to suspected German toxin weapons.[2] Botulism is an acute, afebrile, symmetrical, descending flaccid paralysis that always begins in the bulbar musculature in humans, but is a progressive, symmetrical, ascending paralysis in dogs.[4,5] Botulinum toxin remains a potential terrorist weapon delivered either by contaminating food- or feedstuffs or in an aerosol form. The likelihood of botulinum toxin contaminating municipal water supplies is highly unlikely because the toxin is rapidly inactivated by standard potable water treatments, and large amounts of toxin would be required.[4] There are some doubts whether botulinum toxin could be a weapon because of constraints in concentrating and stabilizing the toxin for aerosol dispersion.[2] A deliberate release of a point-source aerosol botulinum toxin in an urban environment could incapacitate or kill approximately 10% of the exposed human population.[2] At a minimum, the same percent morbidity and mortality could be expected of an exposed animal population.

Sources

The seven distinct botulinum toxins are defined by their antigenicity.[2] In addition to *C. botulinum,* other clostridial strains may produce the toxins. The toxin is a dichain polypeptide weighing approximately 150 kDa, which consists of a 100-kDa "heavy" chain and a 50-kDa "light" chain. Botulinum toxin in solution is colorless, odorless, and, as far as is known, tasteless. It is inactivated by heat (>85° C for 5 minutes).[2] The seven types of botulinum toxins (A–G) do not necessarily cause diseases in all mammals. Types C and D normally occur in domestic animals and wildlife, and type G is a soil isolate from South America. Primates are susceptible to aerosol samples of all three.[2] Types A, B, E, and F have been isolated in food poisoning cases in humans. Exposure to naturally occurring botulinum toxin may occur by consuming poorly preserved food in the case of humans and possibly small animals, dogs and cats ingesting carrion, spoiled meat and compost piles, and animals ingesting decomposing animal carcasses.[5-7]

Toxic Dose

LD_{50}s (IV and intraperitoneal [IP]) of the various botulinum toxins range from 0.1 to 40 ng/kg (1 ng = 0.000001 mg).[8] The cattle IV median lethal dose is 0.388 ng/kg.[7] It is estimated that the oral dose of botulinum toxin is 500 to 700 times greater than the parenteral dose and 77 to 100 times greater than the inhalational dose.[2] The estimated human parenteral lethal dose is 1.3 to 2.4 ng/kg, and the parenteral minimum lethal dose in humans is estimated to be 1 ng/kg. The human inhalational lethal dose is approximately 0.01 mcg/kg, and the oral lethal dose is 1 mcg/kg.[4] Most avian species are affected by botulinum toxin, including domesticated and wild fowl.[9,10] Based on a limited number of birds, the American turkey vulture (*Cathartes aura septentrionalis*) appears to be resistant to the effects of botulinum toxin.[2,4,10]

Toxicokinetics

Botulinum toxins may be absorbed via any mucosal surface but most commonly are absorbed through the gastrointestinal tract following oral exposure.[2] In the case of inhalational exposure, botulinum toxins may be absorbed through the lungs, as has been shown experimentally in primates and humans after a laboratory mishap.[11] The botulinum toxin weapon was developed for this purpose. Botulinum toxins may be absorbed through devitalized wounds containing anaerobic tissue. The toxins do not penetrate through intact skin. The botulinum toxins are distributed by the blood to the various tissues, but they do not penetrate the blood-brain barrier. The biotransformation mechanisms and excretion mechanism of the botulinum toxins are unknown,[2] but neutralizing antibodies play a role in the biotransformation of it.[12] The botulinum toxins are not tightly bound to blood constituents and the elimination $T_{1/2}$ of the botulinum toxins from the blood is 230 to 260 minutes.[12] Although it is not known whether botulinum toxins are excreted in milk, if botulinum toxins were placed in milk and milk products before pasteurization, the pasteurization temperatures would inactivate 99.5% to 99.99% of the toxin.[13]

Mechanism of Toxicity

Botulinum toxin binds to the presynaptic membrane at the neuromuscular synapse, but the structure of the receptor(s) is (are) unknown. The receptor-bound toxin is internalized by a mechanism known as receptor-mediated endocytosis, and the vesicles are transported within the cell.[2,14] The light (50 kDa) chain is cleaved from the heavy chain, leaves the vesicle, and prevents the synaptic vesicle containing acetylcholine from fusing with the neuronal membrane. This action prevents the release of the acetylcholine and results in a flaccid paralysis in which the muscles are unable to contract.[4,7] Interestingly, botulinum toxin A has been demonstrated to have therapeutic efficacy in the treatment of urinary incontinence in female dogs lasting up to 4 months.[15]

Clinical Signs

With naturally occurring botulism, there might be a history of unsupervised animals with access to carrion, garbage, and compost piles.[5] In the case of inhalational exposures, presenting animals may be the first indication of a terrorist action in the area. The chief complaint is a progressive rear end weakness or paresis starting 12 hours to 6 days postexposure. Possible signs include progressive, symmetrical paresis and/or paralysis beginning in the pelvic limbs, and ascending to include the thoracic limbs. Cranial nerve signs include mydriasis, slow pupillary light response, decreased jaw tone, decreased palpebral and gag reflexes, and weak vocalization. Keratitis and conjunctivitis may occur because of weak palpebral reflexes. The respiratory pattern is characterized by diaphragmatic respirations with limited costal respirations. Bradycardia, constipation, and urinary retention are common. As in humans, there is no loss of mental awareness or pain perception. Interestingly, in dogs the tail wag is usually present.[5] Megaesophagus and aspiration pneumonia may be complicating factors.[16]

Minimum Database

There are no common laboratory abnormalities typical of botulism.[5] The occurrence of secondary bacterial infections may cause white blood cell abnormalities, and, depending on the time sequence, an increased packed-cell volume may be seen if dehydration is occurring. An electromyogram (EMG) may or may not be beneficial. Because megaesophagus commonly occurs, thoracic radiographs are indicated.[14]

Confirmatory Tests

The definitive diagnosis depends on toxin identification. In the case of oral exposures, most diagnostic laboratories that offer this analysis require at least 4 mL of serum and 50 g of vomitus, feces, or ingested food samples. It is best to call the laboratory that is doing the testing in advance to find out what samples are most appropriate and how to properly preserve them. In the case of inhalational exposure with botulinum toxins, the toxins cannot be identified in body fluids other than nasal secretions. Therefore the best diagnostic sample for immunological identification is from nasal mucosal swabs obtained within 24 hours of exposure.[2,17]

Treatment

Treatment in cases of botulism normally includes supportive therapy consisting of maintaining hydration and nutritional support.[5] If the animal is hypoxemic, oxygen therapy, including a tracheostomy and intermittent positive pressure ventilation (IPPV), may be indicated. In animals able to swallow, hand feeding and watering may be used. If the animal is unable to swallow, enteral feeding is indicated via a nasogastric, esophagostomy, or gastrotomy tube.[14]

Soft bedding with frequent repositioning is required to prevent decubital ulcers and atelectasis leading to the development of pneumonia. Animals with megaesophagus may develop aspiration pneumonia. Additional nursing care may include eye ointment to prevent keratitis, warm water enemas, and periodic expressing of the urinary bladder.[5,14]

A licensed antitoxin is available but is of no value for toxins already internalized into the neurons.[2] If available, 5 mL of the antitoxin should be administered IV or IM once as early as possible, but within 5 days of exposure.[5] The antitoxin is made from horse serum; therefore, the clinician should administer a test dose of the antitoxin intradermally before administering the antitoxin to determine any hypersensitivity. The clinician should be ready to treat an allergic reaction.

Prognosis

The prognosis for clinically affected animals is guarded to poor.

Gross and Histologic Lesions

No specific gross or histologic changes have been reported.

Differential Diagnoses

Differential diagnoses should include tick paralysis, coonhound paralysis, myasthenia gravis, the dumb form of rabies, coral snake bite, ionophore poisoning, macadamia nut ingestion, and low-dose exposure to some organophosphate insecticides.[5,16]

In the case of tick paralysis, there will be a history of finding either *Dermacentor variabilis* or *D. andersoni* in the United States or *Ixodes holocyclus* in Australia.[5,16] There are no cranial nerve abnormalities as are present in botulism toxicosis. The clinical signs rapidly abate following tick removal and/or treatment with organophosphate insecticide solutions along with appropriate nursing care.

Animals with coonhound paralysis generally have a slower onset of signs (7–9 days).[5,16] Pronounced muscle atrophy is usually present, and cranial nerve signs are either mild or absent.

In animals with myasthenia gravis, the signs are episodic and most commonly related to exercise.[5,16] Edrophonium causes an improvement of clinical signs and may be treated with supportive care and/or anticholinesterase drugs. A large number of these animals may have a spontaneous recovery.[16]

Animals with the dumb form of rabies sometimes exhibit muscular weakness.[5] Immunization status should be confirmed and the possibility of exposure to rabid animals explored. Appropriate safeguards must be instituted until a diagnosis is made.

Coral snake venom causes an ascending flaccid paralysis and depression in dogs and cats.[18] The onset of the clinical signs may be delayed for 10 to 18 hours. This is in contrast to the 12-hour to 6-day delay of onset of signs in botulism. A history of exposure and/or the presence of bite wounds should assist in the diagnosis.[18]

Dogs and especially cats may develop a general neuromuscular weakness syndrome after an acute or chronic exposure to some organophosphate insecticides.[19,20] This syndrome has been characterized as the "intermediate" syndrome.[19,20] Many of these animals respond to appropriate doses of atropine and pralidoxime (2-PAM) for several days.[19,20] Acetylcholinesterase levels may be depressed at the time of presentation.

Ionophore intoxication generally can be confirmed through exposure history and analyzing serum, stomach contents, or suspect feed material for the presence of ionophores. Macadamia nut ingestion is generally confirmed through exposure history.[8]

References

1. Robinson RF, Nahata MC: Management of botulism, *Ann Pharmacother* 37:127–131, 2003.
2. Middlebrook JL, Franz DR: Botulinum toxins. In Sidell FR, Takafuji ET, Franz DR, editors: *Medical aspects of chemical and biological warfare*, Washington, DC, 1997, Office of the Surgeon General at TMM Publications, Borden Institute, Walter Reed Army Medical Center.
3. Lamanna C: The most poisonous poison, *Science* 130:763–772, 1959.
4. Arnon SS, Schecter R, Inglesgy TV, et al: Botulinum toxin as a biological weapon: medical and public health management, *JAMA* 285(8):1059–1070, 2001.
5. Manning AM: Standards of care: emergency and critical care medicine, *Vet Learn Sys* 3(10):1–6, 2001.
6. Kalluri P, Crowe C, Reller M, et al: An outbreak of foodborne botulism associated with food sold at a salvage store in Texas, *Clin Infect Dis* 37:1490–1495, 2003.
7. Moeller RB, Puschner B, Walker RL, et al: Determination of the median toxic dose of type *C. botulinum* toxin in lactating dairy cows, *J Vet Diagn Invest* 15:523–526, 2003.
8. Gill DM: Bacterial toxins: a table of lethal amounts, *Microbiol Rev* 46(1):86–94, 1982.
9. Poppenga RH: Common toxicoses of waterfowl, loons, and raptors. In Kirk RW, Bonagura JD, editors: *Current veterinary therapy XI: small animal practice*, Philadelphia, 1992, Saunders.
10. Levine ND: Listerosis, botulism, erysipelas and goose influenza. In Biester HE, Schwarte LH, editors: *Diseases of poultry*, ed 5, Ames, IA, 1965, Iowa State University Press.
11. Street CS: Experimental botulism in the monkey. In Hassett CC, editor: *Proceedings of a conference on botulinum toxin*, Arsenal, MD, June 28-29, 1965, Edgewood.
12. Ravichandran E, Gong Y, Al Saleem FH, et al: An initial assessment of the systemic pharmacokinetics of botulinum toxin, *J Pharmacol Exp Ther* 318:1343–1351, 2006.

13. Weingart O, Schreiber T, Mascher C, et al: The case of botulinum toxin in milk: experimental data, *Appl Environ Microbiol* 76:3293–3300, 2010.
14. Hackett R, Kam PCA: Botulinum toxin: pharmacology and clinical developments: a literature review, *Med Chem* 3:333–345, 2007.
15. Lew S, Makewski M, Radziszewski P, Kuleta Z: Therapeutic efficacy of botulinum toxin in the treatment of urinary incontinence in female dogs, *Acta Veterinaria Hungarica* 58:157–165, 2010.
16. Shelton GD: Myasthenia gravis and disorders of neuromuscular transmission, *Vet Clin North Am Sm Anim Pract* 32(1):189–206, 2002.
17. Bruchim Y, Steinman A, Markovitz M, et al: Toxicological, bacteriological and serological diagnosis of botulism in a dog, *Vet Rec* 158:768–769, 2005.
18. Peterson ME: Snake bite: coral snake. In Peterson ME, Talcott PA, editors: *Small animal toxicology*, ed 2, Philadelphia, 2006, Saunders.
19. Jaggy A, Oliver JE: Chlorpyrifos toxicosis in two cats, *J Vet Int Med* 4:135–139, 1990.
20. Anonymous: *The Merck veterinary manual*, ed 9, Whitehouse Station, NJ, 2005, Merck.

Bromethalin

David C. Dorman, DVM, PhD, DABVT, DABT

36

- Bromethalin is a neurotoxic rodenticide that produces cerebral edema in dogs, cats, and other species (Color Plate 36-1).
- Minimal oral toxic doses are approximately 0.3 and 2.5 mg/kg in cats and dogs, respectively.
- Extremely high doses produce muscle tremors, increased activity, hyperthermia, and seizures within 2 or more hours after ingestion.
- More frequently bromethalin poisoning develops 12 to 24 hours after ingestion. Poisoned animals develop progressive ataxia, paresis, and hindlimb paralysis and intensifying central nervous system depression that may ultimately result in semicoma or coma. The most prominent lesion is diffuse white matter edema throughout the central nervous system.
- Diagnosis of bromethalin toxicosis is based on a history of exposure, development of compatible clinical signs, and chemical confirmation of bromethalin residues in fat, brain, liver, kidney, or other tissues.
- Treatment is via gastrointestinal tract decontamination, including appropriate use of emetics and repeated administration of oral activated charcoal. Control of cerebral edema is crucial. Mannitol, dexamethasone, and furosemide have been used with variable success. Symptomatic and supportive care, including control of seizures, is recommended.

Introduction

Bromethalin (2,4-dinitro-N-methyl-N-[2,4,6-tribromophenyl]-6-[trifluoromethyl] benzene-amine) was discovered in the mid-1970s[1] and has subsequently been incorporated into a number of rodenticide products. Bromethalin inhibits brain adenosine triphosphate (ATP) production and can be used to control warfarin-resistant rats and mice. Although the incidence of poisoning is not known, widespread use of bromethalin-based products occurs in the United States. As with other commonly used rodenticides, accidental poisoning of dogs, cats, and other companion animals with bromethalin is not uncommon. Malicious poisonings with bromethalin have also been documented.

Sources

Bromethalin-containing rodenticides have been marketed under a variety of trade names including Assault®, Gladiator®, Trounce® (PM Resources, Inc., Bridgeton, MO), Fastrac®, and Tomcat® (Bell Laboratories, Inc., Madison, WI), among others. Because pesticide formulations can change over time, it is critical that the active ingredient be identified whenever an animal consumes a rodenticide. Bromethalin-based products usually contain 0.01% bromethalin and are often manufactured in a pelleted or paraffinized bait block form. Pelletized products are typically sold as individual paper or plastic "place pack" envelopes that contain 16 to 42.5 g (0.57-1.5 oz) of bait. The size and weight of the rodenticide pellets vary depending on manufacturer and product use. Bromethalin is also sold to commercial pest control operators in bulk and in a concentrated (2%-10%) liquid or solid form.

Toxic Dose

Among the common experimental animal species evaluated to date, only guinea pigs have been demonstrated to be relatively resistant to bromethalin toxicosis. The basis for this resistance stems from the decreased ability of guinea pigs to metabolize bromethalin to its more toxic N-demethylated metabolite.[2] The reported median lethal dose (LD_{50}) of bromethalin is greater than 1000 mg/kg in the guinea pig.[2] In all other species examined to date, the acute (single-dose) oral LD_{50} ranges from approximately 1 to 15 mg/kg. Cats appear to be one of the species most sensitive to the toxic effects of bromethalin. For example, the oral LD_{50} of powdered bromethalin bait was found to be 0.54 mg/kg in experimental cats, whereas the LD_{50} in dogs was 3.7 mg/kg.[3,4] The reported oral LD_{50} of technical grade bromethalin ranges from 1.8 mg/kg in the cat to 4.7 mg/kg in the dog.These acute LD_{50}s provide an estimate of the amount of bromethalin required to be ingested to induce toxicity in dogs and cats. It is possible that individual cats and dogs could develop severe clinical signs following exposure to lower doses (e.g., ≥1/10 of an LD_{50}), especially with repeated exposure. Deaths have been reported in dogs ingesting bromethalin at doses as low as 0.95 to 1.05 mg/kg. Cats have shown clinical signs of toxicity after being exposed to dosages as low as 0.24 mg/kg. Secondary poisoning (relay toxicity) of animals resulting from the ingestion of bromethalin-poisoned rodents has not been demonstrated experimentally.[5] However, the author is aware of cases in which relay toxicosis most likely accounted for the animals' exposure.

Toxicokinetics

Most of the information about the metabolism and toxicokinetics of bromethalin has been obtained from experimental studies conducted with rats.[2] On ingestion, bromethalin is rapidly absorbed from the gastrointestinal tract (absorption half-life, approximately 2.7 hours), and peak plasma concentrations occur within 4 hours of ingestion. Bromethalin is rapidly metabolized by liver mixed-function oxygenases to its more toxic N-demethylated metabolite, desmethylbromethalin.

Bioactivation appears to play a crucial role in the development of toxicity because animal species (e.g., guinea pigs) that are unable to metabolize bromethalin to desmethylbromethalin are resistant to its toxic effects. Bromethalin and its metabolite are readily distributed throughout the body and reach their highest concentrations in body fat.[5] Bromethalin is excreted from the body relatively slowly with a plasma excretion half-life of approximately 6 days in the rat.[2] Urinary excretion of bromethalin is minimal and accounts for less than 3% of an oral dose; thus diuresis or other therapies directed at enhancing renal excretion are ineffective at altering bromethalin pharmacokinetics. Excretion of bromethalin occurs primarily through the bile. Total biliary excretion can account for 5% to 25% of an orally administered dose. Reabsorption of bromethalin excreted into the bile by the gastrointestinal tract probably occurs with subsequent cycling between the hepatobiliary system and the gastrointestinal tract. Interruption of the enterohepatic recirculation of bromethalin is a mainstay of decontamination therapy and relies on the repeated oral administration of activated charcoal.

Mechanism of Action

The presumed biochemical mechanism of action of bromethalin and its active metabolite, desmethylbromethalin, is uncoupling of oxidative phosphorylation. Uncoupling of oxidative phosphorylation has been demonstrated to occur in vitro in brain and liver mitochondria isolated from normal rats.[2] Uncoupling of oxidative phosphorylation results in decreased tissue ATP concentrations and reduced activity of ATP-dependent sodium and potassium ion channel pumps. The brain is the primary target site for the biochemical effects of bromethalin, most likely because of its enhanced dependence on oxidative phosphorylation. Inhibition of ATP production leads to impaired ion pump function, subsequent brain electrolyte imbalances, and the associated movement of fluid into the myelinated regions of the brain and spinal cord. Increased cerebral lipid peroxidation also occurs following bromethalin ingestion and may likewise contribute to the development of clinical signs.[6]

Clinical Signs

The primary target for bromethalin is the central nervous system (CNS), and most clinical signs are generally referable to that system. Clinical signs in affected animals can vary tremendously depending on the amount of bromethalin ingested and the stage of intoxication in which the animal is observed. Most animals that ingest a potentially toxic dose of bromethalin remain asymptomatic for the first several hours. The subsequent onset of clinical signs is dose-dependent. Animals that ingest a supralethal dose ($\geq LD_{50}$) of bromethalin often develop clinical signs within 2 to 24 hours of ingestion. This acute-onset syndrome is characterized by severe muscle tremors, hyperthermia, and extreme hyperexcitability, running fits, hyperesthesia, and focal motor and/or generalized seizures that appear to be precipitated by light or noise.[3,4] In many respects, the clinical signs induced by high-dose bromethalin exposure resemble toxic syndromes induced by strychnine or monosodium fluoroacetate (compound 1080) ingestion. Fortunately, such supralethal ingestions infrequently occur, and thus this acute-onset syndrome is rarely reported.

More commonly dogs and cats are exposed to lower doses of bromethalin, which produce a more delayed onset of neurologic signs. In these circumstances, it is not unusual for clinical signs to develop within several days of ingestion and then progress throughout a 1- or 2-week period.[3,4] Clinical signs observed in poisoned dogs and cats with this more typical toxic syndrome usually include hindlimb ataxia and paresis with associated decreased conscious proprioception of the hindlimbs (Figure 36-1). Severely affected animals eventually develop hindlimb paralysis followed by a diminished or absent deep pain response, patellar hyperreflexia, and upper motor neuron bladder paralysis. Mild to severe CNS depression is usually also present in animals presenting with bromethalin-induced ataxia and paresis, with severely affected animals developing semicoma or coma. Abdominal distention is occasionally observed in poisoned cats and has been characterized radiographically by the presence of enlarged bowel loops. Additional clinical signs that can be seen include vomiting, anorexia, anisocoria, behavioral changes ("dementia"), positional nystagmus, abnormal postures (e.g., Schiff-Sherrington, forelimb extensor rigidity), loss of vocalization, opisthotonus, and fine muscle tremors.[3,4,7] Focal motor or generalized seizures also occur in the latter stages of this syndrome. Severely poisoned dogs and cats may develop a decerebrate posture (Figure 36-2) during the terminal phases of the syndrome.

Minimum Database

In general, changes in serum electrolytes and chemistries are unremarkable following bromethalin ingestion. Dogs given bromethalin experimentally developed mild hyperglycemia during the toxic syndrome.[3] Changes in routine serum electrolytes and chemistries consistent with prolonged anorexia and dehydration could also occur during bromethalin toxicosis.

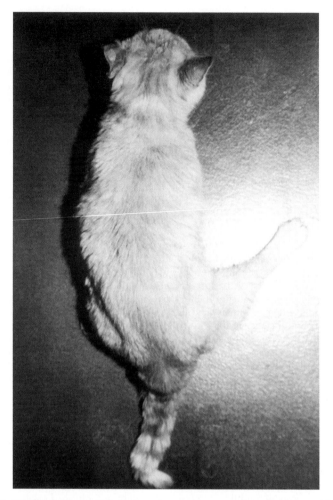

Figure 36-1 Hindlimb ataxia with decreased conscious proprioception in a cat 5 days after administration of bromethalin (0.45 mg/kg). (From Dorman DC: Emerging neurotoxicities. In August JR, editor: *Consultations in feline internal medicine,* ed 2, Philadelphia, 1994, WB Saunders, 429-436.)

As anticipated from the mechanism of action, clinical signs, and lesions, bromethalin toxicosis is associated with the development of increased cerebrospinal fluid (CSF) pressure.[2-4] For example, dogs given a lethal bromethalin dose (6.25 mg/kg) developed a modest elevation in CSF pressure (e.g., mean CSF pressure values observed in bromethalin-exposed dogs were 122 mm CSF versus 80 mm CSF in control dogs). The increase in CSF pressure observed in lethally poisoned dogs is not as severe as that observed with many other causes of cerebral edema (e.g., trauma). Localization of the edema to affected myelin sheaths likely limits the magnitude of the CSF pressure increases that occurs in poisoned animals. Examination of CSF from bromethalin-poisoned dogs revealed normal cytology, protein concentration, specific gravity, and cell count and was thus of limited diagnostic value.[3]

Although not specific for bromethalin toxicosis, electroencephalographic (EEG) abnormalities frequently occur in bromethalin-poisoned dogs and cats.[8,9] Electroencephalographic

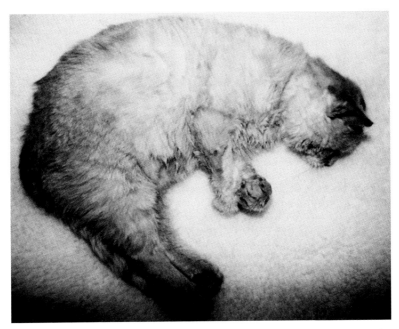

Figure 36-2 Severe CNS depression, recumbency, hindlimb extensor rigidity, and fore-limb flexion present in a cat 14 days after bromethalin (0.45 mg/kg) administration. This posture is often referred to as *decerebrate posture*. Animals placed on their backs demonstrate forelimb as well as hindlimb extensor rigidity. (From Dorman DC: Emerging neurotoxicities. In August JR, editor: *Consultations in feline internal medicine*, ed 2, Philadelphia, 1994, WB Saunders, 429-436.)

abnormalities include increased spike and spike-and-wave activity associated with an irritative or seizure focus, marked voltage depression indicative of cerebral hypoxia, and abnormal high voltage slow wave activities that are associated with the presence of cerebral edema. The reported EEG changes are not pathognomonic for bromethalin toxicosis and provide limited diagnostic utility.

Confirmatory Tests

An antemortem diagnosis of bromethalin poisoning rests on an exposure history to a potentially toxic dose of a bromethalin-based rodenticide and the subsequent development of appropriate clinical signs. Brain imaging studies in poisoned people have revealed the presence of hypodensities and other changes that were suggestive of brain edema that was predominantly affecting the white matter.[10] A postmortem diagnosis of bromethalin poisoning is often suggested by the presence of diffuse white matter vacuolization in CNS samples and can be confirmed by the presence of bromethalin residues in frozen fat, liver, kidney, and brain tissues.[5,10,11] Chemical confirmation of bromethalin residues is not widely available and may have limited clinical application in patients with a delayed presentation.

Treatment

Treatment of the exposed dog or cat is initially directed at reducing gastrointestinal absorption of bromethalin and providing symptomatic and supportive care. Because of its rapid absorption, emesis must be performed quickly after ingestion (1 hour) to produce a clinical benefit. Emetics that can be given safely to alert dogs and cats can include 3% hydrogen peroxide (1 mL/lb given per os [PO]), apomorphine (0.04 mg/kg, given intramuscularly [IM], in dogs), and xylazine (0.4 up to 1.1 mg/kg, IM or subcutaneously [SC], in cats) (see Chapter 10 for more information on emetics). Emetics should not be given to animals that are displaying dyspnea, hypoxia, seizures, CNS depression, or abnormal pharyngeal reflexes.

All animals should be given oral activated charcoal whenever a potentially toxic exposure may have occurred. Activated charcoal powder (1-4 g/kg) combined with sorbitol (70% solution at 3 mL/kg) or sodium sulfate (250 mg/kg) as a suspension in water (10 × volume) can be administered orally or by gastric tube. The use of magnesium sulfate as a saline cathartic is not recommended in animals with bromethalin toxicosis because elevated serum and brain magnesium levels may further exacerbate the development of CNS depression, especially in animals with decreased renal function. Some animals poisoned with bromethalin develop enlarged bowel loops consistent with adynamic (paralytic) ileus, and in these cases cathartics should not be used. Experimental studies conducted in dogs and cats have demonstrated that repeated administration of activated charcoal is more effective than administration of a single activated charcoal dose.[4,12] Smaller subsequent oral doses of activated charcoal (1 g/kg) with reduced sodium sulfate (125 mg/kg) should be given every 4 to 8 hours for at least 2 to 3 days to all animals that may have consumed a potentially lethal dose. The increased efficacy of repeated activated charcoal administration is likely due to its ability to disrupt the enterohepatic recirculation of bromethalin. Unfortunately, even repeated administration of activated charcoal may not be very effective, because delayed deaths were observed in cats 15 to 19 days after bromethalin administration despite the initial administration of four doses of activated charcoal.[4] This observation strongly suggests that prolonged (2-4 days) repeated administration of activated charcoal may be required following ingestion of a potentially lethal dose. Therefore, it is crucial that careful measures be used to maintain hydration status and monitor electrolyte balance after repeated cathartic use, especially when mannitol is used concurrently to control cerebral edema. Single or repeated doses of activated charcoal, particularly in small breed dogs, can lead to clinically significant hypernatremic situations, particularly when the patient is dehydrated or the toxin contains significant amounts of sodium.

It is also vital to control the cerebral edema and elevated intracranial pressure that occur in severe poisoning cases. Diuretic agents may be used to control bromethalin-induced cerebral edema.[2,4,12] Experimental studies conducted in bromethalin-poisoned rats showed that a constant infusion of mannitol or urea or the daily administration of dexamethasone resulted in reduced CSF pressure in rats given a sublethal bromethalin dose. Interestingly, the beneficial effects of mannitol and urea were transient and CSF pressure began to rise once these infusions were stopped. Several experimental studies have examined whether the combined administration of mannitol and dexamethasone could be effective in managing dogs or cats given a lethal dose of bromethalin.[4,12] Unfortunately, these therapies were neither effective in preventing signs from developing nor in reversing the neurotoxic syndrome once it had developed. Observed treatment failures with combined corticosteroid and mannitol therapy in dogs and cats given a lethal dose of bromethalin may indicate that in these species the toxic syndrome is not solely caused by cerebral edema. Alternatively, it is possible that the intramyelinic location of the edema may limit the effectiveness of corticosteroid and mannitol therapy.

Despite the treatment failures observed with mannitol and dexamethasone in research dogs and cats, the use of a hyperosmotic agent such as mannitol (250 mg/kg, given every 6 hours IV) is still indicated for the control of bromethalin-induced cerebral edema. Side effects associated with mannitol use include hypotension, hypernatremia, hyperkalemia, renal failure, and pulmonary edema. Animals receiving several days of mannitol therapy often become dehydrated during treatment. Rehydration of bromethalin-poisoned animals that have been subsequently treated with intravenous mannitol may produce a worsening of neurologic signs, probably because of the development of so-called rebound cerebral and pulmonary edema. Careful maintenance of the animal's hydration status is critical and can be accomplished most safely through the frequent oral administration of small amounts of water.

In many ways, furosemide (1 mg/kg, given IV every 4-6 hours) may be better than mannitol and other hyperosmolar agents because furosemide administration is not associated with rebound cerebral or pulmonary edema, fluctuations in serum osmolarity, or hypernatremia. High doses of dexamethasone (2 mg/kg, every 6 hours IV) can be used in conjunction with either mannitol or furosemide for the management of cerebral edema.

Diazepam (1-2 mg/kg, given IV as needed) and/or phenobarbital (5-15 mg/kg, given IV as needed) may be given to abolish severe muscle tremors and seizures. Many animals recovering from bromethalin toxicosis exhibit prolonged anorexia and may require supplemental feeding to maintain caloric intake. Recumbent animals should be placed in padded cages to prevent the development of decubital ulcers.

Prognosis

Some animals may recover from bromethalin toxicosis. In mild poisoning cases, overt clinical signs usually resolve within several weeks of ingestion, although subtle signs of neurologic dysfunction may persist. Animals with more severe clinical signs, including coma or paralysis, generally have a grave prognosis.

Gross and Histologic Lesions

Lesions are generally confined to the CNS. Gross evidence of cerebral edema may occur but is generally mild. Spongy degeneration of the cerebrum, cerebellum, brainstem, spinal cord, and optic nerve white matter occurs in lethally poisoned dogs and cats.[5,13] The myelin lesion is generally not associated with a leukocytic inflammatory response, gitter cell response, or axonal degeneration and may indeed be reversible. Ultrastructural findings include separation of myelin lamellae at the interperiod lines resulting in apparent intramyelinic edema, spongy changes owing to the rupture and coalescence of these intramyelinic vacuoles, and pronounced cytosolic edema of astrocytes and oligodendroglial cells.

Differential Diagnoses

Bromethalin poisoning in the cat and dog must be distinguished clinically from other neurologic syndromes produced by trauma, neoplasia, cerebral vascular disorders, and infectious and other toxic agents (e.g., macadamia nuts, ionophores, botulism, OP-induced intermediate syndrome, or delayed neuropathy). Similar clinical signs and white matter lesions may occur in hexachlorophene- or trialkyltin-poisoned animals; however, companion animal exposure to these agents is rare.

References

1. Dreikorn BA, O'Doherty GO: The discovery and development of bromethalin, an acute rodenticide with a unique mechanism of action. In Magee PS, Kohn GK, Menn JJ, editors: *Pesticide synthesis through rational approaches*, Washington, DC, 1984, American Chemical Society.
2. VanLier RBL, Cherry LD: The toxicity and mechanism of action of bromethalin: a new single-feeding rodenticide, *Fundam Appl Toxicol* 11:664–672, 1988.
3. Dorman DC, Parker AJ, Buck WB: Bromethalin toxicosis in the dog: I. Clinical effects, *J Am Assoc Anim Hosp* 26:589–594, 1990.
4. Dorman DC, Parker AJ, Dye JA, Buck WB: Bromethalin neurotoxicosis in the cat, *Prog Vet Neurol* 1: 189–196, 1990.
5. Dorman DC, Harlin KS, Simon J, Buck WB: Diagnosis of bromethalin poisoning in the dog, *J Vet Diag Invest* 2:123–128, 1990.
6. Dorman DC, Cote LM, Buck WB: Effects of an extract of *Gingko biloba* on bromethalin-induced cerebral peroxidation and edema, *Am J Vet Res* 53:138–142, 1992.
7. Martin T, Johnson B: A suspected case of bromethalin toxicity in a domestic cat, *Vet Hum Toxicol* 3: 239–240, 1989.

8. Dorman DC, Parker AJ, Schaeffer DJ, Buck WB: Quantitative and qualitative electroencephalographic changes in normal and bromethalin-dosed cats, *Prog Vet Neurol* 1:451–460, 1990.

9. Dorman DC, Parker AJ, Buck WB: Electroencephalographic changes associated with bromethalin toxicosis in the dog, *Vet Hum Toxicol* 33:9–11, 1991.

10. Pasquale-Styles MA, Sochaski MA, Dorman DC, et al: Fatal bromethalin poisoning, *J Forensic Sci* 51:1154–1157, 2006.

11. Braselton WE, Johnson M: Thin layer chromatography convulsant screen extended by gas chromatography-mass spectrometry, *J Vet Diagn Invest* 15:42–45, 2003.

12. Dorman DC, Parker AJ, Buck WB: Bromethalin toxicosis in the dog: II. Treatment of the toxic syndrome, *J Am Assoc Anim Hosp* 26:595–598, 1990.

13. Dorman DC, Zachary JF, Buck WB: Neuropathologic findings of bromethalin toxicosis in cats, *Vet Pathol* 29:139–144, 1992.

Carbon Monoxide

Kevin T. Fitzgerald, PhD, DVM, DABVP

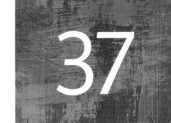

37

- Carbon monoxide is a product of incomplete combustion of hydrocarbons and is produced by fires; automobile exhaust; propane-powered engines; portable generators; kerosene heaters; gas log fireplaces; spray paint; and cigarette, cigar, and pipe smoke.
- The lethal dose is 1000 ppm (0.1%) for all animals. An automobile running in a closed one-car garage for 10 minutes can achieve this level.
- Clinical signs include nausea, vomiting, ataxia, tachypnea, tachycardia, syncope, hypotension, lactic acidosis, seizures, pulmonary edema, and coma.
- Diagnosis is based on history, clinical signs, and response to therapy. No single laboratory test exists to establish carbon monoxide poisoning. Blood levels of carboxyhemoglobin usually have fallen substantially by the time of arrival at the veterinary facility.
- Treatment involves removing the animal from the source of carbon monoxide and immediately administering 100% oxygen.
- Gross and histologic lesions of carbon monoxide poisoning include renal tubular necrosis, myonecrosis, endothelial damage to the blood vessels, and demyelinization injury to the CNS.

Sources

Carbon monoxide (CO) poisoning is the most common form of intoxication in humans in the United States. The molecule is produced by the incomplete combustion (oxidation) of carbon-containing compounds. Possible sources of carbon monoxide include propane-powered engines (e.g., forklifts and chain saws), catalytic radiant heaters, portable generators, kerosene heaters, gas log fireplaces, natural gas appliances, hibachi cookers, automobile exhaust, fires and subsequent smoke inhalation, and paint strippers and spray paints (Box 37-1). An improperly vented natural gas heater can make the air within a small room unsafe to breathe within a matter of minutes. However, several cases of carbon monoxide poisoning have occurred outdoors in association with the use of faulty equipment.

Animals have long been used as sentinels to provide early warning of the risk of human exposure to potentially noxious gases. In the last century, canaries were kept in mines to alert workers to the presence of carbon monoxide and other toxic inhalants. In homes, domestic dogs and cats may likewise serve as sentinels. Pets are at increased exposure risk compared with humans because of their faster breathing rate and smaller volume of distribution. Thus, companion animals may display recognizable signs of toxicosis early enough to allow people to take action to prevent further or prolonged exposure.

Gasoline internal combustion engine exhaust contains from 3% to 7% carbon monoxide. Newer emission standards for new cars in the United States require limitation of carbon monoxide emission to 0.5%. Numerous cases of intoxication of dogs and cats have been reported when they have been inadvertently left in enclosed garages in the wintertime while owners warmed up their cars. Another potent source of carbon monoxide is the smoke of cigarettes, cigars, and pipes, which can contain levels up to 4%. Likewise, diesel engines emit notable levels of CO in their exhaust. In the past decade nonvehicular sources of carbon monoxide exposure, preponderantly from faulty heating and cooking devices, have accounted for a growing number of poisonings. Fire continues to be an important source of exposure. Carbon monoxide is the leading cause of death in fire victims.

Toxic Dose

Lethal concentrations of carbon monoxide can be achieved within 10 minutes from an automobile running in the confines of a closed one-car garage. An ambient CO concentration of 100 ppm (0.01%) produces no clinical signs during an 8-hour exposure. Dogs can tolerate 200 ppm (0.02% CO concentrations) for 90 days with no clinical signs. However, CO concentrations more than 1000 ppm (0.1%) cause unconsciousness, respiratory failure, and death if exposure is continued for 1 hour. Chronic poisoning in the sense of accumulation of carbon monoxide with repeated exposure does not occur. Nevertheless, repeated anoxia from carbon monoxide causes central nervous system (CNS) damage. Carbon monoxide exposure is particularly deleterious to pregnant animals because of fetuses' greater sensitivity to the harmful effects of the gas. Final carboxyhemoglobin levels in the fetus may exceed levels found in the mother. The exaggerated leftward shift of fetal carboxyhemoglobin makes tissue hypoxia more severe because less oxygen is available to fetal tissue. Also, it is estimated that fetal elimination of carbon monoxide takes 3.5 times as long as maternal elimination of the poison. Although the teratogenicity of carbon monoxide is controversial, the risk of fetal injury caused by carbon monoxide is significant. Pregnant animals of many species (farm animals, companion species, and humans) have been shown to be at increased risk when exposed to toxic levels of carbon monoxide.

Box 37-1	Carbon Monoxide Sources

Propane-powered engines
- Forklifts
- Chain saws

Catalytic radiant heaters
Portable generators
Kerosene heaters
Gas log fireplaces
Natural gas appliances
Automobile exhaust
Fires (subsequent smoke inhalation)
Paint strippers
Spray paint
Hibachi cookers
Cigarette, cigar, and pipe smoke

Toxicokinetics and Mechanism of Toxicity

In its pure form, carbon monoxide is undetectable. It is colorless, odorless, and nonirritating, and it disperses readily in room air and does not stratify (Box 37-2). Because it is slightly lighter than air, carbon monoxide tends to rise throughout a building. Carbon monoxide combines with hemoglobin to form carboxyhemoglobin. This molecule is incapable of carrying oxygen (O_2), and tissue hypoxia results. Hemoglobin has an affinity for carbon monoxide that is 240 times greater than that of O_2. In addition, the presence of carbon monoxide increases the stability of the hemoglobin-O_2 bond. Thus the fixation of carbon monoxide on any one of the four oxygen-binding sites of hemoglobin increases the oxygen affinity at the remaining sites. As a result, carbon monoxide reduces the availability of oxygen to tissue in two ways: first, by its direct combination with hemoglobin, which thereby reduces the amount of hemoglobin able to carry oxygen, and second, by preventing the release or unloading of oxygen bound to hemoglobin at peripheral body tissues. This increased affinity for oxygen, known as the Haldane effect, causes the leftward shift of the oxygen hemoglobin dissociation curve. The carboxyhemoglobin molecule is relatively nontoxic. The toxicity of carbon monoxide lies in its capacity to reduce both the oxygen-carrying capacity of hemoglobin and the oxygen-unloading function of the molecule. The net effect of these two processes is decreased availability of oxygen to cells of the body. Levels of carboxyhemoglobin in the blood can help determine overall toxicity of the exposure. Normal levels in nonsmoking humans and normal animals typically are less than 2%; smokers can have chronically elevated levels around 7% to 12%.

In addition to the strong affinity of carbon monoxide for hemoglobin, carbon monoxide has a significant affinity for all iron- or copper-containing sites and competes with oxygen at these active sites. In particular, muscle myoglobin has a selective affinity for carbon monoxide that is 40 times greater than that for oxygen and, like hemoglobin, displays a leftward oxygen dissociation shift when carbon monoxide is present. This binding with myoglobin is further enhanced by hypoxic conditions. Interference with cellular respiration at the mitochondrial level by carbon monoxide also has been demonstrated. Carbon monoxide binds with cytochrome oxidase in conditions of hypoxia and causes the release of mitochondrial-based free radicals. These molecules attract leukocytes that release proteases that activate a cascade of events that damage endothelium, destroy brain microvasculature, and result in lipid peroxidation of brain membranes.

Carbon monoxide toxicity cannot be explained based solely on a carboxyhemoglobin-mediated hypoxia. Clinical effects, tissue destruction, and subsequent neurological deficits cannot be predicted by only the extent of binding between carbon monoxide and hemoglobin. Dogs breathing 13% carbon monoxide die within 1 hour with carboxyhemoglobin levels of 54% to 90%. However, blood transfusions from the dying dogs into healthy dogs produced no deleterious effects. This observation suggests that the carbon monoxide itself is responsible at least partially for its pathological effects. In poisoned animals, 10% to 15% of total body carbon monoxide is found to be extravascular. The delivery of carbon monoxide itself intracellularly, its binding to heme proteins and other molecules other than hemoglobin, the migration and attachment of leukocytes to damaged endothelium and their destructive release of proteases, free radicals, and degradative enzymes all contribute to the toxicity of carbon monoxide in addition to its hypoxic effects.

Clinical Signs

Clinical signs of carbon monoxide poisoning are notoriously nonspecific and may be evident in a wide variety of presentations, depending on the concentration of the poison in air, the duration of the exposure, the ventilation present, the age and size of the animal, and the presence of underlying cardiac or cerebrovascular disease. The earliest clinical signs of carbon monoxide poisoning are easily confused with other illnesses, especially viral syndromes and food poisoning. In humans as many as 5% of those treated for influenza are thought to be actually suffering from the subclinical effects of carbon monoxide exposure. The principal manifestation of carbon monoxide poisoning is dyspnea. However, the earliest signs in mild exposures are nausea, vomiting, and dizziness. In moderate exposures, serious signs appear, including tachycardia, tachypnea, weakness, and ataxia. In more

Box 37-2	Carbon Monoxide Properties

Molecular weight: 28.01 Daltons
Gas density: 0.968 (air = 1)
Odor: none
Color: none
Irritating: no

severe carbon monoxide poisonings, syncope, seizures, hypotension, and coma may ensue (Box 37-3).

Cardiac arrhythmias, such as premature ventricular contractions, atrial fibrillation, heart block, and ischemic changes, may all be present on electrocardiograms. Cardiac signs are frequently observed after carbon monoxide poisoning. At levels of carboxyhemoglobin greater than 6%, there is an increased frequency of premature ventricular contractions. Life-threatening dysrhythmia, myocardial infarction, and cardiac arrest have all been described after carbon monoxide exposure. Acute death from carbon monoxide is usually the result of ventricular dysrhythmia, the cause of which is the underlying devastating hypoxia. Although the heart is readily affected by carbon monoxide, the brain is the most sensitive target organ, and neurological signs may be evident. Continuous exposure to ambient CO concentrations of more than 1000 ppm (0.1%) for more than 1 hour results in unconsciousness, respiratory failure, seizures, and death.

Minimum Database and Confirmatory Tests

For fire victims and animals suffering from smoke inhalation, carbon monoxide poisoning is usually swiftly addressed. However, for the comatose animal having no history, the diagnosis can be easily missed. In one retrospective study in humans, the incidence of misdiagnosis of carbon monoxide poisoning was 30% over a 3-year period. It is important to obtain a detailed toxicologic history, inquiring about the physical surroundings of the animal and about any gas stoves, gas heat, or gas water heaters in use in confined spaces with the animal.

Animals intoxicated with carbon monoxide seldom display bright red gums and mucous membranes and seldom have the classic "cherry red" blood described in textbooks. They may be hypotensive, display arrhythmias on electrocardiograms, and have lactic acidosis. Because carboxyhemoglobin absorbs light at the same wavelength as oxyhemoglobin, a pulse oximeter shows falsely elevated or normal oxyhemoglobin saturation levels. Carboxyhemoglobin levels may be taken from specimens obtained to measure arterial blood gases. Many human hospital lab facilities can run this test fairly quickly. However, an elevated carboxyhemoglobin level is not a reliable indicator of the severity of the poisoning, and a poor correlation exists between the carboxyhemoglobin level and clinical signs. Typically, diagnosis is based on history, clinical signs, blood work, and response to oxygen therapy (Box 37-4).

An accurate predictor of the severity of carbon monoxide intoxication and a better indicator of treatment required and eventual outcome has long been sought. Carboxyhemoglobin levels are a

---

Box 37-3 Clinical Signs of Carbon Monoxide Poisoning

Nausea
Vomiting
Tachycardia
Tachypnea
Arrhythmias
Hypotension
Ataxia
Syncope
Lactic acidosis
Obtundation
Seizures
Pulmonary edema
Coma
Respiratory arrest

Box 37-4 Minimum Database for Carbon Monoxide Poisoning

Vital signs
Electrocardiogram
Pulse oximetry
Doppler blood pressure
Complete blood count
Biochemical profile
Urinalysis
Blood gases (if possible)
Anion gap determination
Radiographs
Carboxyhemoglobin level (if possible)

useful diagnostic tool in suggested poisonings, and high levels may confirm exposure; however, as mentioned, carboxyhemoglobin is not predictive of the severity of the poisoning and correlates poorly in predicting treatment outcome. In addition, carboxyhemoglobin levels can vary with duration of exposure, timing of the measurement, rate of elimination, and concentration of carbon monoxide in the inspired gas. Initial hydrogen ion concentration may be a better index of the severity of poisoning based upon its effect on cellular metabolism as a result of the binding of carbon monoxide to intracellular oxygen-carrying proteins, such as cytochromes, rather than solely to hemoglobin. Poisoning of the cytochrome system results in cellular dysfunction and metabolic acidosis. Hydrogen ion concentration may be a more sensitive and logical marker of tissue poisoning in carbon monoxide toxicity. Measures other than carboxyhemoglobin levels, such as measures of acidemia (hydrogen ion concentration and lactate levels), provide additional information as to the severity of the toxic episode. Furthermore, animals with such an acidosis should be thought to have significant carbon monoxide exposure even if carboxyhemoglobin levels are low.

Finally, a rapid, cheap, and noninvasive diagnostic test for potential carbon monoxide poisoning that could be easily put to use in the veterinary emergency hospital or triage room would be very welcome. Concentration of carbon monoxide in end expiratory breath bears a close relationship to carboxyhemoglobin concentration in the blood. Handheld breath analyzers are commercially available and are suitable for detection of carbon monoxide from any cause. In human beings, breath analysis for carbon monoxide is inexpensive, easy to perform, and fairly accurate and provides an answer in a reasonably short time frame. Breath sampling methods should be further investigated to determine if this might be an effective way of measuring carbon monoxide exposure in animals.

Treatment

The antidote for carbon monoxide poisoning is 100% oxygen administered by endotracheal tube or a tight-fitting mask. Cardiac monitoring should be conducted and any arrhythmias treated. Hypotension should be corrected with administration of intravenous normal saline. Severely poisoned animals should be screened and treated for lactic acidosis if necessary. Animals arriving in emergency situations from closed-space fires with notable metabolic acidosis or elevated lactate levels should also be evaluated for possible concomitant cyanide poisoning.

Use of 100% oxygen facilitates the dissociation of carbon monoxide from hemoglobin. The half-life of carbon monoxide is reduced from more than 240 minutes at room air to 60 minutes when 100% oxygen is delivered via endotracheal tube. Administration of 100% oxygen should not be employed for longer than 18 hours to prevent subsequent oxygen toxicity. This syndrome is thought to be caused by the formation of oxygen radicals that directly damage endothelial and epithelial cells leading to cytotoxicity, increased endothelial permeability, and subsequent inflammation of tissues. For most mammalian species, it has been discovered that prolonged exposure (24 hours or greater) to high concentrations of oxygen is damaging to the lungs. For these reasons, the use of 100% oxygen must be monitored judiciously.

The use of 100% oxygen administered at greater than atmospheric pressure (i.e., hyperbaric oxygen) can shorten the half-life further to about 23 minutes. In several studies hyperbaric oxygen benefits the brain more than normobaric oxygen, because it improves energy metabolism, prevents lipid peroxidation, and decreases neutrophil adherence. In humans hyperbaric oxygen therapy is the treatment of choice for patients severely poisoned by carbon monoxide. Disadvantages of hyperbaric oxygen include risks associated with transport to treatment centers, initiation of hyperoxic seizures, and barotrauma. At present these techniques are not widely available in veterinary medicine. Seizures caused by carbon monoxide poisoning may be treated with appropriate anticonvulsants.

In 1922 carbon dioxide–induced hyperpnea was shown to be effective in treating carbon monoxide poisoning. This technique fell into disfavor in the 1960s with the advent of successful treatment of carbon monoxide poisoning with hyperbaric oxygen. Recently, eucapnic hyperoxic hyperpnea was shown to increase the elimination of carbon monoxide in dogs and in humans by two to three times that of normal breathing of 100% oxygen. With appropriate equipment, this technique could be applied at the time and site of location with a portable circuit. Providing more rapid elimination of carbon monoxide earlier in the course of treatment of this poisoning could dramatically improve prognosis. Because hyperbaric chambers are still relatively rare (only 340 in the United States) and not readily available to veterinary patients, this method of treatment deserves serious reevaluation.

Finally, correction of any underlying acidemia with bicarbonate is controversial because it can result in further cellular hypoxia secondary to a left shift of the oxyhemoglobin dissociation curve. At this time it is not recommended as part of the treatment regimen.

Prevention and Prognosis

All combustion devices must be vented to the outside air. Flame water heaters, gas stoves, gas refrigerators, internal combustion engines, propane- and kerosene-driven tools and vehicles, and paint-stripping devices must all be checked routinely for safety. Animals should not be kept in poorly ventilated areas with such machines, nor should they be kept in confined spaces (such as garages) where owners warm up their automobiles. Animals should not be returned to such enclosed areas until the source of carbon monoxide has been repaired or removed.

Early diagnosis is crucial in preventing much of the morbidity and mortality associated with carbon monoxide toxicity, particularly in nonintentional poisonings. The availability and use of much-improved home carbon monoxide detecting devices should provide an added dimension to prevention of exposure. Identification and treatment of affected cohabitant animals is likewise critical from a standpoint of prevention. Informing owners of the danger to cohabitants and overseeing their swift evaluation may prevent further needless poisonings. In cases of suspected accidental exposure, local fire departments and utility companies can check home equipment and measure ambient levels of carbon monoxide using portable monitoring equipment. Until rescue personnel arrive at sites of accidental poisoning, instruct owners to turn off all portable generators, propane-powered engines, kerosene heaters, and natural gas–fueled appliances; open doors and windows; and evacuate the area.

If the victim recovers, signs of poisoning regress gradually. Signs of CNS damage may be permanent. Complete recovery is unlikely if signs persist for more than 3 weeks. Because of the wide variety of nonspecific clinical signs, diagnosis of carbon monoxide poisoning can be easily missed. However, if the toxicosis is treated early and aggressively, therapy can be successful. The use of hyperbaric oxygen in the management of carbon monoxide-poisoned veterinary cases deserves broader attention. Dogs appear to be more resistant to carbon monoxide intoxication than either human beings or cats. Tabulations for the incidence of carbon monoxide poisonings in dogs and cats (and their outcome) as documented by the American Association of Poison Control Centers (AAPCC) for 2010 are included in Boxes 37-5 and 37-6. Recommendations for the prevention of carbon monoxide intoxication are included in Box 37-7.

Box 37-5	Total Number of Reported Carbon Monoxide Cases—Canine—2010
Confirmed exposures:	32
Outcome	
Death:	0
Moderate effects:	5
Minor effects:	9
Animal recovered:	32

American Association of Poison Control Centers (AAPCC), 2010.

Gross and Histologic Lesions

Carbon monoxide toxicity appears to result from a combination of tissue hypoxia and direct carbon monoxide–mediated damage at the cellular level. After severe poisoning, myonecrosis, retrobulbar optic neuritis with neuroretinal edema, pulmonary edema, damage to the renal tubules, and increased fibrin deposition have all been documented. In addition, carbon monoxide exposure has been shown to cause lipid peroxidation leading to demyelinization of CNS lipids. Exposure to carbon monoxide also may lead to the formation of destructive oxygen radicals that result from the conversion of xanthine dehydrogenase to xanthine oxidase. In humans a delayed neuropsychiatric syndrome (3 to 240 days postexposure) has been described. This may be because of a postischemic reperfusion injury and the effects of carbon monoxide on vascular endothelium and oxygen radical–mediated brain lipid peroxidation.

Severe carbon monoxide poisoning is followed within a few hours by a rise in hydroxyl radicals in the brain. These molecules are responsible for the neural tissue damage and lipid peroxidation of the brain. Necropsy results for several species show decreased density in the central white matter and globus pallidus. Other areas including the cerebral cortex, hippocampus, cerebellum, and substantia nigra are affected by severe exposures. Animal studies have revealed that areas permanently damaged in serious cases of carbon monoxide poisoning are the areas of the brain with the poorest vascular supply. A transitory deafness has been documented in both dogs and cats following carbon monoxide exposure. However, it has been reported to resolve with time.

Box 37-6	Total Number of Reported Carbon Monoxide Cases—Feline—2010
Confirmed exposure:	81
Outcome	
Death:	1
Moderate effects:	17
Minor effects:	21
Animal recovered:	80

American Association of Poison Control Centers (AAPCC), 2010.

Box 37-7	Carbon Monoxide Prevention

- Have heating system, water heaters, and any gas, oil, or coal-burning appliances **serviced yearly** by qualified personnel.
- **Install** battery-operated CO detectors in your home (on each level). Replace all batteries each time you change your clocks every spring and fall. If detector alarm sounds—leave premises immediately and call 911. (Some states now have laws requiring detector installation in new homes and buildings.)
- **Clinical signs** of early carbon monoxide poisoning may include light-headedness, dizziness, and nausea. Seek medical attention if you suspect CO poisoning might be the cause.
- **Never** operate generators, charcoal grills, camping stoves, or gasoline, propane, or charcoal-burning devices inside your home, basement, or garage.
- **Never** run cars or trucks inside a garage—even if the door is open. (Never house pets in garages. It takes 10 minutes in a closed one-car garage housing a running car to achieve lethal CO levels for a 10-pound cat.)
- **Don't burn** anything in a stove or fireplace that is unvented.
- **Don't heat** homes with gas ovens or kerosene heaters.

<table>
<tr><td>Box 37-8</td><td>Differential Diagnoses for Carbon Monoxide Poisoning</td></tr>
</table>

Food poisoning
Heart disease
Alcohol intoxication
Acute solvent intoxication
Barbiturates
Cyanide
Ischemic cerebral disease
Cerebral hemorrhage
Cerebral neoplasia
Viral syndromes
Metabolic disease

Acute changes of the brain after severe exposures can be documented within 12 hours using computed tomography (CT) scans. Loss of density in the globus pallidus, caudate nuclei, and putamen frequently can be observed. Normal initial CT scans generally predict a favorable outcome. Changes in the globus pallidus and subcortical white matter within the first day following poisoning usually indicate a poor outcome. Magnetic resonance imaging appears to be a superior technique in identifying lesions of the basal ganglia. Neuroimaging does not direct treatment choices and should be reserved for animals showing poor response to therapy or who have an equivocal diagnosis. Delayed neurological effects caused by carbon monoxide poisoning involve lesions in the cerebral white matter and basal ganglia. Retinal hemorrhages have been seen in several species following prolonged exposures to carbon monoxide.

Differential Diagnoses

A diagnosis of carbon monoxide intoxication can be easily missed because of a poor history of toxicologic exposure given by the owner and the nonspecific clinical signs characteristic of this toxicosis. A list of differential diagnoses and potential look-alikes is included in Box 37-8. Differentials must include viral syndromes, food poisoning, heart disease, other intoxicants, ischemic cerebral disease, and cerebral neoplasia. The most common signs of carbon monoxide poisoning are nonspecific, such as nausea, dizziness, and syncope. A high index of suspicion is necessary to make the diagnosis of carbon monoxide toxicity, especially when the avenue of exposure is not immediately evident.

Suggested Readings

Barret L, Danel V, Faure J: Carbon monoxide poisoning, a diagnosis frequently overlooked, Clin Toxicol 23:309, 1985.

Kao LW, Nanggs KA: Toxicity associated with carbon monoxide, Clin Lab Med 26(1):99–125, 2006.

Olson KR: Carbon monoxide poisoning mechanisms, presentation, and controversies in management, J Emerg Med 1:233, 1984.

Bronstein AC, Spyker DA, Canitena LR, et al: Annual Report of the American Association of Poison Control Centers National Poison Data System (NPDS): 27th Annual Report 2010, Clin Toxicol 48:979–1178, 2010.

Bartlett R: Carbon monoxide poisoning. In Haddad LM, Shannon MW, Winchester JF, editors: Clinical management of poisoning and drug overdose, ed 3, Philadelphia, 1988, Saunders.

Rosenstock L, Cullen M, Brodkin C, et al: Textbook of clinical occupational and environmental medicine, ed 2, Edinburgh, 2004, Saunders.

Florkowski CM, et al: Rhabdomyolysis and acute renal failure following carbon monoxide poisoning: two case reports with muscle histopathology and enzyme activities, J Clin Toxicol 30:443, 1992.

Penney DG: Hemodynamic response to carbon monoxide, Environ Health Perspect 77:121–130, 1988.

Ernst A, Zibrak JD: Carbon monoxide poisoning, N Engl J Med 330(22):1603–1608, 1998.

Zagami AS, Lethlean AK, Mellick R: Delayed neurological deterioration after carbon monoxide poisoning, J Neurol 240:113–116, 1993.

Aslan S, Karcioglu O, Bilge F, et al: Post interval syndrome after carbon monoxide poisoning, Vet Human Toxicol 46(4):183–185, 2004.

Crocker PJ, Walker JS: Pediatric carbon monoxide toxicity, J Emerg Med 3(6):443–448, 1985.

Cunningham AJ, Hormbrey P: Breath analysis to detect recent exposure to carbon monoxide, Postgrad Med J 78:233–238, 2002.

Goldbaum LR, Ramirez RG, Absalon KB XIII: What is the mechanism of carbon monoxide toxicity? Aviat Space Environ Med 46(10):1289–1291, 1975.

Gorman D, et al: The clinical toxicology of carbon monoxide, *Toxicology* 187(1):25–38, 2003.

Okeda R, et al: Comparative study on pathogenesis of selective cerebral lesions in carbon monoxide poisoning and nitrogen hypoxia in cats, *Acta Neuropathol* 56:265–272, 1982.

Pejsak Z, Zmudski J, Wojnicki P: Abortion in sows associated with carbon monoxide intoxication, *Vet Rec* 162(13):417, 2008.

Piantadosi CA: Carbon monoxide poisoning, *N Engl J Med* 347(14):1054–1055, 2002.

Rabinowitz PM, Conti LA: Carbon monoxide. In Rabinowitz PM, Conti LA, editors: *Human-animal medicine*, St Louis, 2010, Saunders.

Takeuchi A, et al: A simple "new" method to accelerate clearance of carbon monoxide, *Am J Respir Crit Care Med* 161(6):1816–1819, 2000.

Tomaszewski C: Carbon monoxide. In Goldfrank LR, editor: *Goldfrank's toxicologic emergencies*, ed 7, New York, 2002, McGraw-Hill.

Turner M, Esaw M, Clark RJ: Carbon monoxide treated with hyperbaric oxygen: metabolic acidosis as a predictor of treatment requirements, *J Accid Emerg Med* 16(2):96–98, 1999.

Weaver LK, et al: Hyperbaric oxygen for acute carbon monoxide poisoning, *N Engl J Med* 347(14):1057–1067, 2002.

Kent M, Creevy KE, Delahunta A: Clinical and neuropathological findings of acute carbon monoxide toxicity in Chihuahuas following smoke inhalation, *J Am Anim Hosp Assoc* 46(4):259–264, 2010.

Klein J: All clear: laws, codes expanding to help prevent caron monoxide tragedies, *Occup Health Saf* 76(5):82–84, 2007.

United States Environmental Protection Agency: *Carbon monoxide*, 2008, http://www.epa.gov/iaq/co.html.

Cholecalciferol

Wilson K. Rumbeiha, DVM, PhD, DABVT, DABT

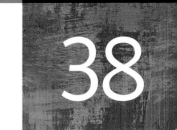

- The most common sources of vitamin D toxicosis in small animals are accidental ingestion of rodenticides containing cholecalciferol and human medications containing vitamin D or its analogues.
- Adulterated pet food has been a source of chronic vitamin D poisoning in dogs.
- A single oral lethal dose of cholecalciferol in a mature dog can be as low as 2 mg/kg (80,000 IU/kg), and signs can been seen at doses as low as 0.1 mg/kg. A single minimum oral toxic dose of calcipotriol or calcipotriene in dogs is as low as 10 mcg/kg body weight and a single oral lethal dose is 65 mcg/kg body weight. Clinical signs of toxicity can be seen at doses of 2.5 ng/kg of calcitriol. One mcg vitamin D_3 equals 40 IU.
- Clinical signs of vitamin D toxicosis arise from hypercalcemia and involve the central nervous, muscular, gastrointestinal, cardiovascular, endocrine, and renal systems. They include depression, weakness, and anorexia. As the disease progresses, vomiting, hematemesis, polyuria, polydipsia, constipation, melena, and dehydration set in.
- Confirmatory tests include serum parathyroid hormone (iPTH), total and ionized calcium, phosphorus levels, $25(OH)D_3$ and $1,25(OH)_2D_3$ levels. In vitamin D toxicosis, iPTH is suppressed. Animals are frequently azotemic. Analysis of bile and kidney for vitamin D metabolites is also available postmortem.
- Treatment may include gastrointestinal decontamination, reduction of hypercalcemia using calcitonin or bisphosphonates, and dietary calcium and phosphorus restriction. Supportive therapy should include fluid therapy, corticosteroids, phosphate binders, antiemetics, and use of gastrointestinal protectants.
- The prognosis is good if treatment is initiated early before persistent hypercalcemia, hyperphosphatemia, and dystrophic mineralization set in.

There are two active forms of vitamin D in mammals—the plant-derived ergocalciferol (vitamin D_2) and the animal-derived cholecalciferol (vitamin D_3). Both vitamin D_2 and vitamin D_3 are prosteroid hormones.[1] In addition to these naturally occurring vitamins, there are several synthetic analogues of 25-hydroxycholecalciferol ($25[OH]D_3$) and 1,25 dihydroxycholecalciferol ($1,25[OH]_2D_3$) that cause effects similar to the corresponding natural metabolites of vitamin D_3.[2] When pet owners call with a complaint that their pet ingested "vitamin D"-containing medications, it is essential that the clinician query the owner about the specific compound and strength.

Sources

Cholecalciferol (vitamin D_3) is naturally synthesized in mammalian skin from its precursor, 7-dehydrocholesterol, in the presence of ultraviolet light.[1] This process is tightly regulated, and toxicosis from natural oversynthesis of cholecalciferol in mammalian skin has not been reported to date. A common source of vitamin D toxicosis in small animals is accidental ingestion of rodenticides containing cholecalciferol as the active ingredient.[3] Rodenticide baits containing cholecalciferol as the active ingredient are sold over the counter. Some common proprietary names of these rodenticides include Muritan, Mouse-B-Gone Mouse Killer, Quintox Mouse Seed, Ceva True Grit Rampage, Quintox Rat and Mouse Bait, and Rampage Rat and Mouse Bait. These products are available in different formulations (e.g., granules, flakes, tablets, cakes, or briquettes) containing 0.075% cholecalciferol.

The other common source of vitamin D toxicosis in small animals is accidental ingestion of human medications.[4] Medications containing vitamin D are currently used for the treatment of a number of human diseases, including hypophosphatemic disorders, hypoparathyroidism, osteomalacia, osteoporosis, and renal failure. Newly discovered functions of vitamin D in cell differentiation and immune function have recently ushered in a new generation of vitamin D medications for prophylactic treatment of cancer and immunosuppression. For example, Dovonex (calcipotriene or calcipotriol), an analogue of $1,25(OH)_2D_3$, is currently used for the treatment of psoriasis in humans. Ingestion of antipsoriasis petroleum-based creams containing calcipotriene has become a potential source of vitamin D intoxication in dogs.[4] Other vitamin D analogues of similar therapeutic uses include $1\alpha(OH)D_3$, $1\alpha(OH)D_2$, dihydrotachysterol, calcitriol (a $1,25(OH)_2D_3$ analogue), and tacalcitol. Some of these vitamin D analogues have potent calcemic and phosphatemic properties and are potentially lethal when ingested at much smaller doses than the parent vitamin D compounds. The recent surge in interest in the therapeutic potential of vitamin D drugs for inflammatory and immune-mediated disorders will likely increase the potential for pet exposure, and these drugs may become the major source of vitamin D toxicosis in pets in the future.

In the past few years there have been outbreaks of vitamin D poisoning in dogs associated with feeding of pet foods that had high levels of vitamin D. One case in 2010 involved dogs that had been fed three Brands of Blue Buffalo pet food that were found to be tainted with 25-hydroxy vitamin D_3 (HyD®). This particular brand of vitamin D is not approved for use in pet food and inadvertently contaminated the pet food as a carryover. However, inadvertent oversupplementation of pet food with cholecalciferol has also sickened or killed dogs in the recent past.[31] In 1999 there was a recall of DVM Nutri-Balance High protein dog food and Golden Sun Feeds Hi-Pro Hunter dog food. In February 2006 there was a recall of ROYAL CANIN Veterinary Diet™. Other sources of vitamin D toxicosis in dogs include iatrogenic oversupplementation of diets in the treatment of dogs with hypoparathyroidism and ingestion of diets containing high concentrations of vitamin D, such as fatty fish, eggs, milk, or liver. Vitamin D_2 and cholecalciferol (vitamin D_3) are fat soluble. Therefore, suckling animals, which are more sensitive to vitamin D toxicosis than adults, are at risk of exposure through milk. To date there has been no report in dogs or cats of an equivalent form of Williams syndrome, an idiopathic form of juvenile hypercalcemia in human infants characterized by exaggerated production of $25(OH)D_3$ in the presence of normal dietary vitamin D content.[5] It is not clear at the present time whether this condition exists in dogs or cats. However, an idiopathic disease in 3- to 10-week-old puppies of several breeds of dogs, characterized histologically by extensive soft tissue mineralization—especially of the lungs, stomach, and kidneys—has been recognized recently. Granulomatous diseases, such as blastomycosis, result in an endogenous increase in $1,25(OH)_2D_3$ in humans and animals. However, these granulomatous disease-related hypercalcemias have not been widely reported in small animals. Vitamin D–containing plants, such as *Solanum malacoxylon* and *Trisetum flavescens,* pose little risk of toxicosis for pets because of the large amount of plant material a pet has to consume to induce a poisoning. There are also reports in the literature of *Cestrum diurnum* (e.g., common names jasmine and jessamine) poisoning. This plant may be used as an ornamental plant and presumably contains 1,25 dihydroxyvitamin D_3.[8]

Toxic Dose

The toxic effects of vitamin D can result from either acute or chronic exposure. In either case, the toxic dose varies depending on the biochemical form of vitamin D involved. Vitamin D_2 and vitamin D_3 parent compounds or their metabolites and analogues have different potencies and are toxic at different doses. Vitamin D_3 is about 10 times more potent than vitamin D_2 on an equimolar basis with respect to enhancing intestinal calcium absorption. One international unit (IU) of vitamin D_3 is equivalent to 0.000025 mg of vitamin D_3. The reported oral LD_{50} for vitamin D_3 in dogs is 88 mg/kg. The single oral lethal dose of cholecalciferol in a mature dog is about 13 mg/kg body weight (520,000 IU/kg); a dose as low as 2 mg/kg (80,000 IU/kg) has been reported to be toxic in dogs.[3,6] In fact, doses around 0.1 mg/kg vitamin D_3 (4000 IU/kg) can cause mild GIT signs, and doses greater than 0.5 mg/kg vitamin D_3 (20,000 IU/kg) can result in hypercalcemia, hyperphosphatemia, and renal failure. For newer compounds, such as calcipotriol (calcipotriene), a potent 1,25(OH)$_2$D$_3$ analogue, the minimum oral toxic dose in dogs is as low as 10 mcg/kg body weight, and the single oral lethal dose is 65 mcg/kg BW.[7] The therapeutic dose for calcitriol (1,25(OH)$_2$D$_3$) is approximately 2.5-3.5 ng/kg once daily. This drug apparently has a very narrow margin of safety, since hypercalcemias have been reported at that dose.

There is limited information available on the chronic toxic dose of vitamin D compounds in dogs and cats. The daily requirement for vitamin D in dogs as stipulated by the National Research Council is 22 IU (0.55 mcg)/kg of body weight. The AAFCO minimum and maximum recommended vitamin D levels in dry dog foods is 500 IU/kg to 5000 IU/kg. In terms of metabolizable energy (ME), the AAFCO maximum guidelines for vitamin D in dog food are 1429 IU/1000 kcal ME. For cats the guidelines recommend a maximum of 2500 IU/1000 kcal ME. Daily intake of 500 to 1000 mcg cholecalciferol/kg of body weight was toxic in dogs in 2 to 3 weeks.[8] Oral ingestion of 15 mg of vitamin D_2 weekly for 2 months was toxic to puppies.[9] A toxic dose for vitamin D in dogs has been reported to be 100,000 IU/kg diet, dry matter.

In general, pups are more sensitive to vitamin D toxicosis than adults, and cats are more sensitive than dogs.[3,10,11] Unfortunately, information on the toxic doses of the several vitamin D biochemical compounds in dogs and cats is incomplete. Practically, it is important to remember that the toxic dose of vitamin D depends on the specific form of the vitamin involved. Some of the newer-generation vitamin D compounds, such as the analogues of 1,25(OH)$_2$D$_3$, are potent calcemic agents and are potentially lethal at much smaller doses than the parent vitamin D compounds. Furthermore, animals with predisposing conditions (e.g., renal disease and hyperparathyroidism) or animals ingesting a high calcium and phosphorus diet are likely more sensitive to vitamin D toxicosis than healthy animals.

Animals with the preexisting diseases listed in Table 38-1 are more susceptible to vitamin D toxicosis than normal animals. In addition, puppies and kittens are more sensitive to vitamin D toxicosis than adult animals, perhaps because young rapidly growing animals have a higher normal serum total calcium concentration than mature adults. High dietary calcium and phosphorus levels and dehydration are other factors that predispose to vitamin D toxicosis. Interestingly, there is a wide individual variation in susceptibility to vitamin D toxicosis, even among mature dogs, for reasons yet unknown. Consequently, the severity of clinical signs in vitamin D toxicosis is not clearly dose related. Dogs given the same toxic dose of cholecalciferol on a body weight basis respond with varying degrees of disease severity. The causes of individual variations in susceptibility to vitamin D intoxication are not clear but may include differences in toxicokinetics, which have yet to be explored in dogs and cats. In serum, vitamin D metabolites are transported bound to vitamin D–binding protein. It has been shown experimentally that the physiologic activity of vitamin D is a result of the active unbound metabolites interacting with receptors.[30] The serum concentration of free metabolites versus bound metabolites may vary among individual animals

Table 38-1 Serum Markers in Differential Diagnosis of Vitamin D Toxicosis and Other Hypercalcemic Disorders in Dogs and Cats

Disease	Ionized Ca	Total P	Intact PTH	25(OH)D$_3$	1,25(OH)$_2$D$_3$	Na/K Ratio
Cholecalciferol, vitamin D$_2$, or 25(OH)D$_3$ toxicosis	↑	↑	↓	↑	N	N
1,25(OH)$_2$D$_3$ or 1α(OH)D$_3$	↑	↑	↓	N	↑	N
Dihydrotachysterol, calcipotriene, and analogues	↑	↑	↓	N	N	N
Malignancy	↑	N	↓	N	↓	N
Primary hyperparathyroidism	↑	N	↑	N	N	N
Granulomatous diseases (e.g., blastomycosis)	↑	↑	↓	N	↑	N
Hypoadrenocorticism	N*	N	**	N	N	↓
Primary renal failure	N*	↑	↑	N	N	N

*Total serum calcium is increased.
**Not known.
N, Normal; ↑, increased; ↓, decreased.

and may affect the severity of the disease. Other possible explanations include variations in numbers of vitamin D receptors in target organs, interindividual differences in biotransformation (activation and degradation) of vitamin D metabolites, and other unknown factors.

Toxicokinetics

Following ingestion, cholecalciferol is rapidly absorbed and transported in plasma to the liver by vitamin D–binding protein.[12] Vitamin D–binding protein also transports all vitamin D metabolites in plasma. In the liver, cholecalciferol is very rapidly metabolized in the endoplasmic reticulum and mitochondria by 25-hydroxylase, a cytochrome P-450 mixed function oxidase enzyme, to 25(OH)D$_3$, the principal circulating metabolite.[1] In dogs the normal range of serum 25(OH)D$_3$ concentration is 60 to 215 nmol/L (24-86 ng/mL).[13] In cats the normal range is 65 to 170 nmol/L (26-68 ng/mL).[13] Following acute ingestion of toxic amounts of cholecalciferol, the concentration of 25(OH)D$_3$ increases at least 15 to 20 times the normal concentration to 3 to 4 μmol/L within 24 hours.[14] The synthesis of 25(OH)D$_3$ from cholecalciferol in the liver is not regulated and is primarily dependent on substrate concentration.[1]

This primary circulating metabolite, 25(OH)D$_3$, is further metabolized primarily to 1,25(OH)$_2$D$_3$ (calcitriol) and 24,25(OH)$_2$D$_3$ in renal proximal convoluted tubule epithelial cell mitochondria by renal 1α-hydroxylase, also a mixed function oxidase enzyme.[1,15] This step, the synthesis of 1,25(OH)$_2$D$_3$ in the kidney from 25(OH)D$_3$ by renal 1α-hydroxylase, is tightly regulated. Calcitriol is the principal active metabolite of cholecalciferol following exposure to physiologic or pharmacologic doses of cholecalciferol in dogs and cats. The normal background serum concentration of 1,25(OH)$_2$D$_3$ is 20 to 50 pmol/L in the dog.[13] In cholecalciferol toxicosis, this metabolite is increased only approximately three times normal to 60 to 150 pmol/L, with peak concentrations reached 48 to 96 hours after a single oral cholecalciferol dose. Because of the tight regulation of its synthesis in the kidneys, the serum 1,25(OH)$_2$D$_3$ concentration falls rapidly to normal or subnormal levels within 1 week of a single oral toxic exposure. In addition to the kidneys, there are other minor extrarenal sources of 1,25(OH)$_2$D$_3$ in mammals, such as the lymphohematopoietic system.[16]

The toxicokinetics of parent vitamin D compounds and their metabolites and analogues has not been widely investigated in dogs and cats. Most of the information on the toxicokinetics and metabolism of these compounds is derived from rodent and/or human studies.

In general cholecalciferol and vitamin D_2 parent compounds are lipid soluble and are extensively stored in the adipose, liver, and muscle tissues. Consequently, the half-life of these parent compounds is measured in months.[17] In comparison, the half-life of $25(OH)D_3$ is 15 days, whereas that of $1,25(OH)_2D_3$ is 4 to 8 hours.[18,19] However, following exposure to cholecalciferol, the half-life (functional) of $25(OH)D_3$ in the dog is 29 days because the ongoing metabolism of the parent compound in the liver adds more metabolite to the pool.[14] For similar reasons, the functional half-life of $1,25(OH)_2D_3$ following cholecalciferol exposure is approximately 3 days. Therefore, identification of the biochemical form of vitamin D involved in each case is important in estimating the duration of therapy required and in rendering an accurate prognosis. There is very little information known on the toxicokinetics of chronic vitamin D intoxication in dogs and cats. As such, the minimum chronic toxic dose of cholecalciferol in dogs and cats is not known and more work is needed in this area.

Mechanism of Toxicity

Vitamin D plays an important role in calcium homeostasis. It enhances calcium and phosphorus absorption from the gut and plays a role in the reabsorption of calcium from the distal tubules in the kidney.[17] Although 90% to 99% of calcium in glomerular filtrate is reabsorbed independent of vitamin D, both vitamin D and parathyroid hormone (PTH) mediate the reabsorption of 1% to 10% of the filtered calcium in the distal tubules. Vitamin D, by enhancing calcium absorption in the gastrointestinal tract and distal renal tubules, helps to maintain optimum serum calcium concentrations and allows proper bone mineralization to proceed. Another major function of vitamin D is to induce mobilization of calcium from bone to prevent hypocalcemia, a potentially life-threatening condition in humans and animals. Calcium plays other vital functions in the body besides skeletal mineralization, including nerve impulse conduction and muscle function, which are also impaired in the presence of subnormal serum calcium concentrations.[17] Hypocalcemia is usually compensated by mobilizing calcium from bones if dietary sources are insufficient to meet the demand. The mobilization of calcium from bones requires both vitamin D and PTH, although the actions of the two hormones are independent of each other.[15] Although the precise mechanisms of bone demineralization are not clear, it is known that vitamin D plays an important role in osteoclastic-mediated bone resorption.[20]

When given in physiologic or pharmacologic doses, the active metabolite of vitamin D is $1,25(OH)_2D_3$. This metabolite binds to an intracellular vitamin D receptor (VDR) within target tissue.[15,18] This calcitriol-receptor complex then binds to DNA to trigger transcriptional events. In intoxications involving ergocalciferol, cholecalciferol, or medications containing $25(OH)D_3$, tissues respond to $25(OH)D_3$, not $1,25(OH)_2D_3$.[18,21] Following ingestion of toxic doses of these compounds, the concentration of $25(OH)D_3$ is increased at least 15 times the normal concentration. This is in contrast to the concentration of $1,25(OH)_2D_3$, which is increased only two to three times normal at most. When present in high concentrations, $25(OH)D_3$ prevails over $1,25(OH)_2D_3$ for binding to the VDR and is the primary cause of biologic effects in target tissues, such as intestines and bone. This explains why the hypercalcemic effects of cholecalciferol toxicosis persist for weeks after the serum concentration of $1,25(OH)_2D_3$ has returned to normal or subnormal concentrations. However, it is known that exogenous administration of calcitriol up-regulates VDR numbers, at least in the gut and kidneys.[18] The biologic activity of calcitriol is proportional to VDR density.[22] Theoretically, it is possible that target tissue responds more efficiently to physiologic amounts of $1,25(OH)_2D_3$ and this may result in notable hypercalcemia because of the increase in receptor density in the course of vitamin D toxicosis.

Clinical Signs

Clinical signs of vitamin D toxicosis result from hypercalcemia (and concurrent hyperphosphatemia) and involve the central nervous, muscular, gastrointestinal, cardiovascular, and renal systems.[3,10,17,23] The latent period between the time of exposure and the appearance of clinical signs depends partly on the form of vitamin D involved. For example, in cases of cholecalciferol intoxication in dogs, clinical signs are usually observed at least 36 to 48 hours after ingestion. However, in intoxications involving $25(OH)D_3$ or $1,25(OH)_2D_3$ and their analogues, clinical signs become apparent only 8 to 24 hours after ingestion. The time lag before the appearance of clinical signs represents the time required for metabolic activation and for overcoming the regular calcium homeostatic mechanisms.

The earliest clinical signs observed in dogs and cats include depression, weakness, and anorexia. As the disease progresses, vomiting, polyuria, polydipsia, constipation, and dehydration become apparent. The high calcium ion concentration alters the action of vasopressin on renal tubules, leading to reduced urinary concentrating ability and polyuria. The specific gravity of urine is hyposthenuric (1.002-1.006). The feces may become dark (melena) because of gastrointestinal bleeding. Hematemesis is a grave sign that is usually observed in the more advanced cases. Hematemesis is a result of gastric ulceration, and if not treated immediately, the animal may die of shock within a few hours. Gastric ulceration is caused by mineralization of the stomach wall. Calciuria is one of the earliest changes noted with vitamin D toxicosis, generally preceding hypercalcemia, but is usually missed because it is not looked for on a routine basis and is difficult to analytically assess. As renal failure progresses, calciuria may be ameliorated because calcium clearance is reduced as a consequence of the reduced glomerular filtration rate. Sometimes bleeding in the lungs may result in dyspnea. Cardiac signs may include bradycardia and other ventricular arrhythmias. Electrocardiographic changes include shortened QT and prolonged PR intervals. Seizures, although not common, have been reported. When the serum calcium × phosphorus product (both in mg/dL) exceeds 60 to 70, metastatic mineralization of tissues tends to occur and this can cause a variety of clinical problems depending on the tissue(s) affected.

Minimum Database

The diagnosis of vitamin D toxicosis is based on a history and clinical signs consistent with vitamin D exposure. Animal owners should be questioned about the use of cholecalciferol rodenticides or vitamin D medications that may be accidentally accessible to pets. In live animals, blood samples should be taken to monitor serum total and ionized calcium, phosphorus, blood urea nitrogen, and creatinine levels, which are elevated in vitamin D toxicosis. The normal range of total blood calcium concentration in a mature dog is about 9.5 to 11.5 mg/dL. However, the normal serum calcium concentration may be as high as 12.5 mg/dL in young, rapidly growing dogs. In vitamin D toxicosis, the total serum calcium concentration increases to at least 13 mg/dL, but is usually as high as 15 to 18 mg/dL or greater. In dogs the normal range of serum ionized calcium is 5.2 to 6.2 mg/dL; this is increased to 6.6 to 8 mg/dL in dogs with vitamin D toxicosis. Total serum phosphorus is increased from the normal range of 3.5 to 5.5 mg/dL to more than 8 mg/dL in dogs. Often the hyperphosphatemia is observed to be elevated up to 12 hours before the serum calcium concentration become elevated. Urinalysis shows a fixed specific gravity and calciuria.

Confirmatory Tests

In live animals, confirmatory tests include serum intact PTH, ionized calcium, $25(OH)D_3$, and $1,25(OH)_2D_3$. In animals with vitamin D toxicosis, intact PTH is suppressed.[24] In acute vitamin D_3 and $25(OH)D_3$ toxicosis, serum $25(OH)D_3$ is increased at least 15 times, and $1,25(OH)_2D_3$ is present at normal to subnormal concentrations. An increase in $1,25(OH)_2D_3$ alone, with no increase in $25(OH)D_3$, suggests that the animal was exposed to 1α $(OH)D_3$ or $1,25(OH)_2D_3$. Unfortunately the competitive protein binding assays currently used for serum $1,25(OH)_2D_3$ are unable to detect analogues of $1,25(OH)_2D_3$ such as calcipotriene (Dovonex®) and dihydrotachysterol.[18] Therefore, intoxications caused by $1,25(OH)_2D_3$ analogues are difficult to confirm at present because test results for $25(OH)D_3$ and $1,25(OH)_2D_3$ are normal. Intoxication involving these products should be considered if both total and ionized calcium are elevated, serum phosphorus is elevated, intact PTH is suppressed, and the history suggests possible exposure to these products.

Confirmation of vitamin D intoxications in dogs at necropsy can be challenging. The current gold standard for confirmation of vitamin D toxicosis is the finding of characteristic histopathologic lesions, such as mineralization of kidneys, lungs, stomach, atria, and major blood vessels (e.g., the aorta). Considering that soft tissue mineralization may result from a number of hypercalcemic disorders, these histologic findings are not pathognomonic. Bile and kidney can be tested for 25-hydroxycholecalciferol levels and reference values are available for these matrices. An alternative diagnostic approach is to perform trace mineral analysis of the kidney. Increased renal calcium and phosphorus concentrations have been reported in primary renal disease and in animals with vitamin D, ethylene glycol, and soluble oxalate toxicoses. The normal renal calcium concentration in dogs is 50 to 200 ppm on a wet weight basis. In dogs that have died of acute vitamin D toxicosis, the renal calcium concentration is generally increased to 2000 to 3000 ppm wet weight. In comparison, dogs that have died of ethylene glycol toxicosis generally have a much higher renal calcium concentration, at least 8000 ppm on a wet weight basis. The calcium to phosphorus ratio of 0.4 to 0.7 in the kidney cortex strongly suggests vitamin D toxicosis. In ethylene glycol poisonings, this ratio is often greater than 2.5. In normal dogs this ratio is less than 0.1. These ratios should be considered as general rules of thumb; exceptions to these criteria have been observed and results of these tests are only suggestive and not confirmatory.

Treatment

Treatment of vitamin D toxicosis depends on how soon postexposure the animal is seen. In general, treatment may include gastrointestinal decontamination, reduction of hypercalcemia and hyperphosphatemia, dietary calcium and phosphorus restriction, supportive therapy to ensure adequate hydration to maintain adequate tissue perfusion and urine flow, and the use of antiemetics.[3,10,17,23]

Gastrointestinal decontamination is recommended if exposure is known to have occurred within the past 6 hours. This involves inducing emesis with apomorphine or 3% hydrogen peroxide in dogs and cats. Following emesis, activated charcoal should be given followed by a saline cathartic, such as sodium sulfate (1 g/kg), 20 to 30 minutes later. The saline cathartic facilitates emptying of the activated charcoal–bound vitamin D from the gastrointestinal tract. Repeated doses of activated charcoal should be performed to decrease enterohepatic recirculation of vitamin D; careful monitoring of sodium levels in small breed patients is recommended. Serum calcium levels (total and ionized) and phosphorus concentrations should be monitored at the time of admission to establish baseline values and every 24 to 48 hours during the first 6 days after exposure.

However, because cholecalciferol toxicosis has a slow onset and clinical signs are not observed until 36 to 48 hours after exposure, usually it is too late for gastrointestinal decontamination to be of any value because absorption is already complete by the time the animal is brought in for treatment. When evaluating a patient showing clinical signs of vitamin D toxicosis, treatment should be considered urgent because persistent hypercalcemia, along with hyperphosphatemia, can be life threatening. Calcitonin has historically been recommended for the treatment of vitamin D–induced hypercalcemia, although controlled studies on the efficacy of calcitonin in vitamin D toxicosis in dogs are lacking. The recommended dosage of salmon calcitonin in dogs is 4 to 6 IU given IM or subcutaneously (SC) every 6-12 hours until the calcium concentration stabilizes.[3] Calcitonin therapy is not only tedious, but is associated with side effects, such as anorexia, anaphylaxis, and emesis, but also has questionable effectiveness. In practice calcitonin therapy or bisphosphonates (see below) is usually combined with corticosteroid and diuretic therapy. Corticosteroids suppress bone resorption, reduce intestinal calcium absorption, and promote calciuresis by reducing distal tubular calcium absorption. The recommended dosage of prednisolone is 2 to 6 mg/kg given IM or per os (PO) every 12 hours. For diuresis, loop diuretics are preferable, and the dose of furosemide in dogs is 2 to 6 mg/kg, and in cats it is 1 to 4 mg/kg given SC, IV, or IM every 8 to 12 hours or as necessary.

Bisphosphonates (a newer class of specific inhibitors of bone resorption) have proved efficacious in the treatment of cholecalciferol toxicosis in dogs.[25] Pamidronate disodium (Aredia) is a drug used for the treatment of hypercalcemia of malignancy and Paget disease in humans. For the treatment of cholecalciferol toxicosis in dogs, pamidronate disodium is given by slow intravenous infusion at a rate of 1.3 to 2 mg/kg of body weight in 0.9% sodium chloride over 2 to 4 hours. Two infusions given 4 days apart were sufficient in treating experimental dogs given one oral dose of 8 mg cholecalciferol/kg of body weight. Pamidronate disodium has the advantage of a long-lasting inhibitory action on bone resorption, therefore requiring only two infusions for the treatment of cholecalciferol toxicosis in dogs. Total serum calcium and blood urea nitrogen should be monitored 48 and 96 hours after the last infusion. Excessive use of pamidronate disodium should be avoided because it has the potential to confound nephrotoxicity. Dietary calcium restriction may be beneficial, but was not necessary when pamidronate disodium was used in test studies.

Supportive therapy in animals with vitamin D toxicosis should include adequate hydration using a 0.9% saline infusion (2-3 times maintenance) to enhance calcium excretion and to ensure adequate tissue perfusion and urine flow. Dehydration confounds hypercalcemia because it causes reduced glomerular filtration. Dietary calcium restriction is recommended to reduce gastrointestinal calcium uptake. Antiemetics such as maropitant in dogs (1 mg/kg SC q24hr) or ondansetron in dogs and cats (0.1-0.2 mg/kg IV, PO q6-12hr) may be required because, if not checked, emesis may cause complications, such as electrolyte and acid-base imbalances. The recommended dosage for metoclopramide is 0.2 to 0.5 mg/kg IM or IV every 8 hours. Treatment for gastrointestinal ulceration should include use of antacids (e.g., H_2 blockers, omeprazole), gastrointestinal protectants, such as sucralfate, and gut rest. The recommended dosage of magnesium hydroxide is 5 to 10 mL/kg PO every 4 to 6 hours; for sucralfate, the total dosage is 0.5 to 1 g PO every 8 to 12 hours in dogs (0.25 g in cats). Orally administered phosphate binders, such as aluminum or magnesium hydroxide, can help lower serum phosphorus levels. Blood urea nitrogen and creatinine should be monitored periodically throughout the course of treatment. Radiographs can be used as a prognostic tool—evidence of soft tissue calcification imparts a poor prognosis.

Prognosis

The prognosis is good if treatment is initiated early before hypercalcemia, hyperphosphatemia, and dystrophic mineralization set in. If treatment is initiated after severe hypercalcemia or hyperphosphatemia has already occurred, prognosis is guarded to poor. Persistent severe hypercalcemia causes disruption of tubular basement membranes, which prevents epithelial cell regeneration. The animal may die of irreversible renal failure. Lung mineralization is also a consequence of persistent calcemia and phosphatemia and may result in hemorrhage. Death may result from dyspnea. The prognosis is grave for animals that have hematemesis. Hematemesis usually signals the terminal phase of the disease, indicating that in addition to renal failure and lung mineralization, severe gastric ulceration has occurred. Anemia and hypovolemia resulting from hematemesis confound renal and respiratory failure. Mineralization of the heart may lead to cardiac failure.

Gross and Histologic Lesions

Dehydration is a frequent finding at necropsy. The stomach is usually empty because the animal has been either vomiting and/or anorexic. In advanced cases, the stomach contents may be bloody because of severe gastric ulceration and bleeding. The gastric mucosa is usually swollen and hyperemic, and ulceration is obvious.[26] Grossly, kidneys may look normal or may have a mottled appearance.[8] The lungs may look normal, edematous, or hemorrhagic. The urinary bladder may contain clear dilute urine.

The major histologic findings of cholecalciferol intoxication include mineralization of the kidneys, heart (particularly the atria), stomach wall, lungs, and major arteries (e.g., aorta). In the kidney, mineralization frequently involves the proximal convoluted tubules, blood vessels, and glomerulus.[26,27] This results in epithelial cell necrosis and exfoliation. Mineralized cellular debris is present along the entire length of the uriniferous tubules. In the glomerulus, mineralization involves the mesangium and the glomerular capsule. In the stomach, mineralization involves the smooth muscles and the lamina propria. Necrosis and erosion of the mucosal epithelium of the stomach wall are evident, and the stomach wall is usually congested. In the lungs, mineralization, hemorrhage, and thickening of the alveolar septa are present.[11] In the major blood vessels, such as the aorta, mineralization usually involves the smooth muscles. There is intimal proliferation and subintimal edema with separation of elastic and collagen fibers. In the heart there is myocardial degeneration.

Differential Diagnoses

The differential diagnosis of vitamin D toxicosis from other causes of hypercalcemia is summarized in Table 38-1. The major differential diagnoses of vitamin D toxicosis in dogs and cats are hypercalcemic diseases, such as pseudohyperparathyroidism in which PTH-like proteins are produced ectopically in neoplasia, primary hyperparathyroidism, acute or chronic renal failure, granulomatous diseases, pheochromocytoma, osteolytic lesions, and hypoadrenocorticism.[18,28,29] Lymphosarcoma and anal sac apocrine gland adenocarcinoma are the most common neoplastic diseases associated with hypercalcemia in dogs.[24,28] Palpation of lymph nodes may help rule out neoplasia. Lymph node enlargement may signal the presence of a neoplastic condition. Primary renal disease can be confirmed by ruling out all other possible causes of hypercalcemia (see Table 38-1). Hypercalcemia and tissue mineralization in the absence of increased serum $25(OH)D_3$ or $1,25(OH)_2D_3$ metabolites is suggestive of primary renal disease. The serum sodium–potassium ratio is decreased in hypoadrenocorticism but normal in vitamin D toxicosis.[28] Granulomatous diseases, such as blastomycosis, are usually associated with elevated serum $1,25(OH)_2D_3$ levels because of the endogenous synthesis of this hormone by the granulomas. Elevated intact PTH in serum characterizes primary hyperparathyroidism. Primary hyperparathyroidism in dogs is especially prevalent in the Keeshond breed.[29] Other diseases or conditions that cause hypercalcemia in humans and may do the same in small animals include immobilization, juvenile hypercalcemia, thiazide diuretics, lithium, estrogens, antiestrogens, testosterone, and vitamin A toxicosis.

References

1. Host RL, Reinhardt TA: Vitamin D metabolism. In Feldman D, Glorieux FH, Pike JW, editors: *Vitamin D*, San Diego, 1997, Academic Press.
2. Binderup L, Binderup E, Godterredsen W: Development of new vitamin D analogs. In Feldman D, Glorieux FH, Pike JW, editors: *Vitamin D*, San Diego, 1997, Academic Press.
3. Dorman DC, Beasley VR: Diagnosis of and therapy for cholecalciferol toxicosis. In Kirk RW, editor: *Current veterinary therapy X, small animal practice*, Philadelphia, 1989, WB Saunders.
4. Campbell DD: Calcipotriol poisoning in dogs, *Vet Rec* 141(1):27–28, 1997.
5. Tylor AB, Stern PH, Bell NH: Abnormal regulation of circulating 25-hydroxyvitamin D in the Williams syndrome, *N Engl J Med* 306:972–975, 1982.
6. Clarke ML, Harvey DG, Humphreys DJ: Vitamins. In Clarke ML, Harvey DG, Humphreys DJ, editors: *Veterinary toxicology*, ed 2, London, 1981, Baillere Tindall.
7. Volmer P: Personal communication, 1998.
8. Spangler WL, Gribble DH, Lee TC: Vitamin D intoxication and the pathogenesis of vitamin D nephropathy in the dog, *Am J Vet Res* 40:73–83, 1979.
9. Clarke EGC, Clarke ML: Vitamins. In Clarke EGC, Clarke ML, editors: *Veterinary toxicology*, Baltimore, 1975, Williams & Wilkins.
10. Moore FM, Kudisch M, Richter K, et al: Hypercalcemia associated with rodenticide poisoning in three cats, *J Am Vet Med Assoc* 193:1099–1100, 1988.

11. Palmer N: Vitamin D poisoning. In Jubb KVF, Kennedy PC, Palmer N, editors: ed 4, *Pathology of domestic animals*, vol 1, San Diego, 1993, Academic Press.
12. Haussler M, McCain TA: Basic and clinical concepts related to vitamin D metabolism and action, *N Engl J Med* 297:1041–1050, 1977.
13. Refsal K: Personal communication, 2010.
14. Rumbeiha WK, Kruger JM, Fitzgerald SF, et al: Use of pamidronate disodium to reverse vitamin D_3-induced toxicosis in dogs, *Am J Vet Res* 60:1092–1097, 1999.
15. Haussler M, McCain TA: Basic and clinical concepts related to vitamin D metabolism and action, *N Engl J Med* 297:974–983, 1977.
16. Mawer EB, Hayes ME: Renal and extrarenal synthesis of 1,25-dihydroxy vitamin D, *Prog Endocrinol* 87:382–386, 1992.
17. Drazner FH: Hypercalcemia in the dog and cat, *J Am Vet Med Assoc* 178:1252–1256, 1981.
18. Thys-Jacobs S, Chan FKW, Koberle LMC, et al: Hypercalcemia due to vitamin D toxicity. In Feldman D, Glorieux FH, Pike JW, editors: *Vitamin D*, San Diego, 1997, Academic Press.
19. DeLuca HF: The vitamin D story. A collaborative effort of basic science and clinical medicine, *FASEB J* 2:224–236, 1988.
20. Suda T, Takahashi N, Abe E: Role of vitamin D in bone resorption, *J Cell Biochem* 49:53–58, 1992.
21. Hughes MR, Baylink DJ, Jones PG, et al: Radioligand receptor assay for 25 hydroxy D_2/D_3 and 1,25-dihydroxyvitamin D_2/D_3: an application to hypervitaminosis D, *J Clin Invest* 58:61–70, 1976.
22. Walters MR, Rosen DM, Norman AW, et al: 1,25 dihydroxyvitamin D receptors in an established bone cell line. Correlation with biochemical responses, *J Biol Chem* 257:7481–7484, 1982.
23. Fooshee SK, Forrester SD: Hypercalcemia secondary to cholecalciferol rodenticide toxicosis in two dogs, *J Am Vet Med Assoc* 196:1265–1268, 1990.
24. Kruger JM, Osborne CA: Canine and feline hypercalcemic nephropathy. Part I. Causes and consequences, *Compend Contin Educ Pract Vet* 16:1299–1324, 1994.
25. Rumbeiha WK, Kruger JM, Fitzgerald SF, et al: *The use of pamidronate disodium for treatment of vitamin D_3 toxicosis in dogs. Proceedings of 40th Annual American Association of Veterinary Laboratory Diagnosticians Meeting*, Louisville, 1997, Kentucky. (Abstract).
26. Gunther R, Felice JL, Nelson KR, et al: Toxicity of vitamin D_3 rodenticide to dogs, *J Am Vet Med Assoc* 193(2):211–214, 1988.
27. Roedner BL, Darr CA, Williamson J: Chronic nephrosis associated with hypervitaminosis D in a 9-month-old bitch, *Vet Med Small Anim Clin* 79(2):205–214, 1984.
28. Kruger JM, Osborne CA: Canine and feline hypercalcemic nephropathy. Part II. Causes and consequences, *Compend Contin Educ Pract Vet* 16:1445–1459, 1994.
29. Dorman D, Osweiler GD: Vitamin D toxicity. In Tilley LP, Smith FWK, MacMurray AC, editors: *The 5-minute veterinary consult*, Baltimore, 1997, Williams & Wilkins.
30. Bouillon R, Van Assche FA, van Baelen H, et al: Influence of vitamin D binding protein on serum concentration of 1,25-dihydroxyvitamin D_3: significance of the free 1,25-dihydroxyvitamin D_3 concentration, *J Clin Invest* 67:589–596, 1981.
31. Rumbeiha W, Morrison J: A review of Class I and Class II pet food recalls involving chemical contaminants from 1996 to 2008, *JMT* 7(1):60–66, 2011.

Christmastime Plants

Sharon M. Gwaltney-Brant, DVM, PhD, DABVT, DABT

- Amaryllis (*Hippeastrum*) ingestion can lead to vomiting, diarrhea, anorexia, and excessive salivation in pets.
- Christmas cactus (*Schlumbergera truncata*), mistletoe (*Phoradendron* spp.), and English holly (*Ilex aquifolium*) ingestions and oral exposures to a wide variety of *evergreen* trees can cause mild to moderate gastrointestinal upset (vomiting, diarrhea, depression, and anorexia).
- Vomiting, depression and lethargy, and diarrhea are the most commonly reported problems seen in pets ingesting Christmas kalanchoe (*Kalanchoe blossfeldiana*). With excessive exposures, cardiac abnormalities may be observed.
- Poinsettias (*Euphorbia pulcherrima*) are highly overrated as to their toxicity. Signs of most exposures are very mild and self-limiting and include contact irritation, hypersalivation, and vomiting.
- Oral exposures to rosemary (*Rosmarinus officinalis*) can lead to gastrointestinal signs, hypotension, renal disease, and seizures.

Christmastime brings with it a large assortment of plants that are used for decorative purposes throughout the holiday season. Because of their novelty, when they seasonally appear in the house, and because these plants are kept primarily indoors, there is increased potential for household pets to be exposed to them. Both dogs and cats have been known to chew on houseplants, with the primary difference between these two species being the amount of plant material ingested. Although cats often only nibble on a few leaves, many dogs will devour the entire plant, including potting soil, if the opportunity arises. Other indoor pets, such as birds and rabbits, may similarly be exposed to these decorative plants. Fortunately, few of the plants common to the Christmas holiday have the potential to cause serious or life-threatening signs in pets if ingested, and the majority are generally expected to cause at most mild gastrointestinal upset.

When dealing with an exposure of a pet to any plant, it is important to determine the identity of the plant (ideally, genus and species name) and whether any plant care products (especially systemic insecticides) may have been applied to the plant or soil.

Amaryllis (*Hippeastrum* spp.)

Sources

Amaryllis (*Hippeastrum* spp.; Color Plate 39-1) is a popular Christmastime plant, native to South America, which blooms from late December until early June. The large blossoms occur in a variety of solid, striped, or variegated colors ranging from white to salmon to red.

Mechanism of Toxicity

Amaryllis and other members of the Amaryllidaceae family contain phenanthridine alkaloids, such as lycorine and tazetine.[1] The alkaloids are primarily concentrated within the bulb and leaves, where they can be present in concentrations up to 0.5%. Lesser amounts of alkaloids are present in the bulbs and flowers. Lycorine, the principal alkaloid responsible for clinical effects, is a centrally acting emetic. In dogs, lycorine acts primarily upon neurokinin-1 receptors, with lesser involvement of 5-hydroxytryptamine (5-HT) receptors.[2] Various other alkaloids found in amaryllis have cholinergic, analgesic, hypotensive, and cytotoxic effects. In most pets, chewing on or ingesting leaves generally only causes mild gastrointestinal upset, although ingestion of parts of the bulb may lead to more severe signs.[1,3]

Toxic Dose and Toxicokinetics

Studies on lycorine in dogs indicated that subcutaneous dosages of 0.5 to 2 mg/kg body weight were sufficient to cause nausea and vomiting in a dose-dependent fashion; at 2 mg/kg, 100% of dogs vomited.[4] The oral bioavailability of lycorine in dogs is 40%. Clinical effects of nausea and vomiting lasted less than 2.5 hours after a single parenteral exposure, but would likely last longer if bulb material was ingested and remained in the gastrointestinal tract.[4]

Clinical Signs

Mild to moderate vomiting, diarrhea, anorexia, and hypersalivation are the most common signs seen when animals ingest leaves, flowers, or small amounts of amaryllis bulb.[2] More severe gastrointestinal upset may be manifested by restlessness, tremors, or dyspnea.[1] Less commonly, hypotension, sedation, or seizures may occur, especially if large amounts of bulb material have been ingested.[3] In humans asthma has been associated with exposure to amaryllis, but this has not been reported in small animals.[5]

Minimum Database

Because protracted vomiting and/or diarrhea may result in dehydration and electrolyte abnormalities, animals showing severe or prolonged gastrointestinal upset should have their hydration and electrolyte status monitored. Hepatopathy has occasionally been reported to be associated with amaryllis ingestion,[3] so measurement of baseline and 72-hour liver enzyme values may also be indicated in more severe cases. Complete evaluation of hematologic and serum biochemical values is usually prudent for aged animals or those with preexisting health problems.

Treatment

Decontamination via emesis and/or administration of activated charcoal should be considered with ingestion of large amounts of leaf material or when parts of the bulb have been ingested. Symptomatic care in animals displaying mild clinical signs might include maintaining the animal with nothing per os for a few hours to allow the stomach to rest. Moderate to severe or persistent vomiting may necessitate the use of antiemetics and/or gastrointestinal protectants. In a study of lycorine-induced vomiting in beagle dogs, maropitant (a neurokinin-1 receptor antagonist) completely blocked vomiting when administered before lycorine administration, whereas ondansetron (a 5-HT$_3$ receptor antagonist) significantly reduced but did not prevent, lycorine-induced vomiting.[2] Other antiemetics such as diphenhydramine, scopolamine, and metoclopramide did not effectively block lycorine-induced vomiting. Based on this study, maropitant appears to be the antiemetic of choice, followed by ondansetron, in managing severe vomiting caused by ingestion of lycorine-containing plant material. Intravenous fluid therapy and correction of electrolyte abnormalities may be required in severe cases. Seizures, should they occur, can usually be managed by the use of diazepam or barbiturates to effect.

Prognosis

In most cases of amaryllis ingestion, the prognosis is very good, and signs usually resolve within 24 hours. Ingestion of large amounts of bulb material or ingestion of amaryllis by animals with prior health conditions may result in more severe signs or prolongation of the course of the toxicosis.

Gross and Histologic Lesions

No significant gross or histopathologic lesions have been reported in association with amaryllis ingestion in small animals.

Differential Diagnoses

Differential diagnoses for the gastrointestinal upset caused by amaryllis ingestion could include ingestion of other gastrointestinal irritants (e.g., other plants, arsenic, lead, zinc, zinc phosphide poisoning), bacterial or viral gastroenteritis (e.g., parvoviral enteritis), and pancreatitis.

Christmas Cactus (*Schlumbergera truncata*)

Sources

Christmas cactus (*Schlumbergera truncata*; Color Plate 39-2), also known as crab's claw cactus, is a member of the cactus family that is native to the jungles of Brazil.[6] These popular cacti have flattened, spineless branches tipped with flowers that range in color from red to pink, white, yellow, or orange.

Mechanism of Toxicity

In humans exposure to Christmas cactus has occasionally been associated with type 1 hypersensitivity, resulting in urticaria and rhinoconjunctivitis.[7] However, in dogs and cats, the primary clinical effects are caused by irritation of the gastrointestinal tract from ingested leaves.[6]

Clinical Signs

Clinical signs following ingestion of Christmas cactus include vomiting (with or without blood), diarrhea (with or without blood), depression, and anorexia.[6,8] In cats ataxia has occasionally been reported as well.[8] These signs are generally mild and rarely require more than withholding of food and water to allow the digestive tract to recover. Aged animals or animals with preexisting health conditions may experience more moderate to severe signs requiring veterinary intervention, including the use of antiemetics or antispasmodics, and correcting any hydration or electrolyte abnormalities.

Minimum Database

In most cases of Christmas cactus ingestion, there is little need for evaluation of clinical laboratory values because signs are generally mild and transient. Animals showing more than mild signs should have clinical laboratory values evaluated to rule out other potential causes for the clinical signs.

Prognosis

The prognosis for complete recovery following ingestion of Christmas cactus is excellent in most cases, with signs often subsiding within a few hours of ingestion.[6]

Gross and Histologic Lesions

No specific lesions would be expected with ingestion of Christmas cactus.

Differential Diagnoses

Differential diagnoses for the clinical signs produced by ingestion of Christmas cactus include dietary indiscretion and other causes of mild, self-limiting gastrointestinal upset. Signs that are persistent or especially severe should lead the clinician to reevaluate the animal to rule out other potential causes of gastrointestinal upset.

Christmas Trees

Sources

A large variety of evergreen trees are sold for use as Christmas trees in the United States. Generally the broad categories of trees that are most commonly used as Christmas trees include the firs (*Abies* spp., *Pseudotsuga menziesii*), pines (*Pinus* spp., Color Plate 39-3), cypresses (*Cupress* spp.), spruces (*Picea* spp.), and cedars (*Juniperus* spp. and *Cedrus* spp.). Christmas trees are most commonly cut before being brought indoors, although occasionally live trees with root-balls will be used as Christmas trees, with the trees planted outdoors after the holiday is over. Indoor pets may ingest needles, cones, branches, or bark from the trees. Cut trees are usually placed in a receptacle into which water is placed, and pets may also be exposed to sap and soluble plant components by drinking the water in the receptacle. (A word about commercial Christmas tree preservatives: These products usually are composed of small amounts of fertilizer and dextrose and are in themselves unlikely to produce more than mild gastric upset if ingested from the water receptacle. However, the potential exists for bacterial or fungal growth over time if the water-fertilizer substance is not routinely changed and could result in more severe gastroenteritis if the contaminated water-fertilizer substance is ingested. The editor is aware of an unpublished case report where an indoor cat succumbed to copper-induced hepatic failure following drinking the water in the receptacle. The owners had placed copper sulfate in the water to prevent fungal growth).

Mechanism of Toxicity

The seed cones from some species of *Juniperus* have been used as food by wildlife and humans, and seed cones and foliage from other *Juniperus* species have been used medicinally for their diuretic and uterine stimulant effects.[1] Juniper berries contain approximately 0.5% to 1.5% essential oils (primarily α-pinene), whereas the leaf of junipers contain approximately 0.25% essential oils (primarily sabinene).[9] Needles, branches, and bark of many of the evergreens used as Christmas trees contain monoterpenes and diterpenes and a variety of essential oils. Some of the terpenes and essential oils have been demonstrated to produce fetal deaths and malformations in laboratory rodents.[10] In livestock, ingestion of green or dry needles, bark, or budding branches of various evergreen plants has been associated with stillbirths, abortions, and other reproductive disorders.[1] Reproductive effects in livestock generally require ingestion of relatively large amounts of plant material over days to weeks. In small animals, where relatively small amounts of evergreen material might be ingested and chronic ingestion is unlikely, reproductive effects should not be expected. Concentrated essential oils of a variety of evergreens (e.g., thujone from cedar oil) have been shown to cause CNS effects, including seizures in animals,[11] but exposure to the level of essential oils in Christmas tree material is unlikely to cause significant CNS effects in pets.

The mechanisms of action for the majority of the constituents of Christmas tree evergreens are not known. Some *Juniperus* species contain podophyllotoxin, which binds tubulin, resulting in arrest of cell division in metaphase and that may contribute to the teratogenic and reproductive disorders seen in livestock ingesting these plants.[1] Some volatile oils in evergreens have been demonstrated to induce hepatic P-450 enzymes, which can alter xenobiotic metabolism.[12] In small animals, ingestion of plant material would be expected to cause gastrointestinal upset, either through mechanical irritation or irritation from terpenes or essential oils. Rarely, ingestion of large quantities of evergreen needles, bark, or cones might result in gastrointestinal foreign body obstruction.

Clinical Signs

In small animals, the most common clinical signs expected with ingestion of evergreen tree material are vomiting, anorexia, abdominal pain, and depression (American Society for the Prevention of Cruelty to Animals [ASPCA] Animal Poison Control Center, unpublished data). Some varieties of evergreens have sharp needles and/or cones, which may cause mechanical trauma to mucous membranes of the alimentary tract. In most cases clinical signs are expected to be mild and self-limiting, although animals with preexisting health problems may be at increased risk for complications, such as dehydration or electrolyte imbalances. Typical signs of gastrointestinal foreign body obstruction (e.g., abdominal discomfort and persistent vomiting) may occur following ingestion of large quantities of plant material.

Minimum Database

Because signs from ingestion of Christmas tree material are expected to be mild, laboratory evaluation is rarely necessary, although monitoring of hydration and electrolyte status is recommended in animals with preexisting health problems. Animals with severe or protracted vomiting should receive a complete laboratory workup to rule out foreign body obstruction and other potential causes of vomiting (e.g., pancreatitis, liver disease, renal disease).

Treatment

In most cases clinical signs associated with ingestion of Christmas tree material are self-limiting and require little treatment beyond withholding food and water to rest the gastrointestinal tract. Antiemetics would be indicated for severe or protracted vomiting, and gastrointestinal protectants (e.g., sucralfate slurries) or antibiotics may be beneficial if there is evidence of mechanical mucosal injury. Correction of hydration and/or electrolyte abnormalities via the use of crystalloid fluid therapy might be required in rare instances. Treatment of foreign body obstruction (e.g., surgical or endoscopic removal of plant material) might be required in rare cases where large amounts of plant material have been ingested.

Prognosis

The prognosis for animals ingesting Christmas tree material is very good, and most signs are expected to be mild and self-limiting. Animals having more severe or protracted signs should be worked up for other potential causes of gastrointestinal distress.

Gross and Histologic Lesions

Other than potential mechanical damage to oral, pharyngeal, and gastric mucosa, no significant lesions are expected from ingestion of Christmas trees by pets.

Differential Diagnoses

Differential diagnoses for ingestion of Christmas tree material would include other causes of gastrointestinal upset, including pancreatitis, ingestion of other irritants, foreign body obstruction, infectious gastroenteritis, and neoplasia.

Holly (*Ilex aquifolium*)

Sources

Ilex aquifolium (Color Plate 39-4), also known as Christmas or English holly, is a popular holiday ornamental plant prized for its shiny green, spiny leaves and bright red berries. As with other Christmas plants, animals that live indoors are at increased risk of exposure to these plants.

Mechanism of Toxicity

In addition to mechanical damage from the spiny leaves, holly contains a variety of potentially injurious substances within the leaves and berries, including saponins, triterpenes, polyphenols, methylxanthines, and cyanogens.[6,9] Fortunately the latter two substances do not appear to contribute significantly to toxicity when holly is ingested by animals. Ethanol leaf extracts of holly were lethal when injected into mice, but fruit extracts caused no toxic effects in mice.[9] The primary toxic effects of holly ingestion are owing to gastrointestinal irritation from the saponins.

Ingestion of holly in small animals generally causes no more than mild to moderate gastrointestinal upset.[6] Ingestion of large amounts of leaves may result in foreign body obstruction, although this is not a common occurrence.

Clinical Signs

In dogs and cats, the most common signs of holly ingestion are hypersalivation, vomiting, anorexia, diarrhea, head shaking, and smacking of the lips.[6] Mechanical injury to the oral mucosa from the leaves is also possible, resulting in mild oral ulceration or lacerations. Foreign body obstruction caused by ingestion of a very large number of leaves could lead to more severe gastrointestinal signs.

Minimum Database

Because signs from ingestion of holly leaves and berries are expected to be mild, laboratory evaluation is rarely necessary, although monitoring of hydration and electrolyte status is recommended in animals with preexisting health problems. Animals with severe or protracted vomiting should receive a complete laboratory workup to rule out foreign body obstruction and other potential causes of vomiting (e.g., pancreatitis, renal disease, liver disease).

Treatment

Most cases of holly ingestion can be managed at home. In cases in which large amounts of leaves and berries have been ingested, bulking the stomach (e.g., bread) and inducing emesis might be recommended to minimize development of more severe vomiting later. Symptomatic animals may be managed by instructing owners to withhold food and water for 1 to 2 hours to allow the stomach to settle, and gradually reintroducing water, and then food. Animals that appear to have oral discomfort (e.g., lip smacking, head shaking) may find relief if the mouth is rinsed with small amounts of water.[6] Antiemetics, although rarely necessary, may be used in cases in which there is protracted vomiting. Animals displaying more than mild gastrointestinal upset should be evaluated by a veterinarian for other potential causes or the presence of foreign body obstruction. Intravenous fluid therapy would be indicated in cases in which protracted vomiting and/or diarrhea have resulted in hydration or electrolyte abnormalities.

Prognosis

The prognosis for animals ingesting holly leaves and/or berries is excellent, with most signs resolving quickly. Animals with prior health issues or those with foreign body obstruction may have a more protracted clinical course.

Gross and Histologic Lesions

Other than potential mechanical damage to oral, pharyngeal, and gastric mucosa, no significant lesions are expected from ingestion of holly by pets.

Differential Diagnoses

Differential diagnoses for the clinical signs produced by ingestion of holly include dietary indiscretion and other causes of mild, self-limiting gastrointestinal upset. Signs that are persistent or especially severe should lead the clinician to reevaluate the animal to rule out foreign body or other potential causes of gastrointestinal upset unrelated to holly ingestion.

Kalanchoe (*Kalanchoe blossfeldiana*)

Sources

Kalanchoe blossfeldiana (Color Plate 39-5), also known as Christmas kalanchoe and flaming Katy, is a member of the Crassulaceae family and a native of Madagascar.[1] Many *Kalanchoe* species have been introduced in the United States and grow wild in the South or are cultivated as landscaping or houseplants. Christmas kalanchoes have bright, vivid flowers ranging from white to orange-gold to red and can be induced to bloom in the winter.

Toxic Dose

All members of *Kalanchoe* are toxic, and losses to livestock occur in South Africa and Australia when these plants are ingested because of scarcity of appropriate forage.[1] Flowers contain the highest levels of cardiotoxic compounds compared with stems, roots, or leaves.[13] Dogs are reported to be particularly sensitive to the cardiotoxic effects of *Kalanchoe*. Toxic doses of *Kalanchoe* spp. other than *K. blossfeldiana* have been determined for livestock and birds, but not for small animals. Death was reported in an iguana that ingested an entire *K. blossfeldiana* plant.[1]

Mechanism of Toxicity

The primary toxic principles of *Kalanchoe* spp. are cardiotoxic bufadienolides that are present in all parts of the plant.[1] These compounds are related to the same cardiotoxic agents responsible for toxicity of *Bufo* spp. toads and have a mechanism of action similar to digoxin. Bufadienolides inhibit Na-K adenosine triphosphatase (ATPase) activity in the myocardial cell membrane, increasing intracellular sodium and decreasing intracellular potassium, which results in reduction of the normal membrane resting potential.[13,14] Normal electrical conduction is inhibited, and there is a decrease in the ability of the myocardium to act as a pacemaker. Ultimately complete loss of normal myocardial electrical function may lead to asystole. Hyperkalemia occurs, especially in severe toxicosis.

Clinical Signs

Clinical signs reported in livestock include depression, anorexia, hypersalivation, and diarrhea.[1] Diarrhea, which may be bloody, is reportedly the most consistent sign in livestock. Cardiac abnormalities include bradycardia, various arrhythmias, and heart block and are manifested by weakness, dyspnea, collapse, and death. Neurologic signs such as nystagmus, delirium, tetany, and mild seizures have been reported in dogs following *Kalanchoe* ingestion.[13] A review of cases from the ASPCA Animal Poison Control Center indicated that the most common signs in dogs and cats ingesting *Kalanchoe* spp. were vomiting (57%), depression and/or lethargy (42%), and diarrhea (29%) (ASPCA Animal Poison Control Center, unpublished data). Other signs included weakness, dyspnea, anorexia, tachycardia, and vocalization. No deaths were reported in dogs or cats following *Kalanchoe* ingestion.

Minimum Database

Animals having clinical signs following *Kalanchoe* ingestion should have the heart rate and rhythm, blood pressure, and electrolyte status closely monitored. Hyperkalemia is a common occurrence in cardiac glycoside toxicosis as a result of the shifting of potassium out of cells. Serum chemistry analysis should be performed to determine the status of liver and kidney function, and renal function should be monitored throughout the toxicosis because hypotension may lead to renal injury. Hyperglycemia has been reported in *Kalanchoe* intoxication, so monitoring of blood glucose is recommended.[1]

Confirmatory Tests

Immunoassays for digoxin or digitoxin cross-react with plant-derived cardiac glycosides.[15] Therefore these assays can be used to aid in confirming a diagnosis of *Kalanchoe* intoxication, provided animals have had no concomitant exposure to other cardiac glycosides (e.g., digoxin). However, serum levels may not necessarily correlate to the degree of toxicity.[15] Most human hospitals have the capability to run these tests on a "stat" basis if necessary.

Treatment

Asymptomatic patients should be decontaminated (emesis and activated charcoal) and monitored for development of gastrointestinal signs. Animals developing more than mild, transient vomiting and/or diarrhea should be brought to a veterinarian for evaluation of cardiac and electrolyte status. Gastrointestinal signs should be managed as necessary, and fluid therapy should be instituted. Cardiac arrhythmias can vary, so it is important to treat the arrhythmia present; atropine may be helpful for bradyarrhythmias, and beta-blockers may be used for tachyarrhythmias. Correction of electrolyte abnormalities, especially hyperkalemia, is important; sodium polystyrene sulfonate (Kayexalate) may be used to aid in reducing serum potassium levels.[16] Management of pulmonary edema, renal failure, ascites, or other complications secondary to cardiac failure may be required.

The use of digoxin-specific immune Fab (Digibind® or Digifab®; d-Fab) is indicated in situations where serum potassium exceeds 5 mEq/L in the face of severe intoxication and/or where severe arrhythmias that are poorly responsive to therapy are present.[17] These antibody fragments bind the cardiac glycosides within the bloodstream, then the glycoside-Fab complexes are removed via glomerular filtration. The use of d-Fab in cardiac glycoside intoxication can result in rapid improvement of cardiovascular status, but recrudescence of signs may occur because of redistribution of the remaining glycoside in the body, requiring additional treatment. Further, animals with impaired renal function may experience relapse as dissociation of the unexcreted glycoside-Fab complexes occurs. Serum potassium levels may drop dramatically following administration of d-Fab because of reactivation of the Na-K ATPase pump, so close monitoring of potassium levels is required. Dosing of d-Fab is generally based on digoxin levels, and there is a formula for determining the recommended dose. In veterinary cases, digoxin levels may not be readily obtainable, and it can be cost prohibitive to administer the initial five vials that are recommended in human cases when digoxin levels are not available. Therefore in these cases it is recommended that one to two vials be used initially and the effects observed.[17] The primary drawback to d-Fab is its cost, which can be several hundred dollars per vial.

Prognosis

The prognosis for animals exhibiting mild gastrointestinal signs following ingestion of *Kalanchoe* is generally good. Animals developing severe gastrointestinal signs are at risk for cardiovascular effects, and the prognosis in animals displaying significant cardiac arrhythmias and/or hyperkalemia is guarded.

Gross and Histologic Lesions

Lesions from animals dying from *Kalanchoe* ingestion are reflective of the cardiac failure. Gross cardiac lesions may be unapparent or mild and may consist of scattered ecchymotic hemorrhages on the epicardium and pale foci within the myocardium.[1] Histopathologic examination of these foci reveals areas of degenerating myofibers, myocardial necrosis, edema, and mononuclear cell infiltrates. Other lesions of cardiac failure, such as pulmonary edema or ascites, may be present depending on the duration and severity of the clinical effects.

Differential Diagnoses

Differential diagnoses for the gastrointestinal signs from *Kalanchoe* include ingestion of other cardiac glycoside–containing products (e.g., pharmaceuticals, plants, toads), other gastrointestinal irritants, foreign body obstruction, pancreatitis, and infectious gastroenteritis. Differential diagnoses for the cardiovascular effects include ingestion of other cardiac glycoside–containing products (e.g., pharmaceuticals, plants, toads), other cardiac drugs (e.g., beta-blockers), sympathomimetics, and primary cardiac disease (e.g., neoplasia, sick sinus syndrome).

Mistletoe (*Phoradendron* spp.)

Sources

Mistletoes are worldwide in distribution, but it is the American Christmas mistletoe (*Phoradendron tomentosum*) that is used as a holiday decoration.[9] European mistletoe (*Viscum* spp.) is used in a variety of folk-medicine products and has been investigated pharmacologically for its immunomodulating properties,[18] but is not commonly used as holiday decoration in the United States. All members of Viscaceae are semiparasitic plants that live on tree branches, and toxicity is thought to vary with the type of host tree on which a particular plant grows.[1] In general the American mistletoes are considered less toxic than the European varieties.

Toxic Dose

Although mistletoe contains a variety of potentially toxic compounds, serious poisonings from mistletoe appear uncommon. Several studies of *Phoradendron* ingestion in humans revealed that the majority of cases remained asymptomatic, with mild gastric upset being the primary clinical finding in humans ingesting leaves, berries, or extracts of the plant.[19] Instances of more serious effects, including hypotension, collapse, ataxia, seizures, and deaths have been reported, but are extremely rare in occurrence.[18-20] Similarly, exposures of animals to *Phoradendron* leaves or berries have not been reported to be associated with serious clinical signs.[18-20]

Mechanism of Toxicity

Mistletoes contain glycoprotein lectins that can inhibit protein synthesis, leading to cell death; although these lectins are of the same class as the very toxic ricin found in castor beans *(Ricinus communis)*, the lectins in *Phoradendron* are much less toxic.[1] Phoratoxins and ligatoxin A found in mistletoe are small proteins that can act as cardiac depressants, causing hypotension, bradycardia, and decreased contractility. Other potential pharmacologic and/or toxicologic agents present in mistletoe include various alkaloids, gamma aminobutyric acid, phenols, phenethylamines, phenylpropanoids, polysaccharides, and flavonoids; however the role of these agents in the toxicity of mistletoe appears to be minimal.[9,20-22]

Clinical Signs

The most common effects seen in animals ingesting mistletoe are vomiting and depression.[6] Diarrhea and hypotension may also be seen, although the latter would not be expected to be a common finding.[1] Serious clinical signs are not expected, and most signs are expected to be mild and self-limiting. Fluid and electrolyte abnormalities could develop in animals with protracted vomiting or with prior health problems.

Minimum Database

Because signs from ingestion of mistletoe leaves and berries are expected to be mild, laboratory evaluation is rarely necessary, although monitoring of hydration and electrolyte status is recommended in animals with preexisting health problems. Animals with severe or protracted vomiting should receive a complete laboratory workup to rule out foreign body obstruction and other potential causes of vomiting (e.g., pancreatitis, renal disease, liver disease). Monitoring for hypotension is recommended in animals showing more mild gastrointestinal upset and depression.

Treatment

As with many of the other Christmastime plants, the majority of cases of mistletoe ingestion by pets can be successfully managed at home by decontamination (if a large amount of plant was ingested) and withholding food and water in the vomiting patient. Animals with more severe vomiting should be evaluated, and fluid and electrolyte abnormalities should be corrected as necessary. Severely affected animals should be evaluated for hypotension.

Prognosis

As with other plants that primarily cause gastrointestinal irritation, the prognosis for full recovery following ingestion of mistletoe is excellent. If signs develop, they are generally mild and self-limiting.

Gross and Histologic Lesions

No specific lesions would be expected with ingestion of mistletoe.

Differential Diagnoses

Differential diagnoses for ingestion of mistletoe would include other causes of gastrointestinal upset, including pancreatitis, ingestion of other irritants, foreign body obstruction, infectious gastroenteritis, and neoplasia.

Poinsettia (*Euphorbia pulcherrima*)

Sources

Poinsettia (*Euphorbia pulcherrima*; Color Plate 39-6) is a very popular Christmas plant that is brought into many households during the holiday season. The uppermost leaves of the plant develop red, white, or pink coloration, resembling a flower. However, the actual flowers are the tiny yellow structures resembling stamens.[6]

Toxic Dose

Historically, poinsettias have received a great deal of negative publicity because of their purported toxicity. However, based on animal and human exposures, it appears that the toxicity of poinsettia is greatly exaggerated because studies of the plant and reviews of incidents of ingestion by humans have failed to show any serious effects.[6] All *Euphorbia* contain milky sap that has irritant properties. Although the sap from some *Euphorbia* species has been associated with serious illness and even death in humans, the sap from poinsettias appears to be much less potent.[1] Feeding 8 to 30 g/kg of poinsettia to cattle caused gastrointestinal irritation of several days duration, and feeding 20 g/kg to sheep produced no effects. When poinsettia sap was administered orally to rats at levels of 125 g/kg for 5 days, no adverse effects were observed, although skin photosensitivity was induced by topical application to the skin of albino rats.[23] In small animals, poinsettia ingestion has been associated with mild and self-limiting signs.[6]

Mechanism of Toxicity

The irritation from the milky sap of poinsettia is thought to be caused by the presence of diterpenoid euphorbol esters and steroids with saponin-like properties that exert a detergent-like effect on tissue.[1] In humans dermal irritation and hypersensitivity from the milky sap has been reported, and humans with latex allergy may react similarly to poinsettia.[24] Anaphylaxis resulting from poinsettia was reported in two infants with atopic eczema and latex allergy.[25]

Clinical Signs

The most common clinical signs expected from poinsettia exposure reflect the irritant nature of the sap.[1] Dermal contact may result in irritation, erythema, and pruritus. Ingestion of the plant material can result in irritation of the mucous membranes of the alimentary tract, causing hypersalivation, vomiting, and rarely, diarrhea. Conjunctivitis caused by ocular exposure to the sap is also possible. Signs are normally expected to be mild and self-limiting, requiring little or no medical treatment. In rare instances, protracted vomiting may result in hydration or electrolyte disorders that may need to be addressed.

Minimum Database

Because signs from ingestion of poinsettia are expected to be mild, laboratory evaluation is rarely necessary, although monitoring of hydration and electrolyte status is recommended in animals with preexisting health problems. Animals with severe or protracted vomiting should receive a complete laboratory workup to rule out foreign body obstruction and other potential causes of vomiting (e.g., pancreatitis, renal disease, liver disease).

Treatment

Induction of emesis should only be considered if very large amounts of plant material have been ingested. In most cases dilution with water and milk and having owners monitor for vomiting is sufficient. Should vomiting develop, food and water should be withheld for a few hours to allow the gastrointestinal tract to settle. If protracted vomiting develops or in animals with significant prior health conditions, monitoring of hydration and electrolyte status is recommended and correction of abnormalities with appropriate fluid therapy may be indicated.

For dermal exposures, bathing with a mild soap and water is recommended. If ocular exposure has occurred, the eye should be flushed copiously with saline or tepid tap water for 15 to 20 minutes followed by thorough examination of the cornea.

Prognosis

The prognosis for complete recovery following ingestion of poinsettia is excellent because signs are generally mild and self-limiting. Deaths from poinsettia ingestion by small animals have not been reported.

Gross and Histologic Lesions

No specific lesions would be expected with ingestion of poinsettia.

Differential Diagnoses

Differential diagnoses for ingestion of poinsettia leaves would include other causes of gastrointestinal upset, including pancreatitis, ingestion of other irritants, foreign body obstruction, infectious gastroenteritis, and neoplasia.

Rosemary (*Rosmarinus officinalis*)

Sources

Rosemary (*Rosmarinus officinalis*; Color Plate 39-7) is a small evergreen shrub with thick aromatic leaves that is used primarily as a culinary herb prized for its rich pungent flavor.[22] Rosemary also has been used extensively as a medicinal herb for its astringent, spasmolytic, antiinflammatory, expectorant, carminative, antirheumatic, analgesic, antimicrobial, and hypotensive properties.[9,26] The use of the rosemary leaf to treat dyspepsia, high blood pressure, and rheumatism was approved by the German Commission E at doses of 4 to 6 g/day.[22] Other pharmacologic effects attributed to rosemary include antimutagenic, anticancer, hepatoprotective, and antioxidant activities.[27–29] Historically, rosemary was a common Christmas plant used for creating wreaths and other aromatic holiday decorations. Recently the use of rosemary for Christmas decorations has undergone a renaissance because many people choose traditional or "old-fashioned" themes for their holiday decorations, thus increasing the opportunity for indoor pets to become exposed to the plant.

Toxic Dose

Rosemary contains a variety of volatile essential oils, including monoterpene hydrocarbons, camphene, limonene, camphor, borneol, cineole, linalool, and verbinol.[22] The plant also contains a variety of flavonoids, diterpenes, polyphenols, and high levels of salicylates. At the low levels of rosemary used in cooking, these agents are of little toxicologic importance, but ingestion of large quantities of rosemary extracts or oils can result in gastrointestinal irritation, renal injury, and neurologic effects. Rosemary is also reportedly an abortifacient.[22]

Mechanism of Toxicity

The mechanism of several of the pharmacologic activities of rosemary have been elucidated (e.g., anticancer properties have been attributed to the induction of anticarcinogenic enzymes, such as quinone reductase, or inhibition of metabolic activation of procarcinogens by P-450 enzymes),[22] but the mechanism of toxicity of rosemary is not as well understood. Gastrointestinal irritation from ingestion of large quantities of rosemary may result from the direct irritant effect of the essential oils on the mucosa. The hypotensive effects of rosemary are considered to be a result of a spasmolytic action on smooth and cardiac muscles. Rosemary can prevent embryonic implantation, but the mechanism of the abortifacient activity of rosemary has not been established.[30] The monoterpene ketones in rosemary are reportedly convulsants.[22] Allergic contact dermatitis has also been reported with dermal exposure to rosemary.[9]

Clinical Signs

The primary clinical signs expected with ingestion of small to moderate amounts of rosemary include nausea, vomiting, and possibly diarrhea.[22] Ingestion of larger amounts may result in hypotension that is characterized by weakness, pale mucous membranes, and depression. Renal injury from ingestion of rosemary may cause polyuria, polydipsia, vomiting, dehydration, weight loss, depression, and in severe cases, signs of uremia (e.g., oral ulceration, neurologic signs). Seizures have been reported in humans ingesting very large doses of rosemary. Reproductive failure and abortion may also result from ingestion of large amounts of rosemary.

Minimum Database

Symptomatic animals that have ingested large amounts of rosemary should be evaluated for hydration, and electrolyte and renal abnormalities. Monitoring of blood pressure, urine output, and neurologic status is indicated in animals displaying more than mild gastrointestinal upset or when large amounts of rosemary have been ingested.

Treatment

Early decontamination via emesis and administration of activated charcoal with a cathartic is recommended when large amounts of rosemary are ingested. Treatment is symptomatic and supportive for those animals showing clinical signs. Antiemetics, fluid therapy, and pressor agents should be used as necessary to maintain blood pressure and hydration. Diuretics may be indicated if oliguria or anuria develops. Seizures should be managed with diazepam or barbiturates.

Prognosis

The prognosis for rosemary ingestion depends on the amount of plant material ingested and the type of clinical signs that develop. In most cases mild gastrointestinal upset is likely to be the extent of the clinical signs, and these animals are expected to make full recoveries. Animals with seizures or renal dysfunction have a more guarded prognosis until response to therapy can be evaluated.

Gross and Histologic Lesions

No specific lesions have been reported associated with ingestion of rosemary.

Differential Diagnoses

Differential diagnoses for the gastrointestinal signs from rosemary include other causes of gastrointestinal upset, including pancreatitis, ingestion of other irritants, foreign body obstruction, infectious gastroenteritis, and neoplasia. Differential diagnoses for hypotension include primary cardiovascular disease, shock, and ingestion of hypotensive pharmaceuticals.

References

1. Burrows GE, Tyrl RJ: *Toxic Plants of North America*, Ames, IA, 2001, Iowa State University Press.
2. Kretzing S, Abraham G, Seiwert B, et al: In vivo assessment of antiemetic drugs and mechanism of lycorine-induced nausea and emesis, *Arch Toxicol*, 2011http://dx.doi.org/10.1007/s00204-011-0718-9.
3. Barr AC: Household and garden plants. In Peterson ME, Talcott PA, editors: *Small animal toxicology*, Philadelphia, 2001, Saunders.

4. Kretzing S, Abraham G, Seiwert B, et al: Dose-dependent emetic effects of the Amaryllidaceous alkaloid lycorine in beagle dogs, *Toxicon* 57:117–124, 2011.
5. Jensen AP, Visser FJ, Nierop G: Occupation asthma to amaryllis, *Allergy* 51:847–849, 1996.
6. Volmer PA: How dangerous are winter and spring holiday plants to pets? *Vet Med* 97:879–884, 2002.
7. Paulsen E, Skov PS, Brindslev-Jensen C, et al: Occupation type I allergy to Christmas cactus, *Allergy* 52:656–660, 1997.
8. ASPCA Animal Poison Control Center: *Household plant reference*, Urbana, IL, 1998, ASPCA APCC.
9. Barceloux DG: *Medical Toxicology of Natural Substances I*, Hoboken, NJ, 2008, Wiley.
10. Pages N, Fournier G, Chamorro G: Teratological evaluation of *Juniperus Sabina* essential oil in mice, *Planta Med* 55:144–146, 1989.
11. Millet Y, Youglard J, Steinmetz MD: Toxicity of some essential plant oils. Clinical and experimental study, *Clin Toxicol* 18:1485–1498, 1981.
12. Burek JD, Schwetz BA: Considerations in the selection and use of chemicals within the animal facility, *Lab Anim Sci* 30:414–421, 1980.
13. Smith G: Toxicology brief: *Kalanchoe* species poisoning in pets, *Vet Med* 99:933–936, 2004.
14. Adams R: *Veterinary pharmacology and therapeutics*, ed 7, Ames, IA, 1995, Iowa State University Press.
15. Klasco RK: POISINDEX® System, Greenwood Village, CO, edition expires 6/2004, Thomson MICROMEDEX.
16. Roder JD: Cardiovascular drugs. In Plumlee KH, editor: *Clinical veterinary toxicology*, St Louis, 2004, Mosby.
17. Gwaltney-Brant SM, Rumbeiha WK: Newer antidotal therapies, *Vet Clin Small Anim* 32:323–339, 2002.
18. Gorter RW, van Wely M: Tolerability of an extract of European mistletoe among immunocompromised and healthy individuals, *Altern Ther Health Med* 5:37–44, 1999. 47–48.
19. Krenzelok EP, Jacobsen TD, Aronis J: American mistletoe exposures, *Am J Emerg Med* 15:516–520, 1997.
20. Hall AH, Spoerke DG, Rumack BH: Assessing mistletoe toxicity, *Ann Emerg Med* 15:1320–1323, 1986.
21. Spiller HA, Willias DB, Gorman SE, et al: Retrospective study of mistletoe ingestion, *J Toxicol Clin Toxicol* 34:405–408, 1996.
22. Der Merderosian A, Beutler JA: *The Review of Natural Products*, ed 3, St Louis, 2000, Facts and Comparisons.
23. Winek CL, Butala J, Shanor SP, et al: Toxicology of poinsettia, *Clin Toxicol* 13:27–45, 1978.
24. Bala TM, Panda M: No poinsettia this Christmas, *South Med J* 99:772–773, 2006.
25. Kimata H: Anaphylaxis by poinsettia in infants with atopic eczema, *Allergy* 62:91–92, 2007.
26. Takaki I, Bersani-Amado LE, Vendruscolo A, et al: Anti-inflammatory and antinociceptive effects of *Rosmarinus officinalis L.* essential oil in experimental animal models, *J Med Food* 11:741–746, 2008.
27. Fahim FA, Esmat AY, Fadel HM, et al: Allied studies on the effect of *Rosmarinus officinalis* L. on experimental hepatotoxicity and mutagenesis, *Int J Food Sci Nutr* 50:413–427, 1999.
28. Sotelo-Felix JI, Martinez-Fong D, Muriel P, et al: Evaluation of the effectiveness of *Rosmarinus officinalis (Lamiaceae)* in the alleviation of carbon tetrachloride-induced acute hepatotoxicity in the rat, *J Ethnopharmacol* 81:145–154, 2002.
29. Johnson JJ: Carnosol: a promising anti-cancer and anti-inflammatory agent, *Cancer Lett* 305:1–7, 2011.
30. Lemonica IP, Damasceno DC, di-Stasi LC: Study of the embryotoxic effects of an extract of rosemary (*Rosmarinus officinalis L.*), *Braz J Med Biol Res* 29:223–227, 1996.

Citrus Oils

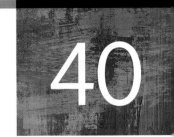

Konnie H. Plumlee, DVM, MS, DABVT, DACVIM

- Citrus oils can be toxic even though they have a natural origin. The primary toxins are limonene and linalool.
- Citrus oils are used in some products marketed for insect control in pets.
- Cats appear to be more sensitive to citrus oils than dogs.
- The most common clinical signs include excessive salivation, hypothermia, muscle tremors, and ataxia.
- Severe cutaneous reactions can also occur.

C itrus oils are derived from botanical sources and so are considered "natural" or "organic" by the consumer, who often has the mistaken belief that the products are completely safe. Most cases of toxicoses are a result of pet owners who fail to follow the dilution directions on the product label. However, severe idiosyncratic skin reactions have also been reported.

Sources

Citrus oil extracts, including d-limonene and linalool, are derived from citrus fruit skin. d-Limonene is a monocyclic terpene with insecticidal properties, especially from the vapor, which primarily acts as a desiccant.[1] d-Limonene is toxic to all life stages of the flea with the order of sensitivity from most to least being eggs, adults, larvae, and pupae.[1]

Several products containing citrus oils are marketed to control ticks, fleas, and other insects. These products include insect sprays, pet dips, shampoos, and soaps. Solvents, fragrances, and cleansers are other types of products that may contain citrus oils.

Toxic Dose

In dogs the oral toxic dose of limonene is 680 g/kg; however, cats appear to be more sensitive than dogs.[2] A dermal study demonstrated that cats had clinical signs when a commercial pet dip containing 78.2% d-limonene was used at five times the recommended dose.[3] In another study, three cats were dipped in a citrus product marketed for dogs. Even though the product was diluted according to label directions, one cat subsequently died, one cat became symptomatic but recovered, and one cat remained asymptomatic.[4] A third study examined the use of a ready-to-use spray containing d-limonene, linalool, and piperonyl butoxide (a mixed function oxidase inhibitor). Mild signs appeared with a single dose in one of six cats.[5] In one case report, a cat had severe clinical signs and was euthanized following the reportedly correct use of a 1% d-limonene–based shampoo labeled for dogs and cats.[1]

Toxicokinetics

Citrus oils are absorbed rapidly both via the dermis and orally, and the distribution within the body is similar to that of other lipid-soluble compounds.[2] d-Limonene reaches maximum blood concentrations 10 minutes after dermal exposure.[1] The urinary tract is the main route of excretion, and less than 10% of excretion is by the fecal route.[2]

Mechanism of Toxicity

The complete mechanism of action for toxic reactions is unknown. However, d-limonene monoxide has a direct vasodilatory effect when given IV to anesthetized dogs.[1] Systemic hypotension in cats may be associated with generalized vasodilation in the skin.[1]

Clinical Signs

Hypersalivation, which may be accompanied by ataxia and/or muscle tremors, develops in cats. The hypersalivation is transient and may be partially or entirely a reaction to the taste of the product following grooming. The brain cholinesterase is not depressed in cats that have hypersalivation.[4] Mild to severe hypothermia often develops.[3,6] Muscle tremors must be differentiated from a shivering reaction caused by the hypothermia. Other reported signs include weakness, lethargy, vocalization, aggressive behavior, recumbency, general paralysis, vasodilation, mydriasis, slowed pupillary response, and hypotension.[1,2,5]

Various skin reactions have been reported. A cat developed acute necrotizing dermatitis and septicemia after being bathed with a limonene-based shampoo labeled for cats and dogs.[1] As the cat's condition progressed, acidemia, hypoglycemia, miosis, and neurologic signs developed consistent with diffuse cerebral edema and possible right vestibular involvement.[1] Excoriation of the scrotal and perineal areas was described in male cats dipped in a d-limonene preparation that was 15 times the recommended concentration.[3] One case report described a dog that exhibited vomiting, anorexia, lethargy, and general cutaneous erythema 24 hours after being dipped in a product containing d-limonene. The dog developed erythema multiforme major and diffuse intravascular coagulation (DIC) before death.[7] In another case a dog developed toxic epidermal necrolysis shortly after being dipped in a d-limonene product. Within 5 minutes of being dipped, the dog exhibited hypersalivation, tonic-clonic seizures, and aggressive behavior. The dog subsequently had focal alopecia, thrombocytopenia, prolonged clotting times, and dark red urine containing blood and protein. A large section of the skin over the thorax and abdomen became necrotic and eventually sloughed.[8]

Confirmatory Tests

No diagnostic laboratory tests are available for citrus oil toxicosis.

Treatment

No antidote is available. Decontamination is best done with a mild dishwashing detergent to remove any product dermally applied. Thermoregulation is frequently necessary to control the hypothermia that may develop. Other treatments are supportive in nature and depend on the clinical signs and their severity.

More aggressive therapy is warranted if cutaneous reactions, such as erythema multiforme or toxic epidermal necrolysis, occur. These conditions can result in loss of the epidermal barrier followed by secondary bacterial infection and sepsis. Antibiotic administration, fluid therapy, wound treatment, and pain control are warranted. Corticosteroids have not been proven beneficial for toxic epidermal necrolysis and may result in increased complications.[1]

Prognosis

Clinical signs can last a few hours to several days. The prognosis is good for most animals that receive appropriate care. However, the survival rate is lower in animals in which a skin reaction develops that compromises the epidermal barrier.

Gross and Histologic Lesions

There are no specific lesions for this toxicosis. Lesions can range from mild excoriation of the skin to severe diffuse epidermal necrosis.[3,7]

Differential Diagnoses

Diagnosis is made from a history of recent exposure to a citrus oil product along with the appropriate signs. Most toxicoses that involve muscle tremors result in a body temperature that is normal or elevated, whereas many cases of citrus oil toxicoses have decreased body temperatures. Affected animals often have a strong citrus odor.

References

1. Lee JA, Budgin JB, Mauldin EA: Acute necrotizing dermatitis and septicemia after application of a d-limonene-based insecticidal shampoo in a cat, *JAVMA* 221:258, 2002.
2. Osweiler GD: Citrus oil extracts. In Osweiler GD, editor: *Toxicology*, ed 2, Philadelphia, 1996, Williams & Wilkins.
3. Hooser SB, Beasley VR, Everitt JI: Effects of an insecticidal dip containing d-limonene in the cat, *JAVMA* 189:905, 1986.
4. Hooser SB: Citrus insecticide hazardous to cats, *JAVMA* 184:236, 1984.
5. Powers KA, Hooser SB, Sundberg JP, et al: An evaluation of the acute toxicity of an insecticidal spray containing linalool, d-limonene, and piperonyl butoxide applied topically to domestic cats, *Vet Hum Toxicol* 30:206, 1988.
6. Hooser SB: D-limonene, linalool, and crude citrus oil extracts, *Vet Clin North Am Small Anim Pract* 20:383, 1990.
7. Rosenbaum MR, Kerlin RL: Erythema multiforme major and disseminated intravascular coagulation in a dog following application of a d-limonene-based insecticidal dip, *JAVMA* 207:1315, 1995.
8. Frank AA, Ross JL, Sawvell BK: Toxic epidermal necrolysis associated with flea dips, *Vet Hum Toxicol* 34:57, 1992.

Copper

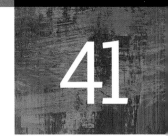

Patricia A. Talcott, MS, DVM, PhD, DABVT

- Acute copper poisoning in dogs and cats is an uncommon occurrence.
- Potential sources include copper-containing coins, copper sulfate solutions and feeds, copper oxide capsules, and miscellaneous copper-containing items (e.g., wire, coils, and jewelry).
- Copper is primarily stored and metabolized by the liver and excreted into the bile. Excess copper that is not excreted is stored in lysosomes.
- Varying degrees of hepatocellular necrosis are seen following acute toxicosis.
- Common signs of illness reported include vomiting, depression, lethargy, inappetence, diarrhea, and abdominal pain. Icterus and hemoglobinemia or hemoglobinuria are less commonly observed.
- Confirmation of poisoning is based primarily on compatible microscopic lesions in liver tissue, along with excessive copper concentrations in liver and kidney tissues. Serum copper concentrations are not necessarily a reliable indicator of excessive copper intake.
- Treatment is primarily supportive in nature, and the prognosis depends on the severity of hepatic damage.

This chapter focuses on "copper" (Cu) poisoning in small animals as opposed to the chronic or inherited form of copper toxicosis (i.e., copper storage disease, chronic active hepatitis) described in Bedlington terriers and other susceptible breeds of dogs. A section at the end of this chapter briefly addresses this disease. Acute copper poisoning in dogs and cats is uncommon, and only a few cases have been documented in the literature. Acute onset of chronic copper exposure is a well-known occurrence in sheep and to a lesser extent in cattle, camelids, and goats. The sources of copper poisoning in small animals are quite different from those in livestock, which most likely contributes to the rarity of this disease in dogs and cats.

Sources

Coins appear to be the primary potential source of excessive oral copper exposure in both dogs and cats. Copper poisoning was documented in a cat following ingestion of 32 Canadian pennies.[1] Canadian pennies minted up to 1997 are composed of 98.5% copper. American pennies (standard weight, 2.5 g) minted up to and including the year 1983 contain 95% copper. Nickels (standard weight, 5 g) contain 75% copper, and dimes (standard weight, 2.268 g), quarters (standard weight, 5.67 g), and half-dollars (standard weight,

11.34 g) contain approximately 91.7% copper. Susan B. Anthony dollars (standard weight, 8.1 g) contain 87.5% copper. Copper poisoning could also conceivably occur as a result of excess copper leaching from copper piping. This would be highly unusual and most likely would not cause an acute intoxication.

Acute copper poisoning was reported in Canada geese following ingestion of water containing excessive copper concentrations following application of copper sulfate to a small, artificial pond.[2] Copper sulfate is a common ingredient in fungicides and algicides and is also used in footbaths or topical solutions for cattle and sheep to control hoof infections. I am aware of an anecdotal report of a cat drinking copper-treated water out of a Christmas tree stand and succumbing to acute liver failure. Copper sulfate is also commonly incorporated into various feeds or drinking water (e.g., for swine, rabbits, cattle, and poultry) to prevent deficiency diseases or to act as a growth promotant or antimicrobial agent. Copper sulfate is also used in some topical wound dressings. Copper oxide–containing capsules intended for oral supplementation for cattle could conceivably be ingested by dogs and cats. I am aware of a dog ingesting an unknown amount of copper-containing wire and exhibiting mild gastrointestinal signs prior to removal. Other miscellaneous sources of copper include jewelry, pipes, toy parts, kitchenware, and numerous household objects.

Toxic Dose and Toxicokinetics

No reported toxic doses for copper in dogs and cats were found in the literature. Approximate normal dietary range of copper in cats and dogs appears to be in the 3 to 10 ppm and 7 to 10 ppm range, respectively, on a dry weight basis. Adequate dietary intake for cats has been reported to be between 0.08 and 0.80 mg Cu/kg body weight/day.[3] The current Association of American Feed Control Officials Food Nutrient Profiles lists the minimum dietary copper requirement for dogs as being 7.3 mg/kg diet, with an upper limit of 250 mg/kg, and for cats, 5 mg/kg diet. I am aware of a case in which a 3.4-g quarter (original weight approximately 5.7 g) was surgically removed from the stomach of a small-breed dog (weight unknown) exhibiting signs of intermittent vomiting, lethargy, and abdominal tenderness associated with elevations of liver enzymes. The serum copper concentration was normal.

Elemental copper is primarily absorbed by the small intestine. The majority of copper is absorbed by active transport, whereas passive diffusion is known to occur at higher concentrations of dietary copper. The bioavailability and eventual uptake of copper can vary with the form of copper (e.g., copper sulfate, copper oxide, copper carbonate). The intestinal mucosal cells regulate copper transfer into the portal circulation in part by the use of intracellular metallothionein. Before being secreted into the general circulation, the copper is mostly bound to albumin. The liver is the primary organ of copper metabolism. In the liver, copper stores are divided into four intercellular pools: the biliary pool, ceruloplasmin, metalloenzymes, and copper-metallothionein complexes. Any excess copper is stored by lysosomes. The normal liver metabolizes copper by excreting excess copper into the bile as a copper-molybdenum-sulfate complex. Small amounts of copper are also normally excreted into the urine.

Mechanism of Toxicity

The specific events occurring in the liver in cases of acute copper poisoning are unclear. Typically, copper accumulates in the liver as a result of excessive intake, or of a primary defect in copper excretion, or secondary to cholestasis. Inherited hepatic copper poisoning has been well described in various breeds of dogs, and this has been attributed to defects in copper excretion and copper-binding proteins. However, in cases of acute poisoning, there seems to be some evidence suggesting that copper is directly cytotoxic to red blood cells or hepatocytes when it is present in high enough concentrations (possibly caused by copper-induced free radical formation) and can cause hemolysis and hepatocyte degeneration and necrosis. However, the hemolytic event is not always seen, and too few cases of acute copper poisoning have been reported in companion animals to accurately estimate the incidence of this occurrence. Various forms of copper, depending on the concentration, can be caustic to the gastrointestinal mucosa.

Clinical Signs

The onset of signs associated with acute copper poisoning can range from a few hours to several days following the initial exposure. This range can mostly be attributed to the form of copper and to the severity of the lesions in the gastrointestinal tract or liver induced by the copper. Typical signs described in cats and dogs following ingestion of copper-containing coins include mild depression and dehydration, anorexia, intermittent vomiting, and mild abdominal pain. Diarrhea can also occur. Copper-containing coins do not appear to be physically altered by the acidic gastric environment as quickly as zinc-containing coins. Therefore the clinical signs of copper poisoning often do not appear initially to be that dramatic, and copper coins seem to be less likely to cause systemic toxicosis. However, I am aware of a case in a cat in which an unknown source and unknown duration of excess copper exposure resulted in a dramatic two-day history of vomiting and depression, which ended in death caused by severe, acute hepatocellular necrosis. Acute intravascular hemolysis was associated with copper poisoning in rabbits; however, the exposure in this case was most likely more chronic.[4] Severe central nervous system depression, lethargy, and icterus were reported in two sibling ferrets with copper poisoning.[5] The authors hypothesized that the disease may have been due to an inherited inability to metabolize copper because histologic examination of the liver tissue indicated a chronic hepatopathy.

Minimum Database

The minimum database should include collection of blood for a complete blood count and serum chemistry panel. Specific values to be evaluated include any evidence of intravascular hemolysis (e.g., anemia, hemoglobinemia), along with elevations in liver enzymes (e.g., alanine transaminase, aspartate transaminase, lactate dehydrogenase) and other evidence of hepatic dysfunction (e.g., hyperbilirubinemia, elevated bile acids). Urinalyses may be run to confirm the presence of hemoglobin or bilirubin. Abdominal radiographs may reveal the presence of radiodense foreign objects in animals that have swallowed coins or metallic items. Lack of visual presence of these objects should not eliminate copper poisoning as a possible cause because vomiting by the patient could have successfully removed the objects before presentation. Histopathologic examination of a liver biopsy tissue sample (e.g., ultrasound guided or exploratory surgery) can be very useful in helping to confirm the presence of abnormal accumulation of copper and compatible histologic lesions.

Confirmatory Tests

Serum copper concentrations may or may not be elevated in cases of acute copper poisoning. A normal serum copper range in cats, generated by our laboratory, was 0.33 up to 1.05 ppm; normal serum range in dogs has been reported as being 0.20 to 0.80 ppm.[3] Liver copper concentrations are much more diagnostic in confirming this type of poisoning. Adequate amounts of liver and kidney tissue (samples ideally should be approximately 1 g but analyses can be done on lesser volumes) are easily collected postmortem for copper quantification, but are much more difficult to collect antemortem. Often insufficient tissue is collected from a biopsy to perform both histopathologic analysis and copper quantification (at least 0.1 to 0.2 g of tissue is necessary, depending on the analytical methodology). Copper staining of formalin fixed tissue can be helpful in identifying excessive copper stores, but this is not definitive, and this should only be considered a screening tool. Adequate copper levels for cats in liver and kidney tissues, respectively, are reported to be 37 to 45 ppm and 2.2 to 2.7 ppm, wet weight.[3] Adequate copper levels reported in dogs for liver and kidney, respectively, are 30 to 100 ppm and 5 to 15 ppm, wet weight.[3] Copper levels that are notably higher than these, accompanied by an appropriate history, clinical signs, clinical pathologic data, and histologic lesions, are compatible with a diagnosis of copper poisoning.

Treatment

There are too few cases in the literature to know exactly what treatments are effective. Surgery to remove foreign objects is generally recommended. Chelation with penicillamine or dimercaprol, or treatment with zinc acetate is most likely not necessary in cases of acute copper poisoning. Basic supportive care is required to treat any patient exhibiting significant hepatic dysfunction or hemolysis (e.g., intravenous fluids [lactated Ringer's solution or 0.9% saline with potassium chloride], B-complex vitamins, glucose, transfusions, SAMe, milk thistle). Because of the potential necrotic effects on the gastrointestinal mucosa, patients may benefit from cytoprotective agents (e.g., sucralfate), parenteral caloric support, and prophylactic broad-spectrum antibiotics.

Prognosis

The prognosis for acutely poisoned patients is guarded to poor, depending on the source and solubility of ingested copper and how rapidly it is absorbed by the gastrointestinal mucosa. The severity of liver dysfunction and possibly hemolysis are the primary factors in determining the outcome.

Gross and Histologic Lesions

Coagulative necrosis of the gastrointestinal mucosa may be observed both grossly and histologically. Varying degrees of hepatocellular degeneration with marked accumulation of rhodanine- or rubeanic acid–positive granules have been described[6] and more severe lesions of centrilobular, midzonal, and diffuse hepatocellular necrosis can be seen. Rhodanine- or rubeanic-positive granular material can also be seen in the epithelium of the proximal convoluted tubules and collecting ducts of the kidney. Hemoglobin casts may be seen within the convoluted tubules and collecting ducts.

Differential Diagnoses

Acute copper poisoning in the dog and cat must be differentiated from acute zinc or lead poisoning and from a multitude of potential hepatotoxic agents (e.g., iron, phenolics, acetaminophen, nonsteroidal antiinflammatory agents, aflatoxin, xylitol, cyanobacteria, mushrooms, sago palm, and pennyroyal oil).

Copper Storage Disease

Numerous canine breeds have been reported as developing copper storage disease, in which the liver abnormally accumulates excessive copper concentrations over time. This is due to an autosomal recessive trait in Bedlington terriers, but the exact mechanism for the copper accumulation has not been worked out for the other breeds (e.g., West Highland white terrier, Skye terrier, Dalmatian, Doberman pinscher, Labrador retriever). Although the onset of clinical signs can be rather abrupt in some of these animals, the accumulation of copper is generally considered a chronic event. Many patients exhibit a chronic waxing and waning of lethargy, anorexia, and weight loss. Massive release of copper from the hepatocytes leading to an intravascular hemolytic event has rarely been reported. This is the primary reason why assessing serum copper levels is not helpful in establishing a diagnosis. The presence of the disease is generally confirmed by compatible histologic changes on a biopsy specimen, along with quantitating liver copper concentrations. Copper levels exceeding 2000 ppm dry weight (400 ppm wet weight) are often considered compatible with a copper storage disease. Readers are recommended to go elsewhere for a more comprehensive description of this disease.[7]

References

1. Poortinga EW: Copper penny ingestion in a cat, *Can Vet J* 36:634, 1995.
2. Henderson BM, Wintefield RW: Acute copper toxicosis in the Canada goose, *Avian Dis* 19(2):385–387, 1975.
3. Puls R: Copper-dog, cat. In Puls R, editor: *Mineral levels in animal health*, Clearbrook, British Columbia, 1994, Sherpa International.
4. Cooper GL, Bickford AA, Charlton BR, et al: Copper poisoning in rabbits associated with acute intravascular hemolysis, *J Vet Diagn Invest* 8:394–396, 1996.
5. Fox JG, Zeman DH, Mortimer JD: Copper toxicosis in sibling ferrets, *J Am Vet Med Assoc* 205(8):1154–1156, 1994.
6. Haynes JS, Wade PR: Hepatopathy associated with excessive hepatic copper in a Siamese cat, *Vet Pathol* 32:427–429, 1995.
7. Twedt DC: Copper storage hepatopathy. In Tilley LP, Smith FWK, editors: *The 5-minute veterinary consult, canine and feline*, Philadelphia, 2004, Lippincott Williams & Wilkins.

Cyanide

Kevin T. Fitzgerald, PhD, DVM, DABVP

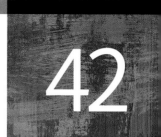

- Hydrogen cyanide (HCN) and cyanide salts are used in a variety of common industrial processes.
- For most species, the lethal dose of HCN is 2 mg/kg. Exposure to cyanide can occur via inhalation, ingestion, or dermal exposure.
- Cyanide disrupts the ability of cells to use oxygen (O_2) in oxidative phosphorylation. The net result is histotoxic tissue hypoxia.
- Clinical signs include vomiting, hyperpnea, tachycardia and cardiac arrhythmias, seizures, coma, and apnea.
- Plasma lactate levels and increased anion gap values may be the best indicators of both the presence and severity of cyanide poisoning. Whole-blood cyanide levels are available in many human laboratories. It may take time to obtain the results, so these tests are often of little use in emergency situations.
- Treatment consists of removing the animal from the source of exposure, initiating supportive measures (100% O_2 and intravenous fluids), decontaminating skin and fur, and, if exposure is certain, administering antidotal therapy. Recently, hydroxocobalamin has been employed as a cyanide antidote in humans and has been shown to reverse cyanide toxicity and reduce mortality in a canine model.
- The classic bitter almond smell and cherry red blood are rarely seen outside of textbooks.
- Differential diagnoses include poisonings with carbon monoxide or acute solvent inhalation, heart disease, cerebral disease, and cerebral neoplasia.

Sources

Small animals may encounter cyanide in a surprisingly broad array of forms. Hydrogen cyanide (HCN) and cyanide salts are used in a wide variety of common industrial processes. Cyanide is used in electroplating techniques, photographic processes, metal cleaning, and gold mining, and HCN gas is used as a fumigant rodenticide. Some fertilizers contain cyanamide. Some coyote traps are still used that fire sodium cyanide baits into the mouths of the animals (i.e., "coyote-getters"). HCN is also known as *prussic acid,* and the nitroprussides are used as hypotensive drugs. Combustion of many plastic compounds produces HCN gas. As a result, many smoke inhalation victims suffer from cyanide toxicity and carbon monoxide poisoning.

Box 42-1	Potential Cyanide Sources or Exposures

Fires
Gold mines
Fumigation
Electroplating and jewelry manufacturing
Photographic chemicals
Manufacture of plastics, rubber, and synthetic fiber
Pesticides (rodenticides, insecticides)
Burning rubber
Certain drugs
Ingestion of certain plants
Terrorist attack

Cyanogenic compounds (e.g., laetrile, amygdalin from plants, and nitriles) can release cyanide during metabolism, which most commonly occurs in the gut. Naturally occurring cyanogenic glycosides, such as amygdalin, are found in numerous plants. Seeds of apples, plums, cherries, apricots, and the jetberry bush all release cyanide on digestion and are dangerous if the seed capsule is broken. As few as 5 to 25 seeds can cause intoxication. Natural oil of bitter almonds contains 4% HCN. In addition, some species of lima bean contain notable amounts of HCN. The dried root of cassava (i.e., tapioca) contains fairly large amounts of cyanide and can cause poisoning when eaten in large amounts or if it is improperly cooked. Other forms of cyanide include glue-on nail removers containing acetonitrile and acrylonitrile, which are used in the production of synthetic rubber. Isocyanates (e.g., methyl isocyanate, toluene diisocyanate, and others) are potent skin and mucous membrane irritants, but do not release cyanide after absorption.

For large animals, the most important source of cyanide is plant material. Frost-damaged, hail-damaged, or freshly trampled dead or wilted plants are more dangerous than intact specimens. The liberation of HCN does not begin until the plant tissue is damaged or starts to decay. In humans the vast majority of cyanide poisonings are intentional. Most involve drinking a sodium cyanide–containing insecticide. The second most common cause of cyanide toxicity in people is smoke inhalation. A list of potential sources of cyanide exposure is included in Box 42-1. Confirmed exposures to cyanide in dogs and cats in 2010 are included in Boxes 42-2 and 42-3.

Toxic Dose

The minimum toxic dose of free HCN and of potassium cyanide given orally in most mammalian species is approximately 2 mg/kg HCN (Box 42-4).

Toxicokinetics and Mechanism of Toxicity

The kinetics of cyanide are not well understood. Cyanide disrupts the ability of cells to use oxygen in oxidative phosphorylation. It does this by binding with the ferric (Fe^{+3}) iron of the mitochondrial cytochrome oxidase system. As a result, a shift to anaerobic metabolism occurs, a decrease in adenosine triphosphate synthesis ensues, and depletion of cellular energy stores and greatly increased lactic acid production follow, causing an anion gap metabolic acidosis. The net effect is a histotoxic tissue hypoxia. In dogs whole blood cyanide levels may be four or five times greater than serum levels because of the concentration of cyanide in erythrocytes. The elimination half-life ($T_{1/2}$) in dogs is 19 hours. The toxic step defining acute cyanide poisoning is that oxygen released by oxyhemoglobin cleavage can no longer be bound. As a result, blockage of cellular respiration results, and respiratory arrest follows within a few minutes. In addition to the development of tissue hypoxia, it has

Box 42-2	American Association of Poison Control Centers 2010

Total number of reported cyanide cases: 2010
Feline confirmed exposures: 0

Box 42-3	American Association of Poison Control Centers 2010

Total number of reported cyanide cases: 2010
Canine confirmed exposures: 6

Outcome: Dogs

Death	1
Moderate effects	1
Minor effects	4
Animal recovered	5

been shown that cyanide also exhibits direct toxic action on cellular membranes, resulting in their necrosis.

Clinical Signs

The clinical signs of cyanide poisoning depend on the dose, route of exposure, and time elapsed since exposure. The primary manifestations of intoxication from cyanide-containing compounds are rapid tachypnea, hypotension, and convulsions leading to coma. Severe acute cyanide poisoning progresses rapidly from convulsions to coma to shock to respiratory failure to death. The process is faster with inhalation than with ingestion. Animals with inhalation exposure in enclosed spaces may lose consciousness after only a few breaths, and death follows rapidly within 1 to 15 minutes. Clinical signs may not develop for up to 30 minutes to 1 hour after exposure in animals ingesting amounts large enough to be fatal. Delayed onset of clinical signs (as late as 12 hours) occurs following ingestion of cyanide-containing compounds, such as laetrile, amygdalin, and the nitroprussides.

Chronic poisoning with cyanide is far less common than acute intoxication. Repeated inhalation of small amounts of cyanogen chloride causes dizziness, hoarseness, conjunctivitis, weakness, loss of appetite, and weight loss. Chronic ingestion of cyanide-containing cassava is reported to cause tropical ataxic neuropathy in people, and chronic ingestion of cyanide-containing fertilizer by animals has been reported to cause neurologic signs.

It has been often stated in previous references that dermal exposure can lead to systemic cyanide intoxication. However, it is difficult to document actual reported cases of poisoning from dermal exposure other than in animals with total body exposure in confined spaces in which inhalation and ingestion also undoubtedly occurred.

In small animals that do not display sudden collapse, the initial signs may resemble anxiety or hyperventilation. Early signs include tachycardia, hyperpnea, and dyspnea. Later signs of cyanide poisoning are nausea and vomiting, hypotension, generalized seizures, coma, apnea, dilated pupils (either sluggish or totally nonreactive), and a host of cardiac effects, including tachycardia, bradycardia, ventricular arrhythmias, erratic supraventricular arrhythmias, ischemic changes on electrocardiography, atrioventricular blocks, and eventual asystole (Box 42-5).

The smell of bitter almonds has been reported often, but the ability to detect this odor is genetically determined, and many people cannot do so. Cyanosis is a late sign that may not be present until the animal is agonal, at the stage of apnea and circulatory collapse. Noncardiogenic pulmonary edema may occur, even after ingestion alone.

Box 42-4	Cyanide
Molecular weight	26.02 D
Airborne	
Immediately fatal	270 ppm
Life threatening	110 ppm
Legal workplace limits	4.7 ppm
Oral	
Lethal dose	200 mg

Box 42-5	Clinical Signs of Cyanide Poisoning

Sudden collapse (inhalation)
Nausea
Vomiting
Dilated pupils
Hypotension
Cardiac signs (electrocardiogram)
Tachycardia
Ventricular arrhythmias
Atrioventricular blocks
Eventual asystole
Hyperpnea
Seizures
Coma
Apnea

To understand the causes of the clinical signs of cyanide poisoning, the mechanism of action of the toxin must be reevaluated. The hallmark of cyanide toxicity is tissue hypoxia based on the disruption of normal oxidative phosphorylation and the ability of cells to use oxygen. Those tissues that most depend on oxidative phosphorylation (e.g., heart and brain) are affected most rapidly and severely. Subsequent central inhibition of the respiratory centers leads to hypoventilation, which produces additional hypoxia. Myocardial depression with decreased cardiac output produces an additional stagnation hypoxia. Until the final stages of respiratory depression or arrest, the blood is normally oxygenated. However, the tissue is unable to extract or use the oxygen because of the cyanide, and this leads to a greater than normal oxygen level on the venous side and the classic "cherry red" color of the superoxygenated blood. Stomach contents may produce a bitter almond smell, and if excessive plant material or fertilizer was ingested, signs of gastroenteritis may be observed.

Minimum Database and Confirmatory Tests

Diagnosis is based on the physical examination and centers on the vital signs and the systems affected (e.g., cardiovascular, respiratory, and the central nervous system). Animals may or may not display the bright red mucous membranes or generate a bitter almond smell. Whole-blood cyanide levels are available in many human laboratories, but the results may take time to be obtained and therefore cannot be relied on to direct therapy in an emergency situation. However, they can contribute to the documentation of the diagnosis and can aid later in any subsequent medicolegal action.

Severe metabolic acidosis occurs in acute cyanide poisoning. Cyanide produces lactic acidosis, which can be determined directly by serum lactate measurements or indirectly on arterial blood gas pH measurements. However, most private veterinary practices do not have blood gas machines. Lactic acidosis may also be reflected in an elevated anion gap on the serum-electrolyte biochemical profile. Normal serum lactate levels are 1 mEq/L (mmol/L) or less. A diagnosis of lactic acidosis can usually be made when serum lactate levels are greater than 2 mEq/L (mmol/L). Plasma lactate levels and increased anion gap values may be the best indicators of both the presence and severity of a potential cyanide poisoning. Continuous vital sign and electrocardiographic monitoring should be performed in any animal with suggested cyanide intoxication.

Treatment

Animals must be swiftly removed from enclosed or confined spaces with high airborne concentrations of cyanide. Rescuers, likewise, must not enter such areas without full protective clothing and proper respirators or self-contained breathing apparatus. Mouth-to-mouth breathing should be avoided, and care must be taken not to inhale the animal's exhaled breath. Exposed skin, fur, and eyes should be copiously flushed with water or normal saline in an attempt to decontaminate the animal.

Many cyanide-exposed animals with only anxiety and hyperventilation can be treated with supportive measures alone without antidotal therapy. All cyanide antidotes are toxic, and therapy may be not only unnecessary but also dangerous. Supportive measures alone may prove to be satisfactory. Appropriate supportive nonantidotal therapy includes administration of 100% supplemental oxygen by tight-fitting mask or endotracheal tube; placement of at least one intravenous line for administration of fluids and sodium bicarbonate if shock and presumed metabolic acidosis are present; decontamination of skin, eyes, and fur with copious amounts of water or normal saline; and administration of antiarrhythmic or anticonvulsant.

Induction of emesis must be closely gauged because the disease process can lead potentially to rapid progression of coma and seizures. Gastric lavage may be beneficial if the material was ingested within the past 60 minutes. Although the older literature questions the efficacy of activated charcoal administration, one dose (1 to 4 g activated charcoal/kg body weight) is recommended for animals known to have ingested cyanide-containing compounds. Amyl nitrite antidotal therapy, which is prominently used in human treatment, is not recommended in animals.

If a diagnosis of cyanide poisoning is certain, sodium nitrite should be given as soon as possible. Sodium nitrite has potentially significant toxicity. This nitrite forms methemoglobin, which combines with cyanide to form cyanmethemoglobin. It is a potent vasodilator, and rapid administration may result in hypotension. Frequent blood pressure monitoring is mandatory during administration of this compound. Another potentially serious adverse effect of sodium nitrite administration is induction of excessive methemoglobin levels. This can be fatal if cyanide poisoning is not present. The usual dose of sodium nitrite is 16 mg/kg IV of a 3% solution. Sodium nitrite is followed by the administration of sodium thiosulfate (1.65 mL of a 25% solution) given intravenously. Thiosulfate converts cyanide to thiocyanate. No cases of significant adverse effects of sodium thiosulfate therapy have been reported in the 50 years this drug has been used clinically. In animals with less severe poisoning, sodium thiosulfate and supportive measures alone may be sufficient. Second doses of sodium nitrite and sodium thiosulfate at one half of the initial amounts may be given 30 minutes after the first dose if a clinical response is not forthcoming. Administering further prophylactic doses to patients that have regained consciousness, are breathing spontaneously, and have stable vital signs is unnecessary and potentially dangerous.

In other parts of the world, alternative antidotes in clinical use include hydroxocobalamin, dicobalt-ethylenediaminetetraacetic (EDTA) acid (Kelocyanor), and 4-dimethylaminophenol. At present there is a lack of international consensus about the definitive treatment of choice.

Hydroxocobalamin was first licensed for treatment of cyanide poisoning in France in 1996 and is currently available in the United States; 50 g of hydroxocobalamin binds 1 g of cyanide, which is then excreted by the kidneys. In humans a dose of 5 g of hydroxocobalamin is administered when cyanide poisoning is suggested, and a second dose may be necessary in response to continued progression of the clinical syndrome. Whether this antidote is able to pass through the blood-brain barrier to potentiate direct detoxification in the central nervous system remains unknown.

Hydroxocobalamin (vitamin B_{12a}) is the precursor molecule of cyanocobalamin (vitamin B_{12}). It is used in the treatment of pernicious anemia in humans. Hydroxocobalamin binds with cyanide on an equimolar basis to form cyanocobalamin and thereby detoxify cyanide. It has less inherent toxicity than other antidotes, has proven effective in restoration and support of cardiovascular function, and in years of foreign clinical experience has been shown to be a safer antidote than either dicobalt edetate or sodium nitrite. Cyanide poisoning has been studied in a variety of species including mice, rats, guinea pigs, rabbits, dogs, and primates. The pharmacokinetics and pharmacodynamics of a cyanide antidote have been elucidated in dogs and the canine model is considered predictive of antidotal effects in humans.

Dicobalt-EDTA (Kelocyanor) is currently used in Europe, particularly in the United Kingdom, but is not currently available in the United States. Dicobalt edetate releases cobalt ions that react with cyanide ions. Highly stable cyanide-cobalt complexes are then released by the kidneys. A 300-mg dose is given over 1 minute, and a further 300-mg dose may be repeated in 5 minutes if no improvement is seen. Numerous side effects have been reported in humans, including vomiting, tachypnea, chest pains, hypotension, ventricular arrhythmias, seizures, urticaria, facial-laryngeal-neck edema, and anaphylactic shock. Each injection of cobalt edetate should be followed immediately by 50 mL of 50-1-glucose. Cobalt-EDTA works faster than the nitrites; however, growing concern about cobalt toxicity led to its recommendation as a second-line antidote.

Finally, 4-dimethylaminophenol, introduced in Germany, also acts by generating methemoglobin. Subsequent intravenous administration of sodium thiosulfate is required to promote the conversion of cyanide to thiocyanate ion, which is then excreted from the body. Side effects to this drug are severe and include reticulocytosis, hemolysis, and nephrotoxicity. A comparative evaluation of currently used antidotes for cyanide poisoning is included in Table 42-1.

Another promising investigational antidote of cyanide is α-ketoglutaric acid. The molecular configuration of this antidote renders it amenable to nucleophilic binding of cyanide. In various animal studies, pretreatment with α-ketoglutarate reduced lethal outcomes and increased efficacy of sodium thiosulfate. The main benefit to α-ketoglutarate is the direct binding of cyanide without the generation of methemoglobin.

Numerous attempts have been made to identify the most effective antidote in cyanide treatment and obtain international consensus. For an antidote to be universally accepted, there are several important prerequisites. First, it must be readily available. Next, it must be demonstrably effective. Finally, it must be safe. *Safe* means that it should not be harmful if given to nonpoisoned patients. Many drugs are effective antidotes to cyanide. At present the selection of antidotes used varies from country to country. In the United States sodium nitrite is the cyanide antidote of choice. It has a wide margin of safety, but if large doses are given, methemoglobin concentrations must be monitored.

Dicobalt edetate is the antidote to cyanide most preferred in the United Kingdom. It has a rapid action, but has a very significant toxicity in its own right. The victim must be confirmed without doubt to be suffering from cyanide toxicity before the drug is given.

Dimethylaminophenol is the most frequently recommended cyanide antidote in Germany. It is responsible for a quick and profound methemoglobinemia. As a result, close monitoring of methemoglobin levels must be performed.

Hydroxocobalamin is the most recommended antidote to cyanide in France. The molecule is a precursor of vitamin B_{12} and has little toxicity. It is a large molecule and binds

Table 42-1	Currently Used Antidotes for Cyanide Poisoning	
Antidote	Advantages	Disadvantages
Methemoglobin formers	Potent	Impairment of O_2 delivery to tissue
Sodium thiosulfate	Efficient Safe	Delayed action
Cobalt-EDTA	Very potent Immediate action Effective if taken	Numerous side effects
Hydroxocobalamin	Less potent Immediate action Safe	Expensive Red discoloration of skin and urine

EDTA, Ethylenediaminetetraacetic acid.

cyanide in an equimolar fashion. The main disadvantage of this antidote is the cost. There is growing consensus that this is the most efficacious and nontoxic cyanide antidote, and it is also relatively safe for administration when unsure of cyanide poisoning. Recently, this cyanide antidote has become available for use in the United States. Studies of cyanide poisoning in dogs has revealed that hydroxocobalamin therapy was efficacious in reducing mortality when compared with a saline vehicle.

Prevention and Prognosis

Because many individuals cannot detect the odor of cyanide, the exposure limit in confined spaces must be closely monitored. Likewise, animals should be restricted from industrial areas where cyanide is used in chemical synthesis. Cyanide-containing compounds should be kept in their original containers listing ingredients and concentrations and should be made pet proof. Most animals that recover from acute cyanide poisoning do not have permanent sequelae.

Asymptomatic animals with apparent minimal exposure should be observed for 6 to 8 hours. If known exposure to a nitroprusside (or to other nitriles) has occurred, the onset of action may be delayed up to 12 hours, and a longer period of observation and monitoring is necessary.

Animals that have suffered from serious signs of cyanide poisoning (e.g., shock, metabolic acidosis, convulsions, coma, cardiac arrhythmias, hypoventilation) and all those receiving antidotes should be hospitalized and monitored for 24 hours following resolution of the clinical signs. Follow-up examinations should be scheduled for several months to screen for the development of rare central nervous system effects. In a few isolated human cases, parkinsonian-like states with memory deficits and personality changes have been reported following cyanide intoxication. This has not been documented in animals.

Hemodialysis cannot be considered standard therapy for cyanide poisoning, but may be of value for treating high thiocyanate levels that have developed in animals (a less toxic compound produced from cyanide metabolism).

Gross and Histologic Lesions

Pathologic findings in cyanide poisonings are not characteristic. Ingestion of potassium cyanide or sodium cyanide causes congestion of the blood vessels and corrosion of the gastric mucosa. The smell of bitter almonds and the cherry red blood color seem to be observed mainly in textbooks.

Box 42-6	Differential Diagnoses for Cyanide Toxicity

Acute solvent inhalation
Carbon monoxide poisoning
Heart disease
Cerebral disease
Cerebral neoplasia

Cyanide poisoning most affects those cerebral structures with the highest oxygen requirement. Magnetic resonance imaging (MRI) studies of the rare individuals that survive acute cyanide intoxication reveal greatest damage to the cerebellum, cerebral cortex, basal ganglia, and sensorimotor cortex. These injuries are manifested as hemorrhagic necrosis in the basal ganglia and pseudolaminar necrosis in the cerebral cortex. The damage is caused by direct toxic action of cyanide and not from the cerebral hypoxia resulting from the acute intoxication cellular process. MRI is the method of choice for determining the exact extent and severity of lesions in cyanide-sensitive areas of the brain in animals that survive the initial toxic exposure.

Differential Diagnoses

A diagnosis of cyanide toxicity is difficult because the clinical signs are nonspecific. Box 42-6 includes a list of differential diagnoses. Differential diagnoses of cyanide poisoning must include any condition that results in loss of consciousness.

Suggested Readings

Baud FJ, Borrow SW, Magarbane B, et al: Value of lactic acidosis in the assessment of the severity of acute cyanide poisoning, *Crit Care Med* 30:2044–2050, 2002.

Beasley DMG, Glass WI: Cyanide poisoning: pathophysiology and recommendations, *Occupational Med* 48:427–431, 1998.

Bhattacharya R, Vijayaraghavan R: Promising role of α-ketoglutarate in protecting against the lethal effects of cyanide, *Human Exp Toxicol* 21:297–303, 2002.

Borron S, Megarbane B, Baud FJ: Hydroxocobalamin is an effective antidote in severe cyanide poisoning in man: abstract, *Int J Toxicol* 23:399–400, 2004.

Borron SW, Barriot P, Imbert M, Baud FJ: Hydroxocobalamin for empiric treatment of smoke-inhalation a-associated cyanide poisoning: results of a prospective study in the prehospital setting: abstract 275, *Am Emerg Med* S77, 2005.

Boron SW, Stonerook M, Reid F: Efficacy of hydroxocobalamin for the treatment of acute cyanide poisoning in adult Beagle dogs, *Clin Toxicol* 44:5–15, 2006.

Breen PH, Isserles SA, Tabac E, et al: Protective effect of stroma-free methemoglobin during cyanide poisoning in dogs, *Anesthesiology* Sep 85(3):558–564, 1996.

Bronstein AC, Spyker DA, Canitena LR, et al: Annual report of the American Association of Poison Control Centers National Poison Data System (NPDS): 27th annual report 2010, *Clin Toxicol* 48:979–1178, 2010.

Campbell A, Jones AL: Cyanide poisoning managed with hydroxocobalamin in the UK, *J Toxicol Clin Toxicol* 39(3):294, 2001.

Cummings TF: The treatment of cyanide poisoning, *Occupational Med* 54:82–85, 2004.

De La Coussaye JE, Houeto P, Sandouk P, et al: Pharmacokinetics of hydroxocobalamin in dogs, *J Neurosurg Anesthesiol* 6:111–115, 1994.

Eyer P: Therapeutic implications of the toxokinetics and toxodynamics in cyanide poisoning, *J Toxicol Clin Toxicol* 38:212–214, 2000.

Firtin JL, Ruttimann M, Domonski L, Kowalski JJ: Hydroxocobalamin: treatment for smoke inhalation associated cyanide poisoning. Meeting the needs of fire victims, *JEMS* 29(Suppl):18–21, 2004.

Forsyth JC, Mueller PD, Becker CE, et al: Hydroxocobalamin as a cyanide antidote: safety, efficacy, and pharmacokinetics in heavily smoking normal volunteers, *Clin Toxicol* 31:277–294, 1993.

Hall AH, Rumack BH: Clinical toxicology of cyanide, *Ann Emerg Med* 15:1067, 1986.

Hall AH, Rumack BH: Cyanide and related compounds. In Haddad LM, Shannon MW, Winchester JF, editors: *Clinical management of poisoning and drug overdose*, ed 3, Philadelphia, 1998, WB Saunders.

Kerns W, Isom G, Kirk MA: Cyanide and hydrogen sulfide. In Goldfrank LR, et al: *Toxicologic emergencies*, ed 7, 2002, McGraw-Hill.

Megarbane B, et al: Antidotal treatment of cyanide poisoning, *J Chin Med Assoc* 66:193–203, 2003.

Megarbane B, Borron SW, Baud F: Hydroxocobalamin versus conventional treatment in cyanide poisoning, *J Toxicol Clin Toxicol* 40(3):314, 2002.

Rachinger J, et al: MR changes after acute cyanide intoxication, *Am J Neuroradiol* 23:1398–1401, 2002.

Rosenthal RE, Bogaert YE, Fiskum G: Delayed therapy of experimental global cerebral ischemia with acetyl-L-carnitine in dogs, *Neurosci Lett* 18(328):82–87, 2005.

Sousa AB, et al: Toxicokinetics of cyanide in rats, pigs, and goats after overdosing with potassium cyanide, *Arch Toxicol* 77:330–334, 2003.

Von Landenberg F, Stonerook M, Judge M, Borron SW: Efficacy of hydroxocobalamin in a canine model of cyanide poisoning: a pilot study: abstract, *Clin Toxicol* 42:692, 2005.

Way JL: Cyanide intoxication and its mechanism of antagonism, *Ann Rev Pharmacol Toxicol* 24:451, 1984.

Cyanobacteria

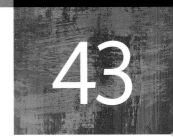

Birgit Puschner, DVM, PhD, DABVT
Caroline Moore, BS

- Cyanobacteria are ubiquitous organisms that pose risks to companion animals all year round.
- Cyanotoxins are either hepatic or neurologic in nature.
- Clinical signs following exposure to the hepatoxic cyanotoxins include lethargy, depression, vomiting, diarrhea, weakness, pallor, shock, and death.
- Clinical signs following exposure to the neurotoxic cyanotoxins include rapid onset of salivation, lacrimation, urination, defecation, muscle rigidity, tremors, seizures, respiratory paralysis, and death.
- Treatment for both syndromes is supportive.
- Confirmation of exposure includes history of exposure to a contaminated water source, identification of cyanobacteria in water or stomach contents, and toxin testing of a variety of biologic specimens (e.g., stomach contents, liver, urine, and bile).

Cyanobacterial proliferations occur in freshwater and saline ecosystems under certain environmental conditions leading to so-called algal blooms (Color Plate 43-1). Of the 2000 species identified based on morphologic criteria, 40 are considered toxigenic. The first scientific report of cyanotoxin poisoning in animals was made in Australia by Francis in 1878.[1] In small animals, blue-green algae poisoning is generally acute, leading to hepato- or neurotoxicosis. Reports of hepatotoxic blue-green algae poisonings are more frequent than reports of neurologic presentations. However, the true frequency of blue-green algae poisonings in animals is unknown and likely greatly underestimated because of a lack of routine diagnostic methods to confirm exposure. In the past, most cases were diagnosed by positive identification of the algae in the suspect water source along with the occurrence of consistent clinical signs and pathologic findings. New analytic methods can now be applied to detect toxins in biologic specimens of animals and humans with suspect exposure to toxic algal blooms. These capabilities will allow for in-depth diagnostic investigations and a better estimate of the true frequency of blue-green algae poisonings in livestock, pets, and wildlife.

Sources

Toxic cyanobacterial (blue-green algae) blooms are found worldwide in fresh and marine waters, including rivers, ponds, lakes, estuaries, and oceans. Several factors, such as nutrient-rich runoff (nitrogen and phosphorus), increased water temperatures, stagnant water conditions, and low rainfall, can increase the production of cyanotoxins in surface waters. Most blooms form during the warm summer months but blue-green algae can proliferate year-round and survive in both arctic and tropical weather, and thus the toxins may be detected year round. Animals and humans can be exposed to cyanotoxins when using surface waters for drinking, in their daily living activities, and during recreation.[2] Additionally, animals might find algae-contaminated water more palatable.[3] Cyanotoxins have also been found in algae health supplements[4] and may move up the food chain because of bioaccumulation.[5]

The most commonly reported deaths of domestic animals have been caused by microcystins, nodularins, and anatoxin-a. These cyanotoxins can be produced by a number of cyanobacterial species, including *Anabaena* spp., *Microcystis* spp., *Aphanizomenon* spp., *Oscillatoria* spp., and *Planktothrix* spp. Some species can produce a variety of cyanotoxins, and thus it is difficult to predict the nature and the level of the toxin production during a bloom event. A 2010 study of 23 lakes in the midwest showed that microcystins were found in all samples, with 95% having multiple microcystin variants and almost half having multiple cyanotoxins.[6] Anatoxin-a, saxitoxins, cylindrospermopsin, and nodularin-R were also detected. Interestingly, there are no documented reports of cyanotoxin poisoning in cats. Possible reasons include lack of exposure, lack of diagnostic work-up, and decreased susceptibility to cyanotoxins by felines.

Hepatotoxins: Microcystins and Nodularins

Toxic Dose

Considering that most microcystin-producing algal blooms contain several of the 80-plus structural variants of microcystins, it is difficult to estimate the toxicity potential of a bloom. To date, the median lethal dose (LD_{50}) of microcystins has not been determined in dogs. In mice, the oral LD_{50} for microcystin-LR is 10.9 mg/kg, whereas the intraperitoneal LD_{50} is 50 mcg/kg, suggesting low bioavailability of microcystins.[7] Currently, there are seven known natural variants of nodularins, yet specifics about each are not well documented and an oral LD_{50} for nodularins in animals is unknown. In rats the intraperitoneal LD_{50} for nodularins is 30-50 mcg/kg.[8]

Toxicokinetics

There is very limited data on the toxicokinetics of microcystins. In mice, microcystins are absorbed by the small intestine and rapidly distributed to the liver, lung, heart, and capillaries.[9] After oral exposure, the liver is the primary target organ, followed by the kidney and gastrointestinal tract.[7,10] As microcystins can cross the blood-brain barrier and enter neurons,[11,12] they may also exhibit neurotoxicity. Laboratory studies have also suggested microcystins are immunotoxic.[13] In dogs, clinical signs of microcystin poisoning are seen as quickly as 1 hour after exposure.[14] Death in dogs may occur within hours of ingestion.[15,16]

From limited data, it is assumed that toxicokinetics of nodularins are similar to those described for microcystins. Nodularins target the liver and kidney[17] after being absorbed in the small intestine. Dogs can develop acute clinical signs as quickly as 5 hours after exposure. Death may occur between 1 and 5 days following exposure.[17-20] There has been some speculation that hepatotoxic cyanotoxins can be immunotoxic; this was confirmed recently in two dogs that died from nodularin poisoning. The dogs had hepatic and renal necrosis along with changes to their lymphoid organs.[18] An analysis of liver, lung, spleen, heart, kidney, stomach, intestine, pancreas, adrenal gland, skeletal muscles, and brain performed 5 days following exposure to nodularins in a dog resulted in only the liver and kidney showing necrosis.

Mechanism of Toxicity

Microcystins and nodularins are cyclic peptides with unique amino acids. After oral exposure, microcystins and nodularins are absorbed in the ileum and enter hepatocytes and nephrons via the bile acid transporter mechanism.[12] They inhibit serine-threonine protein phosphatases 1 and 2A, resulting in disruption of the cytoskeletal components and an associated rearrangement of filamentous actin.[21,22] At high doses this can lead to acute liver necrosis, intrahepatic hemorrhage, and shock.[15,16,18] At low doses, microcystins and nodularins can lead to a slower onset of liver and kidney failure.[14,17,19,20] Microcystins also lead to free radical formation, mitochondrial alterations, intracellular calcium level alterations, and oxidative stress, which can contribute to apoptosis and hepatotoxicity.[23]

Clinical Signs

Microcystin intoxication should be suspected in cases of acute hepatotoxicosis that present with diarrhea, vomiting, weakness, pale mucous membranes, and shock. Although most animals die within a few hours of exposure, some animals may live for several hours to days and develop hyperkalemia, hypoglycemia, nervousness, recumbency and convulsions. A golden retriever vomited blue-green material, had diarrhea, and became lethargic 1 hour after ingesting an unknown amount of stagnant tide pool water in California.[14] Twelve hours later, the dog was icteric, severely depressed, blind, tachypneic, and had mild epistaxis. Despite treatment, the dog became acutely dyspneic and nonresponsive and was subsequently euthanized. Other reports of fatal microcystin poisonings in dogs have no description of clinical findings.[15,16]

Dogs poisoned by nodularins become acutely lethargic and develop vomiting, diarrhea, and inappetence. During the first 24 hours after exposure, dogs may stabilize before developing liver or kidney failure. Melena and hematuria can also be seen. Progression of clinical signs in animals with nodularin poisoning is slower than in microcystin-poisoned animals. In dogs with nodularin poisoning, the time from exposure to death ranges from 1-5 days.[17-20]

Minimum Database

Establishing a history of access to algal-contaminated water is critical when suspecting microcystin poisoning. In some cases, animals may have vomited up algal-containing material or may have algal material on their fur. The key abnormalities when evaluating a serum chemistry panel are related to liver damage: increased alkaline phosphatase (ALP), alanine transaminase (ALT), and aspartate transaminase (AST) activities; hyperbilirubinemia; hypoglycemia; and mild hypokalemia. Other abnormalities may include hyperammonemia, abnormal coagulation parameters, and leukocytosis with a mature neutrophilia, lymphopenia, and monocytosis.[14] Animals that are alive for longer periods after exposure may develop renal failure.

Serum chemistry abnormalities in dogs with nodularin poisoning include elevated ALT, ALP, AST, bilirubin, blood urea nitrogen, creatinine, and phosphorus levels. Thrombocytopenia, anemia, and increased activated partial thromboplastin time, D-dimer, and thrombin time may also be seen.[17-20] However, laboratory findings in individual cases of nodularin poisoning vary, with some dogs displaying all or none of the clinical chemistry abnormalities.

Confirmatory Tests

Identification of microcystin- or nodularin-contaminated water in the environment, on the animal's fur or skin, or in the gastric contents, aids in the diagnosis. Algal samples should be chilled, not frozen, preserved in 10% formalin (v/v 50:50), and submitted to a phycologist for identification. Positive identification, however, does not confirm intoxication. As mentioned earlier, the toxicity of cyanobacteria is strain specific, and morphologic observations alone cannot confirm a suspect diagnosis. Although many assays are available to analyze water samples for microcystins, there are only limited methods available to reliably and accurately detect microcystins or nodularins in biologic specimens (stomach contents, liver) collected from potentially poisoned animals. Veterinary diagnostic laboratories should be consulted to provide confirmatory testing in suspect cases (www.aavld.org).

Treatment and Prognosis

There is no antidote for microcystin intoxication and no specific therapy has been proven effective, especially with the rapid onset of hepatotoxicosis. Further exposure to contaminated water must be stopped immediately and contaminated skin should be washed with a mild detergent. Supportive care should include fluids, plasma transfusions, hepatoprotectants, and vitamin K_1. There are no data on the efficacy of activated charcoal in microcystin exposures in dogs; in fact, in mice dosed with microcystins, activated charcoal did not prove protective. Antioxidants may help reduce oxidative stress, but efficacy data is lacking. Antibiotics such as rifampin, ampicillin, and amikacin have shown mixed effects in animals.[14] Because of the rapid onset of acute hepatotoxicosis, therapeutic intervention is often unrewarding and mortality rates are high. Prognosis is guarded to poor.

Treatment is supportive and may include fluids, antiemetics, vitamin B complex, gastrointestinal protectants, antibiotics, antiinflammatory agents, hepatoprotectants, diuretics, and antioxidants.[17-19] However, there are no successful outcomes of confirmed nodularin poisonings despite therapeutic intervention. Thus nodularin poisoning has a very poor prognosis.

Gross and Histologic Lesions

During necropsy, algal bloom material may be identified in the gastrointestinal tract or on the fur of the animal. Grossly, there is generally only liver enlargement without other lesions. Histopathologic lesions include progressive centrilobular hepatocyte rounding, dissociation, and necrosis, breakdown of the sinusoidal endothelium, and intrahepatic hemorrhage. The kidney may have moderate to severe glomerulosclerosis, shrunken glomerular tufts, and renal casts.[14]

Because animals may be alive for several days after nodularin exposure, icterus may be noted during necropsy. The abdominal cavity may contain large amounts of fluid, and viscera may have subserosal edema. The liver is generally swollen and friable with a prominent reticular pattern.[17,18,20] Petechial hemorrhages can be found in thymus, lungs, and endocardium.[18,20] Kidneys may be swollen and pale.[17] Histopathologically, diffuse centrilobular to panlobular hepatic necrosis and hemorrhage, acute multifocal tubular degeneration and necrosis of the proximal tubules, and scattered necrotic myocardial fibers may be found.[17] Lymphoid depletion of the spleen, lymph nodes, thymus, and gut-associated and bronchus-associated lymphoid tissues can also be observed.[18]

Differential Diagnoses

Other toxic causes of acute hepatic failure include amanitins, cocklebur, cycad palm, aflatoxin, xylitol, certain heavy metals (e.g., copper, iron, zinc), cylindrospermopsin, pennyroyal oil, and acetaminophen. Careful evaluation of the history, food, and environment of the animal can help eliminate most of the toxicant differentials on the list.

Neurotoxins: Anatoxin-A, Homoanatoxin-A, Anatoxin-A(s)

Toxic Dose

The oral LD_{50} for anatoxin-a in dogs is unknown. In mice, the intraperitoneal LD_{50} of anatoxin-a is 200 mcg/kg, whereas the oral LD_{50} is greater than 5000 mcg/kg.[24] Several studies have shown that there are significant species differences with regard to anatoxin-a toxicity. Based on the measured concentration of anatoxin-a in collected biofilm, the estimated amount of algal material that a 2.5- or 25-kg dog would have to ingest to die from anatoxin-a poisoning is 6 and 60 g of algal material, respectively.[25] Homoanatoxin-a is a methyl derivative of anatoxin-a and often co-produced with anatoxin-a by the same species of cyanobacteria.[26] The intraperitoneal LD_{50} of homoanatoxin-a in mice is 250 mcg/kg.[27] Toxicity data for dogs are not known. Anatoxin-a(s) is much more toxic than anatoxin-a or homoanatoxin-a with an intraperitoneal LD_{50} in mice of 20 mcg/kg.[28]

Although toxicity data for dogs is not available, anatoxin-a(s) has been implicated in dog deaths.[29]

Toxicokinetics

Data on the toxicokinetics of anatoxin-a, homoanatoxin-a, and anatoxin-a(s) does not exist. Based on the rapid onset of clinical signs after oral exposure to any of these neurotoxins, rapid absorption is suspected. Dogs exposed to anatoxin-a–contaminated water developed clinical signs as soon as 5 minutes later and died shortly thereafter.[25,30-35] Anatoxin-a is partly excreted unchanged by the kidney and liver as it has been detected in urine and bile in a poisoned dog.[35]

Mechanism of Toxicity

Anatoxin-a and homoanatoxin-a are potent agonists at nicotinic cholinergic receptors in neurons and at the neuromuscular junctions.[36] After initial continuous electrical stimulation, a nerve block will result in respiratory paralysis and death. Anatoxin-a can also trigger dopamine and noradrenaline release.[37,38] Homoanatoxin-a can initiate the opening of endogenous voltage-dependent neuronal L-type Ca^{2+} channels resulting in the release of acetylcholine from peripheral cholinergic nerves.[39] The mechanism of toxicity of anatoxin-a(s) differs from that of anatoxin-a and homoanatoxin-a. Anatoxin-a(s) is a naturally occurring irreversible acetylcholinesterase inhibitor, which leads to persistent stimulation and a neuronal muscular block.[40] This mechanism is very similar to that of organophosphorus and carbamate insecticides, except anatoxin-a(s) is incapable of crossing the blood-brain barrier and its effects are peripheral.

Clinical Signs

Sharing the same mechanism of toxicity, anatoxin-a and homonanatoxin-a poisonings have identical clinical presentations. Clinical signs develop rapidly and include rigidity and muscle tremors, followed by convulsions, paralysis, respiratory failure, cyanosis, and death. Death typically occurs within minutes to a few hours after exposure. Other signs include anxiety, ptyalism, and tachycardia or bradycardia.[25,30-35] Poisoning with anatoxin-a(s) is characterized by a rapid onset of excessive salivation (s stands for salivation), lacrimation, diarrhea, and urination, all of which are clinical signs subsequent to muscarinic overstimulation. Nicotinic overstimulation can result in tremors, incoordination, recumbency, convulsions, and respiratory arrest. Progression is very rapid and animals may die within 30 minutes of exposure.[29]

Minimum Database and Confirmatory Tests

As with other suspect cyanobacteria intoxications, algal identification in water samples or in samples collected from the animal's skin or gastric contents greatly assists with the diagnostic workup. Algal-containing samples should be chilled, not frozen, preserved in 10% formalin (v/v 50:50), and submitted to a phycologist for identification. As toxicity of cyanotoxins is strain-specific, positive identification does not predict the hazard level.

Anatoxin-a, homoanatoxin-a, and anatoxin-a(s) poisonings do not result in specific changes in serum chemistry parameters. In fact, because of the rapid progression and death with these neurotoxins, blood work is rarely performed. If available, possible nonspecific changes are hyperglycemia, acidosis, mild hypophosphatemia, and mild respiratory alkalosis.[30,35] In cases of anatoxin-a(s) poisoning, a depressed blood cholinesterase activity along with an adequate brain cholinesterase activity supports the diagnosis.

Toxicologic analyses for algal toxins in biologic specimens are recommended to establish a diagnosis. Anatoxin-a can be analyzed by liquid chromatography and tandem mass spectrometry[30] in algal material, water, gastrointestinal contents, urine, and bile.[35] Select veterinary toxicology laboratories can perform analysis of biologic specimens for anatoxin-a(s).[41]

Treatment and Prognosis

The treatment plan goals are to prevent further exposure and absorption, to control central nervous system signs, and to provide supportive care. Because of the rapid onset of clinical signs and rapid progression to death, treatment is often impossible or unsuccessful. As with hepatotoxic cyanotoxins, there is no data on the absorptive efficacy of activated charcoal for neurotoxic cyanotoxins. In addition, decontamination procedures are likely contraindicated because of existing neurologic signs. Seizures can be controlled with diazepam, phenobarbital, or pentobarbital. In animals with anatoxin-a(s) poisoning, administration of atropine can alleviate muscarinic signs. The use of 2-pyridine aldoxime methyl chloride (2-PAM; pralidoxime) is not recommended in anatoxin-a(s) poisoned animals.[40]

Cases of recovery from suspected anatoxin-a exposure in dogs have been documented but the amount ingested was not determined.[31,34] In general, neurotoxic cyanotoxin poisonings progress so rapidly that treatment is often too late and prognosis is poor.

Gross and Histologic Lesions

Animals poisoned with anatoxin-a, homoanatoxin-a, or anatoxin-a(s) may have algal material on their fur or skin or in the stomach. Typically, there are no specific gross lesions observed at necropsy. Nonspecific gross findings noted in anatoxin-a–poisoned dogs include hemorrhagic liver, algal material in the stomach, and blood-tinged froth in the upper airways.[30,32,35] Nonspecific histopathologic findings in anatoxin-a–poisoned dogs include patchy eosinophilic fluid in lungs, congestion of the kidneys, and autolytic changes in liver and kidneys.[32]

Differential Diagnoses

Anatoxin-a, homoanatoxin-a, and anatoxin-a(s) poisonings need to be differentiated from other neurotoxicants, such as organophosphorus and carbamate insecticides, strychnine, zinc phosphide, metaldehyde, 4-aminopyridine, ethylene glycol, penitrem A, methylxanthines, amphetamines, saxitoxins, 4-aminopyridine, bromethalin, chlorinated hydrocarbons, certain mushrooms, certain drugs of abuse, and neurotoxic plants.

Other Cyanotoxins

Poisonings with microcystins, nodularins, and anatoxin-a make up the majority of case reports in dogs, but many other cyanotoxins are considered toxic to small animals and may result in illness and death. Thus there are likely many unreported cases because of lack of proper diagnostic workup and confirmatory testing. Without further data it is impossible to estimate the frequency of cyanobacteria poisoning or to better understand the cyanotoxins involved in small animals.

Cylindrospermopsin is hepatotoxic and nephrotoxic and blocks protein synthesis, resulting in possible damage to the liver, kidneys, adrenal glands, intestine, lungs, thymus, and heart.[42] Although there are no confirmed cases in small animals, cylindrospermopsin poisoning has been confirmed in cattle and humans.[42,43]

Saxitoxins belong to the group of paralytic shellfish poisoning toxins, but can also be produced by several freshwater cyanobacteria, especially *Lyngbya wollei*. The toxins are very toxic to mammals by blocking voltage-gated sodium channels, ultimately leading to respiratory arrest, neuromuscular weakness, and cardiovascular shock.[44] In cats, saxitoxin poisoning has resulted in cardiovascular shock that is responsive to adrenergic agonists.[45]

β-*N*-methylamino-L-alanine (BMAA) is a newly confirmed neurotoxic amino acid produced by a cyanobacterial species commonly found in the southeastern United States.[46] In birds, BMAA is associated with avian vacuolar myelinopathy, resulting in ataxia, tilting, weakness, and death. The toxicity potential of BMAA in small animals is not known.

Lyngbyatoxin-a, *debromoaplysiatoxin*, and *aplysiatoxin* are produced by *Lyngbya* spp. in primarily marine waters and have dermonecrotic and tumor-promoting activities. Lyngbyatoxin-a is lipophilic and can penetrate skin, resulting in acute dermatitis. This has been reported in humans swimming in Hawaii's and Florida's ocean waters.[47,48] Debromoaplysiatoxin and aplysiatoxin can cause rashes and skin blisters.[47]

Cyanobacterial *lipopolysaccharides* have been implicated as causing a variety of health effects. However, from what little is known to date, the toxic potential of cyanobacterial lipopolysaccharides is debatable and requires more research. Not all lipopolysaccharides are toxic and the toxicity of lipopolysaccharides in humans differs from animals, resulting in extremely limited data on the toxicity of cyanobacterial lipopolysaccharides in small animals. It is possible that lipopolysaccharides enhance the toxicity of cyanotoxins, although they only possess weak toxicity.[49,50]

References

1. Francis G: Poisonous Australian lake, *Nature* 18:11–12, 1878.
2. Van Apeldoorn ME, van Egmond HP, Speijers GJ, et al: Toxins of *Cyanobacteria*, *Mol Nutr Food Res* 51:7–60, 2007.
3. Lopez Rodas V, Costas E: Preference of mice to consume *Microcystis aeruginosa* (toxin-producing cyanobacteria): a possible explanation for numerous fatalities of livestock and wildlife, *Res Vet Sci* 67:107–110, 1999.
4. Gilroy DJ, Kauffman KW, Hall RA, et al: Assessing potential health risks from microcystin toxins in blue-green algae dietary supplements, *Environ Health Perspect* 108:435–439, 2000.
5. Smith JL, Schulz KL, Zimba PV, et al: Possible mechanism for the foodweb transfer of covalently bound microcystins, *Ecotoxicol Environ Saf* 73:757–761, 2010.
6. Graham JL, Loftin KA, Meyer MT, et al: Cyanotoxin mixtures and taste-and-odor compounds in cyanobacterial blooms from the Midwestern United States, *Environ Sci Technol* 44:7361–7368, 2010.
7. Fawell JK, Mitchell RE, Everett DJ, et al: The toxicity of cyanobacterial toxins in the mouse: I microcystin-LR, *Hum Exp Toxicol* 18:162–167, 1999.
8. Chorus I, Falconer IR, Salas HJ, et al: Health risks caused by freshwater cyanobacteria in recreational waters, *J Toxicol Environ Health Part B, Crit Rev* 3:323–347, 2000.
9. Ito E, Kondo F, Harada K: First report on the distribution of orally administered microcystin-LR in mouse tissue using an immunostaining method, *Toxicon* 38:37–48, 2000.
10. Falconer IR, Dornbusch M, Moran G, et al: Effect of the cyanobacterial (blue-green algal) toxins from *Microcystis aeruginosa* on isolated enterocytes from the chicken small intestine, *Toxicon* 30:790–793, 1992.
11. Feurstein D, Holst K, Fischer A, et al: Oatp-associated uptake and toxicity of microcystins in primary murine whole brain cells, *Toxicol Appl Pharmacol* 234:247–255, 2009.
12. Fischer WJ, Altheimer S, Cattori V, et al: Organic anion transporting polypeptides expressed in liver and brain mediate uptake of microcystin, *Toxicol Appl Pharmacol* 203:257–263, 2005.
13. Shen PP, Zhao SW, Zheng WJ, et al: Effects of cyanobacteria bloom extract on some parameters of immune function in mice, *Toxicol Lett* 143:27–36, 2003.
14. DeVries SE, Galey FD, Namikoshi M, et al: Clinical and pathologic findings of blue-green algae (*Microcystis aeruginosa*) intoxication in a dog, *J Vet Diagn Invest* 5:403–408, 1993.
15. Walker SR, Lund JC, Schumacher DG, et al: Nebraska experience. In Hudnell HK, editor: *Cyanobacterial harmful algal blooms: state of the science and research needs*, 619, Springer New York, NY, 2008, Advances in Experimental Medicine and Biology, pp 139–152.
16. Wood SA, Heath MW, Holland PT, et al: Identification of a benthic microcystin-producing filamentous cyanobacterium (*Oscillatoriales*) associated with a dog poisoning in New Zealand, *Toxicon* 55:897–903, 2010.
17. Simola O, Wiberg M, Jokela J, et al: Pathologic findings and toxin identification in cyanobacterial (*Nodularia spumigena*) intoxication in a dog. Veterinary Pathology OnlineFirst, published on August 8, 2011, as http://dx.doi.org/10.1177/0300985811415703.
18. Algermissen D, Mischke R, Seehusen F, et al: Lymphoid depletion in two dogs with nodularin intoxication, *Vet Rec* 169:15, 2001.
19. Harding WR, Rowe N, Wessels JC, et al: Death of a dog attributed to the cyanobacterial (blue-green algal) hepatotoxin nodularin in South Africa, *J S Afr Vet Assoc* 66:256–259, 1995.
20. Nehring S: Mortality of dogs associated with a mass development of *Nodularia spumigena* (Cyanophyceae) in a brackish lake at the German North Sea coast, *J Plankton Res* 15:867–872, 1993.
21. Falconer IR, Yeung DSK: Cytoskeletal changes in hepatocytes induced by microcystis toxins and their relation to hyperphosphorylation of cell-proteins, *Chem Biol Interact* 81:181–196, 1992.
22. Runnegar M, Berndt N, Kong SM, et al: In vivo and in vitro binding of microcystin to protein phosphatases 1 and 2A, *Biochem Biophys Res Commun* 216:162–169, 1995.

23. Ding WX, Nam Ong C: Role of oxidative stress and mitochondrial changes in cyanobacteria-induced apoptosis and hepatotoxicity, *FEMS Microbiol Lett* 220:1–7, 2003.
24. Stevens DK, Krieger RI: Effect of route of exposure and repeated doses on the acute toxicity in mice of the cyanobacterial nicotinic alkaloid anatoxin-a, *Toxicon* 29:134–138, 1991.
25. Gugger M, Lenoir S, Berger C, et al: First report in a river in France of the benthic cyanobacterium *Phormidium favosum* producing anatoxin-a associated with dog neurotoxicosis, *Toxicon* 45:919–928, 2005.
26. Namikoshi M, Murakami T, Watanabe MF, et al: Simultaneous production of homoanatoxin-a, anatoxin-a, and a new non-toxic 4-hydroxyhomoanatoxin-a by the cyanobacterium-a by the cyanobacterium *Raphidiopsis mediterranea Skuja*, *Toxicon* 42:533–538, 2003.
27. Skulberg OM, Carmichael WW, Andersen RA, et al: Investigations of a neurotoxic oscillatorialean strain (*Cyanophyceae*) and its toxin—isolation and characterization of homoanatoxin-a, *Environ Toxicol Chem* 11:321–329, 1992.
28. Matsunaga S, Moore RE, Niemczura WP, et al: Anatoxin-a(S), a potent anticholinesterase from *Anabaena flos-aquae*, *J Am Chem Soc* 111:8021–8023, 1989.
29. Mahmood NA, Carmichael WW, Pfahler D: Anticholinesterase poisonings in dogs from a cyanobacterial (blue-green algae) bloom dominated by *Anabaena flos-aquae*, *Am J Vet Res* 49:500–503, 1988.
30. Puschner B, Hoff B, Tor ER: Diagnosis of antitoxin-a poisoning in dogs from North America, *J Vet Diag Invest* 20:89–92, 2008.
31. Gunn GJ, Rafferty AG, Rafferty GC, et al: Fatal canine neurotoxicosis attributed to blue-green algae (cyanobacteria), *Vet Rec* 130:301–302, 1992.
32. Wood SA, Selwood AI, Rueckert A, et al: First report of homoanatoxin-a and associated dog neurotoxicosis in New Zealand, *Toxicon* 50:292–301, 2007.
33. Edwards C, Beattie KA, Scrimgeour CM, et al: Identification of anatoxin-a in benthic cyanobacteria (blue-green algae) and in associated dog poisonings at Loch Insh, Scotland, *Toxicon* 30:1165–1175, 1992.
34. Hoff B, Thomson G, Graham K: Neurotoxic cyanobacterium (blue-green alga) toxicosis in Ontario, *Can Vet J* 48:147–147, 2007.
35. Puschner B, Pratt C, Tor ER: Treatment and diagnosis of a dog with fulminant neurological deterioration due to anatoxin-a intoxication, *J Vet Emer Crit Care* 20:518–522, 2010.
36. Thomas P, Stephens M, Wilkie G, et al: (+)-Anatoxin-a is a potent agonist at neuronal nicotinic acetylcholine receptors, *J Neurochem* 60:2308–2311, 1993.
37. Barik J, Wonnacott S: Indirect modulation by alpha 7 nicotinic acetylcholine receptors of noradrenaline release in rat hippocampal slices: interaction with glutamate and GABA systems and effect of nicotine withdrawal, *Mol Pharmacol* 69:618–628, 2006.
38. Campos F, Alfonso M, Duran R: In vivo modulation of alpha 7 nicotinic receptors on striatal glutamate release induced by anatoxin-A, *Neurochem Int* 56:850–855, 2010.
39. Aas P, Eriksen S, Kolderup J, et al: Enhancement of acetylcholine release by homoanatoxin-a from *Oscillatoria formosa*, *Environ Toxicol Pharmacol* 2:223–232, 1996.
40. Hyde EG, Carmichael WW: Anatoxin-a(s), a naturally occurring organophosphate, is an irreversible active site-directed inhibitor of acetylcholinesterase (EC 3.1.1.7), *J Biochem Toxicol* 6:195–201, 1991.
41. Dorr FA, Rodriguez V, Molica R, et al: Methods for detection of anatoxin-a(s) by liquid chromatography coupled to electrospray ionization-tandem mass spectrometry, *Toxicon* 55:92–99, 2010.
42. Griffiths DJ, Saker ML: The Palm Island mystery disease 20 years on: a review of research on the cyanotoxin cylindrospermopsin, *Environ Toxicol* 18:78–93, 2003.
43. Saker ML, Thomas AD, Norton JH: Cattle mortality attributed to the toxic cyanobacterium *Cylindrospermopsis raciborskii* in an outback region of north Queensland, *Environ Toxicol* 14:179–182, 1999.
44. Cestele S, Catterall WA: Molecular mechanisms of neurotoxin action on voltage-gated sodium channels, *Biochimie* 82:883–892, 2000.
45. Andrinolo D, Michea LF, Lagos N: Toxic effects, pharmacokinetics and clearance of saxitoxin, a component of paralytic shellfish poison (PSP), in cats, *Toxicon* 37:447–464, 1999.
46. Bidigare RR, Christensen SJ, Wilde SB, et al: Cyanobacteria and BMAA: possible linkage with avian vacuolar myelinopathy (AVM) in the south-eastern United States, *Amyotroph Lateral Scler* 10(Suppl 2):71–73, 2009.
47. Osborne NJT, Webb PM, Shaw GR: The toxins of *Lyngbya majuscula* and their human and ecological health effects, *Environ Int* 27:381–392, 2001.
48. Burns J: Toxic cyanobacteria in Florida waters. In Hudnell HK, editor: *Cyanobacterial harmful algal blooms: state of the science and research needs*, 619, Springer New York, NY, 2008, Advances in Experimental Medicine and Biology, pp 127–137.
49. Codd GA: Cyanobacterial toxins, the perception of water quality, and the prioritisation of eutrophication control, *Ecol Eng* 16:51–60, 2000.
50. Mohamed ZA: Toxic cyanobacteria and cyanotoxins in public hot springs in Saudi Arabia, *Toxicon* 51, 2008. 1130–1130.

DEET

Konnie H. Plumlee, DVM, MS, DABVT, DACVIM

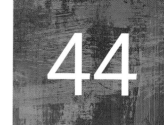

- Insect repellents can contain 5% to 100% DEET.
- The most common clinical signs include hypersalivation, vomiting, hyperexcitability, tremors, ataxia, and seizures.
- No antidote is available, so treatment is supportive.

Sources

N,N-diethyl-m-toluamide (DEET) is an insect repellent marketed for humans and pets to control mosquitoes, flies, and ticks. The various formulations include sprays, sticks, creams, lotions, and gels. Products range in DEET concentration from 5% to 100%, although those marketed for use on pets generally contain less than 10% DEET. Pet products may also contain a pyrethroid insecticide in conjunction with the DEET.

Toxic Dose

Dogs displayed tremors and hyperactivity following each dose when dosed orally with 0.1 to 0.3 mL/kg of 95% DEET isomers daily for 13 weeks.[1,2]

Toxicokinetics

In dogs 7.9% to 12.8% of DEET is absorbed from the skin.[1] Experimentally, 19% to 48% of a topical dose of DEET penetrated intact skin of guinea pigs within 6 hours.[2] Furthermore, topical DEET can accumulate and persist in skin and enhance the dermal absorption of certain chemicals.[2]

The repellent is metabolized in the liver and is excreted chiefly in the urine; there is a small amount of enterohepatic elimination.[1,3]

Mechanism of Toxicity

The toxicologic mechanism of action has not been described.

Clinical Signs

Clinical signs in rabbits and rats include depression, excitation, ataxia, tremors, seizures, and coma.[2] Hypersalivation, vomiting, hyperexcitability, tremors, ataxia, and seizures reportedly can develop in dogs and cats.[1,3]

Minimum Database

Evaluation of the hydration status and urinary function are necessary because the kidneys are the primary site of elimination. Evaluation of liver function may be warranted because the liver is the primary site of metabolism.

Confirmatory Tests

DEET can be detected in serum, urine, liver, bile, and kidney. Greater than 20 ppm DEET in serum is considered diagnostic for poisoning in dogs and cats.[4] Urine concentrations of more than 1 ppm and tissue concentrations of more than 10 ppm support a diagnosis of DEET toxicosis.[4]

Biochemistry panels, complete blood counts, urinalyses, cerebrospinal fluid analysis, and other clinical pathologic tests are not diagnostic for DEET poisoning.

Treatment

If the exposure is dermal, the animal should be washed with a mild dishwashing detergent. Induce emesis if oral exposure is recent and the animal is asymptomatic. Activated charcoal followed by a cathartic can also be used for decontamination. Treat clinical signs with supportive and symptomatic care. No antidote is available.

Prognosis

Sublethally exposed animals usually recover in 24 to 72 hours with timely veterinary care.[3]

Differential Diagnoses

Diagnosis is usually based on a history of recent, excessive exposure to DEET along with the appropriate clinical signs. Diseases to be included on the differential list include any nontoxic conditions that can cause stimulation of the nervous system, such as neoplasia, trauma, infection, metabolic disorders, and congenital disorders.

Toxic agents that should be ruled out include metaldehyde, strychnine, lead, macrolide antiparasitic agents, organochlorine insecticides, and anticholinesterase insecticides (organophosphates and carbamates). Tremorgenic syndromes can be caused by roquefortine, which is a mycotoxin found in moldy blue cheese and other foodstuffs, and by penitrem A, which is a mycotoxin found in moldy English walnuts, cream cheese, and other foods.

References

1. Dorman DC: Diethyltoluamide (DEET) insect repellent toxicosis, *Vet Clin North Am Small Anim Pract* 20:387–391, 1990.
2. Dorman DC, Buck WB, Trammel HL, et al: Fenvalerate/N,N-diethyl-m-toluamide (DEET) toxicosis in two cats, *J Am Vet Med Assoc* 196:100–102, 1990.
3. Osweiler GD: Insecticides and molluscacides. In Osweiler GD, editor: *Toxicology*, Philadelphia, 1996, Williams & Wilkins.
4. Mount ME, Moller G, Cook J, et al: Clinical illness associated with a commercial tick and flea product in dogs and cats, *Vet Hum Toxicol* 33(1):19–27, 1991.

Diethylene Glycol

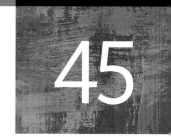

Karyn Bischoff, DVM, MS, DABVT

Motoko Mukai, DVM, PhD, DABT

- Diethylene glycol (DEG) is used as an automotive brake fluid, an industrial lubricant, and a solvent.
- Contamination of pharmaceuticals and health products with DEG have resulted in large-scale human poisoning.
- The kidney is the major target organ of DEG. It also has a direct narcotic effect.
- Clinical signs initially include depression, vomiting, and diarrhea, which are later followed by anuric renal failure.
- Severe oxalate nephrosis does not occur.

Diethylene glycol (DEG), which is composed of two ethylene glycol molecules linked by an ether bond, is a common industrial solvent found in or near the home as an automotive fluid and as a component of chafing fuel such as that marketed by Sterno. Most cases of poisoning in humans have been of epidemic proportions as the result of contamination of pharmaceuticals and healthcare products. The first epidemic of DEG poisoning occurred in the United States in 1937, when DEG was used as a solvent for sulfanilamide elixir. This case was important from a historical perspective in that it resulted in a law requiring safety testing of new drugs in the United States. In the late 1990s, 99 of 109 affected Haitian children died of acute renal failure after ingesting acetaminophen syrup that was contaminated with DEG.[1,2] In 2006 12 of 21 affected adults died from ingestion of DEG-contaminated prescription cough syrup in Panama.[3] Toothpaste imported from China and sold in the United States and in various countries in South America, the Caribbean, and Asia was found to be contaminated with DEG in 2007.[4] During a period from June to August of 2007, several companies recalled products suspected to contain DEG after the Food and Drug Administration issued a warning and an import alert, but thankfully no deaths were reported. As recently as 2008 there were two outbreaks of DEG poisoning: intentional, illegal use of DEG as a solvent in Armillarisin-A in China that resulted in 12 deaths out of 15 affected,[5] and accidental contamination of teething formula in Nigeria resulting in the deaths of 84 children out of 111 affected.[6,7]

Sources

DEG has physical properties similar to those of ethylene and propylene glycol. This solvent is a viscous liquid with a specific gravity of 1.118. It is colorless, nearly odorless, and palatable to children and small animals.[8] It is used as an automotive brake fluid, an industrial lubricant, a solvent, and in liquid chafing fuel. DEG is less toxic than ethylene glycol in most species, but more toxic than propylene glycol. It has occasionally been used as a less expensive substitute for propylene glycol or glycerin in pharmaceutical preparations, resulting in hundreds of human deaths.[1,6,7-17]

Toxic Dose

Accidental DEG toxicosis has been reported in humans.[2,6,10,13-18] Experimental toxicosis has been produced in laboratory animals, cats, dogs, and cattle.[8,19-23] Toxicosis can result from one oral dose or from cumulative dosing.[16,24] The oral median lethal dose (LD$_{50}$) for DEG in dogs, cats, and most laboratory animals is between 3.6 and 11.6 g/kg body weight.[25] Humans seem to be more sensitive to toxicity of DEG. The oral minimum lethal dose in humans, based on several outbreaks, has ranged from 0.014 to 0.35 mL/kg, and the oral LD$_{50}$ is approximately 1.3 mL/kg.[6,26]

Toxicokinetics

DEG is absorbed rapidly in the digestive tract. There is a report of DEG toxicosis resulting from topical exposure to damaged skin in burn patients.[17] A proportion of a dose of DEG is metabolized by hepatic alcohol dehydrogenase and aldehyde dehydrogenase to 2-hydroxyethoxyacetic acid.[6,26] Most is excreted unchanged in the urine.[1,9] Dogs eliminate DEG almost entirely within 36 hours.[25] Like ethylene glycol, the kidney is the target organ of DEG, but unlike ethylene glycol toxicosis, severe oxalate nephrosis is not seen.[1,10,19] The mechanism of DEG toxicosis is not well understood.[1,11,19] Metabolites of DEG are most likely responsible for the clinical toxicosis.[6,26] Like other glycols and alcohols, DEG has a direct narcotic effect.[15]

Clinical Signs

Clinical signs of acute DEG poisoning are similar in most species.[8,16] Animals have signs of CNS depression soon after exposure.[15,27] Dogs sometimes vomit.[16] Initial clinical effects are usually minor unless a large amount has been ingested. When a relatively small amount has been ingested, the initial effects resolve quickly and the animal can appear normal for a day or more. Anuric renal failure, which occurs several days after ingestion and is preceded by polyuria or oliguria, is the hallmark of DEG poisoning.[2] Lumbar pain has been reported in humans.[8,16,18] Vomiting is seen secondary to uremia.[25] Uremic coma precedes death.[1,8-11,16,25] A dog in a recent case report ingested a small amount of tire mounting wax containing DEG and presented after an acute onset of vomiting and diarrhea with oliguria. The dog was markedly azotemic and isosthenuric.[28]

Minimum Database

Unless a large dose is ingested, animals are most likely to present to the veterinarian in the uremic stage of DEG poisoning. Typical clinical pathologic findings associated with uremia include elevated serum urea nitrogen, creatinine, and potassium; lactic acidosis; low urine specific gravity; and erythrocytes present in the urine.[18,29] As with other glycols, the osmolar gap is elevated early in the progression of toxicosis.[26]

Confirmatory Tests

Suspicion of DEG toxicosis is usually based on a history of exposure, evidence of renal failure, and kidney lesions. DEG can be detected in the blood and urine by gas chromatography.[6,20] The osmolar gap is increased early. Because of the rapid elimination rate, this toxicant is unlikely to be detectable in blood or urine for more than a day or two after exposure.

Treatment

Treatment of DEG poisoning is symptomatic, supportive, and depends on early diagnosis. Gastrointestinal evacuation is not warranted unless ingestion was very recent, because gastrointestinal absorption of DEG is rapid and central nervous system (CNS) depression occurs soon after ingestion. Supportive care includes correcting body temperature, electrolyte abnormalities, and acidosis. B vitamins can be added to intravenous fluids.[26] Early fomepizole therapy and peritoneal dialysis or hemodialyses are indicated to treat renal failure in the veterinary patient. Dialysis alone has not been a sufficient treatment in people, but it has been effective when used in conjunction with fomepizole therapy similar to that described for ethylene glycol toxicosis.[2,3,20,26,29] Severe peripheral neuropathy has been described in survivors of DEG poisoning.[3,29,30]

Prognosis

The prognosis is guarded to fair in the early stages, but it is poor for animals in the uremic phase of the toxicosis. Many affected humans have required prolonged dialysis and treatment for peripheral neuropathy, including respiratory support.[26] The continued high mortality rate in human outbreaks has been due both to the age of the affected individuals (who are often small children) and the difficulty in diagnosing DEG toxicosis.[6]

Gross and Histologic Lesions

Renal lesions predominate in animals that have died from DEG poisoning. The kidneys are pale, swollen, and mottled. The renal cortex bulges at the cut surface and hemorrhage is often visible grossly.[16] Microscopic changes include degeneration and necrosis of the proximal convoluted tubular epithelium.[16,19,25] Tubules blocked with protein casts and swollen epithelial cells become ectatic.[16,17,22,25] Calcium deposition in the proximal convoluted tubules has been reported in children.[13] Severe oxalate nephrosis does not occur in DEG poisoning.[10,11,17] Hemorrhagic gastroenteritis lesions, probably secondary to uremia, have been reported.[14,16] Hemorrhage associated with the pericardium, adrenal medulla, lungs, and pleura has been reported in humans.[14,16] Fatty liver, centrilobular hepatocyte degeneration, and necrosis have been seen in some species, but have not been reported in dogs.[23] Central and peripheral nervous lesions have been reported in cattle and humans.[11,14,19,22] Myocardial lesions have been reported in guinea pigs.[21]

Differential Diagnoses

Toxicants causing CNS depression include ethylene glycol, formaldehyde, methanol, propylene glycol, 2-butoxyethanol, ivermectin, amitraz, isopropanol, and other macrolide antiparasitic agents, sedatives, and tranquilizers. Ethylene glycol, grapes and raisins (dogs), paraquat and diquat herbicides, nonsteroidal antiinflammatories, melamine and cyanuric acid, and lily plants (cats) are capable of causing renal damage.

References

1. Malebranche R, Hecdivert C, Lassengue A, et al: Fatalities associated with ingestion of diethylene glycol–contaminated glycerin used to manufacture acetaminophen syrup—Haiti, November 1995-June 1996, *MMWR* 45(30):649–662, 1996.
2. O'Brien KL, Selanikio JD, Hecdivert C, et al: Epidemic of pediatric deaths from acute renal failure caused by diethylene glycol poisoning, *JAMA* 279(15):1175–1180, 1998.
3. Rentz ED, Lewis L, Mujica OJ, Barr DB, Schier JG, Weerasekera G, et al: Outbreak of acute renal failure in Panama in 2006: a case-control study, *Bull World Health Organ* 86(10):749–756, 2008.
4. Bodganich W: Toxic toothpaste made in China is found in US, *New York Times*, 2 June 2007. Available from http://www.nytimes.com/2007/06/02/us/02toothpaste.html.

5. Lin BL, Zhao ZX, Chong YT, Li JG, Zuo X, Tao Y, et al: Venous diethylene glycol poisoning in patients with preexisting severe liver disease in China, *World J Gastroenterol* 14(20):3236–3241, 2008.

6. Alkahtani S, Sammons H, Choonara I: Epidemics of acute renal failure in children (diethylene glycol toxicity), *Arch Dis Child* 95(12):1062–1064, 2010.

7. Bonati M: Once again, children are the main victims of fake drugs, *Arch Dis Child* 94(6):468, 2009.

8. Mathews JM, Parker MK, Matthews HB: Metabolism and disposition of diethylene glycol in rat and dog, *Drug Metab Dispos* 19(6):1066–1070, 1991.

9. Calvery HO, Klumpp TG: The toxicity for human beings of diethylene glycol with sulfanilamide, *South Med J* 32(11):1105–1109, 1939.

10. Wax PM: It's happening again—another diethylene glycol mass poisoning, *J Toxicol Clin Toxicol* 34(5):517–520, 1996.

11. Scalzo AJ: Diethylene glycol toxicity revisited: the 1996 Haitian epidemic, *J Toxicol Clin Toxicol* 34(5):513–516, 1996.

12. Hamif M, Mobarak MR, Ronan A, et al: Fatal renal failure caused by diethylene glycol in paracetamol elixir: the Bangladesh epidemic, *Br Med J* 311(6997):8–91, 1995.

13. Bowie MD, McKenzie D: Diethylene glycol poisoning in children, *S Afr Med J* 46(27):931–934, 1972.

14. Okuonghae OH, Ighogboja IS, Lawson JO, et al: Diethylene glycol poisoning in Nigerian children, *Ann Trop Paediatr* 12(3):235–238, 1992.

15. Heilmair R, Lenk W, Lohr D: Toxicokinetics of diethylene glycol (DEG) in the rat, *Arch Toxicol* 67(10):655–666, 1993.

16. Geiling EMK, Cannon PR: Pathologic effects of elixir of sulfanilamide (diethylene glycol) poisoning, *JAMA* 111(10):919–926, 1938.

17. Cantrell MC, Fort J, Camps S, et al: Acute intoxication due to topical application of diethylene glycol, *Ann Intern Med* 106(3):478–479, 1987.

18. Sing J, Dutta AK, Khare S, et al: Diethylene glycol poisoning in Gurgaon, India, 1998, *Bull World Health Organ* 79(2):88–95, 2001.

19. Winek CL, Shingleton DP, Shanor SP: Ethylene and diethylene glycol toxicity, *J Toxicol Clin Toxicol* 13(2):297–324, 1978.

20. Coppock RW, Mostrom MS, Khan AA, et al: Toxicology of oil field pollutants in cattle: a review, *Vet Hum Toxicol* 37(6):569–576, 1995.

21. Ogbuihi S, Petkovits T, Brinkmann B: Diethylene glycol (DEG)-associated myocardial changes: a pilot investigation of chronic intoxication in guinea pigs, *Int J Legal Med* 104(2):93–97, 1991.

22. Fritz DL, Coppock RW, Khan AA, et al: Toxicopathy of diethylene glycol in cattle, *Toxicologist* 12:119, 1992.

23. Kraul H, Jahn F, Braunlich H: Nephrotoxic effects of diethylene glycol in rats, *Exp Pathol* 42(1):27–32, 1991.

24. Hanzlik PH, Newman HW, Van Winkle W Jr, et al: Toxicity, fate and excretion of propylene glycol and some other glycols, *J Pharmacol Exp Ther* 67(12):101–113, 1939.

25. Hesser L: Diethylene glycol toxicity, *Food Chem Toxicol* 24(3):261–265, 1986.

26. Marraffa JM, Holland MG, Stork CM, et al: Diethylene glycol: widely used solvent presents serious poisoning potential, *J Emerg Med* 35(4):401–406, 2008.

27. Ballantyne B, Meyers RC: The comparative acute toxicity and primary irritancy of the monohexyl ethers of ethylene and diethylene glycol, *Vet Hum Toxicol* 29(5):361–366, 1987.

28. Lewis DH, Goggs RA: Possible diethylene glycol toxicity in a dog, *Vet Rec* 164(4):127, 2009.

29. Borron SW, Baud FJ, Garnier R: Intravenous 4-methylpyrazole as an antidote for diethylene glycol and triethylene glycol poisoning: a case report, *Vet Hum Toxicol* 39(1):26–28, 1997.

30. Rollins YD, Filley CM, McNutt JT: Fulminant ascending paralysis as a delayed sequela of diethylene glycol (Sterno) ingestion, *Neurol* 59:1460–1463, 2002.

Ethanol

Jill A. Richardson, DVM

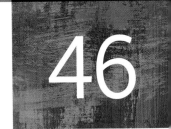

- Ethanol is used therapeutically to treat ethylene glycol poisoning in dogs and cats.
- The most common signs of ethanol toxicity include sedation, weakness, and ataxia.
- Ethanol poisoning has occurred following bread dough ingestion in dogs.
- Ethanol poisoning has also occurred following ingestion of rotten apples in a dog.
- Treatment includes maintaining adequate hydration and correcting any respiratory or CNS depression.

Sources

Ethanol is made by fermentation of sugar or by the hydration of ethene. Ethanol is commonly found in households in the form of alcoholic beverages. The percentage of ethanol found in alcoholic beverages is one half of the value of the drink's proof value. Ethanol is also used for manufacturing paints and varnishes, as a carrier in various medications, as a disinfectant, in some types of thermometers, as a fuel substitute, and in some forms of antifreeze. The principal use of ethanol in veterinary medicine is in the treatment of ethylene glycol antifreeze poisoning (Box 46-1).[1] In humans and nonhuman primates, ethanol is sometimes used to treat methanol poisoning.

Ethanol intoxication has been described in dogs ingesting alcoholic drinks intended for human consumption.[4] Ethanol poisoning in dogs following ingestion of uncooked bread dough has also been reported.[5] Additionally, ethanol intoxication has been reported in a dog from ingestion of rotten apples.[6]

Toxic Dose

The intravenous minimum lethal dose (LD_{LO}) in dogs is 1600 mg/kg, and the oral LD_{LO} is 5500 mg/kg.[7] The oral median lethal dose (LD_{50}) of ethanol in rats is 9000 mg/kg.[7]

Toxicokinetics

Ethanol is well absorbed orally. It rapidly distributes throughout the body and crosses the blood-brain barrier.[1] Ethanol also crosses the placenta.[1] Ethanol is metabolized by hepatic alcohol dehydrogenase, and its metabolites can be excreted in the urine, along with unmetabolized parent compound.

| **Box 46-1** | Doses of Ethanol for Ethylene Glycol Treatment in Dogs and Cats[1,2,3] |

Dogs
1. 5.5 mL/kg of a 20% solution IV q4h for five treatments, then q6h for four additional treatments
2. 22 mL/kg IV of a 5% solution q4h for six treatments, then q6h for four treatments
3. Constant rate IV infusion of 5% solution to run at 5.5 mL/kg/h

Cats
1. 5 mL/kg of a 20% solution IV q6h for five treatments, then q8h for four additional treatments
2. Constant rate IV infusion of 5% solution to run at 5 mL/kg/h
3. 1.3 mL/kg of a 30% ethanol solution given as a bolus, followed by a constant IV infusion of 0.42 mL/kg/hr for 48 hours.

Mechanism of Toxicity

Ethanol is suspected of inhibiting N-methyl-D-aspartate glutamate receptors in brain cells and the related production of cyclic guanosine monophosphate.[8]

Clinical Signs

Clinical signs seen with ethanol treatment and overdose include central nervous system (CNS) depression, ataxia, lethargy, sedation, hypothermia, and metabolic acidosis.[1] Clinical signs (ataxia and depression) would be expected within an hour if the animal ingested a toxic dose. Excessive gas buildup in the gut and flatulence can be noted in animals ingesting fermented bread dough. Adverse effects associated with intravenous therapy include pain and phlebitis.[1]

Minimum Database and Confirmatory Tests

Blood should be collected to monitor fluid and electrolyte status. Most laboratories are capable of determining ethanol levels in blood. In a report, a dog exhibited vomiting, ataxia, tremors, dehydration, and died 48 hours later with an alcoholemia of 300 mg/dL.[4]

Treatment

Alcohols in general are absorbed very quickly via the gastrointestinal tract. Emesis should only be attempted with extreme caution in asymptomatic animals with recent ingestion (less than 15 minutes). Because ethanol can cause depression, inducing emesis in a symptomatic animal may result in aspiration of vomitus. Activated charcoal has been shown not to be effective with ethanol overdoses and is not recommended.[9] Intravenous fluids can be used to correct any dehydration present and to enhance renal ethanol excretion. Feeding ice chips or lavaging the stomach with cold water will help break apart bread dough in the stomach.

Acid-base balance monitoring is recommended in symptomatic animals. Treatment for acidosis may include administration of sodium bicarbonate. Yohimbine has been recommended to treat CNS depression in dogs caused by ethanol poisoning.[5]

Prognosis

Most cases involving mild signs usually will resolve with close monitoring and supportive care within a 24-hour period. The prognosis is guarded in cases involving metabolic acidosis and severe CNS or respiratory system depression.

Gross and Histologic Lesions

There are no specific gross and histologic lesions observed in ethanol-poisoned animals.

Differential Diagnoses

Other toxicants with sedative or CNS-depressant effects include barbiturates, ethylene glycol, propylene glycol, diethylene glycol, methanol, 2-butoxyethanol, isopropanol, benzodiazepines, macrolide antiparasitics, amitraz, xylitol, and marijuana.

References

1. Plumb DC: *Veterinary drug handbook*, ed 4, Ames, 2002, Iowa State University Press.
2. Forrester S, Lees G: Disease of the kidney and ureter. In Birchard SJ, Sherding RS, editors: *Saunders manual of small animal practice*, Philadelphia, 1994, WB Saunders Co.
3. Firth A: Treatments used in small animal toxicoses. *Kirk's current veterinary therapy: XIII small animal practice*, Philadelphia, 2000, WB Saunders.
4. Van Wuijckhuise L, Cremers GG: Alcohol poisoning in dog, *Tijdschr Diergeneeskd* 128(9):284, 2003.
5. Means C: Bread dough toxicosis in dogs, *J Vet Emerg Crit Care* 13(1):39–41, 2003.
6. Kammerer M, Sachot E, Blanchot D: Ethanol toxicosis from the ingestion of rotten apples by a dog, *Vet Hum Toxicol* 43(6):349–350, 2001.
7. *RTECS: Registry of toxic effects of chemical substances*: CD Rom, National Institute for Occupational Safety and Health, Englewood, CO, 2000, MICROMEDEX.
8. Snyder R, Andrews LS: Toxic effects of solvents and vapors. In Klaassen, editor: *Casarett & Doull's toxicology: the basic science of poisons*, ed 5, New York, 1996, McGraw-Hill.
9. Poppenga Robert H: Decontaminating and detoxifying the poisoned patient, *Proceedings of the Western Veterinary Conference*, February 2002.

Ethylene Glycol

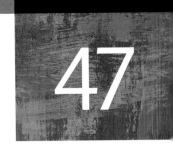

Mary Anna Thrall, DVM, MS, DACVP

Heather E. Connally, DVM, MS, DACVECC

Gregory F. Grauer, DVM, MS, DACVIM

Dwayne W. Hamar, PhD

- Ethylene glycol (EG) has a very high potential for lethal results, but with early recognition of the syndrome and timely institution of therapy, animals can be saved.
- Clinical signs and laboratory findings are very useful in diagnosing the early stage of EG poisoning.
- Treatment of EG toxicosis should be instituted as quickly as possible when EG poisoning is suggested. Prognosis is excellent in dogs treated in less than 5 hours following ingestion and is good in cats treated in less than 3 hours following ingestion.
- Fomepizole, not ethanol, is the therapy of choice for dogs in which EG ingestion is suggested, and data support use of higher doses of fomepizole in cats suspected of ingestion.

thylene glycol (EG) poisoning is common in dogs and cats[1-4] and often results in death if it is not diagnosed and treated promptly.[5] The mortality rate in dogs is reported to range from 59% to 70%[1,5] and is thought to be even higher in cats. EG intoxication is the second most common cause of fatal poisoning in animals according to the American Association of Poison Control Centers.[6] This high incidence is due to the ready availability, possible pleasant taste, and small quantity of EG necessary to induce poisoning. Bittering agents have been added to some EG formulations to deter ingestion. It is not known how effective this has been in reducing the number of poisonings in pets. Although most EG poisonings are accidental, malicious poisonings also occur. The incidence of poisoning is also relatively high in humans, with approximately 5000 episodes reported in the United States each year.[7,8] The vast majority of these are unintentional, and approximately one third of the cases occur in children.[7] EG is the most common cause of human poisoning in some countries, such as Poland.[9] The first reported case of EG intoxication in a human being occurred in 1930,[10] but the toxicity of EG was not fully realized until 1938 when 76 persons died after consuming an elixir of sulfanilamide containing 96% diethylene glycol.[11] Since then many reports of EG poisoning in humans and other animals have been published.[3,12-30]

Sources

EG ($C_2H_6O_2$) is a colorless, odorless, possibly sweet-tasting liquid used primarily as an anti-freeze and windshield deicing agent. Its small molecular weight (62 Da) makes it effective in lowering the freezing point of water. EG is also used as a cryoprotectant for embryo preservation, in the manufacture of polyester compounds, as a solvent in the paint and plastic industries, and as an ingredient in photographic developing solutions, hydraulic brake fluid, motor oil, inks, snow globes, paints, and wood stains.[31] The most readily available source of EG in the home is antifreeze solution, which consists of approximately 95% EG. All dogs and cats that have been brought to Colorado State University Veterinary Teaching Hospital with EG toxicosis are thought to have ingested antifreeze, with the exception of one cat that ingested photographic developing solution.[3] The source of antifreeze is usually an open container or a puddle of antifreeze that has drained from a radiator. Rarely, dogs may chew open a plastic container of antifreeze. Intoxication occurs most commonly in the fall, winter, and spring, the seasons in which antifreeze is most commonly used.[3,26]

Toxic Dose

The minimum lethal dose of undiluted EG is 6.6 mL/kg in the dog[32] and 1.5 mL/kg in the cat.[33]

Toxicokinetics

Following ingestion, EG is rapidly absorbed from the gastrointestinal tract; the rate of absorption is delayed when food is in the stomach.[34] It is then quickly distributed throughout the blood and tissue. The plasma half-life of EG is approximately 3 hours.[35,36] A variable amount, depending on dose and species, is eliminated unmetabolized in the urine.[35,37,38] The remaining EG is metabolized, primarily by the enzyme alcohol dehydrogenase (ADH) and other hepatic enzymes, to glycoaldehydes and organic acids. The elimination system appears to be saturable, with semilogarithmic rates of elimination at low doses giving way to zero-order elimination kinetics at higher doses. Metabolites are present for up to several days, and calcium oxalate is present in tissue for much longer.[31]

The liver is the major site of EG metabolism, although small amounts of ADH are present in other organs, such as the kidney and stomach.[39,40] EG is initially oxidized to glycoaldehyde by ADH, and glycoaldehyde is then oxidized to glycolic acid and then to glyoxylic acid. Glyoxylic acid is primarily converted to oxalic acid but may follow several metabolic pathways; end products may also include glycine, formic acid, hippuric acid, oxalomalic acid, and benzoic acid. EG and glycolic acid are excreted in urine in higher quantities than any other metabolites because their metabolism is rate limiting.[41,42] Calcium is bound to oxalic acid, resulting in calcium oxalate crystal formation. Calcium oxalate crystal deposition is widespread but is most severe in the kidney, and crystalluria is a consistent finding in animals producing urine.[34,43]

Mechanism of Toxicity

Before it is metabolized, EG is no more toxic than ethanol, although EG is a more potent central nervous system (CNS) depressant than is ethanol.[44] EG per se has no major effects other than gastrointestinal irritation, increased serum osmolality, and CNS depression. However, unlike ethanol, EG is biotransformed to highly toxic metabolites that result in severe metabolic acidosis and acute renal failure, which are hallmarks of EG poisoning.[3,31,45]

Cytotoxicity

The cytochrome P450 system is partially responsible for and is inhibited by the metabolism of EG. Electron transfer within the P450 system is affected, resulting in the production of oxygen radicals that are probably toxic to tissue. Moreover, the organic acid metabolites inhibit oxidative phosphorylation, cellular respiration, glucose metabolism, protein synthesis, and deoxyribonucleic acid replication.[46,47] The wide range of tissue toxicities seen in animals with EG toxicosis may be due to the fact that different tissues use different isoenzymes of the cytochrome P450 family.

Gastrointestinal System and Liver

EG is a gastric irritant that commonly results in vomiting in dogs and cats.[26] Nausea, vomiting, hematemesis, abdominal pain, and cramping have been associated with EG ingestion in human beings.[31] Calcium oxalate deposits and focal hemorrhages may be found in the gastric mucosa at necropsy. Ultrastructural evidence of hepatocellular damage has been reported,[48,49] although serum biochemical and histopathologic evidence of hepatotoxicity is not usually associated with EG poisoning in dogs and cats.

Nervous System

Glycoaldehyde is thought to be the metabolite primarily responsible for CNS dysfunction; respiration, glucose, and serotonin metabolism are depressed, and CNS amine concentrations are altered.[19,22] Marked cerebral edema is commonly seen during the later stages of EG poisoning in human beings.[50] Calcium oxalate deposition, hemorrhages, perivascular infiltration, and neuronal degeneration may be present.[51] Hypocalcemia secondary to calcium oxalate deposition may contribute to CNS signs, although the concurrent metabolic acidosis shifts calcium to the ionized active state, reducing the chances of hypocalcemia-associated clinical signs. Acidosis is also thought to lead to altered levels of consciousness and cerebral damage.

Metabolic Acidosis

Metabolic acidosis is often severe and has a deleterious effect on multiple organ systems. Glycolic acid accumulation is the primary cause of the metabolic acidosis associated with EG intoxication,[52] although other acid metabolites also contribute. Glycolic acid accumulates because the lactic dehydrogenase enzyme that metabolizes glycolic acid to glyoxylic acid becomes saturated.

Renal Failure

Renal failure is the most profound consequence of EG poisoning in dogs and cats. In human beings, permanent renal failure, as evidenced by tubular atrophy and interstitial fibrosis, is rare; renal function is usually restored within 2 months after EG ingestion. However, dogs and cats are rarely maintained for this period and are commonly euthanized during the anuric or oliguric stage of acute renal failure.[26]

Although glycoaldehyde and glyoxylate have been suggested as the metabolites responsible for the cytotoxicity, renal epithelial damage has now been shown to be associated with calcium oxalate monohydrate (COM) crystal formation within the renal tubules.[53] The severity of renal damage correlates well with the total accumulation of COM crystals in kidney tissue. Studies in cultured kidney cells have demonstrated that only COM crystals, not the oxalate ion, glycoaldehyde, or glyoxylate, produce cell death. The COM crystals adhere to renal tubular cell membranes, and are then internalized by the cells, where they alter cell membrane structure and function and increase reactive oxygen species and produce mitochondrial dysfunction, resulting in cell death.[54]

Clinical Signs

Clinical signs are dose dependent and can be divided into those caused by unmetabolized EG and those caused by the toxic metabolites of EG. The onset of clinical signs is almost always acute. Early clinical signs are usually observed 30 minutes after ingestion and often last until approximately 12 hours after ingestion; they are primarily associated with EG-induced gastric irritation and high EG blood concentrations. These signs commonly include nausea and vomiting, CNS depression, ataxia and knuckling, muscle fasciculations, decreased withdrawal reflexes and righting ability, hypothermia, and osmotic diuresis with resultant polyuria and polydipsia.[3,26,34] As CNS depression increases in severity, dogs drink less, but osmotic diuresis persists, resulting in dehydration. In dogs CNS signs abate after approximately 12 hours, and patients may briefly appear to have recovered. Cats usually remain markedly depressed and do not exhibit polydipsia. Animals may be severely hypothermic, particularly if housed outside during the winter months.

Clinical signs associated with the toxic metabolites are primarily related to oliguric renal failure, which is evident by 36 to 72 hours following ingestion in dogs and by 12 to 24 hours following ingestion in cats. Clinical signs may include severe lethargy or coma, seizures, anorexia, vomiting, oral ulcers and salivation, and oliguria with isosthenuria. Anuria often develops 72 to 96 hours after ingestion. The kidneys are often swollen and painful, particularly in cats.

Minimum Database

Abnormal laboratory findings can also be divided into those associated with early EG intoxication, which may be related to the presence of EG per se or to its toxic metabolites, and those associated with late EG intoxication, most of which are related to renal failure.

Complete Blood Count

The complete blood count is not particularly useful in the diagnosis of EG poisoning. Hematologic abnormalities, when present, are associated with dehydration (increased packed-cell volume and increased plasma protein concentration) and stress (mature neutrophilia and lymphopenia).[3,26] Erythrocytes occasionally exhibit echinocytosis. The mechanism for this is not understood and may be related to abnormal serum electrolyte concentrations or increased serum osmolality.

Serum Biochemical Profile Abnormalities Associated with Early Ethylene Glycol Intoxication

Abnormalities are primarily due to the presence of acid metabolites of EG in the serum that result in metabolic acidosis and include decreased plasma bicarbonate concentration and an increased anion gap. Additionally, hyperphosphatemia may occur because of ingestion of a phosphate rust inhibitor present in some commercial antifreeze products.[26,34] The decreased plasma bicarbonate (HCO_3^-) concentration (sometimes reported as total CO_2 on biochemical profiles) can be seen as early as 1 hour following EG ingestion.

Metabolites of EG notably increase the pool of unmeasured anions and cause an increased anion gap. The anion gap (the mathematical difference between measured anions and measured cations) is usually reported on biochemical profiles, but if not it can be calculated by subtracting the sum of the HCO_3^- (or total CO_2) and chloride (Cl^-) concentrations from the sum of the sodium (Na^+) and potassium (K^+) concentrations. For example, if a patient has an Na^+ value of 155 mEq/L, K^+ of 6 mEq/L, Cl^- of 110 mEq/L, and HCO_3^- of 10 mEq/L, the anion gap is 41 mEq/L. Under normal conditions, the anion gap for dogs and cats is 8 to 25 mEq/L and 10 to 27 mEq/L, respectively, and is composed of phosphates, sulfates, and negatively charged proteins that are not included in the equation. The anion gap is increased by 3 hours after ingestion, peaks at 6 hours after ingestion, and remains increased for approximately 48 hours.[43]

Biochemical Profile Abnormalities Associated with Late Ethylene Glycol Poisoning

With the onset of renal damage and subsequent decreased glomerular filtration, serum creatinine and blood urea nitrogen (BUN) concentrations increase. In the dog, these increases begin to occur between 24 and 48 hours following EG ingestion. In the cat, BUN and creatinine begin to increase approximately 12 hours after ingestion. Because polydipsia does not develop in cats, this may be in part due to dehydration. Serum phosphorus concentrations increase because of decreased glomerular filtration, but increases as high as 10 mg/dL may also be observed 3 to 6 hours following EG ingestion because of the phosphate rust inhibitors present in antifreeze solutions. In these cases, serum phosphorus concentrations return to normal and then increase again with the onset of azotemia. It is important to realize that hyperphosphatemia in the absence of an increased BUN or creatinine is most likely due to increased intake and is not an indication of compromised renal function. Hyperkalemia develops with the onset of oliguria and anuria.

A decrease in serum calcium concentration is observed in approximately half of patients[3,26] and is due to chelation of calcium by oxalic acid. Clinical signs of hypocalcemia are infrequently observed because acidosis results in a shift to the ionized, physiologically active form of calcium.

Increased serum glucose concentration is also observed in approximately 50% of dogs and cats[3,26] and is attributed to the inhibition of glucose metabolism by aldehydes, increased epinephrine and endogenous corticosteroids, and uremia.

Urinalysis

Dogs are isosthenuric (urine specific gravity of 1.008 to 1.012) by 3 hours following ingestion of EG because of osmotic diuresis and serum hyperosmolality-induced polydipsia.[34,43] The urine specific gravity in cats is also decreased by 3 hours after ingestion, but may be above the isosthenuric range.[55] Animals remain isosthenuric in the later stages of toxicosis because of renal dysfunction and an impaired ability to concentrate urine.

Calcium oxalate crystalluria is a common finding and may be observed as early as 3 and 6 hours after ingestion in the cat and dog, respectively, as a result of oxalic acid combining with calcium.[43,55] COM crystals are variably sized, clear, six-sided prisms (Figure 47-1). In animals and people poisoned with EG, the monohydrate form is observed more frequently than the dihydrate form, which appears as an envelope or Maltese cross.[26,29] Dumbbell or sheaf-shaped crystals are observed infrequently. The monohydrate form was previously considered unusual in EG poisoning and was likely to be misidentified as hippuric acid crystals.[3,56-60] Not only do monohydrate calcium oxalate crystals resemble hippuric acid crystals, theoretical arguments have supported hippuric acid crystal formation in patients with EG toxicosis.[59,60] X-ray diffraction, however, has definitively identified the needle-shaped crystals as the monohydrate form of calcium oxalate rather than hippuric acid.[61-64] The detection of calcium oxalate crystalluria, particularly the monohydrate form, provides strong supporting evidence for the diagnosis of EG poisoning.[65] Thus urine microscopy is an important adjunct in the diagnosis of EG poisoning.

Urine pH consistently decreases following EG ingestion. Inconsistent findings include hematuria, proteinuria, and glucosuria. Granular and cellular casts, white blood cells, red blood cells, and renal epithelial cells may be observed in the sediment of some patients.[3,26]

Confirmatory Tests

Because very few abnormalities may be detected in a minimum database in animals with early EG poisoning, other laboratory tests must be performed when EG poisoning is suggested from the history or clinical signs. These include testing for the presence of EG in the blood or urine or measuring serum osmolality.

Serum Ethylene Glycol Concentration

EG serum concentrations peak 1 to 6 hours following ingestion, and EG is usually no longer detectable in the serum or urine 48 to 72 hours after ingestion.[34,43,66] Inexpensive commercial kits* are available that estimate blood EG concentrations at greater than or equal to 50 mg/dL, and the results correlate relatively well with other established methods of measuring EG concentrations, such as gas chromatography,[67] although the presence of propylene glycol, glycerol, or other compounds in the blood may cause a false-positive test result (some activated charcoal suspensions, formulations of diazepam, and semimoist diets contain propylene glycol). Ethanol and methanol do not result in a false-positive test

---

*Ethylene Glycol Test Kit, PRN Pharmacal Inc, 5830 McAllister Avenue, Pensacola, Florida, 32504 (phone: 800-874-9764).

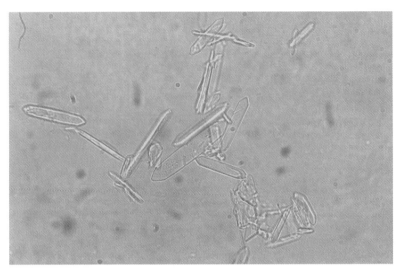

Figure 47-1 Monohydrate calcium oxalate crystals in urine sediment of a dog with ethylene glycol toxicosis.

result. Some hospitals and diagnostic laboratories can determine quantitative concentrations quickly enough to be diagnostically useful using enzymatic assays, although markedly increased concentrations of serum lactate dehydrogenase and lactic acid may result in a false-positive EG concentration result.[29] Laboratory measurement of serum glycolic acid concentration, although diagnostically useful, particularly after EG has been metabolized, is rarely available at reference laboratories.[68] Cats may be intoxicated with a lethal dose of EG that is still less than the 50 mg/dL detectable level of the EG test kit. Therefore, if the test kit result is negative and historical findings and clinical signs are compatible with EG ingestion, the recommendation is to initiate appropriate therapy for EG intoxication and submit a serum sample to a reference laboratory capable of determining a quantitative concentration. It is important to note that whatever kit is used, when EG is detected in serum it confirms exposure only (if it is a true positive), and does not reliably predict whether animals will succumb to clinical signs of intoxication.

Serum Osmolality

Determination of serum osmolality is very useful for diagnosing early EG toxicosis.[69] Serum osmolality is increased by 1 hour after ingestion of EG, increasing in parallel with serum EG concentrations.[43] Hyperosmolality occurs because EG is an osmotically active, small-molecular-weight substance. When measured serum osmolality (by osmometry) is compared with calculated serum osmolality, the difference is referred to as the *osmole gap*. If calculated osmolality is not provided on the biochemical profile printout, osmolality in mosm/kg may be calculated using the following formula:

$$1.86(Na^+ + K^+) + glucose/18 + BUN/2.8 + 9$$

Normal serum osmolality is 280 to 310 mosm/kg, and the normal osmole gap is less than 10 mosm/kg. Serum osmolality as high as 450 mosm/kg serum and an osmole gap as high as 150 mosm/kg serum may be seen 3 hours after ingestion, depending on the quantity of antifreeze ingested.[34,70] Both the gap and the measured osmolality may remain notably high for approximately 18 hours after ingestion. Multiplication of the osmole gap by five yields an approximate serum EG concentration in milligrams per deciliter.[71] More specifically, each 100 mg/dL (16 mmol/L) increment increase in EG concentration contributes approximately

16 mosm/kg of H_2O to the serum osmolality.[29] Simultaneous or sequential increases in osmole and anion gaps are very suggestive of EG intoxication. As EG is metabolized, its contribution to the osmole gap diminishes because the accumulating negatively charged metabolites do not contribute to the osmole gap.[29] Animals presenting with signs of late EG poisoning are likely to have little to no osmole gap increase, but will have an increased osmolality (whether calculated or measured) because of the azotemia.

Two types of instruments are used to measure osmolality: freezing-point osmometers and vapor pressure osmometers. Because EG is nonvolatile (boiling point, 197° C), it is detected by either the freezing-point or vapor-pressure methods. However, methanol, ethanol, and other volatile compounds, although contributing to serum osmolality, may go undetected if assayed by the vapor pressure method. Most clinical laboratories use the freezing-point method.[72] Osmolality can be measured using serum or plasma; if the latter is used, heparin is the preferred anticoagulant. Other anticoagulants, such as ethylenediaminetetraacetic acid, can markedly increase osmolality and can result in spurious increases in the osmole gap.[72]

Other Procedures

Another diagnostic procedure that may be helpful in detecting early EG intoxication is examination of the oral cavity, face, paws, vomitus, and urine with a Wood's lamp to determine whether they appear fluorescent. Many antifreeze solutions manufactured today contain sodium fluorescein, a fluorescent dye that aids in the detection of leaks in vehicle coolant systems. The dye is excreted in the urine for up to 6 hours following ingestion of the antifreeze.[73] A negative test result does not eliminate the possibility of EG ingestion because not all antifreeze solutions contain the dye.

Ultrasonographic patterns in the kidneys of EG-intoxicated dogs and cats may be helpful in diagnosing late EG poisoning. A pattern of greater than normal cortical and medullary echogenicity with persistence of areas of lesser echo intensity at the corticomedullary junction and central medullary regions has been observed concurrent with the onset of clinical anuria and is referred to as the halo sign.[74] Histopathologic examination of kidneys taken at biopsy or necropsy from EG-poisoned animals is usually confirmatory because the renal tubules contain calcium oxalate crystals.

Treatment

Treatment should be instituted before confirmatory tests because EG is metabolized so quickly. Therapy for EG poisoning is aimed at preventing absorption, increasing excretion, and preventing metabolism of EG. Supportive care to correct fluid, acid-base, and electrolyte imbalances is also helpful. Although therapeutic recommendations have traditionally included induction of vomiting, gastric lavage, and administration of activated charcoal,[75,76] it is likely that these procedures are not beneficial because of the rapidity with which EG is absorbed.[31] Moreover, activated charcoal may not be of benefit because large quantities of charcoal are necessary to bind small amounts of EG.[77] Absorption of ethanol can be inhibited to some extent by charcoal. Thus when oral ethanol is used as an emergency antidote, activated charcoal should definitely not be given.[78]

The most critical aspect of therapy is based on prevention of EG oxidation by ADH, which is the enzyme responsible for the initial reaction in the EG metabolic pathway.[19] Historically, treating EG toxicosis has been directed toward inhibiting EG metabolism with ethanol, which is a competitive substrate that has a higher affinity for ADH than EG.[79] Ethanol was first described as an effective antidote for EG intoxication in human beings in 1965 and was the therapy of choice for several years.[80-82] Ethanol therapy was described in dogs and cats in the early to middle 1970s.[16,83-85] Ethanol has numerous disadvantages because it enhances many of the metabolic effects of EG. Both ethanol and EG are CNS depressants, and it is the compounded CNS depression that most limits the usefulness of ethanol as an antidote. The CNS depression produced by high serum ethanol concentrations usually mandates intravenous (IV) fluid therapy for at least 48 hours. Moreover, ethanol, because of its short half-life as a competitive substrate of ADH,[80,84,86] must be administered every 4 hours (IV) or, preferably, as a continuous IV drip, which often results in continuous intensive patient care. One suggested regimen to treat intoxicated dogs is to give 5.5 mL of 20% ethanol/kg body weight IV every 4 hours for five treatments and then every 6 hours for four additional treatments to maintain a serum ethanol concentration of approximately 50 to 100 mg/dL.[87] A lower dosage is suggested for cats: 5 mL of 20% ethanol/kg body weight IV every 6 hours for five treatments and then every 8 hours for four additional treatments.[75,87] Maintenance of more consistent serum levels of ethanol may be safer and more effective; a lower dose of 1.3 mL/kg of a 30% ethanol solution given as a bolus, followed by a constant IV infusion of 0.42 mL/kg/hr for 48 hours, has been shown to be as effective in preventing EG metabolism.[88] Serum ethanol concentrations as low as 50 mg/dL (11 mmol/L) saturate ADH.[82] Older references suggest intraperitoneal (IP) administration of ethanol to cats[85]; however, ethanol is irritating to the peritoneum, and this route of administration offers no advantages over IV drip administration. If pure ethanol for IV administration is unavailable, ethanol can be given orally, but gastric irritation may result in vomiting. An effective dose is approximately 2 to 3 mL/lb of an 80 proof (40% ethanol) alcoholic beverage.

Bolus injections, whether IV or IP, may increase serum ethanol concentrations to the point of suppressing respiration. In a study in which cats were experimentally poisoned with EG and then treated with IP ethanol at a dosage of 5 mL of 20% ethanol/kg of body weight every 6 hours, serum ethanol concentrations ranged from as low as 16 mg/dL at 6 hours after IP ethanol to as high as 240 mg/dL 30 minutes after IP ethanol. Cats with serum ethanol concentrations of more than 200 mg/dL appeared to be near respiratory arrest and were hypothermic.[89] Although severe respiratory depression and coma usually develop when the serum ethanol concentration is 400 to 500 mg/dL, death caused by respiratory arrest has been reported in a human with a serum ethanol concentration of 260 mg/dL.[90] Concentrations of 600 to 800 mg/dL in humans are almost always fatal.[91]

Additional disadvantages of ethanol treatment include its metabolism to acetaldehyde, which impairs glucose metabolism and is a cerebral irritant. Ethanol also contributes to metabolic acidosis by enhancing the formation of lactic acid from pyruvate[92] and may potentiate hypocalcemia.[93] Moreover, ethanol compounds the effects of EG-induced osmotic diuresis and serum hyperosmolality because, like EG, it is a small, molecular weight substance.[72] The recommended therapeutic serum concentration of ethanol, 100 mg/dL (22 mmol/L), contributes 22 mosm/kg of H_2O to the osmole gap.[29] Another substrate with a high affinity for ADH, 1,3-butanediol, has been used experimentally in dogs and rats to prevent the metabolism of EG and has some advantages over ethanol.[66,94] However, it also contributes to the hyperosmolality, and metabolites of 1,3-butanediol contribute to metabolic acidosis.[66] Despite its disadvantages, until recently ethanol has remained the therapy of choice in cats.[55,95]

4-Methyl-1H-pyrazole (fomepizole[66]) has become the preferred antidote in dogs and more recently cats.[24,26,38,43,66,95] Fomepizole is an ADH inhibitor, not a competitive substrate, and it does not induce CNS depression (in dogs), diuresis, or hyperosmolality at the recommended dose. The parent compound, pyrazole, was reported to inhibit ADH in 1963.[96] Fomepizole is a more potent inhibitor of ADH than pyrazole[97] and has none of the toxic effects of pyrazole at recommended doses.[24,26,43,66,98,99] In a study in which the effectiveness of fomepizole therapy was compared with that of ethanol, dogs treated with fomepizole 3 hours after EG ingestion were clinically normal within 24 hours, whereas ethanol-treated dogs remained recumbent for 36 hours and were still severely depressed 72 hours after ingestion. Fomepizole-treated dogs continued to drink water, whereas ethanol-treated dogs were unable to drink, thus necessitating IV fluid therapy.[38] When fomepizole was given to dogs as early as 3 hours following EG ingestion, approximately 90% of EG was excreted unmetabolized[38,43,66] compared with approximately 80% when ethanol was used.[38,66] In the past 30 years, hundreds of dogs examined at Colorado State University's Veterinary Teaching Hospital for suggested or confirmed EG intoxication have been treated with fomepizole.[24,26] Adverse clinical signs associated with the administration of fomepizole are rare. Tachypnea, gagging, excess salivation, and trembling occur occasionally.[26]

The recommended dosage of fomepizole for dogs is 20 mg/kg of body weight IV initially, followed by 15 mg/kg IV at 12 and 24 hours, and 5 mg/kg IV at 36 hours.[26,75,87] For humans receiving concurrent hemodialysis, it is suggested that a continuous infusion of 1 to 1.5 mg/kg/hr of fomepizole be given during the hemodialysis procedure because the drug is lost in the dialysate.[100,101] Presumably, additional fomepizole should be given to dogs if peritoneal dialysis is used as concurrent therapy. The blood concentration of fomepizole can be determined by a high-performance liquid chromatographic assay.[102]

The efficacy of fomepizole treatment in cats was evaluated using the dose for dogs and was found to be ineffective.[55] Results of an in vitro study indicated that canine ADH was more effectively inhibited by fomepizole than feline ADH and suggested that higher doses of fomepizole might be more effective.[103] An in vivo study was then performed in cats to assess the efficacy of high-dose fomepizole compared with ethanol. Six cats were split into two groups: three received high-dose fomepizole and three received ethanol. Of the three cats that received high-dose fomepizole, all survived; however, one developed transient acute renal failure. Of the three that received ethanol (5 mL 20% ethanol/kg IV every 6 hours for 5 treatments, then every 8 hours for 4 more treatments), only one survived: two developed severe acute renal failure and were euthanized.[95] Therefore, we recommend high-dose fomepizole therapy over ethanol to treat EG-intoxicated cats. The recommended dose is 125 mg/kg IV initially, followed by 31.3 mg/kg IV at 12, 24, and 36 hours after the initial dose. If ingestion of a large amount of EG is suspected, repeating serum quantification tests (via a reference laboratory or human hospital) would be advantageous to determine whether continuation of therapy beyond 36 hours is necessary. Alternatively, additional doses of fomepizole can be administered empirically.

Although the advantages of fomepizole therapy in dogs have been recognized since the early 1980s,[66] lack of approval by the Food and Drug Administration (FDA) limited its use in animals because veterinarians were required to obtain an investigational new animal drug (INAD) number from the FDA before purchasing the drug from a chemical supplier. An additional inconvenience was the necessity to prepare a filtered 5% solution of the drug. Fomepizole has now been approved for veterinary use as an antidote for suggested or confirmed EG intoxication and is commercially available as Antizol-Vet,* which can be conveniently reconstituted. Fomepizole is also considered the therapy of choice for EG poisoning in human beings.[36,104-115] Finally, metabolism of glyoxylic acid to nontoxic end products may be enhanced by the administration of thiamine and pyridoxine.[112,113,114,116]

Appropriate supportive therapy consists of IV fluids to correct dehydration, increase tissue perfusion, and promote diuresis. The fluid volume administered should be based on the maintenance, deficit, and continuing loss needs of the patient (Box 47-1). Frequent measurement of urine production, serum urea nitrogen and creatinine, and blood pH, bicarbonate, ionized calcium, and electrolytes daily or twice daily will help guide fluid and electrolyte therapy.[117] Bicarbonate should be given slowly IV to correct the metabolic acidosis (See Box 47-1 for replacement recommendation). Ionized calcium should also be monitored closely, and calcium gluconate or calcium chloride can be supplemented as necessary (see Box 47-1).

Hypothermia, if present, can be controlled with blankets or the use of a pad with circulating warm water.

In animals that are azotemic and in oliguric renal failure when brought to the veterinarian, almost all of the EG has been metabolized, and treatment to inhibit ADH is likely to be of little benefit. However, ADH inhibitors should be given up to 36 hours following

---

*Antizol-Vet (fomepizole) for injection. Orphan Medical Inc, 13911 Ridgedale Drive, Suite 475, Minnetonka, Minnesota 55305. Available through the WA Butler Co (phone 800-551-3861).

ingestion to prevent the metabolism of any residual EG. Fluid, electrolyte, and acid-base disorders should be corrected and diuresis established, if possible. Diuretics, particularly mannitol, may be helpful. The tubular damage caused by EG may be reversible, but tubular repair can take weeks to months. Animals may take up to 1 year following EG toxicosis to regain concentrating ability, and some remain isosthenuric. Supportive care to maintain the patient during the period of renal tubular regeneration is necessary, and peritoneal or pleural dialysis may be useful.[118-120] Hemodialysis has been attempted in dogs with EG-induced renal failure[121] and has been shown to have a relatively good success rate in cats with acute renal failure.[122] Renal transplantation has also been used with variable success in cats with renal failure[123,124] and has been described in dogs.[125] CNS disorders are a common and often fatal complication of renal transplantation in cats.[123,126]

The development of a pharmacologic approach to reduce COM crystal adherence to tubular cells and its cellular interactions would be valuable as this would decrease the renal toxicity in late treated cases of EG poisoning.[53,127]

Prognosis

EG has a very high potential for a lethal outcome, but with early recognition of the syndrome and timely institution of therapy, animals can be saved. The quantity of EG ingested, rate of absorption, and time interval before the institution of therapy are variables that affect the prognosis. The prognosis is excellent in dogs treated with fomepizole within 5 hours of ingesting EG. The importance of early diagnosis and treatment was illustrated in a report of 37 dogs with confirmed EG poisoning that were treated with fomepizole. Of the 18 dogs that had azotemia when initially treated, none survived. Of the 19 dogs that did not have azotemia when initially treated, 17, or approximately 90%, survived.[26] The prognosis for cats is reasonably good if treatment is instituted within 3 hours following ingestion.[55,85]

In contrast, the prognosis in human beings who survive the initial syndrome of severe acidosis is very good. Terminal renal failure in human beings is rare, and most human patients regain renal function by 2 months following EG poisoning.[31] Recovery is very likely because of the effectiveness of hemodialysis therapy in humans[128] and suggests that many more dogs and cats would survive if hemodialysis were more available and economically feasible in animals.

Gross and Histologic Lesions

Histopathologic lesions described in dogs and cats primarily relate to the kidneys. Lesions seen in animals dying of acute renal failure include proximal tubular degeneration and necrosis and intraluminal calcium oxalate deposition. The tubular basement membrane is usually intact, and evidence of tubular regeneration may be present. When chronic renal failure develops in animals, interstitial fibrosis and mononuclear inflammation may be present. Focal hemorrhages may be present in the gastric lining, and calcium oxalate crystal deposition may be found in all organs, including the intestinal mucosa, liver, heart, and brain. CNS lesions may include cerebral edema, focal hemorrhages, neuronal blebbing, and perivascular infiltration by inflammatory cells.

Differential Diagnoses

Ethanol, methanol, propylene glycol, xylitol, barbiturate, ivermectin, and marijuana toxicosis can produce ataxia and other CNS signs similar to those seen in acute EG poisoning.[129-132] These disorders can be differentiated by the diagnostic laboratory tests discussed earlier. Ethanol and methanol toxicosis is rare in domestic animals. Other causes of an increased anion gap include diabetic ketoacidosis and lactic acidosis; these disorders can also be differentiated by appropriate laboratory tests. Other causes of increased

---

| **Box 47-1** | Treatment Recommendations for Ethylene Glycol Intoxication |

Steps to Inhibit EG Metabolism
Dogs*: Use One of the Following Three Therapies:
1. Fomepizole 20 mg/kg IV initially; 15 mg/kg IV 12 and 24 hours after initial bolus; 5 mg/kg IV 36 hours after initial bolus
2. Ethanol as an IV CRI: 1.3 mL of 30% ethanol/kg body weight IV bolus, then CRI of 0.42 mL/kg/hr for 48 hours
3. Ethanol as IV boluses†: 5.5 mL of 20% ethanol/kg body weight IV every 4 hours for five treatments, then every 6 hours for four treatments

Cats*: Use One of the Following Three Therapies:
1. Fomepizole 125 mg/kg IV initially; 31.25 mg/kg IV 12, 24, and 36 hours after initial bolus
2. Ethanol as an IV CRI: 1.3 mL of 30% ethanol/kg body weight IV bolus, then constant rate infusion CRI of 0.42 mL/kg/hr for 48 hours
3. Ethanol as IV boluses†: 5 mL of 20% ethanol/kg body weight IV every 6 hours for five treatments, then every 8 hours for four treatments

Steps to Correct Acid-Base and Electrolyte Imbalances
1. For severe metabolic acidosis (pH <7.2, bicarbonate <12 mEq/L), calculate bicarbonate replacement: base deficit × body weight (kg) × 0.3 = mEq bicarbonate required; base deficit can be obtained from an arterial blood gas or can be calculated using serum bicarbonate [20-measured serum bicarbonate]; replace ⅓ to ½ of this amount over 30 minutes; can give the rest over 4 to 6 hours (in bag of fluids), then reassess blood gas.
2. For severe hypocalcemia (measurement of ionized calcium ideal)
   a. Monitor heart rate, respiratory rate, and heart rhythm during infusion
   b. Dogs: Calcium gluconate 10%, 50-150 mg/kg (0.5-1.5 mL/kg) over 20 to 30 minutes to effect
   c. Cats: Calcium gluconate 10%, 94-140 mg/kg (0.94-1.4 mL/kg) over 20 to 30 minutes to effect

Steps to Correct Fluid Imbalances
1. Estimate dehydration deficit: Estimated degree of dehydration (%) × body weight (kg) × 1000 mL ÷ 12 to 24 hours to replace deficit (Example: 7% dehydrated 10-kg dog: 0.07 × 10 × 1000 mL = 700 mL replaced over 12 hours = 58 mL/hr)
2. Estimate a maintenance rate of fluids: [(30 × body weight [kg]) + 70] ÷ 24 hours
3. Estimate ongoing losses (vomiting): Estimated fluid loss over 4 to 6 hours replaced over the next 4 to 6 hours (total fluid lost ÷ 4 or 6 hours)
4. Calculate fluid rate: Dehydration deficit + maintenance + ongoing losses = total mL/hr to administer

---

CRI, Constant rate infusion; *IV*, intravenous.
*For both dogs and cats, fomepizole is the recommended therapy for EG intoxication.
†Bolus dosing can lead to respiratory depression from acute increases in serum ethanol concentrations and decreases in serum ethanol concentrations below therapeutic levels just before the next dose is administered.

osmolality include ethanol and methanol toxicosis. Ethanol, like EG, can also produce hypocalcemia.[93] Other differential diagnoses for acute renal failure include leptospirosis, ibuprofen and other nonsteroidal antiinflammatory drug toxicoses, aminoglycoside antibiotics, hemolytic uremic syndrome, ingestion of soluble oxalate-containing plants (rare), and lily ingestion, specifically in cats.[133-144] Various members of the lily family, including Easter lily and tiger lily, have been associated with acute renal failure in cats. The toxic principle of lilies that is associated with renal failure is not known.[142,143] Grape and raisin ingestion has also been reported to cause acute renal failure in dogs.[145,146] The majority of the dogs was hypercalcemic, which would not be expected in patients with EG toxicosis. The pathogenesis of grape and raisin toxicosis is not yet understood, nor is it known if the acute renal failure is secondary to the hypercalcemia and mineralization of the kidneys or if the kidney failure leads to the hypercalcemia. Other causes of hypercalcemia in dogs and cats, including cholecalciferol toxicosis,[147-150] will also cause acute renal failure secondary to mineralization of the kidneys.

Acute renal failure must be differentiated from acute decompensation of chronic renal failure. Carbamylated hemoglobin concentration has been shown to be useful in making this differentiation.[151,152] Additionally, animals with chronic renal failure may be anemic and in poor body condition. A history of the duration of clinical signs is also helpful. In children an inherited metabolic disorder, methylmalonic acidemia, has been mistakenly diagnosed as EG poisoning,[153] and conversely, EG poisoning has been misdiagnosed as an inherited metabolic disorder.[154] Methylmalonic acidemia has been reported in a cat but is rare.[155]

Prevention

The taste of EG has long been thought to be an attractant; however, studies have shown that unless dogs are water deprived, they usually will not drink antifreeze solutions, and when given a choice, solutions that contain a lower concentration of EG are preferred.[156] Increasing the awareness of the toxicity of EG will aid in preventing exposure and result in the earlier diagnosis of toxicity in animals. An antifreeze product containing propylene glycol, which is relatively nontoxic, has been marketed and may result in fewer cases of EG poisoning.

Acknowledgment

The authors are grateful to Sarah Freemyer for her assistance in the preparation of this chapter.

References

1. Barton J, Oehme FJ: The incidence and characteristics of animal poisonings seen at Kansas State University from 1975 to 1980, *Vet Hum Toxicol* 23:101–102, 1981.
2. Grauer GF, Thrall MAH: Ethylene glycol (antifreeze) poisoning in the dog and cat, *J Am Anim Hosp Assoc* 18:492–497, 1982.
3. Thrall MA, Grauer GF, Mero KN: Clinicopathologic findings in dogs and cats with ethylene glycol intoxication, *J Am Vet Med Assoc* 184:37–41, 1984.
4. Mueller DH: Epidemiologic considerations of ethylene glycol intoxication in small animals, *Vet Hum Toxicol* 24:21–24, 1982.
5. Rowland J: Incidence of ethylene glycol intoxication in dogs and cats seen at Colorado State University Veterinary Teaching Hospital, *Vet Hum Toxicol* 29:41–44, 1987.
6. Hornfeldt CA, Murphy MJ: American Association of Poison Control Centers report on poisonings of animals, 1993-1994, *J Am Vet Med Assoc* 212:358–361, 1998.
7. Litovitz TL, Smilkstein L, Felberg L, et al: 1996 annual report of the American Association of the Poison Control Centers toxic exposure surveillance system, *Am J Emerg Med* 15:447–500, 1997.
8. Jacobsen D: New treatment for ethylene glycol poisoning (editorial), *N Engl J Med* 340(11):879–881, 1999.
9. Sienkiewicz J, Kwiecinski H: Acute encephalopathy in ethylene glycol poisoning, *Wiadomosci Lekarskie* 45(13-14):536–539, 1992.
10. Anonymous: Possible death from drinking ethylene glycol ("Prestone"). Queries and minor notes, *JAMA* 94:1930, 1940.
11. Geiling EM, Cannon PR: Pathologic effects of elixir of sulfanilamide (diethylene glycol) poisoning. A clinical and experimental correlation: final report, *JAMA* 111(10):919–926, 1938.
12. Hageman PO, Chiffelle TR: Ethylene glycol poisoning: a clinical and pathologic study of three cases, *J Lab Clin Med* 33:573–584, 1948.
13. Kersting EJ, Nielsen SW: Ethylene glycol poisoning in small animals, *J Am Vet Med Assoc* 146:113–118, 1965.

14. Riddell C, Nielsen SW, Kersting EJ: Ethylene glycol poisoning in poultry, *J Am Vet Med Assoc* 150(12):1531–1535, 1967.
15. Durham PJ, Sharman JR: Ethylene glycol poisoning in dogs, *NZ Vet J* 18(4):55–56, 1970.
16. Beckett SD, Shields RP: Treatment of acute ethylene glycol (antifreeze) toxicosis in the dog, *J Am Vet Med Assoc* 158:472–476, 1971.
17. Zenoble RD, Myers RK: Severe hypocalcemia resulting from ethylene glycol poisoning in the dog, *J Am Anim Hosp Assoc* 13:489–493, 1977.
18. Osweiler GD, Eness PG: Ethylene glycol poisoning in swine, *J Am Vet Med Assoc* 160(5):746–749, 1972.
19. Parry MF, Wallach R: Ethylene glycol poisoning, *Am J Med* 57:143–150, 1974.
20. Ettinger SJ, Feldman EC: Ethylene glycol poisoning in a dog, *Mod Vet Pract* 58:237–240, 1977.
21. Walton EW: An epidemic of antifreeze poisoning, *Med Sci Law* 18(4):231–237, 1978.
22. Gordon HL, Hunter JM: Ethylene glycol poisoning, *Anaesthesia* 37:332–338, 1982.
23. Boermans HJ, Ruegg PL, Leach M: Ethylene glycol toxicosis in a pygmy goat, *J Am Vet Med Assoc* 193(6):694–696, 1988.
24. Dial SM, Thrall MA, Hamar DW: 4-Methylpyrazole as treatment for naturally acquired ethylene glycol intoxication in dogs, *J Am Vet Med Assoc* 195:73–76, 1989.
25. Amstrup SC, Gardner C, Myers KC, et al: Ethylene glycol (antifreeze) poisoning in a free-ranging polar bear, *Vet Hum Toxicol* 31(4):317–319, 1989.
26. Connally HE, Thrall MA, Forney SD, et al: Safety and efficacy of 4-methylpyrazole as treatment for suspected or confirmed ethylene glycol intoxication in dogs: 107 cases (1983-1995), *J Am Vet Med Assoc* 209:1880–1883, 1996.
27. Clark P, Henkel K, Swenson C: What is your diagnosis? Ethylene glycol intoxication, *J Small Anim Pract* 38(10):433–450, 1997.
28. Hutchison TW, Dykeman JC: Presumptive ethylene glycol poisoning in chickens, *Can Vet J* 38(10):647, 1997.
29. Eder AF, McGrath CM, Dowdy YG, et al: Ethylene glycol poisoning: toxicokinetic and analytical factors affecting laboratory diagnosis, *Clin Chem* 44(1):168–177, 1998.
30. Wisse B, Thakur S, Baran D: Recovery from prolonged metabolic acidosis due to accidental ethylene glycol poisoning, *Am J Kidney Dis* 33(2):E4, 1999.
31. Davis DP, Bramwell KJ, Hamilton RS, et al: Ethylene glycol poisoning: case report of a record-high level and a review, *J Emerg Med* 15(50):653–657, 1997.
32. Kersting EJ, Nielson SW: Experimental ethylene glycol poisoning in the dog, *Am J Vet Res* 27:574–582, 1966.
33. Milles G: Ethylene glycol poisoning with suggestions for its treatment as oxalate poisoning, *AMA Arch Pathol* 41:631–638, 1946.
34. Grauer GF, Thrall MA, Henre BA, et al: Early clinicopathologic findings in dogs ingesting ethylene glycol, *Am J Vet Res* 45:2299–2303, 1984.
35. McChesney EW, Goldberg L, Parekh CK, et al: Reappraisal of the toxicology of ethylene glycol. II. Metabolism studies in lab animals, *Food Cosmet Toxicol* 9:21–38, 1971.
36. Baud FJ, Bismuth C, Garnier R, et al: 4-Methylpyrazole may be an alternative to ethanol therapy for ethylene glycol intoxication in man, *Clin Toxicol* 24(6):463–483, 1986–87.
37. Gessner PK, Parke DV, Williams RT: Studies in detoxification. The metabolism of ^{14}C-labelled ethylene glycol, *Biochem J* 79:482–489, 1961.
38. Grauer GF, Thrall M, Henre BA, et al: Comparison of the effects of ethanol and 4-methylpyrazole on the pharmacokinetics and toxicity of ethylene glycol in the dog, *Toxicol Lett* 35:307–314, 1987.
39. Coen G, Weiss B: Oxidation of ethylene glycol to glycolaldehyde by mammalian tissue, *Enzymol Biol Clin* 6(4):288–296, 1966.
40. Blair AH, Vallee BL: Some catalytic properties of human liver alcohol dehydrogenase, *Biochemistry* 5(6):2026–2034, 1966.
41. Chow JY, Richardson KE: The effect of pyrazole on ethylene glycol toxicity and metabolism in the rat, *Toxicol Appl Pharmacol* 43:33–44, 1978.
42. Clay KL, Murphy RC: On the metabolic acidosis of ethylene glycol intoxication, *Toxicol Appl Pharmacol* 39:39–49, 1977.
43. Dial SM, Thrall MA, Hamar DW: Efficacy of 4-methylpyrazole for treatment of ethylene glycol intoxication in dogs, *Am J Vet Res* 55:1762–1770, 1994.
44. Berger JR, Ayyar DR: Neurological complications of ethylene glycol intoxication: report of a case, *Arch Neurol* 38:724–726, 1981.
45. Bove KE: Ethylene glycol toxicity, *Am J Clin Pathol* 45:46–50, 1966.
46. Bachman E, Goldberg L: Reappraisal of the toxicology of ethylene glycol. III. Mitochondrial effects, *Food Cosmet Toxicol* 9:39–55, 1971.

47. Voznesensky AI, Schenkman JB: Inhibition of cytochrome P-450 reductase by polyols has an electro-static nature, *Eur J Biochem* 210(3):741–746, 1992.

48. Giermaziak H, Orkisz S: Effects of ethylene glycol on the ultrastructure of hepatocytes, *Exp Toxicol Pathol* 47(5):359–365, 1995.

49. Giermaziak H, Tosik D: Morphometric studies of the hepatocyte mitochondria and endoplasmic reticulum after acute ethylene glycol poisoning, *Exp Toxicol Pathol* 48(4):265–268, 1996.

50. Chung PK, Tuso P: Cerebral computed tomography in a stage IV ethylene glycol intoxication, *Conn Med* 53(9):513–514, 1989.

51. Capo MA, Sevil MB, Lopez ME, et al: Ethylene glycol action on neurons and its cholinomimetic effects, *J Environ Pathol Toxicol Oncol* 12:155–159, 1993.

52. Jacobsen D, Ovrebo S, Ostborg J, et al: Glycolate causes the acidosis in ethylene glycol poisoning and is effectively removed by hemodialysis, *Acta Med Scand* 216:409–416, 1984.

53. De Water R, Noordermeer C, van der Kwast TH, et al: Calcium oxalate nephrolithiasis: effect of renal crystal deposition on the cellular composition of the renal interstitium, *Am J Kidney Dis* 33(4):761–771, 1999.

54. McMartin K: Are calcium oxalate crystals involved in the mechanism of acute renal failure in ethylene glycol poisoning? *Clin Toxicol* 47:859–869, 2009.

55. Dial SM, Thrall MA, Hamar DW: Comparison of ethanol and 4-methylpyrazole as therapies for ethylene glycol intoxication in the cat, *Am J Vet Res* 55:1771–1782, 1994.

56. Scully RE, Galbadine JJ, McNeely BV: Case records of the Mass Gen Hosp, case 38-1979, *N Engl J Med* 30:650–657, 1979.

57. Kramer JW, Bistline D, Sheridan P, et al: Identification of hippuric acid crystals in the urine of ethylene glycol-intoxicated dogs and cats, *J Am Vet Med Assoc* 184(5):584, 1984.

58. Steinhart B: Case report: severe ethylene glycol intoxication with normal osmolal gap—"a chilling thought," *J Emerg Med* 8:583–585, 1990.

59. Gabow PA, Clay K, Sullivan JB, et al: Organic acids in ethylene glycol intoxication, *Ann Intern Med* 105:15–20, 1986.

60. Godolphin W, Meagher EP, Sanders HD, et al: Unusual calcium oxalate crystals in ethylene glycol poisoning, *Clin Toxicol* 16(4):479–486, 1980.

61. Thrall MA, Dial SM, Winder DR: Identification of calcium oxalate monohydrate crystals by x-ray diffraction in urine of ethylene glycol-intoxicated dogs, *Vet Pathol* 22(6):625–628, 1985.

62. Foit FF Jr, Cowell RL, Brobst DF, et al: X-ray powder diffraction and microscopic analysis of crystalluria in dogs with ethylene glycol poisoning, *Am J Vet Res* 46(11):2404–2408, 1985.

63. Jacobsen D, Akesson I, Shefter E: Urinary calcium oxalate monohydrate crystals in ethylene glycol poisoning, *Scand J Clin Lab Invest* 42(3):213–234, 1982.

64. Terlinsky AS, Grochowski J, Geoly KL, et al: Identification of atypical calcium oxalate crystalluria following ethylene glycol ingestion, *Am J Clin Pathol* 76:223–226, 1981.

65. Fogazzi GB: Crystalluria: a neglected aspect of urinary sediment analysis, *Nephrol Dial Transplant* 11(2):379–387, 1996.

66. Thrall MA, Grauer GF, Mero KN, et al: Ethanol, 1,3-butanediol, pyrazole, and 4-methylpyrazole therapy in dogs with experimental ethylene glycol intoxication (abstract), *Proc Am Soc Vet Clin Pathol*, 1982.

67. Dasgupta A, Blackwell W, Griego J, et al: Gas chromatographic-mass spectrometric identification and quantitation of ethylene glycol in serum after derivatization with perfluorooctanoyl chloride: a novel derivative, *J Chromatogr B Biomed Appl* 666(1):63–70, 1995.

68. Fraser AD: Importance of glycolic acid analysis in ethylene glycol poisoning, *Clin Chem* 44(8 Pt 1): 1769–1770, 1998.

69. Ammar KA, Heckerling PS: Ethylene glycol poisoning with a normal anion gap caused by concurrent ethanol ingestion: importance of the osmolal gap, *Am J Kidney Dis* 27(1):130–133, 1996.

70. Jacobsen D, Bredesen JE, Eide I, et al: Anion and osmolal gaps in the diagnosis of methanol and ethylene glycol poisoning, *Acta Med Scand* 212(1–2):17–20, 1982.

71. Burkhart KK, Kulig KW: The other alcohols, *Emerg Med Clin North Am* 8:913–928, 1990.

72. Kruse JA, Cadnapaphornchai P: The serum osmole gap, *J Crit Care* 9(3):185–197, 1994.

73. Winter ML, Ellis MD, Snodgrass WR: Urine fluorescence using a Wood's lamp to detect the antifreeze additive sodium fluorescein: a qualitative adjunctive test in suspected ethylene glycol ingestions, *Ann Emerg Med* 19:663–667, 1990.

74. Adams WH, Toal RL, Breider MA: Ultrasonographic findings in dogs and cats with oxalate nephrosis attributed to ethylene glycol intoxication: 15 cases (1984-1988), *J Am Vet Med Assoc* 199(4):492–496, 1991.

75. Thrall MA, Grauer GF, Dial SM: Antifreeze poisoning. In Bonagura JD, editor: *Kirk's current veterinary therapy XII, small animal practice*, Philadelphia, 1995, WB Saunders.

76. Thrall MA, Connally HE, Grauer GF: Don't freeze up! Quick response is key in ethylene glycol poisoning, *Vet Tech* 19:557–567, 1998.

77. Neuvonen PUJ, Olkkola KT: Oral activated charcoal in the treatment of intoxications: role of single and repeated doses, *Med Toxicol* 3:32–58, 1988.

78. North DS, Thompson JD, Peterson CD: Effect of activated charcoal on ethanol blood levels in dogs, *Am J Hosp Pharm* 38(6):864–866, 1981.

79. Bostrom WF, Li T: Alcohol dehydrogenase enzyme. In Jakoby WB, editor: *Enzyme basis of detoxification*, vol I, New York, 1980, Academic Press.

80. Wacker WEC, Haynes H, Druyan R, et al: Treatment of ethylene glycol poisoning with ethyl alcohol, *JAMA* 194:1231–1233, 1965.

81. Peterson CD, Collins AJ, Keane WF: Ethanol for ethylene glycol poisoning (letter), *N Engl J Med* 305:977, 1981.

82. Peterson CD, Collins AJ, Himes JM, et al: Ethylene glycol poisoning: pharmacokinetics during therapy with ethanol and hemodialysis, *N Engl J Med* 304:21–23, 1981.

83. Nunamaker DM, Medway W, Berg P: Treatment of ethylene glycol poisoning in the dog, *J Am Vet Med Assoc* 159(3):310–314, 1971.

84. Sanyer JL, Oehme FW, McGavin MD: Systematic treatment of ethylene glycol toxicosis in dogs, *Am J Vet Res* 34:527–534, 1973.

85. Penumarthy R, Oehme FW: Treatment of ethylene glycol toxicosis in cats, *Am J Vet Res* 36(2):209–212, 1975.

86. Holman NW, Mundy RL, Teague RS: Alkydiol antidotes to ethylene glycol toxicity in mice, *Toxicol Appl Pharmacol* 49:385–392, 1979.

87. Grauer GF, Thrall MAH: Ethylene glycol (antifreeze) poisoning. In Bonagura JD, editor: *Kirk's current veterinary therapy IX: small animal practice*, Philadelphia, 1986, WB Saunders.

88. Tarr BD, Winters LJ, Moore MP, et al: Low-dose ethanol in the treatment of ethylene glycol poisoning, *J Vet Pharmacol Ther* 8:254–262, 1985.

89. Thrall MA, Dial SM, Hamar DW, et al: Serum ethanol concentrations in ethylene glycol intoxicated cats treated with intraperitoneal ethanol, *Vet Clin Pathol* 17:14, 1988.

90. Maling HM: Toxicology of single doses of ethyl alcohol. In Tremolieres J, editor: *International encyclopedia of pharmacology and therapeutics*, vol II, New York, 1970, Pergamon Press.

91. Mezey E: Ethanol metabolism and ethanol-drug interactions, *Biochem Pharmacol* 25:869–875, 1976.

92. Johnson SE, Osborne CA, Stowe CM, et al: Current status of ethylene glycol toxicity in dogs—a review, *Minnesota Vet* 19:32–43, 1979.

93. Money SR, Petroianu A, Kimura K, et al: Acute hypocalcemic effect of ethanol in dogs. *Alcoholism, Clin Exp Res* 13(3):453–456, 1989.

94. Cox SK, Ferslew KE, Boelen LJ: The toxicokinetics of 1,3 butylene glycol versus ethanol in the treatment of ethylene glycol poisoning, *Vet Hum Toxicol* 34(1):36–42, 1992.

95. Connally HE, Thrall MA, Hamar DW: Safety and efficacy of high-dose fomepizole compared with ethanol as therapy for ethylene glycol intoxication in cats, *J Vet Emerg Crit Care* 20(2):191–206, 2010.

96. Theorell H, Yonetani T: Liver alcohol dehydrogenase-DPN-pyrazole complex: a model of a ternary intermediate in the enzyme reaction, *Biochem Zeitsch* 338:537–553, 1963.

97. Makar AB, Tephly TR: Inhibition of monkey liver alcohol dehydrogenase by 4-methylpyrazole, *Biochem Med* 13:334–342, 1975.

98. Blomstrand R, Ingemansson SO, Jensen M, et al: Normal electroretinogram and no toxicity signs after chronic and acute administration of the alcohol dehydrogenase inhibitor 4-methylpyrazole to the cynomolgus monkey (*Macaca fascicularis*)—a possible new treatment of methanol poisoning, *Drug Alcohol Depend* 13(1):9–20, 1984.

99. Van Stee EW, Harris AM, Horton ML, et al: The treatment of ethylene glycol toxicosis with pyrazole, *J Pharmacol Exp Ther* 192(2):251–259, 1975.

100. Jobard E, Harry P, Turcant A, et al: 4-Methylpyrazole and hemodialysis in ethylene glycol poisoning, *J Toxicol Clin Toxicol* 34(4):373–377, 1996.

101. Jacobsen D, Ostensen J, Bredesen L, et al: 4-Methylpyrazole (4-MP) is effectively removed by haemodialysis in the pig model, *Hum Exp Toxicol* 15(6):494–496, 1996.

102. McMartin KE, Collins TD, Hewlett TP: High pressure liquid chromatographic assay of 4-methylpyrazole. Measurements of plasma and urine levels, *J Toxicol Clin Toxicol* 22(2):133–148, 1984.

103. Connally HE, Hamar DW, Thrall MA: Inhibition of canine and feline alcohol dehydrogenase activity by fomepizole, *Am J Vet Res* 61(4):450–455, 2000.

104. Harry P, Turcant A, Bouachour G, et al: Efficacy of 4-methylpyrazole in ethylene glycol poisoning: clinical and toxicokinetic aspects, *Hum Exp Toxicol* 13(1):61–64, 1994.

105. Harry P, Jobard E, Briand M, et al: Ethylene glycol poisoning in a child treated with 4-methylpyrazole, *Pediatrics* 102(3):E31, 1998.

106. Shannon M: Toxicology reviews: fomepizole—a new antidote, *Pediatr Emerg Care* 14(2):170–172, 1998.
107. Anonymous: Ethylene glycol antidote cleared for marketing (news), *Am J Health Syst Pharm* 55(2):110, 1998.
108. Baud FJ, Galliot M, Astier A, et al: Treatment of ethylene glycol poisoning with intravenous 4-methylpyrazole, *N Engl J Med* 319(2):97–100, 1988.
109. Becker C: Antidotes for methanol and ethylene glycol poisoning—a REAL challenge (editorial), *J Toxicol Clin Toxicol* 35(2):147–148, 1997.
110. Brent J, McMartin K, Phillips S, et al: Fomepizole for the treatment of ethylene glycol poisoning. Methylpyrazole for toxic alcohols study group, *N Engl J Med* 340(11):832–838, 1999.
111. McMartin KE, Heath A: Treatment of ethylene glycol poisoning with intravenous 4-methylpyrazole, *N Engl J Med* 320(2):125, 1989.
112. Porter GA: The treatment of ethylene glycol poisoning simplified (editorial), *N Engl J Med* 319(2):109–110, 1988.
113. Wiley JF: Novel therapies for ethylene glycol intoxication, *Curr Opin Pediatr* 11(3):269–273, 1999.
114. Walder AD, Tyler CK: Ethylene glycol antifreeze poisoning. Three case reports and a review of treatment, *Anaesthesia* 49:964–967, 1994.
115. Buchanan JA, Alhelail M, Cetaruk EW, Schaeffer TH, Palmer RB, Kulig K, Brent J: Massive ethylene glycol ingestion treated with fomepizole alone—a viable therapeutic option, *J Med Toxicol* 6:131–134, 2010.
116. Stokes JB III, Aueron F: Prevention of organ damage in massive ethylene glycol ingestion, *JAMA* 243:2065–2066, 1980.
117. Grauer GF: Fluid therapy in acute and chronic renal failure, *Vet Clin North Am Small Anim Pract* 28(3):609–622, 1998.
118. Fox LE, Grauer GF, Dubielzig RR, et al: Reversal of ethylene glycol-induced nephrotoxicosis in a dog, *J Am Vet Med Assoc* 191(11):1433–1435, 1987.
119. Shahar R, Holmberg DL: Pleural dialysis in the management of acute renal failure in two dogs, *J Am Vet Med Assoc* 187(9):952–954, 1985.
120. Crisp MS, Chew DJ, DiBartola SP, et al: Peritoneal dialysis in dogs and cats: 27 cases (1976-1987), *J Am Vet Med Assoc* 195(9):1262–1266, 1989.
121. DiBartola SP, Chew DJ, Tarr MJ, et al: Hemodialysis of a dog with acute renal failure, *J Am Vet Med Assoc* 186(12):1323–1326, 1985.
122. Langston CE, Cowgill LD, Spano JA: Applications and outcome of hemodialysis in cats: a review of 29 cases, *J Vet Intern Med* 11(6):348–355, 1997.
123. Mathews KG, Gregory CR: Renal transplants in cats: 66 cases (1987-1996), *J Am Vet Med Assoc* 211(11):1432–1436, 1997.
124. Gregory CR, Gourley IM, Kochin EJ, et al: Renal transplantation for treatment of end-stage renal failure in cats, *J Am Vet Med Assoc* 201(2):285–291, 1992.
125. Nemeth T, Toth J, Balogh L, et al: Principles of renal transplantation in the dog: a review, *Acta Vet Hung* 45(2):213–226, 1997.
126. Gregory CR, Mathews KG, Aronson LR, et al: Central nervous system disorders after renal transplantation in cats, *Vet Surg* 26(5):386–392, 1997.
127. Guo C, McMartin KE: Aluminum citrate inhibits cytotoxicity and aggregation of oxalate crystals, *Toxicology* 230(2-3):117–125, 2007.
128. Christiansson LK, Kaspersson KE, Kulling PE, et al: Treatment of severe ethylene glycol intoxication with continuous arteriovenous hemofiltration dialysis, *J Toxicol Clin Toxicol* 33(3):267–270, 1995.
129. Thrall MA, Freemyer FG, Hamar DW, et al: Ethanol toxicosis secondary to sourdough ingestion in a dog, *J Am Vet Med Assoc* 184(12):1513–1514, 1984.
130. Suter RJ: Presumed ethanol intoxication in sheep dogs fed uncooked pizza dough, *Aust Vet J* 69(1):20, 1992.
131. Hurd-Kuenzi LA: Methanol intoxication in a dog, *J Am Vet Med Assoc* 183(8):882–883, 1983.
132. Godbold JC Jr, Hawkins BJ, Woodward MG: Acute oral marijuana poisoning in the dog, *J Am Vet Med Assoc* 175(10):1101–1102, 1979.
133. Vaden SL, Levine J, Breitschwerdt EB: A retrospective case-control of acute renal failure in 99 dogs, *J Vet Intern Med* 11(2):58–64, 1997.
134. Brown CA, Roberts AW, Miller MA, et al: *Leptospira interrogans* serovar *grippotyphosa* infection in dogs, *J Am Vet Med Assoc* 209(7):1265–1267, 1996.
135. Poortinga EW, Hungerford LL: A case-control study of acute ibuprofen toxicity in dogs, *Prevent Vet Med* 35(2):115–124, 1998.
136. Brown SA, Barsanti JA, Crowell WA: Gentamicin-associated acute renal failure in the dog, *J Am Vet Med Assoc* 186(7):686–690, 1985.

137. Spyridakis LK, Bacia JJ, Barsanti JA, et al: Ibuprofen toxicosis in a dog, *J Am Vet Med Assoc* 189(8): 918–919, 1986.
138. Rivers BJ, Walter PA, Letourneau J, et al: Estimation of arcuate artery resistive index as a diagnostic tool for aminoglycoside-induced acute renal failure in dogs, *Am J Vet Res* 57(11):1536–1544, 1996.
139. Holloway S, Senior D, Roth L, et al: Hemolytic uremic syndrome in dogs, *J Vet Intern Med* 7(4): 220–227, 1993.
140. Forrester SD, Troy GC: Renal effects of nonsteroidal antiinflammatory drugs, *Compend Contin Educ Pract Vet* 21(10):910–919, 1999.
141. Adin CA, Cowgill LD: Treatment and outcome of dogs with leptospirosis: 36 cases (1990-1998), *J Am Vet Med Assoc* 216(3):371–375, 2000.
142. Langston CE: Acute renal failure caused by lily ingestion in six cats, *J Am Vet Med Assoc* 220(1):49–52, 2002.
143. Tefft KM: Lily nephrotoxicity in cats, *Compend Contin Educ Pract Vet* 26(2):149–156, 2004.
144. Hovda L: Common plant toxicities. In Ettinger SJ, Feldman EC, editors: *Textbook of veterinary internal medicine*, ed 5, Philadelphia, 2000, WB Saunders.
145. Gwaltney-Brant S, Holding JK, Donaldson CW, et al: Renal failure associated with ingestion of grapes or raisins in dogs, *J Am Vet Med Assoc* 218(10):1555–1556, 2001.
146. Singleton VL: More information on grape or raisin toxicosis, *J Am Vet Med Assoc* 219(4):434–436, 2001.
147. Peterson EN, Kirby R, Sommer M, et al: Cholecalciferol rodenticide intoxication in a cat, *J Am Vet Med Assoc* 199(7):904–906, 1991.
148. Gunther R, Felice LJ, Nelson RK, et al: Toxicity of a vitamin D_3 rodenticide to dogs, *J Am Vet Med Assoc* 193(2):211–214, 1988.
149. Fooshee SK, Forrester SD: Hypercalcemia secondary to cholecalciferol rodenticide toxicosis in two dogs, *J Am Vet Med Assoc* 196(8):1265–1268, 1990.
150. Rumbeiha WK, Braselton WE, Nachreiner RF, et al: The postmortem diagnosis of cholecalciferol toxicosis: a novel approach and differentiation from ethylene glycol toxicosis, *J Vet Diagn Invest* 12(5):426–432, 2000.
151. Vaden SL, Gookin J, Trogdon M, et al: Use of carbamylated hemoglobin concentration to differentiate acute from chronic renal failure in dogs, *Am J Vet Res* 58(11):1193–1196, 1997.
152. Heiene R, Vulliet PR, Williams RL, et al: Use of capillary electrophoresis to quantitate carbamylated hemoglobin concentrations in dogs with renal failure, *J Am Vet Res* 62(8):1302–1306, 2001.
153. Shoemaker JD, Lynch RE, Hoffman JW, et al: Misidentification of propionic acid as ethylene glycol in a patient with methylmalonic academia, *J Pediatrics* 120(3):417–421, 1992.
154. Woolf AD, Wynshaw-Boris A, Rinaldo P, et al: Intentional infantile ethylene glycol poisoning presenting as an inherited metabolic disorder, *J Pediatrics* 120(3):421–424, 1992.
155. Vaden SL, Wood PA, Ledley FD, et al: Cobalamin deficiency associated with methylmalonic academia in a cat, *J Am Vet Med Assoc* 200(8):1101–1103, 1992.
156. Doty RL, Dziewit JA, Marshall DA: Antifreeze ingestion by dogs and rats: influence of stimulus concentration, *Can Vet J* 47(4):363–365, 2006.

Grapes and Raisins

Michelle S. Mostrom, DVM, MS, PhD, DABVT, DABT

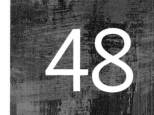

- Raisins, grapes, sultanas, and currants may be toxic to some dogs—no apparent dose response exists between the exposure dose and development of renal disease.
- Clinical signs of toxicosis include vomiting, anorexia, diarrhea, lethargy, abdominal pain, oliguria, and subsequent anuria.
- Clinical pathologic changes are of acute renal failure and include elevated blood urea nitrogen and creatinine concentrations, along with hypercalcemia and hyperphosphatemia.
- Treatment includes early implementation of gastrointestinal decontamination and aggressive fluid therapy for up to 72 hours postingestion to support renal function. Prognosis for animals with clinical oliguria or anuria is poor and requires prolonged aggressive supportive care (e.g., hemodialysis, peritoneal dialysis).
- Histopathologic changes observed in the kidney include proximal renal tubule degeneration or necrosis (with intact basement membranes) and tubular debris or proteinaceous casts in the tubules and collecting ducts. Intracellular and intraluminal pigment has been observed in some cases.

Sources

A grape is the fruit of a vine of the genus *Vitis*. Raisins are dried grapes, and grapes do not become raisins until their moisture content is reduced to approximately 15%. Raisin colors can vary as a result of the different drying processes; a dark purple or black raisin is sun-dried, a light brown raisin is mechanically dehydrated, and yellow raisins are mechanically dried and treated with sulfur dioxide. Grapes and raisins have been reported to cause poisoning in dogs since the mid- to late 1990s. No confirmed cases of raisin and grape toxicosis have been described in cats, although there have been anecdotal reports suggesting cats and ferrets may be susceptible as well.[1] The toxic syndrome is observed with consumption of varying amounts of fresh grapes (all types and colors) from stores or private yards, grape crushings, fermented grapes from wineries, and commercially available raisins.[2] A sultana is a white to pale green, oval, seedless grape variety. The term currant can also refer to a grape or raisin.

Toxic Dose

There appears to be large variability in dogs' tolerance for the *Vitis* fruits; dried fruit seems to be more likely to cause adverse effects as compared with grapes.[1] The estimated quantity of raisins causing toxicity ranges between 0.1 to 1.3 oz/kg (2.8 to 36.4 g/kg) and the estimated quantity of grapes causing toxicity ranges between 0.7 to 5.3 oz/kg (19.6 to 148 0.4 g/kg).[3] Other reports have calculated toxic, and potentially fatal, doses as ranging from 0.16 to 0.7 oz raisins, as is, per kg of body weight; and four to five grapes, as is, was toxic to an 8.2-kg dog.[4] In a review of more than 150 dogs following acute ingestion of *Vitis* fruits, data indicate that toxicity increases with increasing amounts ingested; however, some animals were asymptomatic after ingesting 1 kg of raisins.[1]

Toxicokinetics

The toxic principle have not been identified. Ochratoxin, flavonoids, tannins, polyphenolics, and monosaccharides have all been hypothesized as potential toxic principles; to date, none has been proven. Toxicities generally have a fairly rapid onset of clinical signs (generally within 24 hours following ingestion) and probable excretion of a toxin through the kidneys. There does not appear to be a dose-response relationship between the amounts of grapes and raisins ingested and the resultant renal lesions, implying some variation in the number of toxic principles or varying sensitivities in individual dogs.[5]

Mechanism of Toxicity

The mechanism of toxicity is not known at this time. It appears to involve a nephrotoxic agent or idiosyncratic reaction leading to hypovolemic shock and renal ischemia.[4]

Clinical Signs

Typical clinical signs include vomiting within 24 hours of ingestion; vomiting may begin within a few hours of ingestion in some dogs. It is not clear whether the vomiting is due to some direct effect of the grapes, raisins, or the toxin on the gastrointestinal tract or whether it is the result of the uremia secondary to renal failure. Partially digested raisins or grapes have been reported in the vomit, fecal material, or both.[1-3] Subsequently, clinical signs of diarrhea, anorexia, lethargy, and abdominal pain have been reported. Some of the initial diarrhea observed can be directly due to the high sugar content. These clinical signs may have a duration of days to weeks after ingestion. Within 24 hours to several days postingestion, dogs may appear dull and dehydrated with oliguria or anuria, with or without isosthenuria.[1-3] The onset of azotemia is not known in many cases because of a lack of recognition of the problem by the owners and subsequent delayed referral to a veterinary facility. The acute renal failure may progress to severe metabolic abnormalities and anuria, resulting in death or euthanasia as a result of poor treatment response.

Minimum Database

Clinical pathologic findings reflect renal failure—hypercalcemia, hyperphosphatemia, hyperkalemia, an elevated Ca × P product, and high concentrations of blood urea nitrogen and creatinine may develop within 24 hours to days after ingestion.[1,2] Mild elevations in alanine aminotransferase, and hyperamylasemia have also been reported.[4]

Confirmatory Tests

Because the toxic principles are unknown, an analytic diagnosis cannot be used for raisin and grape poisoning. The diagnosis is based on history of exposure, clinical signs, and histopathologic findings. Mineral analysis of two kidneys collected from a poisoned dog indicated a slightly elevated calcium to phosphorus ratio of 0.12 and 0.29 (normal: <0.1).[6]

Treatment

The ingestion of raisins and grapes in dogs (and perhaps other species due to anecdotal reports of poisoning in cats and ferrets) should be handled aggressively. Following recent ingestion, prompt decontamination of the gastrointestinal tract through emesis, lavage, and activated charcoal is highly recommended. Induction of emesis more than 2 hours following ingestion may be warranted because *Vitis* fruits remain in the gut for some time. Fluid therapy should be administered for a minimum of 48 to 72 hours and serum chemistry values monitored for at least 72 hours for indications of acute renal failure.[1-3] Careful monitoring of central venous pressure and urine output is imperative to prevent possible fluid overload.[4] Other treatments to combat potential renal failure may include furosemide, dopamine, mannitol, furosemide, H_2-antagonists, and hemodialysis or peritoneal dialysis.[1,4]

Prognosis

Clinical signs of ataxia, weakness, and oliguric or anuric renal failure in dogs indicate a poor prognosis. Aggressive fluid therapy or hemodialysis and peritoneal dialysis may be inadequate to overcome the anuria at this stage. Disseminated intravascular coagulation has occurred in some dogs during the treatment phase.

Gross and Histologic Lesions

Proximal renal tubule degeneration or necrosis associated with an intact basement membrane, along with less severe degeneration of the distal convoluted tubules are described in dogs following raisin and grape ingestion.[4-6] Proximal and distal tubule regeneration has been observed in several cases, along with tubular debris or granular to proteinaceous casts in the tubules and collecting ducts. Some minimal mineralization within the renal tubules has also been reported. Intracellular and intraluminal pigment, irregular in shape and golden-brown in color, was observed in several poisoning cases. This pigment did not stain with Von Kossa (calcium stain) or bile stains, but reacted variably with Prussian blue (iron stain).[6] Several cases of poisoned dogs had vascular lesions involving arteritis in the colonic lamina propria, myocardium, and aortic adventitia.[6]

Differential Diagnoses

Differential diagnoses associated with acute renal failure and tubular necrosis may include ethylene glycol, heavy metals (e.g., lead, cadmium, arsenic, mercury), antibiotics (e.g., aminoglycosides, β-lactams, sulfonamides, tetracycline), hemoglobinuria, myoglobinuria, nonsteroidal antiinflammatories, leptospirosis, mushrooms, and cholemic nephrosis. Ethylene glycol–poisoned dogs may display vomiting, anorexia, depression, dehydration, and oliguria. Typically, ethylene glycol poisoned dogs have elevated serum anion gaps, blood pH values less than 7.3, and calcium oxalate monohydrate crystals in the urine and convoluted tubules. Lead-poisoned dogs show clinical signs associated with the gastrointestinal tract, such as vomiting, and the central nervous system, such as tremors, seizures, or depression, in association with an elevated blood lead level. Cadmium poisoning in dogs is uncommon and usually is a result of chronic exposure. Clinical signs can be associated with the development of anemia and kidney and hepatic failure; affected patients often have high urinary cadmium levels. Arsenic poisoning is uncommon as well, and potentially can be ruled out by assessing blood or urine (liver and kidney postmortem) arsenic concentrations. An evaluation of the clinical history could indicate a possible aminoglycoside- or antibiotic-related renal failure. Hemoglobinuria, myoglobinuria, and cholemic nephrosis could be distinguished by pigmented casts in renal tubules and the presence of hepatic lesions to explain the cholemia or bile pigments in the blood. Further examination for changes in hemoglobin, creatine phosphokinase, and liver enzymes could differentiate among these latter causes of acute renal failure. Most mushroom poisonings are ruled out based on history of exposure, and finding mushroom fragments in the vomit or feces.

References

1. Sutton NM, Bates N, Campbell A: Factors influencing outcome of *Vitis vinifera* (grapes, raisins, currants and sultanas) intoxication in dogs, *Vet Record* 164:430–431, 2009.
2. Gwaltney-Brant S, Holding JK, Donaldson CW, et al: Renal failure associated with ingestion of grapes or raisins in dogs, *J Am Vet Med Assoc* 218:1555, 2001.
3. Eubig PA, Brady MS, Gwaltney-Brant SM, et al: Acute renal failure in dogs after the ingestion of grapes or raisins: a retrospective evaluation of 43 dogs (1992-2002), *J Vet Intern Med* 19:663–674, 2005.
4. Mazzaferro EM, Eubig PA, Hackett TB, et al: Acute renal failure associated with raisin or grape ingestion in 4 dogs, *J Vet Emerg Crit Care* 14(3):203–212, 2004.
5. Morrow CK, Valli VE, Volmer PA: Renal pathology associated with grape or raisin ingestion in canines: 10 cases, *American Association of Veterinary Laboratory Diagnosticians 46th Annual Proceedings*. San Diego, 2003.
6. Morrow CMK, Valli VE, Volmer PA, Eubig PA: Canine renal pathology associated with grape or raisin ingestion: 10 cases, *J Vet Diagn Invest* 17(3):223–231, 2005.

Insects—Hymenoptera

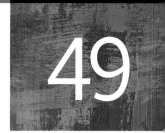

Kevin T. Fitzgerald, PhD, DVM, DABVP

- The medically important groups of Hymenoptera are the Apoidea (bees), Vespoidea (wasps, hornets, and yellow jackets), and Formicidae (ants).
- These insects deliver their venom by stinging their victims.
- Bees lose their barbed stinger after stinging and die. Wasps, hornets, and yellow jackets can sting multiple times.
- Most deaths related to Hymenoptera stings are the result of immediate hypersensitivity reactions, causing anaphylaxis.
- Massive envenomations can cause death in nonallergic individuals. The estimated lethal dose is approximately 20 stings/kg in most mammals.
- Anaphylactic reactions to Hymenoptera stings are not dose dependent or related to the number of stings.
- Bee and wasp venoms are made up primarily of protein. Conversely, fire ant venoms are 95% alkaloids.
- Four possible reactions are seen following insect stings: local reactions, regional reactions, systemic anaphylactic responses, and less commonly a delayed-type hypersensitivity.
- Clinical signs of bee and wasp stings include erythema, edema, and pain at the sting site. Occasionally, animals develop regional reactions.
- Onset of life-threatening anaphylactic signs typically occur within 10 minutes of the sting.
- Diagnosis of bee and wasp stings stems from a history of potential contact matched with onset of appropriate clinical signs.
- The composition and lethality of venom is similar between European and Africanized bees. The main reason for the seriousness of African bee attacks is high number of stings rather than difference in potency or amount of venom per bee.
- Treatment of uncomplicated envenomations (stings) consists of conservative therapy (antihistamines, ice or cool compresses, topical lidocaine or corticosteroid lotions).
- Prompt recognition and initiation of treatment is critical in successful management of anaphylactic reactions to Hymenoptera stings.
- Imported fire ants both bite and sting, and envenomation only occurs through the sting. Anaphylaxis following imported fire ant stings is treated similarly to anaphylactic reactions following honeybee and vespid stings.
- The majority of Hymenopteran stings are self-limiting events, which resolve in a few hours without treatment. Because life-threatening anaphylactic reactions can progress rapidly, all animals stung should be closely monitored and observed.

Bees, Wasps, Hornets, Yellow Jackets

Sources

The stinging insects are members of the order Hymenoptera of the class Insecta. These venomous insects possess the capability to sting using a modified ovipositor found on the terminal end of their abdomen. The three medically important groups are the Apoidea (bees, with 20,000 species), Vespoidea (wasps, hornets, and yellow jackets, with 15,000 species) and Formicidae (ants, with 15,000 species). The fire ants are considered separately in this discussion.

The family Apoidae includes the social honeybees, the solitary bees, and bumblebees. Honeybees are herbivorous and live on nectar and pollen. Wasps, hornets, and yellow jackets (Vespoidae) are predaceous carnivores and live on other insects and sweet substances, such as sap and nectar. Feeding cues for bees emanate from flowers among which they forage. The feeding cue for the vespids comes from flesh and the smell of sugars. There is often a great deal of misidentification between bees and their vespid cousins. However, the two groups differ tremendously in their behavior and body type and can be readily identified. Honeybees are social insects and build their nests (hives) in hollow trees or other cavities. Yellow jackets are usually ground dwellers, whereas the hornets and wasps live in shrubs and trees, and are not ground nesting. Unlike bees, vespids can be frequently found near open cans of soft drinks and sweet food and garbage.

The stinger of these insects is another method of identification.[1,2] Honeybees can only sting once; they possess a barbed stinger that stays behind in the victim's skin after they sting. The stinger and the venom sac are pulled out of the bee's abdomen and soon after the insect dies. Wasp, hornet, and yellow jacket stingers are not barbed and each insect is capable of delivering multiple venom-injecting stings without dying.[3] Vespids are much more aggressive, whereas bees are generally more docile. However, honeybees vigorously defend their hives against intruders. Worker honeybees use their venom only in defense of the colony against invaders, even large mammalian and other vertebrate predators. Queen honeybees do not sting in defense; they only sting and use venom in the killing of rival queens. Typically, people and animals are stung accidentally when they step on bees or otherwise disturb the insects. An exception to this is the aggressive behavior of the more recently introduced Africanized honeybee. These bees attack more readily than their European and North American counterparts, potentially inflicting hundreds of stings.[4,5] If the offending specimen causing the sting is not available, learning the circumstances of the stinging incident, looking for the presence of a stinger in a victim, knowing the differences in body types, and understanding the behavioral differences between bees and wasps can be instrumental in correctly identifying the stinging insect.[6] The taxonomy and relationship of hymenopterans is illustrated in Figure 49-1.

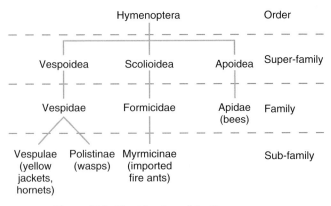

Figure 49-1 Classification of the Hymenoptera.

Toxic Dose

Most deaths related to Hymenoptera stings are the result of immediate hypersensitivity reactions causing anaphylaxis. However, death may also occur from severe local reactions, particularly if involving the airways with subsequent respiratory obstruction. Massive envenomation, as seen in swarm attacks, can likewise cause death in nonallergic individuals. In humans, the estimated lethal dose is approximately 500 stings for adults.[7,8] The estimated lethal dose is approximately 20 stings/kg in most mammals.[9,10]

It has been estimated that the European honeybee injects 147 mcg of venom per sting, the Africanized honeybee injects an average of 94 mcg of venom per sting, and most wasps approximately 17 mcg of venom each sting.[11-13] It does not appear that stinging insects can meter their venom like some venomous snakes and spiders; each Hymenoptera sting delivers a relatively standard venom volume. Anaphylactic reactions are not dose-related and death can occur following a single sting. Death from anaphylactic reactions results from acute bronchoconstriction airway collapse and respiratory arrest. Death as a result of massive envenomations is a consequence of hepatic necrosis, renal degeneration, and cardiac arrest.[14]

Toxicokinetics and Mechanism of Toxicity

Hymenoptera venoms are composed of complex mixtures of allergic proteins, active antigens, and peptides.[15] Both bee and wasp venoms are made up primarily of protein. Bee venom is a complex mixture of biologically active components, primarily consisting of proteins, enzymes, and amines.

Bee Venom

The major component of honeybee venom is mellitin, which acts as a detergent to disrupt cell membranes and liberate biogenic amines and potassium.[15,16] Mellitin is a protein that hydrolyzes cell membranes, alters cellular permeability, and causes histamine release. Mellitin is considered the agent most responsible for local pain. In addition, it induces catecholamine release, which acts with phospholipase A_2 to cause intravascular hemolysis. Large doses of mellitin cause irreversible contraction of the heart and rapid death.

Peptide 401 (or mast cell degranulating peptide) causes mast cells to degranulate, releasing histamine and vasoactive amines. Histamine release by bee venom is mainly mediated by mast cell degranulation peptide.

Phospholipase A_2 is the major allergenic component of bee venom and acts in concert with mellitin to cause intravascular hemolysis. Phospholipase A_2 appears to represent the major antigen or allergen in bee venom. Phospholipase readily forms antibodies, is the main allergen in bee venom, and is probably responsible for many anaphylactic deaths.

Hyaluronidase causes changes in cell permeability by altering cell membranes and disrupts collagen, allowing other venom components to penetrate into the victim's tissues; it is called the "spreading factor." Hyaluronidase is allergenic. The chief enzymes found in bee venom are hyaluronidase and phospholipase A.

The venom also contains vasoactive amines, such as histamine, dopamine, and norepinephrine, and other unidentified proteins.[7,17]

Apamin in bee venom is a neurotoxin that acts on the spinal cord. Adolapin inhibits prostaglandin synthetase and has antiinflammatory actions, and it has been postulated that it may be useful in the treatment of arthritis. The two most lethal factors in honeybee venom are phospholipase A_2 and mellitin. These two peptides account for 70% of the venom. Mellitin has been shown to produce cardiotoxicity and result in cardiac failure and toxic death in massive honeybee envenomations. The allergen phospholipase is probably the factor most responsible for anaphylactic deaths. The effects of the two venom components have not been shown to be synergistic. Furthermore, unlike phospholipase, mellitin is a poor antigen and antimellitin antibodies are not readily produced. As a result, antivenom produced by injection of a whole honeybee venom is not likely to be of much effect in saving lives of victims massively envenomated by honeybees. The most beneficial research efforts for saving the lives of massively envenomated victims focus on neutralizing or blocking the cardiotoxic effects of mellitin.[13]

Wasp and Hornet Venom

The venom of the vespids contains three major proteins that act as allergens and also a wide variety of vasoactive amines and peptides.[18] Mellitin is not found in vespid venom. The intense pain of vespid stings is due to serotonin, wasp kinins, and acetylcholine. The major allergen in vespid venom is called antigen 5. Its biologic activity has not been fully determined. The mastoparans are similar to the mast cell degranulation peptide in bee venom, but its action is weaker. Phospholipase A may account for some of the coagulation abnormalities caused by wasp venom. A comparison of Hymenoptera venoms is included in Box 49-1.

Response to Envenomation

Four primary reactions may be seen following a Hymenoptera envenomation. First and most commonly seen is local pain and swelling. This reaction occurs in all envenomated (stung) individuals to some degree and is caused by vasoactive components of bee venom rather than by an allergic mechanism. Second is a larger, regional reaction, mediated by allergic mechanisms, involving parts of the body in continuity with the sting site. The third and more severe type of reaction is a systemic, anaphylactic response characterized by varying degrees of urticaria, angioedema, nausea and vomiting, hypotension, and dyspnea, caused by an immediate hypersensitivity reaction. This type of reaction occurs in individuals who have specific immunoglobulin (Ig) E antibodies to allergenic components of bee venom and occurs within a few minutes of the sting. The fourth possible reaction is uncommon and consists of skin rashes and serum sickness–like symptoms occurring within 3 days to 2 weeks after envenomation. This type of response is thought to be mediated by circulating immune complexes or a delayed hypersensitivity reaction.

The exact incidence of anaphylactic reactions to bee or vespid stings is unknown in companion animals. In humans the incidence is somewhere between 1% and 3%. Anaphylactic signs usually are apparent within 15 minutes of the sting. For dogs, if a severe systemic allergic reaction has not occurred within 30 minutes, it is unlikely to begin.

Anaphylaxis is IgE mediated.[17] In individuals who have previously been sensitized to bee venom, IgE antibodies attach to tissue mast cells and basophils. Once these cells are activated, the progression of the cascade reaction increases vasoactive substances, which stimulate release of leukotrienes, histamine, and eosinophil chemotactic factor-A. Anaphylactic reactions do not depend on the number of stings. Animals allergic to bee and vespid venom develop a wheal and flare reaction at the site of the inoculum. The shorter the interval between the sting and the onset of signs, the more severe the anaphylactic reaction will be. A fulminant cascade of reactions can quickly follow initial mild clinical signs. Death can occur within several minutes.

The accidental introduction of the native African bee *Apis mellifera scutellata* into Brazil in 1957 and its subsequent displacement and hybridization with the long-established European bee *Apis mellifera mellifera* has resulted in the highly aggressive Africanized honeybee.[19] The Africanized

---

Box 49-1   Comparison of Hymenoptera Venom

Apids (Bees)
Phospholipase A
Hyaluronidase
Mellitin
Apamin
Biogenic amines
Acid phosphatase
Mast cell degranulating peptide
Minimine

Vespids (Wasps, Yellow Jackets, Hornets)
Phospholipase A
Hyaluronidase
Biogenic amines
Kinins
Acid phosphatase
Antigen 5
Mast cell degranulating peptide

Formicides (Fire Ants)
Phospholipase
Hyaluronidase
Biogenic amines
Piperidines

bees attack in larger numbers, are ready to sting much faster and with much less provocation, and are more persistent in their attacks than their European counterparts. The Africanized hybrids are better adapted to warmer climates than European bees and as a result have been very successful and have spread rapidly throughout Latin America. By 1992 the African hybrid bees crossed the border into the United States and are now found in Texas, Arizona, New Mexico, and southern California. Based on weather and seasonal temperatures, they are predicted to eventually be distributed as far east as North Carolina. Despite the Africanized bees' tendency to attack and sting more quickly and in much greater numbers (victims may be stung by dozens if not hundreds of these bees), the venom of the African hybrids is no more toxic than the venom of European varieties. In view of the almost identical nature of their venom, the greater toxic reaction seen in animals stung by Africanized hybrids is a direct result of the higher venom dose to the victim because of the greater number of stings inflicted. Investigations have shown the lethalities of the two venoms to be indistinguishable, and in fact the venoms of the different species of honeybees are remarkably similar in their lethal activity to mice[20-23] or in cases in which venoms vary in activity in regard to body size. The giant honeybee releases more venom per sting compared with the Asian and dwarf honeybees.

Clinical Signs

Typically, honeybee stings are manifested as localized edema without a systemic reaction. Unlike venomous spider bites, venom of all Hymenoptera causes some degree of local swelling and pain, and victims know that they have been stung. Generally the small local reaction of erythema, edema, and pain at the site of the sting is a self-limiting, non–IgE-mediated condition, which spontaneously resolves within 24 hours. Occasionally, animals develop more extensive regional reactions. These more severe regional responses involve erythema and local edema and may involve an entire extremity. The regional reaction is thought to occur from local mast cell degranulation and may not develop until up to 24 hours after the envenomation. This reaction is often termed *cellulitis*; however, infection rarely follows insect stings. A less common reaction to envenomating stings is edema of the oropharynx, which can result in compromise of the airways. Fatalities can result from airway occlusion from stings inside the oral cavity.

Systemic anaphylactic signs caused by insect stings are no different from other anaphylactic reactions. Onset of life-threatening signs occurs rapidly (often within 10 minutes of the sting). Although it is not understood, signs of anaphylactic reaction may vary in severity.[24] Mild anaphylactic signs include urticaria, pruritus, and angioedema.[25] Other non–life-threatening signs include vomiting and diarrhea. More serious signs of anaphylactic reaction include the respiratory and cardiovascular systems.[26] Wheezing, dyspnea, cough, and bronchoconstriction[23] may occur and lead to hypoxia and respiratory arrest. Local upper airway edema can cause congestion of the larynx, epiglottis, and surrounding tissue. The majority of insect sting fatalities are the result of severe respiratory compromise.

The unusual delayed reactions reported include serum sickness, vasculitis, glomerulonephritis, neuropathy, disseminated intravascular coagulation, and arthritis.[24] Direct toxic effects of Hymenoptera venom independent of immune mechanisms are venom volume–dependent reactions. Animal victims of such multiple stings may demonstrate rhabdomyolysis, hemolysis, and acute renal failure from direct tubular toxicity.[25-29] Myocardial infarction has been documented in victims of insect stings.

Bee and wasp stings typically cause only local redness, erythema, and transient pain in dogs. Urticaria may or may not accompany the swelling. Dogs may cry out when stung, and they may rub their mouth and eyes on the ground. These cutaneous reactions appear quickly and will spontaneously regress.

Potential allergen mediators of anaphylaxis include phospholipase A, hyaluronidase, acid phosphatase, and mellitin.[1] Vespid venoms share much more similarity in allergens with other vespids than with bee venoms. This may explain the cross-sensitivity in allergic reactions seen in people stung by various vespids. Furthermore, cross-sensitivity to both bee and wasp venom has been documented in humans.

The signs of anaphylaxis in dogs include urination, vomiting, defecation, muscular weakness, depressed respiration, and finally seizures.[25-29] Signs typically are seen within 15 minutes of the sting and if a systemic reaction has not started within the first 30 minutes, it is unlikely to occur. Fatalities typically occur within 60 minutes of the initial sting. Anaphylaxis in cats is manifested by pruritus, salivation, incoordination, and collapse.[22-27] The signs of anaphylaxis are attributable to antigen-induced IgE release and formation of chemical mediators that target smooth muscle and blood vessels.

Animals receiving massive envenomations (many stings) are usually febrile and visibly depressed. Facial paralysis, ataxia, seizures, and neurologic signs may be observed. Dark brown or red urine, bloody feces, and bloody or dark brown vomitus may also be seen.[14,25] A complete blood count may reveal a leukocytosis. Animals may be thrombocytopenic, particularly if disseminated intravascular coagulation is imminent. Granular casts may be detected on urinalysis reflecting renal tubular damage as a result of the nephrotoxic nature of Hymenoptera venom. Acute renal failure can be caused by acute tubular necrosis (the result of hemolysis) or direct renal toxic effects of the venom.[25-29] Dogs suffering multiple stings may develop a secondary immune-mediated hemolytic anemia.[18] Animals suffering massive envenomations should be hospitalized and monitored closely. Clinical signs of insect stings are listed in Box 49-2.

Minimum Database and Confirmatory Tests

Accurate diagnosis of Hymenoptera stings stems from a history of potential contact with stinging insects and the clinical signs displayed by the victim. It has been reported that certain dog breeds (bull terriers, Staffordshire terriers, and boxers) have a higher incidence of severe reactions to insect stings.[25]

The circumstances surrounding the sting episode may reveal clues as to the offending insect. Yellow jackets are attracted to and are frequently found near open sweet soft drink cans. Bees usually are not. Honeybees are more commonly found foraging among flowers. They are often stepped on as they work through clover. Honeybees can sting only once, leaving their stinger behind in the victim. Wasps and other vespids can sting multiple times and do not lose the stinger. Thus if the attacker is not seen or found, the presence or absence of a stinger, the conditions surrounding the sting incident, and knowing something of the different behavior between bees and wasps can be helpful in narrowing the index of suspicion and identifying the stinging insect.[6]

Other diagnostic aids include skin testing, isolation of specific IgE or IgG antibodies, assay for histamine release, and actual sting challenges. Most insect stings cause small, self-limiting local reactions and victims rarely are taken to veterinary hospitals for treatment. Dense fur may mask local clinical signs of Hymenoptera stings. The true incidence of insect stings in companion animals is unknown as many incidents probably go unrecognized.

Box 49-2	Clinical Signs of Insect Stings

Mild
  Swelling
  Urticaria
  Erythema
  Pruritus
  Pain
Severe (anaphylaxis)
  Vomiting
  Defecation
  Urination
  Swelling
  Muscle weakness
  Respiratory depression
  Seizures
  Death

Treatment

The majority of small local reactions to honeybee and wasp stings resolve completely without treatment within a few hours. On account of their dense coats, time-consuming and meticulous searches for and removal of embedded stingers in animals should not be attempted. Vespids do not leave stingers behind. Honeybee venom sacs continue to contract even after the stinging apparatus is torn from the bee's body and 100% of its contents is delivered within 60 seconds of the sting.[30] Victims should be watched closely because animals with anaphylaxis can deteriorate rapidly, without warning, and catastrophically. Access to cardiac monitoring, supplemental oxygen, crash cart drugs, and airway intubation equipment must be readily available in veterinary hospitals treating Hymenoptera stings.

More severe, regional reactions and those involving multiple stings should be initially treated as the small local reactions. However, the animal should be hospitalized and monitored closely for onset of more devastating progression of the envenomation syndrome. Corticosteroids may benefit these patients (prednisolone sodium succinate 10 mg/kg IV and followed by prednisolone orally at 1 mg/kg twice daily, then tapered over 3 to 5 days). An intravenous bolus of normal saline is indicated if hypotension is present. Continuous intravenous fluid infusion ensuring constant urine output is usually indicated for these animals. For severe reactions of this type, administration of fluids and electrolytes, correction of hypovolemia, and prevention of vascular stasis is a cornerstone of therapy. Toxic reactions to massive envenomations from multiple stings require early aggressive stabilization and therapy with fluids, corticosteroids, and topicals, and may require vigilant monitoring of hematologic, cardiac, respiratory, and renal parameters for several days. Animals suffering this type of insect attack may require hospitalization and supportive therapy until stable. Septicemia is a possible sequela of massive envenomations and administration of broad-spectrum antibiotics may be justified. Most single stings do not become infected.[2,10]

Because most anaphylactic deaths from insect stings occur within 1 hour of the initial sting, early aggressive monitoring, treatment, stabilization, and intervention are mandatory. Death may ensue quickly if the anaphylactic reaction is not managed expeditiously and appropriately. Anaphylaxis following insect stings has been reported in companion animals and when diagnosed, epinephrine 1:1000 (0.1 to 0.5 mL) should be given subcutaneously immediately.[10,25] Administration can be repeated every 10 to 20 minutes. When epinephrine must be given intravenously, it must be diluted to 1:10,000 and 0.5 to 1 mL should be administered. Intravenous epinephrine must be administered cautiously and slowly infused while the patient is carefully scrutinized for signs of improvement or adverse effects (arrhythmia). Vigilant monitoring is required of heart rate, heart rhythm, and blood pressure. Epinephrine stabilizes mast cells and thereby terminates continued propagation of anaphylaxis. Intravenous fluids are crucial to prevent vascular collapse, and shock volumes of crystalloid solutions (90 mL/kg dog and 60 mL/kg cat) should be given rapidly in anaphylactic animals. Antihistamines and corticosteroids may need to be administered. Aggressive airway management may be necessary and intubation equipment and supplemental oxygen should be readily available. Dogs displaying discomfort or pain following a bee sting may be treated with carprofen (2.2 mg/kg every 12 hours PO) or tramadol (2-4 mg/kg every 8 hours PO).

Delayed reactions characterized by rashes, serum sickness, low-grade fever, general malaise, polyarthralgias, and lymphadenopathy can occur within 2 weeks of the sting.[26] Unless the initial sting is witnessed or identified, the actual cause of the reaction may not be recognized, and the diagnosis of a delayed reaction is easily missed.

Because of their potential for anaphylaxis and subsequent rapid deterioration and life-threatening destabilization, all insect stings should be taken seriously. Any animal sustaining multiple stings (massive envenomations) and any animal exhibiting clinical signs of anaphylaxis should be hospitalized, treated aggressively, and kept for 24 hours following cessation of signs.

Certain protocols, products, and principles of immunotherapy for insect stings have been taken from human medicine and applied to dogs who have previously demonstrated severe systemic reactions.[31,32] At present this therapy regimen is not widely available in veterinary medicine.

Prevention and Prognosis

Bees are attracted to dark colors and strong fragrances. Mammalian sweat seems to agitate them, attacks can be triggered by CO_2 from the victim's breath, and they are defensively stimulated by dark colors.[10,17] Avoiding areas with flowering plants where bees are feasting

---

Box 49-3	Prevention of Insect Stings

Avoid scented lotions, soaps, or perfumes.

Avoid large areas of flowering plants.

Do not leave open cat food or dog food dishes outside.

Keep all garbage cans tightly closed.

Do not leave open soft-drink cans outside.

Bees are attracted to dark colors.

Keep picnic foods tightly covered.

Quickly dispose of freshly fallen fruit.

Have only professional exterminators remove hives and insect nests.

---

on nectar and keeping outdoor eating areas and garbage cans clean (because wasps are attracted to food waste) lowers an animal's risk of being stung. Avoid scented shampoos and soaps for your dog. Do not leave canned cat or dog food in dishes outside in warm weather because this may also attract hungry wasps. Antihistamines should be part of any animal first aid kit. Animals that have demonstrated severe or anaphylactic reactions following insect stings should be identified with bee anaphylaxis identification collar tags. A number of ways to decrease insect stings is included in Box 49-3.

Stinging bees deposit an alarm pheromone that triggers other bees to sting at the same site. The pheromone has an odor that smells like ripe bananas. The odor stems from isopentyl acetate found both in bananas and the bee pheromone secretion. This alarm pheromone, when released, signals other bees where to sting. As a result, bananas must be kept away from bee hives and picnic outings so as not to attract and upset the bees.[10]

The prognosis for most victims of insect stings is excellent. Most of these episodes are self-limiting and will resolve within a few hours without treatment. The majority of deaths occur within the first hour, primarily from anaphylaxis. If anaphylactic signs are not apparent within 30 minutes of the sting they are unlikely to occur. Animals suffering from anaphylaxis or from severe reactions as a result of multiple stings may be successfully stabilized if aggressive therapy is instituted early and appropriately applied. These therapies would involve intravenous volume support, drugs, and intubation with supplemental oxygen. Many dogs do not seem to learn about insect stings and are repeatedly stung over multiple summers.

Gross and Histologic Lesions

Histopathologic lesions following simple, single, nonreactive local stings are either absent, undetectable, extremely mild, or nonspecific. Even following fatal anaphylaxis, there are no pathognomonic findings on necropsy and pathologic changes are very general.[1,7] In necropsy after suspected fatal anaphylactic reactions, particular attention must be paid to the larynx for the presence of hyperemia, edema, and hemorrhage.[17] Histologic examination of the larynx can be helpful in confirming a diagnosis of anaphylaxis. In cases of mass envenomation, evidence of acute renal tubular necrosis; fatty degeneration of the kidneys, liver, and myocardium; presence of hyaline membrane disease; and splenic hemorrhage and infarction may be documented.[15]

Tryptase is a mast cell–specific enzyme that is released from mast cells on degranulation; in human victims it is almost 100% specific for anaphylaxis.[17] The peak of tryptase activity occurs 1 to 2 hours following anaphylaxis, and then declines fairly rapidly with a half-life of approximately 2 hours. Studies in postmortem human cases have demonstrated that venom-specific IgE and tryptase were elevated in anaphylactic death but not in other causes of death. Further studies are needed to establish the usefulness of a serum tryptase test in animals.

The majority of deaths related to insect stings are the direct result of the immediate hypersensitivity reaction mediated by IgE and resulting in anaphylaxis. However, death can occur from severe local reactions (regional) involving airways and resultant respiratory obstruction. The primary pathologic finding in wasp and bee sting deaths is found in the respiratory tract, such as massive edema, obstructive secretions, and total collapse or severe reduction in functional airway diameter. Massive envenomation from swarm stings can

Box 49-4	Differential Diagnoses for Insect Stings

Infection
Cat fight abscess
Trauma
Neoplasia
Allergy
Abscessed tooth
Foreign object

also cause death in nonallergic individuals. Deaths from multiple stings result from three major mechanisms: direct venom toxicity, intravascular hemolysis mediated by mellitin, and the profound hypotension resulting from massive histamine release.[17] Together these mechanisms have a cumulative, cascading effect, resulting in multiorgan failure represented by acute tubular necrosis and renal failure, respiratory distress, rhabdomyolysis, myoglobinemia, myocardial cell damage, hepatocellular necrosis, disseminated intravascular coagulation, and hemorrhage. The kidney tubular degeneration and necrosis comes from direct venom activity against the tubules, renal hypotension stemming from venom ischemic-toxic effect, and lesions caused by myoglobin and hemoglobin.[33-36]

In summary, even with catastrophic fatal systemic responses, there may be little or very nonspecific histologic evidence on necropsy. As a result, such causes of death are probably underreported in our companion animals. Insect stings must remain on the list of differentials for a variety of clinical presentations and more specific ways of documenting their actual incidence in companion animals need to be researched.

The incidence of infection following insect stings is extremely low. The abdomen of the honeybee is covered with numerous hairs, most of them branched and plumelike, to which pathogenic bacteria can attach. Vespids lack these hairs. It is known that bees may be attracted to garbage, which may contaminate these hairs. Potentially, the act of stinging could inoculate either bacteria from the bee or bacteria from the victim's skin surface under the epidermis. In addition, scratching because of pruritus commonly associated with insect stings can cause further traumatic epidermal injury and lead to intradermal implantation of pathogenic bacteria. Nevertheless, infection following insect stings is rare.

Differential Diagnoses

Because the initial stinging incident is rarely witnessed, and the clinical signs can be notoriously nonspecific, a diagnosis of insect sting can be easily missed by both owners and clinicians. A correct diagnosis depends on a high index of suspicion for possible insect stings, presenting clinical signs, and attempts to understand the conditions surrounding the episode. A list of differential diagnoses and potential look-alikes for insect stings is included in Box 49-4.

Fire Ants

Sources

Fire ants are members of the order Hymenoptera, family Formicidae, subfamily Myrmicinae, and genus *Solenopsis*. There are native fire ants in the United States, but two imported species, *Solenopsis richteri* (the black imported fire ant) and *Solenopsis invicta* (the red imported fire ant), are of major medical importance.[17] The black imported fire ant (*S. richteri*) is originally from eastern Argentina and Uruguay.[37] The red imported fire ant (*S. invicta*) is a native of the Mato Grosso region of Brazil, where its range extends into northern Argentina. Both species appear to have entered the United States on produce through the port of Mobile, Alabama, the black imported fire ant in about 1918 and the red imported fire ant species around 1939. The black imported species (*S. richteri*) has been contained to a small area of Alabama and Mississippi. However, the red imported fire ant (*S. invicta*) has colonized more than 310 million acres in 12 southern states (Alabama, Arkansas, Florida, Georgia, Louisiana, Mississippi, North Carolina, Oklahoma, South Carolina, Tennessee, Texas, and Virginia).[38] The red imported fire ant is also found in Puerto Rico. Populations have recently been found in California, Arizona, New Mexico, and up the eastern coast to Washington, D.C.[39] Highly adaptive insects, the red imported fire ant has both supplanted and interbred with local native ants. Red imported fire ants and their hybrids now account for more than 90% of ants in some parts of some southern states.

Initially, it was estimated that the spread of the ants would be limited by a minimum climatic temperature of −12.5° C (10° F).[40] However, it appears that the hybrids are more cold tolerant than the original species. Also the hybrids have been seen to use concrete and human habitations as heat sumps and successfully overwinter. It is currently estimated that the ants could expand into areas with a minimum temperature of −17.8° C (0° F). If these predictions are accurate red imported fire ants and their hybrids could ultimately colonize at least 25% of the continental United States. These ants are very mobile and have a capacity to exploit diverse habitats in setting up new colonies, allowing a westward migration rate of approximately 120 miles per year. Because of their ability to interbreed with native species, it may take several years before the presence of the new ants is first detected.

Fire ants are aggressive and venomous. They have definite adverse effects on agriculture as their mounds can damage farming equipment and the ants can attack livestock and food crops. Reports of attacks on livestock and native wildlife (including the decimation of some ground-nesting birds, turtles, frogs, and arthropod species) are not uncommon. Accounts of attacks indoors on both companion animals and debilitated humans (nursing home patients) have become more frequent.

Fire ant workers range in size from 1.8 to 6 mm in length (average 3 to 4 mm).[41] Fire ants are similar in appearance to ordinary, native house and garden ant species. The life span of worker fire ants is 2 to 6 months. Queens are larger than workers and measure approximately 1 centimeter in length. Queens also have wings used during the nuptial flight. Recently, single mounds have been found with 40 to 300 egg-laying queens. Fire ant mounds measure up to 1 meter in diameter and half a meter in height. In heavily infested areas, mound density can range from 40 to 200 mounds per acre. Tunnels between mounds can extend more than 40 meters. A single queen mound may have more than 200,000 worker ants, whereas multiple queen colonies can have more than 500,000 workers. Queens are capable of producing 100 to 200 eggs per hour for up to 6 years.[42] Four castes of fire ants exist: fertile females (queens) with wings before mating, winged males, major workers, and minor (smaller) workers. All fire ants have efficient chemical tracking capabilities, which allow them to quickly locate food sources. It has been reported that fire ants get to injured and dead people at automobile accident scenes faster than rescue squads. In addition to finding food, the major (larger) ants also aggressively swarm and defend their nest and will sting anything unfortunate enough to disturb their mound. Workers have powerful mandibles with four teeth. Fire ants contain magnetite, which functions as a compass and orients them to a north-south axis. The magnetite senses other electric fields and fire ants have been shown to be attracted to underground power lines.

Imported fire ants are omnivorous and sting and kill invertebrates as their primary food source; they also scavenge dead animals and eat plants, ripe fruit, and seeds. Worker ants ingest sugars, fats, and oils, and return solid food to be fed to the immature brood ants. Fire ants are fast and can move 1.6 cm per second. They accumulate on victims in large numbers before detection. They then sting simultaneously using chemical pheromone cues. The majority of sting encounters involve worker ants.

Fire ants are named for the burning pain they inflict. The sting of the fire ant is a two-stage maneuver. Before stinging prey or intruders, the fire ant latches itself on to the victim with its prominent mandibles and thus anchors by biting. It then tucks up its abdomen under its body and stings. The nonbarbed stinger of the imported fire ant is a modified ovipositor, with an associated venom gland at the posterior portion of the abdomen. After the first sting, while still secured to the victim by its mandibles, the imported fire ant withdraws the stinger, rotates one step sideways, and stings again. Typically, they sting six or seven times in a circular pattern pivoting around the attached head. Unlike bees, wasps, and hornets, fire ants inject their venom slowly. Each sting takes 20 to 30 seconds. As a result, the onset of pain is delayed. Humans describe an initial burning sensation, but the majority of those stung by fire ants report it is less painful than a bee sting.

Toxic Dose

Imported fire ants represent a significant health hazard for people and animals living in endemic areas. Sting reactions range from local pustules to anaphylaxis. Anaphylaxis is the main cause of fatal response to fire ant stings. Anaphylactic reactions are not dose dependent and do not correlate with the number of stings.

Systemic toxic reactions to envenomations by fire ants have been reported after 50 to 100 simultaneous stings.[9] Fatal toxic reactions have been reported in dogs and other small animals following massive envenomation (multiple stings).[42] In humans, nonallergic subjects have survived hundreds of stings with only supportive therapy. However, there are reports of death related to direct venom toxicity. In general, death caused by direct venom toxicity following massive envenomations occurs more than 24 hours after the stings, whereas death caused by anaphylaxis typically occurs a short time after the sting.

On stinging, each imported fire ant delivers approximately 0.11 mcL of venom and they can deliver venom in 20 consecutive stings before depleting their venom store.[40,43] A lethal number of fire ant stings has not been reported for mammals. However, most fatalities following fire ant stings are thought to be caused by anaphylaxis and do not depend on the number of stings.

Toxicokinetics and Mechanism of Toxicity

Imported fire ant venom differs from the venoms of bees, wasps, and hornets, which are composed largely of protein-containing aqueous solutions. Fire ant venom is made up of 95% water-insoluble alkaloid.[43,44] The alkaloid portion consists primarily of 2,6 di-substituted piperidines, which have cytotoxic, hemolytic, antibacterial, and insecticidal properties. The alkaloids produce sterile pustules, but do not induce the IgE response that is the hallmark of anaphylaxis. The aqueous phase of fire ant venom contains four major allergenic proteins that are responsible for the specific IgE response of allergic animals. In addition, the small protein fraction contains hyaluronidase and phospholipase, which may explain why fire ant venom antigenetically cross-reacts with vespid venom (especially yellow jackets). Venoms from the two imported fire ant species are highly cross-reactive. The piperidine alkaloids found in fire ant venom have local necrotic and hemolytic effects and are responsible for pain.

The usual response to fire ant stings for most individuals is an immediate development of a 25- to 50-mm dermal flare. A wheal forms within 1 minute and papules within 2 hours. Vesicles develop within 4 hours and are first filled with a clear fluid that is cloudy by 8 hours and then develops into sterile pustules by 24 hours.

The fire ant pustule results from tissue inflammation caused by the venom alkaloids. The presence of this pustule is almost pathognomonic for the sting of the imported fire ant. The superficial pustule is infiltrated with activated neutrophils and platelets, with necrosis at the base in 24 hours.

A small percentage of those bitten (17%) also develop extensive local reactions adjacent to the bite, with induration, erythema, and pruritus that may last up to 7 days.[37] Large, regional reactions to fire ant venom have been shown to be mast-cell dependent, IgE-mediated, late-phase reactions. Systemic reactions and direct toxic effects of massive envenomations have also been documented. It has been reported that systemic nonallergic responses (direct venom effects) often exhibit a large number of pustules, rhabdomyolysis, disseminated intravascular coagulation, and seizures.[40] Anaphylactic reactions to fire ant stings have been observed in both humans and animals. Anaphylactic reactions usually happen shortly after the sting occurs. Anaphylactic reactions may include general urticaria, cutaneous or laryngeal edema, bronchospasm, or cardiovascular collapse. Untreated, these anaphylactic reactions can become life threatening. Secondary infection may follow imported fire ant stings, particularly those involving regional reactions.

Clinical Signs

Reactions to imported fire ant stings range from minor skin lesions to anaphylaxis and death. Typical stings cause an annoying burning sensation. Three types of local reactions may be present: a wheal and flare reaction, a sterile pustule, and a large regional reaction. Local reactions alone occur in nonallergic animals.

The typical local reaction to a sting, the wheal and flare, is followed by immediate pain, inflammation, and intense pruritus. The wheal and flare reaction usually resolves within 30 minutes to 1 hour. A papule forms and evolves into a fully developed sterile pustule at the site of the sting within 24 hours. These sterile pustules may last up to 2 to 3 weeks before spontaneously involuting. The pustules are usually accompanied by significant pruritus. Occasionally, the pustules become secondarily infected (usually from self-trauma by scratching) and can progress from cellulitis to sepsis. By 24 hours, the pustule contains necrotic tissue with cellular infiltration of lymphocytes, eosinophils, and polymorphonuclear cells. Usually after 72 hours, the epidermis covering the pustule sloughs and then healing takes place, leaving a scar or macule.

A smaller number of victims display regional reactions at the site of the sting. These lesions are erythematous, edematous, indurated, and extremely pruritic. Regional reactions to fire ant stings are mast cell–dependent, IgE-mediated, late-phase reactions. Regional reactions may lead to enough tissue edema to compromise blood flow to an extremity.

Systemic or anaphylactic reactions are IgE-mediated reactions that involve clinical signs occurring remote from the initial sting site. The signs include urticaria, cutaneous or laryngeal edema, bronchospasm, and vascular collapse. Most deaths resulting from imported fire ant stings are due to systemic anaphylaxis. However, it is possible that secondary infection of large reaction sites can also lead to death. The direct toxic effect of the venom of multiple fire ant stings can result in the death of the victim. In general, deaths caused by anaphylaxis occur a short time after the sting, whereas deaths caused by venom toxicity occur greater than 24 hours following the sting. The exact incidence of fire ant anaphylaxis is unknown. The mechanism of anaphylaxis following fire ant stings is identical to the pathway of anaphylaxis from other causes. The systemic reaction to fire ant venom is similar to those experienced with other Hymenoptera venoms, except the pathognomonic pustule almost always enables identification of the imported fire ant as the stinging insect. Clinical signs following fire ant stings are listed in Box 49-5.

Box 49-5	Clinical Signs of Fire Ant Stings

Simple, Local Sting
Wheal and flare
Erythema
Warmth
Pain
Intense itching

Large, Regional Reaction
Erythema
Warmth
Pain
Itching

Anaphylactic Reaction
Urticaria
Cutaneous edema
Laryngeal edema
Bronchospasm
Vascular collapse

Minimum Database and Confirmatory Tests

Helpful clinical clues in determining a diagnosis of fire ant stings include development of a classic pustule after 24 hours, actual identification of the stinging insect, and the presence of typical fire ant mounds in the vicinity of the stinging incident. There are no laboratory tests to determine fire ant exposure. Veterinary clinicians should familiarize themselves with stinging insects found in their region.

Treatment

Currently no treatment has been shown to be beneficial in preventing or resolving local reactions, including the characteristic pustules. However, various therapies may provide symptomatic relief. Local sting reactions may benefit from antihistamines, topical corticosteroids, application of cool compresses (water or alcohol), ice, and topical treatment with camphor and menthol (Sarna lotion). Topical lidocaine preparations have also been suggested. Some dogs stung by fire ants appear to feel much better after warm baths. Although widely proposed, topical application of aluminum sulfate and meat tenderizer (papain) is ineffective in relieving the pain and itching of imported fire ant stings.[45,46]

Severe, regional reactions are less commonly encountered, but these should be treated supportively and therapy may include antihistamines, corticosteroids, analgesics, and intravenous volume support. Secondary infections to fire ant stings should be treated with broad-spectrum antibiotics.

Anaphylactic reactions to fire ant stings have been documented both in humans and animals. They are typically seen not long after the initial sting incident. Anaphylaxis after a fire ant sting should be treated similarly to anaphylactic reactions seen following honeybee and vespid stings and may require epinephrine, endotracheal intubation, and the administration of oxygen, corticosteroids, antihistamines, and supportive fluid therapy. Prompt recognition and initiation of treatment is crucial in the successful management of anaphylaxis. Companion animals showing severe, regional reactions or anaphylaxis following fire ant stings should be hospitalized until stable enough to be released for treatment and subsequent observation at home. Research is currently being done examining the merits of treating hypersensitivity to fire ant stings with immunotherapy regimens.

Prevention and Prognosis

Reaction to imported fire ant stings is best prevented by avoidance. Yards, exercise areas, and playing fields must be routinely inspected for the presence of ant mounds. Many attempts have been made to eradicate fire ants from an area, but none have been shown to be completely successful. Basic methods currently used are broadcast applications of toxic baits that are carried back to the mound by workers and fed to the queen, and individual mound treatments with chemicals to kill the queen and other ants.[40] The chemicals used are generally insecticides and formulated as drenches, granules, dusts, aerosols, or liquid fumigants. If the queen is not destroyed, she will continue to produce eggs and the treated mound will recover. Baits used usually contain slow-acting toxicants dissolved in an attractive food source like soybean oil. The toxicant-containing oil is then absorbed into corn grits, a carrier that permits easy handling and application. The slow action of the poison allows the workers to carry it back to the mound and feed it to the queen, to immature ants, and to other workers before they die. Toxic bait eliminates the need to locate mounds because it relies on foraging workers who bring the bait back and feed the poison to the rest of the colony.

Baits using insect growth regulators are also marketed.[39] These growth-inhibiting substances are placed in baits to be carried back to the mound to prevent the development of adult worker ants. A major drawback of these growth regulators is that they act slowly over days to months. Additionally, they are not specific for fire ants and can have environmental consequences for other sensitive insects, some of which are beneficial to humans. Other methods under study for more specific and effective control of fire ants include the use of various parasites, including nematodes and microsporidians that directly feed on ants and infect ant blood cells.[39]

The prognosis for animals stung by fire ants depends on the nature of the reaction displayed following the sting. Simple local reactions are painful and itch, but resolve with supportive measures and time. Regional reactions require more aggressive therapy, but typically resolve. Anaphylactic reactions to fire ant stings can be fatal if untreated. Prompt recognition and initiation of treatment is critical in the successful management of anaphylactic reactions.

Finally, in endemic areas, companion animals should not be left outdoors unsupervised for long periods and should be examined often for signs of ant stings. Older, more debilitated animals and very young animals should be even more vigilantly observed. Particular attention should be paid to garbage containers, uncovered food dishes, and outside feeding areas, all of which may attract ants. Methods of prevention of imported fire ant stings are listed in Box 49-6.

Box 49-6	Methods of Prevention for Imported Fire Ant Stings

Companion animals must be closely supervised in endemic areas.

Yards, exercise areas, and playing fields must be routinely inspected for ant mounds.

Old, debilitated, and very young animals deserve particular attention in endemic areas.

Garbage containers, outside feeding areas, and uncovered food dishes may attract ants.

Ant mounds must be vigorously treated (the queen must be killed) for eradication attempts to be successful.

Gross and Histologic Lesions

The intense inflammatory response and pustule that develops at the fire ant sting site has been shown to result from potent cytotoxins and hemolytics found in the alkaloid venom fraction. These toxins cause localized necrosis of the dermis and underlying connective tissue that creates the characteristic sterile pustule that develops within 24 hours of most stings.[44] In the continental United States, the pustule is only caused by imported fire ant stings. An erythematous flare follows the sting followed in minutes by a wheal. The wheal-flare resolves within 2 hours. A central vesicle containing clear fluid begins to form within 4 hours. The fluid becomes cloudy and the pustule appears, generally surrounded by a red halo and an area of edema.

Histologic studies have demonstrated that imported fire ant venom causes histamine release at the sting site.[44] Edema, painful necrosis, and infiltration of histiocytes, plasma cells, and lymphocytes occurs within minutes. By 24 hours, the pustule contains many polymorphonuclear cells, lymphocytes, and neutrophils. At 72 hours, plasma cells and eosinophils can also be found. The pustule's central core becomes obliterated, and the pustular infiltrate extends into surrounding necrotic tissue. At this point the pustule fluid is composed of primarily neutrophils and necrotic debris.

The pustule usually heals and resolves spontaneously; however, the intense pruritus may cause an animal to scratch off the epidermal covering, establishing a microhabitat compatible with secondary bacterial infection, which can potentially become systemic. Undisturbed pustules resolve unremarkably in 3 to 10 days, leaving a small macule with little scarring. Secondarily infected stings may leave a significant scar.

Large regional reactions are not uncommon in many Hymenoptera stings. It has been shown that the size of the wheal-flare response at 20 minutes correlates directly with the size of the regional reaction at 6 hours. Pathologically, the regional reaction resembles late-phase IgE-mediated reactions developing after intradermal injections of ragweed or insulin. These reactions are characterized by development of dense fibrin deposits, with trapping of edema in the reticular dermis around the pustule. Eosinophils are present in the pustular fluid. This is not the same as the systemic allergic (anaphylactic) reaction.

In the United States, fatal anaphylactic reactions to imported fire ant stings are less frequent than other Hymenoptera stings; however, this may change as the range of the ants increases.[44] Like other Hymenopterans, true anaphylactic reactions to imported fire ant envenomations do not depend on the number of stings inflicted. Necropsy findings, although nonspecific, are typical of Hymenoptera-induced pathologic changes. Primary findings include acute pulmonary changes and cerebrovascular congestion.[44] In many cases congestion can also be seen in the kidneys, liver, spleen, and adrenal glands.

Other histologic changes following fire ant stings include serum sickness, nephrotic syndrome, and mononeuritis. Some animals have been reported to have seizures following multiple stings. It should be noted that cross-reactivity and similar sequences of histologic reactions occur between imported fire ant venom and the venom of other Hymenopterans.

Box 49-7	Differential Diagnoses of Fire Ant Stings

Trauma
Infection
Allergy
Neoplasia
Self-trauma
Other causes of anaphylaxis

Differential Diagnosis

Potential differential diagnoses and possible look-alikes to imported fire ant stings are listed in Box 49-7. These include any conditions leading to immediate swelling, pain, and pruritus. Differential diagnoses include trauma, infection, neoplasia, allergy, self-trauma, or other causes of anaphylaxis.

References

1. Tunney FX: Stinging insects. In Haddad LM, Shannon MW, Winchester JF, editors: *Clinical management of poisoning and drug overdose*, ed 3, Philadelphia, 1998, WB Saunders.
2. Reisman RE: Insect stings, *N Engl J Med* 321:523, 1994.
3. Goddard J: *Physician's guide to arthropods of medical importance*, ed 3, Philadelphia, 2000, WB Saunders.
4. Minton SA, Hechtel HB: Arthropod envenomation. In Auerbach PS, editor: *Wilderness medicine: management of wilderness and environmental emergencies*, St Louis, 1995, Mosby.
5. Schmidt JU, Hassen LV: When Africanized bees attack: what you and your clients should know, *Vet Med* 10:923–928, 1996.
6. Degrondi-Hoffman G, Hoffman RF: Bee sting dysphagia, *Ann Intern Med* 130(11):943, 1999.
7. Vetter RS, Visscher PK: Bites and stings of medically important venomous arthropods, *Int J Dermat* 37:481–496, 1998.
8. Vetter RS, Visscher PK, Camazine S: Mass envenomations by honey bees and wasps, *West J Med* 170:2223–2227, 1999.
9. Manoquerra AS: Hymenoptera stings. In Ling LJ, et al: *Toxicology secrets*, 2001, Hanley and Belfus.
10. Fitzgerald KT, Flood AA: Hymenoptera stings, *Clin Tech Small Anim Pract* 21(4):194–204, 2006.
11. Franca FOS, et al: Severe and fatal mass attacks by "killer" bees in Brazil: clinicopathological studies with measurement of serum venom concentrations, *Q J Med* 87:269–282, 1994.
12. Winkler B, et al: Allergen specific immunosuppression by mucosal treatment with recombinant Ves v. 5, a major allergen of Vespula vulgaris venom, in a murine model of wasp venom allergy, *Immunology* 110:376–385, 2003.
13. Schmidt JO: Toxinology of venoms from the honey bee genus, *Apis, Toxicon* 33(7):917–927, 1995.
14. Oliveira EC, Pedroso PM, Meirelles AE, et al: Pathological findings in dogs after multiple Africanized bee stings, *Toxicon* 49:1214–1218, 2007.
15. Banks BEC: the composition of Hymenoptera venoms with particular reference to venom of the honeybee. In Kornalik F, Mebs D, editors: Prague, 1986, Proceedings of the 7th European Symposium on Animal, Plant and Microbial Toxins.
16. Ownby CL, Powell JR, Jiang MS, et al: Melittin and phospholipase A_2 from bee (*Apis mellifera*) venom cause necrosis of murine skeletal muscle in vivo, *Toxicon* 35:67–80, 1997.
17. Hahn I, Lewin NA: Arthropods. In Goldfrank LR, et al: *Goldfrank's toxicologic emergencies*, ed 7, New York, 2002, McGraw-Hill.
18. Lichtenstein LM, Valentine MD, Sobotka AK: Insect allergy: the state of the art, *J Allergy Clin Immunol* 64:5–12, 1979.
19. Jones RGA, et al: A novel fab-based antivenom for treatment of mass bee attacks, *Am J Trop Med Hyg* 61(3):361–366, 1999.
20. Schmidt JO, Yamane S, Matsuura M: Hornet venoms: lethalities and lethal capacities, *Toxicon* 24:950–954, 1986.
21. Schumacher MJ, Schmidt JO, Egen NB: Lethality of "killer" bee stings, *Nature* 337:413, 1989.
22. Schumacher MJ, Schmidt JO, Egen NB, et al: Quantity, analysis, and lethality of European and Africanized honey bee venoms, *Am J Trop Med Hyg* 43:79–86, 1990.
23. Schumacher MJ, Schmidt JO, Egen NB, et al: Biochemical variability of venoms from individual European and Africanized honey bees (*Apis mellifira*), *J Allergy Clin Immunol* 90:59–65, 1992.
24. Ludolph-Hauser D, Rueff F, Fries C, et al: Constitutively raised serum concentrations of mast-cell tryptase and severe anaphylactic reactions to Hymenoptera stings, *Lancet* 357:361–362, 2001.
25. Cowell AK, Cowell RL: Management of bee and other Hymenoptera stings. In Bonagura JD, Kirk RW, editors: *Kirk's veterinary therapy XII: small animal practice*, Philadelphia, 1995, WB Saunders.
26. Kocer U, et al: Skin and soft tissue necrosis following Hymenoptera sting, *J Cutan Med Surg*133–135, 2003.
27. Riches KJ, Gillis D, James RA: An autopsy approach to bee sting related deaths, *Pathology* 34:257–262, 2002.

28. Antin JP: Fatal anaphylactic reaction of a dog to bee sting, *J Am Vet Med Assoc* 142:775, 1963.

29. Cowell AK, Cowell RL, Tyler RD, et al: Severe systemic reactions to Hymenoptera stings in three dogs, *J Am Vet Med Assoc* 198:1014–1016, 1991.

30. Schumacher M, Treten M, Egen R: Rate and quantity of delivery of venom from honeybee stings, *J Allergy Clin Immunol* 93:831, 1994.

31. Baker E: *Small animal allergy: a practical guide*, Philadelphia, 1990, Lea and Febiger.

32. Weiss K: *The little book of bees*, Gottingen, 2002, Copernicus.

33. Hommel D, Bollandard F, Hulin A: Multiple African honey bee stings and acute renal failure, *Nephron* 78:235–236, 1998.

34. Bresolin NL, Carvalho FL, Goes JC, et al: Acute renal failure following massive attack by Africanized bee stings, *Pediatr Nephrol* 17:625–627, 2002.

35. Betten DP, Richardson WH, Jong TC, et al: Massive honey bee envenomation induced rhabdomyolysis in an adolescent, *Pediatrics* 117:231–235, 2006.

36. Shimada A, Nakai T, Morita T, et al: Systemic rhabdomyonecrosis and acute tubular necrosis in a dog associated with wasp stings, *Vet Rec* 156:320–322, 2005.

37. Stafford CT: Hypersensitivity to fire ant venom, *Ann Allergy Asthma Immunol* 77:87–95, 1996.

38. Kemp SF, de Shazo RD, Moffitt JE, et al: Expanding habitat of the imported fire ant (*Solenopsis invicta*): a public health concern, *J Allergy Clin Immunol* 105(4):683–691, 2000.

39. Hoffman DR: Fire ant venom allergy, *Allergy* 50:535–544, 1995.

40. DeShazo RD, Soto-Aguilar M: Reactions to imported fire ant stings, *Allergy Proc* 14(1):13–16, 1993.

41. Stafford CT: Fire ant allergy, *Allergy Proc* 13(1):11–16, 1992.

42. Prahlow JA, Barnard JA: Fatal anaphylaxis due to fire ant stings, *Am J Forensic Med Pathol* 19(2):137–142, 1998.

43. Schmidt JO: Chemistry, pharmacology, and chemical ecology of ant venoms. In Pier T, editor: *Venoms of the Hymenoptera*, London, 1986, Academic Press, pp 425–508.

44. Lockey RF: The imported fire ant: immunopathological significance, *Hosp Pract* 25(3):109–124, 1970.

45. Bruce S, Tschen EH, Smith EB: Topical aluminum sulfate for fire ant stings, *Internat J Derm* 23(3):211, 1984.

46. Ross EV Jr, Badame AJ, Dale SE: Meat tenderizer in the acute treatment of imported fire ant stings, *J Amer Acad Derm* 16(6):1189–1192, 1987.

Ionophores

Jeffery O. Hall, DVM, PhD, DABVT

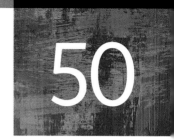

- Ionophores can be present as a contaminant in dog or cat food. Alternatively, companion animals can be exposed by consuming premixes or feed designed for other species.
- Mechanism of toxicity includes disruption of intracellular to extracellular ion gradients and disruption of intramitochondria to extramitochondria ion gradients.
- Clinical signs include a neuromuscular paralytic syndrome that progresses in a caudal to cranial direction.
- Biochemical abnormalities include increases in creatine phosphokinase, lactate dehydrogenase, aspartate transaminase, and urine protein; myoglobinuria may or may not occur.
- Confirmatory tests include detection of the ionophore in the diet or tissue.
- Treatment includes good supportive care, including possible positive pressure ventilation.
- Prognosis is fair to good, depending on the severity of clinical signs.
- Gross and histologic lesions may include gross paling of skeletal and cardiac muscles and necrosis of skeletal and cardiac tissue, as well as potential peripheral neuropathy.
- Differential diagnoses include botulism, tick paralysis, polyradiculoneuritis, myasthenia gravis, organophosphate and carbamate insecticides, macadamia nuts, and amitraz or macrolide parasiticides (e.g., ivermectin) poisoning.

Sources

Several polyether carboxylic antibiotics (ionophores) are extensively used as anticoccidials in several species and as growth promotants in ruminants. The name *ionophore* has been used to denote this group of compounds because of their ability to transport ions across biologic membranes and down concentration gradients. The ion transport capability is the key to their anticoccidial activities and their antibacterial activities. In ruminants, the antibacterial effects result in changed ruminal microflora and growth promotant effects. Although these compounds have proved very effective for therapeutic use as growth promotants in ruminants and as anticoccidial agents, they also have proved to be toxic in a variety of species. Most cases of small-animal poisonings have resulted from inadvertent inclusion of ionophores in dog or cat foods, but pet exposure to feed premixes or bolus products can also occur.

Several ionophores are in common use and more will likely gain market approval in the near future. Generic and trade names of several marketed ionophores are as follows: laidlomycin propionate (Cattlyst), lasalocid (Avotec, Bovatec), maduramicin (Cygro), monensin (Coban, Rumensin), narasin (Maxiban, Monteban), and salinomycin (Coxistat, Biocox, Saccox).[1,2] These ionophorous drugs are marketed in finished feed products, in which their concentrations are generally in the parts per million range or in milligrams per kilogram quantities. However, they also are marketed at much higher concentrations in the form of premixes or concentrates intended for mixing into finished feeds or for use as a top dressing on feeds, as well as in sustained-release bolus products.

Because of the variety of concentrations and preparations of products in which ionophores are marketed, there are numerous potential sources of exposure to small animals. Field cases of ionophore poisoning have been reported in which premixes were inadvertently included in cat,[3] dog,[4,5] and rabbit[6] foods. In another case, dog food was stored in the same bin that had previously been used to store a monensin premix.[7] In Hungary, rabbits were poisoned with high concentrations of narasin in their pellets.[8] A dog was also poisoned by ingestion of a sustained release bolus product.[9] Thus ionophore poisonings in small animals can be caused by food mixing errors or storage contamination, or possibly by ingestion of feeds or premixes intended for other species.

Toxic Dose

Species susceptibility is quite varied to the toxic effects of the ionophores. The toxicity also is affected by the duration of exposure to ionophores, the daily dose that produces toxic effects being lower with subacute or chronic exposures than the toxic dose for a single acute exposure. Table 50-1 summarizes the literature on the toxicity and clinical signs of several ionophores in small animals. Although toxicity information is available for most ionophores with regard to dogs and rabbits, very little information is available for cats. No toxicity studies and only two clinical reports were found for cats.[3,10]

Toxicokinetics

Although little true kinetic data is available, some toxicokinetic information can be gleaned from the field cases and premarket safety studies. The onset of clinical signs can be either acute or somewhat delayed. With acutely toxic concentrations of ionophores, the onset of clinical signs generally occurs within 6 to 24 hours.[4,5,7,16] However, with lower concentrations, clinical signs may not occur for 2 weeks or more.[15,16] Thus the onset of toxic effects is dose dependent.

As with the onset of clinical effects, the duration of effects is quite varied. Once ionophore exposure stops, clinical signs may continue for as little as a few days or as long as 3 months.[4,5,7,15,16] But persistent effects from peripheral neuropathy have also been reported.[10] The duration of clinical signs is thought to correlate with the severity of the clinical signs at the time exposure was terminated. Because ionophores are lipid soluble and clinical severity is dose related, it is likely that there is either a long terminal elimination phase from the tissue compartments or a long period of tissue repair in the more severely affected animals.

Ionophores appear to be extensively metabolized and are primarily eliminated in the feces in dogs.[12] Less than 2% of a dose of laidlomycin propionate was eliminated in the urine as either the parent drug or its metabolites. Dogs metabolize laidlomycin propionate to at least 11 different metabolites.[12] However, it is not known whether the ionophore metabolites retain any of their ionophore transport capability.

Mechanism of Toxicity

Translocation of ions and disruption of ion gradients are responsible for the therapeutic and toxic effects of ionophores.[17,18] Translocation of ions across the mitochondria disrupts

Table 50-1		Toxicity of Various Ionophores and Resultant Clinical Signs	
Ionophore	Species	Toxic Dose	Clinical Signs
Laidlomycin propionate[11,12]	Canine	No observed effect: 2 mg/kg of diet for 91 days	
	Canine	Acute: 60 mg/kg; Chronic: 1.5 mg/kg/day	Labored breathing, salivation, paleness, abnormal gait, loss of peripheral reflexes, and collapse
Lasalocid[4,5,12,29]	Canine	Field cases: 166-210 mg/kg of dog food (ingestion of approximately 10-15 mg/kg/day)	Muscle weakness, depression, paresis, ataxia, dysuria, dyspnea, quadriplegia
	Canine	Chronic: 2-year study No observed effect: 35 ppm (1 mg/kg/day)	
	Rabbit	Acute LD_{50}: 40 mg/kg	
Maduramicin[14]	Canine	No observed effect: 12 mg/kg of diet for 30 days; 6 mg/kg of diet for 1 year	
	Canine	≥24 mg/kg of diet for 28 days	Hindlimb weakness, stiffness, ataxia, hindlimb paralysis
Monensin[7,15]	Canine	Acute oral LD_{50}: >20 mg/kg (males); >10 mg/kg (females)	
	Canine	≥5 mg/kg for 1 year	Anorexia, weakness, hypoactivity, weight loss, labored breathing, ataxia
	Canine	Field case: 165 mg/kg in dog food	Weakness, ataxia, urinary incontinence, paresis
	Rabbit	Acute LD_{50}: 41.7 mg/kg	
Narasin[6,8,16]	Canine	No observed effect: 1.5 mg/kg of diet for 30 days; 1 mg/kg of diet for 6 months	
	Canine	Acute oral LD_{50}: >10 mg/kg Subacutely toxic: ≥2 mg/kg/day Chronically toxic: ≥1 mg/kg/day	Anorexia, leg weakness, diarrhea, ataxia, hypoactivity, depression, salivation, labored breathing, recumbency, weight loss
	Rabbit	Acute oral LD_{50}: 15.5 mg/kg; Subacutely toxic: >1 mg/kg/day	Anorexia, leg weakness, ataxia, incoordination, hypoactivity
	Rabbit	Field cases: 140-150 mg/kg in feed; 30 mg/kg in feed	Anorexia, incoordination, weakness, paralysis, recumbency, diarrhea, opisthotonus, labored breathing
Salinomycin[3]	Feline	Field case: 440 mg/kg in cat food	Dyspnea, weakness, hyporeflexia, paresis, paralysis, recumbency

LD_{50}, Median lethal dose.

mitochondrial energy production and causes mitochondrial swelling and fragmentation.[19-21] This loss of energy production is at least partially responsible for the cell death and tissue necrosis associated with ionophore poisoning.

The translocation of ions across the plasma membrane by ionophores also inhibits the activity of excitable tissues. The disruption of potassium, hydrogen, calcium, and sodium concentrations in excitable cells alters resting potentials, action potentials, and contractility.[22-28] In rat neuronal cell cultures, lasalocid causes neuronal cell damage and death but spares the nonneuronal cells.[29] The alteration in excitable tissues can decrease or halt neurologic, cardiac, and skeletal muscle functions.

Clinical Signs

Presenting clinical signs are suggestive of a neurologic or neuromuscular disorder (see Table 50-1). Feed refusal, a common finding in ionophore-poisoned livestock, has not been consistently reported in companion animal poisonings. In acutely toxic ionophore exposures, there is generally a history of a sudden onset of depression, weakness, and incoordination, with some animals exhibiting hypersalivation.[3-7,10,12,14] The weakness and incoordination begin in the hindlimbs and progress to include the front limbs. With more chronic lower exposure rates there can be a more gradual onset of signs.[10,12-16] Both the acute and chronic syndromes progress to include recumbency, paresis, paralysis, loss of reflexes, dyspnea, and apnea. Even in the presence of quadriplegia, cutaneous sensitivity remains intact.[5] Some quadriplegic dogs retain the ability to wag their tails and follow movement with their eyes. Respiratory paralysis is the life-threatening sequela.

Although myocardial necrosis can be found in ionophore-poisoned animals, electrocardiographic (ECG) abnormalities were absent in salinomycin-poisoned cats[3] and monensin-poisoned dogs.[7] However, one must remember that ECG changes may occur in ionophore-poisoned animals that develop myocardial necrosis. In addition, the extent and type of ECG changes are directly related to the location and severity of the myocardial necrosis.

Minimum Database

Clinicopathologic changes have been found to be inconsistent between animals and across time. Changes associated with ionophore-poisoned dogs include increased creatine phosphokinase, lactate dehydrogenase, and aspartate transaminase levels; proteinuria; and myoglobinuria.[4,5,7,15,16] However, these changes occurred in only some of the animals and only periodically during the evaluations. Although it is inconsistent, increased creatine phosphokinase appears to be the most common alteration identified in dogs. In a field case of salinomycin poisoning in cats, one of the seven affected cats had a slight hypokalemia and leukocytosis,[3] but no clinicopathologic abnormalities were noted in the other cats. Thus clinicopathologic changes are quite inconsistent, and their absence does not rule out ionophore toxicosis.

Confirmatory Tests

Analytic verification of the presence of an ionophore drug is currently the most valid confirmatory test. The most diagnostic analytical test is serum analysis to verify that the drug is in the body, but currently analytic sensitivities and diagnostic laboratory capabilities do not permit this type of testing on a routine basis. Thus analytic verification of the presence of ionophores in the food or stomach contents of live animals and in the food or tissues (e.g., gastrointestinal contents, feces, bile, liver) of dead animals is the next best option.

Treatment

In cases of known recent exposure, general decontamination procedures should be implemented. These procedures include evacuation of the gastric contents by induction of emesis and administration of activated charcoal along with a cathartic. However, this may be contraindicated in animals with severe clinical signs, because emesis or administration of adsorbents could result in aspiration in animals exhibiting the paralytic effects. When implemented early after exposure, decontamination procedures minimize the absorption of the drug and thus the potential for clinical effects. Administration of selenium and vitamin E has been shown to provide some protection against monensin poisoning in swine; this treatment might be of potential benefit in companion animals.

In animals with clinical signs of ionophore poisoning, good general supportive care is the only effective treatment. Nutritional intake must be maintained, and the animal must be kept warm and hydrated. Recovery has even occurred in animals that developed respiratory paralysis by maintaining them on positive-pressure ventilation. In lasalocid-poisoned dogs that developed apnea, spontaneous respiration returned after 6 to 12 hours.[4] Recovery time was reported to be as long as 50 days in severely affected lasalocid-poisoned dogs. In contrast, some salinomycin-poisoned animals exhibited clinical signs as long as 7 weeks after the intoxication or had permanent neurologic effects.[3,10]

Prognosis

Although recovery occurs with good supportive care, in severely affected animals a fair to guarded prognosis is advised. For mildly affected animals, a fair to good prognosis is warranted. However, owners must be advised that the recovery process may be extended, and if severe cardiac or skeletal muscle damage has occurred or there is severe neuromuscular involvement, the animal may experience some permanent deficits.[3,10]

Gross and Histologic Lesions

Gross lesions may or may not be present in animals that die from ionophore poisoning. The gross lesion that is most commonly found is a paling or pale spotting of the heart.[3,6] Similar gross lesions have been observed in the skeletal musculature in several ionophore-poisoned food animal species,[6,30] but this finding has not been reported in dogs or cats.

Ionophore-induced microscopic pathologic lesions generally involve the cardiac musculature, skeletal musculature, and peripheral nerves, but in some animals it may be absent. Although there are limited numbers of reports, dogs tend to have more necrosis of the skeletal muscles than of cardiac muscle.[7,10,14-16] Cats, on the other hand, have more cardiac lesions.[3] In contrast, rabbits more commonly have histologic lesions in both the skeletal and cardiac musculature. In both skeletal and cardiac muscle, lesions comprise fibrillar degeneration and necrosis.[6-8,12,14-16] In animals that live long enough, there may be evidence of cellular repair and fibrosis. In addition to the muscular lesions, vacuolization and degeneration of peripheral sensory and motor nerves have been identified.[3,12,16]

Differential Diagnoses

Most clinical conditions included in a differential with ionophore toxicosis can be ruled out based on the history and a clinical examination. Absence of ticks and wounds can aid in ruling out tick paralysis and polyradiculoneuritis. Normal serum mineral concentrations can be used to rule out calcium and magnesium abnormalities. Rear-limb to front-limb progression and rapid onset can be used to rule out myasthenia gravis. Macrolide parasiticides (i.e., ivermectin) and amitraz poisoning can present as a severe central nervous system depression, recumbency, or a paralytic syndrome and must be ruled out by lack of previous exposure. The most difficult differential that must be ruled out is botulism. Botulism is not common in dogs and cats, but mimics ionophore poisoning in many ways. Laboratory analysis that is negative for the organism and toxin serve to rule out botulism. Other differential diagnoses may include macadamia nut ingestion in dogs, bromethalin poisoning, and organophosphate-induced intermediate syndrome or delayed neuropathy.

References

1. Bennett K: *Compendium of veterinary products*, ed 3, Port Huron, MI, 1995, North American Compendiums.
2. McDougald LR, Roberson EL: Antiprotozoan drugs. In Booth NH, McDonald LE, editors: *Veterinary pharmacology and therapeutics*, ed 6, Ames, 1988, Iowa State University Press.
3. Van Der Linde-Sipman JS, VanDen Ingh TSGAM, Van Nes JJ, et al: Salinomycin-induced polyneuropathy in cats: morphologic and epidemiologic data, *Vet Pathol* 36:152–156, 1999.
4. Safran N, Aizenberg I, Bark H: Paralytic syndrome attributed to lasalocid residues in a commercial ration fed to dog, *J Am Vet Med Assoc* 202:1273–1275, 1993.
5. Segev G, Baneth G, Levitin B, et al: Accidental poisoning of 17 dogs with lasalocid, *Vet Rec* 155:174–176, 2004.
6. Salles MS, Lombardo de Barros CS, Barros SS: Ionophore antibiotic (narasin) poisoning in rabbits, *Vet Hum Toxicol* 36(5):437–444, 1994.
7. Wilson JS: Toxic myopathy in a dog associated with the presence of monensin in dry food, *Can Vet J* 21:30–31, 1980.
8. Osz M, Salyi G, Malik G, et al: Narasin poisoning in rabbits, *Vet Bull* 59:416, 1989 (Abstract 2985).
9. Condon FP, McKenzie RA: Fatal monensin toxicity in a dog after chewing a bovine intra-ruminal slow-release device, *Aust Vet Pract* 32(4):179–180, 2002.
10. Pakozdy A, Challande-Kathman I, Doherr M, et al: Retrospective study of salinomycin toxicosis in 66 cats, *Vet Med Int*, 2010.
11. Syntex: *Material safety data sheet*, Palo Alto, CA, July 1991, Syntex Inc.
12. Food and Drug Administration: *Laidlomycin propionate*. NADA Number 141-025, Rockville, MD, 1994, Freedom of Information Office, Center for Veterinary Medicine.
13. Galitzer SJ, Oehme FW: A literature review on the toxicity of lasalocid, a polyether antibiotic, *Vet Hum Toxicol* 26:322–326, 1984.
14. Food and Drug Administration: *Maduramicin ammonium*. NADA Number 139075, Rockville, MD, 1989, Freedom of Information Office, Center for Veterinary Medicine.
15. Todd GC, Novilla MN, Howard LC: Comparative toxicology of monensin sodium in laboratory animals, *J Anim Sci* 58:1512–1517, 1984.
16. Novilla MN, Owen NV, Todd GC: The comparative toxicology of narasin in laboratory animals, *Vet Hum Toxicol* 36(4):318–323, 1994.
17. Pressman BC: Induced active transport of ions in mitochondria, *Proc Nat Acad Sci* 53:1076–1083, 1965.
18. Pressman BC: Ionophorous antibiotics as models for biological transport, *Fed Proc* 27:1283–1288, 1968.
19. Estrada OS, Celis H, Calderon E, et al: Model translocators for divalent and monovalent ion transport in phospholipid membranes: the effects of ion translocator X-537A on the energy-conserving properties of mitochondrial membranes, *J Membr Biol* 18:201–218, 1974.
20. Mitani M, Yamanishi T, Miyazaki Y, et al: Salinomycin effects on mitochondrial ion translocation and respiration, *Antimicrob Ag Chem* 9:655–660, 1976.
21. Wong DT, Berg DH, Hamill RH, et al: Ionophorous properties of narasin, a new polyether monocarbox-ylic acid antibiotic, in rat liver mitochondria, *Biochem Pharmacol* 26:1373–1376, 1977.
22. Haeusler G: The effects of the ionophore X-537A (lasalocid) on the heart and on vascular smooth muscle, *Experientia* 32:779, 1976 (Abstract).
23. Levy JV, Cohen JA, Inesi G: Contractile effects of a calcium ionophore, *Nature* 242:461–463, 1973.
24. Lattanzio FA Jr, Pressman BC: Alterations in intracellular calcium activity and contractility of isolated perfused rabbit hearts by ionophores and adrenergic agents, *Biochem Biophys Res Commun* 139:816–821, 1986.
25. Satoh H, Uchida T: Morphological and electrophysiological changes induced by calcium ionophores (A23187 and X-537A) in spontaneously beating rabbit sino-atrial node cells, *Gen Pharmacol* 24:49–57, 1993.
26. Devore DI, Nastuk WL: Effects of "calcium ionophore" X537A on frog skeletal muscle, *Nature* 253:644–646, 1975.
27. Murakami K, Karaki H, Nakagawa H, et al: The inhibitory effect of X537A on vascular smooth muscle contraction, *Naunyn-Schmiedeberg's Arch Pharmacol* 325:80–84, 1984.
28. Levy JV, Cohen JA, Inesi G: Contractile effects of a calcium ionophore, *Nature* 242:461–463, 1973.
29. Safran N, Haring R, Gurwitz D, et al: Selective neurotoxicity induced by the ionophore lasalocid in rat dissociated cerebral cultures, involvement on the NMDA receptor/channel, *Neurotox* 17:883–895, 1996.
30. Novilla MN: The veterinary importance of the toxic syndrome induced by ionophores, *Vet Hum Toxicol* 34:66–70, 1992.
31. Food and Drug Administration: *Lasalocid*. NADA Number 096-298, Rockville, MD, 1982, Freedom of Information Office, Center for Veterinary Medicine.

Iron

Jeffery O. Hall, DVM, PhD, DABVT

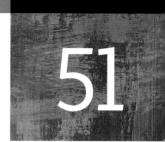

- Sources include gestational supplements, multivitamins or minerals, fertilizers, iron-EDTA slug and snail baits, hand warmers, and oxygen absorber sachets (for spoilage prevention).
- Toxic dose: less than 20 mg/kg absorbable elemental iron is generally not systemically toxic; 20 to 60 mg/kg absorbable elemental iron can be mildly to moderately toxic; more than 60 mg/kg absorbable elemental iron can cause severe intoxication.
- Iron is a highly reactive metal, when not protein bound, that induces free radical production and lipid peroxidation in biologic systems.
- Clinical signs include gastrointestinal distress, shock, and cardiovascular collapse.
- Confirmatory tests include analytical confirmation of serum iron concentrations that surpass the iron binding capacity.
- Treatment should include early gastric decontamination, good supportive care (fluids, electrolytes, acid-base correction), and chelation therapy.
- Prognosis is fair to good depending on the severity of clinical signs.
- Gross and histologic lesions include gross erythema or necrosis of the gastrointestinal mucosa, hepatic swelling, systemic edema or hemorrhage, and damage to hepatocytes or vascular epithelium.
- Differential diagnoses are garbage intoxication, gastric torsion, caustic or corrosive intoxication, snake bite, heat prostration, and bacterial and viral enteritis.

Iron is an essential mineral, but when a large amount is ingested, it also can be lethal. This type of acute poisoning occurs primarily in dogs because of their often indiscriminate eating habits. Although cats are also susceptible to the toxic effects of large doses of iron, there are no reported cases in the literature. Ingestion of large doses of soluble iron overwhelms the body's protective defense mechanisms and results in free circulating iron, which causes severe tissue damage.

Sources

Numerous products contain iron in some form, but the more soluble salt forms of iron pose the greatest risk of toxicosis. This type of soluble iron is commonly found in numerous over-the-counter multivitamin-mineral preparations, gestational iron supplements, some types of slug and snail baits (iron-EDTA baits), some types of oxygen absorbing sachets (used in products to prevent spoilage), hand warming pads, and some fortified lawn and garden fertilizers. Because dietary or nutritional supplements are often sugar coated, dogs may eat large numbers of tablets. In addition, pet owners frequently think that vitamin or mineral supplements are not dangerous and leave this type of material in locations where animals can gain easy access. Although many other products contain iron in some form, its solubility is often so low that toxicosis would not occur. For example, metallic iron and ferric oxide (rust) are so poorly soluble that they are not considered a threat for a toxic ingestion. This type of insoluble iron may be the type found in some fertilizers, so identification of the iron's chemical form is important.

Toxic Dose

The dose of soluble, absorbable iron necessary to induce an iron toxicosis in the dog follows that reported for humans.[1] Ingestion of less than 20 mg/kg is generally not a threat for systemic intoxication, although a mild gastric upset may occur. With ingestion of 20 to 60 mg/kg, a mild to moderate intoxication can be expected. Ingestion of more than 60 mg/kg is a serious threat for severe intoxication. Without early intervention, ingestion of greater than 100 mg/kg is potentially fatal. However, it is important to remember that these toxic doses are based on soluble, bioavailable forms of iron and would greatly overestimate the toxicity of an insoluble iron form.

In evaluating the potential for toxicosis, one must calculate the amount of elemental iron ingested. This is accomplished by multiplying the amount of the iron salt (mg) by the percentage of elemental iron (0.10 for 10%). Table 51-1 lists the more common salt forms of iron and their relative percentages of elemental iron. For tablet ingestions, this information will provide the amount of elemental iron per tablet because most tablets are labeled with the amount of iron salt per tablet. Because iron ingestion can be underestimated if the label lists elemental iron instead of iron salt, one must be certain about whether the amount of iron is listed as the elemental or salt form. In addition, the ferrous salt forms of iron are more bioactive and more rapidly absorbed, but their overall toxicity is more dependent on the total soluble concentration of elemental iron.

Toxicokinetics

Because free elemental iron is deleterious to tissue, mammals have mechanisms to bind and store iron. As iron enters the systemic circulation, it is rapidly bound to transferrin, the primary iron transport protein.[2] This protein transports iron to the peripheral tissue where iron is needed. Serum transferrin concentrations greatly exceed those necessary to bind iron under normal physiologic conditions. This reserve binding capacity provides protection against iron becoming free in systemic circulation. In cases of intoxication, this protein-binding capacity becomes saturated, thus allowing nonbound iron to interact with cellular constituents. Cellular iron that is not necessary for production of proteins is bound into ferritin, an iron-storage protein of the tissues.[3] Chronic exposure to excess iron induces the production of additional transferrin and ferritin, but in acute exposures iron can overwhelm the binding capacity of these proteins.[4]

The kinetics of iron absorption are quite complex and do not follow the normal pattern for most nutrients. The overall body load of iron is regulated at the point of absorption because there is no mechanism for actively eliminating excess iron. The absorption of iron from the gastric lumen into the systemic circulation involves a two-step regulation. First, the iron must be transferred into the gastric mucosal cells. It is thought that this involves a carrier-mediated process, but may include multiple iron transporter proteins.[5] Next the iron is either transferred from the mucosal

Table 51-1 Percentage of Elemental Iron in Common Soluble Iron Salts	
Salt	Percentage of Elemental Iron
Iron (as ferric salt)	100
Iron (as ferrous salt)	100
Ferric ammonium citrate	15
Ferric chloride	34
Ferric EDTA	13
Ferric hydroxide	63
Ferric phosphate	37
Ferric pyrophosphate	30
Ferriglycine sulfate	16
Ferrous fumarate	33
Ferrous carbonate	48
Ferrous gluconate	12
Ferrous lactate	24
Ferrous sulfate (anhydrous)	37
Ferrous sulfate (hydrate)	20
Peptonized iron	16

cell into the circulation, or it is lost when the cells are sloughed through normal cellular turnover.[6] It is interesting that much more iron is absorbed into the gastric mucosal cells than is eventually transferred into the systemic circulation. This retained cellular iron is bound in ferritin. In animals with large acute exposures, the gastric mucosal cells' ability to sequester the iron into ferritin probably becomes saturated, allowing nonbound iron to damage the cells and enter systemic circulation, where it is bound to transferrin until that also becomes saturated. Damage to the gastric mucosal cells may also allow for the direct entry of iron into systemic circulation, bypassing this normal limiting barrier.

In nonlethal exposures, the excess iron is sequestered into tissue. Iron elimination from the body occurs at a fairly constant rate. Even with large doses of iron, there is no increase in the rate of elimination.[7] Thus the excess is stored in the body in ferritin or hemosiderin, a mineralized iron deposit in tissues.

Mechanism of Toxicity

Iron is a very reactive transition metal that can change valence states, from ferrous to ferric and then back to the ferrous form, very rapidly. This is one reason why iron plays a major role in biologic redox reactions. This same characteristic is responsible for the toxic nature of nonbound iron. Iron's toxicity centers on its ability to act as and produce free radicals (also commonly referred to as reactive oxygen species), molecules with one or more unpaired electrons.[3] Free radicals seek to scavenge electrons and in doing so produce additional free radicals. These free radicals can initiate autooxidation of polyunsaturated fatty acids (lipid peroxidation).[8] Thus free iron can either directly or indirectly result in tissue damage and necrosis. Because free iron is so reactive, the primary tissues that are damaged are those that have first contact with absorbed free iron: the gastrointestinal, vascular, hepatic, and cardiac tissues. However, all tissues are susceptible to the toxic effects of free iron.

In addition to direct cellular damage, metabolic disorders can also occur. With severe systemic tissue damage, coagulopathies can appear. Severe metabolic acidosis is common because of fluid and electrolyte loss resulting from vascular and gastrointestinal damage, and from direct mitochondrial damage. The mitochondrial damage, along with decreased tissue perfusion, causes increases in lactic acid. The direct tissue damage and resultant metabolic disruption combine to result in gastrointestinal distress, hepatic necrosis, cardiovascular collapse, and occasionally death.

Clinical Signs

Clinical signs that are commonly reported are associated with gastrointestinal damage, cardiovascular damage, and neurologic effects. These signs can include depression, vomiting, hematemesis, diarrhea, bloody stools, abdominal pain, muscle tremors, shock, and death.[1,9,10] The progression of clinical effects in domestic animals closely follows the four stages described in humans. The first stage, 0 to 6 hours after ingestion, primarily involves gastrointestinal upset and depression resulting from damage to the gastrointestinal mucosa. Bloody vomitus or stool can occur in this stage. The second stage, 6 to 24 hours post ingestion, is one of apparent recovery. The gastrointestinal effects subside, and the animal becomes more alert. This stage can lead to a false sense of security that the animal is out of danger. The third stage, 12 to 96 hours following ingestion, involves a return of the gastrointestinal effects plus metabolic acidosis, shock, hepatic failure, cardiovascular collapse, coagulation disorders, and in some cases, death. The fourth stage, which occurs at 2 to 6 weeks post exposure, is one of gastrointestinal obstruction secondary to the fibrosing repair of the gastrointestinal damage. This stage is not seen as commonly as the other stages, but can occur.

Minimum Database

The database necessary to evaluate an exposure or clinical condition includes estimating the potential iron exposure and performing a thorough clinical evaluation. However, estimation of exposure is often difficult because numbers of tablets or amounts can often only be estimated. When pets are symptomatic or exposures are potentially large, one should evaluate the total serum iron concentration and serum iron binding capacity (these tests are often available at most human hospitals and some veterinary clinical pathology laboratories), and perform complete blood count, serum chemistry profile, and abdominal radiographs. On abdominal radiographs, precipitated iron or tablets remaining to be dissolved and absorbed can often be observed, and it is not uncommon for the tablets to adhere to the gastric mucosa or form a mass that will slowly dissolve and be absorbed over time.

Confirmatory Tests

Measurements of total serum iron concentration and serum iron binding capacity are the most reliable tests for the presence of iron poisoning. Systemic poisoning does not occur until the serum iron binding capacity has been exceeded. Because iron binding capacity varies greatly among dogs, it is recommended that both serum iron concentration and serum iron binding capacity be measured. Caution must be observed in the timing of sample collection because the rate of tablet dissolution can vary and iron has multicompartmental kinetics of disposition. Thus the serum iron concentration can vary greatly in the first few hours. It is therefore recommended that serum iron concentration and iron binding capacity be measured 4 to 6 hours after ingestion. Although serum iron may peak by 6 hours post exposure, one must also remember that masses of tablets will dissolve and be absorbed over much greater periods of time. These tests should be repeated in 2 to 4 hours if the results show serum iron concentration below but near the total iron binding capacity. If there has been a large ingestion or if the patient is clinically symptomatic, earlier serum iron measurements may be indicated. Iron concentrations greater than 300 to 500 mcg/dL in properly collected and preserved serum samples where there is no evidence of hemolysis should raise a concern about a possible iron intoxication.

Treatment

With acute ingestions in asymptomatic animals, gastric decontamination is recommended by means of induction of emesis (Fig. 51-1). Ingestion of a large quantity of tablets, adverse clinical signs, or failure of tablets to be removed by induction of emesis, as indicated by densities on abdominal radiographs, are indications for gastric lavage under anesthesia, with an endotracheal tube in place. A gastrotomy is indicated when radiographic observation indicates a tablet bezoar or adherent tablets. Activated charcoal is not indicated because it does not bind iron. In addition, gastric administration of salt solutions to precipitate the iron and render it nonbioavailable has not been successful.

Careful management of fluid load, electrolytes, and acid-base status, along with symptomatic care, is necessary in the care of an iron-poisoned animal. Fluid replacement is necessary to combat circulatory shock and fluid loss. The amount of replacement fluids should be based on replacement of the fluid deficit plus fluids necessary for maintenance. Electrolytes should be monitored and added to the fluids as necessary to correct deficits. Blood gas analysis aids in determining whether treatment is necessary for the correction of a metabolic acidosis. The use of gastrointestinal protectants, such as sucralfate, is also indicated in patients that have indications of potential or ongoing gastrointestinal damage.

In animals that are experiencing severe toxicosis or in animals that have serum iron in excess of the iron binding capacity, chelation therapy is indicated. If serum iron binding capacity is not available, chelation should be considered in cases for which serum iron is greater than 300 mcg/dL. It is imperative that *only* clean serum samples be tested for serum iron, as hemolysis can result in artificially increased readings for serum iron with some testing methodologies. Using a regimen originally based on human treatment protocols, the Animal Poison Control Center has successfully used deferoxamine (Desferal) to chelate

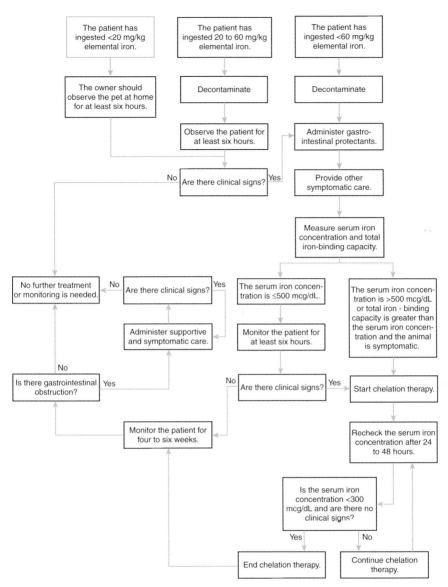

Figure 51-1 Management of iron toxicosis. (From Albretsen J: The toxicity of iron, an essential element. *Vet Med* 82-90, 2006.)

iron (other chelating agents include deferasirox and deferiprone). This chelation agent has a very high binding affinity for iron. Chelation therapy should be started early in the clinical course of the intoxication because it usually has little benefit when started more than 12 hours after ingestion. Deferoxamine should be given by continuous intravenous (IV) infusion at a rate of 15 mg/kg/hour. Faster rates of infusion are associated with arrhythmias and a worsening of existing hypotension. If continuous infusion is not possible, intramuscular administration of 40 mg/kg every 4 to 8 hours is recommended. However, this method is not as effective as the IV infusion. Chelation therapy should be continued until the serum iron concentration is below either 300 mcg/dL or the measured serum iron binding capacity, whichever is lower.

Prognosis

For most asymptomatic patients that receive early decontamination, the prognosis is good. However, in animals that are symptomatic the prognosis can range from guarded to good depending on the severity of the clinical effects, the amount of iron ingested, and how early chelation and supportive therapies were started.

Gross and Histologic Lesions

Gross and histologic lesions are primarily the result of damage to the gastrointestinal tract, vascular system, and liver. Gastrointestinal damage can range from mild erythema to severe necrosis and sloughing of the mucosal epithelium with severe hemorrhage. Damaged vascular epithelium leads to the development of edema, which can occur at any site. In animals with a coagulopathy, hemorrhage can be observed in any organ. Gross hepatic lesions can range from mild capsular swelling to severe friability and hemorrhage. Histologic lesions follow the gross lesions and can include cellular swelling and/or necrosis of the mucosal epithelial cells, myocardial cells, vascular epithelium, and hepatocytes. Vascular leaking and hemorrhage are also observed.

Differential Diagnoses

There are not many differential diagnoses to consider if an iron-poisoned dog develops the full spectrum of clinical effects, but as with most clinical conditions, this spectrum is not often encountered. Primary considerations include any cause of gastrointestinal distress that also causes shock, such as garbage intoxication, gastric torsion, caustic or corrosive intoxication, snake bite, heat prostration, bacterial enteritis, or viral enteritis.

References

1. Greentree WF, Hall JO: Iron toxicosis. In Bonagura JD, editor: *Kirk's current veterinary therapy small animal practice*, ed 12, Philadelphia, 1995, Saunders.
2. Adrian GS, Korinek BW, Bowman BH, et al: The human transferrin gene: 5′ region contains conserved sequences which match the control elements regulated by heavy metals, glucocorticoids, and acute phase reaction, *Gene* 49:167–175, 1986.
3. Ponka P, Schulman HM, Woodworth RC: *Iron transport and storage*, Boca Raton, FL, 1990, CRC Press.
4. McKnight GS, Lee DC, Hemmaplardh D, et al: Transferrin gene expression: effects of nutritional iron deficiency, *J Biol Chem* 255(1):144–147, 1979.
5. Simovich M, Hainsworth LN, Fields PA, et al: Localization of the iron transport proteins mobilferrin and DMT-1 in the duodenum: the surprising role of mucin. *Am J Hematol* 74:32–45, 2003.
6. Whebey MS, Cosby WH: The gastrointestinal tract and iron absorption, *Blood* 22(4):416–428, 1963.
7. Smith A, Morgan WT: Haem transport to the liver by haemopexin, *Biochem J* 1983:47–54, 1979.
8. O'Connell MJ, Ward RJ, Baum H, et al: The role of iron in ferritin- and hemosiderin-mediated lipid peroxidation in liposomes, *Biochem J* 229:135–139, 1985.
9. Haldand SL, Davis RM: Acute toxicity in five dogs after ingestion of a commercial snail and slug bait containing iron EDTA, *Austr Vet J* 87(7):284–286, 2009.
10. Brutlag AG, Flint CTC, Puschner B: Iron intoxication in a dog consequent to the ingestion of oxygen absorber sachets in pet food treat packaging, *J Med Toxicol* 8:76–79, 2012.

Ivermectin: Macrolide Antiparasitic Agents

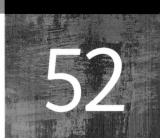

Katrina L. Mealey, DVM, PhD, DACVIM, DACVCP

- Ivermectin, selamectin, moxidectin, doramectin, eprinomectin, abamectin, and milbemycin are potential sources of toxicity caused by accidental overdose or access or when used in susceptible breeds.
- Some collies and other herding breeds lack a functional P-glycoprotein that renders them more susceptible to the neurotoxic effects of these drugs.
- Clinical signs typically include disorientation, ataxia, hyperesthesia, hypersalivation, vocalization, blindness, recumbency, and coma.
- Most animals will recover following appropriate supportive care, but recovery may take hours, days, or even weeks.

Ivermectin, selamectin, moxidectin, and milbemycin are macrolides (or macrocyclic lactones) that are used to treat a variety of parasitic diseases in dogs and cats.[1] In the United States, each of these agents is licensed for use as a heartworm preventive in dogs. In cats, macrolide antiparasitic agents are licensed for use as heartworm preventives, and some are licensed for the treatment of otodectes and hookworms, *Ancylostoma braziliense* and *Ancylostoma tubaeforme*. In an extralabel manner, and at doses greatly exceeding the recommended label dose, macrolide antiparasitic agents are also used to treat scabies, lice, cheyletiella, demodecosis, gastrointestinal nematodes, and the microfilaria of *Dirofilaria immitis*.[1] Macrolide antiparasitic agents are generally considered to have a wide margin of safety.[2] However, a percentage of collies and other herding breeds harbor a mutation in the *MDR1* (*ABCB1*) gene that renders them exceptionally susceptible to toxicity from most, if not all, of these agents.[3] It is important to note that at the labeled doses for heartworm prevention, the macrolide antiparasitic agents are safe for use in herding breeds, even those dogs with the mutant *MDR1* genotype. Although toxicosis in nonherding dog breeds and cats generally results from an extreme overdose (i.e., when a product marketed for livestock is used off-label in small animals), the author is aware of reports of suspected toxicosis in a dog (moxidectin) and cat (topical ivermectin) receiving the approved label dose of the particular macrolide.

Doramectin and eprinomectin are macrolides approved for use in cattle only.[4] The manufacturers of these agents do not recommend their use in other species.

Clinical signs associated with macrolide toxicity reflect the actions of these drugs on the central nervous system.[1] A specific antidote is not available, but most animals experiencing toxicosis from exposure to these drugs will have a complete recovery if appropriate supportive care is provided.

Sources

Ivermectin (Heartguard, others) is a mixture of 22,23-dihydroavermectin B_1a (>80%) and B_1b (<20%), formulated to control a number of internal and external parasites in animals.[1]

It is produced from the fungus *Streptomyces avermitilis* and is marketed for dogs and cats (tablets, chewables, and an otic solution [cats]), with some formulations also containing pyrantel pamoate. Ivermectin is also marketed for cattle (injectable, pour-on, bolus), swine (injectable, premix), horses (liquids and pastes), and sheep (drench).

Moxidectin (Proheart) is approved for use in dogs (tablet, injectable), cattle (pour-on), and horses (oral gel). Proheart 6 is an injectable, sustained-release (6-month duration) heartworm prevention product labeled for dogs. Moxidectin products are also available in Australia, Canada, and Europe. Like ivermectin, moxidectin is used to control many types of internal and external parasites. Moxidectin is a chemically altered product of *Streptomyces aureolacrimosus noncyanogenus.*[1]

Selamectin (Revolution) is marketed as a topical solution for use in dogs and cats for the control of both internal and external parasites. Selamectin, a macrolide antibiotic, is a fermentation product of *Streptomyces avermitilis.*[1]

Milbemycin (Interceptor) oral tablets are approved for use in dogs and cats for the prevention of *Dirofilaria*, and for treatment of some internal parasites. Milbemycin is a fermentation product *of Streptomyces hygroscopicus aureolacrimosus.*[1]

Doramectin (Dectomax) is marketed as an injectable or pour-on formulation for the control of endoparasites and ectoparasites in cattle. Doramectin is a fermentation product of *Streptomyces avermitilis.*[5]

Eprinomectin (Eprinex) is marketed as a pour-on formulation for the control of endoparasites and ectoparasites in cattle.[5]

Abamectin (Avert cockroach bait; Kraft[TM]; others) is an environmental insecticide/pesticide that is frequently used for insect control. It is licensed for use on crops, yards, and within buildings (including homes, offices, and restaurants).

Relatively high concentrations of macrolide antibiotics can be excreted in the feces in their active form. Toxicosis has occurred in dogs that have ingested the feces of sheep and/or horses that were treated with some macrolides.

Toxic Dose

Ivermectin is approved for use in dogs and cats for the prevention of dirofilariasis at oral doses of 0.006 and 0.024 mg/kg, respectively, once a month. Most dogs tolerate oral ivermectin dosages up to 2.5 mg/kg before clinical signs of toxicity occur.[6] The LD_{50} for beagle dogs is 80 mg/kg.[7] Some dogs, especially collies and other herding breeds, are more sensitive to ivermectin and can only tolerate doses up to 0.1 mg/kg, which is sixteenfold higher than the label dose.[3,8,9] There are numerous reports of ivermectin toxicity in collies and other herding breeds receiving "antiparasitic" doses of ivermectin (0.2 to 0.6 mg/kg).[6,10-13] Two Australian shepherd dogs receiving ivermectin at oral dosages of 0.17 mg/kg and 0.34 mg/kg, respectively, developed clinical signs of toxicosis,[12] as did an old English sheepdog mix that received 0.15 mg/kg ivermectin orally (PO).[13] However, at the recommended dosage for heartworm prevention (0.006 mg/kg per month), ivermectin is safe for all dog breeds.

Cats generally tolerate dosages of 0.2 to 1.3 mg/kg ivermectin given orally or subcutaneously (SQ).[1,14] The apparent no-effect level for oral ivermectin in cats is approximately 0.5 to 0.75 mg/kg of body weight. Toxicosis has been reported in a limited number of cats and kittens exposed to lower doses (0.30 to 0.40 mg/kg SQ).[15]

Moxidectin is available in tablet form for monthly oral administration at a dose of 0.003 mg/kg, and as a sustained release injectable formulation at a dose of 0.17 mg/kg administered every 6 months.[5] The manufacturer's package insert states that moxidectin was administered orally to dogs at doses 300-fold greater than the label dose without producing signs of toxicity. However, at 0.09 mg/kg (30× label dose), clinical signs of moxidectin toxicosis were observed in a collie.[1] Furthermore, moxidectin toxicosis has been reported in a Jack Russell terrier (a breed not known to harbor the *MDR1* mutation) that consumed the equine product[16] and a Shetland sheepdog that received an injection of the sustained release product labeled for use in dogs.

Milbemycin is available in tablet form for monthly administration at a dose of 2 mg/kg (cats) and 0.5 mg/kg (dogs).[5] Beagles have received doses 200 times greater than the label dose, with no apparent signs of toxicity.[1] In a study involving collies, hypersalivation, ataxia, mydriasis, and central nervous system depression were observed in 2 of 5 collies treated with 5 mg/kg (10× label dose), and 5 of 5 collies treated with 10 mg/kg (20× label dose).[17] According to some dermatologists, milbemycin can be used at a dose of 0.5 to 1.6 mg/kg daily to treat canine demodecosis.[18] However, toxicosis has been reported in dogs with the *MDR1* mutation when milbemycin has been used according to this protocol.

According to the manufacturers, selamectin was proven safe when given at 10 times its recommended dose to puppies and kittens and 5 times its recommended dose when administered to collies (a 10× topical dose in collies caused ataxia).[5,19] Oral administration of selamectin at the recommended topical dose in young beagle dogs did not cause any noticeable adverse reactions.[1,5] When selamectin was administered orally at dosages of 2.5, 10, or 15 mg/kg to ivermectin-sensitive collies, only one animal showed ataxia at the 15-mg/kg exposure dosage (oral dose of 2.5 times the label dose for topical administration). Oral administration of selamectin to cats at the recommended topical dose (6 mg/kg) caused salivation and vomiting.[1,5] There is one report of a kitten (0.3 kg) that died 8 hours after receiving a single topical dose of selamectin. However, this young kitten was malnourished and underweight for its age.

Doramectin has been used safely for treating spirocercosis in dogs at a dose of 0.4 mg/kg injected subcutaneously at 2-week intervals for 6 treatments. Beagles treated with this protocol demonstrated no signs of toxicity.[20] However, doramectin toxicosis has been reported in a collie.[21]

Limited information exists in the literature on the toxic dose of eprinomectin for dogs and cats. It is likely that eprinomectin has a safety profile similar to those of other macrolides.

Toxicokinetics

Up to 95% of ivermectin is absorbed after oral administration in monogastric animals.[1] It is primarily excreted unchanged in the feces likely by a P-glycoprotein–dependent mechanism. A fraction of the dose is metabolized in the liver through oxidation. The terminal elimination half-life in MDR1 wild-type dogs is about 2 days.

Bioavailability of selamectin after topical administration to dogs and cats is 5% and 75%, respectively, with peak plasma concentrations occurring in 3 days (dogs) and 15 hours (cats).[1] The terminal elimination half-life after topical administration is reported to be approximately 11 days for dogs and 8 days for cats.[5] These likely represent sustained release from a depot site, such as the skin, because the terminal half-life after intravenous administration was shorter.

Moxidectin is absorbed rapidly after oral administration, with peak plasma concentrations occurring within a few hours of administration. The terminal half-life after oral administration is reported to be approximately 19 days.[22]

Specific pharmacokinetic information regarding milbemycin, doramectin, and eprinomectin in dogs and cats is not available. It is reasonable to assume that these agents also have long elimination half-lives in dogs and cats. Consequently, patients suffering from toxicosis after exposure to one of these agents may require a fairly prolonged course of treatment.

Mechanism of Toxicity

The macrolides were originally thought to act as a γ-aminobutyric acid (GABA) agonist, but more recent evidence suggests that the actions of macrolides against parasites and nontarget animals are mediated through glutamate-gated chloride channels in the central nervous system.[1,2] Macrolides bind with high affinity to these channels, triggering the influx of chloride ions that results in hyperpolarization of the neuron and prevention of action potential initiation or propagation.[1,2] The ultimate result is paralysis and death of the target parasite.

Mammals are generally protected from the effects of macrolides because their central nervous system, the site of action for macrolides, is generally not exposed to high concentrations of these agents.[1,3] Although these agents tend to be highly lipid soluble, which favors entry into the central nervous system, the mammalian blood-brain barrier prevents accumulation of high concentrations of these agents in brain tissue. Some of these agents have been shown to be substrates of P-glycoprotein, the product of the *MDR1* (*ABCB1*) gene. Based on structural similarities, it is suspected that all of the currently available macrolides are P-glycoprotein substrates. P-glycoprotein, an integral component of the blood-brain barrier, is expressed on the luminal aspect of brain capillary epithelial cells.[23] There it functions as an efflux pump for a large number of substrate drugs (Box 52-1), binding the drug and transporting it back into the capillary lumen. Animals that lack functional P-glycoprotein, including MDR1(-/-) knockout mice and herding breeds with the *MDR1* mutation, accumulate much higher (i.e., fiftyfold greater) concentrations of P-glycoprotein substrate drugs in brain tissue, and are therefore more susceptible to neurologic toxicity from these drugs. In addition to increased sensitivity to macrolide antiparasitic agents, collies and other herding breeds harboring the *MDR1* mutant genotype have severe neurotoxicity develop after treatment with standard doses of loperamide (Imodium),[24] and are extremely sensitive to adverse effects caused by standard doses of vincristine and doxorubicin.[25]

Clearly, functional P-glycoprotein is crucial for protecting mammals from macrolide-induced neurologic toxicity. P-glycoprotein dysfunction in mammals can be genetic (involving a polymorphism of the *MDR1* gene) or acquired. The *MDR1* mutation in herding breeds is a four-base-pair deletion mutation. The frame shift that results from this deletion mutation generates several premature stop codons such that P-glycoprotein synthesis is prematurely terminated.[3] Less than 10% of the P-glycoprotein product is synthesized in dogs with the *MDR1* mutation, and the truncated P-glycoprotein is nonfunctional. Acquired P-glycoprotein dysfunction can occur as a result of drug interactions. A number of drugs can inhibit P-glycoprotein function (Box 52-2).[26] When drugs that inhibit P-glycoprotein function are administered concurrently with P-glycoprotein substrates (such as macrolide antiparasitic agents), increased susceptibility to neurologic toxicity can occur. Ketoconazole has been shown to inhibit P-glycoprotein function, thereby enhancing CNS penetration and blunting biliary excretion of P-glycoprotein substrate drugs in MDR1 wild-type dogs.[27] Similarly, concurrent administration of the flea preventive spinosad (Comfortis) and ivermectin (extralabel dose used for treating demodex) has been reported by the FDA to cause neurologic toxicity (http://www.fda.gov/AnimalVeterinary/NewsEvents/CVMUpdates/ucm047942.htm).

Clinical Signs

Most signs of macrolide toxicity are associated with the central nervous system.[1,8,10,17] In an acute overdose, clinical signs may occur within a few hours of administration. However, in some animals that are being treated daily (i.e., for demodecosis), clinical signs of toxicity may occur after several days of treatment. Animals are typically depressed and commonly display disorientation, ataxia, hyperesthesia, and hypersalivation and/or vocalization.[10,17] Depending on the dose, the animal may become progressively weaker and then may become recumbent and possibly comatose. Other reported neurologic signs include muscle fasciculations, tremors, and seizures. Affected animals may have normal or exaggerated reflexes. Many animals have apparent blindness, with a decreased or nonexistent menace response and/or pupillary light reflex. Miosis, mydriasis, and strabismus have been reported.

Other reported signs in severely depressed dogs include hypothermia, decreased heart rate, slow shallow breathing, vomiting, mild diarrhea, and sinus arrhythmia. Clinical signs can persist for several days to several weeks, and the severity of the signs may not correlate with their persistence.[1,8,10,17]

Box 52-1	Examples of Drugs That

Are Proven P-Glycoprotein Substrates

Macrolide Antiparasitic Agents*
Ivermectin
Selamectin

Antineoplastic Agents
Doxorubicin
Vinca alkaloids
Taxanes
Epipodophyllotoxins

Immunosuppressants
Cyclosporine A
Tacrolimus

Gastrointestinal Drugs
Loperamide (Imodium)
Ondansetron

Cardiac Drugs
Digoxin
Quinidine

*Others are likely to be substrates but have not yet been tested.

Box 52-2	Examples of Drugs That

Inhibit P-Glycoprotein Function

Cyclosporine A
Ketoconazole
Verapamil
Tamoxifen

Confirmatory Tests

Ivermectin and other macrolides can be detected in liver, adipose tissue, or serum to confirm exposure to the drug.[28] However, there is little correlation between macrolide concentrations in the blood and the development of clinical signs because it is the concentration of drug in the brain that is of clinical importance.[29] Administration of physostigmine (1 mg intravenously) has been used to temporarily reverse neurologic clinical signs in dogs suffering from ivermectin toxicosis.[30] Physostigmine is an anticholinesterase agent that has been used in humans to reverse central nervous system depression caused by sedative-hypnotics. Therefore, response to physostigmine does not confirm a diagnosis of macrolide toxicosis but may support such a diagnosis.

Recently, a DNA-based test has become available to determine if a dog harbors the mutant *MDR1* genotype. Anticoagulated blood or cheek cells (using a cytology brush) are obtained from the dog and submitted to the laboratory.* After extraction of DNA a fragment containing the site of the *MDR1* mutation is amplified using the polymerase chain reaction and sequenced. Although this test does not confirm a diagnosis of macrolide toxicosis, it will identify dogs that are at increased risk of macrolide toxicity.

Treatment

There is no specific antidote for treating patients suffering from macrolide toxicity. In cases of overdoses of macrolide antiparasitic agents, emesis is indicated if ingestion of the drug has occurred within 2 hours. Repeated doses of activated charcoal plus one or two doses of a cathartic are recommended because the majority of ivermectin, and possibly other macrolides, are excreted unchanged in the feces.[1] Although physostigmine may be of some benefit in dogs suffering from ivermectin toxicosis,[30] its use is not recommended because it is not a specific antagonist; it causes only transient improvement in clinical signs and can be associated with a variety of adverse effects. Furthermore, in one study, dogs with ivermectin toxicosis treated with adequate supportive care experienced complete recoveries.[10] Neostigmine methylsulfate, 25 and 150 mcg, and 5% dextrose, 100 mL, was used intravenously according to a recent report on ivermectin poisoning in two 4-week-old kittens.[31] One kitten died, and the second survived after multiple treatments over a 2-day period. Picrotoxin, a GABA antagonist, has been administered to a collie with

---

*Veterinary Clinical Pharmacology Laboratory, College of Veterinary Medicine, Washington State University, Pullman, WA 99164-6610.

ivermectin toxicity, but seizures occurred shortly after its administration.[32] For reasons similar to those listed for physostigmine, its use is also not recommended.

Recently the use of intravenous fat or lipid emulsion (ILE) has been demonstrated to be beneficial in the treatment of toxicoses involving lipid-soluble drugs such as local anesthetics in human patients.[33] Because macrocyclic lactones are lipophilic, they constitute potential targets for ILE therapy. Although ILE has been reported to be effective for a case of moxidectin toxicity in a Jack Russell terrier (*MDR1* status not assessed),[16] it was not effective in treating ivermectin toxicoses in three Australian shepherds that were homozygous for the *MDR1* deletion mutation.[34]

Appropriate supportive care may include fluid and electrolyte therapy, nutritional support, and prevention of decubital ulcers because the patient may be recumbent and even comatose for several days to weeks. Arterial blood gases may be indicated to determine if ventilatory support is needed because the respiratory center may be affected.

Prognosis

The prognosis for macrolide toxicosis depends largely on the exposure dose. Animals may require supportive care for 1 day, several days, or even several weeks. One dog fully recovered after being comatose for 7 weeks.[14] Animals that recover usually have no long-term sequelae.[10]

Gross and Histologic Lesions

Macrolide antiparasitic agents do not result in specific lesions.

Differential Diagnoses

Many diseases affect the nervous system and produce clinical signs similar to all or some of those described for toxicity associated with macrolide antiparasitic agents. Specific toxicants that must be differentiated include lead, anticholinesterase insecticides (e.g., organophosphate and carbamate insecticides), tremorgenic mycotoxins, ethanol, methanol, ethylene glycol, diethylene glycol, propylene glycol, xylitol, isopropanol, amitraz, and drugs with central nervous system depressing properties (e.g., opiates, phenothiazines, benzodiazepines, and barbiturates).

References

1. Lynn RC: Drugs for the treatment of helminth infections. In Boothe DM, editor: *Small animal clinical pharmacology and therapeutics*, ed 1, Philadelphia, 2001, Saunders.
2. Kohler P: The biochemical basis of anthelmintic action and resistance, *Int J Parasitol* 31(4):336–345, 2001.
3. Mealey KL, Bentjen SA, Gay JM, et al: Ivermectin sensitivity in collies is associated with a deletion mutation of the MDR1 gene, *Pharmacogenetics* 11(8):727–733, 2001.
4. Dorny P, Demeulenaere D, Smets K, et al: Persistent efficacy of topical doramectin and eprinomectin against *Ostertagia ostertagi* and *Cooperia oncophora* infections in cattle, *Vet Rec* 147(5):139–140, 2000.
5. Plumb D: *Veterinary drug handbook*, ed 20, Ames, IA, 2000, Iowa State University Press.
6. Bauck S: Ivermectin toxicity in small animals, *Can Vet J* 28(9):563, 1987.
7. Paul AJ, Tranquilli WJ: Ivermectin. In Kirk RW, editor: *Current veterinary therapy X*, Philadelphia, 1989, Saunders.
8. Paul A, Tranquilli W, Seward R, et al: Clinical observations in collies given ivermectin orally, *Am J Vet Res* 48(4):684, 1987.
9. Fassler P, Tranquilli W, Paul A, et al: Evaluation of the safety of ivermectin administered in a beef-based formulation to ivermectin-sensitive collies, *J Am Vet Med Assoc* 199(4):457, 1991.
10. Hopper K, Aldrich J, Haskins SC: Ivermectin toxicity in 17 collies, *J Vet Intern Med* 16:89–94, 2002.
11. Nelson OL, Carsten E, Bentjen SA, et al: Ivermectin toxicity in an Australian Shepherd dog with the MDR1 mutation associated with ivermectin sensitivity in collies, *J Vet Intern Med* 17(3):354–356, 2003.

12. Hadrick M, Bunch S, Kornegay J: Ivermectin toxicosis in two Australian shepherds, *J Am Vet Med Assoc* 206(8):1147, 1995.
13. Houston D, Parent J, Matushek K: Ivermectin toxicosis in a dog, *J Am Vet Med Assoc* 191(1):78, 1987.
14. Lovell R: Ivermectin and piperazine toxicosis in dogs and cats, *Vet Clin North Am Small Anim Pract* 20(2):453, 1990.
15. Frischke H, Hunt L: Suspected ivermectin toxicity in kittens, *Can Vet J* 32:245, 1991.
16. Crandell DE, Weinberg GL: Moxidectin toxicosis in a puppy successfully treated with intravenous lipids, *J Vet Emerg Crit Care* 19:181–186, 2009.
17. Tranquilli WJ, Paul AJ, Todd KS: Assessment of toxicosis induced by high-dose administration of milbemycin oxime in collies, *Am J Vet Res* 52(7):1170–1172, 1991.
18. Mueller RS, Bettenay SV: A proposed new therapeutic protocol for the treatment of canine mange with ivermectin, *J Am Anim Hosp Assoc* 35:77–80, 1999.
19. Jacobs DE: Selamectin—a novel endectoside of dogs and cats, *Vet Parasit* 91:161–162, 2000.
20. Lavy E, Aroch I, Bark H: Evaluation of doramectin for the treatment of experimental spirocercosis, *Vet Parasit* 109:65–73, 2002.
21. Yas-Natan E, Shamir M, Kleinbart S: Doramectin toxicity in a collie, *Vet Rec* 153:718–720, 2003.
22. Vanapalli SR, Hung YP, Fleckenstein L: Pharmacokinetics and dose proportionality of oral moxidectin in beagle dogs, *Biopharm Drug Dispos* 23(7):263–272, 2002.
23. Nobmann S, Bauer B, Fricker G: Ivermectin excretion by isolated functionally intact brain endothelial capillaries, *Br J Pharmacol* 132(3):722–728, 2001.
24. Sartor LL, Bentjen SA, Trepanier L: Loperamide toxicity in a collie with the MDR1 mutation associated with ivermectin sensitivity, *J Vet Intern Med* 18(1):117–118, 2004.
25. Mealey KL, Northrop NC, Bentjen SA: Increased toxicity of P-glycoprotein-substrate chemotherapeutic agents in a dog with the MDR1 deletion mutation associated with ivermectin sensitivity, 1434, *J Am Vet Med Assoc* 223(10):1453–1455, 2003.
26. Ford JM: Modulators of multidrug resistance, preclinical studies, *Hematol Oncol Clin North Am* 9(2):337–361, 1995.
27. Coelho JC, Tucker R, Mattoon J, Roberts G, Waiting DK, Mealey KL: Biliary excretion of technetium-99m sestamibi in wildtype dogs and in dogs with intrinsic (MDR1 mutation) and extrinsic (ketoconazole treated) P-glycoprotein deficiency, *J Vet Pharmacol Ther* 32(5):417–421, 2009.
28. Smith R, Stronski E, Beck B, et al: Death of a rough collie exposed to an ivermectin-based paste, *Can Vet J* 31:221, 1990.
29. Tranquilli W, Paul A, Seward R: Ivermectin plasma concentrations in collies sensitive to ivermectin-induced toxicosis, *Am J Vet Res* 50(5):769, 1989.
30. Tranquilli W, Paul A, Seward R, et al: Response to physostigmine administration in collie dogs exhibiting ivermectin toxicosis, *J Vet Pharmacol Therap* 10:96, 1987.
31. Muhammad G, Jabbar A, Khan MX, et al: Use of neostigmine in massive ivermectin toxicity in cats, *Vet Human Toxicol* 46(1):28–29, 2004.
32. Sivine F: Picrotoxin, the antidote to ivermectin in dogs? *Veterinary Record* 116:195, 1985.
33. Jamaty C, Bailey B, Larocque A: Lipid emulsions in the treatment of acute poisoning: a systematic review of human and animal studies, *Clin Tox* 48:1–27, 2010.
34. Wright HM, Chen AV, Talcott PA, Poppenga RH, Mealey KL: Intravenous fat emulsion as a treatment for ivermectin toxicosis in three dogs homozygous for the ABCB1-1D gene mutation, *J Vet Emerg Crit Care* (in press).

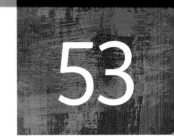

Lead

Tina Wismer, DVM, DABVT, DABT

- Sources include lead-based paint, solder, sinkers, toys and trinkets, and lead projectiles.
- Lead, a multisystem poison, is a serious human and animal health hazard.
- Absorption of lead can be rapid and quite variable depending on its physical and chemical form.
- Lead is tightly bound to the surface of red blood cells; it has a wide tissue distribution and, long term, is stored in bone. Excretion of lead occurs primarily via the urine.
- Clinical signs include gastrointestinal disturbances and nervous system dysfunction.
- Minimum database should include a complete blood count, radiographs, and chemical analysis of tissues (whole blood antemortem; liver and kidney postmortem).
- Treatment can include removal of the source, chelation therapy, gastrointestinal protectants, and seizure control.
- Prognosis is generally favorable in dogs and cats; less so for avian patients.

Sources

Lead toxicosis has been reported in many species of mammals, birds, and reptiles.[1] Lead is distributed throughout the environment and found in various forms (elemental, inorganic, and organic). Elemental lead is a heavy, silvery-gray metal that is soft and malleable.[2] Inorganic compounds such as metallic lead or lead salts are the most common forms. Inorganic salt sources include industrial effluents (mostly lead oxide), solder (metallic), lead paint, and lead containing soldering fluxes. Organic lead (organoleads) includes tetramethyl and tetraethyl lead. Tetraethyl lead had been widely used as an antiknock agent in gasoline, but has been phased out by the Environmental Protection Agency.[1,2]

Dogs and cats can be exposed to lead from many sources: automotive batteries, bone meal supplements, ceramic glazes (found on pottery, earthenware, bone china, porcelain), lead weights (fishing sinkers, curtain weights), lead-based paints (old houses, artist's paints, some agricultural and marine paints), lead solder, putty and caulk, leaded gasolines, linoleum, electronic equipment, roofing felt, lead arsenate pesticides, and wine cork covers.[3] Lead also may be found in the plastic coating wire. Soil contaminated with lead can be another source but this is more common in grazing animals.[1] Lead bullets and shot can be ingested from carcasses or firing ranges. Animals that are shot can develop lead poisoning if the retained bullet is in an acidic environment (synovial joint, area of inflammation).[4]

Toxic Dose

In dogs, the acute toxic dose of lead is 191 to 1000 mg/kg. The chronic cumulative toxic dose for dogs is 1.8-2.6 mg/kg/day.[1] Since 1977, household paint can contain no more than 0.06% (600 ppm) lead by dry weight. However, a chip of lead-based paint the size of a thumbnail may contain 50 to 200 mg of lead. Because of preventive measures in recent years (e.g., removing lead from gasoline, banning lead-based paint), the average blood lead level for children and human adults has decreased.[5]

Toxicokinetics

Lead is absorbed primarily from the gastrointestinal tract. Gastrointestinal absorption of lead in adult animals varies from 5% to 15% depending on the physical form, whereas young animals absorb lead more readily, with up to 50% being absorbed.[1,6] Organolead is most readily absorbed, followed by lead salts and then metallic lead.

After ingestion, lead is ionized in the acidic environment of the stomach. Ionization increases absorption.[7] Absorption is also increased in animals with deficiencies of iron, zinc, vitamin D, or calcium.[6] Lead may also be inhaled if the dust is in a fine particulate state (sanded lead paint). Once deposited in the lungs, lead is almost completely absorbed.[8] Dermal absorption of inorganic lead is poor. However, grooming behavior of cats and even dogs can make a dermal exposure into an oral exposure.[8,9]

Once absorbed, more than 90% of lead is bound to red blood cells. Unbound lead is distributed widely with the highest concentrations in bone, teeth, liver, lung, kidney, brain, and spleen.[1,7] Lead precipitates as insoluble salts in bone and forms a long-term storage depot. Bone remodeling or chelation can release stored lead, resulting in clinical signs long after the original lead exposure.[1]

Lead is excreted from the body in various ways. A majority of ingested lead is excreted in the feces without being absorbed.[10] If lead is absorbed, it is filtered across the glomeruli and can accumulate in the renal tubular epithelium. Chelating agents will enhance the urinary excretion of lead. Small amounts of lead are secreted by the pancreas and some lead is excreted in milk.[7] Lead has a triphasic half-life in dogs of 12, 184, and 4591 days.[1]

Mechanism of Toxicity

Lead interferes with multiple processes within the body. It affects various cell types, enzymes, tissues, and organ systems. Lead competes with calcium ions, resulting in substitution for calcium in bone. Lead mimics or inhibits many cellular actions of calcium and alters calcium flux across membranes, ultimately increasing levels of cytoplasmic calcium in many cell types.[11,12] Acute calcium-mediated cell death and chronic impairment in neuronal differentiation and synaptogenesis result.[13] Increases in intracellular calcium in the cerebrovascular endothelium disturb microfilaments and/or other cellular components responsible for the integrity of tight junctions and contribute to cerebral edema.[14] A chronic feeding study in rats demonstrated a significant increase of lead in capillaries and synaptosomes in the brain.[15] This suggests a blood-brain barrier dysfunction. It is proposed that altered lipid composition of membranes may cause a change in membrane permeability. The increased susceptibility of juvenile animals to lead encephalopathy may be a result of the diminished ability of immature brain astrocytes to sequester lead.[16]

Lead's inhibition of calcium flux is responsible for some of its myriad effects on central and peripheral neurotransmission.[11] Lead can substitute for calcium in the activation of protein kinase C, which contributes to lead's amplification of glutamate-induced oxidative stress in the brain and other tissues.[17] Lead toxicosis can lead to inhibition of cytochrome P-450, which in turn results in inhibition of tryptophan pyrrolase, increased plasma tryptophan levels, elevations in brain serotonin levels, and ultimately, aberrant neurotransmission of serotonergic pathways.[1] Lead exposure has been associated with impaired growth hormone secretion and increased catecholamine levels.[18]

Lead may also alter many enzymes via its competing effects with other cations, such as ferrous iron and zinc. Interruption of zinc-dependent enzyme processes can interfere with gamma-aminobutyric acid (GABA) production or activity in the CNS.[19]

Lead interferes with cellular energy and metabolism in mitochondria. It affects calcium-sensitive mitochondrial permeability transition pores, which causes mitochondrial depolarization and the initiation of the cytochrome-*c*-caspase cascade resulting in apoptosis.[20]

Lead is especially toxic to the fetus and young animals because it inhibits dendritic arborization in the brain of the developing animal. Rat studies have demonstrated that lead exposure may alter the phosphorylation and binding activity of cyclic-AMP response element binding protein. This affects development of the hippocampus and cerebral cortex at certain stages of development.[21]

By binding with –SH (sulfhydryl) groups of enzyme systems, lead interferes with enzymes involved in heme synthesis, such as δ-aminolevulinic acid dehydratase (ALAD) and ferrochelatase. Lead causes a reduction in glutathione (GSH), and an increase in zinc protoporphyrin (ZPP), by altering the heme synthesis pathway. This results in red blood cell abnormalities and anemia.[1] Damage to membrane-associated enzymes such as sodium-potassium pumps results in red blood cell fragility and a shortened life span. The basophilic stippling of red blood cells is caused by accumulated ribosomal RNA aggregates. There is no degradation or dephosphorylation of RNA by pyrimidine-5′-nucleotidase (P5NT), because lead inhibits the activity of P5NT.[22] Increased serum ALAD levels themselves can be neurotoxic by interfering with GABA transmission.[1]

Lead-induced alterations in synaptic transmission at the neuromuscular junction of visceral smooth muscle can lead to altered intestinal motility and tone leading to lead colic.[23] Lead colic is from spasmodic contractions of the smooth muscles of the intestinal wall.[24]

Clinical Signs

Dogs and cats with lead poisoning show neurologic and gastrointestinal signs most commonly.[25] Acute lead poisoning is characterized by anorexia, vomiting, abdominal pain, behavior changes, ataxia, tremors, hyperexcitability, and seizures.[25] Chronic lead poisoning is somewhat more vague, with abdominal discomfort, vomiting, diarrhea, anorexia, lethargy, weight loss, anemia, behavior changes, intermittent seizures, and megaesophagus (cats; rare) reported.[25]

Lead easily crosses the placenta and is concentrated in breast milk.[26] Exposure during pregnancy has shown a preferential accumulation of lead in fetal rather than maternal bone in cynomolgus monkeys.[27] Inorganic lead salts have been shown to be teratogenic in experimental animals.[28] Prenatal lead exposure can affect reproductive function in the offspring (prolonged and irregular diestrous, reduced sperm counts).[29,30] Multiple animal studies have demonstrated behavioral abnormalities following intrauterine lead exposure.[31] Mobilization of lead from the maternal skeleton during pregnancy can also result in clinical signs in the dam.[32]

Minimum Database

Hematologic abnormalities may occur with lead toxicosis, but none is pathognomonic. Anemia may develop as lead affects heme synthesis at several enzymatic steps causing a shortened RBC lifespan and decreased erythrocyte replacement. With acute poisoning, lead-induced anemia is microcytic and hypochromic; as it becomes more chronic, it often changes to normochromic and normocytic.[9] Some lead salts can cause hemolysis.

Basophilic stippling and the presence of large numbers of nucleated red blood cells (5 to 40 per 100 white blood cells) without evidence of severe anemia are suggestive of lead toxicosis in small animals.[25] Basophilic stippling may be found with other disease processes.[25]

Leukocytosis is occasionally seen with lead toxicosis. Serum chemistry elevations of kidney and liver parameters may be seen in acute cases.[33] Lead objects are radio-opaque and can be found in the gastrointestinal tract or less commonly as embedded lead projectiles.

Confirmatory Tests

The diagnosis of lead poisoning is made by measuring whole blood lead levels. Whole blood is the preferred sample as more than 90% of circulating lead is bound to erythrocytes. Although an ideal blood lead level is zero (lead has no biologic value) in most species blood lead levels above 0.3 to 0.35 ppm (30-35 mcg/dL) indicate significant lead exposure. With appropriate clinical signs, these levels support the finding of lead toxicosis.[7,25] Blood lead levels greater than 0.6 ppm (60 mcg/dL) are diagnostic for lead toxicosis.[25] Blood lead levels change rapidly in response to acute lead intake, and blood levels may not necessarily correlate with severity of clinical signs.

Anemia, nucleated red blood cells, and basophilic stippling suggest lead intoxication but have other causes, and their absence does not rule out lead poisoning. Other confirmatory laboratory tests available for the live patient include measurement of erythrocyte ALAD activity, erythrocyte porphyrin assay, urinary ALA levels, and zinc protoporphyrin levels; these analyses, however, are rarely offered by veterinary diagnostic laboratories.

Radiographs may reveal radio-opaque lead objects. In chronic lead poisoning radio-opaque lines can be seen in the metaphyseal regions. For confirmatory testing postmortem, toxic levels of lead in canine tissues are liver (5-10 ppm, wet weight) and kidney (50-200 ppm wet weight).[34] Generally speaking, lead levels in liver and kidney that exceed 5 ppm wet weight indicate excessive lead exposure.

Treatment

Treatment of lead toxicosis consists of several steps. Animals should be stabilized first, followed by elimination of lead from the gastrointestinal tract, and then chelation therapy if needed. Symptomatic animals need to be stabilized. Seizuring animals should be treated with diazepam. Fluid and electrolyte abnormalities secondary to gastrointestinal signs should be corrected and antiemetics given if needed. If a dermal exposure has occurred, wash the animal thoroughly with liquid dish detergent and rinse with copious amounts of water.

Radiographs may be used to determine if there is any lead still in the digestive tract. Lead should be removed before chelation as many chelating agents may actually enhance gastrointestinal absorption of lead.[25,33] Induce emesis in dogs with hydrogen peroxide or apomorphine if lead is still in the stomach. Small objects or flakes of paint may be removed by gastric lavage with tap water or normal saline. Endoscopy or surgery may be employed to remove larger objects. Activated charcoal does not bind well to heavy metals and is not recommended.[35]

Enemas or cathartics may be used to help empty the gastrointestinal tract of lead. Sulfate-containing cathartics (magnesium or sodium sulfate) may bind with lead to form lead sulfate, which is poorly absorbed from the gastrointestinal tract.[25] Lead-containing shot or bullets in or adjacent to synovial joints should be surgically removed.

Various lead chelation agents have been used in domestic animals. Calcium disodium ethylene diamine tetraacetate (Ca-EDTA), BAL (British-Anti-Lewisite), d-penicillamine (cuprimine), and succimer (DMSA, Chemet) all have advantages and disadvantages to their use (Table 53-1). However, CaEDTA and succimer are generally speaking the most commonly used chelators in veterinary medicine.

The lead chelator of choice for several decades has been Ca-EDTA and it is the most efficient parenteral chelating agent. It is used off label in animals. It removes lead from blood and osseous tissues. The removal of lead from the bone can result in increases in blood lead levels and precipitate clinical signs during chelation. Ca-EDTA is nephrotoxic. Reduced doses must be used in patients with preexisting renal disease.[36] Other side effects include vomiting, diarrhea, anorexia, depression, and injection site pain. CA-EDTA may also bind essential minerals such as zinc, copper, iron, and calcium.[37] Dogs are dosed at 100 mg/kg/day for 2 to 5 days. Each dose is divided into four portions and diluted to a final concentration of 10 mg Ca-EDTA per mL of 5% dextrose before being administered at

Table 53-1	The Pros and Cons of Various Lead Chelators	
Chelator	**Pros**	**Cons**
CaEDTA	Most efficient	Nephrotoxic Painful injections Chelates essential minerals
BAL	Removes lead from brain	Nephrotoxic Painful injections
Penicillamine	Oral	Vomiting Nephrotoxic Chelates essential minerals
DMSA	Oral (rectally if vomiting) Does not chelate essential minerals Can use with lead in GI tract	Expensive

different subcutaneous sites. The daily dose of Ca-EDTA should not exceed 2 g per dog to decrease the risk of nephrotoxicosis.[25] The animal is rested for 5 days, and then treatment is repeated if needed. Improvement is normally seen within 24 to 48 hours. Concurrent zinc supplementation should be given. The recommended dose for cats is 27.5 mg/kg diluted in 15 mL of 5% dextrose subcutaneously every 6 hours for 5 days.[25] Monitor closely for nephrotoxicity.[35] Sodium EDTA should not be used for chelation, because of the risk of hypocalcemia.[37]

British-Anti-Lewisite (BAL or dimercaprol) is used alone or in conjunction with Ca-EDTA; adsorbs lead from the erythrocytes, removes lead from parenchymatous tissues (particularly the brain), and increases both urinary and biliary excretion of lead;[25] and is nephrotoxic and very painful on injection. It is reported that renal toxicity can be reduced by alkalinization of the urine,[38] but BAL should not be used in animals with hepatic dysfunction.[38] Side effects include vomiting, tachycardia, hypertension, mercaptan odor to breath, and seizures. Animals are dosed at 3 to 6 mg/kg intramuscularly 3 to 4 times daily.[35]

Penicillamine is another lead chelator. Penicillamine has the advantage that it is given orally and patients can be treated at home. Disadvantages include nephrotoxicity and that it cannot be started until all lead has been removed from the gastrointestinal tract. It also binds dietary copper, iron, and zinc. Dogs are dosed at 30 to 110 mg/kg/day PO divided q 6 hours for 7 days followed by 7 days of rest. Cats are given 125 mg/cat PO (not per kg) q 12 hours for 5 days.[35] Vomiting is the most common adverse effect. Premedicating with an antiemetic or by dividing the dose may decrease the gastrointestinal side effects. Penicillamine should not be used in pregnant animals because of teratogenesis.[39]

Succimer (2,3-dimercaptosuccinic acid, DMSA) is an orally administered chelator approved for use in children with lead poisoning.[40] It is a structural analogue to BAL. Succimer has been shown to be an effective off-label chelator of lead in animal studies.[41] It has fewer side effects and is more efficacious than penicillamine. Succimer is administered orally or rectally if the patient is vomiting. It is less likely to cause vomiting, nephrotoxicosis and does not bind essential minerals such as zinc, copper, calcium, and iron.[37] Succimer also has the advantage of not enhancing lead absorption from the gastrointestinal tract.[37,41] Dogs are dosed at 10 mg/kg PO or PR three times daily for 10 days and the dose can be repeated as needed.[37] Combining DMSA with taurine (50-100 mg/kg) increases depleted blood glutathione (GSH) levels, increases the activity of ALAD, and reduces the blood ZPP levels to near normal.[42] Succimer may be used alone and following EDTA and/or BAL.

Blood lead levels may rise following chelation and this could be caused by either re-exposure or "rebound," which consists of rising blood lead levels because of reequilibration with the bone. History and environmental investigation may be needed to ensure re-exposure is not occurring.

Prognosis

Prognosis in most cases is good with an early diagnosis and appropriate therapy. The source of the lead must be removed from the environment.

Gross and Histologic Lesions

Few gross lesions are reported in dogs and cats. Lead objects may be found in the gastrointestinal tract. On histopathology, there can be damage to brain capillaries and interstitial edema of white matter, particularly in the cerebellum and spinal cord, when there are signs of lead encephalopathy.[43] Myelin degeneration within the cerebellum and cerebrum and spongiosis of deep cerebral structures have also been reported.[44] Intranuclear inclusion bodies may be found in the renal tubular epithelium and degenerative changes may be seen in the liver and kidney of dogs with chronic lead toxicosis. Intranuclear inclusion bodies are rare in the hepatocytes of dogs with chronic toxicosis. Swelling of proximal renal tubular cells occurs early in lead toxicosis followed by tubular dilation, atrophy of the tubular lining cells, and interstitial fibrosis. Glomerular sclerosis and interstitial scarring develop after months of lead exposure.[38]

Differential Diagnoses

Some differential diagnoses for acute lead poisoning includes rabies, canine distemper, other viral encephalitides, toxoplasmosis, hepatic encephalopathy, idiopathic epilepsy, and gastrointestinal disorders.

Prevention

Dogs and cats can be sentinels for human exposure. Pet owners should be counseled about the potential for human exposure to lead in the household.[45] Local public health officials may be contacted for more information. If there is no obvious source of exposure, analysis of water and soil may be needed.

References

1. ATSDR: US Public Health Service, Agency for Toxic Substances and Disease Registry, Toxicological Profile for Lead. Agency for Toxic Substances and Disease Registry, US Department of Health and Human Services. Atlanta, GA, 2007. Available from http://www.atsdr.cdc.gov/toxprofiles/tp.asp?id=96&tid=22. Accessed 2011.
2. Lewis RJ: *Sax's dangerous properties of industrial materials*, ed 9, New York, 1996, Van Nostrand Reinhold.
3. Keogh J: Lead. In Sullivan J, et al: *Hazardous materials toxicology*, Baltimore, 1992, Williams & Wilkins.
4. Akhtar AJ, Funnye AS, Akanno J: Gunshot-induced plumbism in an adult male, *J Nat Med Assoc* 95(10):900–986, 2003.
5. ATSDR: *Lead toxicity*. Environmental alert: Course SS3059, US Department of Health and Human Services, Atlanta, GA, 2000, Agency for Toxic Substances and Disease Registry. Division of Health Education and Promotion.
6. Mahaffey KR: Nutritional factors in lead poisoning, *Nutr Rev* 39:353–365, 1981.
7. Schmitz DG: Toxicologic problems. In Reed SM, et al, editors: *Equine internal medicine*, Philadelphia, 1998, Saunders.
8. Harbison RM: *Hamilton and Hardy's industrial toxicology*, ed 5, St Louis, 1998, Mosby.
9. Zenz C: *Occupational medicine*, ed 3, St Louis, 1994, Mosby-Year Book.
10. Lewis RJ: *Hawley's Condensed Chemical Dictionary*, ed 14, New York, 2001, Wiley.
11. Bressler JP, Goldstein GW: Mechanism of lead neurotoxicity, *Biochem Pharmacol* 41:479–484, 1991.
12. Simmons TJB: Lead-calcium interactions in cellular lead toxicity, *Neurotoxicology* 14:77–86, 1993.
13. Shanne FAX, Kane AB, Young FE, et al: Calcium dependence of toxic cell death: a final common pathway, *Science* 206:700, 1979.
14. Hariri RJ: Cerebral edema, *Neurosurg Clin North Am* 5:687–706, 1994.
15. Struzynska L, Walski M, Gadamski R: Lead induced abnormalities in blood-brain barrier permeability in experimental chronic toxicity, *Mol Chem Neuropathol* 31:207–224, 1997.

16. Tiffany-Castiglioni E, Sierra EM, Wu JN, et al: Lead toxicity in neuroglia, *Neurotoxicology* 10:417–443, 1989.
17. Naarala JT, Loikkanen JJ, Ruotsalainen M, et al: Lead amplifies glutamate-induced oxidative stress, *Free Rad Biol Med* 19:689–693, 1995.
18. Huseman CA, Varma MM, Angle CR: Neuroendocrine effects of toxic and low blood lead levels in children, *Pediatrics* 90:186–189, 1992.
19. Gwaltney-Brant SM: Heavy metals. In Hascheck-Hock W, et al, editors: *Handbook of toxicologic pathology*, ed 2, San Diego, 2002, Academic Press.
20. He L, Poblenz AT, Medrano CJ, et al: Lead and calcium produce rod photoreceptor cell apoptosis by opening the mitochondrial permeability transition pore, *J Biol Chem* 275:12175–12184, 2000.
21. Toscano CD, McGlothan JL, Guilarte TR: Lead exposure alters cyclic-AMP response element binding protein phosphorylation and binding activity in the developing rat brain, *Dev Brain Res* 145:219–228, 2003.
22. George JW, Duncan JR: Pyrimidine-specific 5′ nucleotidase activity in bovine erythrocytes: effect of phlebotomy and lead poisoning, *Am J Vet Res* 43:17, 1982.
23. Janin Y, Couinuad C, Stone A, et al: The "lead-induced colic" syndrome in lead intoxication, *Surg Ann* 17:287–307, 1985.
24. Anzelmo V, Bianco P: Gastrointestinal and hepatic effect of lead exposure. In Castellino N, Castellino P, Sannolo N, editors: *Inorganic lead exposure*, Boca Raton, FL, 1995, CRC Press.
25. Kowalczyk DF: Lead poisoning. In Kirk RW, editor: *Current veterinary therapy IX*, Philadelphia, 1986, Saunders.
26. Hallen IP, Jorhem L, Oskarsson A: Placental and lactational transfer of lead in rats: a study on the lactational process and effects on offspring, *Arch Toxicol* 69:596–602, 1995.
27. Inskip MJ, Franklin CA, Subramanian KS: Sampling of cortical and trabecular bone for lead analysis: method development in a study of lead mobilization during pregnancy, *Neurotoxicology* 13:825–834, 1992.
28. Schardein JL: *Chemically induced birth defects*, ed 2, New York, 1993, Marcel Dekker.
29. McGivern RG, Sokol RZ, Berman NG: Prenatal lead exposure in the rat during the third week of gestation: long-term behavioral, physiological, and anatomical effects associated with reproduction, *Toxicol Appl Pharmacol* 110:206–215, 1991.
30. Coffigny H, Thoreux-Manlay A, Pinon-Lataillade G: Effects of lead poisoning of rats during pregnancy on the reproductive system and fertility of their offspring, *Human Exp Toxicol* 13:241–246, 1994.
31. Rodrigues AL, Rocha JB, Mello CF: Effect of perinatal lead exposure on rat behavior in open-field and two-way avoidance tasks, *Pharmacol Toxicol* 79:150–156, 1996.
32. Gulson BL, Jameson CW, Mahaffey KR: Pregnancy increases mobilization of lead from maternal skeleton, *J Lab Clin Med* 130:51–62, 1997.
33. Shannon M: Lead. In Shannon MW, Borron SW, Burns MJ, editors: *Haddad and Winchester's clinical management of poisonings and drug overdosage*, ed 4, Philadelphia, 2007, Saunders.
34. Puls R: *Mineral levels in animal health*, Clearbrook, British Columbia, 1988, Sherpa International.
35. Plumb DC: *Veterinary drug handbook*, ed 7, Ames, IA, 2011, Wiley-Blackwell.
36. Product information: *Calcium disodium versenate, edetate calcium disodium injection*, Northridge, CA, 2004, 3M Pharmaceuticals.
37. Ramsey D, et al: Use of orally administered succimer (meso-2, 3-dimercaptosuccinic acid) for treatment of lead poisoning in dogs, *J Am Vet Med Assoc* 208:37, 1996.
38. Casteel SW: Lead. In Peterson ME, Talcott PA, editors: *Small animal toxicology*, ed 2, St Louis, 2006, Saunders.
39. Linares A, Zarranz JJ, Rodrigues-Alarcon J: Reversible cutis laxa due to maternal d-penicillamine treatment, *Lancet* 2:43, 1979.
40. Product information: *CHEMET(R) oral capsules, succimer oral capsules*, Deerfield, IL, 2005, Ovation Pharmaceuticals, Inc.
41. Kapoor S, et al: Influence of 2,3-dimercaptosuccinic acid on gastrointestinal lead absorption and whole body retention, *Toxicol Appl Pharmacol* 97:525, 1989.
42. Flora SJS, Pande M, Bhadauria S, et al: Combined administration of taurine and meso 2,3-dimercaptosuccinic acid in the treatment of chronic lead intoxication in rats, *Human Exper Toxicol* 23:157–166, 2004.
43. Goldstein GW, Asbury AK, Diamond I: Pathogenesis of lead encephalopathy: uptake of lead and reaction of brain capillaries, *Arch Neurol* 31:382–389, 1974.
44. Jubb KVF, Huxtable CR: Pathology of domestic animals. In Jubb KVF, et al, editors: ed 4, San Diego, 1993, Academic Press.
45. Dowsett R, Shannon M: Childhood plumbism identified after lead poisoning in household pets, *N Engl J Med* 331:1661, 1994.

Lilies

Jeffery O. Hall, DVM, PhD, DABVT

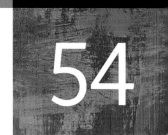

54

- *Lilium* spp. and *Hemerocallis* spp. plants are common ornamentals that are used as potted holiday houseplants and common constituents of flower arrangements.
- The true mechanism of toxicity is unknown, but it involves damage to the renal tubular epithelium resulting in renal failure in cats.
- Clinical signs include lethargy, vomiting, anorexia, and polyuria followed by anuria, weakness, and death.
- Clinicopathologic abnormalities include increases in creatinine and BUN, isosthenuria, glucosuria, proteinuria, and urinary casts.
- Confirmatory tests include identification of plant exposure, as well as clinical and pathologic compatible abnormalities.
- Treatment includes early decontamination, early aggressive fluid diuresis, and good supportive care. Once anuria develops, dialysis can be used.
- Prognosis is fair to good, depending on the timing of treatment initiation.
- Gross and histologic lesions include renal congestion, +/- perirenal edema, and renal tubular nephrosis with significant tubular casts.

Sources

The first report of *Lilium* spp. nephrotoxicity was presented in 1992 and was based on data generated at the ASPCA Animal Poison Control Center (ASPCA-APCC) in Urbana, Ill.[1] The first report involved *Lilium longiflorum* (Easter lily), but further observations now suggest that all species of the *Lilium* genera and plants in the *Hemerocallis* genera (day lilies) should be viewed as potentially nephrotoxic in cats.[1-7] It is of special note that the only animal to date that is known to be susceptible to the nephrotoxicity of these plants is the domestic cat.

The principal source of *Lilium* spp. and *Hemerocallis* spp. exposure in cats is via household entry of potted ornamental plants and floral arrangements. And since both the leaves and the flowers are associated with poisoning, corsages of these flowers also pose a risk. Although outdoor cats could be exposed to these plants in flowerbeds, currently there have only been reports of lethal indoor ingestions.

The key in first identifying the *Lilium* spp. as being toxic stemmed from the fact that some of these plants are more commonly introduced into houses during specific holiday seasons. The Easter lily is a common plant introduced into houses from 1 week before to 3 weeks after Easter and has resulted in clusters of cases being reported to the ASPCA-APCC.[8] Following these clusters, using past years' data, and following up on past reported exposures from previous years, it was found that this plant had a high risk of causing renal damage.

Toxic Dose

Species susceptibility to the toxic effects of *Lilium* spp. and *Hemerocallis* spp. lilies is quite distinct. The toxic effects of these plants have only been manifest in cats. After the original identification of suspected toxicity, rats, mice, and rabbits were fed plant material at up to 1.5% of their body weight without any adverse effects.[8] In addition, cases of ingestion by dogs have only resulted in gastrointestinal upset, without any renal effects.

Small amounts of plant ingestion can be toxic to cats. Ingestion of as little as 2 to 3 leaves or part of a flower has resulted in lethal effects in cats. The rapid onset of clinical signs, especially vomiting, likely limits the amount of plant ingestion. It has been found that the toxin(s) in the Easter lily is in the water-soluble fraction of the plant.[9]

Toxicokinetics

No true kinetic data are available for the toxin(s) in the *Lilium* spp. and *Hemerocallis* spp., since the toxin(s) have yet to be identified. However, it is likely that the toxic constituent of the plants is rapidly absorbed. This observation is based on the common finding that early emesis of the plant material may lessen the clinical effects,[8] but renal damage still occurs without other supportive treatment. In addition, clinical signs can begin as early as 5 to 10 minutes post ingestion.

The elimination of the toxin(s) from the body likely occurs within the first 48 hours, although the duration of clinical effects can last for several days. The longer duration of effects after the toxin(s) are eliminated is the result of acute renal tissue damage and secondary effects from the renal failure. Early fluid diuresis initiated before the onset of renal shutdown and continued for 24 to 72 hours can significantly prevent renal failure–associated death. These data suggest a relatively rapid elimination of the toxin(s), especially in the presence of fluid diuresis.

Metabolism of the toxin(s) of *Lilium* spp. and *Hemerocallis* spp. is unknown. But one potential cause for the sensitivity of cats could be a differing metabolism of the toxin(s), as compared with dogs, rats, mice, and rabbits, resulting in a toxic metabolite. This would be supported by the fact that direct application of the water-soluble plant components was not toxic to cultured feline renal tubular epithelial cells (unpublished data).

Mechanism of Toxicity

The exact mechanism of lily toxicity in cats is not known. However, it is known that it directly involves damage to the renal tubular epithelium and subsequent renal failure. Based on clinical field cases, it has been found that the mechanism of toxicity requires two components to result in the acute renal failure associated with anuria and death. The first component is the direct action of the plant toxin(s) on the renal tubular epithelium resulting in cellular damage and an initial polyuric renal failure. The second component is the development of severe dehydration caused by polyuric renal failure. This is based on the fact that fluid therapy and fluid diuresis before the onset of the anuric renal failure will prevent complete renal shutdown from developing.[1,3,5,8]

A study of Easter lily poisoning found that the water-soluble plant fraction was nephrotoxic. This study identified changes in the renal tubular epithelium consisting of swollen mitochondria, megamitochondria, edema, and lipidosis.[9] However, this study dosed quantities of extracted plant materials that would greatly exceed reported clinical ingestions and may or may not represent the mechanism in cases of much smaller ingestions.

Clinical Signs

Presenting clinical signs can differ, depending on the timing of presentation relative to the ingestion.[1,3,5,6-9] The first clinical signs are vomiting, salivation, anorexia, and depression and develop within the first 1 to 3 hours post ingestion. The vomiting and salivation will last for 2 to 6 hours, but the anorexia and depression last throughout the syndrome. The next observed clinical signs are the development of polyuria at 12 to 30 hours post ingestion, followed by a resulting dehydration at 18 to 30 hours. The polyuria lasts until the onset of anuria, which can develop by 24 to 48 hours. As the renal shutdown causes buildup of metabolic waste, the vomiting reoccurs, along with the onset of weakness by 30 to 72 hours. This is generally followed by recumbency and death. Deaths have been reported to occur by 3 to 7 days post ingestion. Seizures have also been reported, but they may be a secondary effect of severe uremia or caused by an extremely large ingestion, which would not be seen with the more typical case presentation.[6,9]

Minimum Database

Clinical signs and clinicopathologic changes can aid in establishing the clinical phase at presentation, allowing a more accurate prognosis and treatment regimen. Serum chemistry profiles to identify increases in BUN, creatinine, and potassium are necessary to establish the current degree of renal effects. In addition, urinalysis for identification of renal casts, isosthenuria, proteinuria, and glucosuria can be helpful. Early in the syndrome, the renal tubular casts that result from a complete sloughing of the tubular epithelium are so significant that cellular detail and nuclei can still be discerned in the cells of the casts.[8] Abnormalities in the urinalysis can occur as early as 12 hours post ingestion. In comparison, changes in the serum chemistry parameters do not generally occur until after 18 to 24 hours. Some cases develop increased aspartate transaminase (AST) and alanine aminotransferase (ALT) later in the syndrome, but this is likely due to the pronounced anorexia and associated hepatic stress. Increased creatinine kinase was identified in a dosing study with exaggerated doses compared with field case ingestions.[9]

Confirmatory Tests

Analytic verification of lily ingestion is currently not available. The most definitive confirmations are recognition of lily ingestion, compatible clinical syndrome, compatible clinicopathologic data, and lesions in the cats that die.

Treatment

In cases of known recent exposure, general decontamination procedures should be implemented. These procedures include evacuation of the gastric contents by induction of emesis (the editor is aware of endoscopy being employed to both visualize and remove plant material) and administration of activated charcoal along with a cathartic. However, in cases where significant vomition has already occurred, antiemetics followed by activated charcoal and a cathartic should be used. When implemented early after exposure, decontamination procedures will minimize the absorption of the toxin(s) and thus the potential for clinical effects.

In cats with clinical signs of lily poisoning that are not anuric, the best treatment to date is correction of the dehydration and the use of 2 to 3 times maintenance fluids to cause fluid diuresis. Fluid diuresis should be maintained for 48 to 72 hours. The exact duration of fluid diuresis necessary is not known, but before the onset of anuric renal failure, this protocol in cats has resulted in prevention of the anuric renal failure and survival in the vast majority of cases. Serum chemistry panels and urinalyses should be run every 12 to 24 hours throughout the treatment period.

Once anuric renal failure is present, the treatment options are limited. I am personally aware of two individual cases in which dialysis was performed on cats with lily-associated renal failure. Both cats survived and regained renal function by 10 and 14 days. However, both positive and negative outcomes have been reported for peritoneal dialysis.[6,8-11] Drugs that are normally used to stimulate renal output, such as furosemide, hypertonic dextrose, thiazides, and mannitol, have not been very successful in cases of anuric renal failure from lily poisoning. Thus, peritoneal dialysis and hemodialysis are the only potential treatments once anuria develops.

Prognosis

Prognosis should be based on the severity of effects at the onset of treatment. Early presentation followed by decontamination and fluid diuresis results in an excellent prognosis. However, presentation at the point of anuric renal failure warrants a guarded to poor prognosis. Since so few animals have been treated with dialysis, the true recovery potential is not known.

Gross and Histologic Lesions

Gross lesions are consistent with renal effects. Renal congestion and perirenal edema have been observed. Pulmonary congestion, gastrointestinal congestion, and paleness of the liver also have been reported and are thought to be secondary to severe uremia from the anuria and hepatic lipidosis from the anorexia.

Histologic lesions are primarily limited to the renal tissue. Severe renal tubular degeneration with luminal accumulation of cellular and proteinaceous debris is common. Collecting ducts are often occluded with casts. Pulmonary edema has been reported in some cases. In cats that survive past 3 to 5 days, it is not uncommon to find mitotic figures in the renal tubules suggestive of early repair. And, because the basement membrane is not affected, this is suggestive that dialysis would be successful in allowing return of renal function over time. Two cases have reported chronic fibrosing pancreatitis or pancreatic acinar cell vacuolization.[6,9] However, in the dosing study serum chemistry analysis did not find increased amylase.[9]

Differential Diagnoses

The clinical conditions that would be included in a differential diagnosis with lily poisoning include any cause of acute renal failure or gastrointestinal upset early in the syndrome. Other differential diagnoses may be ethylene glycol poisoning, ingestion of soluble oxalate-containing plants, boric acid poisoning, nephrotoxic mushrooms, aminoglycosides, NSAIDs, leptospirosis, acute presentation of a chronic renal failure, melamine-cyanuric acid poisoning, infectious renal disease, or metabolic renal disease.

References

1. Hall J: Nephrotoxicity of Easter lily (*Lilium longiflorum*) when ingested by the cat, *Proc Annu Meet Am Vet Int Med* 6:121, 1992.
2. Carson TL, Sanderson TP, Halbur PG: *Acute nephrotoxicosis in cats following ingestion of lily (Lilium sp.), proceedings of the 37th AAVLD meeting*, 1994.
3. Groff RM, Miller JM, Stair EL, et al: Toxicoses and toxins. In Norsworthy DG, editor: *Feline practice*, Philadelphia, 1993, Lippincott.
4. Gulledge L, Boos D, Wachsstock R: Acute renal failure in a cat secondary to Tiger lily (*Lilium tigrinum*) toxicity, *Feline Pract* 25:38–39, 1997.
5. Hall JO: Lily nephrotoxicity. In August JR, editor: *Consultations in feline internal medicine*, ed 4, Philadelphia, 2001, Saunders.
6. Langston CE: Acute renal failure caused by lily ingestion in six cats, *J Am Vet Med Assoc* 220:49–52, 2002.
7. Volmer P: Easter lily toxicosis in cats, *Vet Med* 94(4):331, 1999.
8. Hall JO: Nephrotoxicity of Easter Lily (*Lilium longiflorum*). In Panter KE, Wierenga TL, Pfister JA, editors: *Poisonous plants: global research and solutions*, Wallingford, UK, 2007, CABI.
9. Rumbeiha WK, Francis JA, Fitzgerald SD, et al: A comprehensive study of Easter lily poisoning in cats, *J Vet Diagn Invest* 16:527–541, 2004.
10. Cooper RL, Labato MA: Peritoneal dialysis in cats with acute kidney injury: 22 cases (2001–2006), *J Vet Internal Med* 25:14–19, 2011.
11. Dorval P, Boysen SR: Management of acute renal failure in cats using peritoneal dialysis: a retrospective study of six cases (2003–2007), *J Fel Med Surg* 11:107–115, 2009.

Poisonous Lizards

Michael E. Peterson, DVM, MS

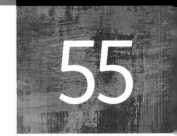

- Poisonous lizards are primarily located in the southwestern United States and Mexico.
- The median lethal intravenous dose (LD_{50} IV) of the venom is estimated to be 8 mg/kg in humans, 0.5 to 1 mg/kg in mice.
- Clinical signs include sudden onset of pain and bleeding at the bite site and local swelling. Marked hypotension and cardiac irregularities may be present.
- The minimum database includes blood pressure, respiratory rate, heart rate, hematocrit, and total protein. One may need a complete blood count, coagulation profile, serum chemistries, and electrocardiogram.
- Treatment includes the use of crystalloid fluids, pain control, and exploration of the wound for fractured lizard teeth.

Sources

There are two species of venomous lizards in the world. Both species belong to the genus *Heloderma* and are found in the Americas. Two *Heloderma* (gila monster) species, *H. suspectum* and *H. cinctum,* are found in the United States in an area extending from southern Utah through most of Arizona, areas of New Mexico and Nevada, and a small part of California. They are also found in Sonora, Mexico, west to the Gulf of California. The other species of *Heloderma, H. horridum* (the Mexican beaded lizard), is significantly larger than other Helodermatids and occupies parts of Mexico and Guatemala.[1]

These lizards are heavy bodied, large (adult gila monsters can reach 55 cm in length), and generally slow moving, but can strike relatively quickly. Their tails are blunt and rounded and may measure one-half of the lizard's total body length. They have tough, bead-like skin scales, which on gila monsters form a dark reticular pattern on a yellowish-orange background. The head is held low, has a rounded muzzle, and is flat and large. They have heavy mandibular musculature and a short neck. The feet are handlike and clawed.

The venom from these lizards is used for defense only because these animals raid burrows and nests, consuming eggs and preying on the young of birds and small mammals. The venom is excreted from venom glands located on the lower jaw. The venom delivery apparatus is poorly developed and relies on the grasping and chewing action of the lizard.[2] The venom apparatus consists of bilateral venom glands connected by a venom duct to the gums at the base of the teeth in the lower jaw. The venom is pulled up along grooves in these teeth by capillary and chewing action. Gila monsters bite tenaciously, and victims may be presented for veterinary care with the lizard still firmly attached.

621

Toxic Dose

The low end of the toxic dose for humans has been estimated at 8 mg venom (dry weight).[3] The average gila monster has a venom yield of 15 to 20 mg of venom (dry weight). The intravenous (IV) median lethal dose (LD_{50}) of venom in mice is 0.5 to 1 mg/kg of body weight. As a point of reference, the IV LD_{50} of western diamondback rattlesnake venom in mice is 2.18 mg/kg of body weight. The toxic dose for dogs and cats is unknown. Because of the poor venom delivery system of the lizard, the degree of envenomation is most likely a function of the duration of the bite. The author is aware of at least one fatal bite in a 20-kg dog. The dog was found agonal with the lizard still firmly attached; the duration of the bite was unknown.

Toxicokinetics

The toxicokinetics have not been extensively studied.

Mechanism of Toxicity

In animal studies, IV administration of Helodermatid venom into dogs and cats induced an initial tachypnea followed by a decrease in rate and depth of respiration, and eventual respiratory collapse. Increases in both lacrimation and salivation were noted, coupled with vomiting and polyuria. No confirmed evidence of coagulopathy has been identified, although there still is some suspicion that this may occur. Tachycardia, cardiac irregularities, and marked hypotension have also been described.[4]

Heloderma venom contains multiple fractions, which include hyaluronidase, arginine hydrolase, kallikrein-like enzymes, and phospholipase. Additionally, several other proteins have been identified. These include a pancreatic secretory protein exhibiting phospholipase activity, gilatoxin, helothermine, and a toxin that inhibits a contraction response to direct stimulation of isolated mouse diaphragm.[5]

Hyaluronidase, called the "spreading factor," facilitates the uptake of the venom by decreasing the viscosity of connective tissue through catalyzing the cleavage of internal glycoside bonds of some acid mucoglycosides. Destruction of the hyaluronic acid barrier permits the other venom components to penetrate deeper into the victim's tissue.[6]

Arginine hydrolase directs its activity toward hydrolysis of the peptide linkage to which an arginine residue contributes to a carboxyl group. The exact impact of this venom component has not been well defined, but it may have a bradykinin releasing–like effect.[5]

Kallikrein-like enzymes mimic the action of kallikrein by causing vasodilatation, increased capillary permeability, edema, and contraction or relaxation of extravascular smooth muscles. These enzymes also attract leukocytes and induce pain when injected subcutaneously.

Phospholipase has been identified in many types of venoms and exists as a variety of isoenzymes. One action of phospholipase is to uncouple oxidative phosphorylation, thereby inhibiting cellular respiration. Phospholipase can also contribute to the release of other active enzymes by causing membrane destruction along with other compounds like histamine, kinin, serotonin, acetylcholine, and slow-reacting substance.

Gilatoxin is an acidic neurotoxic protein.[7] Helothermine depresses the body temperature in mice that have been injected with this toxin.[8]

Clinical Signs

Poisonous lizards most commonly affect dogs. They are usually bitten on the lower lip, and the lizard may still be attached when the dog is presented. Human victims who have experienced previous pit viper bites claim that gila monster bites are more painful.

The pugnacious manner of the bite combined with the aggressive chewing action of the lizard often cause profuse hemorrhage at the bite site. Additionally, the teeth are brittle and may break off in the wound. These bites are intensely painful and usually reach peak pain levels within 1 hour after envenomation. This local pain may last for 24 hours. Although there may be some delay, edema generally occurs when venom has been injected. The area around the bite site is very tender, and regional lymphangitis can occur. Tissue necrosis is rare. However, ecchymoses may be evident.

In humans, systemic signs that may develop include weakness, dizziness, nausea, vomiting, tinnitus, muscle fasciculations, tachycardia, and hypotension. In canine and feline patients, increased respirations, vomiting, polyuria, salivation, lacrimation, and aphonia (in cats only) can occur.[9] There is no evidence that the venom has any effect on coagulation. However, because of the limited database available, this possibility cannot be ruled out. Bolus injection of *Heloderma* venom into dogs and cats has been shown to induce tachycardia, hypotension, and respiratory distress. Pulmonary congestion and edema have also been described.

Minimum Database

Pretreatment laboratory values should be obtained for the following parameters: blood pressure, respiratory rate, heart rate, hematocrit, and total protein. If the syndrome progresses or if the patient exhibits evidence of systemic envenomation, this database should be expanded to include a complete blood count with platelet count, coagulation profile (e.g., prothrombin time, partial thromboplastin time, and fibrinogen), serum electrolytes, electrocardiography, and urinalysis. Any abnormal values should be repeated as often as needed to monitor the progression of that parameter adequately.

Confirmatory Tests

In the United States no confirmatory tests are commercially available.

Treatment

Extraction of the lizard may be necessary if it is still attached. Placing a prying instrument between the jaws of the lizard and pushing against the back of the mouth can achieve this (be aware these lizards are toxic to humans and, it should be noted, federally protected). All patients bitten by Helodermatids should be hospitalized for several hours and monitored for evidence of and/or progression of envenomation.

The bite site should be irrigated (not infused) with lidocaine, cleaned, and gently probed with a 25-gauge needle to search for fractured teeth fragments. Because of the wide variety of pathogenic bacteria cultured from reptile mouths, broad-spectrum systemic antibiotics should be administered.

There is no specific antivenin available for lizard bites, and treatment consists primarily of supportive care. Intravenous fluid therapy should be started when hypotension is evident. Pain control can be obtained with carprofen. In general, nonsteroidal antiinflammatory agents, which can affect coagulation factors or platelets, should be avoided. Diazepam can reduce the need for analgesics.

Prognosis

Prognosis is generally guarded, given the toxicity of the lizard venom.

Gross and Histologic Lesions

Bleeding bite wounds with possible fractured lizard teeth are the only gross lesions visible.

Differential Diagnoses

Trauma and venomous snakebite are the two primary differential diagnoses.

References

1. Bogert CM, del Carpo RM: The gila monster and its allies. The relationships, habits, and behavior of the lizards of the family Helodermatidae, *Bull Am Mus Nat Hist* 1:109, 1956.
2. Fox H: Anatomy of the poison gland of *Heloderma*. In Loeb L, editor: *The venom of* Heloderma, Washington, DC, 1953, Carnegie Institution.
3. Phisalix M: Note sur les effects mortels reciproques des morsures de l'*Heloderma* suspectum cope et de la vipera aspis laur et sur les caracte'res diffe'rentiels de leurs venins, *Bull Mus Hist Nat Paris* 17:485, 1911.
4. Cooke E, Loeb L: General properties and actions of the venom of *Heloderma*, and experiments in immunization. In Loeb L, editor: *The venom of* Heloderma, Washington, DC, 1953, Carnegie Institution.
5. Alagon AC, Maldonado ME, Julia JZ: Venom from two species of *Heloderma horridum* (Mexican beaded lizard): general characterization and purification of N-benzoyl-L-arginine ester hydrolase, *Toxicon* 20:463–475, 1982.
6. Stybolva Z, Kornalik F: Enzymatic properties of *Heloderma suspectum* venom, *Toxicon* 5:139, 1967.
7. Hendon RA, Tu AT: Biochemical characterization of the lizard toxin gilatoxin, *Biochemistry* 20:3517–3522, 1981.
8. Mochca-Morales J, Martin BM, Possani LD: Isolation and characterization of helothermine, a novel toxin from *Heloderma horridum horridum* (Mexican beaded lizard) venom, *Toxicon* 28:299–309, 1990.
9. Patterson RA: Smooth muscle stimulating action of venom from the gila monster, *Heloderma suspectum*, *Toxicon* 5:5, 1967.

Macadamia Nuts

Sharon M. Gwaltney-Brant, DVM, PhD, DABVT, DABT

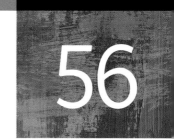

- Ingestion of macadamia nuts in dogs has been associated with weakness, depression, vomiting, ataxia, hind limb paresis/paralysis, joint and muscle pain, and joint swelling.
- The toxin is unknown, and treatment is supportive and symptomatic care.
- Most nuts are high in fat, and large exposures can pose a risk for the development of gastrointestinal upset and pancreatitis.
- Prognosis is excellent, and signs generally subside within 24 to 48 hours.

Sources

Macadamia integrifolia and *Macadamia tetraphylla* trees are members of the family Proteaceae that originated in Australia. The trees have been cultivated in the United States, primarily in Hawaii and California, since the late 1800s.[1] The majority of commercial macadamia nuts in the United States originate from Hawaii. Macadamia nuts contain 75% fat by weight, of which 80% is monounsaturated. Ingestion of a high-monounsaturated-fat diet based on macadamia nuts in humans has been shown to lower serum cholesterol and low-density lipoprotein levels.[2,3] Proteins (27% to 30%) and sugars (6% to 8%) comprise the majority of the oil-free components of macadamia nuts.[1] One novel protein (MiAMP1) found in macadamia nuts is being investigated for its potential antimicrobial activity.[4,5]

Macadamia nuts are popular snack foods, both as plain nuts and when incorporated into candies, cakes, and cookies. Ingredients other than macadamia nuts, such as chocolate, xylitol, and grapes/raisins, may also need to be considered as potential toxicants in cases where candies or baked goods containing the nuts have been ingested. Macadamia nut toxicosis has to date only been reported in dogs, who will readily ingest the nuts or products made from them.[6]

Toxic Dose

In dogs, ingestion of 2.2 grams of raw or roasted nuts per kilogram of body weight has been associated with the development of clinical signs.[7] Another source out of Australia cited a toxic dose, from field cases, as being between 0.7 and 4.9 g/kg body weight (5 to 40 nuts for a 20-kg dog).[8] In experimental trials, weakness was associated with doses ranging from 2.4 to 62.4 g/kg, whereas vomiting occurred with doses ranging from 7 to 62.4 g/kg. Based on these numbers, and assuming that a roasted macadamia nut weighs between 2.1 and 3 g (Gwaltney-Brant, personal observation), the minimum toxic dose of macadamia nuts for dogs is approximately 1 nut/kg BW. In four dogs experimentally dosed with a slurry of commercially available macadamia nuts at 20 g/kg, all dogs developed significant clinical signs of toxicosis.[6]

Toxicokinetics

No toxicokinetic studies have been reported in dogs. In dogs experimentally dosed with macadamia nuts, serum triglyceride levels peaked in 3 to 8 hours and returned to normal within 12 hours following dosing,[6] which suggests relatively rapid absorption of the lipid component of the nuts. The peak triglyceride levels mirrored most of the peak clinical effects seen in the experimental dogs.

Mechanism of Toxicity

Allergic reactions to macadamia nuts have been reported in humans; these allergies are IgE-driven and are thought to be similar to other nut allergies.[9] The mechanism of action for toxic reactions to macadamia nuts in dogs is currently not known.

Clinical Signs

Clinical signs in dogs generally develop within 6 to 24 hours of ingestion of macadamia nuts. The most common signs from field cases of macadamia nut ingestion by dogs, in descending order, are weakness (55%), depression (32%) vomiting (21%), ataxia (18%), tremors (18%), and hyperthermia (7%).[7] Joint and muscle pain, and swelling have also been reported.[8] Weakness in dogs experimentally dosed with macadamia nuts was noted within 6 hours of dosing and was characterized by difficulty in rising or inability to rise, reluctance to remain in a standing position, and/or decreased height when jumping in recovering dogs.[6] Some dogs have shown slightly exaggerated patellar and cranial tibial reflexes. Ataxia and tremors, not recorded in experimental cases but common in field cases, may have been related to weakness. The weakness peaked by 12 hours, improved greatly within 24 hours, and was completely resolved by 48 hours after dosing. Mild depression developed in most dogs within 3 hours of dosing, peaked at about 8 hours, and appeared resolved by 24 hours. Hyperthermia peaked by 8 hours with a range of 39.8° C to 40.5° C (103.6° F to 104.9° F) and returned to normal within 36 hours following dosing.

Minimum Database

Clinical laboratory evaluation of dogs experimentally dosed with macadamia nuts revealed a marked twofold to fivefold increase in serum lipase by 24 hours and return to normal by 48 hours postdosing.[6] Moderate increases in serum triglycerides (125 to 235 mg/dL; normal 20 to 150 mg/dL) were also noted within 6 hours of dosing. Serum alkaline phosphatase had slight elevations above baseline values (122 to 220 U/L; normal 1 to 88 U/L) that peaked at 24 hours postdosing (293 to 424 U/L) and remained elevated at 48 hours (237 to 308 U/L). Serum cholesterol and amylase remained unchanged from predosing values.

White blood cell (WBC) counts were elevated in all experimentally dosed dogs (18,400-26,500 cells/μL) within 24 hours following dosing, primarily because of significant increases in segmented neutrophils (15,640 to 23,585 cells/μL).[6] By 48 hours, the WBC counts of all but one of the dogs had returned to normal.

Confirmatory Tests

There are no specific tests to confirm exposure to macadamia nuts, so the diagnosis is based on history of exposure along with consistent clinical findings. Observation of feces may be beneficial in confirming exposures because many nut fragments pass through the GIT undigested.

Treatment

In asymptomatic dogs with recent ingestion of macadamia nuts, induction of emesis should be considered. Emesis may be followed by administration of activated charcoal with a cathartic, although the efficacy of activated charcoal in preventing absorption of the toxic principle(s) has not been established.

In most cases, dogs developing clinical signs subsequent to ingesting macadamia nuts can be managed with symptomatic care at home. Very young, old or debilitated dogs or dogs with significant preexisting medical conditions, may be best managed by symptomatic care and monitoring at a veterinary clinic. Intravenous fluid therapy and antiemetics may be considered in such dog, or in dogs presenting with signs that are more than mild to moderate in severity. Dogs coingesting chocolate, xylitol, or grapes/raisins may require treatment for these other toxicoses depending on the amount ingested.

Prognosis

The prognosis for recovery of dogs that develop clinical signs from ingesting macadamia nuts is usually excellent, and resolution of signs within 24 to 48 hours with minimal veterinary intervention is expected in the majority of cases.[7] Dogs with preexisting medical conditions or those that have co-ingested other toxicant(s) (e.g., chocolate, xylitol, grapes/raisins) may have slower or more complicated recoveries.

Gross and Histologic Lesions

As fatalities have not been reported with macadamia nut exposure, no gross or histopathologic lesions have been reported.[10] Given the transient nature of the clinical effects of macadamia nut toxicosis, it is unlikely that significant gross or histopathologic lesions related strictly to the nuts would be found in intoxicated dogs.

Differential Diagnoses

Other potential toxic causes of rear limb weakness, depression, and hyperthermia might include bromethalin, metaldehyde, ionophores, salicylates, hops (*Humulus lupulus*), and delayed neuropathy or intermediate syndrome associated with organophosphate insecticide exposure. Conditions not related to toxicosis that might have similar signs may include systemic infection, neoplastic syndromes, myasthenia gravis, coonhound paralysis, polyradiculoneuritis, botulism, spinal trauma, and pancreatitis.

References

1. California Rare Fruit Growers Inc: *Macadamia fruit facts*: http://www.crfg.org/pubs/ff/macadamia.html. 1997. Accessed September 13, 2011.
2. Curb JD, Wergowske G, Dobbs JC, et al: Serum lipid effects of a high-monounsaturated fat diet based on macadamia nuts, *Arch Intern Med* 160:1154–1158, 2000.
3. Garg ML, Blake RJ, Willis RB: Macadamia nut consumption lowers plasma total and LDL cholesterol levels in hypercholesterolemic men, *J Nutr* 133:1060–1063, 2003.
4. McManus AM, Neilsen KJ, Marcus JP, et al: MiAMP1, a novel protein from *Macadamia integrifolia* adopts a Greek key beta-barrel fold unique amongst plant antimicrobial proteins, *J Mol Biol* 293:629–638, 1999.
5. Stephens C, Harrison SJ, Kazan K, Smith FW, Goulter KC, Maclean DJ, et al: Altered fungal sensitivity to a plant antimicrobial peptide through over-expression of yeast cDNAs, *Curr Genet* 47(3):194–201, 2005.
6. Hansen SR, Buck WB, Meerdink G, et al: Weakness, tremors and depression associated with macadamia nuts in dogs, *Vet Hum Toxicol* 42:18–21, 2000.
7. Hansen SR: Macadamia nut toxicosis in dogs, *Vet Med* 97:275–276, 2002.
8. Gwaltney-Brant SM: Garbage ingestion, *Clinician's Brief* June:45–46, 2007.
9. Herbst RA, Wahl R, Frosch PJ: Specific IgE reactivity and identification for potential allergens in macadamia allergy, *J Eur Acad Dermatol Venereol* 24(11):1361–1363, 2010.
10. Sebastian MM: Role of pathology in diagnosis. In Gupta RC, editor: *Veterinary toxicology: basic and clinical principles*, New York, 2012, Academic Press, pp 100–1136.

Mercury

John H. Tegzes, VMD, MA, DABVT

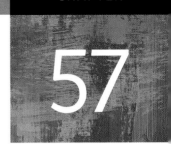

- Mercury is a naturally occurring metal. There are three primary forms: elemental, inorganic, and organic, each with its own distinct characteristics.
- Elemental mercury can be found in fluorescent lightbulbs, batteries, thermometers, barometers, lubrication oils, dental amalgams, and pressure-sensing devices. Inorganic mercury can be found in topical blistering agents, stool fixatives, latex paints, skin-lightening creams and soaps, laxatives, and old disinfectant and pesticide formulations. Organic mercury may be found in fish-based diets. Mercury toxicosis can result from acute high-dose exposures and from chronic low-dose exposures.
- Elemental mercury is not well absorbed from the stomach and will generally not cause poisoning in a healthy person except when high-dose exposures occur. Most forms of mercury are not well absorbed from the skin.
- Inhalation of elemental mercury vapors is the main cause of toxicity, followed by oral ingestion of inorganic or organic mercury–containing products. Once absorbed, mercury is directly cytotoxic. Following a one-time exposure, the gastrointestinal tract, lungs, and kidneys are the primary targets. Chronic inhalation exposure can cause selective damage to the central nervous system.
- Treatment includes decontamination, supportive care, and chelation to enhance elimination.
- Though renal and neurologic lesions are often irreversible, improvement has been seen several months after exposure ceases in some cases.

Sources

Mercury is a metal that exists in several physical and chemical forms. It occurs naturally in the earth's crust as inorganic mercury. Through a natural process of degassing from the earth's surface, it is released into the atmosphere as mercury vapor.[1] Mercury also enters the environment through volcanic activity.[2]

Human activity has generated sources of environmental mercury since Roman times, when the mining of mercury ore began.[1] Today, coal burning power stations and municipal waste incinerators liberate mercury vapor when household and commercial products that contain mercury are disposed of by this method. Elemental mercury can be found in fluorescent lightbulbs, batteries, thermometers, barometers, lubrication oils, dental amalgams, and pressure-sensing devices. Inorganic mercury can be found in topical blistering agents, stool fixatives, latex paints, skin-lightening creams and soaps, laxatives, and old disinfectant and pesticide formulations.

From whatever source, mercury vapors emitted into the atmosphere can reside there for many months and be distributed over vast geographical areas.[1] In fact, mercury contamination is a worldwide problem.

Once in the atmosphere, mercury vapor is slowly transformed to a water-soluble, inorganic form.[1] Water-soluble inorganic mercury is then precipitated back to the surface and accumulates in fresh and marine water bodies by direct contamination and through runoff into rivers and streams. Inorganic mercury is methylated to organic mercury by methanogenic bacteria, which are present in both fresh and marine waters.[1]

The methylated, or organic, form of mercury could potentially pose a threat to both humans and companion animals, such as dogs and cats. Methylated mercury readily enters the aquatic food chain by first diffusing into forms of zooplankton. Bottom-feeding fish consume zooplankton. Bottom-feeding fish are eaten by other fish, and mercury continues up the aquatic food chain reaching highest concentrations in the largest, long-lived carnivorous fish in both fresh and marine waters.[1] In this manner, mercury is biomagnified from environmental contamination of water approximately 1 million-fold by the time it reaches the top of the aquatic food chain.[1]

Fish-based diets therefore represent a potential source of mercury exposure for dogs and cats. There are many commercial and prescription veterinary diets that contain fish. Fish oil supplements are also frequently used in therapeutic regimens for a variety of conditions for dogs and cats. However, recent work has shown that commercial human-grade fish oil supplements contain very low concentrations of mercury, ranging from less than 6 mcg/L to 12 mcg/L.[3]

Another potential dietary mercury source could occur when food animals are inadvertently fed seed grain that has been treated with a methylmercury fungicide. These types of fungicides have been used on seed destined for planting, but not for seed used as feed. When the meat from these exposed animals is fed to pets, severe mercury poisoning could occur. This type of scenario has been reported in a family that ate the meat from a hog that was accidentally fed treated seed grain. The family members who ate the meat over a 3-month period developed long-term neurologic effects.[4]

Another potential source of mercury may be from ingestion of folk medicines. Nontraditional remedies may sometimes be used by animal owners on their pets and should be considered when taking a history in cases with unusual presentations. Some folk medicines contain inorganic mercury compounds, and some Latin American and Caribbean communities have used elemental mercury in religious and cultural rituals.[5] Animals may be exposed intentionally or inadvertently.

Inhalation of elemental mercury vapors could conceivably happen in pets where mercury has contaminated a household through broken thermometers, barometers, or fluorescent lightbulbs. Poisonings could also potentially occur in pets ingesting products containing the inorganic mercury forms, such as mercuric chloride (e.g., stool fixatives, latex paint, laxatives, old disinfectants and pesticides, topical therapeutic agents, and blistering agents).

Toxic Dose

When determining exposure doses in pet animals, it is important to consider whether the exposures have been acute or chronic. This information can be correlated with data from the primary literature, as both acute and chronic dosing studies have been performed in cats. Cats given oral doses of methylmercuric hydroxide at 1.29 and 0.86 mg/kg per day began exhibiting clinical signs after 15 days of daily exposure.[6] Chronic doses of methylmercury at 0.25 mg/kg per day produced clinical signs between 76 and 100 days of daily dosing.[7] In this chronic study, a total dose of between 19 and 25 mg/kg was required before clinical signs were observed.[7] In a long-term diet study using fish contaminated with methylmercury, cats did not develop clinical signs or damage to the central nervous system (CNS) when doses were below 46 mcg/kg/day, even after 1175 to 1227 days.[8] Clinical signs referable to the nervous system and notable pathologic findings in the CNS were found in cats dosed with 176 mcg/kg/day for 92 to 119 days and in cats dosed with 74 mcg/kg/day after 276 to 526 days.[8,9]

It is possible for the veterinary clinician to estimate the mercury exposure from fish diets. Edible tissues from swordfish and shark can contain 1 mcg/g of mercury, whereas tuna, trout, pike, and bass can contain about 0.1 to 0.5 mcg/g. Invertebrates, such as shellfish, have even lower concentrations.[3] Unfortunately, the specific fish and concentrations included in commercial pet foods are usually not known.

Because there are several possible sources of mercury exposure in companion animals, it is difficult to determine the toxic dose from chronic, possibly lifelong, exposure. Background exposure levels to pet animals do tend to mimic human exposure rates in certain geographic regions.[6] So if this information is known from regional public health data, it may be possible to estimate potential exposure levels.

Toxicokinetics

Mercury poisoning can occur after ingestion, inhalation, injection, or dermal absorption of various forms of mercurials.[10] Mercury vapor is absorbed by the lungs and dissolves in the systemic circulation, where it travels to all tissues.[1] It readily crosses the blood-brain and placental barriers. Excretion is mostly in the urine and feces, though a small amount is excreted by the lungs.[1]

Ingested elemental mercury is generally poorly absorbed. Absorption of inorganic mercury depends on its solubility, because soluble inorganic compounds can be sufficiently absorbed orally and cause severe poisoning.[1] Inorganic mercury can also be absorbed by the lungs after inhalation, and by the skin after integumentary exposure.[1] Following distribution, inorganic mercury accumulates in greatest concentrations in the kidneys. Excretion is via the feces and urine.

Organic mercury is well absorbed from the gastrointestinal tract after ingestion.[1] After absorption, it is carried by erythrocytes to various tissues throughout the body.[11] It readily crosses the blood-brain and placental barriers.[1] Excretion is primarily in the feces.

Mechanism of Toxicity

Inhaled mercury vapor is highly diffusible and lipid soluble and readily crosses cell membranes. Once inside the cell, it is converted to Hg^{++} ion (mercuric ion) and is directly cytotoxic.[1] The central nervous system and kidneys are the primary targets.

Inorganic mercury attaches to thiol-containing molecules, such as cysteine and glutathione, in cells.[1] In the presence of organic ligands, it releases Hg^{++} ion, which is the toxic species of mercury.[1] The primary target organ of acute poisoning with inorganic mercury is the gastrointestinal tract. Chronic exposures lead to kidney dysfunction; the pars recta of the proximal tubule is the most vulnerable segment of the nephron to toxic injury.[12] Through molecular interactions at nucleophilic sites,[13] the Hg^{++} ion directly damages the epithelial cells of the proximal tubule, resulting in the failure of solute and water reabsorption.[1]

Methylmercury also has a high affinity for thiol-containing molecules.[1] Over time, it is slowly degraded to inorganic mercury, probably by the action of phagocytic cells.[1] This conversion results in the presence of inorganic mercury in the kidney, brain, and other tissues, even when the source of exposure was from organic mercury.[1] There is selective damage to the central nervous system that has not yet been explained.[1] In severe poisoning, the peripheral nervous system is also affected. Extensive loss of neuronal cells occurs in the granular layer of the cerebellum, in the visual cortex, and other focal areas. Consistent with this pathology, clinical signs include ataxia and constriction of the visual fields.[1]

Clinical Signs

Because mercury can affect multiple organ systems, the clinical effects seen are varied. The clinical presentation also depends on the form of mercury, the concentration, and whether it is an acute or chronic exposure. In general, the most consistent signs of mercury poisoning in mammals are anorexia, nervous dysfunction, renal dysfunction, gastrointestinal signs, shock, and death.[14] Nervous signs include ataxia, decreased conscious proprioception, blindness, paresis, tremors, and seizures.[14] Gastrointestinal signs include vomiting, diarrhea, abdominal pain, and hypersalivation.[14]

Inhaled mercury vapor can cause direct lung damage and pneumonitis.[1] In humans, a syndrome of mercurialism has been described after chronic exposures of weeks or more to mercury vapor. This syndrome is characterized by tremors, erethism, and gingivitis. Erethism is evidenced by extreme shyness, hallucinations, or aggressive behavior.[1]

Clinical signs seen in cats with chronic methylmercury poisoning include anorexia, ataxia, intention tremors, impaired righting reflex, hypermetria, proprioceptive deficits, blindness, vertical nystagmus, and tonic-clonic seizures.[6,7] In terms of behavior, cats fed a fish diet were less active than similar cats fed a beef diet. On necropsy, the cats fed the fish diets had significantly higher brain, kidney, liver, and muscle mercury concentrations. It was speculated that the mercury content of the fish diet caused the behavior changes.[15]

Clinical signs seen in dogs with acute mercury poisoning include intermittent or persistent vomiting (with or without blood), diarrhea, ataxia, reluctance to walk, horizontal nystagmus, and progressive depression with seizure activity.[14] After a 7-year exposure to a daily fish diet, a dog that developed ataxia and behavioral changes slowly improved and returned to normal months after the fish diet was withdrawn.[16]

Minimum Database

Because mercury can affect multiple organ systems, the minimum database should include a chemistry profile that includes electrolytes, glucose, BUN, and creatinine to assess renal function and electrolyte balance; liver transaminases (aspartate and alanine), alkaline phosphatase, and total bilirubin to assess liver function; and a complete blood count to assess red blood cell morphology and number. A urinalysis is also indicated to assess the renal function. In addition to clinical pathology, a thorough neurologic examination is warranted along with a thorough history to help determine possible sources of mercury exposure.

Confirmatory Tests

Mercury exposure can be confirmed by measuring whole blood and urine mercury concentrations. Urine mercury concentrations are not usually elevated following exposure to organic mercury, so if the source of exposure is to the organic form, then whole blood analysis is the preferred sample. Whole blood mercury and urine concentrations exceeding 6.0 ppm and 1.5 ppm, respectively, indicate excessive mercury exposure.

To confirm mercury exposure in deceased animals, liver and kidney samples can be collected and analyzed for mercury.[17] Additionally, brain and skeletal muscle may also contain elevated concentrations of mercury in animals chronically exposed.[15]

Histochemical visualization of mercury in tissue can be done when the mercury present in the tissue is chemically bound to either sulfide or selenide ions.[17] Histopathology of the brain and kidneys can often confirm the presence of associated lesions.

Treatment

Decontamination after acute oral exposures to all forms of mercury includes the oral administration of activated charcoal. In cases of very recent large ingestions, gastric lavage may be performed before administering activated charcoal. Administering a bulk laxative to pets ingesting energy-saving lightbulbs and thermometers and following its movement via radiography are warranted.

Treatment of acute and chronic exposures to inorganic and organic mercury is largely symptomatic and supportive. In cases of mercury vapor exposure, supplemental oxygen may be indicated when acute pneumonitis is present. Acute ingestion of inorganic mercury salts may precipitate severe gastroenteritis, renal failure, and shock. Intravenous fluid therapy to replace fluids and maintain urine output is indicated, along with the use of gastrointestinal protectants and antiemetics.

Chelation therapy may be indicated to enhance mercury excretion after both acute and chronic exposures. Oral succimer (meso-2,3-dimercaptosuccinic acid [DMSA]) is protective against the acute lethal and nephrotoxic effects of inorganic mercuric salts in animals and also increases the urinary excretion of mercury.[5] A suggested dosage of succimer would be the one recommended for lead poisoning (see Chapter 53). D-Penicillamine may also be given orally after the intestinal tract has been cleared of inorganic mercury salts. There is limited data that oral succimer and oral N-acetylcysteine may be effective in decreasing mercury concentrations in tissues, including the brain, after organic mercury exposure.[5]

Prognosis

Although most of the renal and neurologic lesions produced by mercury toxicosis are irreversible, there are reports of improvement once exposure ceases.[16] However, several months of supportive care may be necessary before improvements are seen.

Gross and Histologic Lesions

Grossly, gastrointestinal lesions can include gastric ulcers, necrotic enteritis, and colitis, especially after acute ingestion of mercury salts.[18] The kidneys may be pale and swollen. Histologically, there may be renal tubular cell degeneration and necrosis with proteinaceous cast formation. Nervous system lesions may be present in the cerebrum, cerebellum, brainstem, and spinal cord.[14] Changes consist of loss of nerve cells with replacement by reactive and fibrillary gliosis.[7] Neuronal necrosis and perivascular cuffing within the cerebrum, cerebellum, and brainstem have been reported after chronic methylmercury feeding studies in cats.[6]

Differential Diagnoses

Differential diagnoses would include other toxic causes of renal tubular disease, such as acute ethylene glycol toxicosis, and causes that are not toxic in nature, such as infectious agents like leptospirosis. Nervous system clinical signs may also be caused by other heavy metals, such as lead, or other nervous system disorders, such as encephalitis and distemper. The gastrointestinal signs associated with mercury poisoning are nonspecific and differentials can include numerous toxic (e.g., lead, thallium, inorganic arsenic, zinc phosphide, zinc, vomitoxin) and nontoxic (e.g., pancreatitis, gastrointestinal obstruction, liver disease, renal disease) causes.

References

1. Clarkson TW: The toxicology of mercury, *Crit Rev Clin Lab Sci* 34(3):369–403, 1997.
2. Fitzgerald WF, Clarkson TW: Mercury and monomethyl mercury: present and future concerns, *Environ Health Perspect* 96:159–166, 1991.
3. Foran SE, Flood JG, Lewandrowski KB: Measurement of mercury levels in concentrated over-the-counter fish oil preparations, *Arch Pathol Lab Med* 127:1603–1605, 2003.
4. Davis LE, Kornfeld M, Mooney HS, et al: Methylmercury poisoning: long-term clinical, radiological, toxicological, and pathological studies of an affected family, *Ann Neurol* 35:680–688, 1994.
5. Kosnett MJ: Mercury. In Olson KR, editor: *Poisoning and drug overdose*, ed 4, New York, 2004, Lange Medical Books/McGraw-Hill.
6. Davies TS, Nielsen SW: Pathology of subacute methylmercurialism in cats, *Am J Vet Res* 38(1):59–67, 1977.
7. Munro IC, Moodie A, Willes RF, et al: Toxic effects of methylmercury in the cat, *Toxicol Appl Pharmacol* 22(2):294–295, 1972.
8. Nera EA, Charbonneau SM, Munro IC: Chronic toxicity of methylmercury in the adult cat, *Toxicol Appl Pharmacol* 23(1):192, 1976.

9. Charbonneau SM, Munro EA, Nera EA, et al: Chronic toxicity of methylmercury in the adult cat, *Toxicology* 5:337–349, 1976.

10. Graeme KA, Pollack CV: Heavy metal toxicity, part I: arsenic and mercury, *J Emerg Med* 16(1):45–56, 1998.

11. Doi R, Tagawa M: A study on the biochemical and biological behavior of methylmercury, *Toxicol Appl Pharmacol* 69(3):407–416, 1983.

12. Zalups RK: Molecular interactions with mercury in the kidney, *Pharmacol Rev* 52(1):113–143, 2000.

13. Yeh J-H, Chung H-M, Ho C-M, et al: Mercury-induced Ca2+ increase and cytotoxicity in renal tubular cells, *Life Sci* 74:2075–2083, 2004.

14. Farrar WP, Edwards JF, Willard MD: Pathology in a dog associated with elevated tissue mercury concentrations, *J Vet Diagn Invest* 6:511–514, 1994.

15. Houpt KA, Essick LA, Shaw EB, et al: A tuna fish diet influences cat behavior, *J Toxicol Environ Health* 24:161–172, 1988.

16. Hansen JC, Reske-Nielsen E, Thorlacius-Ussing O, et al: Distribution of dietary mercury in a dog; quantitation and localization of total mercury in organs and central nervous system, *Sci Total Environ* 78:23–44, 1989.

17. Hansen JC, Danscher G: Quantitative and qualitative distribution of mercury in organs from arctic sledgedogs: an atomic absorption spectrophotometric and histochemical study of tissue samples from natural long-termed high dietary organic mercury-exposed dogs from Thule, Greenland, *Pharmacol Toxicol* 77(3):189–195, 1995.

18. Osweiler GD: Mercury toxicosis. In Osweiler GD, editor: *Toxicology*, Philadelphia, 1996, Lippincott Williams & Wilkins.

Metaldehyde

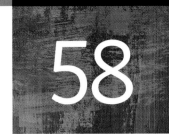

Ahna G. Brutlag, DVM, MS
Birgit Puschner, DVM, PhD, DABVT

- Metaldehyde, a common molluscicide, is widely used for the control of slugs and snails.
- The target organ of toxicity is the central nervous system. Clinical signs of acute exposure to metaldehyde include tremors, seizures, hyperthermia, salivation, restlessness, panting, vomiting, and ataxia.
- Metaldehyde toxicity results in the disruption of the GABAergic system. Monoamine oxidase, serotonin or 5-hydroxytryptamine, and norepinephrine may also be involved in the toxic mechanism.
- Treatment aims to decontaminate the poisoned animal, stabilize vital signs, control muscle tremors and seizure activity, and correct metabolic acidosis.
- Accurate diagnosis must be made via careful correlation of data collected from the history, clinical signs, clinical abnormalities, and toxicologic analysis.
- Animals that survive the first 24 hours of intoxication have a good prognosis and spontaneous recurrent seizures are not expected.

In the United States, metaldehyde is most commonly encountered as the active ingredient in slug and snail baits. If ingested, it can result in severe neurologic signs with tremors, seizures, and secondary hyperthermia being the most notable. This common collection of clinical signs has given rise to the informal name for this poisoning: "shake and bake syndrome."

Poisoning from metaldehyde has been frequently reported in dogs, livestock, horses, and humans. Dogs often eat baits voraciously, whereas cats in contrast are more selective in their eating behavior. Although cats are quite susceptible to this agent, few toxicoses have been documented. Metaldehyde, a tetramer of acetaldehyde, has been used as a molluscicide worldwide for more than 60 years. Preparations of snail baits made in the 1960s and early 1970s were attractive not only to snails but also to dogs and may account for the large number of dog poisonings reported during that time period. Such poisonings are less common now because some formulations are made to be less attractive to dogs. In some countries other than the United States, it is also used as a solid fuel. In general most exposures to metaldehyde are acute and require immediate treatment. Dogs and cats can be exposed to other neurotoxicants that cause similar clinical signs, and only careful correlation and evaluation of data collected from the history, clinical signs, clinical abnormalities, and chemical analysis will lead to an accurate diagnosis.

Sources

Metaldehyde is primarily used to kill slugs and snails to protect horticultural crops and household gardens. Baits are commonly available in the form of granules (often dyed), but can also be obtained as liquid, powder, meal, gels/pastes, or pellets that can release metaldehyde for approximately 10 to 14 days under moderately moist conditions. Baits are sometimes mixed with other herbicides and pesticides, most commonly with carbamate insecticides (e.g., carbaryl, 5%). Bran or molasses is commonly added to the bait to increase its attractiveness to snails and slugs, causing this form of bait to be attractive and palatable to dogs as well. Regulatory action requiring that snail baits be unattractive to dogs exists in some countries and states.[1,2]

The concentration of metaldehyde in baits sold for domestic use in the United States is generally between 2% and 5%. The product trade names most commonly reported to the Pet Poison Helpline include Ortho Bug-Geta Snail & Slug Killer (metaldehyde, 3.25%); Ortho Bug-Geta Plus Snail, Slug, & Insect Killer (metaldehyde, 2% and carbaryl, 5%); Corry's Slug & Snail Death (metaldehyde, 3.25%); RainTough Deadline Slug & Snail Killer (metaldehyde, 4%); Force II Deadline Slug & Snail Killer (metaldehyde, 4%); and Lily Miller Slug, Snail & Insect Killer Bait (metaldehyde, 2% and carbaryl, 5%).[3] Other trade names of metaldehyde-containing products available in the United States include Antimilace, Cekumeta, Meta, Metason, OR-CAL, Slugger Snail & Slug Bait, Ortho Metaldehyde 4% Bait, Slug Pellets, Slugit Pellets, and Slug-Tox. In Europe baits can contain up to 50% metaldehyde, and metaldehyde is also used as a fuel in small heating systems, such as camping stoves and lamps.[4] Trade names for metaldehyde fuel are Meta-fuel and Meta-Brennstoff, which are available in the form of tablets, solid blocks, or powder. In Japan metaldehyde is an ingredient in color flame tablets that are ignited for entertainment.[4]

Toxic Dose

Metaldehyde is moderately toxic when ingested. Acute oral median lethal dose (LD_{50}) values range from 210 to 600 mg/kg of body weight for dogs and 207 mg/kg of body weight for cats.[5-7] To be conservative, decontamination and/or medical observation is typically recommended in healthy adult cats or dogs ingesting more than 1/10 to 1/5 of the lowest reported LD_{50}. Inhalation exposure is unlikely but can occur with exposure to dusts of commercial pesticide products. Inhalation LD_{50} values (4 hours) of 203 mg/m^3, 203 mg/m^3, and 175 to 700 mg/m^3 are reported for rats, mice, and guinea pigs, respectively.[8]

Toxicokinetics

The solubility of metaldehyde in water is poor, which may limit the rate of absorption; however, metaldehyde is absorbed intact from the gastrointestinal tract.[9] In the stomach, metaldehyde may undergo some acid hydrolysis to acetaldehyde. The half-life of metaldehyde at 24° C is 0.75 and 4 hours, in 0.1 and 0.01 mol/L aqueous hydrochloric acid, respectively.[10] In 0.18 mol/L physiological gastric hydrochloric acid, metaldehyde is unlikely to hydrolyze extensively in the stomach before absorption. Once absorbed, the metabolic fate of metaldehyde is largely unknown, although a rapid metabolism is suspected. The involvement of cytochrome P450 enzymes has been suggested because P450 inducers protect against metaldehyde toxicity.[11] In mice it was reported that only 8% of an oral dose was excreted unmetabolized in urine and feces.[11] Urinary excretion in dogs dosed with metaldehyde was less than 1%.[5] The apparent elimination half-life derived from a human metaldehyde poisoning case was approximately 27 hours.[12] Although data on elimination kinetics in animals are not available, it is presumed that the hydrolysis product acetaldehyde is rapidly converted to carbon dioxide and eliminated via expiration.

Mechanism of Toxicity

Studies have suggested that acetaldehyde is unlikely to be the toxicant in metaldehyde poisoning since acetaldehyde is extremely unstable and is rapidly oxidized to carbon dioxide.[13] This finding is supported by several studies in which acetaldehyde was not detected in plasma or urine of metaldehyde-treated dogs[6] or brains of mice poisoned with metaldehyde.[10] Thus, the toxicity of metaldehyde is not mediated by or perhaps is only partly mediated by the degradation product acetaldehyde. Instead metaldehyde itself may be the actual toxicant that acts on the γ-aminobutyric acid (GABA)-ergic system.

Metaldehyde readily crosses the blood-brain barrier and was detected in the brain, blood, and liver of mice given metaldehyde orally at toxic and nontoxic doses.[10] It was also found in the serum and urine of a human for up to 3 to 4 days following exposure.[12] Decreased brain concentrations of GABA, norepinephrine (NE), and serotonin or 5-hydroxytrypta-mine (5-HT) and increased monoamine oxidase (MAO) activity were seen in mice dosed with metaldehyde.[14,15] GABA has an inhibitory role in neuronal excitation, and a decrease in GABA levels may lead to convulsions. The mechanism of disruption of the GABAergic system by metaldehyde is still unknown, but inhibition of glutamic acid decarboxylase as the cause of reduction of GABA concentrations is unlikely.[10] Depletion of central stores of NE and 5-HT is correlated with a decreased threshold of convulsions.[16] Because MAO is an important enzyme in the metabolism of NE and 5-HT, these may interact to contribute to the mode of action, in addition to GABA.

Hyperthermia can play a major role in the pathophysiology of metaldehyde toxicosis, and it is assumed that the muscle tremors often seen in metaldehyde-poisoned animals are the primary cause of body temperatures in excess of 41° C to 42° C (106° F to 107° F). At body temperatures of 42° C to 43° C (107° F to 109° F), cellular necrosis may begin to occur within a few minutes in all organ systems.[17] Hyperthermia may alter electrolyte balances, and metaldehyde is reported to cause severe acid-base derangements. The resulting metabolic acidosis is associated with hyperpnea and central nervous system (CNS) depression.

Clinical Signs

In dogs the main clinical features of metaldehyde poisoning involve the central nervous system with common signs including muscle tremors, seizures, secondary hyperthermia (often exceeding 41° C to 42° C or 106° F to 107° F), tachypnea or hyperpnea, tachycardia, excessive salivation, and ataxia.[18,19] Other reported signs include depression, vomiting, diarrhea, hyperesthesia, incoordination, and nystagmus. Opisthotonos and convulsions may occur in severely poisoned patients.[6,20] Clinical signs often develop within 30 minutes to 3 hours of ingestion of a toxic dose but a longer duration for onset of clinical signs is possible.[18] Convulsions are often continuous, sometimes elicitable by external stimuli in dogs, and give way to CNS depression and narcosis. Death from disseminated intravascular coagulation (DIC) and/or respiratory failure may occur within 4 to 24 hours or later after exposure.[19] Animals may recover if narcosis does not become too deep. If the animal survives the acute period, it may suffer from liver damage within 2 to 3 days after exposure (although serious, this is not commonly observed in clinical cases). Liver damage and cirrhosis may lead to delayed death. However, if the animal has not been lethally poisoned, full recovery may occur within a few weeks. In one case a dog that survived metaldehyde toxicosis was blind initially, but regained normal vision within 3 weeks after exposure.[21]

In cats metaldehyde poisoning may cause locomotor signs, dyspnea, hyperthermia, muscle spasms, mydriasis, and opisthotonos.[22] Perhaps more pronounced than in dogs, nystagmus may develop in cats, and external stimuli may evoke convulsions. Recovery may take approximately 2 weeks in cats with no sequela. Secondary illness, such as liver disease, has not been reported in cats.

Metaldehyde is often used in combination with carbaryl or methiocarb, carbamates that may cause muscarinic and nicotinic signs in animals upon ingestion. In this type of scenario, the clinical signs may be more complicated.

Confirmatory Tests

Chemical analysis for metaldehyde of the stomach contents (best), serum, urine, and liver is available at many veterinary diagnostic laboratories. Samples must be kept frozen for analysis. Bait material can also be tested for metaldehyde, and this may add important information.

Treatment

There is no antidote for metaldehyde intoxication and, given the potential for severe intoxication, rapid treatment is critical and should focus on decontamination; controlling hyperthermia, tremors, and seizures; maintaining adequate organ perfusion; and monitoring for the development of metabolic acidosis.

Emetics, gastric lavage, and enemas are recommended for removal of metaldehyde from the gastrointestinal tract. Prompt but appropriate decontamination results in a high survival rate and a significant reduction in the duration of treatment.[20] Careful evaluation of each patient is required before a specific method of decontamination is chosen. Emetics are recommended only in patients that are asymptomatic, with little risk for developing aspiration pneumonia, and that have recently ingested the material (<1-2 hours). The induction of emesis at home is not always advisable due to the rapid onset of CNS stimulation and, often, is most safely performed in a veterinary setting.

In cases of very recent ingestion, the induction of emesis may be attempted at home in dogs (not cats) by administering fresh 3% hydrogen peroxide (1 mL/pound, PO). If the dog has not vomited within 5 to 10 minutes and remains asymptomatic, a second dosage may be administered. Offering a small amount of food prior to the administration of hydrogen peroxide may increase its effectiveness. Unfortunately, there are currently no safe and effective at-home emetic agents for cats. Products such as table salt, mustard, and syrup of ipecac are no longer recommended in any veterinary species.

If emesis cannot be safely induced at home, apomorphine (0.03-0.04 mg/kg, IV, IM, or place the tablet directly into the subconjunctival sac) may be used in dogs. If subconjunctival apomorphine is used, the subconjunctival sac must be flushed thoroughly after emesis or protracted vomiting may occur. The use of apomorphine in cats is not recommended due to poor efficacy and the potential for CNS stimulation. Instead, xylazine (0.44 mg/kg, IM) or dexmedetomidine may be administered. Reversal with yohimbine (0.1 mg/kg, IM, SQ, or slowly IV) or atipamezole (Antisedan, 25-50 mcg/kg, IM or IV) should be performed if severe CNS and/or respiratory depression develop.

Gastric lavage is indicated when massive ingestion has occurred (greater than LD_{50}) or when emesis is unproductive or contraindicated. Typically, gastric lavage is recommended following a recent (<1-2 hours) ingestion; however, there are two case reports in which a productive lavage was performed 36 hours after ingestion due to persistent neurologic signs.[19]

Following lavage or the induction of emesis, the administration of one dose of activated charcoal (1-5 grams/kg, PO) with a cathartic such as sorbitol is indicated. In order to reduce the risk of aspiration, administration via an orogastric tube is advised in any symptomatic patient. Due to the lack of evidence for enterohepatic recirculation, multiple doses of activated charcoal are not typically recommended. Finally, enemas with tepid water can further help with the decontamination. Anecdotally, this method of decontamination has been reported to be of great benefit for metaldehyde, specifically.

Controlling tremors and seizures with muscle relaxants and anticonvulsants is critical as persistent signs can result in severe hyperthermia, rhabdomyolysis with secondary acute renal failure (rare), and DIC. For tremors, methocarbamol (55-220 mg/kg, IV to effect, repeat PRN; not to exceed 330 mg/kg/day) is the drug of choice and large doses may be necessary. Diazepam (0.5-1 mg/kg, IV repeat in 5 minutes if no effect) is the initial drug of choice for seizure control. Diazepam has a short duration of action ranging from 20 to 60 minutes and can be repeated if necessary. If initial diazepam treatment has no effect or seizures continue once the drug wears off, continuous rate infusion of diazepam or midazolam may be used. Additionally, phenobarbital has excellent anticonvulsant properties and is generally recommended to supplement diazepam. The onset of the drug occurs about 15 to 30 minutes after administration and should therefore be administered simultaneously with diazepam. In order to effectively load the patient give four dosages of 4 mg/kg, IV q 4 hours. Alternatively, a single dose of 16 to 20 mg/kg may be given IV, especially in cases of severe poisoning. Be alert to the potential development of severe CNS depression and hypoventilation. As mentioned earlier, metaldehyde degradation may be regulated by cytochrome P450 enzymes. Phenobarbital is an inducer of hepatic microsomal enzymes and can be of benefit in metaldehyde poisoning cases by potentially increasing the metabolic degradation of metaldehyde. If adequate doses of methocarbamol, benzodiazepines, or barbiturates are not sufficient to control the patient's seizures, inhalant anesthetics may be used. All patients under general anesthesia require endotracheal intubation and ventilation.

Because of the severe hyperthermia resulting from tremors and seizures, direct and evaporative cooling measures are often needed including ice baths, cold IV fluids, the use of fans, and application of alcohol to the pinna and paw pads. Cooling measures should be stopped once the body temperature has been reduced to 39.7° C (103.5° F) to avoid hypothermia and the body temperature should be monitored every 1-2 hours thereafter.

Intravenous fluid therapy should be instituted to control hyperthermia, maintain perfusion, and prevent or correct dehydration. Fluid administration and control of seizures may also correct metabolic acidosis that is often seen with metaldehyde poisoning. If venous blood gas analysis reveals a severe metabolic acidosis (pH <7.1, base excess <-15, HCO_3 <11 mEq/L), alkalinization therapy with sodium bicarbonate may be required (0.5-1 mEq/kg, IV slowly over 1-3 hours).

Intensive laboratory monitoring is required, especially in patients with severe clinical signs. Venous blood gas analysis should be performed to note acid-base disturbances (especially metabolic acidosis), coagulation parameters should be monitored for the development of DIC, renal and electrolyte parameters monitored for the onset of acute renal failure secondary to rhabdomyolysis, and blood glucose concentrations for the presence of hyper- or hypoglycemia. Hepatic damage is a rare but possible sequela to metaldehyde intoxication so hepatic parameters should be rechecked 2 to 3 days following clinical resolution. Additionally, hepatoprotectants such as SAMe (20 mg/kg, PO q 24 h for 2 weeks) can be considered.

Prognosis

The prognosis is good if the animal survives the first 24 hours after exposure and receives treatment as soon as possible. Initially, treatment is directed toward removing metaldehyde from the gastrointestinal tract and controlling seizures, hyperthermia, and respiratory depression. After the acute clinical signs have been controlled, treatment must focus on minimizing possible liver damage. Death is frequently due to DIC or respiratory failure so laboratory and clinical monitoring are paramount. In cases where adequate treatment and monitoring is provided, a full recovery is generally expected within 2 to 3 days.

In dogs suffering prolonged periods of status epilepticus (SE), concern regarding the development of epilepsy later in life has been raised as this has been observed in other species. In rodent models of epilepsy chemoconvulsant agents were administered in order to achieve SE of greater than 30 minutes' duration. This duration of SE is typically sufficient to induce epileptogenesis, resulting in spontaneous recurrent seizures following a latency period of one month.[23,24] Similar results have been reported in humans where febrile seizures during childhood have been associated with the development of epilepsy.[25] Recent studies have explored the potential for epileptogenesis in dogs following SE induced by specific toxicants including metaldehyde.[26,27] A population of 20 dogs (metaldehyde = 17) experiencing SE for greater than 30 minutes' duration (range 0.8 to more than 36 hours) was monitored for a median of 757 days (range 66-1663 days). None of the dogs in this study developed spontaneous recurrent seizures following intoxication. Likewise, from a group of 14 dogs that also suffered SE following intoxications (metaldehyde = 3), none developed spontaneous recurrent seizures.[27] These studies support the notion that no long-term neurologic sequela are expected following metaldehyde intoxication and that the use of anticonvulsant medications following discharge is not indicated.

Gross and Histologic Lesions

Metaldehyde has a characteristic odor of formaldehyde that may be present in the stomach contents along with bait material. No consistent and pathognomonic gross or histologic lesions occur in metaldehyde-poisoned animals. Necropsy findings in dogs may include hepatic, renal, and pulmonary congestion.[28] The lung tissue may show edema and interstitial hemorrhage. Petechial and ecchymotic hemorrhages may be present in the gastrointestinal mucosa. Also, severe subepicardial and subendocardial hemorrhages may be found. In animals that survive the acute phase of poisoning, degeneration of liver and ganglion cells in the brain may occur. Most reported necropsy findings date from the 1970s, and only a few postmortem reports are available. The high survival rate (close to 100% with optimal treatment) of metaldehyde-poisoned animals is most likely the reason why limited information is available on gross and histopathologic lesions. No data on necropsy findings in cats poisoned with metaldehyde are available.

In rats poisoned with metaldehyde, necropsy findings may reveal a fracture or dislocation of the vertebrae and subsequent compression of the spinal cord.[29] The definitive cause of the lesion remains unknown, and it may be secondary to posterior paralysis.

Differential Diagnoses

Table 58-1 describes the most important toxicology differential diagnoses and their clinical signs. It is evident that a definite diagnosis of metaldehyde poisoning can be difficult. One of the crucial clinical signs of metaldehyde poisoning that requires special attention is hyperthermia because it is not as commonly observed in other neurotoxicoses. In addition to the listed toxicants, neurotoxic mushrooms, cyanide, neurologic pharmaceuticals (e.g., antidepressants, anxiolytics, sleep aids), and illicit drugs should also be considered.

Other differential diagnoses of seizures in small animals include metabolic diseases (involving hypoglycemia, uremia, and hypocalcemia), neoplasms, thiamine deficiency, bacterial or viral encephalitis, severe head trauma, and congenital disorders (e.g., hydrocephalus, portosystemic shunt, idiopathic epilepsy, and lysosomal storage diseases). Breed or species predisposition, age of onset, and a complete history are important for each animal and will help establish an accurate diagnosis.

Table 58-1	Differential Diagnoses of Metaldehyde Poisoning
Toxicant	**Common Clinical Signs**
4-Aminopyridine (avicide)	Acute onset, salivation, tremors, tachycardia, ataxia, seizures
Amphetamines (commonly prescribed for ADD/ADHD)	Acute onset, restlessness, hyperactivity, tachycardia, mydriasis, tachypnea, tremors, seizures
Blue-green algae — cyanobacteria (anatoxin-A and saxitoxins)	Peracute onset, hypersalivation, vomiting, diarrhea, cyanosis, limb twitching, rigors, coma, seizures
Bromethalin (rodenticide)	Acute or delayed onset (until several days after ingestion), muscle tremors, hyperexcitability, hind limb ataxia, paresis, or paralysis, running fits, seizures (potentially evoked by external stimuli), vocalization (cats)
Chocolate (theobromine) and caffeine	Acute onset, hyperactivity, vomiting, diarrhea, PU/PD, tachycardia, hypertension, ataxia, tachypnea, muscle tremors, seizures
Hops (*Humulus* spp.)	Acute onset, severe hyperthermia, tachypnea, panting, tachycardia, anxiety, vomiting
Ivermectin and related drugs	Acute or delayed onset, depression, blindness, comatose, seizures
Methionine (urine acidifier)	Acute onset, vomiting, salivation, abdominal pain, ataxia, seizures, agitation, restlessness, pacing, hyperactivity, disorientation

Table 58-1	Differential Diagnoses of Metaldehyde Poisoning—*cont'd*
Toxicant	**Common Clinical Signs**
Organochlorine insecticides (e.g., DDT, lindane)	Acute onset, hypersalivation, tremors, hyperactivity, ataxia, circling, hyperthermia, clonic-tonic seizures potentially evoked by external stimuli
Organophosphorus and carbamate insecticides	Acute onset, acetylcholinesterase depression (blood and brain), nicotinic, muscarinic and central nervous system signs
Penitrem A (moldy walnuts and dairy products) and roquefortine (blue cheese and decaying organic matter)	Acute onset, frequent defecation and urination, muscle tremors, ataxia, polypnea, hyperthermia, seizures (potentially evoked by external stimuli)
Pyrethrin and pyrethroid insecticides	Acute onset, hypersalivation, anorexia, vomiting, ataxia, depression, muscle tremors, weakness, dyspnea, seizures, temporary blindness
Sodium chloride (e.g., table salt, play dough)	Acute onset, vomiting, diarrhea, anorexia, ataxia, tremors, seizures, coma, dehydration, hyperthermia, tachypnea, tachycardia, blindness
Sodium fluoroacetate (compound 1080)	Acute onset, vomiting, diarrhea, frequent urination, restlessness, pulmonary edema, hyperirritability, running fits, opisthotonos, paddling, tonic-clonic seizures
Strychnine (rodenticide)	Acute onset, muscle tremors, extensor rigidity, hyperesthesia, opisthotonos, sawhorse stance (tetany), seizures (potentially evoked by external stimuli)
Xylitol (in chewing gum, breath mints, dental products, etc.)	Acute onset, vomiting, signs secondary to hypoglycemia (weakness, depression, ataxia, tremors, collapse, seizures)
Zinc phosphide (rodenticide)	Acute onset, anorexia, vomiting, weakness, lethargy, tachypnea, pulmonary edema, recumbency, hyperesthesia, running fits, seizures

References

1. Kitchell RL, Schubert TA, Mull RL, et al: Palatability studies of snail and slug poison baits, using dogs, *J Am Vet Med Assoc* 173(1):85–90, 1978.
2. Firth AM: Treatment of snail bait toxicity in dogs: literature review, *Vet Emerg Crit Care* 2(1):25–30, 1992.
3. Shintani S, Goto K, Endo Y, et al: Adsorption effects of activated charcoal on metaldehyde toxicity in rats, *Vet Hum Toxicol* 41:15–18, 1999.
4. Pet Poison Helpline. Unpublished data. Pet Poison Helpline and SafetyCall International, PLLC, Bloomington, MN. Accessed January 4, 2011.
5. Hatch RC: Poisons causing nervous stimulation or depression. In Booth NH, McDonald LE, editors: *Veterinary pharmacology and therapeutics*, Ames, IA, 1988, Iowa State University Press.
6. Booze TF, Oehme FW: An investigation of metaldehyde and acetaldehyde toxicities in dogs, *Fund Appl Toxicol* 6:440–446, 1986.
7. von Burg R, Stout T: Toxicology update-metaldehyde, *J Appl Toxicol* 11(5):377–378, 1991.
8. Registry of Toxic Effects of Chemical Substances (RTECS): *Computerized database*, Cincinnati, OH, 1991, National Institute for Occupational Safety and Health.
9. Keller KH, Shimizu G, Walter FG, et al: Acetaldehyde analysis in severe metaldehyde poisoning, *Vet Hum Toxicol* 33:374, 1991.
10. Sparks SE, Quistad GB, Cole LM, et al: Metaldehyde molluscicide action in mice: distribution, metabolism, and possible relation to GABAergic system, *Pest Biochem Physiol* 55:226–236, 1996.
11. Tardieu D, Thouvenat N, Fargier C, et al: Phenobarbital-type P450 inducers protect rats against metaldehyde toxicity, *Vet Hum Toxicol* 38(6):454–456, 1996.

12. Moody JP, Inglis FG: Persistence of metaldehyde during acute molluscicide poisoning, *Hum Exp Toxicol* 11:361–362, 1992.
13. Zaleska MM, Gessner PK: Metabolism of [^{14}C] paraldehyde in mice in-vivo, generation and trapping of acetaldehyde, *J Pharm Exp Ther* 224(3):614–619, 1983.
14. Homeida AM, Cook RG: Pharmacologic aspects of metaldehyde poisoning in mice, *J Vet Pharmacol Ther* 5:77–81, 1982.
15. Homeida AM, Cook RG: Anticonvulsant activity of diazepam and clonidine on metaldehyde-induced seizures in mice: effects on brain gamma-amino butyric acid concentration and monoamino oxidase activity, *J Vet Pharmacol Ther* 5:187–190, 1982.
16. Kilian M, Frey HH: Central monoamines and convulsive thresholds in mice and rats, *Neuropharmacology* 12:681–692, 1973.
17. Morgan RV: Heat prostration. In Morgan RV, editor: *Handbook of small animal practice*, New York, 1998, Churchill Livingstone.
18. Richardson JA, Welch SL, Gwaltney-Brant SM, et al: Metaldehyde toxicoses in dogs, *Compend Conti Educ Vet* 25(5):376–380, 2003.
19. Yas-Natan E, Segev G, Aroch I: Clinical, neurological and clinicopathological signs, treatment and outcome of metaldehyde intoxication in 18 dogs, *J Small Anim Pract* 48:438–443, 2007.
20. Firth AM: Treatment of snail bait toxicity in dogs: retrospective study of 56 cases, *J Vet Emerg Crit Care* 2(1):31–36, 1992.
21. Bishop CH: Blindness associated with metaldehyde poisoning, *Vet Rec* 96:438, 1975.
22. Jacquier C: Guerison de deux chats intoxiques au meta, *Arch Tierheilk* 120:47–50, 1978.
23. Cavalheiro EA, Leite JP, Bortolotto ZA, et al: Long-term effects of pilocarpine in rats: structural damage of the brain triggers kindling and spontaneous recurrent seizures, *Epilesia* 32:778–782, 1991.
24. Stafstrom CE, Thompson JL, Holmes GL: Kainic acid seizures in the developing brain: status epilepticus and spontaneous recurrent seizures, *Brain Res* 65:227–236, 1992.
25. Wallace RH, Marini C, Petrou S, et al: Mutant GABA(a) receptor gamma2-subunit in childhood absence epilepsy and febrile seizures, *Nat Genet* 28:49–52, 2001.
26. Jull P, Risio LD, Horton C, et al: Effect of prolonged status epilepticus as a result of intoxication on epileptogenesis in a UK canine population, *Vet Rec* 169:361–364, 2011.
27. Zimmermann R, Hulsmeyer VI, Sauter-Louis C, et al: Status epilepticus and epileptic seizures in dogs, *J Vet Intern Med* 23:970–976, 2009.
28. Maddy KT: Poisonings of dogs with metaldehyde in snail and slug poison bait, *Calif Vet* 29(4):24–25, 1975.
29. Verschuuren HG, Kroes R, Den Tonkelaar EM, et al: Long-term toxicity and reproduction studies with metaldehyde in rats, *Toxicology* 4:97–115, 1975.

Methanol

Karyn Bischoff, DVM, MS, DABVT

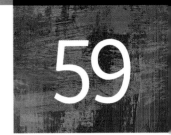

- Methanol (methyl alcohol) is found in windshield washer fluid, gasoline antifreeze, rubbing alcohol, Sterno, model airplane fuel, and paint remover. It is also used as an industrial solvent.
- Methanol toxicosis in most domestic animals is not as severe as in primates, and blindness does not occur.
- Clinical signs include CNS depression and behavioral abnormalities.
- Treatment is mainly symptomatic and supportive. Therapy using fomepizole or ethanol is unlikely to be of benefit and could be harmful in most veterinary patients, with the exception of primates.

Methanol is commonly found in automotive windshield washer fluid, some gasoline additives, and other solvents and household products. Although methanol causes severe acidosis and blindness in humans, other primates, and a few laboratory animals, clinical signs in most domestic animals are less severe and are similar to ethanol toxicosis.

Sources

Methanol, or methyl alcohol, is a colorless, nearly flavorless solvent with a specific gravity of approximately 0.80 at 0° C. Methanol is found in automotive products, including windshield washer fluid, gasoline antifreeze, and alternative fuels. It is a common industrial solvent and is sometimes present in household products such as paint removers, Sterno, model airplane fuel, and rubbing alcohol.

Toxic Dose

The toxicity of methanol to humans and other primates is well known, but it is considerably less toxic to other mammalian species.[1,2] Lethal human toxicosis has been reported at doses as low as 0.1 mL/kg.[3] However, the toxic oral dose for methanol in dogs is much higher: approximately twice that of ethanol.[4] The oral median lethal dose (LD_{50}) of methanol in dogs is reported to be between 5 and 11.25 mL/kg.[1,4] Methanol toxicosis in mammals other than primates is due to direct central nervous system (CNS) depressant effects and is similar to ethanol toxicosis.[1,4]

Toxicokinetics and Mechanism of Toxicity

Methanol is rapidly absorbed from the digestive tract.[1,5] Toxic dermal and inhalation exposures have been reported in humans.[6] It is believed that half of the dose of methanol is eliminated by the lungs in dogs.[5] A small amount is eliminated unchanged by the kidneys.[7] The rest is metabolized.

Methanol is oxidized in the liver to formaldehyde.[1] The enzyme responsible for this process varies from species to species. Alcohol dehydrogenase is preponderant in most primates, and a catalase peroxidase complex predominates in rodents, humans, and possibly some other species.[1,3,4,8,9] Formaldehyde is rapidly oxidized to formic acid by formaldehyde dehydrogenase.[4] Formic acid is responsible for the delayed clinical signs of methanol toxicosis in humans and other primates.[2,3,4,6,8,9] Formic acid causes acidosis directly and indirectly in primates through cytochrome C oxidase inhibition, which interferes with aerobic metabolism.[3,8-12] Inhibition of mitochondrial cytochrome is also responsible for the CNS effects.[3] Formic acid is metabolized relatively rapidly to carbon dioxide and water by an enzyme system that depends on tetrahydrofolate in most domestic species, but this enzyme system is deficient in humans and some primates.[4] Toxicity of methanol is enhanced in folic acid–deficient animals.[4]

Clinical Signs

Clinical signs of methanol toxicosis in dogs and other nonprimates are similar to those of ethanol toxicosis. CNS depression, possibly narcosis, and behavioral changes are the dominant signs. The depressive effects usually last <12 hours and have no residual effects. Methanol is teratogenic in laboratory rodents, causing impairment of neural tube closure.[9,13]

The first stage of methanol toxicosis in primates is a brief period of CNS depression or inebriation, similar to the narcotic effects seen in other species. Primates then undergo a latent period of 12 or more hours, during which formic acid accumulates to high concentrations in the circulation. The second stage is marked by more severe CNS signs and the beginning of visual disturbances.[4,11] Primates are the only mammals known to accumulate enough formic acid after methanol ingestion to produce acidosis.[14] Bilaterally reduced pupillary light reflexes and retinal and optic disk edema are common in methanol-intoxicated humans and monkeys but have not been reported in nonprimate mammals.[14] The nervous and ocular effects associated with formic acid in humans are irreversible in one tenth to one third of affected patients.[3,6]

Minimum Database and Confirmatory Tests

No consistent clinical pathology findings have been reported in nonprimate mammals exposed to methanol. The osmolal gap can be elevated early, but it decreases as the methanol is metabolized.[3,6] Primates in the second phase of methanol toxicosis have an increased anion gap and severe metabolic acidosis due to formic acid accumulation.[3,6]

Diagnosis of methanol poisoning in small animals is based on clinical signs and a history of exposure. Methanol concentrations in blood can be determined by gas chromatography if required.

Treatment

Treatment of methanol toxicosis in humans is similar to treatment of ethylene glycol toxicosis, and includes antidotal use of fomepizole or ethanol and correction of acidosis.[1,3,5,8,12] Folinic acid is a reduced form of folic acid that is rapidly converted to bioactive folate and is used during treatment of methanol toxicosis to enhance formic acid metabolism in humans.[12] Hemodialysis is also used to remove methanol and formic acid from the circulation.[3,6,12]

Treatment of methanol toxicosis in nonprimates is based on detoxification and symptomatic therapy. Dermal exposure should be treated with a mild detergent bath. Activated charcoal and cathartic treatment are unlikely to be helpful because of the rapid uptake of methanol from the gastrointestinal tract.[6,12] Correct dehydration and any electrolyte abnormalities is a necessity. Except in primates, there is no evidence that fomepizole or ethanol administration is beneficial in methanol toxicosis. Ethanol treatment would likely cause further CNS impairment and prolong clinical toxicosis in most domestic animals.

Prognosis

The prognosis for methanol ingestion in companion animals is usually good, but it depends on the extent of CNS depression. The prognosis in primates is much more guarded, with human mortality rates reported over 10%.[15]

Gross and Histologic Lesions

There are no specific lesions associated with methanol poisoning in nonprimate mammals. Changes reported in humans who died from methanol toxicosis include retinal and optic disk edema.[2,4] The most common CNS lesion is hemorrhage and necrosis of the putamen, though the optic nerve and other areas of the brain also can be affected.[15-17]

Differential Diagnoses

Some toxicants that could mimic this clinical presentation include ethanol, ivermectin and other macrolide antiparasitic agents, ethylene glycol, propylene glycol, diethylene glycol, 2-butoxyethanol, isopropanol, sedatives and tranquilizers, marijuana, xylitol, and amitraz.

References

1. Valentine WM: Short-chain alcohols, *Vet Clin North Am Small Anim Pract* 20(2):515–523, 1990.
2. Eells JT: Methanol-induced visual toxicity in the rat, *J Pharmacol Exp Ther* 257(1):56–63, 1991.
3. Jammalanadaka D, Raissi S: Ethylene glycol, methanol, and isopropyl alcohol intoxication, *Am J Med Sci* 339(3):276–281, 2010.
4. Wimer WW, Russell JA, Kaplan HL: *Alcohol toxicology*, Park Ridge, NJ, 1983, Noyes Data Corp.
5. Herd-Kuenzi LA: Methanol intoxication in a dog, *J Am Vet Med Assoc* 183(8):882–883, 1983.
6. Kraut JA, Kurtz I: Toxic alcohol ingestions: clinical features, diagnosis, and management, *Clin J Am Soc Nephrol* 3(1):208–225, 2008.
7. Lund A: Metabolism of methanol and formic acid in dogs, *Acta Pharmacol* 4:108–121, 1948.
8. Sullivan-Mee M, Solis K: Methanol-induced vision loss, *J Am Optom Assoc* 69(1):57–65, 1998.
9. Dorman DC, Dye JA, Nassise MP, et al: Acute methanol toxicity in minipigs, *Fund Appl Toxicol* 20(3):341–347, 1993.
10. Jacobsen D, Bredesen JE, Eide I, et al: Anion and osmolal gaps in the diagnosis of methanol and ethylene glycol poisoning, *Acta Med Scand* 212(1–2):17–20, 1982.
11. McMartin KE, Ambre LJ, Tephly TR: Methanol poisoning in human subjects: role of formic acid accumulation in the metabolic acidosis, *Am J Med* 68(3):414–418, 1980.
12. Barcelous DG, Bond GR, Krenzelok EP, et al: American Academy of Clinical Toxicology practice guidelines on the treatment of methanol poisoning, *Clin Toxicol* 40(4):415–446, 2002.
13. Medinsky MA, Dorman DC: Recent developments in methanol toxicity, *Toxicol Lett* 82/83:707–711, 1995.
14. Roe O: Species differences in methanol poisoning, *Crit Rev Toxicol* 10(4):275–286, 1982.
15. Ley CO, Gali FG: Parkinsonian syndrome after methanol intoxication, *Eur Neurol* 22(6):405–409, 1983.
16. Andresen H, Schmoldt H, Matschke J, et al: Fatal methanol intoxication with different survival times—morphological findings and postmortem methanol distribution, *Forensic Sci Internat* 179(2-3):206–210, 2008.
17. Karayel F, Turan AA, Sav A, et al: Methanol intoxication: pathological changes of the central nervous system (17 cases), *Am J Forensic Med Pathol* 1(1):34–36, 2010.

Methylxanthines: Caffeine, Theobromine, Theophylline

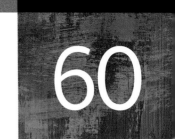

Linda K. Dolder, DVM

- Dogs are most commonly poisoned by ingestion of chocolate, caffeine and weight loss tablets, and cacao bean mulch.
- Clinical signs observed include acute onset of CNS excitation and cardiac stimulation (e.g., vomiting, hyperactivity, excitement, tremors, seizures).
- Marked tachycardia, premature ventricular contractions, and arrhythmias are commonly seen. Hypertension can be seen as well.
- Treatment includes evacuation of the gastrointestinal tract, use of activated charcoal, and cathartics/enemas.
- Diazepam is commonly used to control excitement and seizures.
- Propranolol (or other beta blocker) is used for tachycardia/tachyarrhythmias, atropine for bradycardia.

Caffeine, theobromine, and theophylline are methylated xanthine alkaloids of plant origin commonly found in a variety of foods, beverages, human medical preparations, and other products around the home. These closely related alkaloids share several pharmacologic actions, including stimulation of the central nervous system (CNS); stimulation of cardiac muscle; relaxation of smooth muscle, most notably bronchial muscle; and diuresis of the kidney. Toxicosis is most common in dogs ingesting concentrated sources of these compounds, resulting in acute cardiac and CNS stimulation.

Sources

Caffeine is found in coffee (from the fruit of *Coffea arabica*) and tea (from the leaves of *Thea sinensis*) and is an additive in many soft drinks. In addition to its use as a stimulant in popular beverages, the CNS-stimulating effect of caffeine is used in medications to increase mental alertness. Human cold preparations, analgesics, and diet pills often contain caffeine but can contain other stimulants (examples are ephedrine, guarana, *Hoodia gordonii*, 5-hydroxytryptophan). Over-the-counter stimulant tablets can easily cause small animal toxicosis because they often contain from 100 to 200 mg of caffeine per tablet (Table 60-1). Caffeine poisoning has also been seen in dogs ingesting herbal medications containing guarana.[1]

Table 60-1 Selected Sources of Caffeine

Product	Concentration
OTC stimulants (i.e., Vivarin)	200 mg/tablet
Dexatrim diet pill	200 mg/tablet
Excedrin	65 mg/tablet
Coffee beans	280-570 mg/oz
Coffee	
Drip	85-80 mg/5-oz cup
Instant	30-90 mg/5-oz cup
Decaffeinated	2-4 mg/5-oz cup
Tea	20-90 mg/5-oz cup
Cola soft drinks	40-60 mg/8 oz
Chocolate products	Often contain from 2-40 mg caffeine/oz

OTC, over-the-counter.

Table 60-2 Selected Sources of Theobromine

Product	Concentration (mg/oz)
Cacao beans	300-1500
Unsweetened baking chocolate	390-450
Cacao powder	400-737
Dark semisweet chocolate	135
Milk chocolate	44-60
White chocolate	0.25
Cacao bean hulls	150-255
Cacao bean mulch	56-900

Theobromine occurs naturally in cacao beans (the seeds of *Theobroma cacao*) and in chocolate candy and other products manufactured from these seeds. A few of the most concentrated sources are unsweetened baking chocolate and cocoa, which often contain more than 400 mg of theobromine/oz. Milk chocolate usually contains from 44 to 60 mg of theobromine/oz.[2] The concentrations of theobromine in other products are listed in Table 60-2. Determining the theobromine content of food products can be challenging and can change over time. There are many websites and programs that can assist the practitioner in determining the risk to pets (e.g., chocolate toxicity calculator - Veterinary Information Network, Hershey website, ChocToxVM Lite, Dogs and Chocolate Wheel - ASPCA-APCC). Toxicosis is often associated with the availability of chocolate products in the home, especially at holiday times, and often occurs in dogs consuming large amounts of chocolate. Dogs and other animals may also be poisoned from ingesting cacao bean hulls used as landscaping mulch or bedding.[3,4]

Theophylline is found in tea and in human asthma medications in which it is used as a bronchodilator. Although these concentrated preparations may present a risk, animal poisoning with these products has not been commonly reported.

Toxic Dose

The minimum lethal dose of caffeine in the dog is 140 to 150 mg/kg of body weight. Cats are slightly more sensitive than dogs, with the minimum lethal dose of caffeine ranging from 100 to 150 mg/kg of body weight.[5] Toxicosis is infrequent in cats apparently because of their more selective eating habits.

Theobromine was once used in veterinary practice as a diuretic and cardiac stimulant, with the therapeutic dose in the dog being 20 mg/kg body weight.[6] The LD_{50} of theobromine in dogs ranges from 250 to 500 mg/kg body weight and the LD_{50} in a cat is 200 mg/kg.[5] Consequently a 10-kg dog could be poisoned by consuming 2.25 oz of baking chocolate or 20 oz of milk chocolate.[7] Dogs can readily eat a toxic dose of chocolate.

Toxicokinetics

Caffeine is quickly absorbed after ingestion and reaches peak serum levels in 30 to 60 minutes; it is distributed throughout the organ systems in proportion to body water. Caffeine crosses the blood-brain barrier and into the placenta and the mammary gland. It is rapidly metabolized by the liver where microsomal enzymes promote the metabolism of caffeine by *N*-demethylation and phase II conjugation reactions. There is evidence that methylxanthines are excreted in the bile and then undergo enterohepatic recirculation.[7] About 10% of caffeine is excreted unchanged in the urine. The serum half-life is reported to be 4.5 hours in the dog.[8]

Dogs, reaching peak plasma levels at approximately 10 hours, absorb theobromine from chocolate more slowly; however, in humans peak plasma levels from the same amount of theobromine occur at 3 hours.[9] As with caffeine, theobromine is metabolized primarily in the liver. Dogs excrete theobromine slowly; the plasma half-life is about 17.5 hours, a fact that likely predisposes dogs to theobromine poisoning.[8] In comparison the theobromine plasma half-life in humans is between 6 and 10 hours.[10]

Peak serum levels of theophylline are reached at 1.5 hours in the dog and cat after ingestion of regular-release formulations, and the elimination half-life is 5.7 hours in the dog and 7.8 hours in the cat. Absorption may be much slower with ingestion of a sustained-release product, where peak levels may not be reached until 16 hours. Most theophylline elimination depends on hepatic microsomal enzyme metabolism, and only 10% of a dose is excreted unchanged in the urine.[11]

Mechanism of Toxicity

The methylxanthines inhibit cyclic nucleotide phosphodiesterases and antagonize receptor-mediated actions of adenosine. These combined actions result in cerebral cortical stimulation and seizures, myocardial contraction, smooth muscle relaxation, and diuresis. Caffeine appears to stimulate the synthesis and release of catecholamines, especially norepinephrine. Caffeine stimulates the medullary, respiratory, vasomotor, and vagal centers and the spinal cord at high doses. In comparison with theobromine, caffeine has less effect on cardiac stimulation and coronary artery dilation. However, skeletal muscles are stimulated more by caffeine than by other methylxanthines.[12]

Clinical Signs and Minimum Database

Caffeine

Onset of clinical signs usually occurs within 2 hours of ingestion; however, with ingestion of chocolate products, signs can be delayed for several hours. Initially, restlessness, hyperactivity, abnormal behavior, and vomiting may be noted. As the syndrome rapidly progresses, panting, strong forceful tachycardia, weakness, ataxia, diuresis, diarrhea, hyperexcitability, hyperactivity, muscle tremors, and clonic convulsions are common. Heart rate is often more than 200 beats per minute, and premature ventricular contractions can be noted as well as hypertension. Animals are often hyperthermic and dehydrated. Hypokalemia commonly develops. Hypertension, cyanosis, and coma can precede death from cardiac arrhythmias or respiratory failure.

Theobromine

Initial signs can be seen 2 to 4 hours after ingestion and include restlessness, panting, vomiting, urinary incontinence (diuresis), and perhaps diarrhea. Polydipsia may be seen as well. Patients are often brought for treatment in an excited state with marked tachycardia and hyperthermia. As the syndrome advances during the next few hours, cardiac arrhythmias, premature ventricular contractions, muscular rigidity, hyperreflexia, ataxia, terminal seizures, and coma are observed. Death may occur 18 to 24 hours after the onset from cardiac arrhythmias or respiratory failure or may be delayed for several days and then occur suddenly from cardiac failure.[12] In the author's experience, death caused by respiratory failure is quite uncommon in chocolate toxicosis.

Theophylline

Nausea, vomiting, abdominal pain, mild metabolic acidosis, leukocytosis, and tachycardia characterize acute theophylline overdose. Serum potassium, phosphorus, and magnesium concentrations are low, and serum glucose is commonly elevated. In human subjects, severe effects, such as seizures, hypotension, or hemodynamically significant dysrhythmias, generally do not develop unless serum concentrations reach 80 to 100 mg/L.

Confirmatory Tests

Much of the time confirmatory tests will not be done because the history, along with clinical signs, is sufficient to treat the problem and the patient. However, laboratory tests can be run to help confirm an exposure, if desired. Elevated levels of the methylxanthines may be detected in the stomach contents, plasma, serum, urine, and liver of poisoned animals. Theobromine may be detected in serum for 3 to 4 days after the initial exposure. These compounds are stable in plasma or serum for 7 days at room temperature, 14 days if refrigerated, and 4 months if frozen.[8] In one report, a serum concentration of 133 mg of theobromine/L was associated with death in a dog;[9] however, another dog ingesting cacao powder had a theobromine concentration of 250 mg/L in the blood and 140 mg/L in the serum.[13] The liver of a dog dying from acute caffeine poisoning contained more than 5000 mg of caffeine/kg on a wet weight basis.[14]

Treatment

The goals of treatment for methylxanthine poisoning include (1) sustain basic life support, (2) decrease further absorption, (3) increase excretion of absorbed alkaloid, and (4) provide symptomatic relief of seizures, respiratory difficulties, and cardiac dysfunction. There is no specific antidote for methylxanthine poisoning.

A presumptive diagnosis is based on a history of exposure and clinical signs. One should try to determine the type of product consumed, the amount of exposure (e.g., chocolate toxicity calculator, ChocToxVM Lite, etc.), and the time since ingestion.

Initially the respiratory and cardiac function of the patient should be assessed. If necessary the airway should be secured, and artificial respiration and/or intravenous (IV) fluids for shock should be provided.

If exposure has occurred within the past 2 hours and clinical signs are not present, emetics should be used to induce the patient to vomit. Typically, preexisting heart problems, a history of seizures, or a recent abdominal surgery may alter whether emesis is recommended. With chocolate ingestions, sometimes this time frame for induction can be extended out to approximately 6 hours postexposure, because the chocolate can form a ball in the stomach and it may still be possible to expel the chocolate at that late time. Apomorphine will generally produce vomiting quickly (can administer IV, IM, subconjunctival). Plumb references 0.03 mg/kg IV or 0.04 mg/kg IM or crush a portion of a tablet and dissolve with a few drops of water and administer into the conjunctival sac (after vomiting occurs, rinse sac of the apomorphine).[15] Another option is 3% hydrogen peroxide at 1 mL/pound per os and may repeat once after 15 minutes if vomiting has not occurred.[15] In dogs, bloody vomiting can occur with use of hydrogen peroxide, though in the author's experience it is uncommon. In cats, bloody vomiting is more common and the author does not typically recommend the use of hydrogen peroxide. If, however, the patient is showing marked excitement, is comatose, or has lost the postural or gag reflex, appropriate sedation, placement of an endotracheal tube (with the cuff inflated), and gastric lavage could be used to remove the stomach contents.

The decision to administer activated charcoal is based on the initial dose of methylxanthines ingested, the effectiveness of emesis, and what the likely remaining methylxanthine dose risk is to the patient. Activated charcoal (with sorbitol) is often used to prevent further absorption and increase excretion. A low-end therapeutic dose of activated charcoal PO or by stomach tube should be given. Electrolyte abnormalities can occur and monitoring should be done before and after activated charcoal dosing. If hypernatremia is seen, symptomatic measures are indicated (warm water enemas, low sodium containing fluids, etc.). In some very high methylxanthine exposures, repeated activated charcoal doses may be considered.

IV fluid therapy is often used to maintain adequate renal perfusion, increase urinary excretion of the alkaloid, and correct electrolyte imbalances. Frequent bladder emptying is preferred to prevent reabsorption of the alkaloids and their metabolites from the urine across the bladder wall. There may be an advantage in catheterizing the urinary bladder in some cases.

Additional treatment of the methylxanthine-poisoned animal is symptomatic. Tremors can be managed with methocarbamol or diazepam. Seizures and hyperactivity can generally be controlled with diazepam (0.5 to 2 mg/kg IV) or midazolam (0.1 to 0.25 mg/kg IV, IM). However, when seizures are not responsive to diazepam, phenobarbital or other general anesthetics/anticonvulsants may be used.

Heart function should be monitored closely. Tachycardia is commonly treated with propranolol at 0.02-0.06 mg/kg IV slowly. Persistent tachyarrhythmias may require the use of an oral beta-blocker, such as metoprolol (Lopressor or Betaloc), at an initial dose of 0.1 mg/kg repeated three times a day; this dose can be increased up to 0.3 mg/kg if needed. Frequent premature ventricular contractions in dogs should be treated with lidocaine (without epinephrine) at an initial loading dose of up to 2 mg/kg IV followed by maintenance with an IV drip at a 0.025 to 0.08 mg/kg per minute infusion rate. Lidocaine should be used with caution in cats as they are reportedly sensitive to the CNS effects.[15] For the few patients that have bradycardia, atropine at 0.022 to 0.044 mg/kg given IV, IM, or subcutaneously is recommended.[15] (Caution: reflex bradycardia can be the result of hypertension. In this situation, the hypertension should be managed.)

Prognosis

Signs of methylxanthine poisoning usually last for 12 to 36 hours, depending on the dose of the alkaloid and the effectiveness of decontamination and treatment measures. If effective oral decontamination is obtained within 2 to 4 hours of ingestion, the prognosis is generally favorable. However, in animals presenting with severe seizures or arrhythmias, the prognosis should be guarded.[16]

Gross and Histologic Lesions

Gross examination at necropsy may reveal evidence of chocolate material or stimulant tablets in the stomach. Generally, no specific lesions are associated with methylxanthine poisoning, although gastroenteritis and congestion of organs has been reported. A severely irritated gastric mucosa was reported in one fatally poisoned dog.[12] A degenerative fibrotic cardiomyopathy was found in the right atrial appendage of several dogs chronically dosed with theobromine.[17]

Differential Diagnoses

Conditions that produce the acute onset of strong cardiac and/or CNS stimulation may have to be differentiated from methylxanthine poisoning. These include other alkaloids, such as strychnine, nicotine, amphetamine, or 4-aminopyridine. Chlorinated hydrocarbons, organophosphorus, and carbamate anticholinesterase pesticides; metaldehyde; tremorgenic mycotoxins, such as penitrem A or roquefortine; acute psychedelic drugs, such as LSD or cocaine; fluoroacetate; or cardioactive glycosides, such as those from *Digitalis* spp. or *Nerium oleander;* as well as guarana, 5-hydroxytryptophan, phenylpropanolamine, pseudephedrine, and phenylephrine should also be considered.

References

1. Ooms TG, Khan SA, Means C: Suspected caffeine and ephedrine toxicosis resulting from ingestion of an herbal supplement containing guarana and ma huang in dogs: 47 cases (1997-1999), *J Am Vet Med Assoc* 218(2):225–229, 2001.
2. Zoumas BL, Kreiser WR, Martin RA: Theobromine and caffeine content of chocolate products, *J Food Sci* 45:314, 1980.

3. Drolet R, Arendt TD, Stowe CM: Cacao bean shell poisoning in a dog, *J Am Vet Med Assoc* 185(8):902, 1984.
4. Hovda LR, Kingston RL: Cacao bean mulch poisoning in dogs (abstract), *Vet Hum Toxicol* 36(4):357, 1994.
5. Albretson JC: Methylxanthines. In Plumlee KH, editor: *Clinical veterinary toxicology*, St Louis, 2004, Mosby.
6. Jones LM: *Veterinary pharmacology and therapeutics*, Ames, IA, 1953, Iowa State College Press.
7. Beasley VR, Dorman DC, Fikes JD, et al: *A systems affected approach to veterinary toxicology*, ed 2, Urbana, IL, 1994, University of Illinois.
8. Hooser SB: VR Beasley: Methylxanthine poisoning (chocolate and caffeine toxicosis). In Kirk RW, editor: *Current veterinary therapy IX: small animal practice*, Philadelphia, 1986, Saunders.
9. Glauberg A, Blumenthal HP: Chocolate poisoning in the dog, *J Am Anim Hosp Assoc* 19:246–248, 1983.
10. Shively CA, Tarka SM Jr, Arnand MJ, et al: High levels of methylxanthines in chocolate do not alter theobromine disposition, *Clin Pharmacol Ther* 37:1415–1424, 1985.
11. Papich MG: Bronchodilator therapy. In Kirk RW, editor: *Current veterinary therapy IX: small animal practice*, Philadelphia, 1986, Saunders.
12. Iserson KV: Caffeine and nicotine. In Haddad LM, Winchester JF, editors: *Clinical management of poisoning and drug overdose*, ed 2, Philadelphia, 1990, Saunders.
13. Strachan ER, Bennett A: Theobromine poisoning in dogs, *Vet Rec* 134(11):284, 1994.
14. Vig MM, Dalvi RR, Kufuor-Mensah E: Acute caffeine poisoning in a dog, *Compend Contin Educ Pract Vet* 8(2):82–83, 1986.
15. Plumb DC, editor: *Veterinary drug handbook*, ed 6, Ames, IA, 2008, Wiley-Blackwell.
16. Osweiler GD: Chocolate toxicity. In Tilley LP, Smith FWK, editors: *The 5 minute veterinary consult canine and feline*, Baltimore, 1997, Williams & Wilkins.
17. Gans JH, Korson R, Cater MR, et al: Effects of short-term and long-term theobromine administration to male dogs, *Toxicol Appl Pharmacol* 53:481, 1980.
18. Serafin WE: In Hardman JG, Limbird LE, editors: *Goodman and Gilman's the pharmacological basis of therapeutics*, ed 9, New York, 1995, McGraw-Hill.

Metronidazole

Kevin T. Fitzgerald, PhD, DVM, DABVP

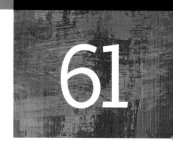

- Metronidazole is widely used in humans and animals in the treatment of protozoal and bacterial infections and is also employed as a therapy for inflammatory bowel disease.
- Metronidazole toxicity is closely dose related, following inappropriately high doses, inappropriate long-term administration, or both.
- In dogs dosages as low as 60 mg/kg/day may cause neurotoxicity in 3 to 14 days. Cats can show clinical signs with 58 mg/kg given daily. The half-life of metronidazole in most mammalian plasma is approximately 8 hours.
- Clinical signs include anorexia, vomiting, ataxia, tremors, peripheral neuropathies, and seizures.
- Treatment for metronidazole poisoning includes withdrawal of the drug and supportive therapy. Diazepam has shown promise in hastening recovery.
- Prognosis is excellent in metronidazole intoxication, with most animals showing complete recovery in 14 days.

Sources

The 1950s saw the discovery and biologic testing of the 5-nitroimidazole group. These drugs have both antiprotozoal and antibacterial effects. In 1959 the effective trichomonacidal activity of 1-(β-hydroxy-ethyl) 2-methyl-5-nitroimidazole (metronidazole) was first reported.[1] Before this time female trichomoniasis patients were treated with a variety of topical drugs with limited success. A large number of infections became chronic and persisted. Males did not respond at all to topical treatment. Metronidazole proved effective for these infections and also in treating infections of the protozoan *Giardia*.

Currently, metronidazole is widely employed in humans and animals for the treatment of trichomoniasis, giardiasis, amebiasis, and obligate anaerobic bacteria, including *Bacteroides* species.[2] Metronidazole has also been shown to be beneficial in the management of inflammatory bowel disease.[3]

Toxic Dose

Metronidazole is available as 250- and 500-mg tablets, various strengths of compounded suspensions (some flavored), and as a 5-mg/mL injectable. The canine recommended oral dosage for anaerobic bacterial infections is 15 mg/kg every 12 hours.[4] Recommendations for the same microbial infections in cats is a once-daily oral treatment of 10 to 25 mg/kg.[4] The canine dosage considered effective for infections with the protozoan *Giardia* is 12 to 15 mg/kg given orally every 12 hours.[4] The recommended oral dosage for feline giardial infections is 17 mg/kg (approximately one third of a tablet per cat) once a day.[4] The maximum daily dosage that is thought to be safe for any species should not exceed 50 mg/kg/day.

There is a strong correlation between dosage and duration of treatment and the time of onset and severity of clinical signs associated with toxicity. In dogs, doses as low as 60 mg/kg have been shown to cause neurotoxicity when treated for as short a time as 3 to 14 days.[5,6] Doses of more than 250 mg/kg will show acute signs of poisoning shortly after metronidazole therapy is initiated. Most dogs showing neurotoxic signs receive lower dosages over a prolonged period. Cats have shown clinical signs of metronidazole poisoning at doses of 111 mg/kg daily for 9 weeks, and 58 mg/kg given daily for 6 months.[7,8]

Although fetal abnormalities have not been documented at suggested dosages, metronidazole has been shown to be mutagenic and genotoxic in some species.[2,9] As a result, metronidazole is not recommended for use during pregnancy. Metronidazole is contraindicated in animals with liver disease, active neurologic diseases, and blood dyscrasias.

Finally, the drug is bitter tasting. Tablets broken up or crushed are generally found to be unpalatable (particularly by cats). As mentioned, various flavored suspensions (citrus, fish, and chicken) are presently available through compounding pharmacies. Unfortunately, use of such flavored medications may actually increase the incidence of poisonings in children and animals because they may mistakenly ingest too much of a pleasant-tasting mixture that contains a potentially dangerous drug.

Toxicokinetics

Metronidazole is synthesized as pale yellow crystals that are slightly soluble in water and alcohol. Metronidazole is well absorbed from the gastrointestinal tract, and high concentrations of the drug are achieved in plasma, bone, peripheral tissue, and in the central nervous system (CNS).[10] The half-life of metronidazole in most mammalian plasma is approximately 8 hours. The half-life in dogs is 3 to 13 hours. Metronidazole can be found in high concentrations in the cerebrospinal fluid.[11]

Metronidazole is metabolized in the liver by oxidation and by glucuronide formation. It is excreted primarily by the kidneys. Urine of some patients may show reddish-brown color caused by water-soluble pigments derived from the drug. During exposure low concentrations of metronidazole can be found in both saliva and milk.[10]

Mechanism of Toxicity

The mechanism of action of metronidazole follows four successive steps.[12] First, it enters susceptible organisms (anaerobic or microaerophilic microorganisms and hypoxic or anoxic cells). Next, the nitro group of metronidazole is reduced by electron transport proteins and deprives the cell of required reduction mechanisms. Following this reductive activation step, the reduced intermediate molecule binds to microbial deoxyribonucleic acid (DNA), causing loss of helical structure, strand breakage, and impairment of normal DNA function. Cell death is caused by this disruption and degradation of the cellular DNA and by the release of inactive and nonfunctional cellular end products. Through these mechanisms metronidazole kills *Giardia*, trichomonads, various amebae, and the anaerobic bacteria *Bacteroides*. The exact nature of metronidazole poisoning remains unknown; however, the types of adverse neurologic effects caused implicate central vestibular and cerebellar dysfunction.

Finally, metronidazole can produce reactions similar to disulfiram (Antabuse) if given simultaneously with ethanol. This drug or chemical interaction results in production of acetaldehyde in the blood. Acetaldehyde is hepatotoxic, cardiotoxic, and arrhythmogenic. Toxic reactions and fatalities have been reported as a result of metronidazole or ethanol interactions in humans; this is not likely to occur in pets.

Clinical Signs

Clinical signs of metronidazole toxicity typically follow prolonged exposure or administration of inappropriately high doses. Clinical signs and their severity may vary and reflect the dose given and duration of treatment.

Toxic side effects of metronidazole reported include anorexia, vomiting, stomatitis, and glossitis.[5,6] The more severe neurotoxic effects observed include ataxia, hypermetric gait, inability to walk, peripheral neuropathies, spasms of lumbar and hind limb musculature, dorsiflexion of the tail, vertical nystagmus, head tilt, and seizures.[5,6] Many species show neutropenia.[2] Metronidazole causes a sensory axonopathy characterized by sensory ataxia as a result of large fiber proprioceptive involvement. Neurologic effects in cats tend to implicate forebrain dysfunction (disorientation and seizures) rather than brainstem involvement.[7,8]

Minimum Database and Confirmatory Tests

The most definitive test in diagnosing metronidazole toxicity is establishing blood concentrations for the drug. This is not commonly done in private practice, but the test is available to practitioners. Most diagnoses of metronidazole toxicity rely heavily on a good history, appearance of clinical signs compatible with the syndrome, absence of other diseases, and subsequent recovery of the animal after withdrawal of the drug. Early determination of any and all medications the animal has been given recently is essential. Generally, clinicians learn from the owner about current or recent use of metronidazole. However, further diagnostics, such as complete blood count, biochemical profile, and neurologic imaging such as computed tomography or magnetic resonance imaging (MRI), may be necessary to rule out other conditions, such as infection, metabolic disease, other toxins, neurologic disorders, or neoplasia, which may resemble metronidazole poisoning.

Treatment

Treatment for metronidazole toxicity is generally supportive and includes discontinuation of the drug. Most animals show total recovery within 14 days of withdrawal of metronidazole therapy.[2] Ataxic animals must be protected from falling, and anorexic animals must be identified and supported appropriately.

Diazepam has been reported as a potentially successful treatment for the neurologic signs associated with metronidazole poisoning.[5] Diazepam is believed to exert its reversal of adverse effects by facilitation of the potent inhibitory neurotransmitter γ-aminobutyric acid (GABA) within the vestibular system. When diazepam was given (0.43 mg/kg orally every 8 hours for 3 days), signs of response decreased in 4.25 days in untreated dogs to 13.4 hours in treated dogs.[5] In addition, recovery was reduced from 11 days to 38.8 hours in treated dogs. Diazepam therapy appears promising for treatment of metronidazole toxicosis. Metronidazole treatment should be discontinued immediately if any signs of ataxia or neurologic involvement are observed.

Prevention and Prognosis

Most animals demonstrating signs of intoxication from metronidazole treatment either received an inappropriate dose, were given the drug for an inappropriate duration, or both. Subsequently, the single most important safeguard is always double checking dosages and length of recommended treatment. Furthermore, certain animals—those with existing cerebral disease, hepatic disorders, pregnant females, and those with preexisting blood dyscrasias—should not be given metronidazole. Pleasantly flavored, compounded medications should always be stored safely out of the reach of animals and children. Outdated or unused medication should never be flushed down the toilet and never discarded in trash cans where inquisitive animals may blunder across them. Out-of-date drugs can be returned to pharmacies in some states where they can be destroyed or disposed of properly and not end up in the environment.

The prognosis for most metronidazole poisonings is excellent. Most animals will recover totally within 2 weeks. However, those suffering from severe CNS signs may take months to recover. Animals exhibiting clinical signs when exposed to dosages greater than 250 mg/kg may show permanent CNS signs; however, this is rare. Withdrawal of the drug, supportive care, and the possible use of diazepam will all facilitate the recovery of the animal. A reasonable prognostic indicator is the dosage the animal received, the duration of the treatment provided, and the severity of the clinical signs observed.

Gross and Histologic Lesions

Histologic examination of brains of dogs with metronidazole poisoning reveals Purkinje cell loss and axonal degeneration of vestibular tracts.[6] Brains of mice treated with toxic metronidazole doses show cerebellar Purkinje cell loss and degenerative changes in the vestibular, cochlear, deep cerebellar, and olivary nuclei and in the rostral colliculi.[2] These nuclei and their associated tracts help to regulate fine motor control, equilibrium, and hearing. Also, these nuclei, especially Purkinje cells, exert an inhibitory influence on postsynaptic receptors. The major neurotransmitter of these nuclei is GABA, which is the principal inhibitory neurotransmitter of the CNS. Activation of the GABA receptor by GABA or by GABA mimetics (such as diazepam) increases chloride conduction of the postsynaptic membrane, resulting in hyperpolarization. Metronidazole either inhibits the effects of GABA or actively destroys the cells releasing the neurotransmitter. Whatever the mechanism, it is the GABA-dependent interactions of the cerebellar and central vestibular system that are affected.

Vestibulocerebellar axonal generation with no loss of neurons has been reported in dogs given 63 mg/kg/day.[6] Although these dogs recovered, the potential exists for permanent, subclinical damage to neurons and to white matter tracts in all cases of metronidazole poisoning. As a result of such permanent changes, animals previously poisoned with metronidazole may be more susceptible to subsequent toxic exposures. Consequently, it is not recommended that animals once having shown signs of metronidazole toxicosis be treated with the drug again.

Metronidazole toxicity appears to be a result of a predominantly sensory axonopathy caused by large fiber proprioceptive involvement.[13,14] The tracts damaged by metronidazole have a prevalence of GABAergic receptors. It is speculated that this interference of the GABA receptor at the postsynaptic membrane results in the ataxia, tremors, seizures, and neurotoxic effects seen with metronidazole intoxication. It is believed that diazepam acts to offset the poisoning by competing with metronidazole for receptor sites or directly stimulating GABA synthesis. Diazepam thus causes an inhibitory effect on excitatory neurons and counters the adverse actions of metronidazole. Typically, MRI abnormalities seen with metronidazole-induced toxicity are symmetrical and bilateral and involve cerebellar dentate nuclei, midbrain, dorsal pons (vestibular nucleus, abducens nucleus, and superior olivary nucleus), the splenium of the corpus callosum, and dorsal medulla. MRI abnormalities have been postulated to be reversible mitochondrial dysfunction in susceptible animals.

Finally, advanced imaging studies have revealed that, except for the most severe cases of metronidazole toxicity, drug-induced CNS histologic changes resolve following discontinuation of therapy.[15-18] MRI performed at the time of clinical signs of poisoning and followed up by imaging studies performed 6 and 8 weeks after the initial episode demonstrated that changes first seen in the cerebellum and deep cerebellar nuclei (areas most sensitive to metronidazole toxicity and the most specific imaging manifestations of such poisoning) are nearly completely resolved 6 to 8 weeks after cessation of the drug.[19] MRI represents yet another way to diagnose metronidazole toxicity and provides an indication of the severity of the poisoning episode.[20]

Differential Diagnoses

Correct diagnosis of metronidazole intoxication may be overlooked if current, recent, or accidental administration of the drug is not uncovered or suspected. Differential diagnoses and potential look-alikes include metabolic disease, infectious disorders of the CNS, neoplasia, and other subacute or chronic neuropathies (e.g., arsenic, ethanol, mercury, organophosphate- and carbamate acetylcholinesterase–inhibiting pesticides). Metronidazole must remain within the clinician's index of suspicion whenever an animal demonstrates sensory ataxia.

References

1. Cosar C, Julou L: Activité de 1-(hydroxy-2-ethyl) 1-methyl-2-nitro-5 imidazole vis-à-vis des infections experimentales à *Trichomonas vaginalis, Ann Instit Pasteur (Paris)* 96:238–241, 1959.
2. El-Nahas AF, El-Ashmawy IM: Reproductive and cytogenetic toxicity of Metronidazole in male mice, *Basic Clin Pharmacol Toxicol* 94:226–231, 2004.
3. Tams TR: Feline inflammatory bowel disease. In Kirk RW, editor: *Current veterinary therapy IX*, Philadelphia, 1986, WB Saunders.
4. Papich MG: *Handbook of veterinary drugs*, Philadelphia, 2002, WB Saunders.
5. Evans J, et al: Diazepam as a treatment for metronidazole toxicosis in dogs: a retrospective study of 21 cases, *J Vet Int Med* 17:304–310, 2003.
6. Dow SW, LeCouteur RA, Poss ML, et al: Central nervous system toxicosis associated with metronidazole treatment of dogs: five cases (1984-1987), *J Am Vet Med Assoc* 195:365–368, 1989.
7. Saxon B, Magne M: Reversible central nervous system toxicosis in three cats, *Prog Vet Neurol* 4:25–27, 1993.
8. Caylor KB, Cassimatis MK: Metronidazole neurotoxicosis in two cats, *J Am An Hosp Assoc* 37:258–262, 2001.
9. Bost RG: Metronidazole: mammalian mutagenicity. In Finegold JA, McFazeam JA, Roe FIC, editors: *Metronidazole: proceedings of the international metronidazole conference*, Montreal, Quebec, 1977, Canada.
10. Rollo IM: Miscellaneous drugs used in treatment of protozoal infections. In Gilman AG, Goodman LS, Gilman A, editors: *The pharmacological basis of therapeutics*, New York, 1980, Macmillan Press.
11. Finegold SM: Metronidazole, *Ann Intern Med* 93:585–587, 1980.
12. Finegold SM, Mathisen GE: Metronidazole. In Mandell GL, Douglas RG, Bennett JE, editors: *Principles and practice of infectious disease*, ed 3, New York, 1990, Churchill Livingstone.
13. Gallagher EJ: Neurologic principles. In Goldfrank LR, et al: *Toxicologic emergencies*, New York, 2002, McGraw-Hill.
14. Bradley WG, Karlsson IJ, Russo ICG: Metronidazole neuropathy, *BMJ* 2:610–611, 1977.
15. Heaney CJ, Campeau NG, Lindell EP: MR imaging and diffusion-weighted imaging changes in metronidazole (flagyl)-induced cerebellar toxicity, *Am J Neuroradiol* 24:1615–1617, 2003.
16. Woodruff BK, Wijdicks EF, Marshall WF: Reversible metronidazole-induced lesions of the cerebellar dentate nuclei, *N Eng J Med* 346:68–69, 2002.
17. Cecil KM, Halsted MJ, Schapiro M, et al: Reversible MR imaging and MR spectroscopy in abnormalities in association with metronidazole therapy, *J Comput Assist Tomoyr* 26:948–951, 2002.
18. Kim E, Noi DG, Kim EY, et al: MR imaging of metronidazole-induced encephalopathy: lesion distribution and diffusion-weighted imaging findings, *AJNR Am J Neuroradiol* 28:1652–1658, 2007.
19. Puri V: Metronidazole neurotoxicity, *Neurol India* 59:4–5, 2011.
20. Park K, Chung JM, Kim JY: Metronidazole toxicity: sequential neuroaxis involvement, *Neurol India* 59:104–107, 2011.

Mushrooms

Birgit Puschner, DVM, PhD, DABVT

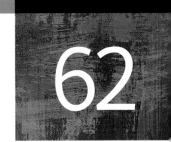

- Mushroom ingestion can occur all year round, but is most frequently reported in September and October.
- The northeastern United States has the highest incidence of reported mushroom poisonings in small animals, followed by the western, midwestern, southeastern, and southwestern U.S. regions.
- Signs of gastrointestinal distress (e.g. vomiting, diarrhea) are commonly observed following ingestion of mushrooms.
- Mushrooms can contain a variety of potential toxic substances, capable of affecting the gastrointestinal tract, nervous system, kidney, and liver.
- Treatment is primarily supportive, aimed at decontaminating the patient and addressing the clinical problems.
- Treatment options following exposures to unknown mushrooms in asymptomatic patients should include consideration of: complete blood work assessments, decontamination procedures, and gastrointestinal and liver protectants.
- A confirmed diagnosis can be difficult, and an accurate diagnosis relies very heavily on toxicologic analysis and accurate identification of a well-preserved mushroom specimen.

Reporting Mushroom Poisonings

Mushroom poisoning is a real problem in veterinary clinical toxicology because of the high mortality rate. The most reported and serious mushroom intoxications in small animals are caused by amanitin-containing mushrooms. Until recently, diagnosis of mushroom poisoning was primarily presumptive, and many cases were likely undiagnosed. But recent advancements in toxicologic analysis allow for a more comprehensive approach to reach a confirmed diagnosis of mushroom poisoning. This will, over time, help to assess the true frequency of mushroom poisonings in small animals. In addition, practitioners are encouraged to report animal mushroom poisonings to the North American Mycological Association's Mushroom Poisoning Case Registry at http://www.namyco.org/toxicology/index .html. Reports may be submitted online (http://namyco.org/toxicology/email_report_form .html) or by mail. The website provides a list of volunteers willing to assist in the identification of mushrooms (http://www.namyco.org/toxicology/identifiers.html). The volunteers are listed by region. Alternatively, many universities and colleges have lists of mycologists available for assistance.

Collection and Identification

There is no simple test to differentiate a poisonous from a nonpoisonous mushroom. If a mushroom ingestion is suspected, thoroughly examine the area where the animal may have been exposed and collect any mushrooms in the area for identification by an experienced mycologist. Place the mushrooms in paper, not plastic, bags. The most useful collection technique is to place the mushroom with cap gills down on a white sheet of paper that has the site and conditions (e.g., moisture, nearby trees, and substrate) written on it, and then wrap each type of mushroom in wax paper. In small-animal poisoning cases it may be very difficult to obtain a complete sample set of mushrooms if the animal has ranged over a wide area. Accurate mushroom identification requires consultation with an experienced mycologist. Several important factors aid in this process.

Mushrooms grow on various substrates. A mushroom growing on wood is lignicolous, one on the ground is terrestrial, one on another plant or animal is parasitic, and one growing on dung is coprophilous. Knowledge of the substrate helps identify the mushroom and, if possible, this information should be provided along with the collected specimen. Certain mushrooms are commonly associated with specific trees. Knowledge of the surrounding trees can aid in identification (Table 62-1).

Mushroom spores are also important for identification. The spores are microscopic and may only be seen as a mass. Before dispersal they may be located under the mushroom cap in structures that look like a pincushion, sponge, or gills. Some mushrooms do not have a specific cap and bear their seeds inside the mushroom (Figure 62-1). As the mushroom matures and the spores ripen, the surface of the mushroom opens and the spores are blown out, providing a "puffball." Some spores are borne on cap wrinkles or folds, as in a false morel mushroom (Color Plate 62-1), or inside pits, like in the true morel mushroom (Color Plate 62-2).

A spore print is also very helpful in identification. A spore print consists of a mass of spores deposited on white paper. The color of the spores is specific to a species and is usually listed in most field guides used for identification. The spore print is obtained by cutting the stem of the mushroom off just under the cap. The mushroom is placed with the gills or spongy area down on a white sheet of paper. The spores fall out of the cap and onto the paper to provide the color. Colors include brown, reddish brown, chocolate brown, white, cream, black, purple-black, green, and yellow. The pattern of the spore print is not important because it is determined by the shape of a single mushroom and may vary considerably. If the mushroom has greatly raised edges or is irregular in shape, a bowl may be placed over the mushroom to get a better concentration of spores (Color Plate 62-3).

Mushrooms have many different shapes. Structures with some importance in poisoning cases are the annulus, universal veil remnants, volva, and stem and cap shape (Color Plate 62-4). Imagine a mushroom as it comes out of the ground as an egg. As it increases in size, it splits horizontally. In some types of mushrooms the universal veil, or "egg shell," that once was the outer surface breaks into smaller and smaller pieces, often sticking to the surface of the actual mushroom growing underneath. These spots, or splotches, are called *universal veil remnants* and are helpful in identifying various species, many of which are poisonous. Part of that outside veil may separate from the cap and stay with the stem to form a ring on the stem, called an *annulus.* The annulus may be large, small, fleshy, or threadlike, characteristics that are useful for identification. The shape of the stipe (stem) is important; it may be equal in size from top to bottom, wider at the top, or wider at the bottom. The stem base may be directly attached to the mycelium and substrate or enclosed within a cuplike sheath called a *volva.* As an example of how these characteristics are used, a poisonous *Amanita* mushroom looks a lot like an edible white button mushroom *Agaricus,* but the *Amanita ocreata* has white spores, a volva, and an annulus (Color Plate 62-5), whereas the *Agaricus* has brown spores and an annulus only. The overall color of the mushroom is of some importance, but considerable biologic variation makes identification by color alone unreliable.

Table 62-1	Mushrooms Found in Association with Various Trees
Tree Type	**Mushroom**
Alder	*Clitocybe candicans*
	Clitocybe clavipes
	Inocybe dulcamara
Balsam	*Gyromitra esculenta*
Beech	*Amanita citrina*
	Amanita gemmata
	Amanita phalloides
	Boletus satanas
	Clitocybe candicans
	Clitocybe clavipes
	Cortinarius orellanus
	Cortinarius splendens
	Entoloma sinuatum
	Inocybe patouillardii
	Ramaria formosa
Birch	*Amanita citrina*
	Amanita muscaria
	Clitocybe candicans
	Clitocybe clavipes
	Inocybe dulcamara
	Lactarius helvus
	Lactarius torminosus
	Leccinum atrostipitatum
	Leccinum scabrum
Chestnut	*Amanita verna*
	Omphalotus olearius
Fir	*Amanita pantherina*
	Gyromitra esculenta
	Inocybe spp.
	Suillus lakei
Hornbeam	*Amanita phalloides*
	Cortinarius orellanus
	Entoloma sinuatum
Larch	*Clitocybe candicans*
	Fuscoboletinus spectabilis
	Suillus cavipes
Madrona	*Amanita calyptroderma*
	Amanita muscaria
Oak	*Agaricus xanthodermus*
	Amanita citrina
	Amanita phalloides
	Amanita verna
	Boletus satanas
	Clitocybe clavipes
	Cortinarius orellanus
	Entoloma sinuatum
	Inocybe dulcamara
	Lepiota spp.
	Omphalotus olearius
Olive	*Omphalotus olearius*
Pine	*Amanita citrina*

Continued

Table 62-1	Mushrooms Found in Association with Various Trees—cont'd
Tree Type	**Mushroom**
	Amanita muscaria
	Amanita gemmata
	Amanita pantherina
	Amanita regalis
	Armillaria mellea
	Armillaria ponderosa
	Armillaria zelleri
	Chroogomphus vinicolor
	Clitocybe candicans
	Cortinarius orellanus
	Hebeloma crustuliniforme
	Inocybe dulcamara
	Lactarius helvus
	Ramaria pallida
	Suillus brevipes
	Suillus granulatus
	Suillus luteus
	Suillus pictus
Poplar (aspen)	Hebeloma crustuliniforme
	Flammulina velutipes
	Lactarius controversus
	Leccinum insigne
	Pleurotus ostreatus
Spruce	Amanita citrina
	Amanita regalis
	Amanita virosa
	Armillaria mellea
	Gyromitra esculenta
	Lactarius helvus
	Ramaria pallida

Data from references 70-73.

Mushrooms have many different toxin types (Table 62-2). Some toxins result in very specific clinical presentations, whereas others have nonspecific presentations. Some toxins are destroyed by cooking, whereas others are stable, which is less of a criterion for small animals ingesting raw mushrooms in the environment.

Hepatotoxic Mushrooms

Death in amanitin intoxications is caused by acute liver failure. Amanitin-containing mushrooms are commonly found in North America and have resulted in deaths in dogs and cats.[1,2] *Amanita phalloides* is also known as the *death cap* or *death angel* and is common in the San Francisco Bay area, the Pacific Northwest, and the northeast. It is often commonly found in association with oaks, birch, and pine during wet and warm years. *A. phalloides* has a yellowish-green, smooth cap; white gills; a white veil around the upper part of the stem; and a white volva. *Amanita ocreata* (see Color Plate 62-5), also called *Western North American destroying angel,* is generally found in sandy soils along the Pacific coast from Baja California, Mexico, to Washington. *A. ocreata* has a white or cream-colored

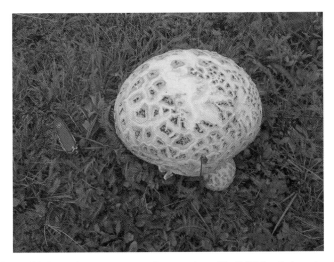

Figure 62-1 Mushroom spore surface inside puffball (*Calvatia booniana*).

cap; white, short gills; a partial veil on a white stem; and a white, thin cup around the base of the stem. In addition to *Amanita* spp., *Lepiota* and *Galerina* spp. contain hepatotoxic amanitins. Although infrequently reported, *Galerina autumnalis, Lepiota josserandii,* and *Amanita bisporigera* have been associated with fatalities in animals and humans in North America.[3]

Amanitins

The principal toxins of hepatotoxic mushrooms are amanitins. Although other toxic cyclo-peptides (amatoxins, virotoxins) and proteins (lectins, toxovirin) have been identified, they are unlikely to contribute to poisonings.[4] Amanitins are bicyclic octapeptides that are not degraded under acidic conditions in the stomach or by heat and thus pose a risk to animals and humans in fresh and cooked form.[5] Once ingested, amanitins are taken up by cells in the gastrointestinal tract where first damaging effects can occur.[2,6] Bioavailability is considered greatest in humans, followed by dogs, rabbits, and mice. Cats have died from amanitin poisoning. Amanitins must be sufficiently absorbed to result in poisoning. After reaching the systemic circulation, an organic anion-transporting polypeptide, OATP1B3, mediates the amanitin uptake into hepatocytes.[7] Amanitins' well-known toxic mechanism of action is the binding to and inhibition of nuclear ribonucleic acid polymerase.[8] The effects are particularly severe in hepatocytes, but can also be seen in the intestinal mucosa and proximal renal tubules. Alpha-amanitin also induces p53-dependent apoptosis, a mechanism that may play a major role in the pathogenesis of liver damage.[9] Hepatocytes excrete aminitins via the bile, but only to a small extent. More than 85% of amanitins are eliminated via the kidneys, where subsequent reabsorption by renal tubules can lead to acute tubular necrosis.

Toxicity and Clinical Signs

The oral LD_{50} for methyl-γ-amanitin in dogs is 0.5 mg/kg body weight. In humans, the esti-mated oral LD_{50} of α-amanitin is 0.1 mg/kg body weight. A single *A. phalloides* or *A. ocreata* can contain lethal concentrations of amanitins.

It is absolutely critical that the veterinarian closely monitor liver and kidney functions in any animal with possible mushroom exposure to diagnose potentially lethal amanitin intoxication in a timely manner. Following exposure to amanitin-containing mushrooms, the poisoned animal will not develop clinical signs of illness for approximately 6 to 12 hours.

Table 62-2	Mushrooms by Toxin Type
Toxin	**Mushroom**
Amanitins (cyclopeptides)- Hepatic, gastrointestinal, and renal effects	*Amanita bisporigera* *Amanita ocreata* *Amanita phalloides* *Amanita verna* *Amanita virosa* *Conocybe filaris* *Galerina autumnalis* *Galerina marginata* *Galerina venenata* *Pholiotina filaris*
Coprine type—rare	*Boletus luridus* *Clitocybe clavipes* *Coprinus atramentarius* *Coprinus micaceus*
Gastrointestinal irritants	*Amanita xanthodermus* *Amanita volvata* *Boletus eastwoodiae* *Boletus pulcherrimus* *Boletus satanas* *Cantharellus floccosus* *Chlorophyllum molybdites* *Entoloma lividum* *Hebeloma crustuliniforme* *Gomphus floccosus* *Laccaria amethystina* *Lactarius spp.* *Lampteromyces japonicus* *Omphalotus illudens* *Psalliota campestris* *Ramaria formosa* *Rhodophyllus rhodopolius* *Rhodophyllus sinuatus* *Russula emetica* *Scleroderma spp.* *Suillus tomentosus* *Tricholoma species* *Tylopilus felleus*
Hydrazines- Gastrointestinal, CNS, and RBC effects	*Gyromitra ambigua* *Gyromitra esculenta* *Gyromitra gigas* *Gyromitra fastigiata* *Gyromitra infula* *Helvella crispa* *Helvella lacunosa* *Helvella elastica* *Verpa bohemica* *Peziza badia*
Ibotenic acid and muscimol- Gastrointestinal and CNS effects	*Amanita muscaria* *Amanita pantherina* *Amanita strobiliformis* *Amanita gemmata* *Amanita smithiana* *Tricholoma muscarium*

Table 62-2	Mushrooms by Toxin Type—cont'd
Toxin	**Mushroom**
Psilocybin and psilocin- CNS effects	*Conocybe spp.* *Gymnopilus spp.* *Panaeolus spp.* *Psilocybe spp.*(many) *Stropharia spp.*
Muscarine- Cholinergic (peripheral) effects	*Boletus* spp. *Clitocybe dealbata* *Chlorophyllum molybdites* *Clitocybe rivulosa* *Clitcybe illudens* *Clitocybe truncicola* *Entoloma rhodopolium* *Inocybe lacera* *Inocybe fastigiata* *Inocybe patouillardii* *Inocybe phaeocomis* *Inocybe pudica* *Mycena pura* *Rubinoboletus* spp.
Nephrotoxic	*Cortinarius orellanus* *Cortinarius speciosissimus* *Amanita smithiana*

Data from references 67, 68, 70, and 72.
CNS, Central nervous system; *RBC*, red blood cell.

This latency period often leads to a delay of diagnostic and therapeutic intervention, because the owners do not consult their veterinarian until clinical signs develop. Approximately 6 to 24 hours after exposure, poisoned animals develop abdominal pain, vomiting, and diarrhea. After a 12- to 24-hour period of "false recovery," the terminal phase of fulminant liver failure develops.[1] At that time, significant elevations in serum aspartate aminotransferase, alanine aminotransferase, alkaline phosphatase, and bilirubin are found. Hepatic failure will become evident clinically and biochemically approximately 36 to 48 hours after exposure. Hepatocellular damage will lead to coagulopathy, encephalopathy, and renal or multiorgan failure at several days after exposure. Severe hypoglycemia as a result of breakdown of liver glycogen can also occur and is associated with mortality. Of dogs given lethal doses of amanitins or pieces of *A. phalloides,* 50% died from hypoglycemia 1 to 2 days after exposure.[10] Puppies, or dogs that ingest significant amounts of amanitins, can die of amanitin poisoning within 24 hours but most animals die within several days of exposure.

Findings at necropsy may include a swollen liver with a reticular pattern, and mucosal hemorrhages in the gastrointestinal mucosa.[1,2] In some cases, there may be no significant gross abnormalities. Histopathologic findings include submassive to massive acute hepatic necrosis, renal proximal tubular epithelial necrosis, and foci of necrosis and inflammation in the gastrointestinal tract.

Confirmatory Testing

Detection of amanitins in biologic specimens is confirmatory, and these tests are now more commonly available at veterinary toxicology laboratories. Rapid confirmation of amanitins in suspect exposures assists in the early recognition of exposure, whereas a negative result can prevent unnecessary hospitalization.

If vomitus, gastric lavage fluid, or a suspect mushroom were saved, identification can be useful, and analysis for amanitins or deoxyribonucleic acid can be performed to determine the presence of amanitins.[11,12] In any suspect case it is best to freeze and save gastrointestinal contents for further analysis.

Amanitins are detectable in serum and urine well before any clinical sign of poisoning, whereas routine laboratory tests such as complete blood cell count and serum chemistry profiles are unremarkable until liver or kidney damage has occurred. As amanitins are primarily excreted unchanged in urine, urine is a very useful specimen antemortem. In fact, urine is of diagnostic value for up to 72 hours following exposure.[13] In contrast, serum is only diagnostically useful for a maximum of 24 hours after exposure because of the short plasma half-life. Plasma and urine amanitin concentrations do not seem to correlate with the clinical severity or outcome.

Postmortem, liver and kidney samples, along with bile, are suitable for confirmatory testing. Human cases showed that kidney amanitin concentrations are higher than concentrations in liver in patients who were alive for up to 3 weeks following exposure. Thus it is best to save both liver and kidney, frozen, for toxicologic analysis. Limited data showed that analysis of formalin-fixed tissues for amanitin is unreliable; only positive results can be interpreted; negative results cannot rule out amanitin exposure.

The well-known newspaper test to identify the presence of amanitin, also known as the *Meixner* or *Wieland test,* has limitations and cannot be relied on to identify amanitin-containing mushrooms.[14]

Treatment

Despite the evaluation of numerous therapeutic approaches for animals and humans, the mortality rate of amanitin intoxications is high, especially in young animals and children.[15,16] The essential components of treatment are close monitoring, fluid replacement, and supportive care, as there is no specific antidote. However, optimal management of animals after ingestion of amanitin-containing mushrooms is still not determined as data on the clinical efficacy of these recommended treatment approaches do not exist. Rapid administration of activated charcoal at 1 g/kg orally followed by two to three doses at 0.5 g/kg within 24 hours of exposure is recommended. In the past multidose activated charcoal over the course of several days was recommended, but recent data no longer supports this practice.[13] At approximately 16 to 24 hours after exposure, intestinal reuptake of amanitins is negligible, making long-term administration of activated charcoal unnecessary. At that time (16 to 24 hours after exposure), amanitin concentrations have also dropped below levels considered appropriate to initiate hemodialysis or hemoperfusion.

Because most animals with amanitin poisoning are not presented until 1 to 2 days after ingestion, therapeutic options are clearly limited at that time. Dextrose, vitamin K_1, blood products, and intravenous (IV) fluids must be considered as beneficial therapeutic agents for case management.

Hepatocyte protection with antioxidants and silymarin must also be considered. Silibinin (Legalon-SIL), the main component of silymarin (milk thistle extract) is an approved and effective treatment for amanitin poisoning in humans that reduces the uptake of amanitins into hepatocytes.[17,18] Previous studies in beagles showed that IV administration of 50 mg/kg silibinin at 5 and 24 hours after intoxication with *A. phalloides* was effective and prevented death.[19] Commercially available silibinin preparations for small animals vary in content and bioavailability, are often combined with S-adenosylmethionine, and are marketed as nutritional supplements to maintain and improve liver function. Clinical studies documenting the effectiveness of these available supplements in dogs and cats with amanitin poisoning do not exist. Penicillin antibiotics are also effective in reducing the uptake of amanitins into hepatocytes by serving as OATP1B3 substrates.[20] IV administration of 1000 mg/kg (1 million units = 1000 mg Pen GK) of penicillin G at 5 hours after dogs were exposed to *A. phalloides* was protective. Although there is no conclusive data on the efficacy of *N*-acetylcysteine in amanitin-poisoned animals, it is known to be useful in other toxicant-induced hepatic injury, such as acetaminophen poisoning. Thus administration of *N*-acetylcysteine should be considered. Other compounds that may boost the hepatocyte antioxidant capacities include vitamin E, vitamin C, and zinc. However, whether any of these antioxidants provide rapid hepatoprotection, as necessary in an acute, severe amanitin intoxication, is unknown. Draining the gallbladder (via needle) was a procedure recently employed in an *Amanita phalloides* intoxicated dog — more studies need to be done to see how efficacious this treatment really is.

Animal Exposures

Amanitin poisoning has been reported in cats.[2,21] Reported clinical signs include initial lethargy and vomiting, followed by rapid development of neurologic signs. There are numerous publications describing the clinical, clinicopathologic, and postmortem findings of amanitin poisoning in dogs.[1,22-26] There is limited information on the incidents of amanitin poisoning in large animals. An 18-year-old horse died after apparently ingesting one or more *Amanita verna* mushrooms. The horse had meningioangiomatosis, which may have altered its normal eating behavior.[27] Amanitin intoxication was confirmed in two calves that were found dead without showing any signs of illness prior to death.[28] It is important to note that the limited availability of confirmatory testing for amanitins has likely led to severe underreporting of amanitin poisonings in animals. In fact, because animals are at much greater risk to be exposed to toxic mushrooms than humans, mushroom poisonings in animals are likely to be quite common.

Differential Diagnoses

Other toxicants that can results in gastrointestinal upset and hepatic failure in dogs and cats include microcystins in cyanobacteria, cocklebur, cycad palm, aflatoxin, xylitol (dogs only), ricin, abrin, gyromitrin, copper, zinc, and acetaminophen overdose. The history and geographic environment of the animal can help to eliminate most of the toxicant differentials on the list.

Neurotoxic Mushrooms

Hydrazines

Hydrazines are found in false morels, such as *Gyromitra gigas, Gyromitra esculenta, Gyromitra infula, Verpa bohemica, Helvella elastica, Helvella crispa,* and *Helvella lacunosa;* in common brown cup fungi such as the *Peziza badia;* and likely in several other genera. False morels are often found under conifers, aspens, and sometimes around melting snow banks. Gyromitrin (acetaldehyde *N*-methyl *N*-formylhydrazone), the compound found in these mushrooms, is a direct irritant to the gastrointestinal tract. Gyromitrin hydrolysis in the stomach yields *N*-methyl-formylhydrazine, which is further metabolized to monomethylhydrazine and reactive metabolites. Monomethylhydrazine is partly responsible for the neurologic signs as it decreases pyridoxal 5-phosphate with subsequent decrease in γ-aminobutyric acid (GABA) synthesis.[29] Pyridoxine is not the total answer because injection of pyridoxine will terminate some but not all of the clinical signs. Oxidative damage to the red blood cells and liver and kidney injury can develop from reactive metabolites.

Toxicity and Clinical Signs

Hydrazines are degraded by heat and drying. Although humans usually eat cooked mushrooms, animals eat them raw and can be seriously poisoned by hydrazine-containing mushrooms. The concentration of gyromitrin varies by species, locality, and season, leading to considerable variation in the degree of poisoning. In humans, the estimated lethal dose of gyromitrin is 20 to 50 mg/kg for adults and 10 to 30 mg/kg for children. There is no data on the toxicity for small animals.

Within 6 to 12 hours of gyromitrin exposure, vomiting and watery diarrhea will begin. In humans, a delayed onset of clinical signs of 53 hours after exposure has been reported. The gastrointestinal effects may last up to 2 days in humans. Tremors, weakness, and ataxia may also develop in the first 2 days. In serious yet rare cases, jaundice, methemoglobinemia, hemolysis, seizures, and coma (including hepatic coma) can develop several days after exposure.[30] Hemolysis may lead to rhabdomyolysis and impaired renal function (rare).

Diagnostic Workup

As with all suspect mushroom intoxications, identification by an experienced mycologist is critical in reaching a diagnosis. In case of *Gyromitra* poisoning, it is especially important to accurately differentiate between false morels (toxic) and edible, true morels. The analysis of suspect poisonous mushrooms or biologic specimens from animals for gyromitrin or its toxic metabolites is not routinely available.[31] Thus diagnosis is primarily based on mushroom identification and compatible clinical signs and laboratory abnormalities.

Treatment

Gyromitrin poisoning is managed with supportive care. Decontamination is only recommended if animals present within a few hours after exposure. As most animals have vomited voluntarily, inducing emesis is generally not necessary. Activated charcoal may be given, and the animals must be carefully monitored for electrolyte imbalances, hemolysis, and methemoglobinemia. Pyridoxine is recommended for serious neurologic signs in humans, such as seizures and coma, but there are inadequate clinical efficacy data in animals. In humans, 25 mg/kg of pyridoxine is given intravenously over 15 to 30 minutes. Recurring neurologic signs may require additional doses, up to a maximum of 15 to 20 g/day. As pyridoxine toxicity has occurred in human patients, large doses should be administered with caution and for limited periods. Because these mushrooms may affect several organ systems, blood glucose, methemoglobin levels, free hemoglobin, and hepatic and renal function should be monitored. If serious liver injury has occurred, therapeutic measures require the same supportive treatment as described for amanitin poisoning.

Animal Exposures

There are very few reports of gyromitrin poisoning in the veterinary literature. A 10-week-old dog who chewed on a *G. esculenta* started to vomit 2 to 3 hours later.[32] The dog became lethargic and comatose 6 hours after exposure and died 30 minutes later. Histopathologic findings included renal tubulonephrosis, periascinar hepatic degeneration, and erythrophagocytosis. Rabbits poisoned with gyromitrin developed anorexia, depression, tonic-clonic seizures, hemoglobinuria, proteinuria, bilirubinuria, decreased urinary pH, and weight loss. Postmortem findings were fatty degeneration of the liver and tubular degenerative changes.[33]

Isoxazoles—Ibotenic Acid and Muscimol

Toxins that have psychotropic properties have been found in *Amanita muscaria, Amanita pantherina, Amanita strobiliformis, Amanita gemmata, Amanita smithiana,* and *Tricholoma muscarium.* Many of these mushrooms are cosmopolitan species found all over the United States. Some are used intentionally for recreational purposes. The major isoxazoles are ibotenic acid and muscimol, which are not degraded by heat. Decarboxylation of ibotenic acid during drying or digestion can result in the formation of muscimol. Their neurotoxic properties are based on their ability to cross the blood-brain barrier and their structural similarity with glutamic acid and GABA.[34] Ibotenic acid is an agonist of N-methyl-D-aspartate glutamate receptors, whereas muscimol is a potent GABA$_A$ agonist. When muscimol is given to rats, it affects brain serotonin, noradrenalin, and dopamine levels in a manner similar to that characteristic of lysergic acid diethylamide (LSD), psilocybin, and mescaline.[35]

Toxicity and Clinical Signs

Although concentrations of ibotenic acid and muscimol can vary considerably, ingestion of a single *A. pantheriana* can be deadly to a dog.[23] In humans, a minimum of 6 mg of muscimol and 30 mg of ibotenic acid result in psychoactive effects.[36] *A. muscaria* (Color Plate 62-6) can contain 100 mg/kg (fresh weight) of ibotenic acid. Thus an average-size (60 to 70 g) fruiting body of *A. muscaria* can result in intoxication. The reported oral LD_{50} in mice is 22 mg/kg for muscimol and 38 mg/kg for ibotenic acid.

In humans, isoxazole poisoning has been termed the "pantherine-muscaria" syndrome. First clinical signs of poisoning appear 30 to 90 minutes after ingestion and include unsteadiness, drowsiness, confusion, nausea, vomiting, diarrhea, hallucinations, disorientation in place and time, euphoria or depression, anxiety, and mystical experiences. In severe cases, coma, convulsions, and respiratory and circulatory collapse may occur; fatalities can occur but are not common. In most cases there is complete recovery within 24 hours.[37] Anticholinergic effects, such as mydriasis and cycloplegia may also occur. Clinical signs are generally maximal 2 to 3 hours after ingestion. In dogs and cats, clinical signs of poisoning are disorientation, opisthotonus, paresis, seizures, paddling, chewing movements, miosis, vestibular signs, respiratory depression, and in severe cases coma.

Diagnostic Workup

To confirm an isoxazole intoxication, analysis of urine for muscimol and ibotenic acid is possible.[38] The toxins can be detected in urine within 1 hour of ingestion. Severity of intoxication does not correlate with urinary isoxazole alkaloid levels, as peak clinical signs may still be present more than 5 hours after peak excretion. Accurate mushroom identification can aid in the diagnosis.

Treatment

There is no specific antidote or treatment. Atropine is not recommended. Care is generally symptomatic and supportive, and special attention must be given to medications for seizure control. As mentioned, muscimol interferes with $GABA_A$ receptors. Therefore administration of GABAergic anticonvulsants such as diazepam, midazolam, or phenobarbital may result in respiratory or central nervous system depression, and thus the lowest effective therapeutic dose should be used. Extremely drowsy or unconscious animals have to be carefully monitored and treated accordingly. In small animals, recoveries are expected within 24 hours of ingestion and accompanying therapeutic measures including mechanical ventilation during periods of respiratory depression.

Animal Exposures

In the North American Mycological Associations Case Registry, the most commonly ingested mushrooms by dogs were the *A. muscaria* and *A. pantherina* species. The signs most frequently reported were lethargy, staggering, whining, panting, agitation, dizziness, and hyperactivity.

A severe but transient neurologic disorder similar to that seen in humans following ingestion of *A. pantherina* developed in three 5-week-old German shepherd puppies. The exact quantity of poison ingested was unknown.[39] *A. muscaria* ingestion resulted in vomiting, diarrhea, panting, labored breathing, muscle spasms, collapse, cyanosis, and eventual death in a 4-year-old, 13-kg male Cairn terrier. The dog aspirated vomitus on the way to the veterinarian, which probably contributed to its death.[21] *A. pantherina* was ingested by a 6-kg female West Highland white terrier of unknown age.[40] The animal vomited several pieces of mushroom later and was taken to the veterinarian, where the presenting signs included tachycardia, muscular tremors, incoordination, head pressing, and salivation. Hypercalcemia was the only notable serum chemistry abnormality. A dog consumed mushrooms (thought to be *A. muscaria* or *A. pantherina*) and became disoriented. This dog habitually ingested mushrooms.[41]

A cat ingested a small piece of an owner's stash of dried *A. muscaria* and vomited but eventually recovered.[42] Cats with *A. pantherina* exposures developed sedation within 15 to 30 minutes of exposure, followed by a 4-hour period of muscle spasms and excitement.[43] They fully recovered within a day.

Psilocin and Psilocybin

Mushrooms in the psilocin and psilocybin group are often referred to as "magic mushrooms" because of their psychoactive properties. The psychotropic compounds have been isolated from four genera of mushrooms: *Psilocybe, Panaeolus, Gymnopilus,* and *Conocybe*; some *Stropharia* species in the United States are also thought to contain this toxin. They are common in the northwestern and southeastern United States, and many are coprophilic. The majority of mushrooms contain only psilocybin, but some, such as *Psilocybe cyanescens, Psilocybe cubensis,* and *Psilocybe semilanceata,* contain psilocybin and psilocin. Both compounds are classified as schedule I drugs in the United States.

Psilocybin and psilocin are classic 4-substituted tryptamine hallucinogens. It appears that psilocybin acts as a prodrug as esterases rapidly convert it to its hydroxyl metabolite psilocin. Psilocin is considered the major pharmacologically active compound derived from "magic mushrooms." Although the effect on neurotransmitter systems is not fully understood, it is known that psilocin's structural similarity to serotonin results in stimulation of serotonin receptors.[44] In addition, dimethyltryptamines also have peripheral effects by being substrates at the plasma membrane serotonin transporter and the vesicle monoamine transporter.[45]

Toxicity and Clinical Signs

Concentrations of greater than 115 mcg/kg psilocybin result in psychological effects in humans.[46] Psychedelic effects are seen if the psilocybin dose exceeds 8 to 10 mg. Depending on the concentrations of psilocin and psilocybin, 1 to 20 mushrooms may be required to produce psychological effects. There is no data on toxicity for dogs or cats.

In humans, a dysphoric hallucinogenic state similar to LSD begins approximately 20 to 30 minutes after ingestion; however, onset of clinical signs may be delayed for up to 3 hours. Clinical signs include an altered state of consciousness, sweating, alterations in mood, changes in perception of time and space, illusions, visual hallucinations, speech alterations, compulsive movements, panic attacks, flash-backs, and acute psychoses.[47] Effects usually last for 4 to 8 hours, with the peak activity occurring after approximately 1 hour. Some nonpsychological effects, such as mydriasis (18 hours), hypertension (18 hours), and drowsiness (24 hours) may persist for longer periods. Nausea and vomiting occur in approximately 20% of reported cases. In dogs, exposure to psilocybin containing mushrooms can result in aggression, ataxia, vocalization, nystagmus, seizures, and increased body temperature.[48]

Diagnostic Workup

Exposure can be confirmed by detection of psilocin and psilocybin in urine, serum, or gastrointestinal contents. The analysis by liquid chromatography-mass spectrometry is offered only by select veterinary diagnostic laboratories. It is important to note that macroscopic identification of dried hallucinogenic mushrooms is very difficult. Thus it is especially critical to submit suspect mushrooms to an experienced mycologist for identification.

Treatment

Inducing emesis may not alter the clinical course. In addition, emetics are recommended only in patients that are asymptomatic, with little risk for developing aspiration pneumonia, and that have recently ingested the mushrooms. Most cases are managed with supportive care. Patients should be placed in a stimulus-free environment. If severe neurologic signs occur, diazepam (0.5-1 mg/kg IV, repeat in 5 minutes if no effect) is the initial drug of choice. Diazepam has a short duration of action ranging from 20 to 60 minutes and can be repeated if necessary. IV fluid therapy should be instituted to maintain perfusion and to prevent or correct dehydration.

Animal Exposures

A colt developed pyrexia, tremors of the triceps, dilated pupils, and hyperexcitability, followed by recumbency or seminarcosis and generalized weakness. The animal was euthanized 48 hours later. The pasture had large numbers of *Psilocybe* mushrooms.[49] Seizures developed in puppies intraperitoneally injected with 15 mg/kg of pure psilocybin.[50] A dog developed aggression, ataxia, vocalization, nystagmus, seizures, and had an increased body temperature after ingestion of "magic mushrooms" (species unidentified).[48] The dog had an uneventful recovery on day 3.

Mushrooms Resulting In Gastrointestinal Distress

Muscarine

Mushrooms in the genera *Inocybe* and *Clitocybe* spp. contain the highest concentrations of muscarine, but *Entoloma* spp., *Mycena* spp., *Boletus* spp., *Rubinoboletus* spp., and *A. muscaria* also contain muscarine, yet in much lower concentrations. *Inocybe* and *Clitocybe* spp. are frequently found worldwide in forested areas and grasslands.

Muscarine is thermostable and not degraded by digestive enzymes. As it is a quarternary ammonium compound, it is poorly absorbed from the gastrointestinal tract and does not cross the blood-brain barrier. Thus the effects of muscarine on cholinergic receptors are predominantly peripheral, with smooth muscles, glands, and the cardiovascular system representing the major targets.

Toxicity and Clinical Signs

In humans, the oral lethal dose of muscarine is estimated between 40 mg and 495 mg. Based on the muscarine concentrations of between 0.1% and 0.33% (dry weight) in *Inocybe* and *Clitocybe* spp., ingestion of a single mushroom can be lethal. To produce clinical signs, mushrooms usually must contain a minimum of 0.01% muscarine. Therefore ingestion of *A. muscaria,* which contains only approximately 0.0003% muscarine, does not lead to a cholinergic syndrome, but can result in isoxazole poisoning.

Clinical signs of cholinergic overstimulation usually develop between 0.5 and 2 hours after ingestion. When high concentrations of muscarine are present, signs may appear in as little as 15 to 20 minutes. A delay in onset of clinical signs appears to be directly related to the amount of mushroom ingested and its muscarine concentration. Humans with muscarine poisoning develop excessive perspiration, lacrimation, and salivation (so-called PSL syndrome) within 15 to 30 minutes after ingestion. The combination of these symptoms is diagnostic and is generally seen only with this type of mushroom poisoning.[51] The patient may also develop blurred vision, miosis, vomiting, abdominal pain, increased peristalsis, watery diarrhea, bradycardia, lowered blood pressure, dyspnea, congested pulmonary circulation, bronchorrhea, urinary incontinence, and nasal discharge. Peripheral vasodilation, mild hypotension, and flushing may also be seen. Dogs develop typical signs of muscarinic overstimulation, including salivation, diarrhea, vomiting, depression, and collapse.[52] The clinical signs—salivation, lacrimation, urination, diarrhea, dyspnea, and emesis—are often described using the acronym SLUDDE.

Diagnostic Workup

Muscarine can be detected in urine and gastrointestinal contents, but analysis is not routinely offered by veterinary diagnostic laboratories. In addition, response to treatment with atropine is an important diagnostic parameter.

Treatment

If the animal has not already vomited, emesis is probably indicated. Activated charcoal may also be of some use, but, because of the rapid onset of clinical signs, decontamination is often not feasible. Because muscarine causes increased gastric tract peristalsis and diarrhea in many patients, administration of a cathartic is probably unnecessary. If life-threatening cholinergic clinical signs occur, atropine should be administered. If there are no signs of atropinization after a low-dose test dose of atropine, additional atropine may be administered. The end point is not mydriasis but the cessation of respiratory secretions. IV fluid therapy should be instituted as needed to maintain perfusion and to prevent or correct dehydration.

Animal Exposures

A 14-year-old springer spaniel was found eating mushrooms. *Coprinus micaceus, Hygrocybe ceracea, Laccaria laccata,* and *Inocybe phaeocomis* (containing muscarine) were found in the gastric lavage fluid. Salivation, capillary refill time of more than 3 seconds, drowsiness, increased intestinal activity, vomiting, diarrhea, body temperature of 36.1° C, and a heart rate of 100 beats per minute were observed. The dog improved with symptomatic treatment within 24 hours and was released 48 hours after exposure.[52] A 10-year-old Maltese dog ate 5 to 10 *Inocybe fastigiata.*[53] Within 1 hour, the dog developed marked salivation, frequent vomiting, lacrimation, diarrhea, respiratory difficulty, and weakness. The dog recovered within 48 hours after a gastric lavage was performed and atropine was given.

Other Gastrointestinal Irritants

Agaricus xanthodermus, Amanita volvata, Boletus satanas, Chlorophyllum molybdites, Entoloma lividum, Gomphus floccosus, Lactarius spp., *Lampteromyces japonica, Rhodophyllus rhodopolius, Rhodophyllus sinuatus, Scleroderma* spp., and *Tricholoma* spp. are all mushrooms that can cause gastrointestinal irritation. This group includes a variety of mushrooms and toxins. It is a "catch-all" category for cases that present primarily with gastrointestinal signs. For most of the mushrooms, the specific toxins are unknown. It is obvious that gastrointestinal distress is a very common clinical presentation in small animals and that, in most instances, a specific cause is not identified. Additionally, not all of the gastrointestinal reactions are due to mushroom toxins. Occasionally spoiled mushrooms (contaminated by bacteria) are ingested and cause illness. When evaluating cases of gastrointestinal mushroom "poisonings," bacterial infections and other causes for gastrointestinal distress must be included in the list of differential diagnoses.

Poisonings by mushrooms of this category are rarely fatal; however, a few fatalities have been reported in Europe. Nausea, vomiting, abdominal pain, and diarrhea occur relatively soon, within 15 minutes to 2 hours, after ingestion. Weakness, dizziness, paresthesia, tetany, headache, and sweating have also been reported in humans. Some of these neurologic clinical signs, such as paresthesia and tetany, may be due to fear and hyperventilation.[54] Usually the clinical signs resolve spontaneously within a few hours, but they may last a day or two. There are few serious sequelae. It is important to carefully evaluate the lag period between suspected exposure to mushrooms and onset of gastrointestinal signs: onset is within minutes to a few hours with mushrooms in this category, whereas onset is delayed by 6 to 12 hours in potentially lethal amanitin intoxications.

Omphalotus illudens is common in North America and is also known as *Jack O'Lantern mushroom.* The toxin is thought to be illuden S.[55] *Omphalotus olearius* and *Lampteromyces* spp. also contain this toxin and have been reported to cause illness. Treatment is generally limited to rehydration and correction of any electrolyte abnormalities.

C. molybdites, commonly known as the *false parasol,* is widespread and can cause significant nausea, vomiting, and diarrhea. It is a gray-green, spored mushroom that superficially looks like the meadow mushroom *Agaricus campestris.* The toxin is unknown. Vomiting can be extensive and hospitalization may be required for fluid and electrolyte replacement.[54] A human case of hypovolemic shock has been reported.[56]

The chemicals leading to gastrointestinal distress are as diverse as the mechanisms. *Albatrellus* species have been shown to contain irritant monoterpenes.[57] *Gomphus* toxicity is due to norcaperatic acid, an aconitase inhibitor.[58] *Hebeloma crustuliniforme* contains the cytotoxic triterpene hebelomic acid A,[59] and *Hebeloma vinosophyllum* contains various cucurbitane triterpene glycosides.[60] *Laccaria amethystine* contains lectins that may contribute to gastroenteritis in a manner similar to that seen with the lectins in castor bean intoxications.[61] *Russula* and *Lactarius* species contain marasmane or lactarane sesquiterpenes[62]; *Laetiporus sulphureus* and *Meripilus* species contain phenolethylamines such as tyramine. It is unknown what specific contribution all these compounds make to gastroenteritis.

Diagnostic Workup

Diagnosis is essentially based on history, clinical signs, mushroom identification, and laboratory abnormalities or lack thereof (i.e., no elevation in liver enzymes). Because for most mushrooms in this group, specific toxin analysis is not possible, any sample that contains parts of the suspect mushroom (vomitus, mushroom pieces, whole mushrooms) should be saved and submitted for identification. This is critical in reaching a diagnosis.

Treatment

The severity of illness depends on the type of mushroom, amount ingested, and individual sensitivity. Many cases are self-limiting and resolve without treatment. However, the need for treatment must be made on a case-by-case basis after careful evaluation and examination. There are no specific antidotes, and treatment is symptomatic and supportive. Emesis is generally not needed because most mushrooms in this group result in rapid onset of vomiting. In fact, administration of antiemetics may be needed. Activated charcoal can be considered. Administration of IV fluids is important to maintain hydration and electrolyte balance. Gastrointestinal protectants may be given. In most cases, the prognosis is good and full recovery is expected within a few hours to days.

Animal Exposures

Bloody vomiting developed in a cat after ingesting some mushrooms in the owner's yard.[63] Several of the mushrooms were presumptively identified as a *Russula* species. The mushrooms had a shellfish odor that may have attracted the animal. The animal was examined by a veterinarian, but no confirmed diagnosis was made.

A 1-year-old cat ingested part of an unknown species of *Agaricus* and developed diarrhea, disorientation, foaming at the mouth, and vomiting. The amount consumed was thought to be approximately half of a cap.[21] A 7-month-old pet potbellied pig ate a *Scleroderma citrinum* and died 5 hours later.[64] Within 20 minutes the pig started vomiting, and by 1 hour it was depressed, weak, recumbent, hypothermic, tachycardic, and tachypneic, in addition to having continuous vomiting.

Nephrotoxic Mushrooms

Cortinaria spp. are commonly known as "web-caps" and are difficult to identify; the edibility of many species is unknown. The presence of the nephrotoxin orellanine has been confirmed in some *Cortinarius* mushrooms.[65] In addition, these mushrooms also contain cortinarin, a nephrotoxic cyclopeptide that may contribute to the nephrotoxic effects. Poisonings have been reported in humans, especially in Europe, and there are no reports of accidental poisonings in dogs or cats. Diagnosis is difficult, because clinical signs may not appear for 2 to 20 days after ingestion, and orellanine can only be detected for approximately 24 hours after exposure.[66] Onset of signs and severity of illness are dose-dependent. Animals may exhibit anorexia, vomiting, diarrhea, polydipsia, polyuria, abdominal pain, paresthesia, depression, and renal failure. Decontamination methods are useful if the ingestion is recognized in the first few hours. There is no specific antidote and treatment consists of supportive care for renal failure and gastrointestinal signs. IV fluids, gastrointestinal protectants, and antiemetics may be used. In humans, chronic hemodialysis is often necessary. Kidneys recover slowly but return to normal function. Dialysis can be helpful during this period of renal failure and renal transplantation is necessary only in severe cases.

Amanita smithiana grows along the Pacific coast from British Columbia to California. It has characteristic *Amanita* spp. features, such as a white cap, a veil, and a volva, and has been mistaken for the edible matsutake mushroom (*Tricholoma magnivelare*). At this time, there are no confirmed reports in animals. Poisonings have been reported in humans and are characterized by gastrointestinal and renal effects.[67] In contrast to amanitin poisoning, there is no liver damage with *A. smithiana* intoxication. *A. smithiana* intoxication differs from orellanine poisoning by a much shorter latency period until renal failure develops. Typically, initial clinical signs of vomiting, nausea, abdominal pain, and diarrhea develop approximately 5 hours after ingestion, but signs may develop earlier. Thus *A. smithiana* exposure may initially look like a poisoning from a "gastrointestinal irritant" mushroom. Renal failure develops 1 to 4 days after exposure and may require several weeks of hemodialysis before recovery. The toxin is allenic norleucine and routine diagnostic testing is not available. Thus diagnosis is based on history, clinical signs, and mycologic identification. Treatment is focused on supportive care for renal failure and gastrointestinal signs, and a complete recovery is expected within several days to weeks.

Animal Exposures

A cat, guinea pig, and mouse were experimentally given *Cortinarius orellanus* orally and clinical signs developed similar to those seen in humans. The tubular epithelium of the kidney was the primary target.[68] Sheep grazing a field with *Cortinarius speciosissimus* developed severe renal damage.[69]

Conclusions

Today, emergency and critical care clinicians have increasing occasions to treat mushroom poisonings. Availability of specific toxicology testing will provide much needed data on the frequency and type of mushroom poisonings in dogs and cats. Toxicology testing will also help establish confirmed diagnoses, which may ultimately lead to the development of prognostic markers. There are also gaps in knowledge about the efficacy of treatment regimens for mushroom poisonings in animals. Having confirmed diagnoses will allow better comparison of therapeutic approaches.

There are many types of mushrooms that can be ingested by animals and there is the potential for acute and severe clinical signs and death. Accurate identification of mushrooms collected from the environment or found in stomach contents by nonmycologists is challenging. Thus it is safest to assume that any mushroom exposure is potentially toxic and a complete clinical assessment should be performed. Particular attention must be given to animals that may have ingested amanitin-containing mushrooms.

Ackowledgment

I wish to acknowledge the exceptional contribution of David Spoerke, who authored this chapter for the previous edition of the book.

References

1. Puschner B, Rose HH, Filigenzi MS: Diagnosis of Amanita toxicosis in a dog with acute hepatic necrosis, *J Vet Diag Invest* 19:312–317, 2007.
2. Tokarz D, Poppenga R, Kaae J, et al: Amanitin toxicosis in two cats with acute hepatic and renal failure, *Vet Pathol OnlineFirst*, December 19, 2011.
3. Beug M: NAMA toxicology committee report for 2009. North American mushroom poisonings, *McIlvainea* 19:1–5, 2009.
4. Li C, Oberlies NH: The most widely recognized mushroom: chemistry of the genus, *Amanita Life Sci* 78:532–538, 2005.
5. Himmelmann A, Mang G, Schnorf-Huber S: Lethal ingestion of stored *Amanita phalloides* mushrooms, *Swiss Med Wkly* 131:616–617, 2001.
6. Gundala S, Wells LD, Milliano MT, et al: The hepatocellular bile acid transporter Ntcp facilitates uptake of the lethal mushroom toxin alpha-amanitin, *Arch Toxicol* 78:68–73, 2004.
7. Letschert K, Faulstich H, Keller D, et al: Molecular characterization and inhibition of amanitin uptake into human hepatocytes, *Toxicol Sci* 91:140–149, 2006.
8. Lindell TJ, Weinberg F, Morris PW, et al: Specific inhibition of nuclear RNA polymerase II by alpha-amanitin, *Science* 170:447–449, 1970.
9. Arima Y, Nitta M, Kuninaka S, et al: Transcriptional blockade induces p53-dependent apoptosis associated with translocation of p53 to mitochondria, *J Biol Chem* 280:19166–19176, 2005.
10. Faulstich H, Fauser U: The course of Amanita intoxication in beagle dogs. In Faulstich H, Kommerell B, Wieland T, editors: *Amanita toxins and poisoning*, Baden-Baden, Germany, 1980, Verlag Gerhard Witzstrock, pp 115–123.

11. Harper KA, Smart CD, Davis RM: Development of a DNA-based macroarray for the detection and identification of *Amanita* species, *J Forensic Sci* 56:1003–1009, 2011.
12. Filigenzi MS, Poppenga RH, Tiwary AK, et al: Determination of alpha-amanitin in serum and liver by multistage linear ion trap mass spectrometry, *J Agric Food Chem* 55:2784–2790, 2007.
13. Thiel C, Thiel K, Klingert W, et al: The enterohepatic circulation of amanitin: kinetics and therapeutical implications, *Toxicol Lett* 203:142–146, 2011.
14. Beuhler M, Lee DC, Gerkin R: The Meixner test in the detection of alpha-amanitin and false-positive reactions caused by psilocin and 5-substituted tryptamines, *Ann Emerg Med* 44:114–120, 2004.
15. Trabulus S, Altiparmak MR: Clinical features and outcome of patients with amatoxin-containing mushroom poisoning, *Clin Toxicol (Phila)* 49:303–310, 2011.
16. Enjalbert F, Rapior S, Nouguier-Soule J, et al: Treatment of amatoxin poisoning: 20-year retrospective analysis, *J Toxicol Clin Toxicol* 40:715–757, 2002.
17. Abenavoli L, Capasso R, Milic N, et al: Milk thistle in liver diseases: past, present, future, *Phytother Res* 24:1423–1432, 2010.
18. Karlson-Stiber C, Persson H: Cytotoxic fungi—an overview, *Toxicon* 42:339–349, 2003.
19. Vogel G, Tuchweber B, Trost W, et al: Protection by silibinin against Amanita phalloides intoxication in beagles, *Toxicol Appl Pharmacol* 73:355–362, 1984.
20. Magdalan J, Ostrowska A, Piotrowska A, et al: Benzylpenicillin, acetylcysteine and silibinin as antidotes in human hepatocytes intoxicated with alpha-amanitin, *Exp Toxicol Pathol* 62:367–373, 2010.
21. Trestrail JHI: Mushroom poisoning case registry: NAMA report 1994, *McIlvainea* 12:68–73, 1995.
22. Tegzes JH, Puschner B: Amanita mushroom poisoning: efficacy of aggressive treatment of two dogs, *Vet Hum Toxicol* 44:96–99, 2002.
23. Hunt RS, Funk A: Mushrooms fatal to dogs, *Mycologia* 69:432–433, 1977.
24. Kallet A, Sousa C, Spangler W: Mushroom (*Amanita phalloides*) toxicity in dogs, *Calif Vet 42* 9-11(22):47, 1988.
25. Liggett AD, Weiss R: Liver necrosis caused by mushroom poisoning in dogs, *J Vet Diagn Invest* 1:267–269, 1989.
26. Cole FM: A puppy death and *Amanita-phalloides, Aust Vet J* 70:271–272, 1993.
27. Frazier K, Liggett A, Hines M 2nd, et al: Mushroom toxicity in a horse with meningioangiomatosis, *Vet Hum Toxicol* 42:166–167, 2000.
28. Yee MM, Woods LW, Poppenga RH, et al: Amanitin intoxication in two beef calves in California, *J Vet Diagnost Invest* 24(1):241–244, 2012.
29. Lheureux P, Penaloza A, Gris M: Pyridoxine in clinical toxicology: a review, *Eur J Emerg Med* 12:78–85, 2005.
30. Michelot D, Toth B: Poisoning by *Gyromitra esculenta*—a review, *J Appl Toxicol* 11:235–243, 1991.
31. Arshadi M, Nilsson C, Magnusson B: Gas chromatography-mass spectrometry determination of the pentafluorobenzoyl derivative of methylhydrazine in false morel (*Gyromitra esculenta*) as a monitor for the content of the toxin gyromitrin, *J Chromatogr A* 1125:229–233, 2006.
32. Bernard MA: Mushroom poisoning in a dog, *Can Vet J* 20:82–83, 1979.
33. Niskanen A, Pyysalo H: Short-term peroral toxicity of ethylidene gyromitrin in rabbits and chickens, *Food Cosmet Toxicol* 14:409–415, 1976.
34. Michelot D, Melendez-Howell LM: *Amanita muscaria*: chemistry, biology, toxicology, and ethnomycology, *Mycol Res* 107:131–146, 2003.
35. Konig-Bersin P, Waser PG, Langemann H, et al: Monoamines in the brain under the influence of muscimol and ibotenic acid, two psychoactive principles of *Amanita muscaria, Psychopharmacologia* 18.1–10, 1970.
36. Theobald W, Buch O, Kunz HA, et al: Pharmacological and experimental psychological studies with 2 components of fly agaric (*Amanita muscaria*), *Arzneimittelforschung* 18:311–315, 1968.
37. Satora L, Pach D, Butryn B, et al: Fly agaric (*Amanita muscaria*) poisoning, case report and review, *Toxicon* 45:941–943, 2005.
38. Stribrny J, Sokol M, Merova B, et al: GC/MS determination of ibotenic acid and muscimol in the urine of patients intoxicated with *Amanita pantherina, Int J Legal Med* 126(4):519–524, 2012.
39. Naude TW, Berry WL: Suspected poisoning of puppies by the mushroom *Amanita pantherina, J South African Vet Assoc* 68:154–158, 1997.
40. Shaw M: Reported case of an *Amanita pantherina* ingestion in a dog. In Trestrail JHI, editor: *North American Mycological Association report*, Grand Rapids, MI, 1994, Grand Rapids Poison Center.
41. Shaw M: Reported case of an *Amanita pantherina* or muscaria ingestion in a dog. In Trestrail JHI, editor: *North American Mycological Association report*, Grand Rapids, MI, 1994, Grand Rapids Poison Center.
42. Shaw M: Reported case of an *Amanita muscaria* ingestion in a cat, *North American Mycological Association report*, Grand Rapids, MI, 1993, Grand Rapids Poison Center.
43. Ridgway RL: Mushroom (*Amanita pantherina*) poisoning, *J Am Vet Med Assoc* 172:681–682, 1978.

44. Halberstadt AL, Koedood L, Powell SB, et al: Differential contributions of serotonin receptors to the behavioral effects of indoleamine hallucinogens in mice, *J Psychopharmacol* 25:1548–1561, 2011.
45. Cozzi NV, Gopalakrishnan A, Anderson LL, et al: Dimethyltryptamine and other hallucinogenic tryptamines exhibit substrate behavior at the serotonin uptake transporter and the vesicle monoamine transporter, *J Neural Transm* 116:1591–1599, 2009.
46. Studerus E, Kometer M, Hasler F, et al: Acute, subacute and long-term subjective effects of psilocybin in healthy humans: a pooled analysis of experimental studies, *J Psychopharmacol* 25:1434–1452, 2011.
47. Van Amsterdam J, Opperhuizen A, van den Brink W: Harm potential of magic mushroom use: a review, *Regul Toxicol Pharmacol* 59:423–429, 2011.
48. Kirwan AP: "Magic mushroom" poisoning in a dog, *Vet Rec* 126:149, 1990.
49. Jones J: "Magic mushroom" poisoning in a colt, *Vet Rec* 127:603, 1990.
50. McCawley EL, Brummett RE, Dana GW: Convulsions from psilocybe mushroom poisoning, *Proc West Pharmacol Soc* 5:27–33, 1962.
51. Lurie Y, Wasser SP, Taha M, et al: Mushroom poisoning from species of genus *Inocybe* (fiber head mushroom): a case series with exact species identification, *Clin Toxicol (Phila)* 47:562–565, 2009.
52. Yam P, Helfer S, Watling R: Mushroom poisoning in a dog, *Vet Rec* 133:24, 1993.
53. Lee S, Nam SJ, Choi R, et al: Mushroom poisoning by *Inocybe fastigiata* in a Maltese dog, *J Anim Vet Adv* 8:708–710, 2009.
54. Smith CW: Mushroom poisoning by *Chlorophyllum molybdites* in Hawaii, *Hawaii Med J* 39:13–14, 1980.
55. Vanden Hoek TL, Erickson T, Hryhorczuk D, et al: Jack o'lantern mushroom poisoning, *Ann Emerg Med* 20:559–561, 1991.
56. Stenklyft PH, Augenstein WL: *Chlorophyllum molybdites*—severe mushroom poisoning in a child, *J Toxicol Clin Toxicol* 28:159–168, 1990.
57. Vrkoc J, Budesinsky M, Dolejs L: Phenolic meroterpenoids from basidiomycete *Albatrellus ovinus*, *Phytochemistry* 16:1409–1411, 1977.
58. Carrano RA, Malone MH: Pharmacologic study of norcaperatic and agaricic acids, *J Pharm Sci* 56:1611, 1967.
59. Bocchi M, Garlaschelli L, Vidari G, et al: Fungal metabolites .27. New farnesane sesquiterpenes from *Heboloma senescens*, *J Nat Prod* 55:428–431, 1992.
60. Fujimoto H, Hagiwara H, Suzuki K, et al: New toxic metabolites from a mushroom, *Hebeloma vinosophyllum*. 2. Isolation and structures of Hebevinoside-VI, Hebevinoside-VII, Hebevinoside-VIII, Hebevinoside-IX, Hebevinoside-X, and Hebevinoside-Xi, *Chem Pharm Bull* 35:2254–2260, 1987.
61. Guillot J, Genaud L, Gueugnot J, et al: Purification and properties of 2 hemagglutinins of the mushroom *Laccaria amethystina*, *Biochem* 22:5365–5369, 1983.
62. Ayer WA, Browne LM: Terpenoid metabolites of mushrooms and related basidiomycetes, *Tetrahedron* 37:2199–2248, 1981.
63. Shaw M: Reported case of Russula ingestion in a cat, In Trestrail JH III, editor: *North American Mycological Association report*, Grand Rapids, MI, 1986, Grand Rapids Poison Center.
64. Galey FD, Rutherford JJ, Wells K: A case of scleroderma-citrinum poisoning in a miniature Chinese potbellied pig, *Vet Human Toxicol* 32:329–330, 1990.
65. Frank H, Zilker T, Kirchmair M, et al: Acute renal failure by ingestion of *Cortinarius* species confounded with psychoactive mushrooms—a case series and literature survey, *Clin Nephrol* 71:557–562, 2009.
66. Short AI, Watling R, MacDonald MK, et al: Poisoning by *Cortinarius speciosissimus*, *Lancet* 2:942–944, 1980.
67. West PL, Lindgren J, Horowitz BZ: Amanita smithiana mushroom ingestion: a case of delayed renal failure and literature review, *J Med Toxicol* 5:32–38, 2009.
68. Michelot D, Tebbett I: Poisoning by members of the genus *Cortinarius*—a review, *Mycol Res* 94:289–298, 1990.
69. Overas J, Ulvund MJ, Bakkevig S, et al: Poisoning in sheep induced by the mushroom *Cortinarius speciosissimus*, *Acta Vet Scand* 20:148–150, 1979.
70. Bresinsky A, Besl H: *A colour atlas of poisonous fungi. A handbook for pharmacists, doctors, and biologists*, London, 1990, Wolfe.
71. Kibby G: *Mushrooms and other fungi*, New York, 1992, Smithmark.
72. Smith AH, Smith-Weber N: *The mushroom hunter's field guide*, Ann Arbor, MI, 1980, University of Michigan Press.
73. Rambousek V, Janda J, Sikut M: [Severe *Amanita phalloides* poisoning in a 7-year-old girl], *Cesk Pediatr* 48:332–333, 1993.

Mycotoxins

Patricia A. Talcott, MS, DVM, PhD, DABVT

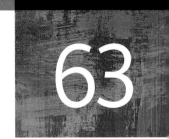

Aflatoxin

- Aflatoxin residues can be found on moldy food items and in dog food made with contaminated cereal grain (e.g., corn). The liver is the primary target organ.
- Commonly reported clinical signs include weakness, lethargy, depression, anorexia, vomiting and diarrhea, abdominal pain, and icterus.
- Clinical pathologic changes can include elevations in serum hepatic enzymes, hypoalbuminemia, hyperbilirubinemia, hyperbilirubinuria, hyperammonemia, anemia, thrombocytopenia, and increased clotting times.
- Confirmation of exposure includes detection of aflatoxin in the suspect feed; if large amounts were ingested and the intoxication is acute, detection of residue in liver collected postmortem may be possible.
- Treatment aims are supportive in nature, and prognosis depends on the extent and severity of liver damage.

Vomitoxin (Deoxynivalenol; DON)

- Vomitoxin can be found in dog foods made with contaminated cereal grain (e.g., wheat).
- Abrupt onset of refusal to eat preferred feed and vomiting are the most commonly observed signs in exposed dogs.
- Prognosis is excellent, and clinical signs cease abruptly once the contaminated food is removed. There are no long-term sequelae.

Penitrem A and Roquefortine

- Penitrem A and roquefortine can be found in moldy food items and decaying organic material, such as compost.
- Both mycotoxins are rapidly absorbed orally and cause excessive salivation, restlessness, muscle tremors, and seizures.
- Either methocarbamol or diazepam is a treatment option, coupled with appropriate symptomatic and supportive measures.
- Confirmation of exposure can best be accomplished by analysis of vomitus, lavage washings, gastric contents, serum, and urine.

Mycotoxins can cause significant losses in livestock. Because of differences in housing, feeding, and behavior of dogs and cats, poisonings in these species are much less common. Experimentally, however, dogs and cats are also susceptible to these toxins. For the purposes of this chapter, only those mycotoxins that have actually been reported in clinical poisoning cases are included.

Aflatoxin

Sources

Aflatoxins (the most prevalent of which is aflatoxin B_1) are specific chemical compounds produced by some toxicogenic strains of the *Aspergillus* group (e.g., *Aspergillus flavus, Aspergillus parasiticus,* and *Aspergillus nomius*) of fungi. These fungi grow when the moisture content of the substrate is 25% to 35% and air temperatures are 24° C to 35° C.[1] Aflatoxin contamination can be additive in foods, beginning in the preharvest crop and accumulating further during harvest, drying, storage, and processing.[2] Dogs have been poisoned by eating moldy food items (e.g., bread)[3,4] or contaminated grains (e.g., corn) used in the production of food.[5,6] There have been several instances in the past decade in which commercial pet foods have been contaminated with aflatoxins that have led to animal illnesses and death and pet food recalls.[7]

Toxic Dose

Dogs have been poisoned through the ingestion of dog food containing 100 to 300 ppb of aflatoxin[5] or moldy bread that was reported to contain 6.7 or 15 ppm of aflatoxin.[3,4] As observed in other species, young males and pregnant females may be more susceptible to the effects of aflatoxin. Experimentally, cats (oral median lethal dose [LD_{50}] = 0.55 mg/kg) are reported to be approximately as sensitive as dogs (oral LD_{50} = 0.80 mg/kg) to purified aflatoxin.[8]

Toxicokinetics

Following ingestion, aflatoxins are absorbed from the intestine and are largely taken up by the liver. Metabolic activation of aflatoxin to its 8,9-epoxide by a cytochrome P450 is necessary for toxicity.[9] This activation occurs in hepatocytes, proximal renal tubular epithelial cells, and, to a lesser extent, in other cells throughout the body. The highly reactive 8,9-epoxide then binds to and damages macromolecules (including deoxyribonucleic acid [DNA] and proteins) throughout the cell. Detoxification in the liver occurs largely through binding to glutathione and some biliary excretion.[10]

Mechanism of Toxicity

Following cytochrome P450 activation of aflatoxin to its reactive epoxide, binding to various intracellular macromolecules (e.g., DNA, ribonucleic acid, and proteins) is thought to be responsible for injury to and necrosis of hepatocytes and other metabolically active cells. This damage can ultimately lead to biliary hyperplasia, hepatic fibrosis, and decreased liver function.[8]

Clinical Signs

Dogs are very sensitive to the hepatotoxic effects of aflatoxin, and the clinical signs primarily reflect varying degrees of liver damage. In most reported cases, relatively short exposures of 1 to several days are thought to be involved, as opposed to the chronic exposures of weeks to months often seen in livestock and avian species. Acute poisoning with large dietary concentrations of aflatoxin results in weakness, depression, lethargy, severe gastrointestinal disturbances (e.g., vomiting and diarrhea), bleeding (sometimes with hemorrhage into the lumen of the intestine and elsewhere throughout the body), and icterus. Death can occur suddenly or within several days following the onset of clinical signs. Chronic exposure to lower levels of aflatoxin can result in anorexia, depression, vomiting, diarrhea, bleeding disorders (e.g., melena, epistaxis, and hemarthrosis), and icterus.[1,4,6]

Minimum Database

A minimum database should include a complete blood cell count, serum chemistry panel, urinalysis, and ammonia and bile acid levels. The most commonly reported alterations are increases in the serum activity of hepatic enzymes (e.g., alanine aminotransferase, aspartate aminotransferase, and alkaline phosphatase). Hypoalbuminemia, hyperbilirubinemia, hyperbilirubinuria, and elevations in serum or plasma ammonia concentrations can also occur. In severely affected dogs, prolongation of bleeding times, thrombocytopenia, elevation in bile acids, and anemia may be observed.

Confirmatory Tests

The most common confirmatory test is analysis of the suspected contaminated food items for aflatoxins.[11] Histologic examination of a liver biopsy sample can be useful to assist in ruling out other causes of hepatic disease. If the amount of ingested aflatoxin was recent and very large, liver analysis may be of value. Analysis of fresh liver (50 g) for aflatoxin residue is offered by some diagnostic laboratories.

Treatment

Treatment aims include prevention of further absorption by identification and removal of the contaminated feed and supportive care (e.g., maintenance of adequate caloric intake with a high-quality protein diet and intravenous fluids supplemented with dextrose and vitamins K_1 and B_{12}). Supplementation with liver protectants, such as *S*-adenosylmethionine, milk thistle, selenium, and vitamin E, should be highly considered.

Prognosis

In one reported outbreak, approximately 50 dogs ingested food containing aflatoxins for 13 to 17 days. Many died within 48 to 96 hours after the onset of clinical signs, although some did survive for several weeks to months. A few recovered after the contaminated food was eliminated.[6] The prognosis depends on the extent and severity of the liver damage.

Gross and Histologic Lesions

On gross examination, icterus, widespread petechial and ecchymotic hemorrhages, hepatic damage (fine red mottling with red to orange discoloration), ascites, and subserosal edema of the gallbladder may be seen. Microscopically, areas of hepatic necrosis and fatty change with proliferation of bile ducts and areas of regenerating liver parenchyma (nodular hyperplasia) were described in a dog following a 1- to 2-week history of aflatoxin exposure. Dogs that are acutely exposed to high aflatoxin concentrations in the diet often have widespread hemorrhage and massive hepatic necrosis. As exposure concentrations decline, histologic lesions vary greatly in severity (e.g., focal hepatocellular or periacinal necrosis, fatty change, varying degrees of inflammatory changes, megalocytosis, and biliary hyperplasia). Renal proximal tubular necrosis can also be present.[6,12]

Differential Diagnoses

Similar clinical signs can occur in dogs suffering from acute or chronic liver disease caused by a wide array of causative agents (e.g., congenital, infectious, neoplastic, chemical, or drug induced). Some toxic differentials include acetaminophen, microcystin from cyanobacteria (blue-green algae), xylitol, copper, zinc, pennyroyal oil, sago palm, iron, and amanitin and phalloidin from mushrooms.

Vomitoxin (Deoxynivalenol)

Sources

Vomitoxin (deoxynivalenol [DON]), one of many structurally related trichothecene mycotoxins, has been found in dog foods made with corn, wheat, barley, and oats contaminated with toxicogenic *Fusarium* spp.[1,13] Vomitoxin appears to remain stable through the high temperatures and pressures reached during the manufacturing of pet foods. Fungal infection of the cereal grain typically occurs in the field, and its presence is commonly associated with times of heavy rainfall and high humidity and delays in harvesting the crop.

Toxic Dose

In feeding trials testing beagles and Brittany spaniels, feed refusal was reported at 4 to 5 ppm DON in the feed. Cats showed feed refusal at 7.5 ppm DON.[14] Vomiting in dogs and cats was reported to be frequent at an 8- to 10-mg/kg concentration range.[14] Anecdotal incidences of vomiting and feed refusal (breeds not specified) have been reported with feed vomitoxin concentrations of approximately 1 to 4 ppm.

Toxicokinetics

In general, for most species, vomitoxin is thought to be rapidly absorbed in the gastrointestinal tract. Metabolism and excretion of DON seems to be species dependent and differs dramatically between monogastrics and ruminants. Swine metabolize very little of an absorbed vomitoxin dose and excrete it mainly unchanged through the urine. Ruminants and poultry, on the other hand, metabolize an orally administered dose of DON both in the rumen and in the liver. Very little of the parent form or metabolites are excreted via the milk.

Mechanism of Toxicity

DON is thought to initiate vomiting by directly affecting the chemoreceptor trigger zone. It also can cause gastrointestinal lesions that perhaps can affect the absorption of necessary nutrients. Vomitoxin has also been associated with skin irritation, cardiotoxicity, and immune system abnormalities in various species.

Clinical Signs

Clinical signs in exposed animals include an abrupt onset of feed refusal and vomiting, generally within 2 to 3 hours of ingestion. Diarrhea or abdominal tenderness are not common features of DON poisoning but can occur.

Minimum Database and Confirmatory Tests

A complete blood cell count, serum chemistry panel, abdominal radiographs or ultrasound, intestinal biopsies, and fecal analysis can help rule out other causes of anorexia and vomiting. These tests are often not necessary because signs abruptly subside once the contaminated food is removed. Exposure is confirmed by analyzing the suspected contaminated feed. Analysis for DON is performed by most veterinary diagnostic laboratories.

Treatment and Prognosis

Changing the diet, including removing the offending source and replacing with palatable, good-quality feed when vomiting has ceased, and basic supportive care (e.g., attending to the vomiting and diarrhea and any complications that could arise from these problems) should lead to a favorable prognosis. Few fatalities have been reported in small animals.

Gross and Histologic Lesions

There are no specific gross or histologic lesions, other than perhaps some congestion and edema of the gastrointestinal mucosal lining.

Differential Diagnoses

Other differentials should include causes of abrupt onset of vomiting, anorexia, and diarrhea. These should include viral, bacterial, or parasitic infections, pancreatitis, ethylene glycol, phenoxy herbicides, arsenic, copper, zinc, lead, zinc phosphide, neoplasia, and inflammatory bowel disease.

Tremorgens (Penitrem A and Roquefortine)

Sources

Penitrem A poisoning has been reported in dogs that have ingested moldy food items (e.g., moldy cheese, bread, and English walnuts). The mold *Penicillium crustosum* producing penitrem A has been incriminated most often.[15-17] Roquefortine poisoning has also been reported in dogs following ingestion of moldy food (e.g., moldy blue cheese) or decaying organic material (e.g., compost pile). *Penicillium roquefortii* and other *Penicillium* species producing roquefortine have been incriminated as sources.[18-23]

Toxic Dose

A dose of 0.5 mg/kg of purified penitrem A given intraperitoneally to dogs resulted in the onset of acute tremors.[24] In one case report, tremors were described in a small-breed dog following ingestion of one moldy piece of bread.[16]

Toxicokinetics

Both penitrem A and roquefortine are readily absorbed following ingestion, and both are excreted principally through the bile.[19] Very small amounts are found in the urine.

Mechanism of Toxicity

The mechanism of toxicity is unknown, but penitrem A may act as an antagonist to central nervous system glycine production by centrally inhibiting inhibitory neurons, or it may influence presynaptic neurotransmitter release.[16] It is still unclear whether both mycotoxins are independently toxic, whether they act synergistically, or whether one (roquefortine) is merely a biomarker for the presence of the other (penitrem A).

Clinical Signs

Clinical signs typically begin to appear within 30 minutes of toxin ingestion, but can be delayed for several hours (rare). Early signs of restlessness, panting, and excessive salivation often progress to include mild to moderate whole-body muscle tremors. In high-dose exposures, the tremors may become severe, and seizure activity is not uncommon. Poisoned patients often display hyperresponsiveness to external stimuli (e.g., touch and noise). Untreated muscle tremors lead to hyperthermia, exhaustion, and dehydration, along with possible metabolic acidosis (mild) and rhabdomyolysis (rare).

Minimum Database and Confirmatory Tests

The minimum database should include a complete blood cell count, serum chemistry panel, urinalysis, and acid-base assessment. Exposure to either penitrem A or roquefortine can be confirmed by analysis of suspect feed or compost, vomitus, gastric lavage washings, or stomach contents; these analytes have also been detected in very low levels in urine and serum.[25,26] Analysis of bile may be rewarding if vomitus or stomach contents are not available postmortem.[19]

Treatment

In asymptomatic animals, decontamination procedures should include induction of emesis followed by oral administration of activated charcoal and an osmotic cathartic. Symptomatic patients should be sedated or anesthetized and gastric lavage performed to remove the ingested material. This procedure should be followed by instillation of activated charcoal and a cathartic. Diazepam can be used to control agitation, muscle tremors, or seizure activity. Methocarbamol (either intramuscularly or intravenously) or barbiturates have been used successfully to control tremors and seizures when the patient does not respond to diazepam. A venous port should be established to provide intravenous fluids for the first 24 hours.

Prognosis

The majority of poisoned patients recovers uneventfully following aggressive therapy within 24 to 48 hours; however, with excessive exposures, clinical signs can be prolonged for up to 4 to 5 days.

Gross and Histologic Lesions

No significant gross or histologic lesions have been reported in animals that have died following either penitrem A or roquefortine exposure.

Differential Diagnoses

Differential diagnoses that should be considered include poisoning with strychnine, metaldehyde, theobromine, caffeine, pyrethroids, 1080, nicotine, recreational drugs, mushrooms, chlorinated hydrocarbon insecticides, bromethalin, or organophosphorus or carbamate acetylcholinesterase-inhibiting insecticides and eclampsia in a pregnant animal.

References

1. Osweiler GD, Carson TL, Buck WB, et al: *Clinical and diagnostic veterinary toxicology*, ed 3, Dubuque, Iowa, 1985, Kendall/Hunt Publishing.
2. Wilson DM, Payne GA: Factors affecting *Aspergillus flavus* group infection and aflatoxin contamination of crops. In Eaton DL, Groopman JD, editors: *The toxicology of aflatoxins: human health, veterinary and agricultural significance*, San Diego, 1994, Academic Press.
3. Bailly JD, Raymond I, Le Bars P, et al: Canine aflatoxicosis: reported case and review of the literature, *Rev Med Vet* 11:907–914, 1997.
4. Ketterer PJ, Williams ES, Blaney BJ, et al: Canine aflatoxicosis, *Aust Vet J* 51:355–357, 1975.
5. Bastianello SS, Nesbit JW, Williams MC, et al: Pathological findings in a natural outbreak of aflatoxicosis in dogs, *Onderstepoort J Vet Res* 54:635–640, 1987.
6. Thornburg LP, Raisbeck MF: A study of canine hepatobiliary diseases. Part 9: Hemolytic disease, mycotoxicosis, and pregnancy toxemia in the bitch, *Comp Anim Pract* 2(12):13–17, 1988.
7. Rumbeiha W, Morrison J: A review of class I and class II pet food recalls involving chemical contaminants from 1996-2008, *J Med Toxicol* 7(1):60–66, 2011.
8. Cullen JM, Newberne PM: Acute hepatotoxicity of aflatoxins. In Eaton DL, Groopman JD, editors: *The toxicology of aflatoxins: human health, veterinary and agricultural significance*, San Diego, 1994, Academic Press.
9. Eaton DL, Ramsdell HS, Neal GE: Biotransformation of aflatoxins. In Eaton DL, Groopman JD, editors: *The toxicology of aflatoxins: human health, veterinary and agricultural significance*, San Diego, 1994, Academic Press.
10. Hsieh DPH, Wong JJ: Pharmacokinetics and excretion of aflatoxins. In Eaton DL, Groopman JD, editors: *The toxicology of aflatoxins: human health, veterinary and agricultural significance*, San Diego, 1994, Academic Press.
11. Trucksess MW, Wood GE: Recent methods of analysis for aflatoxins in foods and feeds. In Eaton DL, Groopman JD, editors: *The toxicology of aflatoxins: human health, veterinary and agricultural significance*, San Diego, 1994, Academic Press.
12. Carlton WW, Szczech GM: Mycotoxicoses in laboratory animals. In Wyllie TD, Morehouse LG, editors: *Mycotoxic fungi, mycotoxins, mycotoxicoses*, vol 2, New York, 1978, Marcel Dekker.
13. Murphy M: *Common animal poisons*, Ames, 1996, Iowa State University Press.
14. Hughes DM, Gahl MJ, Graham CH, et al: Overt signs of toxicity to dogs and cats of dietary deoxynivalenol, *J Anim Sci* 77:693–700, 1999.
15. Arp LH, Richard JL: Intoxication of dogs with the mycotoxin penitrem A, *J Am Vet Med Assoc* 175(6):565–566, 1979.
16. Hocking AD, Holds K, Tobin NF: Intoxication by tremorgenic mycotoxin (penitrem A) in a dog, *Aust Vet J* 65(3):82–84, 1988.
17. Richard JL, Bacchetti P, Arp LH: Moldy walnut toxicosis in a dog caused by the mycotoxin penitrem A, *Mycopathologia* 75(3):55–58, 1981.
18. Puls R, Ladyman E: Roquefortine toxicity in a dog, *Can Vet J* 29:569, 1988.
19. Lowes NR, Smith RA, Beck BE: Roquefortine in the stomach contents of dogs suspected of strychnine poisoning in Alberta, *Can Vet J* 33:535–538, 1992.
20. Young KL, Villar D, Carson TL, et al: Tremorgenic mycotoxin intoxication with penitrem A and roquefortine in two dogs, *J Am Vet Med Assoc* 222:52–53, 2003.
21. Boysen SR, Rozanski EA, Chan DL, et al: Tremorgenic mycotoxicosis in four dogs from a single household, *J Am Vet Med Assoc* 221:1441–1444, 2002.
22. Naude TW, O'Brien OM, Rundberget T, et al: Tremorgenic neuromycotoxicosis in 2 dogs ascribed to the ingestion of penitrem A and possibly roquefortine in rice contaminated with, *Penicillium crustosum, J South African Vet Assoc* 73:211–215, 2002.
23. Walter SL: Acute penitrem A and roquefortine poisoning in a dog, *Can Vet J* 43:372–374, 2002.
24. Hayes AW, Presley DB, Neville JA: Acute toxicity of penitrem A in dogs, *Toxicol Appl Pharmacol* 35(2):311–320, 1976.
25. Braselton WE, Rumler PC: MS/MS screen for the tremorgenic mycotoxins roquefortine and penitrem A, *J Vet Diagn Invest* 8:515–518, 1996.
26. Braselton WE, Johnson M: Thin layer chromatography convulsant screen extended by gas chromatography-mass spectrometry, *J Vet Diagn Invest* 15:42–45, 2003.

Nicotine

Konnie H. Plumlee, DVM, MS, DABVT, DACVIM

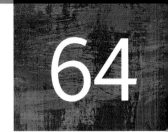

64

- Pets can be exposed to a variety of nicotine sources such as tobacco products, insecticides, and smoking cessation aids.
- Onset of clinical signs is rapid.
- Clinical signs vary with the dose of nicotine exposure. Vomiting, excitement, tremors, or convulsions may be evident after low-dose exposures and initially after high-dose exposures. The patient becomes depressed and a descending paralysis can occur following high-dose exposures.
- Prognosis is poor with high-dose exposures unless the animal can be stabilized quickly.

Sources

Animals can be exposed to nicotine from a variety of sources. Tobacco products include cigarettes, chewing tobacco, cigars, and snuff. Cigarette and cigarette-butt ingestions have been reported in domestic animals, with the vast majority by dogs, followed by cats, and occasionally by birds.[1] Cigarettes have been reported to contain varying levels of nicotine: 9 mg,[2] 15 to 20 mg,[3] 20 mg,[4] and 20 to 30 mg.[5] This disparity may reflect a difference in nicotine content among the various brands of cigarettes. One source reports that a regular cigar contains five times the amount of nicotine as a cigarette.[4] Each gram of moist snuff contains 12.9 to 16.6 mg of nicotine.[2] Chewing tobacco is palatable to dogs because it contains flavoring agents, such as honey, molasses, licorice, syrups, or sugar.[4]

Other sources of nicotine include smoking cessation aids such as skin patches and gums. Nicotine patches can contain 7 to 114 mg of nicotine. Gums can contain 2 to 4 mg of nicotine per piece.

Nicotine sulfate is present at concentrations of 0.05% to 4% in insecticidal dusts or sprays and also as a 40% concentrated solution known as Black Leaf 40.[6] Nicotine has also been used as an immobilizing agent for wild animals but has a very narrow margin of safety.

Toxic Dose

Clinical signs have been reported at 1 mg/kg nicotine.[1] The oral median lethal dose (LD_{50}) for nicotine in dogs is 9.2 mg/kg.[7]

Toxicokinetics

Nicotine is a water-soluble alkaloid that is readily absorbed via the gastrointestinal tract, skin, and mucous membranes.[5] Alkalinization of the stomach increases absorption. In humans nicotine has a half-life of 2 hours, and excretion is completed by 16 hours after exposure.[4] Nicotine is excreted via the kidneys and is pH dependent. Excretion is decreased when the urine pH is alkaline.[4]

Mechanism of Toxicity

At low doses, nicotine mimics acetylcholine and stimulates the postsynaptic nicotinic receptors of the central nervous system, sympathetic ganglia, parasympathetic ganglia, and neuromuscular junctions of skeletal muscle. Nicotine stimulates the emetic chemoreceptor trigger zone and can result in vomition. But at high doses, the initial stimulatory effects are followed by blockage of the nicotinic receptors caused by persistent depolarization.[6,8]

Clinical Signs

According to data from the American Society for the Prevention of Cruelty to Animals Animal Poison Control Center, between 2005 and 2010, 55% of dogs believed to have ingested tobacco products were vomiting and 25% were ataxic. Lethargy, hypersalivation, bradycardia, and tremors were also commonly reported.[1]

Signs often occur within 1 hour of exposure. Animals often vomit spontaneously because of stimulation of the emetic center.[4,5] Other digestive tract effects can include increased salivation and peristalsis and repeated defecation.[6] Miosis has been reported in dogs.[4]

Small doses of nicotine stimulate all autonomic ganglia. Bradycardia results from stimulation of the vagus nerve. Stimulation of the sympathetic ganglia results in peripheral vasoconstriction. After the nicotinic receptors become blocked as the absorbed dose of nicotine increases, the heart rate returns to normal and may become elevated. Vasodilation also occurs following high-dose exposures.[6]

At low-dose exposures and initially after high-dose exposures, stimulation of the central nervous system results in excitement, tremors, and possibly convulsions. At high doses, these signs progress to depression. Descending paralysis and depolarizing block of the neuromuscular junctions results in paralysis of the diaphragm and chest muscles, which is the cause of death.[6,8]

Confirmatory Tests

Urine, gastric contents, kidney, liver, and blood can be tested for nicotine.[4]

Treatment

No specific antidote for nicotine toxicosis is available. Decontamination by induced emesis or gastric lavage should be performed. Many animals vomit soon after nicotine ingestion, which aids in decontamination. Activated charcoal decreases further absorption of nicotine. Intravenous fluids will hasten elimination from the body. Acidification of the urine can be used to increase excretion as long as the animal is not acidotic. Antacids should not be administered because they can increase nicotine absorption from the stomach.

The heart rate and blood pressure should be monitored and the animal treated accordingly. Artificial respiration and oxygen therapy are warranted if the animal is suffering from respiratory paralysis. Seizures can be controlled with diazepam or barbiturates.

Prognosis

Exposures to high levels of nicotine warrant a poor prognosis. Patients that can be stabilized for the first 4 hours after intoxication have a much better chance of survival.[4]

Gross and Histologic Lesions

Necropsy and histopathologic findings are nonspecific.[4]

Differential Diagnoses

At low doses of nicotine and initially after high doses, the animals may exhibit signs similar to anticholinesterase insecticide poisoning: tremors, bradycardia, miosis, vomiting, hypersalivation, and increased defecation. The latter stages of high-dose nicotine poisoning are similar to those caused by many other depressants.

References

1. Novotny TE, Hardin SN, Hovda LR, et al: Tobacco and cigarette butt consumption in humans and animals, *Tobacco Control* 20(Suppl 1):i17, 2011.
2. Olson BL, Livingston GK, Potter RH, et al: Assessment of salivary cotinine levels in college students using smokeless tobacco, *Biol Monitoring* 1:53, 1991.
3. Kaplan B: Acute nicotine poisoning in a dog, *Vet Med* 63:1033, 1968.
4. Vig MM: Nicotine poisoning in a dog, *Vet Hum Toxicol* 32:573, 1990.
5. Saxena K, Scheman A: Suicide plan by nicotine poisoning: a review of nicotine toxicity, *Vet Hum Toxicol* 27:495, 1985.
6. Adams HR: Cholinergic pharmacology: autonomic drugs. In Adams HR, editor: *Veterinary pharmacology and therapeutics*, ed 7, Ames, 1995, Iowa State University Press.
7. *RTECS Registry of toxic effects of chemical substances.* National Institute for Occupational Safety and Health, Cincinnati, CD-ROM version, vol 43, Englewood, CO, MICROMEDEX Inc.
8. Manoguerra AS, Freeman D: Acute poisoning from the ingestion of *Nicotiana glauca*, *J Toxicol Clin Toxicol* 19:861, 1982-1983.

Nonsteroidal Antiinflammatories

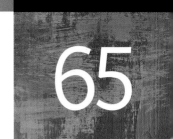

65

Patricia A. Talcott, MS, DVM, PhD, DABVT

Sharon M. Gwaltney-Brant, DVM, PhD, DABVT, DABT

- Nonsteroidal antiinflammatory drugs (NSAIDs) are popular drugs in human and veterinary medicine that are readily available to the pet population and can be harmful, if not deadly, to pets with improper use or accidental access.
- Because of species differences in pharmacokinetics, many NSAIDs are more toxic in cats and dogs than in humans.
- Gastrointestinal toxicity is the most common adverse effect of NSAID administration in animals.
- Clinical signs include vomiting, depression or stupor, diarrhea, anorexia, ataxia or incoordination, bloody stool and melena, polyuria, polydipsia, tachypnea, and panting.
- Idiosyncratic hepatopathy is possible with chronic NSAID administration.
- The minimum laboratory database may include a complete blood cell count, reticulocyte count, chemistry panel, blood gases, contrast studies, ultrasound, renal studies, bleeding times, and coagulation panel.
- Therapeutic options include the use of emetics, gastric aspiration and lavage, activated charcoal, intravenous fluid diuresis, correction of acidemia, gastric acid reducers, sucralfate, misoprostol, blood transfusions, hemoglobin-based oxygen-carrying solutions, or surgery (if indicated).
- Misoprostol (a prostaglandin E_1 analogue) is a key therapeutic drug for the prevention of NSAID-induced gastrointestinal lesions.

Sources

Nonsteroidal antiinflammatory drugs (NSAIDs) are very popular human and veterinary drugs, either prescription or sold as over-the-counter medications, and they are readily available to the pet population through misuse or accidental consumption (Table 65-1). These drugs are used for the treatment of pain, inflammation, and pyrexia. NSAIDs are classified according to their chemical structure: salicylates (e.g., aspirin), indoles (e.g., indomethacin), propionic acids (e.g., ibuprofen, naproxen, ketoprofen, and carprofen), fenamates (e.g., meclofenamic acid), azole derivatives (e.g., phenylbutazone, tepoxalin, and dipyrone), sulfonamides and sulfones (e.g., deracoxib and firocoxib), and oxicams (e.g., piroxicam and tenoxicam) (Table 65-2).[1,2] Certain drugs (e.g., diclofenac, ibuprofen, and naproxen) that have relatively safe profiles in humans can induce serious toxicoses in dogs.[1-8] Metabolism and half-lives of NSAIDs have species differences, and doses in dogs and cats should not be

Table 65-1	Examples of Veterinary and Human Food and Drug Administration–Approved Nonsteroidal Antiinflammatory Drugs
Veterinary Approved	**Human Approved**
Carprofen (dogs)	Celecoxib
Deracoxib (dogs)	Diclofenac
Diclofenac (horses)	Diflunisal
Etodolac (dogs)	Etodolac
Firocoxib (dogs, horses)	Fenoprofen
Flunixin meglumine (cattle, horses, swine)	Flurbiprofen
Ketoprofen (horses)	Ibuprofen
Meclofenamic acid (dogs, horses)	Indomethacin
Meloxicam (cats, dogs)	Ketoprofen
Naproxen (horses)	Ketorolac
Phenylbutazone (dogs, horses)	Meclofenamate
Robenacoxib	Mefenamic acid
Tepoxalin (dogs)	Meloxicam
	Nabumetone
	Naproxen
	Oxaprozin
	Piroxicam
	Rofecoxib
	Salsalate
	Sulindac
	Tolmetin

Table 65-2	Chemical Classification of Nonsteroidal Antiinflammatory Drugs
Oxicams	Piroxicam, meloxicam
Azole derivatives	Phenylbutazone, tepoxalin
Phenylacetic acid	Diclofenac, diclofenac, eltenac, robenacoxib
Salicylates	Acetylsalicylic acid, diflunisal
Propionic acids	Carprofen, fenoprofen, ibuprofen, ketoprofen, naproxen, tiaprofenic acid, vedaprofen
Fenamates	Meclofenamic acid, mefenamic acid, tolfenamic acid
Aminonicotinic acid	Flunixin meglumine
Pyrrolopyrrole	Ketorolac
Naphthylalkanone	Nabumetone
Indoleacetic acids	Indomethacin, sulindac, tolmetin, etodolac
Oxindoles	Tenidap
Sulfonamides and sulfones	Deracoxib, firocoxib, mavacoxib, nimesulide

extrapolated from recommended human doses.[1,2,4,5,8-13] The following section relates mostly to the toxic effects of ibuprofen; other NSAIDs are discussed separately at the end of the chapter.

Toxic Dose

The American Society for the Prevention of Cruelty to Animals (ASPCA) Animal Poison Control Center (APCC) lists ibuprofen as first in its top 10 incidences of poisonings in dogs, based on calls received between 2001 and 2005.[14] In cats ibuprofen and other NSAIDs were the seventh most common poisonings reported to the ASPCA APCC during the same time, with accidental ingestion of chewable formulations designed for dogs being a common scenario.[15]

Pharmacokinetic studies of ibuprofen administration in canines revealed that gastric lesions were produced in dogs given 8 mg/kg/day.[13] These lesions were produced by parenteral and oral administration, thus revealing that the ulcerogenic action of ibuprofen is partly systemic. All dogs receiving 16 mg/kg/day of ibuprofen were found to have gastric ulcers on postmortem examination.[13] A case report exists of a dog receiving 3 mg/kg every other day for 6 weeks that died of a perforated gastric ulcer.[16] As a single exposure, 25-125 mg/kg body weight BW of ibuprofen has been associated with gastrointestinal signs in dogs; ulceration is likely at doses exceeding 50 mg/kg. Doses of more than 100 to 175 mg/kg BW have resulted in renal failure; older dogs or dogs with preexisting renal disease may develop renal issues at lower doses.[14,16] Doses exceeding 400 mg/kg may result in central nervous system effects such as depression, seizures, and coma.[16] The acute minimum lethal dose of ibuprofen in dogs is 600 mg/kg, although dogs can die of complications from renal failure or gastrointestinal perforation at much lower doses. Cats are considered to be approximately twice as sensitive as dogs to the toxic effects of ibuprofen.

Toxicokinetics and Mechanism of Toxicity

NSAIDs are a group of drugs with very different chemical structures that share many physiologic activities. The analgesic, antipyretic, and antiinflammatory actions of NSAIDs are caused by direct inhibition of cyclooxygenase (COX), an enzyme system that catalyzes the formation of prostaglandins and thromboxane.[12,17,18] NSAIDs (other than aspirin) produce reversible COX inhibition by competing with the substrate arachidonic acid for the active site of the enzyme.[18] Thus NSAIDs reduce the production of prostaglandins and thromboxane.

NSAIDs differ from glucocorticoids in that glucocorticoids inhibit phospholipase, which is higher up in the inflammatory cascade. Glucocorticoids therefore inhibit lipoxygenases as well.[1,12,18,19] As Maddison notes, "There is no clinical situation where the concurrent use of corticosteroids and NSAIDs has any rational basis."[19] Tepoxalin, a newer veterinary NSAID (no longer sold in the United States), is unique in that it inhibits both COX and 5-lipoxygenase, yet has low gastrointestinal toxicity.[20]

COX exists in two isoforms. Constitutive COX-1 is responsible for physiologic functions and is expressed in most tissues. It functions in synthesizing prostaglandins that regulate normal cell activity. Inducible COX-2 is involved in inflammation. COX-2 is an enzyme that is rapidly induced at the site of inflammation and is responsible for the production of proinflammatory prostaglandins.[19,21-23] Most NSAIDs (including ibuprofen) are nonselective COX inhibitors, thus contributing to gastrointestinal and renal side effects.[19,20-23]

A group of NSAIDs that inhibit COX-2 selectively is still receiving significant attention in the human literature,[24-27] and COX-2–selective NSAIDs are continually being introduced into the veterinary market. As previously stated, the selective inhibition of COX-2 may be the cause of the favorable antiinflammatory, analgesic, and antipyretic effects of NSAIDs, whereas inhibition of COX-1 may result in unwarranted gastrointestinal, renal, and possibly other side effects. COX selectivity is species specific; for example, meloxicam is considered to be COX-2 selective in dogs, but not for cats.[24] In humans nimesulide,[25] meloxicam,[26,27] flosulide,[28] and etodolac[29] apparently produce the therapeutic effects of NSAIDs without the adverse side effects. In dogs, carprofen, deracoxib, etodolac, firocoxib, meloxicam, and robenacoxib are considered to be COX-2 selective (or COX-1 sparing) NSAIDs,[30,31] and robenacoxib is COX-2 selective in cats.[32] However, it is important to note that all NSAIDs, whether they are labeled as COX-1 or COX-2 selective, will alter both pathways in cases of excessive exposure. There is information to suggest that many human-approved NSAIDs are not well metabolized in companion animals; information regarding metabolism and excretion of many human-approved NSAIDs is not available for dogs and cats.

NSAIDs are weak acids and are well-absorbed following oral administration.[11,13] Because of their different chemical structures, differences in drug distribution and dissolution may lead to differences in the bioavailability of these drugs.[1,2] Because NSAIDs are largely ionized at physiologic pH, they are primarily confined to plasma and extracellular fluid.[1,33] However, the lipid solubility of NSAIDs enhances their penetration of cell membranes, and the acidic pH of inflamed tissue draws them to target tissue.[1]

Serum protein binding varies among different NSAIDs.[34] Many NSAIDs are highly protein bound, often exceeding a rate of 99% binding to serum albumin.[1,11,12,33] Therefore the volume of distribution is small, often less than 10% of body weight. Only the unbound portion of the drug is pharmacologically active.[1,33] The rate of plasma drug clearance in small animals depends on the rate of protein binding. Plasma protein binding slows the rate of clearance.[1,33]

In dogs orally administered ibuprofen is rapidly absorbed. Maximum plasma concentrations were found ½ to 3 hours after administration. Ninety-six percent of the drug is bound to serum proteins. The elimination half-life of ibuprofen in dogs ranges from 2.5 to 5.8 hours.[11,13]

Clearance of NSAIDs varies among species and among individuals within species and by age.[1,2,12,13,35-38] Very young animals (younger than 6 weeks of age) and older patients metabolize these drugs more slowly and therefore have delayed clearance.[12] NSAIDs are excreted at varying rates, depending on their metabolic pathway and enterohepatic circulation.[9,11,13,39]

In contrast to humans, many NSAIDs (e.g., ibuprofen, naproxen, carprofen, indomethacin, piroxicam, flunixin, and tolfenamic acid) undergo enterohepatic recycling in the dog.[2,9,11-13,39] In toxicity studies of ibuprofen in dogs, no metabolites of ibuprofen were demonstrated in plasma; however, high levels were demonstrated in the bile.[13] Biliary excretion of NSAIDs allows for reabsorption and repeated exposure and is a critical factor in the pathogenesis of NSAID-induced small intestinal injury.[40] This difference may partially explain the gastrointestinal sensitivities apparent in dogs compared with humans with the use of ibuprofen and other NSAIDs.[2,9,11,13]

Clearance of some NSAIDs (e.g., aspirin and phenylbutazone) requires two phases of metabolism. The lipid-soluble drug, which is difficult to excrete, is metabolized to a water-soluble form that is more easily excreted. Phase I metabolism is catalyzed by enzymes in the endoplasmic reticulum in hepatocytes. These metabolites are usually more susceptible to phase II metabolism than the parent compound. A large molecule (glucuronic acid, glutathione, or sulfate) is added to the metabolite or sometimes to the parent compound. Usually this renders the drug "inactivated," and it becomes more water-soluble and is readily excreted in the urine.[1,34] Renal elimination of NSAID metabolites is pH dependent. Drug elimination usually occurs at a faster rate in alkaline urine.[1,34]

Drug interactions can alter the elimination rate of NSAIDs because of changes in hepatic metabolism or renal excretion. Phenobarbital, a hepatic enzyme inducer, speeds the clearance of NSAIDs, and chloramphenicol and cimetidine, hepatic enzyme inhibitors, delay the clearance.[1,12] Drug interactions that alter renal elimination usually result when NSAIDs must compete with other weak acids for renal tubular secretory proteins. Drugs that alter urinary pH may alter renal elimination.[1] Dietary supplements and additives should be thoughtfully considered before administering NSAIDs.

Ibuprofen and other NSAIDs have the potential to cause multiorgan toxicities (Table 65-3). Adverse effects involving the gastrointestinal tract, kidneys, liver, and hematopoietic system have been documented. Risk factors that may predispose animals to side effects and drug interactions with NSAIDs exist.

Gastrointestinal Adverse Effects

In humans NSAID damage to the gastrointestinal tract most commonly becomes manifest as ulcers in the stomach and duodenum, and there is some risk of injury in the esophagus, small bowel, and colon as well.[41-47] The mechanism of action may not be the same throughout the gastrointestinal tract.

The causes of the ulcerogenic effects of NSAIDs in the stomach are thought to be twofold.[46] The first is the ability of these drugs to suppress prostaglandin synthesis.

Table 65-3	Adverse Reactions to Nonsteroidal Antiinflammatory Drugs
Site	**Effect**
Gastrointestinal tract	Decreased appetite, emesis, hematemesis, abdominal pain, diarrhea, melena, superficial erosions, ulceration, hemorrhage, perforation, inflammation, stricture, protein-losing enteropathy
Kidney	Decreased renal flow, decreased glomerular filtration rate, fluid and sodium retention, hyperkalemia, azotemia, acute renal insufficiency, papillary necrosis
Liver	Rise in liver enzymes, icterus
Hemostatic system	Decreased platelet aggregation, increased bleeding time
Hematopoietic system	Bone marrow depression, aplastic anemia, hemolytic anemia, thrombocytopenia, neutropenia, pancytopenia, methemoglobinemia
Central nervous system	Depression, seizure, coma, behavioral changes
Immune system	Allergic reactions

From Isaacs JP: Adverse effects of nonsteroidal anti-inflammatory drugs in the dog and cat, *Aust Vet Practit* 26:180-186, 1996.

Gastrointestinal mucosal defense mechanisms are influenced or mediated by prostaglandins, including mucus and bicarbonate secretion, blood flow, epithelial cell turnover and repair, and mucosal immunocyte function.[40,41,45,46] Inhibition of prostaglandin synthesis leads to a reduction in the ability of the gastrointestinal mucosa to defend itself.

The second mechanism of action is the topical irritant properties of NSAIDs. Epithelial damage may be related in part to ion trapping, a phenomenon that allows accumulation of NSAIDs in these cells, and in part to the ability of NSAIDs to decrease the hydrophobicity of the mucous layer in the stomach (the primary barrier to damage induced by acid).[46] Most NSAIDs have been shown to impair gastric mucosal microcirculation and cause gastric mucosal damage.[47] After NSAID administration, neutrophils can be attracted to mucosal capillaries, where they form thrombi and obstruct capillaries.[46,48]

Parenteral or rectal administration of NSAIDs has failed to prevent topical mucosal injury.[40,46] In humans, drug dose, increased age, and the influence of food and beverages contribute to the mucosal injury associated with NSAIDs.[44,49-52] In rats a low dose of a parenterally administered NSAID (e.g., indomethacin or diclofenac) impaired the physicochemical barrier against luminal acidity and rendered the mucosa susceptible to injury.[52] Oral administration of ibuprofen to rats induces increased bowel permeability.[53] In humans an increased risk of emergency admission to the hospital for colitis caused by inflammatory bowel disease, particularly among patients with no previous history of this disease, has been associated with the use of NSAIDs.[43]

In dogs the most common side effect of NSAIDs is gastrointestinal irritation and ulceration. As described earlier, dogs are more susceptible because of the enterohepatic recycling of many of these drugs. Enterohepatic recirculation of NSAIDs is of critical importance in the pathogenesis of NSAID enteropathy. Gastrointestinal ulceration is due to inhibition of the prostaglandins normally responsible for inhibiting the secretion of gastrin (prostaglandin E_2 [PGE_2]) and hydrochloric acid (PGE_2 and PGI_1). NSAIDs also inhibit the prostaglandins responsible for stimulating the secretion of mucus and bicarbonate.[42,46]

Ibuprofen appears to cause gastric irritation and ulcers more frequently in dogs than in humans.[1-6,11,13,54,55] Most NSAID-induced ulcers were found in the pyloroantral region,[54] although lesions were also apparent in the cardia, lesser curvature, and fundus and diffusely throughout the stomach.[50] Gastric perforation associated with the administration of ibuprofen has been reported.[3]

Renal Adverse Effects

In humans analgesic nephropathy is widely acknowledged because of the chronic use of these drugs in older adults for arthritic conditions.[56-61] Under normal conditions, NSAIDs have little effect on the kidney because of the low renal production of prostaglandins. In the kidney, vasodilatory prostaglandins modulate vasoconstrictive stimulants (e.g., epinephrine and angiotensin II), which would otherwise impair renal blood flow.

"Classic" analgesic nephropathy is the result of habitual NSAID use and is characterized by chronic interstitial nephritis. Other NSAID-related nephrotoxicoses include vasoconstrictive acute renal failure, acute interstitial nephritis associated with the nephrotic syndrome, fluid and electrolyte abnormalities, interactions with antihypertensive and other medications, renal papillary necrosis, and chronic renal failure.[56,61]

In dogs and cats, renal injury is most commonly seen in overdose situations, but may also occur with chronic use at therapeutic levels. Significant renal toxicity can result if NSAIDs are administered when the animal is volume depleted, is avidly retaining sodium (e.g., congestive heart failure or hepatic cirrhosis), or has preexisting renal dysfunction.[2,26,39] Patients experiencing any hypotensive condition, such as anesthesia[60-62] or posttraumatic shock, and animals with significant gastrointestinal disease resulting in dehydration and volume depletion are also at increased risk.[2,4,20,39]

The concurrent administration of NSAIDs and nephrotoxic medications (e.g., gentamicin) is contraindicated.[63] The concurrent use of two NSAIDs should be avoided, and a 5-7 day "washout" period is sometimes recommended when switching from one NSAID to another (though few studies have been performed that support this recommendation).[64-67] Renal papillary necrosis may occur secondary to NSAID use, especially in dehydrated hypovolemic patients or if nephrotoxic agents are being administered.[68] Renal dysfunction has been reported in dogs and cats in association with the use of many NSAIDs.

Hematologic Adverse Effects

NSAIDs inhibit COX activity in platelets. COX is essential for the formation of thromboxane, a potent vasoconstrictor and stimulus for platelet aggregation. Prolongation of bleeding times can occur with the use of NSAIDs.[2,8,45,69] With most NSAIDs, the alteration in platelet function occurs during the dosing time of the NSAID, but aspirin irreversibly inhibits platelet function for the lifetime of the platelet, which can result in prolonged bleeding times many days after aspirin therapy has been discontinued.[62] The most important bleeding problems in humans occur in individuals with coexisting coagulopathies or those who are concomitantly using alcohol or receiving anticoagulant medication.[45] NSAIDs should be used with caution in dogs with bleeding problems (e.g., von Willebrand's disease).[20]

Hepatic Adverse Effects

Hepatotoxicity can occur following administration of labeled doses of most NSAIDs, regardless of COX selectivity.[63] In humans NSAIDs account for approximately 10% of total cases of drug-induced hepatopathy worldwide. The overall incidence of NSAID-induced liver disease ranges from one to nine cases per 100,000 persons exposed. Concurrent use of other potentially hepatotoxic drugs increases the risk of NSAID-induced hepatopathy. As with humans, hepatotoxicity induced by ibuprofen and similar NSAIDs in veterinary patients is not a common occurrence. A 30-day study in dogs receiving 16 mg/kg/day of ibuprofen showed no significant biochemical abnormalities, and sulfobromophthalein retention remained normal. Abnormal postmortem results were confined to ulcerative lesions in the gastrointestinal tract.[13] However, hepatotoxicity has been reported following the approval of several veterinary NSAIDs.

Hepatic injury from NSAIDs is thought to develop by a variety of mechanisms, and recent work has shown that genetic polymorphisms in activation and detoxification enzymes can influence the susceptibility of an individual to drug-induced liver injury.[70] Proposed mechanisms of drug-induced liver injury include formation of reactive metabolites that cause hepatocellular injury by binding to cellular macromolecules or disrupting organelle functions, activation of cellular apoptotic mechanisms, haptenization of hepato-cellular membrane components that triggers an immune-mediated attack, and release of drug-modified macromolecules that trigger an immune response.[63,70]

Although NSAID-induced hepatopathy can occur after weeks, months, or years of NSAID use, hepatopathies in dogs are most often seen within the first 3 weeks of NSAID administration.[62] When detected early and the drug discontinued, most patients make full recoveries, but continued NSAID administration in the face of hepatopathy may lead to liver failure and death. For patients on chronic NSAID therapy, baseline liver enzyme values should be obtained, followed by recheck 2 weeks after initiation of NSAID therapy; periodic rechecks are recommended thereafter.[62]

Risk Factors

A number of risk factors may predispose animals to the side effects of NSAIDs (Box 65-1). These risk factors parallel published human risk factors. They include high doses of NSAIDs, decreased renal function, gastrointestinal disease, dehydration, hypovolemia, hypotension, kidney disease, heart disease, stress, severe trauma, spinal injury, surgery or anesthesia, age, and drug interactions.[1,2,37,38,42,49,50,53,55-57,59,61]

Additionally, a possible link between NSAID therapy and acute necrotizing fasciitis was reviewed in the human literature. Group A beta-hemolytic streptococci were isolated in most of the cases associated with NSAID use.[71] Usually the disease process developed spontaneously or after minor trauma for which NSAIDs were prescribed for pain. The progression of the disease was quick, occurring in less than 1 week in most cases. Nearly all patients required extensive surgical debridement because in most cases intravenously administered antibiotics failed to slow the progression of the disease. The authors concluded that "NSAIDs should be administered with caution, if at all, to patients with inflammatory soft-tissue lesions, especially if concurrent infection is likely."[71]

Drug Interactions

NSAIDs can interact with many other drugs (Table 65-4). Clinicians should be aware of any other medications their patients are receiving. It is not uncommon for veterinarians to administer corticosteroids and NSAIDs simultaneously. Because corticosteroids have the potential to induce gastric ulcers and perforation, concurrent use with NSAIDs is likely to compound the gastrointestinal toxicity.

A study in canines of the use of flunixin and flunixin with prednisolone revealed endoscopically apparent gastric lesions after 4 days of flunixin therapy. Lesions occurred much earlier and were more severe in patients receiving dual medications.[72] Additionally, in the latter group, lesions consistent with coagulative necrosis of the superficial epithelium were found in the small intestinal and colonic mucosa. In another reported case, one dog received a different combination of NSAIDs and corticosteroids for a spinal lesion. The

Box 65-1	Factors Predisposing to Side Effects of Nonsteroidal Antiinflammatory Drugs	
High doses of NSAIDs		Kidney disease
Decreased renal function		Heart disease
Gastrointestinal disease		Stress, severe trauma, spinal injury
Dehydration		Surgery, anesthesia
Hypovolemia		Age
Hypotension		Other drugs

From Isaacs JP: Adverse effects of nonsteroidal anti-inflammatory drugs in the dog and cat, *Aust Vet Practit* 26:180-186, 1996.

Table 65-4	Drug Interactions with Nonsteroidal Antiinflammatory Drugs
Drug	**Effect**
ACE inhibitors	May reduce response to these drugs
Aminoglycosides	Increase risk of renal injury
Beta-blockers	May reduce antihypertensive effect
Cisplatin	Increase risk of cisplatin toxicosis
Corticosteroids	Increase risk of gastrointestinal ulceration and renal injury
Digoxin	Increase risk of digoxin toxicosis if renal function is decreased
Diuretics	May reduce response to diuretics
Heparin	Increase risk of bleeding
Methotrexate	Increase risk of methotrexate toxicosis
Oral anticoagulants	Increase anticoagulant effect
Pentosan	Increase risk of gastrointestinal bleeding

From Isaacs JP: Adverse effects of nonsteroidal anti-inflammatory drugs in the dog and cat, *Aust Vet Practit* 126: 180-186, 1996.

ACE, Angiotensin-converting enzyme; *NSAID*, nonsteroidal antiinflammatory drug.

dog collapsed on the fourth day and was brought to the veterinarian recumbent with hemorrhagic diarrhea and tetraparesis.[73] There is no medical reason to administer corticosteroids and NSAIDs simultaneously. This practice poses significant risk of severe consequences.

Because NSAIDs are highly protein bound, they can interact with a number of drugs, displacing other protein-bound drugs.[74] This displacement can result in increased levels of unbound drugs, which can be clinically important with drugs that have a narrow therapeutic index. Drugs of significance in this group are digoxin, oral anticoagulants, and some cytotoxic agents. NSAIDs have been shown to decrease the effectiveness of diuretics, angiotensin-converting enzyme inhibitors, and beta-blockers.[2,33,35,38,50,61,66]

Clinical Signs

The clinical signs of ibuprofen toxicosis in canines (listed in order of decreasing frequency) are vomiting, depression or stupor, diarrhea, anorexia, ataxia and incoordination, bloody stool and melena, polyuria, and polydipsia. Hemorrhagic gastroenteritis seems to develop less often in cats than in dogs, but cats may display tachypnea and panting somewhat more frequently.[16]

Published clinical reports of ibuprofen toxicosis show that one dog had hematemesis only.[5] Another dog had a history of lethargy, vomiting, and anorexia for 2 weeks and was dehydrated when brought in.[3] A third dog came in with a history of infrequent vomiting and melena, severe depression, anorexia, weight loss, polyuria, and polydipsia.[6] An elevated rectal temperature, depression, and a distended abdomen are suggestive of peritonitis from a perforated gastrointestinal lesion.[3] Abdominal pain was apparent in two separate canine cases of naproxen-induced gastrointestinal perforation.[75-76] Collapse and pallor may also be presenting clinical signs.

In one canine study, repeated ibuprofen administration resulted in consistent vomiting.[11] In another canine study of ibuprofen, gastrointestinal signs (e.g., frequent vomiting, diarrhea with the passage of fresh blood, anorexia, and weight loss) were apparent in the eighth week of dosing.[13] In this same study, dogs given 16 mg/kg/day for 30 days showed no overt signs of toxicosis; however, postmortem examination revealed gastric erosions or ulcers and intestinal inflammation in all the dogs.[13] These results suggest that patients with a history of NSAID administration but without clinical signs may nevertheless benefit from medical intervention.

Minimum Database

When ibuprofen toxicosis is suspected, a complete blood cell count, reticulocyte count, chemistry panel, and urinalysis should be included in the diagnostic plan. Depending on the extent of the poisoning, laboratory results may be either within normal reference ranges or abnormal.

In seven canine cases with confirmed gastric ulcerations secondary to NSAID administration, all dogs had normocytic, normochromic anemias consistent with short-term blood loss.[55] A reticulocyte count was performed in six dogs, revealing a nonregenerative anemia in two and mild to moderate regeneration relative to the anemia in the other four. In a dog with peracute bleeding, the animal may be brought to the veterinarian before there is an adequate bone marrow response, and the reticulocyte count may be low. If there is prolonged bleeding, a microcytic hypochromic anemia caused by iron deficiency may be apparent.[77-79]

Evaluation of serum proteins (albumin and globulin) can support a diagnosis of blood loss anemia. A decrease in both proteins occurs as a result of gastrointestinal bleeding because both proteins are lost equally.[79] Low serum proteins, however, were apparent in only three of seven dogs with confirmed NSAID-induced gastrointestinal bleeding.[55] Serum total protein concentration was normal (6.8 g/dL) in a dog with ibuprofen-induced gastric perforation.[3]

Leukocytosis, especially with a left shift, mandates further evaluation for the presence of a gastrointestinal perforation and peritonitis.[75,76] Serum biochemical analyses may be normal. However, results above the normal reference ranges in blood urea nitrogen (BUN), creatinine, phosphorus, and possibly calcium, plus isosthenuria, help confirm a diagnosis of renal toxicosis.[80]

Abdominal radiographs may show no visible gastrointestinal lesions. However, in patients with gastrointestinal perforation, radiographs of the abdomen may reveal poor visualization of the serosal surfaces of the abdominal organs, free gas in the peritoneal cavity, or intestinal ileus.[3,75,76] If a perforation is suggested, water-soluble contrast agents should be used, because barium sulfate suspension is a complication of peritonitis that results in higher mortality.[76]

Gastrointestinal imaging by ultrasound can be a quick, noninvasive way to examine the stomach and proximal duodenum.[81] Adding water through a stomach tube can help to identify the features of gastric ulceration. These features are thickening of the gastric wall, possible loss of the normal five-layer architecture, disruption of the mucosa by crater formation, and accumulation of gas bubbles (bright echoes with typical "ring-down" or "comet-tail" gas artifacts).[81] Additionally, abdominal ultrasound can identify fluid accumulation and may help in obtaining fluid (abdominal paracentesis) in a dog in which a perforation is suggested.[82] Evaluation of this fluid would reveal a purulent exudate.[3,83]

Other diagnostic procedures that may be considered include coagulation profiles, platelet counts, and bleeding times. In seven dogs with confirmed NSAID-induced ulceration, coagulation profiles were normal.[55] Acquired disorders of platelet dysfunction have been attributed to NSAID use. Bleeding time can be prolonged, platelet aggregation may be poor to absent, and thrombocytopenia may be present. These effects are reversible (in contrast to those caused by aspirin) and last only as long as the NSAIDs are in circulation.[84] However, in a canine study comparing the gastroduodenal lesions that occurred after 7 days of different NSAID administration, bleeding times were normal.[85]

Fecal occult blood testing can aid in the diagnosis of gastrointestinal bleeding; however, false-positive results can occur if red meat has been ingested in the 3 days prior to testing.[86] The fecal occult blood test result was negative, however, in a canine study in which hemorrhagic gastrointestinal lesions were seen on endoscopic examination. The authors concluded that the blood loss was too small to be detected.[85]

Confirmatory Tests or Procedures

Serum NSAID concentrations may be used to confirm absorption of the drug following an unknown exposure or an unknown ingested dose, to evaluate the success of emesis or of adsorptive or cathartic therapy, and to monitor symptomatic therapy.[5] Serum ibuprofen concentrations greater than 130 mcg/mL may fall to less than 10 mcg/mL within 48 hours in dogs receiving aggressive symptomatic treatment.[5]

Endoscopy is the most sensitive and specific diagnostic procedure for detecting gastroduodenal ulcers in patients receiving NSAIDs.[39,54,55,85] Ulcers, however, may be missed on endoscopy. Because an anesthetic is required, these patients need to be hemodynamically stable.

Treatment

For patients presenting soon (<2 hours) following NSAID overdose, therapy may involve emetics, activated charcoal, and a saline or osmotic cathartic to minimize absorption; decontamination should be omitted or delayed if there is evidence of significant neurologic signs or prior vomiting.[5,10,16] Because of the long half-life of ibuprofen in dogs and cats, repeated administration of activated charcoal should be considered in large overdoses.[16] Intravenous fluids facilitate perfusion of target organs and help support renal function. In patients ingesting sufficient ibuprofen to be concerned with acute renal injury, or in patients showing signs of renal insufficiency caused by more chronic NSAID exposure, intravenous crystalloids should be administered at twice the daily maintenance rate for at least 48 hours; fluid ins and outs should be monitored closely and fluid rates adjusted accordingly.[16] If renal function tests are normal at 48 hours, fluid rate may be reduced to maintenance rate for 24 hours and discontinued if renal values remain normal. If renal values elevate, then diuresis should be continued until renal values stabilize or normalize. Vomiting should be controlled with an appropriate antiemetic. Patients with perforated gastrointestinal lesions require surgical intervention.

Extremely anemic patients may require blood transfusions.[55] Specific measurements to look for in dogs and cats with acute blood loss include acute loss of more than 30% of blood volume (30 mL/kg), packed-cell volume (hematocrit) of less than 20%, plasma protein concentration of less than 3.5 g/dL, and ongoing blood loss.[87] In one study, four of seven dogs that had received NSAIDs required whole blood transfusions because they showed clinical signs of anemia or continued blood loss.[55] A blood replacement therapy, Oxyglobin (Biopure Corporation, Cambridge, Mass.), offers an alternative to blood for oxygen-carrying support. This product allows immediate and efficient oxygen delivery to tissues and also has colloidal properties that allow expansion of circulatory volume. However, this product has limited availability to U.S. veterinarians.

Neurologic signs should be managed symptomatically.[16] Diazepam or a barbiturate may be used to manage seizures; refractory cases may require general anesthesia. Comatose animals should be provided with thermoregulation, respiratory support, and general nursing care as needed.

The goal of medical therapy in dogs and cats with NSAID-induced gastroduodenal lesions is to restore the normal mucosal defense mechanisms. Various drug therapies are recommended to prevent gastroduodenal ulcers or to promote ulcer healing. Drug therapy may include the use of histamine H_2 receptor antagonists (e.g., cimetidine or famotidine), a proton pump inhibitor (e.g., omeprazole), sucralfate (an aluminum salt of sucrose sulfate), and misoprostol (a PGE_1 analogue). Gastrointestinal protectants should be administered for a minimum of 7-14 days following acute NSAID overdose (exact duration depends on NSAID, dose ingested, and patient risk factors).[16]

Many studies have been conducted on the prevention and treatment of gastric and duodenal ulcers. A study of the effects of cimetidine on aspirin-induced gastric hemorrhage in dogs revealed that cimetidine treatment did not prevent gastric lesions or reduce gastric hemorrhage.[88] In the dog, famotidine reduces gastric acid secretion and increases gastric pH, whereas ranitidine does not.[89] Furthermore, famotidine has been found to alleviate the reduction of gastric blood flow caused by the NSAID diclofenac.[90] For these reasons, famotidine may be the superior H_2 receptor antagonist to use in cases of NSAID-induced gastrointestinal injury.

Omeprazole, a proton pump inhibitor, profoundly suppresses gastric acid secretion in dogs and cats.[89,91] Pantoprazole and lansoprazole, newer proton pump inhibitors, have been shown to have similar effects on gastric acid secretion as omeprazole.[89,92] In humans, studies have revealed a decrease in gastric and duodenal NSAID-induced ulcers with the use of omeprazole versus a placebo.[93,94] However, in a comparative study, neither omeprazole nor ranitidine provided significant protection against naproxen-induced gastric damage, but both agents protected against duodenal damage.[95] Omeprazole has been shown to speed healing of NSAID-induced gastric (and perhaps duodenal) ulcers when NSAID use is continued.[96] Omeprazole was successful in treating a dog with NSAID-induced gastric ulcers when treatment with other medications (e.g., cimetidine, sucralfate, and ranitidine) had failed.[54]

Sucralfate, an aluminum salt of sucrose sulfate, acts by forming a complex with exposed proteins on the surface of the ulcer, protecting the ulcer from gastric acid and pepsin. Sucralfate may also induce prostaglandin-mediated cytoprotection.[97,98] Additionally, sucralfate adsorbs pepsin and bile acids and can interfere with the absorption of other drugs.[97,99] If concurrent oral medications are prescribed, staggering the times of drug administration may be indicated. In a canine study of dogs with NSAID-induced gastric ulceration, five of six dogs responded positively following the use of cimetidine and sucralfate, and the sixth dog responded positively with the use of sucralfate alone.[55] This dog had a grossly normal gastric mucosa when endoscopy was performed 9 days later.

Misoprostol, a PGE_1 analogue, has been shown to prevent the development of NSAID-induced gastric and duodenal ulcers and to reduce the risk of their complications as well. It is an appropriate choice for prophylaxis in at-risk patients requiring NSAID therapy.[42] In a canine study, misoprostol was discovered to be an appropriate preventive treatment for NSAID-induced gastrointestinal hemorrhage and ulceration.[100] Notably less gastrointestinal hemorrhage and ulceration were documented endoscopically in the misoprostol-treated dogs. There was notably less vomiting in the treated group. The dose of misoprostol administered was 2.3 to 5 mcg/kg per os (PO) every 8 hours. Misoprostol dosed at 3 mcg/kg PO every 12 hours was found to be as effective as 3 mcg/kg PO every 8 hours in preventing aspirin-induced gastric injury in dogs.[101] Because of misoprostol's uterogenic effects, its use is contraindicated in pregnant animals.[42] The concurrent use of misoprostol in patients receiving high doses of gentamicin may exacerbate renal dysfunction.[102]

Drug doses for all the medications described earlier are listed in Table 65-5.[103]

Prognosis

The prognosis varies with the dose ingested, severity of signs, and time to initiation of appropriate treatment. Medical intervention has led to positive results.[5-7,16,54,55] One dog

---

Table 65-5 Medical Therapy for Dogs and Cats with Nonsteroidal Antiinflammatory Drug–Induced Gastroduodenal Lesions

Drug	Dosage
Cimetidine	10 mg/kg every 6-8 hours IV, IM, PO (with renal failure: 2.5 mg/kg every 12 hours IV, PO)
Famotidine	0.5 mg/kg every 12-24 hours PO
Ranitidine	Dog: 2 mg/kg every 8 hours IV, PO Cat: 2.5 mg/kg every 12 hours IV, 3.5 mg/kg every 12 hours PO
Omeprazole	Dog: 20 mg/dog or 0.5-1 mg/kg PO once daily Cat: 0.7-1 mg/kg PO q24h
Sucralfate	Dog: 0.5-1 g every 8-12 hours PO Cat: 0.25 g every 8-12 hours PO
Misoprostol	Dog: 2.5 mcg/kg every 8 hours PO

IV, Intravenous; *IM,* intramuscular; *PO,* per os.

with ibuprofen-induced renal failure had a persistent decrease in creatinine clearance 2 months after the initial therapy.[6] Surgical intervention was successful in three cases of dogs with NSAID-induced gastric perforation.[3,75,76]

Gross and Histologic Lesions

In one study, dogs receiving NSAID treatment tended to have pyloroantral ulcers,[54] and a similar finding plus intestinal inflammation was confirmed at postmortem examination in a research study involving ibuprofen administration in dogs.[13] In another study, the lesser curvature and fundus and the pyloric antrum were involved, and there were diffuse lesions throughout the stomach.[55] The latter report described lesions consisting of petechiation, mucosal erosions, small bleeding ulcers, and craterlike ulcers.

Histologically, gastric ulceration is defined as a break in the mucosa with a fibrous base.[42] An erosion is a defect that does not extend that far into the mucosa.[16] Renal failure involving necrosis of the collecting ducts and loop of Henle in dogs anesthetized with methoxyflurane that were also receiving flunixin has been described.[104] Renal papillary necrosis was detected on postmortem examination in 2 of 25 dogs receiving piroxicam therapy for transitional cell carcinoma of the urinary bladder.[105]

Differential Diagnoses

The clinical signs and laboratory data can mimic those characteristic of other metabolic derangements in canines and felines. The rule-out list can include hemorrhagic gastroenteritis, hypoadrenocorticism (Addison's disease), gastrointestinal foreign objects, severe inflammatory bowel disease, gastrointestinal neoplasia, hemangiosarcoma, anticoagulant rodenticide toxicosis, ethylene glycol poisoning, hepatic failure, and renal failure. Therefore a complete history and diagnostic plan are imperative for medical management of these patients. Owners may have to be asked direct questions about any NSAID administration because the majority of pet owners do not understand the risk that medications pose to their pets.

Other NSAIDs

Aspirin

Acetylsalicylic acid was the first synthetic NSAID to be sold commercially. It was synthesized in 1899, but not until 1971 was it discovered that aspirin specifically blocks prostaglandin synthesis. Aspirin is readily absorbed from the stomach and upper small intestines of dogs and cats.[106] Aspirin undergoes hepatic metabolism before it enters the circulation as salicylic acid, which is the active form. Salicylic acid is 70% to 90% protein bound (primarily to albumin), significantly less than other NSAIDs.[106] Therefore salicylic acid is distributed to most tissues.[1] Plasma elimination of salicylic acid depends on phase II conjugation with glucuronic acid. Rates of elimination vary among species, the half-life of salicylates ranging from 8 hours in the dog to 38 hours in the cat.[2,106,107]

Cats have a relative deficiency of glucuronate, which accounts for the prolonged elimination in this species. At high doses of aspirin, the capability of the glucuronide conjugation system is overwhelmed. Thus the rate of drug clearance drops, and the drug begins to accumulate, leading to toxicity.[1]

By acetylating COX, aspirin irreversibly inhibits the activity of thromboxane and prostacyclin.[45,108] Thromboxane causes vasoconstriction, which promotes platelet aggregation. Prostacyclin causes vasodilation, which inhibits platelet aggregation. A dose-related response permits the use of aspirin to selectively inhibit thromboxane formation. Lower doses of aspirin result in irreversible acetylation of COX in platelets while still allowing endothelial cells to produce prostacyclin.[108] An aspirin dose of only 3 mg/kg once every 6 days may be sufficient to inhibit platelet function in dogs.[1]

The most common side effect of aspirin administration is gastric irritation.[1,38,106,108] Local irritation and damage resulting from the hydrolysis of aspirin to salicylic acid can also contribute to the formation of gastroduodenal ulcers.[107,109] A study of 10 beagle dogs receiving 250 mg of aspirin three times per day for 30 days revealed that five dogs had gastric lesions (four ulcerative and one hemorrhagic) after the fourth dosing period (endoscopy was performed 26 hours after the initial medication).[110] In a study comparing ketoprofen, copper and indomethacin, prednisolone and cinchophen, and aspirin administration in dogs, the aspirin group showed significantly more severe gastric lesions.[111] Additionally, in another study performed in canine arthritic patients that compared aspirin administration and aspirin and misoprostol administration, the aspirin and misoprostol group showed notably less gastroduodenal hemorrhage and clinical signs of vomiting than the aspirin-only group.[100] Fecal occult blood test results were generally negative despite endoscopically apparent gastroduodenal hemorrhage. Buccal mucosal bleeding times in dogs remained normal in one study.[84]

Dogs dosed at 25-35 mg/kg PO every 8 hours developed increased fecal hemoglobin levels and had evidence of gastric ulceration on endoscopy.[8] Dogs receiving 50 mg/kg PO every 12 hours developed vomiting and similar dosing resulted in perforating gastric ulcers within 4 weeks.[112] Severe metabolic disturbances (metabolic acidosis, seizures, coma) have been associated with aspirin doses of 450 mg/kg or higher in dogs.[113] In cats, doses of 100-110 mg/kg/day have been associated with death within 7 days.[112]

Because aspirin is an NSAID, renal adverse effects similar to those seen with other NSAIDs might be expected.[106,108] However, in human medicine, oliguria has rarely been a complication of salicylate poisoning,[111] and in veterinary medicine, hepatic injury is more commonly encountered in aspirin overdoses.[114] Salicylate-induced seizures have been reported in a dog.[115] Animal studies suggest that the seizures may be the result of hyperventilation or reduced brain glucose concentrations.[116] Cerebral edema has been reported on rare occasions.[116]

In animals the clinical signs of aspirin toxicosis are attributed to respiratory alkalosis secondary to hyperpnea, which is then followed by a marked metabolic acidosis, which is responsible for the majority of the clinical signs.[117] In cats aspirin toxicoses have primarily been the result of overdoses. Reported adverse effects in cats are nausea, vomiting, depressed respiration, metabolic acidosis, seizures, and coma.[2,106] Aspirin-induced hepatitis has been observed at excessive doses in cats.[117]

Fluid retention and pulmonary edema have been sequelae of salicylate poisoning in humans.[116] Because pulmonary capillary wedge pressures remain normal, the edema is considered noncardiogenic and not the result of fluid overload. In sheep, salicylates increased the rate of pulmonary lymph flow and lymph protein clearance, indicating increased lung vascular permeability, perhaps as a result of impaired platelet function, a direct toxic effect on capillary endothelium, or inhibition of prostaglandin synthesis. In children with salicylate poisoning and pulmonary edema, a high anion gap acidosis was noted to be a predisposing factor.[116]

Hyperpyrexia has been a reported common complication of salicylate intoxication in children. It may be the result of metabolic stimulation caused by the uncoupling of oxidative phosphorylation, but it may also reflect the illness for which the salicylate was prescribed. Hyperpyrexia is a very uncommon complication of salicylate poisoning in adults but is a serious prognostic sign.[116] Aspirin should not be administered to patients with coagulation disorders and should be discontinued in any patient 1 week before surgery to prevent the risk of excessive bleeding.[106] Risk factors are similar to those described for other NSAIDs. Concurrent administration with other NSAIDs or corticosteroids is contraindicated.

Management of aspirin toxicosis is directed at managing clinical signs, correcting acid-base imbalances, and preventing and treating liver injury. In patients with recent aspirin ingestion, induction of emesis is recommended.[114] Activated charcoal is indicated in the management of salicylate poisoning to reduce salicylate absorption. It is most effective if it is administered immediately after ingestion of the salicylate and probably has little effect if administered 2 hours after exposure.[116]

In human patients with salicylate toxicosis, measures are taken to enhance elimination of the drug if acidemia, impaired consciousness, pulmonary or cerebral edema, or cardiac or renal failure is present. Techniques for increasing elimination of salicylate in humans include forced alkaline diuresis, administration of alkali alone, exchange transfusion, peritoneal dialysis, hemodialysis, charcoal hemoperfusion, and administration of repeated doses of activated charcoal. These procedures require close patient monitoring to prevent circulatory overload, pulmonary edema, dangerous alkalemia and hyperosmolality or hypernatremia.[116] Acetazolamide, a carbonic anhydrase inhibitor, effectively alkalinizes the urine, but may exacerbate metabolic acidosis and should not be used.

Gastrointestinal protectants should be initiated as outlined in the Treatment section of this chapter. One canine study revealed that a group of dogs receiving aspirin and misoprostol had notably less gastroduodenal hemorrhage and clinical signs of vomiting than dogs receiving aspirin alone.[100]

Baseline liver enzyme values should be obtained and monitored following large aspirin overdoses.[114] In general, elevations in liver enzymes will begin within 12-24 hours following exposure and will peak approximately 72 hours later. Patients with rapid or severe liver enzyme elevations should be managed for liver injury (e.g., hepatoprotectants, dextrose, dietary alterations, etc.).

Published therapeutic doses for aspirin are:[103]

As an antiinflammatory: dog: 10 to 25 mg/kg every 12 hours; cat: 10 to 20 mg/kg every 48 hours
For antiplatelet use: dog: 5 to 10 mg/kg every 24 to 48 hours; cat: 80 mg every 48 hours

Carprofen

Carprofen is a drug of the propionic acid class. Carprofen is COX-2 selective in dogs, but not in cats.[31] The current recommended dose for canines is 2.2-4.4 mg/kg/day PO, intramuscularly or subcutaneously; in the United Kingdom, carprofen is approved for one-time administration in cats at a dose of 4 mg/kg, subcutaneously or intravenously. Carprofen is extensively and rapidly absorbed from the gastrointestinal tract in dogs following oral administration.[118,119] The mean half-life of carprofen ranges from 6.7 (±1.5) to 9.3 (±1) hours, and it shows good correlation with single exponential elimination kinetics.[119] The majority of an absorbed dose is excreted in the bile and undergoes enterohepatic recirculation. Although exposures of 25 mg/kg/day for 42 days and 40 mg/kg/day in dogs were reported to cause no adverse effects in preclinical trials, the ASPCA APCC reports that, based on overdoses reported in dogs, doses more than 20 mg/kg could result in severe gastrointestinal signs and renal injury may occur at doses of more than 40 mg/kg (mild elevations in liver enzymes may also occur at this exposure dose).[120] According to the ASPCA APCC database, cats are at risk of gastrointestinal injury at doses of 4 mg/kg or more and doses of 8 mg/kg or more may result in acute renal failure.[112] Management of carprofen overdoses is the same as for ibuprofen overdose: decontamination, gastrointestinal protection, and fluid diuresis, as indicated by degree of exposure.[114]

Carprofen-associated hepatic toxicosis is believed to be idiosyncratic and host dependent.[121] Clinical signs associated with carprofen-induced hepatic toxicosis included inappetence, vomiting, and icterus. Biochemical abnormalities included increased serum activity of hepatic enzymes and hyperbilirubinemia. Liver biopsies in 18 of these dogs revealed a spectrum of multifocal to extensive hepatocellular necrosis that was characterized by ballooning degeneration (i.e., vacuolar change), lytic necrosis, and apoptosis. Most dogs recover uneventfully after discontinuation of carprofen and administration of supportive care.

Deracoxib

Deracoxib is a selective COX-2 inhibitor in dogs.[122] Deracoxib is rapidly absorbed, with 90% bioavailability and peak plasma levels occurring 2 hours following oral exposure in dogs.[123] Deracoxib is more than 90% protein bound in the serum. Deracoxib is metabolized in the liver and excreted primarily in the feces as a parent compound or one of four main metabolites. The half-life of deracoxib increases with increasing dosage: at 2-3 mg/kg the half-life in dogs is 3 hours, and it increases to 19 hours at 20 mg/kg. Deracoxib is approved for use in dogs of more than 4 pounds at 1-2 mg/kg PO once daily as needed for arthritis pain and 3-4 mg/kg/day PO for no more than 7 days for postoperative pain.[124] It has also been used off label at 3 mg/kg/day PO for treatment of transitional cell carcinoma in dogs.[125]

The most commonly reported adverse effects of deracoxib with therapeutic use are vomiting, anorexia, lethargy, and depression.[126] Proximal duodenal perforation was reported in 3 dogs following therapeutic dosing of deracoxib at 2-3 mg/kg PO every 24 hours.[127] Two of the three dogs had received deracoxib per the labeled dosing scheme. A retrospective study of 29 cases of gastrointestinal tract perforation subsequent to therapeutic use of deracoxib in dogs revealed that 90% of the dogs had received doses higher than labeled, had received an additional NSAID or corticosteroid in close temporal association with deracoxib therapy, or both.[122] Of those, 20 (69%) died or were euthanized. The authors concluded that approved dosage regimens should be followed carefully and that deracoxib should be used cautiously in dogs likely to have gastrointestinal tract injury.

Acute deracoxib overdoses of more than 15 mg/kg may produce significant gastrointestinal injury, and doses of more than 30 mg/kg may result in renal injury in dogs.[114] In cats, gastrointestinal injury may be seen at 4 mg/kg or more, whereas 8 mg/kg or more may result in renal injury. Management of deracoxib overdoses is the same as for ibuprofen overdose: decontamination, gastrointestinal protection, and fluid diuresis, as indicated by degree of exposure.[1]

Etodolac

Etodolac is approved for oral use in dogs 11 pounds and larger.[128] The labeled dosage for dogs is 10-15 mg/kg bw PO once daily. In dogs etodolac is rapidly absorbed following oral administration and undergoes enterohepatic recycling. The plasma half-life of etodolac is 7 hours in fasted dogs and 12 hours in unfasted dogs.

Keratoconjunctivitis sicca (KCS) has been reported in dogs receiving therapeutic doses of etodolac.[129] Dogs with etodolac treatment intervals of less than 6 months prior to the development of KCS were more than four times more likely to regain tear production than those with etodolac treatment intervals of 6 months or more. The authors conclude that monitoring of tear production prior to and during etodolac administration be considered.

Dogs receiving 10 mg/kg BW for 12 months or 15 mg/kg BW for 6 months exhibited mild weight loss, diarrhea, hypoproteinemia, and gastrointestinal erosions.[128] Dogs receiving greater than 40 mg/kg/day displayed gastrointestinal ulceration, emesis, and weight loss. Death, accompanied by gastrointestinal and renal problems, was documented in dogs receiving greater than 80 mg/kg/day. Management of etodolac overdoses is the same as for ibuprofen overdose: decontamination, gastrointestinal protection, and fluid diuresis, as indicated by degree of exposure.[114]

Firocoxib

Firocoxib has been shown to be a highly selective COX-2 inhibitor using in vitro studies on canine blood.[130] Firocoxib has relatively low bioavailability (38%) in dogs when administered orally, and is 96% protein bound. The half-life of firocoxib in dogs is 7.8 hours. Firocoxib is approved for oral use in dog for control of pain and inflammation associated with osteoarthritis and postoperative pain. The recommended dose is 5 mg/kg PO once daily as needed.

Dosing of adult beagle dogs at 15 and 25 mg/kg/day for 180 days resulted in transient decreases in serum albumin levels, and gastrointestinal lesions including inflammation and ulceration were seen in the 25 mg/kg group.[130] Administration of firocoxib to juvenile (10-13 weeks) beagle dogs at 15 and 25 mg/kg/day for 180 days resulted in decreased weight gain, hepatic lesions, pancreatic edema, duodenal ulceration, and death or euthanasia of 4 out of 12 dogs in the high-dose group by day 72. In a separate study, doses of 50 mg/kg/day for 22 days caused intestinal erosion or ulceration in three out of four dogs. In a clinical study of dogs with osteoarthritis dosed at 5 mg/kg/day PO for 52 days, 5.1% were withdrawn from the trial because of gastrointestinal side effects.[131] The most common adverse effects of firocoxib reported to the U.S. Food and Drug Administration are vomiting, anorexia, elevated BUN, and depression.[126] Management of acute firocoxib overdoses is the same as for ibuprofen overdose: decontamination, gastrointestinal protection, and fluid diuresis, as indicated by degree of exposure.[114]

Indomethacin

The reported minimum toxic dose in canines of indomethacin is 0.5 mg/kg/day.[9] This drug, like ibuprofen, undergoes extensive enterohepatic recycling.[9] The effects of indomethacin on the postoperative course following experimental orthopedic surgery in dogs was studied.[132] At a dose of 25 mg given twice daily, indomethacin was discontinued on day 1 postoperatively because signs of toxicosis were observed in all the dogs (e.g., lethargy, vomiting, and bloody stool). All patients had by then received a total dose of 125 mg of indomethacin. One dog died the fifth day postoperatively. Postmortem examination revealed intestinal ulcers in all dogs receiving this dose. When indomethacin was administered at a lower dose (5 mg twice daily) only one dog showed adverse effects (bloody stool on postoperative day 5). All dogs in the study, however, showed evidence of healing intestinal ulcers at postmortem examination. Because of the narrow margin of safety of indomethacin, any exposure in dogs or cats merits a minimum treatment of decontamination and gastrointestinal protection.

Ketoprofen

In dogs ketoprofen has been used for short-term anti inflammatory/analgesic use (up to 5 days).[2] Ketoprofen caused no adverse effects and was effective in cats at a dose of 2 mg/kg given subcutaneously, followed by 1 mg/kg PO every 24 hours for 4 days.[133] The antipyretic effect of ketoprofen in cats was rapid and persisted for at least 8 hours but less than 24 hours, and the authors reported no drug side effects based on clinical observation. The published dose for dogs is 2 mg/kg, followed by 1 mg/kg/day for 4 to 5 days.[38] Exposure doses of ketoprofen greater than 20 mg/kg may be associated with adverse effects. Management of ketoprofen overdoses is the same as for ibuprofen overdose: decontamination, gastrointestinal protection, and fluid diuresis, as indicated by degree of exposure.[114]

Meloxicam

Meloxicam is approved for oral and parenteral (intravenous or subcutaneous) use in dogs and for subcutaneous use in cats. In dogs, meloxicam is dosed at 0.2 mg/kg BW intravenously or subcutaneously followed in 24 hours by 0.1 mg/kg/day PO.[134] Cat dosing is a one-time subcutaneous dose of 0.3 mg/kg BW; additional doses are contraindicated.[135] In dogs, orally administered meloxicam has nearly 100% bioavailability when administered with food.[136] Meloxicam is approximately 97% protein bound in dogs and cats.[135,136] Terminal half-lives for dogs and cats are 24 and 15 hours, respectively, regardless of route of administration.

In safety studies, dogs were dosed orally at 0.1, 0.3, and 0.5 mg/kg/day for 180 days. All dogs developed vomiting or diarrhea during the testing interval.[136] Two thirds of dogs dosed at 0.3 mg/kg/day and one half of dogs dosed at 0.5 mg/kg/day had decreases in red blood cell counts, and regenerative anemia was identified in some of the dogs. BUN values showed increasing trends in two of the high-dose dogs, but values remained within the reference range. No changes in coagulation parameters were noted during the study.

In feline efficacy studies, 8.3% of cats administered meloxicam subcutaneously prior to surgery (onychectomy or onychectomy and surgical neuter) developed elevated posttreatment elevations of BUN (compared with 0% in butorphanol-treated cohorts), and 12.5% developed posttreatment anemia (compared with 4% in butorphanol-treated cohorts).[135] Cats administered 0.9 and 1.5 mg/kg (three and five times the recommended dose) subcutaneously once daily for 3 days developed gastrointestinal and renal adverse effects. Cats given 0.3 or 0.6 mg/kg subcutaneously followed by 0.3 mg/kg/day orally for 10 days developed severe signs of gastrointestinal and renal injury; one cat in each dose group died on day 8.

Based on the safety studies, it appears that meloxicam has a fairly narrow margin of safety, especially in cats, so any overdoses should be managed promptly and measures taken to protect against gastrointestinal and renal injury as described in the Treatment section previously.

Naproxen

In the dog, naproxen has a half-life of 35 to 72 hours and is eliminated primarily through the feces.[137] In a 30-day tolerance trial in dogs, naproxen given at 15 mg/kg/day (1.3 times the high end of the recommended human juvenile dose) caused gastrointestinal lesions and hematologic changes, and some dogs eventually died.[138] When dogs were given only 5 mg/kg/day, gastrointestinal lesions were also common.

Naproxen-associated duodenal ulcer, perforation, and peritonitis were reported in a dog receiving 22 mg/kg/day for 3 days and 5.5 mg/kg/day for 2 to 3 weeks.[85] A transmural pyloric perforation in a 25-kg dog was the result of periodic administration by the owner of 250 mg of naproxen once or twice daily for several weeks before the dog was brought to the veterinarian.[84] Single acute doses of more than 5 mg/kg BW may result in gastrointestinal toxicity and doses of more than 25 mg/kg have been associated with renal injury in dogs.[112] Acute doses of more than 50 mg/kg may result in neurologic signs. Management of naproxen overdoses is the same as for ibuprofen overdose: decontamination, gastrointestinal protection, and fluid diuresis, as indicated by degree of exposure.[114]

Phenylbutazone

Phenylbutazone is not commonly used in dogs anymore. The recommended dose is listed as 14 mg/kg PO three times daily initially (maximum of 800 mg/day regardless of weight) and then titrate the dose down to the lowest effective dose.[38] The average lethal dose reported in the dog is 150 mg/kg, with an oral median lethal dose (LD_{50}) of 332 mg/kg.

Piroxicam

When administered on an empty stomach, piroxicam in dogs is rapidly absorbed and undergoes enterohepatic recycling.[35,139] The mean elimination half-life is 40.2 hours; however, a half-life of 35 hours in beagles and a half-life of 74 hours in mongrel dogs have been reported.[35]

In a two-phase clinical trial, piroxicam was administered to dogs at a dose of 0.6 mg/kg/day.[140] The drug was administered in various regimens. These dosing schedules included 7 days only; two 7-day periods with a 3-day wash-out period between treatments; and discontinuous administration of 7 days on, 3 days off for four consecutive periods with a 7-day wash-out period, which was extended to 169 days. Only two dogs experienced gastric upset. The authors concluded that a discontinuous schedule of piroxicam at 0.6 mg/kg/day in dogs with no existing diseases involving the gastrointestinal tract, kidneys, or liver may be safe. However, an almost perforated ulcer in the distal pylorus of a dog after 17 days of piroxicam therapy at a dose rate of 0.8 mg/kg on alternate days has been reported.[139] Additionally, gastrointestinal reactions in 6 and renal papillary necrosis in 2 of 34 dogs treated with piroxicam for transitional cell carcinoma of the urinary bladder at 0.3 mg/kg/day has been reported.[105] Management of piroxicam overdoses is the same as for ibuprofen overdose: decontamination, gastrointestinal protection, and fluid diuresis, as indicated by degree of exposure.[114]

Tepoxalin

Tepoxalin is considered a dual inhibitor of arachidonic acid metabolism as it inhibits both COX and 5-lipoxygenase.[141] Tepoxalin is rapidly absorbed following oral administration and the presence of food enhances bioavailability. The parent compound, tepoxalin, is rapidly converted to an active metabolite that has a half-life of 12-13 hours. Tepoxalin and its metabolite are almost exclusively eliminated via the bile.

Tepoxalin is approved for use in dogs 3 pounds or larger at an initial dose of 10-20 mg/kg PO followed by daily maintenance doses of 10 mg/kg. The most common adverse effects reported with tepoxalin in dogs are vomiting, anorexia, and diarrhea.[126] Doses of 300 mg/kg/day for 180 days resulted in gastric ulceration in dogs; lower doses of 20 mg/kg/day and 100 mg/kg/day caused gastric irritation. Although safety studies on tepoxalin have suggested a wider margin of safety than some other veterinary NSAIDs, it would be prudent to manage tepoxalin overdoses in the same fashion as ibuprofen overdoses: decontamination, gastrointestinal protection, and fluid diuresis, as indicated by degree of exposure.[114]

Conclusion

Because of their antiinflammatory, analgesic, and antipyretic properties, NSAIDs have a role in therapy in dogs and cats. Judicious administration is warranted. Risk factors, elimination half-lives of the various NSAIDs, and concurrent administration of other medications should be considered before prescribing any NSAID. Pet owners must be made aware that over-the-counter NSAID medications can be harmful and even deadly if they are administered improperly to their pets.

Acknowledgment

The editors wish to acknowledge the exceptional contribution of Dr. Marilyn Mikiciuk, who authored this chapter for the original edition of the book. Her contribution served as the foundation for the material appearing in this edition.

References

1. Boothe DM: Controlling inflammation with nonsteroidal anti-inflammatory drugs, *Vet Med Sept* 875–883, 1989.
2. Isaacs JP: Adverse effects of non-steroidal anti-inflammatory drugs in the dog and cat, *Aust Vet Pract* 26(4):180–186, 1996.
3. Godshalk CP, Roush JK, Fingland RB, et al: Gastric perforation associated with administration of ibuprofen in a dog, *J Am Vet Med Assoc* 201(11):1734–1736, 1992.
4. Rubin SI, Papich MG: Clinical uses of nonsteroidal anti-inflammatory drugs in companion animal practice. Part II, drugs, therapeutic uses and adverse effects, *Canine Pract* 15(2):27–33, 1992.
5. Jackson TW, Costin C, Link K, et al: Correlation of serum ibuprofen concentration with clinical signs of toxicity in three canine exposures, *Vet Hum Toxic* 33(5):486–488, 1991.
6. Spyridakis LK, Bacia JJ, Barsanti JA, et al: Ibuprofen toxicosis in a dog, *J Am Vet Med Assoc* 188(9):918–919, 1986.
7. Cosenza SF: Drug-induced gastroduodenal ulceration in dogs, *Mod Vet Pract Dec* 923–925, 1984.
8. McKellar QA, May SA, Lees P: Pharmacology and therapeutics of non-steroidal anti-inflammatory drugs in the dog and cat: two individual agents, *J Small Anim Pract* 32:225–235, 1991.
9. Duggan DE, Hooke KF, Noll RM, et al: Enterohepatic circulation of indomethacin and its role in intestinal irritation, *Biochem Pharmacol* 25:1749–1754, 1975.
10. Nap RC: Nonsteroidal anti-inflammatory drugs (NSAIDs) in companion animal medicine, *Tijdschr Diergeneeskd* 118(Suppl 1):6S–8S, 1993.
11. Scherkl R, Frey HH: Pharmacokinetics of ibuprofen in the dog, *J Vet Pharmacol Ther* 10:261–265, 1987.
12. Lees P, May SA, McKellar QA: Pharmacology and therapeutics of nonsteroidal anti-inflammatory drugs in the dog and cat. General pharmacology, *J Small Anim Pract* 32:183–193, 1991.
13. Adams SS, Bough RG, Cliff EE, et al: Absorption, distribution, and toxicity of ibuprofen, *Toxicol Appl Pharmacol* 15:310–330, 1969.
14. Meadows I, Gwaltney S: The 10 most common toxicoses in dogs, *Vet Med* 101:82–90, 2006.
15. Merola V, Dunayer E: The 10 most common toxicoses in cats, *Vet Med* 101:339–342, 2006.
16. Dunayer EK: Toxicology brief: ibuprofen toxicosis in dogs, cats, and ferrets, *Vet Med* 99:580–586, 2004.
17. Willard MD: Diseases of the stomach. In Ettinger SJ, Feldman EC, editors: *Textbook of veterinary internal medicine*, ed 4, vol 2, Philadelphia, 1995, WB Saunders.
18. Vane JR, Botting RM: Mechanism of action of anti-inflammatory drugs, *Scand J Rheumatol* 25(Suppl 102):9–21, 1996.
19. Maddison JE: Corticosteroids and non-steroidal anti-inflammatory drugs, *Proc Annu Semin Eq Branch Comp Anim Soc, NZ Vet Assoc* 158:91–106, 1994.

20. Knight EV, Kimball JP, Keenan CM, et al: Preclinical toxicity evaluation of tepoxalin, a dual inhibitor of cyclooxygenase and 5-lipoxygenase, in Sprague-Dawley rats and beagle dogs, *Vundam Appl Toxicol* 33(1):38–48, 1996.
21. Masferrer JL, Isakson PC, Seibert K: Cyclooxygenase-2 inhibitors, *Gastroenterol Clin North Am* 25(2):363–372, 1996.
22. Brideau C, Kargman S, Liu S, et al: A human whole blood assay for clinical evaluation of biochemical efficacy of cyclooxygenase inhibitors, *Inflamm Res* 45:68–74, 1996.
23. Frolich JC: A classification of NSAIDs according to the relative inhibition of cyclooxygenase isoenzymes, *Trends Pharmacol Sci* 18(1):30–34, 1997.
24. Bergh MS, Budsberg SC: The coxib NSAIDs: potential clinical and pharmacological importance in veterinary medicine, *J Vet Intern Med* 19:633–643, 2005.
25. Famaey JP: In vitro and in vivo pharmacological evidence of selective cyclooxygenase-2 inhibition by nimesulide: an overview, *Inflamm Res* 46:437–446, 1997.
26. Engelhardt G: Pharmacology of meloxicam, a new non-steroidal anti-inflammatory drug with an improved safety profile through preferential inhibition of COX-2, *Br J Rheumatol* 35(Suppl):4–12, 1996.
27. Donnelly MT, Hawkey CJ: Review article: COX-2 inhibitors—a new generation of safer NSAIDs? *Aliment Pharmacol Ther* 11:227–236, 1997.
28. Hayllar J, Bjarnason I: Gastroduodenal tolerability of highly specific cyclooxygenase-2 inhibitor, *Ital J Gastroenterol* 28(Suppl 4):30–32, 1996.
29. Wallace JL: NSAID gastroenteropathy: past, present and future, *Can J Gastroenterol* 10(7):451–459, 1996.
30. King JN, Arnaud JP, Goldenthal EI, et al: Robenacoxib in the dogs: target species safety in relation to extent and duration of inhibition of COX-1 and COX-2, *J Vet Pharmacol Ther* 34:298–311, 2011.
31. Clark TP: The clinical pharmacology of cyclooxygenase-2-selective and dual inhibitors, *Vet Clin Small Anim* 36:1061–1085, 2006.
32. Schmid VB, Seewald W, Lees P, King JN: In vitro and ex vivo inhibition of COX isoforms by robenacoxib in the cat: a comparative study, *J Vet Pharmacol Ther* 33:444–452, 2010.
33. Conlon PD: Nonsteroidal drugs used in the treatment of inflammation, *Vet Clin North Am Small Anim Pract* 18:1115–1131, 1988.
34. Borga O, Borga B: Serum protein binding on nonsteroidal antiinflammatory drugs: a comparative study, *J Pharmacokinet Biopharm* 25(1):63–77, 1997.
35. Galbraith EA, McKellar QA: Pharmacokinetics and pharmacodynamics of piroxicam in dogs, *Vet Rec* 128:561–565, 1991.
36. McKellar QA, Galbraith EA, Simmons RD: Pharmacokinetics and serum thromboxane inhibition of two NSAIDs when administered to dogs by the intravenous or subcutaneous route, *J Small Anim Pract* 32:335–340, 1991.
37. Cunningham FM, Lees P: Advances in anti-inflammatory therapy, *Br Vet J* 150:115–134, 1994.
38. Papich MG: Principles of analgesic drug therapy, *Semin Vet Med Surg (Small Anim)* 12(2):80–93, 1997.
39. Pearson SP, Kelberman I: Gastrointestinal effects of NSAIDs, *Postgrad Med* 100(5):131–143, 1996.
40. Seitz S, Boelsterli UA: Diclofenac acyl glucuronide, a major biliary metabolite, is directly involved in small intestinal injury in rats, *Gastroenterology* 115(6):1476–1482, 1998.
41. Hawkey CJ: Non-steroidal anti-inflammatory drug gastropathy: causes and treatments, *Scand J Gastroenterol* 31(Suppl 220):124–127, 1996.
42. Champion GD, Feng PH, Azuma T, et al: NSAID-induced gastrointestinal damage, *Drugs* 53(1):6–19, 1997.
43. Evans JMM, McMahon AD, Murray FE, et al: Non-steroidal anti-inflammatory drugs are associated with emergency admission to hospital for colitis due to inflammatory bowel disease, *Gut* 40:619–622, 1997.
44. Gutthan SP, Garcia Rodriguez LA, Raiford DS: Individual nonsteroidal anti-inflammatory drugs and other risk factors for upper gastrointestinal bleeding and perforation, *Epidemiology* 8(1):18–24, 1997.
45. Matzke GR: Nonrenal toxicities of acetaminophen, aspirin, and nonsteroidal anti-inflammatory agents, *Am J Kidney Dis* 28(1 Suppl 1):S63–S70, 1996.
46. Wallace JL: Nonsteroidal anti-inflammatory drugs and gastroenteropathy: the second hundred years, *Gastroenterology* 112(3):1000–1016, 1997.
47. Kawano S, Tsuji S, Sato N, et al: NSAIDs and the microcirculation of the stomach, *Gastroenterol Clin North Am* 25(2):299–314, 1996.
48. Strom H, Thomsen MK: Effects of non-steroidal anti-inflammatory drugs on canine neutrophil chemotaxis, *J Vet Pharmacol Ther* 13:186–191, 1990.
49. Hansen JM, Hallas J, Lauritsen JM, et al: Non-steroidal anti-inflammatory drugs and ulcer complications: a risk factor analysis for clinical decision-making, *Scand J Gastroenterol* 31:126–130, 1996.

50. Faucheron JL, Parc R: Non-steroidal anti-inflammatory drug-induced colitis, *Int J Colorect Dis* 11:99–101, 1996.

51. Peterson WL: The influences of food, beverages and NSAIDs on gastric acid secretion and mucosal integrity, *Yale J Biol Med* 69:81–84, 1996.

52. Lugea A, Antolin M, Mourelle M, et al: Deranged hydrophobic barrier of the rat gastroduodenal mucosa after parenteral nonsteroidal anti-inflammatory drugs, *Gastroenterology* 112:1931–1939, 1997.

53. Davies NM, Wright MR, Russell AS, et al: Effect of the enantiomers of flurbiprofen, ibuprofen, and ketoprofen on intestinal permeability, *J Pharmaceut Sci* 85(11):1170–1173, 1996.

54. Stanton ME, Bright RM: Gastroduodenal ulceration in dogs, *J Vet Intern Med* 3:238–244, 1989.

55. Wallace MS, Zawie DA, Garvey MS: Gastric ulceration in the dog secondary to the use of nonsteroidal anti-inflammatory drugs, *J Am Anim Hosp Assoc* 26:467–472, 1990.

56. Wen SF: Nephrotoxicities of nonsteroidal anti-inflammatory drugs, *J Formos Med Assoc* 96(3):157–171, 1997.

57. Gutthann SP, Garcia Rodriguez LA, Raiford DS, et al: Nonsteroidal anti-inflammatory drugs and the risk of hospitalization for acute renal failure, *Arch Intern Med* 156:2433–2439, 1996.

58. de Leeuw PW: Nonsteroidal anti-inflammatory drugs and hypertension, *Drugs* 51(2):179–187, 1996.

59. Evans AM: Pharmacodynamics and pharmacokinetics of the profens: enantioselectivity, clinical implications, and special reference to S(+)-ibuprofen, *J Clin Pharmacol* 36:7S–15S, 1996.

60. Nuutinen LS: Risk/benefit evaluation of NSAIDs in postoperative pain therapy, *Acta Anaesth Belg* 47:129–133, 1996.

61. Murray MD, Brater DG: Effects of NSAIDs on the kidney, *Prog Drug Res* 49:155–171, 1997.

62. Lascelles BD, McFarland J, Swann HS: Guidelines for safe and effective use of NSAIDs in dogs, *Vet Ther* 6(3):237–251, 2005.

63. Bessone F: Non-steroidal anti-inflammatory drugs: what is the actual risk of liver damage? *World J Gastroenterol* 16(45):5651–5661, 2010.

64. Editorial Board: Effects of two non-steroidal anti-inflammatory drugs (NSAIDs) and gentamicin on renal function (comment), *Clin Sci (Colch)* 91(2):119, 1996.

65. Elwood C, Boswood A, Simpson K, et al: Renal failure after flunixin meglumine administration, *Vet Rec* 130(26):582–583, 1992.

66. Smitherman P: Intra-operative use of flunixin meglumine, *Vet Rec* 131(20):471, 1992.

67. Boydell P: Drug combination side effects, *Vet Rec* 130(14):307, 1992.

68. Rubin SI, Papich MG: Nonsteroidal anti-inflammatory drugs. In Kirk RW, editor: *Current veterinary therapy X, small animal practice*, Philadelphia, 1989, WB Saunders.

69. Harder S, Thurmann P: Clinically important drug interactions with anticoagulants, *Clin Pharmacokinet* 30(6):416–444, 1996.

70. Stirnimann G, Kessebohm K, Lauterburg B: Liver injury caused by drugs: an update, *Swiss Med Wkly* 140:w13080, 2010.

71. Browne BA, Holder EP, Rupnick L: Nonsteroidal anti-inflammatory drugs and necrotizing fasciitis, *Am J Health Syst Pharm* 53:265–269, 1996.

72. Dow SW, Rosychuk R, McChesney AE, et al: Effects of flunixin and flunixin plus prednisolone on the gastrointestinal tract of dogs, *Am J Vet Res* 51:1131, 1990.

73. Butterworth SJ, Weaver BMQ: Drug combination side effects, *Vet Record* 130(12):251–252, 1992.

74. Verbeeck RJ: Pharmokinetic drug interactions with nonsteroidal anti-inflammatory drugs, *Clin Pharmacokinet* 19:44, 1990.

75. Daehler MH: Transmural pyloric perforation associated with naproxen administration in a dog, *J Am Vet Med Assoc* 189(6):694–695, 1986.

76. Gfeller RW, Sandors AD: Naproxen-associated duodenal ulcer complicated by perforation and bacteria- and barium sulfate-induced peritonitis in a dog, *J Am Vet Med Assoc* 198(4):644–646, 1991.

77. Mahaffey EA: Disorders of iron metabolism. In Kirk RW, editor: *Current veterinary therapy IX*, Philadelphia, 1986, WB Saunders.

78. Weiser MG: Erythrocyte responses and disorders. In Ettinger SJ, Feldman EC, editors: *Textbook of veterinary internal medicine*, ed 4, vol 2, Philadelphia, 1995, WB Saunders.

79. Rogers K, Anemia: In Ettinger SJ, Feldman EC, editors: *Textbook of veterinary internal medicine*, ed 4, vol 2, Philadelphia, 1995, WB Saunders.

80. Grauer GF, Lane IF: Acute renal failure. In Ettinger SJ, Feldman EC, editors: *Textbook of veterinary internal medicine*, ed 4, vol 2, Philadelphia, 1995, WB Saunders.

81. Pennick DG, Matz M, Tidwell A: Ultrasonography of gastric ulceration in the dog, *Vet Radiol Ultrasound* 38:308–312, 1997.

82. Owens JM: Gastrointestinal diagnostic imaging. In Bonagura JD, editor: *Kirk's current veterinary therapy XII*, Philadelphia, 1995, WB Saunders.

83. Ettinger SE, Barrett K: Ascites, peritonitis, and other causes of abdominal distension. In Ettinger SJ, Feldman EC, editors: *Textbook of veterinary internal medicine*, ed 4, vol 1, Philadelphia, 1995, WB Saunders.

84. Feldman BF: Disorders of platelets. In Kirk RW, editor: *Current veterinary therapy X, small animal practice*, Philadelphia, 1989, WB Saunders.

85. Forsyth SF, Guilford WG, Lawoko CRO: Endoscopic evaluation of the gastroduodenal mucosa following non-steroidal anti-inflammatory drug administration in the dog, *N Z Vet J* 44:179–181, 1996.

86. Strombeck DR, Guilford WG: Procedures for the evaluation of pancreatic and gastrointestinal tract diseases. In Strombeck DR, Guilford WG, editors: *Small animal gastroenterology*, ed 2, Davis, Calif., 1990, Stonegate Publishing Co.

87. Lagutchik MS: Blood transfusions. In Wingfield WE, editor: *Veterinary emergency medicine secrets*, Philadelphia, 1997, Hanley & Belfus.

88. Boulay JP, Lipowitz AJ, Klausner JS: Effect of cimetidine on aspirin-induced gastric hemorrhage in dogs, *Am J Vet Res* 47:1744–1746, 1986.

89. Bersenas AME, Mathews KA, Allen DG, Conlon PD: Effects of ranitidine, famotidine, pantoprazole and omeprazole on intragastric pH in dogs, *Am J Vet Res* 66:425–431, 2005.

90. Hata J, Kamada T, Manabe N, et al: Famotidine prevents canine gastric blood flow reduction by NSAIDs, *Aliment Pharmacol Ther* 21(Suppl 2):55–59, 2005.

91. Coruzzi G, Bertaccini G: Antisecretory activity of omeprazole in the conscious gastric fistula cat: comparison with famotidine, *Pharmacol Res* 21(5):499–506, 1989.

92. Coruzzi G, Adami M, Bertacciini G: Gastric antisecretory activity of lansoprazole in different experimental models: comparison with omeprazole, *Gen Pharmacol* 26(5):1027–1032, 1995.

93. Loeb DS, Ahlquist DA, Talley MJ: Management of gastroduodenopathy associated with the use of non-steroidal anti-inflammatory drugs, *Mayo Clin Proc* 67(4):354–364, 1992.

94. Ekstrom P, Carling L, Wetterhus S, et al: Omeprazole reduces the frequency of gastroduodenal lesions and dyspeptic symptoms during NSAID treatment, *Gastroenterology* 108:A87, 1995.

95. Oddsson E, Gudjonsson A, Thjodleifsson B: Protective effect of omeprazole or ranitidine against naproxen induced damage to the human gastroduodenal mucosa (abstract), *Scand J Gastroenterol* 176(Suppl 25):25, 1990.

96. Whalan A, Bader JP, Classen M, et al: Effect of omeprazole and ranitidine on ulcer healing and relapse rates in patients with benign gastric ulcers, *N Engl J Med* 320(2):69–75, 1989.

97. Tarnowski AJ, Hollander D, Gerglely MS, et al: Comparison of antacid, sucralfate, cimetidine, and ranitidine in protection of the gastric mucosa against ethanol injury, *Am J Med* 79(Suppl 2C):8–14, 1985.

98. Tarnowski A, Hollander D, Krause WJ, et al: Does sucralfate affect the normal gastric mucosa? *Gastroenterology* 90:893–905, 1986.

99. Pedrazzoli Junior J, de Almeida Pierossi M, Muscara MN, et al: Short-term sucralfate administration alters potassium diclofenac absorption in healthy male volunteers, *Br J Clin Pharmacol* 43(1):104–108, 1997.

100. Murtaugh RJ, Matz ME, Labato MA, et al: Use of synthetic prostaglandin E1 (misoprostol) for prevention of aspirin-induced gastroduodenal ulceration in arthritic dogs, *J Am Vet Med Assoc* 202(2):251–256, 1993.

101. Ward DM, Leib MS, Johnston SA, Marini M: The effect of dosing interval on the efficacy of misoprostol in the prevention of aspirin-induced gastric injury, *J Vet Intern Med* 17(3):282–290, 2003.

102. Davies CD, Forrester D, Troy GC, et al: Effects of a prostaglandin E1 analogue, misoprostol, on renal function in dogs receiving nephrotoxic doses of gentamicin, *Am J Vet Res* 59(8):1048–1054, 1998.

103. Papich M: Table of common drugs: approximate dosages. In Bonagura JD, editor: *Kirk's current veterinary therapy XII, small animal practice*, Philadelphia, 1995, WB Saunders.

104. Matthews KA, Doherty T, Dyson DH, et al: Nephrotoxicity in dogs associated with methoxyflurane anaesthesia and flunixin meglumine analgesia, *Can Vet J* 31:766–771, 1990.

105. Knapp DW, Richardson RC, Chan TCK, et al: Piroxicam therapy in 34 dogs with transitional cell carcinoma of the urinary bladder, *J Vet Intern Med* 8:273, 1994.

106. Davis LE: Clinical pharmacology of salicylates, *J Am Vet Med Assoc* 176:65, 1980.

107. Kauffman G: Aspirin-induced gastric mucosal injury: lessons learned from animal models, *Gastroenterology* 96:606–614, 1989.

108. Holland M, Chastain CB: Uses and misuses of aspirin. In Bonagura JD, editor: *Kirk's current veterinary therapy XII, small animal practice*, Philadelphia, 1995, WB Saunders.

109. Guslandi M: Gastric toxicity of antiplatelet therapy with low-dose aspirin, *Drugs* 53(1):1–5, 1997.

110. Haggert G, McCormick G, Frank P, et al: Temporal pattern of gastric mucosal damage in beagle dogs dosed daily with aspirin over a four week period (abstract). *Proceedings of the 12th American College of Veterinary Internal Medicine Forum*, San Francisco, 1994.

111. Brater DC: Clinical pharmacology of NSAIDs, *J Clin Pharmacol* 28:518–524, 1988.
112. Bischoff K: Toxicity of over-the-counter drugs. In Gupta RC, editor: *Veterinary toxicology: basic and clinical principles*, New York, 2007, Academic Press.
113. Villar D, Buck WB: Ibuprofen, aspirin and acetaminophen toxicosis and treatment in dogs and cats, *Vet Human Toxicol* 40(3):156–161, 1998.
114. Gwaltney-Brant SM: Toxicology of pain medications, *Proceedings of the Central Veterinary Conference (CVC)*, Baltimore, MD, 2010.
115. Schubert TA: Salicylate-induced seizures in a dog, *J Am Vet Med Assoc* 185:1000, 1984.
116. Proudfoot AT: Salicylates and salicylamide. In Haddad LM, Winchester JF, editors: *Clinical management of poisoning and drug overdose*, Philadelphia, 1990, WB Saunders.
117. Cribb AE: Adverse effects of NSAIDs. In Dowling PM, editor: *Clinical pharmacology, principles and practice*, Monograph Series 982, Western Veterinary Conference, Las Vegas, 1998.
118. McKellar QA, Delatour P, Lees P: Stereospecific pharmacodynamics and pharmacokinetics of carprofen, *J Vet Pharmacol Ther* 17:447–454, 1994.
119. McKellar QA, Pearson T: Bogan JA: Pharmacokinetics, tolerance and serum thromboxane inhibition of carprofen in the dog, *J Small Anim Pract* 31:443–448, 1990.
120. Mensching D, Volmer P: Managing acute carprofen toxicosis in dogs and cats, *Vet Med* 104(7):325–333, 2009.
121. MacPhail C, Lappin MR, Meyer DJ, et al: Hepatocellular toxicosis associated with administration of carprofen in 21 dogs, *J Am Vet Med Assoc* 212(12):1895–1901, 1998.
122. Lascelles DX, Blikslager AT, Fox SM, Reese D: Gastrointestinal tract perforation in dogs treated with a selective cyclooxygenase-2 inhibitor: 29 cases (2002-2003), *J Am Vet Med Assoc* 227:112–117, 2005.
123. Deramaxx (deracoxib) Chewable Tablets [package insert]: Greensboro, 2006, Novartis Animal Health.
124. Plumb DC: Deracoxib. In *Veterinary drug handbook*, ed 6, Ames, IA, 2008, Blackwell.
125. McMillan SK, Boria P, Moore GE, et al: Antitumor effects of deracoxib treatment in 26 dogs with transitional cell carcinoma of the urinary bladder, *J Am Vet Med Assoc* 239(8):1084–1089, 2011.
126. U.S. Food and Drug Administration: *Animal & veterinary adverse drug experience reports.* Retrieved 01/2012 from 1987-2011, http://www.fda.gov/AnimalVeterinary/SafetyHealth/ProductSafetyInformation/ucm055369.htm.
127. Case JB, Fick JL, Rooney MB: Proximal duodenal perforation in three dogs following deracoxib administration, *J Am Anim Hosp Assoc* 46(4):255–258, 2010.
128. EtoGesic (etodolac) tablets [package insert]: *Fort Dodge, Fort Dodge Animal Health*, 2004.
129. Klauss GI, Giuliano EA, Moore CP, et al: Keratoconjunctivitis sicca associated with administration of etodolac in dogs: 211 cases (1992-2002), *J Am Vet Med Assoc* 230(4):541-547.
130. Previcox (firocoxib) chewable tablets [package insert]: Duluth, 2007, Merial Ltd.
131. Autefage A, Palissier FM, Asimus E, Pepin-Richard C: Long-term efficacy and safety of firocoxib in the treatment of dogs with osteoarthritis, *Vet Rec* 168(23):617.
132. Mbugua SW, Skoglund A, Lokken P: Effects of phenylbutazone and indomethacin on the post-operative course following experimental orthopaedic surgery in dogs, *Acta Vet Scand* 30(1):27–35, 1989.
133. Glew A, Aviad AD, Keister DM, et al: Use of ketoprofen as an antipyretic in cats, *Can Vet J* 37:222–225, 1996.
134. U.S. Food and Drug Administration: Metacam [meloxicam 5 mg/mL solution for injection], *Freedom of Information Summary*, 2003. Retrieved 01/2012 from http://www.fda.gov/downloads/AnimalVeterinary/Products/ApprovedAnimalDrugProducts/FOIADrugSummaries/ucm118006.pdf.
135. U.S. Food and Drug Administration: Metacam [meloxicam 5 mg/mL solution for injection], *Freedom of Information Summary*, 2004. Retrieved 01/2012 from http://www.fda.gov/downloads/AnimalVeterinary/Products/ApprovedAnimalDrugProducts/FOIADrugSummaries/ucm118027.pdf.
136. U.S. Food and Drug Administration: Metacam [meloxicam oral suspension], *Freedom of Information Summary*, 2004. Retrieved 01/2012 from http://www.fda.gov/downloads/AnimalVeterinary/Products/ApprovedAnimalDrugProducts/FOIADrugSummaries/ucm118008.pdf.
137. Runkel R, Chaplin M, Boost G, et al: Absorption, distribution, and excretion of naproxen in various laboratory animals and human subjects, *J Pharm Sci* 61:703–708, 1972.
138. Hallesy D, Shotts L, Hill R: Comparative toxicology of naproxen, *Scand J Rheumatol* 2(Suppl):20–28, 1973.
139. Thomas NW: Piroxicam-associated ulceration in a dog, *Compend Cont Ed* 10:1004, 1987.
140. Sumano H, DeVizcaya A, Brumbaugh G: Tolerance and clinical evaluation of piroxicam in dogs, *Israel J Vet Med* 51(1):27–29, 1996.
141. U.S. Food and Drug Administration: Zubrin [tepoxalin rapidly-disintegrating tablets for dogs], *Freedom of Information Summary*, 2003. Retrieved 01/2012 from http://www.fda.gov/downloads/AnimalVeterinary/Products/ApprovedAnimalDrugProducts/FOIADrugSummaries/ucm117603.pdf.

Organochlorine Pesticides

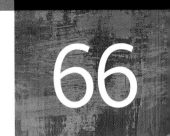

66

Merl F. Raisbeck, DVM, MS, PhD, DABVT

- The most likely source of acute organochlorine poisoning in small animals is improperly stored stockpiles of outdated pesticides. With the exception of a very few, very limited applications, most organochlorine insecticides have not been used in more than 30 years.
- Clinical signs of organochlorine poisoning are best summarized as neurologic. Poisoned animals become hyperesthetic and exhibit motor tremors and convulsions. Treatment is symptomatic and supportive in nature.
- Most pesticides of this class are extremely persistent in body fat. Poisoned animals should be monitored for several weeks for recurrences.
- Most of the modern environmental guidelines ("toxic levels") are based on theoretical human cancer considerations or on endocrine effects in nonmammals. Clinicians should be aware when evaluating possible sources of exposure that such guidelines are very low compared with the exposure required for clinical poisoning.

Sources

After the introduction of dichlorodiphenyltrichloroethane (DDT) in 1940, a number of halogenated organic compounds were created for use as pesticides. Although there are many toxic chlorinated organic compounds, the term *chlorinated hydrocarbons* or *organochlorines* (OCs) usually refers to this group of insecticides. The OCs may be classified according to either their intended principal use (e.g., insecticides, nematocides, and fungicides) or their chemical structure (e.g., chlorinated aryl hydrocarbons, cyclodiene, diphenyl aliphatics, and so on). The latter scheme is most useful from the standpoint of mammalian metabolism and toxicology. With only a few exceptions, the OCs are refractory to metabolism and are lipophilic. As such, they tend to be readily absorbed, but only slowly eliminated and thus accumulate in humans, domestic animals, and wildlife, and bioconcentrate in the food chain. Many are suspect or known carcinogens and endocrine disruptors. As a result, the class has been largely replaced by less persistent agents, such as the organophosphates and pyrethroids. Some examples of OCs include aldrin, dieldrin, endrin, lindane, chlordane, endosulfan, heptachlor, toxaphene, and methoxychlor.

The OCs were heavily used for pest control from the 1950s through the 1970s. Thus contaminated soils or leakage from old dump sites are possible sources of exposure for wildlife and domestic carnivores, especially given the propensity of the OCs to bioconcentrate in the food chain. Because one of the few remaining legal applications of the OC is ectoparasite control, accidental overdose is also a possible source of acute toxicosis. The most likely source of poisoning in companion animals, however, is old stockpiles of insecticides and improper waste disposal.

Toxic Dose

The acutely toxic dose varies considerably with the specific OC. In general the OCs are less acutely toxic than organophosphates or carbamates used for similar purposes. For example, the most potent OCs have a mammalian acute median lethal dose (LD_{50}) of approximately 50 mg/kg body weight, 10-fold to 100-fold larger than the LD_{50} of the carbamate, aldicarb. Within the class, the cyclodienes (e.g., heptachlor, chlordane, and dieldrin) are generally most toxic, followed by the aryl hydrocarbons (e.g., lindane and methoxychlor), and finally by the diphenyl aliphatics (DDT, etc.). Because of their lipophilicity, both oral and dermal exposures may result in notable systemic effects. Their low volatility usually precludes significant respiratory exposure unless aerosolized. Most of the OCs have an offensive odor.

Toxicokinetics

After exposure the OCs are rapidly redistributed via plasma lipoproteins to liver, brain, and other lipid-rich tissues. Adipose tissue serves as a "sink" for the OC, competing with critical organs, such as the brain, for circulating OC in a fashion similar to the short-acting barbiturates. Thus, after acute oral exposure to an OC, the blood concentration peaks and then declines relatively quickly as redistribution and elimination at first equal and then exceed absorption. Later, as the OC concentrations in fat exceed those in blood, stored pesticide is slowly released back into the systemic circulation, and the rate of decline in blood concentration slows dramatically. The initial period, in which both elimination and redistribution serve to decrease blood concentration, is referred to as the *alpha* phase. During the later, or *beta*, phase, redistribution from adipose tissue tends to sustain circulating levels and greatly prolongs the half-life. The beta phase half-life of most OCs is measured in months.

Body fat may also serve as a source of OC poisoning. During prolonged low-dose exposure, the adipose OC concentration increases in a logarithmic manner, eventually approaching a plateau in which the relationship between tissue concentrations, blood levels, and excretion rates is in equilibrium with uptake. At this point, the total amount of OCs in the body may be several times greater than a toxic dose, but because it is sequestered in fat, poisoning does not occur. However, if the animal is forced to lose weight rapidly, the potentially toxic dose stored in adipose tissue becomes available to the general circulation and may result in acute intoxication.

Lipophilic compounds, such as the OCs, are readily passed from blood to mammary cell lipid, which are subsequently secreted as milk fat. Transfer of the OC body burden to milk fat is ensured by the large perfusion of the mammary gland and the favorable concentration gradient created by constant synthesis and secretion of milk. Because milk is a major elimination route of persistent OCs, it is a potential source of exposure for neonates. In practice the likelihood of acute poisoning from milk of an asymptomatic dam is relatively low, but the possibility should be considered if a lactating animal has been exposed to an OC.

Metabolism of most OCs contributes little to elimination and may actually produce more toxic metabolites. For example, the cyclodienes (e.g., heptachlor) are rapidly converted to their epoxides, and the diphenyl aliphatics are partially dechlorinated, but in both cases the end product is stable, lipophilic, and at least as toxic as its parent. Metabolites are released slowly from the lipid storage depot and transported through the blood to liver, where they are excreted in the bile. However, after excretion into the intestine, many OCs are reabsorbed. This enterohepatic recycling also serves to prolong the persistence of the OC in the body.

Mechanism of Toxicity

With the possible exception of DDT, the biochemical and cellular mechanisms of acute OC insecticide toxicity are incompletely understood in mammals. In sufficiently high doses, most OCs interfere with the axonal transmission of nerve impulses and therefore disrupt nervous system functions. DDT, specifically, inhibits the mechanism whereby the influx of sodium is stopped and the outflux of potassium is started during an action potential, thereby rendering the fiber hyperactive. DDT metabolites (specifically mitotane) also inhibit the output of the adrenal gland by causing selective necrosis of the zona fasciculata and reticularis.

The mechanisms of action of the other OCs are poorly understood. Dieldrin, aldrin, and lindane apparently enhance neurotransmitter release at cholinergic synapses and may increase brain ammonia concentrations by impairing glutamine synthesis. Heptachlor and lindane have been shown to inhibit binding of the inhibitory neurotransmitter γ-aminobutyric acid. Clinically, however, all compounds cause intense nervous stimulation and hypersensitivity, a fact that is responsible for the most dramatic signs of acute poisoning.

A number of nonneurotoxic syndromes have been attributed to some OCs, especially the polynuclear aromatic OCs, such as polybrominated biphenyls. These syndromes are particularly likely to occur after long-term chronic exposure. A brief catalog of such effects includes altered hepatic steroid metabolism, male infertility, bone marrow suppression, cutaneous hypersensitivity, hyperestrogenism, eggshell thinning, hepatic necrosis and nephrosis, and immunosuppression. However, most of these effects are of only marginal significance to small-animal practice. Readers interested in chronic OC toxicity are referred to reviews by Matsumura,[1] Murphy,[2] and Safe.[3]

Clinical Signs

Although a variety of clinical and subclinical toxic effects have been attributed to the OC insecticides, the clinical signs of acute poisoning are best summarized as neuromuscular. Signs may begin within a few minutes or may occur as much as 1 to 2 days after exposure to an acutely toxic dose. Mammals exposed to an acutely toxic dose typically exhibit an early period of apprehension and hypersensitivity, during which they become increasingly agitated, incoordinated, and aggressive. This phase in turn is followed by fasciculations of the head and neck that progressively involve the rest of the body. There may be abnormal posture, a spastic gait, and continuous chewing movements. Finally, there are tonic-clonic convulsions that progress to coma and death or that alternate with intermittent periods of severe depression. Animals that remain comatose for prolonged periods (i.e., more than a few hours) will probably die. The occurrence of clinical signs may be slowly progressive or explosive in nature. Other signs may include disorientation, weakness, paresthesia, vomiting, and respiratory depression.

Minimum Database

The diagnosis of acute OC insecticide poisoning hinges on (1) a history of exposure to a particular OC insecticide; (2) clinical signs as described previously; and (3) demonstration of diagnostic concentrations of that particular OC or its metabolites in brain, liver, fat, or blood. However, tremors or convulsive seizures in animals that have been potentially exposed to a pesticide and do not exhibit parasympathomimetic signs are sufficient to justify emergency therapy.

Confirmatory Tests

Detection of OC residues in blood or tissue does not in itself confirm poisoning. Given the persistent nature of the OCs, their widespread use in the past, and the incredible sensitivity of modern analytical instrumentation, it is not unusual to detect OCs in apparently healthy animals. Adipose tissue is especially likely to contain OCs. Definitive diagnosis requires demonstrating concentrations of a specific OC in a specific tissue consistent with poisoning. Unfortunately, various tissue concentrations vary with the time since exposure, and critical concentrations have not been determined for all compounds in all species. Thus in many instances it is necessary to extrapolate from other species or similar compounds. Table 66-1 summarizes the tissue concentrations reported from acute poisonings in several species.

Table 66-1	Blood and Tissue Concentrations Associated with Acutely Toxic Effects		
Species	**Compound**	**Concentration**	**Effect**
Waterfowl	Heptachlor epoxide	40-50 ppm brain	Acute intoxication
Swine	Aldrin	4 ppm brain (dieldrin)	Acute intoxication
Chicken	Aldrin	3 ppm brain (dieldrin)	Acute intoxication
Waterfowl	DDE	250 ppm brain	Acute lethality
Human	Dieldrin	0.2 mcg/mL blood	Toxic threshold
Human	Endrin	0.05-0.1 mcg/mL blood	Toxic threshold
Rat	Endrin	0.05-0.1 mcg/mL blood	Toxic threshold
Horse	Heptachlor epoxide	38 ppm brain	Acute intoxication
Waterfowl	Heptachlor epoxide	3 ppm brain	Acute lethality
Calves	Lindane	15 ppm brain	Acute lethality
Calves	Pentachlorophenol	40-50 ppm brain	Acute intoxication
Human	Telodrin	0.015 mcg/mL blood	Acute intoxication
Human	Toxaphene	4 ppm liver	Acute intoxication

DDE, Dichlorodiphenyldichloroethylene.

Sample contamination is another common problem in OC diagnosis. Many organic compounds, such as plasticizers, may interfere with the chemical analysis of OC in tissue. Thus every effort should be made to collect diagnostic samples from acutely affected animals in clean glass or metal containers.

Treatment

There are no specific antidotes for OC intoxication. Practical therapeutic regimens are based on symptomatic and supportive therapy and on preventing further absorption of the toxicant. Poisoned animals should be lightly sedated with anesthetics (e.g., barbiturates) or given muscle relaxants (e.g., methocarbamol) to minimize convulsions. Only the minimum amount necessary to control convulsions should be given. Phenothiazine tranquilizers, epinephrine, and other adrenergic amines are contraindicated. Phenothiazines tend to lower the seizure threshold further; the adrenergic amines may result in cardiac arrhythmias because of the enhanced myocardial sensitivity associated with the OC.

Because many OC insecticides are respiratory depressants, possible additive effects of anesthetics on respiration should be considered. Supplemental oxygen may be given through an intranasal tube or an oxygen cage or, if the animal is comatose, via tracheal intubation. As with any poison that induces convulsions or coma, establishing and maintaining a patent airway is very important to prevent aspiration. Administration of a small amount of parenteral nutrition (e.g., electrolytes and dextrose) may be considered if the animal is unable to eat or drink.

If oral exposure is suspected, the animal should be given an adsorbent, such as activated charcoal (AC) or cholestyramine, and a saline cathartic. Mineral oil should be given if AC is not available. Gastric lavage may be useful in some cases. If topical exposure is suspected, the animal should be thoroughly washed with soap and water, taking care that the individuals doing the washing are not themselves exposed to hazardous doses.

Adsorbents should also be considered to prevent enterohepatic recycling of the OC. Given the biologic persistence of the OC, it is probably wise to continue the use of adsorbents for several days to a month after the acute episode to maximize elimination. Because these compounds are lipid soluble, consideration should be given to the use of IV lipid therapy as a treatment option (Intralipid®, Liposyn®, Intravenous Lipid Emulsion). Current dose recommendations for IFE 20% are extrapolated from human medicine (1.5 mL/kg bolus IV over 1-3 minutes and then 0.25-0.50 mL/kg/min for 30-60 min) with a goal not to exceed 8 mL/kg/day. For patients who are still symptomatic, one author has recommended considering additional doses of 1.5 mL/kg IV over 30 minutes q4-6h for 24 to 36 hours until clinical signs resolve or maintaining a CRI of 0.5 mL/kg/h until signs resolve.[4]

Prognosis

The prognosis is guarded to good, depending on the dose received and how quickly detoxification is initiated. Animals that remain comatose for more than a few hours have a poor prognosis. Animals that show only a few mild clinical signs and that receive prompt antidotal treatment have a good prognosis.

Gross and Histologic Lesions

There are no diagnostically useful lesions of OC insecticide intoxication. Some individuals may have evidence of prolonged convulsions, such as bruising and hyperthermia. Hepatocellular degeneration and necrosis and renal tubular degeneration have been reported occasionally with certain OCs, but such lesions are more frequently associated with prolonged exposure than with acute poisoning.

Differential Diagnoses

Convulsive seizures in animals that have possibly been exposed to a pesticide and that do not exhibit parasympathomimetic signs warrant a tentative diagnosis of OC intoxication for purposes of emergency therapy. Other differentials, which must be ruled out on the basis of pathologic changes and chemical analysis, include infectious encephalitis, lead poisoning, rabies, eclampsia, canine distemper, and convulsant poisons (e.g., strychnine, metaldehyde, penitrem A and roquefortine, theobromine, caffeine, sodium monofluoroacetate [1080], nicotine, organophosphates, carbamates).

References

1. Matsumura F, editor: *Differential toxicities of insecticides and halogenated aromatics*, New York, 1984, Pergamon Press.
2. Murphy SD: Toxic effect of pesticides. In Klassen C, Amdur M, Doull J, editors: *Toxicology: the basic science of poisons*, New York, 1986, Macmillan.
3. Safe S: Environmental estrogens: roles in male reproductive tract problems and in breast cancer, *Rev Environ Health* 17:249–252, 2002.
4. Lee, JA: Advances in toxicology: the use of intra-lipid therapy & high dextrose insulin therapy, *Proceedings: ACVIM*. Accessed by Veterinary Information Network (VIN).

Organophosphate and Carbamate Insecticides

67

Dennis J. Blodgett, DVM, PhD, Diplomate, ABVT

Charlotte Means, DVM, MLIS, DABVT, DABT

- Organophosphate and carbamate insecticides are common pesticides used in agriculture, around the home, and on and around domestic animals.
- Both groups of insecticides inhibit acetylcholinesterase (AChE) activity.
- Clinical signs of acute poisoning are generally divided into three major categories. Muscarinic signs include salivation, lacrimation, urination, defecation, miosis, bronchospasm, bradycardia, and emesis. Nicotinic signs include muscle tremors, ataxia, weakness, and paralysis. Central nervous system signs can range from severe depression to hyperactivity and seizures.
- Exposures in dogs and cats to lipophilic organophosphates may lead to an "intermediate syndrome," characterized mostly by a delayed onset of anorexia, depression, generalized weakness, muscle tremors, ventroflexion of the neck, and abnormal behavior.
- Blood or brain AChE activity should be assessed and is an excellent screening tool to determine exposure in clinically affected patients or postmortem.
- Treatment options include decontamination, use of atropine sulfate, 2-pyridine aldoxime methyl chloride, diazepam, and respiratory support.

Sources

Organophosphate (OP) insecticides are marketed for control of insects on plants, animals, soils, and around the house. A few OP products are sold as anthelmintics. Many OPs are designed to remain on the surface of objects to which they are applied; others are meant to be absorbed by plants or animals and to become systemic. Labels on the products have the term *phosphate, phos, phoro,* or *phosphor* somewhere in the long chemical name of the ingredients. Most OPs are insoluble in water and are often formulated with oily vehicles or organic solvents. Others are sold as dusts, wettable powders, emulsions, or adsorbed to clay particles. The OPs used to combat fleas are sold as sprays, dips, shampoos, flea collars, or flea bombs. As newer classes of insecticides are marketed for flea control, OPs are involved in fewer cases of poisoning associated with intentional applications. Agricultural uses of OPs are varied, but many are used for control of corn rootworms. Many of these corn rootworm insecticides are very toxic. As such, agricultural OPs have begun to replace strychnine as the malicious pesticide of choice for killing dogs in some areas of the United States.[1] Baits are often mixed with food items (e.g., meat, bread, carcasses, and tuna fish) in cases of malicious poisoning.

Carbamate insecticides were designed for purposes similar to those described for OPs (Color Plate 67-1). Carbamates are similar in structure to physostigmine and neostigmine. The use of carbamates in flea products is also declining with the advent of safer classes of insecticides. Carbamates are still used abundantly for household and agricultural applications. Not all pesticides having the word *carbamate* in their chemical name are acetylcholinesterase (AChE) inhibitors. Care should be taken to obtain the entire chemical name of a product when working up a possible pesticide exposure. Carbamates, as in the case of OPs, have also gained in popularity as malicious pesticides of choice. Onset times are often shorter than OPs, and the poisoned animal may die within yards of the bait. Some carbamates, such as *Tres Pasitos,* are imported and sold illegally. This literally means "three steps" and frequently contains aldicarb.

Toxic Dose

The toxicity of the insecticides is as varied as the types of insects they were formulated to control. Little is known about the lethal doses of OPs and carbamates for dogs and cats. The median lethal dose (LD_{50}) in rats ranges from less than 1 mg/kg to more than 4 g/kg. There is also a large species variation in susceptibility. In general cats, fish, and birds seem to be more susceptible. The indiscriminate tastes of dogs make them likely candidates for insecticide toxicoses, however. Younger animals are usually more susceptible to toxicosis than mature animals. Because OPs and carbamates have similar mechanisms of action, multiple exposures to these types of insecticides are usually additive, especially if the longer-acting OP was encountered before the shorter-acting carbamate.

A general list of carbamates, in order from most to least toxic, includes aldicarb, carbofuran, methomyl, propoxur, and carbaryl.

A general list of OPs, from most to least toxic, includes disulfoton, terbufos, phorate, parathion, chlorpyrifos, fenthion, diazinon, malathion, and tetrachlorvinphos. Chlorpyrifos is especially toxic for cats, with an oral minimum lethal dose of 10 to 40 mg/kg.[2]

Toxicokinetics

Carbamate and OP insecticides may be absorbed through the skin, respiratory tract, or gastrointestinal tract. Most of the OP insecticides must be metabolized in the body by cytochrome P450 enzymes or flavin monooxygenase enzymes to become active.[3] OP insecticides are formulated with either sulfur or an oxygen atom attached via a double bond to the phosphorus atom. Sulfur products are often denoted by a *thio* in the name of the insecticide (e.g., *phosphorothionate*). Sulfur products are inactive until cytochrome P450 enzymes in the liver or other organs (e.g., lungs and brain) replace the sulfur with oxygen. In massive exposures, this time lag for activation is not noticeable and may require only 5 to 10 minutes to activate sufficient amounts of OP to cause a toxicosis. OP products that have oxygen attached to the phosphorus are active as soon as they are absorbed into the body. Carbamates do not require liver activation and are active cholinesterase (ChE) inhibitors as absorbed. Typical metabolic routes for OPs and carbamates are the cytochrome P450 routes, hydrolysis (enzymatic and nonenzymatic), and various conjugation mechanisms.[4,5] Distribution occurs throughout the body. The OPs tend to be more lipid soluble than carbamates. Therefore OPs are more likely to cross the blood-brain barrier. However, many carbamates can and do cause dramatic central nervous system (CNS) signs in animals. Metabolites of OPs and carbamates tend to be primarily eliminated in the urine.[5]

Mechanism of Toxicity

The OP and carbamate insecticides interfere with the metabolism or breakdown of acetylcholine (ACh) at cholinergic sites. ACh is the neurotransmitter found between preganglionic and postganglionic neurons of the autonomic nervous system; at the junction of postganglionic parasympathetic neurons in smooth muscle, cardiac muscle, or exocrine glands; at neuromuscular junctions of the somatic nervous system; and at cholinergic synapses in the CNS. Acetylcholinesterase (i.e., AChE, true ChE) is the enzyme responsible for breaking down ACh at these sites. It is also located on the surface of red blood cells (RBCs). AChE has an anionic and an esteratic site in which ACh is temporarily bound until hydrolysis initially releases choline from the anionic site and then acetate from the "acetylated" esteratic site. AChE is inhibited by both OP and carbamate insecticides at these cholinergic sites, so that ACh keeps depolarizing the postsynaptic membrane and cannot be broken down by synaptic AChE, which is inactive because it is "phosphorylated" or "carbamylated." Depolarization of postsynaptic membranes begins as a stimulatory process that may progress to paralysis because repolarization of the membranes is inadequate.

The OP insecticides were designed to emulate the structure of ACh and occupy both the anionic and esteratic sites of AChE. The OP moiety that fills the anionic site is quickly hydrolyzed away, leaving the phosphorus atom with multiple attached groups bound to the esteratic site. In the case of OP insecticides, binding of the phosphorus atom with its attached groups to the esteratic site of AChE is considered "irreversible" binding because the half-life may be hours or days compared with the microsecond binding of ACh.[3,4] The OPs with dimethoxy groups tend to have shorter half-lives than OPs with diethoxy groups. At some point, the organic carbon groups (i.e., methyl or ethyl) attached to the phosphorus may be hydrolyzed away and replaced by hydrogen. This makes the bond between the phosphorus atom and the esteratic site unbreakable. At this point, the enzyme has undergone "aging" and will never be functional again. The body will have to synthesize new AChE at the rate of approximately 1% per day.[6] The OPs with dimethoxy groups tend to age faster than OPs with diethoxy groups.[3]

Carbamate insecticides initially occupy both the anionic and esteratic sites of AchE also. The moiety attached to the carbonyl structure is quickly hydrolyzed away, leaving AChE "carbamylated" at the esteratic site. Carbamylation is considered a "reversible" inhibition of AChE and has a half-life of approximately 30 to 40 minutes.[4] No aging of AchE is possible with carbamate insecticides. Although the half-life of AChE inhibition by carbamates is shorter than that of OPs, the time is long enough for clinical signs and sometimes death to occur.

Other esterase enzymes in the body act for the most part as a cushion or prevention against clinical signs. Most of these enzymes can be inhibited or can hydrolyze OPs and carbamates without producing any noticeable clinical signs. Arylesterases or type A esterases hydrolyze OPs and carbamates without being inhibited in the process. Type B esterases, consisting of AChE, pseudocholinesterase (pChE), carboxylesterase, and neuropathy target esterase (NTE), are inhibited. PChE, located in serum, liver, pancreas, and nervous tissue,[7] and carboxylesterase (aliesterase), located in serum, liver, muscle, and nervous tissue, can both be inhibited without causing clinical signs. Inhibition of NTE correlates with a loss of myelin and axons in the spinal cord approximately 2 to 3 weeks after exposure to some OP compounds. The resulting syndrome is called *delayed neuropathy* or *OP-induced delayed neurotoxicity*. This effect is monitored in a chicken test model before any insecticide can be registered. Therefore delayed neuropathy is very rare and is reported only occasionally with exposure to industrial OP chemicals (e.g., tri-*o*-tolyl phosphate, found in hydraulic fluid).

Death from either OPs or carbamates is associated with respiratory problems resulting from massive respiratory tract secretions, bronchiolar constriction, intercostal and diaphragm muscle paralysis, and respiratory paralysis from CNS effects in the medulla.

Clinical Signs

Acute Syndrome

Clinical signs can be grouped under three broad categories: muscarinic, nicotinic, and CNS signs. Muscarinic signs are usually the first to appear, followed by nicotinic and then CNS effects. Usually the progression of signs is hard to differentiate, however. All of the clinical signs listed here are not necessarily seen in every case. Not all OP and carbamate toxicoses look alike, and the same toxicosis may look much different in different species, at different doses, with different routes of exposure, or at different stages in the toxicosis. Major systems in the body that are affected include the pulmonary and gastrointestinal systems and the CNS.

Onset of clinical signs depends on the dose, formulation, and route of exposure. Massive oral doses often produce clinical signs within 10 minutes and can cause death easily within 30 minutes. Dermal exposures or ingestion of delayed-release products may take 12 to 24 hours or sometimes longer to produce clinical signs.

Muscarinic Signs

Muscarinic signs are sometimes attenuated by sympathetic stimulation via ganglia. They include the following: salivation, lacrimation, urination (micturition), defecation (i.e., SLUD); anorexia; coughing; miosis; dyspnea; bradycardia; abdominal pain and distress; and vomiting (emesis).

In place of the mnemonic SLUD, the mnemonic DUMBELS is also sometimes used to describe the diarrhea, urination, miosis, bronchospasm (bradycardia), emesis, lacrimation, and salivation.[8]

Nicotinic Signs

Nicotinic signs include muscle tremors of the head and then of the general body, generalized muscle tetany, stiffness (i.e., sawhorse stance), weakness with paresis, and paralysis caused by the inability of membranes to repolarize adequately before the next action potential. Tachycardia and mydriasis are possible because of stimulation of sympathetic ganglia with release of epinephrine and norepinephrine from the postganglionic sympathetic neurons; this is more likely observed with massive oral exposures.

Central Nervous System Signs

CNS signs also occur: anxiety, restlessness, hyperactivity, depression, clonic-tonic seizures, depressed respiration, and coma.

Intermediate Syndrome

A different syndrome from the classic acute syndrome is sometimes seen in both dogs and cats, usually with exposure to lipophilic OP insecticides. Prolonged dermal exposure from a single dose of insecticide, repetitive exposures to low doses of OP or carbamate insecticides, or a single oral dose of a very lipophilic OP insecticide may produce an intermediate syndrome. The intermediate syndrome may follow an acute crisis within 24 to 72 hours or may be the first syndrome to be noticed after exposure. This syndrome has been associated with the production of tolerance in cholinergic receptors resulting from prolonged bombardment with ACh.[3] Persistent exposure to the ACh agonist is believed to cause down-regulation of cholinergic receptors through an internalization of receptors into cells. Muscarinic receptors are especially prone to down-regulation in tolerance situations.[9-11] Long-term accumulation of ACh at muscarinic receptors may induce tolerance, causing an intermediate syndrome that lacks the more dramatic muscarinic signs of the acute syndrome. Nicotinic receptors at skeletal muscle sites, which cannot develop tolerance to the ACh bombardment, are primarily involved in the intermediate syndrome. Dermal exposure of cats to chlorpyrifos used around the house has historically been the most common cause of the intermediate syndrome. Fortunately, indoor and outdoor residential uses of chlorpyrifos have been canceled or phased out by the EPA. Often, clinical signs were not apparent until 3 to 10 days after chlorpyrifos was used. Clinical signs of the intermediate syndrome in dogs or cats include anorexia, diarrhea, generalized weakness, muscle tremors, abnormal posturing, abnormal behavior, cervical ventroflexion, depression, and death.[2,12,13] Severely affected animals may have clonic-tonic convulsions. Pupil size in affected animals may range from miotic to mydriatic.[2] The chlorine groups on chlorpyrifos make it more lipid soluble than many other OPs. This property may change its toxicokinetics in the body, resulting in a slower stepwise but persistent lowering of AChE levels in the body. Other very lipophilic OPs with long half-lives (e.g., fenthion, dimethoate, chlorpyrifos, and phosmet) have been associated with a similar intermediate syndrome in humans.[14,15] An intermediate syndrome in dogs was recognized after oral exposure to an insecticide used on roses, probably disulfoton.[13] Long-term dietary exposure to carbaryl has been associated with a similar syndrome in swine.[16]

Minimum Database

Typically, a history of access to or treatment with an OP or carbamate insecticide within 24 hours before the onset of classic signs of ChE inhibition is enough to begin supportive treatment. Usually, there is not enough time to wait for a ChE assay before administering atropine to an animal showing clinical signs of acute OP or carbamate toxicosis. Acute signs require emergency action. An atropine test dose (see later section on treatment of suggestive ChE inhibitor toxicosis) is an excellent field test.

The intermediate syndrome requires a thorough work-up of the patient because of its nondescript clinical signs. A full complete blood cell count, chemistry panel, and electrolyte values are advisable. A blood ChE assay may lead the clinician to a diagnosis and may also suggest a prognosis and treatment of choice. Pancreatitis has been reported in dogs exposed to some of the more lipophilic organophosphate insecticides.

Confirmatory Tests

In a live animal, OP or carbamate insecticide toxicosis can be diagnosed by ChE activity of heparinized whole blood. This activity is a combination of true AChE activity of RBCs and pChE activity of serum. The activity of blood ChE differs among species and is reported in different units based on the type of enzyme assay used. Because of the difference in species and enzyme assays, the diagnostic laboratory should provide a normal reference range. Many laboratories use an Ellman assay on heparinized blood; normal whole blood activities for most species using this assay are 1 µmol/mL/min or higher. Blood ChE activities that are less than 50% of normal are suspicious, and activities that are less than 25% of normal are fairly diagnostic. Blood ChE activities correlate fairly well with brain AChE activities, but the correlation is not always perfect. Blood should be kept refrigerated to prevent the loss of enzyme activity. AChE activity can also be depressed when anemia is present; it is recommended to assess a packed cell volume on blood samples for AChE testing. Diagnosis in a live animal is also sometimes based on the animal's response to treatment (see later section, Suggestive Cholinesterase Inhibitor Toxicosis). Stomach content, vomitus, hair, or suspected baits can also be submitted to the laboratory for an OP or carbamate residue screen.

In a dead animal, brain ChE can be used to gauge exposure to OP or carbamate insecticides. Usually the brain is cut in half in sagittal sections; one half is frozen for ChE analysis, and the other half is fixed in formalin. Normal brain ChE values again vary with species, but usually are 1 µmol/g/min or more. The same percentage depressions in ChE activity necessary for diagnosis of blood apply to the brain also. Because OP and carbamate insecticides are metabolized so rapidly in the body, neither body organs (e.g., liver and kidney) nor urine are routinely analyzed for insecticides, but such analysis can be done when stomach content is unavailable. Because chlorpyrifos is more persistent than most OPs, it is sometimes detected in body tissue, such as liver and fat.

Measurements of ChE activity in blood or brain from actual cases of carbamate toxicoses are sometimes within the normal range and are not depressed. Just as carbamates bind reversibly with AChE in the body, they may also dissociate from AChE or pChE in a blood tube or brain specimen during transit. Keeping blood refrigerated and brain frozen will help to minimize this dissociation, but ChE inhibition assay results may still be falsely negative with carbamate toxicoses. Some ChE assays also have a long incubation time before enzyme activity is measured, which can also cause false-negative results for carbamate toxicoses. Carbamate screens on stomach content are necessary to absolutely rule out carbamate toxicoses associated with oral ingestions. Some OPs and carbamates do not cross the blood-brain barrier as readily as others, thereby leading to a possible false-negative result on the brain ChE test.

Additional biochemical indices that may be altered include hyperamylasemia, hyperlipasemia, hyperglycemia, hypokalemia, acidosis, leukocytosis with or without a left shift, and increased creatine kinase and aspartate transaminase levels.[7]

Treatment

Known Organophosphate or Carbamate Toxicosis

Both OP and carbamate toxicoses that produce severe muscarinic signs should be treated with atropine sulfate. Atropine relieves muscarinic and some CNS-related signs but not nicotinic signs (i.e., muscle fasciculations, paralysis, and weakness). The initial dose of atropine for a known OP or carbamate toxicosis is 0.1 to 0.5 mg/kg, with one fourth of this dose given intravenously (IV) and the rest given intramuscularly (IM) or subcutaneously (SC) (some individuals administer the entire dose slowly IV). The dose is based on the severity of the muscarinic signs. Tachycardia is not a contraindication for initial use of atropine in acute OP or carbamate toxicoses. Repeat doses should be lower (0.1 mg/kg) and given as needed based on a combination of signs, including heart rate and wet lung sounds. Pupil size and degree of salivation are indicators of toxicosis but are not life threatening. Atropine acts as a noncompetitive antagonist to protect the ACh receptors from excessive bombardment by the accumulating ACh and is a specific physiologic antidote for both OP and carbamate toxicoses. The primary goal of atropine is to control bradycardia and bronchial secretions.

In animals poisoned by OP insecticides, AChE can be reactivated with oximes if aging has not occurred. The oxime in greatest use is 2-pyridine aldoxime methyl chloride (2-PAM; pralidoxime chloride [Protopam]). Oximes are generally not necessary in carbamate toxicoses because the inhibition of AChE is very reversible. The dose is 20 mg/kg (some recommend up to 50 mg/kg) given IM, SC, or very slowly IV according to the product label. The dose may be repeated once or twice at 12-hour intervals if the previous dose appeared to be beneficial (i.e., caused relief of some nicotinic signs or loss of anorexia). Do not give more than three doses if no improvement is noted. Reactivation of ChE may also be monitored by analysis of heparinized blood. The oxime settles into the unoccupied anionic site of AChE, and a bond is formed with the OP moiety in the esteratic site. The combination leaves the reactivated enzyme and is excreted in the urine. Muscarinic, nicotinic, and CNS signs may all be somewhat ameliorated by 2-PAM.[6]

Other treatments are mostly symptomatic and should be given after the patient has been stabilized. An emetic (e.g., 3% hydrogen peroxide or apomorphine in dogs) can be administered to animals with recent oral ingestions if this is not contraindicated (i.e., by the presence of mental depression, convulsions, or loss of gag reflex) and if the animal has not vomited on its own. Activated charcoal mixed with sorbitol is useful for decontamination, depending on the amount and toxicity of the compound ingested. Emesis should not be induced if highly toxic compounds, like methomyl, were ingested more than ½ hour earlier because of the risk of acute onset of seizures. Enterogastric lavage or just gastric lavage may be appropriate in some cases if a large amount of poison has been ingested and emesis has not occurred or induction of emesis is contraindicated. Anesthesia is induced with a short-acting barbiturate, and an endotracheal tube is placed before gastric lavage is attempted. When the stomach has been lavaged several times with water, activated charcoal and a saline cathartic are left in the stomach. If more than 2 to 3 hours have passed since ingestion, the risks of emesis or anesthesia may outweigh the questionable benefit of minimal recovery of poison from the stomach.[17] Activated charcoal with a saline cathartic or sorbitol should be administered without emesis or lavage in these cases of delayed presentation. Animals with dermal exposures are washed with a mild dishwashing detergent (e.g., Dawn) and water. The individuals bathing the animals should wear protective gloves and aprons. The detergent should be rinsed off immediately after lathering the animal to prevent further absorption of the insecticide. The necessity for fluid therapy to correct possible dehydration, electrolyte imbalances, and acidosis should be evaluated. Convulsions are treated with diazepam or a short-acting barbiturate. Artificial respiration may be necessary in cases of respiratory paralysis. Seizures and severe hypoxia have priority in the treatment protocol.

The use of antihistamines in cases of ChE inhibition is controversial. Although antihistamines, such as diphenhydramine, have some effect against muscarinic signs,[18] antihistamines are not as specific a physiologic antidote as atropine, a muscarinic antagonist. Diphenhydramine purportedly relieves nicotinic signs in some cases of ChE inhibition.[19] This alleged antinicotinic action is not commonly recognized in pharmacology texts[18] and, in addition, antihistamines are listed as contraindicated for the treatment of ChE inhibition.[8,20] Because of the potential adverse CNS effects of antihistamines, diphenhydramine should probably not be administered when ChE inhibition is present.[21]

Other drugs that are contraindicated include phenothiazine tranquilizers, opiates, local anesthetics, aminoglycoside antibiotics, clindamycin, lincomycin, theophylline, and neuromuscular blockers.[7]

Unknown Cholinesterase Inhibitor Toxicosis

Animals frequently are admitted with *classic* signs of acute ChE inhibition, but the type of insecticide exposure (OP versus carbamate) is unknown. These animals should be treated with atropine as described previously for known OP or carbamate toxicoses. The decision then becomes whether or not to give 2-PAM. The use of 2-PAM has been beneficial in some carbamate toxicoses, but is definitely contraindicated in carbaryl toxicosis.[22,23] Because carbaryl is fairly safe (the rat oral LD_{50} is approximately 0.5 g/kg), the chance that an unknown ChE inhibitor toxicosis is associated with carbaryl is remote. Therefore, in addition to known OP toxicoses, 2-PAM is recommended for (1) these unknown ChE inhibitor toxicoses, (2) ChE inhibitor toxicoses associated with dual exposure to both OP and carbamates, and (3) severe carbamate toxicoses that do not respond favorably to atropine alone.[8]

Suggestive Cholinesterase Inhibitor Toxicosis

In animals with suggestive but not classic clinical signs of acute ChE inhibition and no history of insecticide exposure, a test dose of atropine can be given IV. The test dose should be low, corresponding to a preanesthetic dose of 0.02 mg/kg. If eyes dilate maximally, heart rate increases dramatically, or salivation stops within 10 to 15 minutes, the original problem was not an OP or carbamate toxicosis. If none of the suggestive clinical signs improves significantly, the disease is very likely an OP or carbamate toxicosis. A dose of 0.1 to 0.2 mg/kg of atropine can then be administered as described previously. Administration of 20 mg/kg of 2-PAM given IM, SC, or very slowly IV is also advisable. If the high dose of atropine (0.1 to 0.5 mg/kg) was administered first and the problem was not an insecticide toxicosis, the animal would very likely experience an atropine toxicosis. Excessive atropine use causes hyperthermia, redness of the skin, decreased salivation, belligerency, intestinal stasis, and possible convulsions (i.e., "hot as a pistol, red as a beet, dry as a bone, and mad as a hatter"). Atropine toxicosis is treated symptomatically with cool water baths, fluids, diazepam, and possibly physostigmine hydrochloride (which should be reserved for heroic circumstances only).

Intermediate Syndrome

Because the intermediate syndrome lacks the typical muscarinic signs of the acute syndrome, atropine is not indicated. Anorexia and neuromuscular weakness are the most dramatic problems seen in these animals. Supportive care measures depend on the severity and duration of the anorexia. Parenteral nutrition or pharyngostomy tubes may be necessary. Electrolyte imbalances (e.g., hypokalemia) and dehydration if present must be addressed. The animal should be bathed with a mild detergent and water if the exposure was dermal. A ventilator may be required for hypoxemia.[13] Typically, AChE values in these animals are severely depressed. Contrary to the insert information provided with 2-PAM, many of these animals respond to 2-PAM many days after the initial OP exposure. Unlike atropine, 2-PAM is capable of working at nicotinic skeletal muscle sites (e.g., diaphragm and cervical muscles) that are primarily affected by the intermediate syndrome. Although 2-PAM has been a miracle worker in some of these animals, anecdotal reports of death in some cats following 2-PAM administration have also surfaced. Administration of 20 mg/kg of 2-PAM IM or SC is indicated in animals that need heroic intervention. The same dose of 2-PAM should be repeated once 12 hours later. These animals probably have blood AChE values of less than 10% of normal. Animals with blood AChE values of more than 25% of normal that are eating reasonably well on their own will probably survive with supportive care only, and their AChE values will regenerate during a few weeks of convalescence. Administration of 2-PAM in some of these less affected animals could speed recovery and cut owner expenses, but again it carries a risk of an adverse reaction.

Prognosis

Prognosis depends very much on the dose and time of exposure to the insecticide. Because atropine is a specific physiologic antidote, it can bring about dramatic and rapid changes in an animal that seems close to death. On the other hand, many of the acute toxicoses progress so rapidly that the animal is dead before it arrives at the clinic. Anecdotal reports of malicious cases of carbamate toxicosis document death within a few minutes of ingestion of a bait. Animals with the intermediate syndrome often respond slowly to supportive care. Owners may not have the financial resources or the patience to go through days or weeks of supportive care. In the absence of aspiration pneumonia or other rare occurrences of brain anoxia, animals that come through the acute syndrome should experience no chronic problems.

Gross and Histologic Lesions

Animals should be examined closely for any signs of excessive parasympathomimetic stimulation, such as excessive salivation on the muzzle or in the trachea and diarrhea in the perineal area. Hair and stomach contents should be examined for unusual odors that smell like petroleum products, sulfur, or garlic.[6] Internally, often there are no visible gross lesions. Potential gross lesions include foreign substances in the stomach, diarrhea, an empty bladder, or pulmonary edema. Nonspecific petechial hemorrhages associated with an agonal death may be found on the endocardial and epicardial surfaces. Petechial hemorrhages are also sometimes seen on the subserosal surface of the gastrointestinal tract. Histologically, only pulmonary edema is likely to be seen. However, even pulmonary edema is not a consistent finding. Pancreatitis is also a rare but potential histologic finding in dogs but not in cats; it is associated with pChE inhibition of the pancreas.[24]

Differential Diagnoses

Tremorgenic Mycotoxicoses

Roquefortine and penitrem A are tremorgenic mycotoxins associated with decaying organic matter, moldy walnut hulls, and spoiled dairy products. These toxicoses are associated with muscle tremors, salivation, vomiting, and clonic-tonic convulsions. Differential features are the lack of miosis and the general absence of respiratory signs.

Amitraz Toxicosis

The client should be questioned about the pet's access to a flea collar and whether the collar was also formulated for ticks. Typically, dogs with amitraz toxicosis have muscle weakness, muscle tremors, vomiting, and possible CNS signs. The best differential feature is mydriasis versus the more typical miosis present with OP and carbamate toxicoses.

Pyrethrin and Pyrethroid Toxicosis

Pyrethrin and pyrethroid toxicoses often are marked by some salivation, muscle tremors, muscle weakness, depression, and possibly seizures. Usually, pyrethroid toxicoses are associated with known dermal application of a product. Asking the client to bring the preparation to the clinic so that the label can be read will help with the differential diagnosis.

Cationic Surfactant Toxicosis

Cationic surfactants are components found in some disinfectants, potpourri oils, and dermal pet sprays. Generic names include *benzalkonium chloride, benzethonium chloride,* and *cetylpyridinium.* These compounds can cause neuromuscular and ganglionic blockade. Typical clinical signs include vomiting, salivation, muscle tremors, depression, and clonic-tonic convulsions. Cationic surfactants are more likely to cause oral and gastric irritation and ulcers than are OP and carbamate insecticides.

Pancreatitis

Pancreatitis lacks the life-threatening respiratory signs characteristic of an acute OP or carbamate toxicosis. Amylase and lipase may be elevated in OP or carbamate toxicoses, but usually not to the same extent as in acute pancreatitis.

Garbage (Endotoxin) Intoxication

Endotoxins may affect multiple systems in the body and mimic many diseases. Typically, endotoxins would not cause the severe miosis, salivation, or muscle tremors associated with ChE inhibitions. Endotoxins may cause some CNS depression, but would not cause seizures.

Blue-Green Algae

Anatoxin-a(s) is produced by some strains of *Anabaena* spp., a blue-green algae species. Anatoxin-a(s) is the only known naturally occurring organophosphorus ChE inhibitor. It appears to primarily inhibit peripheral cholinsterases and is not likely to cross the blood-brain barrier.

Muscarinic Mushrooms

Primarily *Inocybe* spp. and *Clitocybe* spp. contain muscarine. Muscarine does not cross the blood-brain barrier. Muscarine binds to muscarinic (ACh) receptors in the parasympathetic nervous system. These mushrooms do not inhibit AChE. Clinical signs are SLUD. Atropine dislodges muscarine from receptor sites.

References

1. Smith RA, Tramontin RR, Poonacha KB, et al: Carbofuran (Furadan) poisoning in animals, *Canine Pract* 20(2):8, 1995.
2. Fikes JD: Feline chlorpyrifos toxicosis. In Kirk RW, Bonagura JD, editors: *Current veterinary therapy XI: small animal practice*, Philadelphia, 1992, WB Saunders.
3. Sultatos LG: Mammalian toxicology of organophosphorus pesticides, *J Toxicol Environ Health* 43:271, 1994.
4. Fukuto TR: Mechanism of action of organophosphorus and carbamate insecticides, *Environ Health Perspect* 87:245, 1990.
5. Dorough HW: Metabolism of insecticidal methylcarbamates in animals, *J Agric Food Chem* 18(6):1015, 1970.
6. Aaron CK, Howland MA: Insecticides: organophosphates and carbamates. In Goldfrank LR, Flomenbaum NE, Lewin NA, editors: *Goldfrank's toxicologic emergencies*, ed 5, Norwalk, Conn., 1994, Appleton & Lange.
7. Fikes JD: Organophosphate and carbamate insecticides, *Clin North Am Small Anim Pract* 20(2):353, 1990.
8. Ellenhorn MJ, Schonwald S, Ordog G, et al, editors: *Ellenhorn's medical toxicology: diagnosis and treatment of human poisoning*, ed 2, Baltimore, 1997, Williams & Wilkins.
9. Schwab BW, Costa LG, Murphy SD: Muscarinic receptor alterations as a mechanism of anticholinesterase tolerance, *Toxic Appl Pharmacol* 71:14, 1983.
10. Costa LG, Schwab BW, Murphy SD: Differential alterations of cholinergic muscarinic receptors during chronic and acute tolerance to organophosphorus insecticides, *Biochem Pharmacol* 31(21):3407, 1982.
11. Costa LG, Schwab BW, Murphy SD: Tolerance to anticholinesterase compounds in mammals, *Toxicology* 25:79, 1982.
12. Levy JK: Chronic chlorpyrifos toxicosis in a cat, *J Am Vet Med Assoc* 203(12):1682, 1993.

13. Hopper K, Aldrich J, Haskins SC: The recognition and treatment of the intermediate syndrome of organophosphate poisoning in a dog, *J Vet Emerg Crit Care* 12(2):99, 2002.
14. De Bleecker J, Lison D, Van Den Abeele K, et al: Acute and subacute organophosphate poisoning in the rat, *Neurotoxicology* 15(2):341, 1994.
15. Guadarrama-Naveda M, Calderon de Cabrera L: Intermediate syndrome secondary to ingestion of chlorpiriphos, *Vet Human Toxicol* 43(1):34, 2001.
16. Smalley HE, O'Hara PJ, Bridges CH, et al: The effects of chronic carbaryl administration on the neuromuscular system of swine, *Toxic Appl Pharmacol* 14:409, 1969.
17. Hansen SR: Management of organophosphate and carbamate toxicoses. In Bonagura JD, Kirk RW, editors: *Current veterinary therapy XII: small animal practice*, Philadelphia, 1995, WB Saunders.
18. Babe KS, Serafin WE, et al: Histamine, bradykinin, and their antagonists. In Hardman JG, Limbird LE, Molinoff PB, editors: *Goodman and Gilman's the pharmacological basis of therapeutics*, ed 9, New York, 1996, McGraw-Hill.
19. Clemmons RM, Meyer DJ, Sundlof SF, et al: Correction of organophosphate-induced neuromuscular blockade by diphenhydramine, *Am J Vet Res* 45(10):2167, 1984.
20. Fernandez G, Gomez MID, Castro JA: Cholinesterase inhibition by phenothiazine and nonphenothiazine antihistaminics: analysis of its postulated role in synergizing organophosphate toxicity, *Toxic Appl Pharmacol* 31:179, 1975.
21. Blodgett D, Neer TM, Coates JR: How do I treat? Organophosphate toxicity, *Prog Vet Neurol* 7(2):56, 1996.
22. Natoff IL, Reiff B: Effect of oximes on the acute toxicity of anticholinesterase carbamates, *Toxic Appl Pharmacol* 25:569, 1973.
23. Lieske CN, Clark JH, Maxwell DM, et al: Studies of the amplification of carbaryl toxicity by various oximes, *Toxicol Lett* 62:127, 1992.
24. Frick TW, Dalo S, O'Leary JF, et al: Effects of the insecticide, diazinon, on pancreas of dog, cat and guinea pig, *J Environ Pathol Toxicol Oncol* 7(4):1, 1987.

Oxalate-Containing Plants

68

Sharon M. Gwaltney-Brant, DVM, PhD, DABVT, DABT

- There are two types of oxalate-containing plants: those that contain insoluble oxalates (i.e., calcium oxalate) and those that contain soluble oxalates (i.e., sodium and potassium oxalate).
- Insoluble calcium oxalates are found in many common household plants.
- Ingestion of these plants typically causes oral, pharyngeal, and upper gastrointestinal irritation and discomfort. Fatalities are rare and are the result of airway obstruction.
- Soluble oxalate–containing household plants are much less common; toxicoses in pets are rare.
- Large oral exposures can lead to vomiting and, if excessive, could potentially lead to renal impairment.

Introduction

Calcium oxalate crystals are present in a large number of plants, including some used as food (e.g., spinach contains both soluble and insoluble calcium oxalate [IO] crystals).[1] Several calcium oxalate–containing plants are toxic, but the degree of toxicity varies depending on the type and amount of oxalate crystals present. Plants containing large amounts of soluble oxalates have the potential to cause systemic illness, whereas IO-containing plants are of concern primarily for their local effects on the alimentary tract.[2] As with other toxins found in plant material, the amount of oxalate in plants can vary with individual plants, growing season, and plant portion.[3]

Whenever presented with an animal that has been exposed to a plant, it is important to attempt to positively identify the plant so that appropriate risk assessments may be made. Because common names may be shared by several unrelated plants, genus and species names should be obtained whenever possible to avoid confusion.

Insoluble Oxalates

Sources

A wide variety of common house and landscape plants contain IOs in sufficient quantity to cause clinical signs if chewed on or ingested (Table 68-1). Many of the IO-containing plants most commonly associated with ingestion by small animals tend to have broad, often shiny leaves and do not produce flowers.[4] The family *Araceae* contains a large number of plants that are popular as ornamentals and that contain IOs. Introduction of these plants to a pet's environment may result in the pet "exploring" the plant with its mouth, often with painful consequences.

Table 68-1	Common Plants Containing Insoluble Calcium Oxalate Crystals[2,4]
Scientific Name	**Common Names**
Aglaonema modestum	Chinese evergreen
Alocasia macrorrhiza	Alocacia, giant elephant ear, giant taro
Anthurium spp.	Flamingo plant
Arisaema triphyllum	Jack-in-the-pulpit
Arum italicum	Arum
Arum maculatum	Cuckoo pint
Caladium bicolor	Caladium, elephant ear
Calla palustris	Wild calla, wild arum
Colocasia esculenta	Taro, dasheen, cocoyam
Dieffenbachia spp.	Dumb cane, American arum (see Color Plate 27-7)
Epipremnum (Scindapsus) spp.	Devil's ivy, pothos, marble queen, variegated philodendron, taro vine
Lysichiton americanum	Yellow skunk cabbage
Philodendron spp.	Philodendrons
Pistia stratiotes	Water lettuce, shellflower
Spathiphyllum spp.	Peace lily, white sails
Symplocarpus foetidus	Skunk cabbage
Syngonium podophyllum	Nephthytis
Xanthosoma spp.	Blue tannia, blue taro, caladium, elephant ears, malanga, tannia, yautia
Zantedeschia aethiopica	Calla lily, arum lily

Toxicity

Despite the fact that even a single bite of IO plants has the potential to cause immediate and intense clinical signs, many exposures result in no apparent clinical effects in dogs and cats.[5] The severity of signs depends on the concentration and type of oxalate crystals in the plant and the extent of exposure. Fortunately, immediate pain often results in cessation of chewing, limiting exposure. In humans, ingestion of *Dieffenbachia* leaves has occasionally been associated with pharyngeal obstruction resulting in potentially fatal respiratory compromise.[6] Airway obstruction in dogs caused by chewing on oxalate-containing plants has been reported, and a single case report exists of a dog fatality caused by airway obstruction following ingestion of *Dieffenbachia picta* (dumb cane) (see Color Plate 27-7).[7,8] However, because the relatively large pharyngeal area in species such as dogs and cats makes complete obstruction from tissue swelling uncommon, most cases of ingestion of IO plants by these pets are rarely serious or life threatening. One case report associated the development of gastric ulcers in a cat with ingestion of *Dieffenbachia*.[9] A few early anecdotal reports on *Philodendron* spp. suggested that nephrotoxicity or neurotoxicity was possible, especially in cats, but attempts to reproduce these clinical effects in experimental felines have not been successful.[2] In canaries, orally administered suspensions of *Dieffenbachia* leaves resulted in acute death, but no adverse effects were reported when budgerigars were similarly dosed.[10]

Mechanism of Toxicity

IO crystals (raphides) resembling dual-pointed needles are arranged and packed in bundles and located within specialized cells (idioblasts) found throughout the plant.[4] Damage to the tip of the idioblast, such as during chewing, allows water to enter the cell, causing swelling of a gelatinous material surrounding the raphides. This stimulates the forceful propulsion of the raphides from the cell and into the surrounding environment (Figure 68-1). This "darting" of alimentary soft tissue by the needlelike crystals is responsible for much of the discomfort associated with chewing on IO plants. The idioblasts may continue to expel

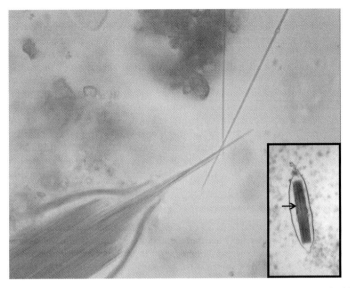

Figure 68-1 Raphides being ejected from tip of idioblast, 450×. Inset: Intact idioblast with a sheaf of raphides (*arrow*) 100×.

raphides for some time after the plant material has been swallowed, extending the irritation to the throat, esophagus, and stomach. Barbs found on raphides of some species of IO plants are responsible for prolongation of the irritation from the crystals, and some *Aracaea* plants have raphides with grooves that deposit proteolytic enzymes, which activate kinins and histamines, further potentiating the irritant effect through stimulation of an intense inflammatory reaction.[2,4]

Clinical Signs

The onset of clinical signs from ingestion of IO plants is generally immediate but may be delayed up to 2 hours following exposure.[4] Immediate pain on chewing may present as head shaking, pawing at the mouth, intense drooling, vocalization, depression, and anorexia. Dysphonia may result if pharyngeal tissues are affected. Erythema, swelling, and edema of the oral mucosa may occur. In very rare instances, dyspnea may result from severe swelling of the oropharyngeal tissues. If plant material has been swallowed, or if pain is intense, vomiting or hematemesis may occur. Diarrhea is also possible, depending on the degree of exposure. Severe vomiting and diarrhea may result in fluid and electrolyte imbalances. Although reports exist of cardiac arrhythmia, coma, and death in humans, these are rare occurrences. In most cases signs are expected to be relatively mild and self-limiting, and veterinary intervention is rarely indicated.

Ocular exposures to IO plants have been reported in humans.[11] In these cases, epiphora, blepharospasm, conjunctivitis, severe pain, and nodularity of the corneal surface (interpreted as "very fine needles" embedded in the cornea) have been reported. Permanent ocular injury has not been reported.

Diagnosis

Diagnosis is based on evidence of exposure and appropriate clinical signs.

Treatment

If massive amounts of plant material have been ingested and the animal is asymptomatic, induction of emesis may be considered. The primary goals of treatment of symptomatic

IO plant exposure are to prevent further exposure, relieve pain and swelling, and provide symptomatic and supportive care. The oral cavity should be rinsed with water or milk; calcium-containing foods, such as yogurt and cottage cheese, are said to aid in relief of the discomfort from the IO crystals.[4] Eugenol (4-alil-2-metoxiphenol) has been shown to reduce tongue edema caused by *Dieffenbachia* exposure in mice; its topical use might be considered if severe oral tissue swelling is present following exposure to IO-containing plants.[13] Antihistamines, analgesics, antispasmodics, or gastrointestinal protectants such as sucralfate and gastric acid reducers may also be of benefit in cases in which severe oral or gastric irritation are present. Animals should be monitored at home for several hours for respiratory compromise, and veterinary care should be sought if dyspnea develops. Supportive treatment includes management of fluid and electrolyte abnormalities that may develop subsequent to protracted vomiting. For ocular exposures, irrigation is recommended with sterile saline followed by topical application of an antibiotic.[2]

Prognosis

In most cases involving exposure to IO crystals, the prognosis is good and full recovery is expected with minimal veterinary intervention required. Ocular injuries may take several weeks to resolve.[11]

Gross and Histologic Lesions

In severe cases there may be erythema and edema of the oral cavity, pharynx, esophagus, and possibly stomach.[2] Ocular exposure may result in erythema and edema of the conjunctiva, scleral injection, and a nodular appearance to the surface of the cornea.[11]

Differential Diagnoses

Differential diagnoses for the clinical effects produced by IOs include corrosive injury (e.g., alkalis or acids), thermal burns, uremic stomatitis, trauma, and severe periodontal disease. The transient nature of the signs from IO exposure should aid in differentiating this type of exposure from more serious conditions.

Soluble Oxalates

Sources

Intoxication by soluble oxalate–containing plants is most commonly associated with livestock, but companion animals may potentially be affected by ingestion of household or garden plants containing high levels of soluble oxalates. Rhubarb (*Rheum rhabarbarum*) is a popular garden plant with petioles (stems) used in cooking. Shamrock (*Oxalis* spp.) is a houseplant that is especially popular during the March holiday of Saint Patrick's Day in the United States (Color Plate 68-1).[13] [Note: Some species of white clover (*Trifolium repens*) are also marketed as "shamrocks"; these plants have little appreciable oxalate content (Color Plate 68-2).]

Toxicity

Rhubarb stems are edible, but the leaf blades contain approximately 0.28% soluble sodium and potassium oxalates. No reports of toxicosis from rhubarb in dogs or cats were found in the literature, but there have been occasional reports of human illness and death following ingestion of rhubarb leaves.[12] Ingestion of 10 to 20 g of fresh leaves has been reported to cause immediate vomiting, and renal insufficiency has been associated with ingestion of 20 to 100 g of fresh leaves. *Oxalis* species, such as sorrels and dock, have been reported to contain 7% to 10% soluble oxalates, but the amount of oxalates in shamrocks used as houseplants has not been established.[2] Sheep have developed hypocalcemia following acute ingestion of 600 g of *Oxalis* species, and chronic ingestion of smaller amounts has resulted in renal calcium oxalate deposition.[14]

Toxicokinetics

Soluble oxalates are generally well absorbed orally, although co-ingestion of high calcium foods, such as dairy products, can significantly reduce absorption.[1]

Mechanism of Toxicity

Soluble oxalates bind serum calcium to form calcium oxalate.[14] Hypocalcemia may result if large amounts of soluble oxalates are rapidly absorbed, although hypocalcemia from soluble oxalate ingestion has only been reported in livestock. In the kidney, calcium oxalate may precipitate to form large crystals, resulting in renal tubular damage and renal insufficiency. Oxidative injury caused by generation of free radicals may exacerbate the renal tubular injury.[14]

Clinical Signs

Acute ingestion of large amounts of soluble oxalate–containing plant material by dogs or cats may result in rapid onset of vomiting. This is especially true for rhubarb because of the cathartic effect of anthroquinones within the leaves. Hypocalcemia, if it occurs, is expected within a few hours of ingestion and presents as weakness, tetany, and seizures. The development of acute renal failure may be associated with vomiting, anorexia, lethargy, polydipsia, and polyuria. Oliguria or anuria may develop. Chronic renal failure caused by chronic low-level exposure to soluble oxalate plants generally displays a more insidious onset of polyuria, polydipsia, weight loss, anorexia, and vomiting.[2]

Minimum Database

In symptomatic animals, evaluation of serum biochemistry, electrolytes, and urinalysis are recommended. Evidence of hypocalcemia should be present within 6 hours after ingestion of soluble oxalate plants.[2] Elevations in blood urea nitrogen and creatinine can occur within 4 to 24 hours following ingestion. Urinalysis may reveal the presence of calcium oxalate crystals in the urine; absence of crystals does not exclude the possibility of an oxalate nephrosis.

Diagnosis

Diagnosis of soluble oxalate toxicosis is based on history, appropriate clinical signs, and laboratory confirmation of hypocalcemia or renal insufficiency.

Treatment

Recent exposure to soluble oxalate–containing plants may be managed by induction of emesis. The efficacy of activated charcoal in adsorbing oxalates is not known. However, oral administration of dairy products (e.g., milk, yogurt) may reduce the bioavailability of the oxalates. Profoundly hypocalcemic animals should be treated with intravenous calcium gluconate as necessary. Animals displaying evidence of renal insufficiency should be treated with intravenous fluid therapy and general supportive care (e.g., antiemetics, gastrointestinal protectants, H_2-antagonists).

Prognosis

Most exposures of pets to soluble oxalate–containing plants result in little more than mild gastrointestinal upset. Animals that ingest large quantities of these plants are at risk of developing severe hypocalcemia and renal failure and have a more guarded prognosis because response to treatment may be poor.[2]

Gross and Histologic Lesions

The kidneys from animals acutely affected by soluble oxalates may be enlarged, pale, and swollen on gross examination.[2] Histologically, the presence of large numbers of intratubular calcium oxalate crystals and associated tubular degeneration and necrosis would aid in confirming the diagnosis. In chronic cases, the kidneys may be small, firm, and fibrotic, and histopathological changes could include interstitial fibrosis, loss of nephrons, and scattered calcium oxalate crystals within the tubules.

Differential Diagnoses

Differential diagnoses for acute hypocalcemia include eclampsia, ethylene glycol toxicosis, and hypoparathyroidism. Differential diagnoses for oxaluria and oxalate nephrosis include toxicosis caused by ethylene glycol or other sources of oxalate (e.g., oxalic acid).

References

1. Brogren M, Savage GP: Bioavailability of soluble oxalate from spinach eaten with and without milk products, *Asia Pac J Clin Nutr* 12:219–224, 2003.
2. Burrows GE, Tyrl RJ: *Toxic plants of North America*, Ames, 2001, Iowa State University Press.
3. Knight MW, Dorman DC: Selected poisonous plant concerns in small animals, *Vet Med* 92:260–272, 1997.
4. Means C: Insoluble calcium oxalates. In Plumlee KH, editor: *Clinical veterinary toxicology*, St Louis, 2004, Mosby.
5. Beasley VR, Trammel HL: Incidence of poisonings in small animals. In Kirk RW, editor: *Current veterinary therapy X*, Philadelphia, 1989, Saunders.
6. Cumpston KL, Vogel SN, Leikin JB, et al: Acute airway compromise after brief exposure to a Dieffenbachia plant, *J Emerg Med* 25:391–397, 2003.
7. Loretti AP, da Silva Ilha MR, Riberio RE: Accidental fatal poisoning of a dog by *Dieffenbachia picta* (dumb cane), *Vet Hum Toxicol* 45:233–239, 2003.
8. Peterson K, Beymer J, Rudoff E, O'Brien M: Airway obstruction in a dog after *Dieffenbachia* ingestion, *J Vet Emerg Crit Care* 19:635–639, 2009.
9. Arai M, Stauber E, Shropshire CM: Evaluation of selected plants for their toxic effects in canaries, *J Am Vet Med Assoc* 200:1329–1331, 1992.
10. Muller N, Glaus T, Gardelle O: Extensive stomach ulcers due to *Dieffenbachia* intoxication in a cat, *Tierarztl Prax Ausq K Kleintiere Heintiere* 26:404–407, 1998.
11. Frohne D, Pfander HJ: *A colour atlas of poisonous plants*, London, 1983, Wolfe Publishing Ltd.
12. Dip EC, Pereira NA, Fernandes PD: Ability of eugenol to reduce tongue edema induced by *Dieffenbachia picta* Schott in mice, *Toxicol* 43:729–735, 2004.
13. Spoerke DG, Smolinske SC: *Toxicity of houseplants*, Boca Raton, FL, 1990, CRC Press.
14. Pickerell JA, Oehme F: Soluble oxalates. In Plumlee KH, editor: *Clinical veterinary toxicology*, St Louis, 2004, Mosby.

Paraquat

Caroline Donaldson, DVM, DABT

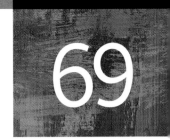

- Paraquat is a contact herbicide widely used as an agricultural chemical.
- When used according to the manufacturer's application instructions, paraquat is a safe compound; however, it is extremely toxic to companion animals and all mammals when ingested or excessively applied topically.
- Initial signs following oral exposures include severe gastrointestinal distress: abdominal pain, vomiting, and diarrhea (oral-esophageal-gastrointestinal ulceration may be present).
- Once in the systemic circulation, paraquat is selectively taken up by alveolar epithelial cells through an energy-dependent carrier mechanism and results in severe and progressive pulmonary toxicity.
- There are no antidotes currently available to effectively treat paraquat poisoning, and most often ingestions or other absorption of toxic doses leads to death.
- Various treatment modalities have been and continue to be tried for paraquat toxicity with little or only moderate success.

Sources

Paraquat (1,1'-dimethyl-4,4'-bipyridyl) was first synthesized in 1882, but its herbicidal action was not discovered until 1959.[1] Paraquat dichloride has been marketed commercially since 1965 and is formulated in many countries. It is a nonselective herbicide and has rapid contact action when applied as a postemergent herbicide. Paraquat is used as an herbicide, defoliant, desiccant, and plant growth regulator. It is sold worldwide under the trade names *Cekupat, Dextron X, Dextrone, Gramoxone, Herbaxon, Herboxone, Pillarxone, Pillarquat, Total,* and *Toxer* and was previously sold under the trade names *Esgram, Goldquat, Dexuron, Sweep,* and *Weedol.* It is also known by the code names *PP-148* and *PP-910.*

The usual paraquat formulation available is as the dichloride salt form. Other forms of the compound are the cationic form (bipyridylium ion) and the dimethyl sulfate form. To increase the herbicidal action, it is often formulated with surface-acting agents as an aqueous solution. Commercial products are available as granular, solid, and soluble concentrate preparations. In some commercial preparations paraquat is combined with diquat and sold under the trade names *Actor, Herbaxon, Pregalone, Priglone,* and *Weedol.* In these preparations paraquat is present as the dichloride or dimethyl sulfate salt and is very stable under alkaline conditions. It has no appreciable vapor pressure.

Paraquat is one of the most specific pulmonary toxicants known. It has been the subject of intensive international scrutiny because it has been responsible for severe and often fatal poisonings in humans. Many countries have effectively banned or severely restricted paraquat use because of the large number of reported accidental and suicidal fatalities. Diquat, the analogue of paraquat, is considerably less potent than paraquat as a pulmonary toxicant, but it may also cause severe acute and chronic poisoning.

If used according to the manufacturer's instructions on the label, paraquat is a safe agricultural chemical because with routine agricultural or commercial use little of the diluted material is absorbed across intact skin or becomes systemic by inhalation of the spray. The aerosol particles generated are too large to enter into the lower airways. The most common ailments resulting from inhalation of the aerosol are sore throat and nosebleeds, but systemic toxicity is rare. Injury can become severe if prolonged and excessive contact with the chemical occurs. Most occupational injuries reported are caused by irritation and corrosive effects to the mucous membranes, cornea, and skin.

Toxic Dose

In animals, paraquat shows a moderate degree of toxicity. The oral median lethal dose (LD_{50}) for various species ranges from 22 to 262 mg/kg. Specifically, the oral LD_{50} for dogs is 25 to 50 mg/kg, and for cats it is 40 to 50 mg/kg.[2] Most cases of poisoning in domestic animals are caused by ingestion of paraquat via access to spills or improperly stored or disposed of material, or as a result of malicious poisoning.[3] Ingestion of paraquat in toxic doses causes similar clinical signs and pathologic lesions in humans, monkeys, rats, dogs, and cats.[4] Most of the accidental or suicidal poisonings have been reported in humans, whereas most of the experimental data on paraquat toxicosis have come from animal studies.

Paraquat causes rapid leaf desiccation when applied to plants. Photochemical degradation occurs on plant surfaces rather than in plant metabolism. Methylamine hydrochloride and 4-carboxyl-1-(methyl) pyridinium chloride are identified products of paraquat photodegradation.[5] No cases of residual toxicity have been reported from ingestion of paraquat-treated plant products in either humans or animals. Once paraquat has reached the soil, absorption by soil components makes it biologically unavailable, and it is then considered of little toxic consequence to plants or animals.

Toxicokinetics

Oral Absorption

Various studies have shown that in dogs low oral doses of paraquat are rapidly but incompletely absorbed, the peak plasma concentration being attained 75 minutes after dosing.[6] Dose-dependent data from dogs and whole-body autoradiography suggest that absorption is facilitated in the small intestine. A liquid formulation enters the small intestine quite rapidly, particularly if the stomach is empty. Approximately 25% to 28% of the oral paraquat is absorbed with the remainder excreted unchanged in feces.[7]

Once absorbed, paraquat is distributed to most organs in the body; the highest concentrations are found initially in the kidney, the major organ of elimination, and the lungs. Paraquat does not bind to plasma proteins. Several organs, significantly the lungs, act as reservoirs for paraquat, slowly releasing the unchanged paraquat back into the bloodstream. This compartmentalization and subsequent sustained release by the various organs at least partly accounts for the continued renal excretion of the compound for many weeks after ingestion.

Pulmonary Absorption

Paraquat is selectively sequestered in the lung's type I and II alveolar cells and in Clara cells by an active energy-dependent process (Figure 69-1), resulting in the lungs having the highest paraquat retention; at 4 hours, the concentration is 10 times higher than in other selective sites, and by 4 to 10 days after exposure paraquat concentrations in the lungs are 30 to 80 times greater than in the plasma.[7] Experimental studies have shown a diphasic efflux of the paraquat in lungs with a rapid-phase half-life of 2.6 minutes and a slow-phase half-life of 356 minutes. The slow phase represents the storage pool of paraquat in the lungs and is probably responsible for its pulmonary toxicity.

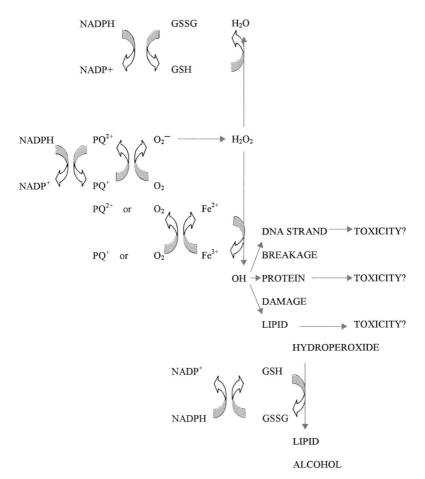

Figure 69-1 Proposed biochemical mechanism of paraquat toxicity. (Modified from Lewis CPL, Nemery B: Pathophysiology and biochemical mechanisms of the pulmonary toxicant of paraquat. In Bismuth C, Hall A, editors: *Paraquat poisoning,* New York, 1995, Marcel Dekker.)

Metabolic Transformation and Excretion

Paraquat undergoes cyclic reduction-oxidation reactions to a considerable extent. After undergoing a single electron reduction in tissues, the resultant free radical is readily oxidized by molecular oxygen to the parent compound. This leads to an overall excretion of essentially unchanged paraquat in urine after oral administration. Thus most absorbed paraquat is excreted unchanged in the urine within the first 24 hours, even in animals that develop renal failure.[1] Before the onset of acute renal failure, the clearance of paraquat is higher than that of creatinine because of net tubular secretion. As renal failure develops, the renal clearance of paraquat decreases and the plasma half-life increases from less than 12 hours to 120 hours or longer. This also contributes to the prolonged urinary excretion of paraquat.

Mechanism of Toxicity

The mechanisms of toxic action of paraquat have been extensively studied in animals. Paraquat participates in cyclic reduction-oxidation reactions in biologic systems. The compound readily undergoes a single-electron reduction in tissues (plant and animal), forming a free radical. In an aerobic environment the generated free radical is soon oxidized by molecular oxygen, generating the superoxide radical (O_2^-). The reoxidized paraquat again accepts another electron, and the reaction continues in a catalytic manner (see Figure 69-1).

Lung tissue acquires much higher concentrations of paraquat in all animal species studied, including humans. Biochemical studies have shown that paraquat is actively taken up by the alveolar cells through a diamine-polyamine transport system,[8] where it undergoes the one-electron reduction described previously. This reaction leads to two partially toxic consequences. The first is the generation of the superoxide radical, and the second is the oxidation of cellular nicotinamide adenine dinucleotide phosphate (NADPH), which is the major source of reducing equivalences for the intracellular reduction of paraquat.

Generation of the superoxide radical can lead to more toxic forms of reduced oxygen, hydrogen peroxide, and hydroxyl radicals. Hydroxyl radicals have been implicated in the initiation of the membrane damage by lipid peroxidation, depolymerization of hyaluronic acid, inactivation of proteins, and damage to deoxyribonucleic acid (see Figure 69-1). The resulting cellular membrane damage effectively reduces the functional integrity of the cell, affects efficient gas transport, and damages respiratory exchange, causing respiratory impairment. In the lung tissue, this toxic damage is further exacerbated by the availability of oxygen.

Clinical Signs

Paraquat is an irritant and a vesicant and thus can cause severe local toxicity by topical exposure; it causes erythema, blistering, irritation, and ulceration of the skin. Eczematous dermatitis has been reported in paraquat-exposed experimental animals. Direct contact with concentrated paraquat solutions produces localized discoloration or a transverse band of white discoloration affecting the nail plate. If paraquat is splashed in the eyes, severe corneal inflammation can occur and proceeds to corneal ulceration and secondary bacterial infection. In uncomplicated cases full recovery is possible.

Acute poisoning in animals is almost always the result of ingestion of the compound. The signs of toxicosis vary widely depending on the dose ingested. The course of the disease can be divided into three phases.

In the initial phase lesions from the caustic action of the herbicide are seen. These lesions lead to the development of pain associated with the gastrointestinal tract. Vomiting always occurs in dogs, even in the absence of the emetic additives often found in herbicide formulations. The corrosive action of the compound can lead to abdominal pain and diarrhea. Animals with lesions in the oral cavity and gastrointestinal tract are aphagic and may require parenteral nutrition. Experimental studies using fiber optic esophagogastroscopy have documented instances of gastric perforation and massive gastrointestinal hemorrhage following oral paraquat exposures.

The second phase typically starts the second to third day following ingestion and includes development of renal failure and hepatocellular necrosis. Renal insufficiency is caused partly by hypovolemic conditions resulting from fluid loss (diarrhea and vomiting), and also from direct renal injury from paraquat itself. The renal injury is generally a pure tubulopathy and can progress to full recovery without sequel. In some paraquat-poisoned animals, full return to normal renal function can occur by the time of death caused by other organ damage. The liver lesions seen in these animals are centrilobular hepatocellular necrosis.

Delayed development of pulmonary fibrosis is the characteristic and hallmark lesion of the third phase of paraquat poisoning; it is responsible for the poor prognosis in acute poisoning cases. Both clinically and radiographically, this effect appears several days after ingestion. In experimental animals, the weight of the lung is increased after a single paraquat exposure.

The acute pulmonary toxicity of paraquat seen in animals occurs in two stages. Initially, alveolar epithelial cells are severely damaged, and their disintegration results in a completely denuded alveolar basement membrane. Pulmonary edema sets in, leading to severe respiratory impairment that usually results in death. Animals that survive this initial destructive stage progress to a proliferative stage in which extensive fibrosis of the lung tissue occurs.[7]

In subacute or chronic paraquat poisoning, low doses can induce hyperplasia of the type II cells through which the lung attempts to repair the damaged epithelium. With ingestion of a single high dose of paraquat, the earlier structural changes occur in type I alveolar cells and are characterized by cellular and mitochondrial swelling, increased numbers of mitochondria, and the appearance of dark granules in the cytoplasm. In these animals interstitial lesions extend inexorably. The diagnosis of pulmonary fibrosis in humans can in fact be made by pulmonary function testing well before PO_2 decreases become evident.

Radiologic changes do not always parallel the severity of clinical effects.[7] Thus thoracic radiographs of poisoned animals may be normal, particularly in animals that die acutely from multiorgan failure following ingestion of paraquat. Development of pulmonary fibrosis leads to refractory hypoxemia, resulting in death over a period of a few days to several weeks. Various therapeutic modalities, including spontaneous and artificial ventilation, have little success in delaying the fatal outcome in animals.

In the final stages of fatal paraquat poisoning, when sepsis has not set in, decerebration occurs during mechanical ventilation, characterized by an inspired oxygen fraction (FiO_2) of 100% and an arterial oxygen tension (PaO_2) of less than 30 mm Hg.

In cases of massive ingestion of the compound (>55 mg/kg), animals survive less than 4 days and die of cardiogenic shock. Acidosis develops in such cases. Alveolitis is also observed, with clinical signs of acute noncardiogenic pulmonary edema. At necropsy, lesions are often seen in the gastrointestinal tract, adrenal glands, renal tubules, and hepatocytes.[7]

Minimum Database and Confirmatory Tests

Paraquat poisoning of companion animals can present as acute or chronic pulmonary disease. Because treatment is not effective in the chronic stages of the disease, successful management of paraquat toxicosis requires institution of treatment within hours of the exposure. Therefore rapid diagnosis is vital for the successful outcome of therapy.

Clinical signs of acute paraquat poisoning include diarrhea, vomiting, and ulceration of the oral and gastrointestinal tracts. In all cases of acute poisoning, acute respiratory distress develops because of pulmonary edema. Days to weeks after exposure, progressive respiratory insufficiency occurs because of severe pulmonary fibrosis. Radiographic changes are often minimal and frequently do not correlate with the severity of clinical signs.[7] One of the earliest changes reported in paraquat-poisoned dogs is pneumomediastinum. Dogs that enter the chronic stage of the disease do not respond to treatment and eventually die from respiratory failure. All these factors point to the importance of early diagnosis and treatment of paraquat poisoning.[9]

Measurement of plasma paraquat concentrations is the most reliable method of assessing the severity and predicting the outcome of paraquat poisoning. However, measurement of plasma paraquat is not available in most veterinary practices and is rarely performed even in teaching institutions. Therefore other reliable methods of detection of paraquat must be employed.[7]

The dithionate spot test may detect paraquat in tissue or bait samples. Methods for the quantification of paraquat have been developed using visible light spectrophotometry[5] and liquid chromatography-mass spectrometry. In acute poisoning cases, stomach contents, vomit, or suspected bait are the samples of choice, and lung and kidney tissue are the organs of choice for paraquat testing. Urine samples may contain paraquat up to 48 hours after ingestion. In chronic poisoning cases, the lung is the sample of choice, but the liver and kidney may also contain sufficient quantities of the compound for testing to be valuable. Within 30 hours of oral ingestion, lung tissue contains the highest concentration of the compound.[8]

The half-life of paraquat in lung tissue is approximately 30 hours.[10] In rats exposed to paraquat, the compound could be detected only in the lung tissue after 4 days.[11] Because of its rapid excretion and tissue storage, paraquat concentrations in body fluids and tissues may be below the limit of detection in animals that die from pulmonary fibrosis.

Treatment

Treatment of paraquat-poisoned patients must be instituted as early as possible because delaying treatment often results in fatal outcomes. Although various treatment approaches have been described by various authors, most of these were designed for human patients. The validity and relevance of these treatments in companion animals are not well established. One promising aspect of these treatments is that they all were developed by studying the effect in experimental animals.

There is no specific and effective antidote for paraquat poisoning, and measures designed to enhance the elimination of paraquat from the body have not altered mortality significantly in human patients. The prognosis is extremely guarded, especially in companion animal practice, where treatment is frequently delayed.[7]

Attention has been given to gastrointestinal decontamination in an attempt to reduce the absorption of ingested paraquat. Gastric emesis followed by gastric lavage and activated charcoal administration is mandatory in all cases of acute paraquat exposure. Paraquat absorption from the gut is often incomplete, but is rapid, as evidenced by the early development of peak plasma concentrations. Energy-dependent accumulation of paraquat in lung tissue and subsequent development of toxicity occur once a crucial plasma concentration has been reached. This accumulation is time dependent. Therefore every early intervention procedure available that will reduce adsorption must be employed to prevent the rapid rise in plasma concentration to the critical level. In 1977 the manufacturer of paraquat (Imperial Chemical Industries, Fernhurst, Haslemere, Surrey, England) added a potent emetic to its liquid and solid preparations because experiments conducted in primates demonstrated a fivefold decrease in toxicity following emesis. A significant reduction in mortality from paraquat poisoning after the introduction of this emetic-containing formulation has not yet been reported for human paraquat exposure cases.

There is little experimental information about the use of gastric lavage alone for the treatment of paraquat poisoning. However, studies have demonstrated that reduced blood levels of paraquat occur in the cat following gastric lavage.[12] Whether these low plasma paraquat levels have any beneficial influence on the outcome of toxicosis is still questionable.

There are obvious drawbacks to the use of these procedures. Ulceration of oropharyngeal and esophagogastric mucosal surfaces because of contact with the concentrated paraquat is likely to make these procedures hazardous. In addition, unnecessary waste of valuable time may go into the efforts, delaying deployment of alternative forms of treatment that may have greater value. There is no definite evidence that gastric lavage has any value in paraquat poisoning in humans.[12] It may also be of limited value in companion animal practice unless initiated in the first few hours following exposure. Whole-bowel lavage can also be used soon following ingestion to reduce the amount of paraquat absorbed from the gut.

Administration of oral adsorbents followed by cathartics may reduce the severity of the disease. The common oral adsorbents used are bentonite, fuller's earth, and activated charcoal. Of these, activated charcoal is preferred because it is more effective in reducing mortality than is either fuller's earth or bentonite. In vitro adsorption of paraquat to the different activated charcoals occurs to a greater degree in the presence of sodium chloride, suggesting that saline should be used as the carrier vehicle for the activated charcoal.[13]

In general, published reports in human cases of paraquat ingestion do not support the efficacy of gastrointestinal decontamination. The relevance of this observation to companion animal practices is difficult to confirm.

Once gastrointestinal decontamination has been performed, two other possible treatment modalities are still available. The first is to alter the distribution of paraquat in the body, and the second is to modify the herbicide's effect on various biologic target organs.

Paraquat is poorly absorbed from the intestinal tract in all animal species. It is not metabolized but is excreted unchanged in the urine. Paraquat reaches higher concentrations in body tissue than in plasma. This has led to therapeutic interventions aimed at removing paraquat from blood by increasing its renal clearance or by using extracorporeal elimination routes.

Administration of large volumes of fluids to establish and maintain a diuretic urine flow is beneficial because the kidney is the major route of paraquat elimination. The increased urine flow in diuresis will increase the glomerular filtration and tubular secretion of paraquat. Fluid administration has additional benefits in paraquat poisoning cases because most clinically affected animals are severely dehydrated because of the gastrointestinal loss of fluids.

Paraquat also causes vasodilatation apart from the fluid losses described earlier. Both of these mechanisms can account for a functional adverse component in the early stages of paraquat-induced acute renal failure. This functional impairment can be corrected by administering sufficient fluids to cause plasma volume expansion and maintain adequate renal perfusion, thus allowing maximal clearance of the systemically absorbed and circulating paraquat.

Diuretics can also be administered to increase urinary flow; however, renal excretion of paraquat is often not accelerated by diuretics because tubular reabsorption is very limited. Experimental therapies have been proposed to protect renal tubular cells from the direct effects of absorbed paraquat. A combination of free superoxide dismutase (SOD), liposomal SOD, and glutathione peroxidase is being evaluated for this purpose.[13]

Peritoneal dialysis is of little value in paraquat poisoning because it dialyzes paraquat very poorly, even in the presence of elevated paraquat plasma concentrations. Substantial amounts of paraquat can be cleared by hemodialysis, with as much as 150 mL cleared per minute.[13] However, because plasma concentrations in animals with paraquat poisoning tend to be low compared with the concentrations in tissue compartments, the actual amount of paraquat removed by this procedure is clinically insignificant. Another drawback of this procedure is that paraquat clearance with hemodialysis drops considerably when plasma concentrations fall to less than 0.5 mg/L.[13]

Charcoal hemoperfusion is considered the most efficient extracorporeal procedure for removing paraquat, offering plasma clearances as high as 170 mL/min. One study using Hemocol cartridges reported paraquat clearance from plasma at rates between 113 and 156 mL plasma/min, even when the plasma concentration was only 0.2 mg/L. Hemodialysis and hemoperfusion have also been used in series to increase total paraquat removal.[13]

The aim of all these procedures is to increase the elimination of paraquat from the circulation and to prevent its uptake by pneumocytes. Studies conducted in dogs showed that the survival time of exposed animals was longer when the animals underwent charcoal hemoperfusion for 4 hours, beginning 12 hours after ingestion.[13]

The poor total paraquat body clearance by these methods and the rise in plasma concentrations for several hours following the cessation of such therapy can be explained by the extensive paraquat tissue distribution and its slow and sustained redistribution back into the circulation following the termination of extracorporeal procedures. One way to overcome this is to institute continuous hemoperfusion. This procedure is reported to be successful in paraquat poisoning cases in which lethal concentrations of the compound have been ingested. The exact clinical value of this procedure has not been convincingly demonstrated, although animal studies have shown improved survival rates with this technique.

Continuous arteriovenous hemofiltration is a procedure more easily instituted than hemodialysis or hemoperfusion. Unfortunately, definitive clinical data on the clinical benefits in humans and animals are lacking.

Supportive care has improved the prognosis of paraquat-poisoned human patients and holds the same unfulfilled promise in veterinary practice.[7] The most useful management techniques still include protection of the airway, maintenance of cardiovascular circulation, frequent monitoring of vital signs and blood gases, prompt and timely treatment of secondary infections, adequate pain relief, prevention and management of renal failure, replacement of blood losses, and treatment of cardiac complications and neurologic signs.

Supplemental oxygen is contraindicated, even when the animal shows signs of respiratory difficulty. Reduction of the oxygen supply has even been attempted because there is evidence that a positive relationship exists between the inspired oxygen concentration in inspired air and the severity of pulmonary damage. Mechanical ventilation may therefore not be a treatment option to a patient who is in impending respiratory failure caused by pulmonary fibrosis.

There is no effective antidote available for paraquat poisoning. Research into the mechanisms of paraquat toxicity and the development of antidotes has yielded mixed results. Although efforts to understand the mechanisms of free radical generation, lipid peroxidation, and polyamine-mediated uptake of the compound into tissue have generated productive information, the development of an effective antidote remains as elusive today as it was a decade ago.

Certain compounds have shown promising results in animal studies if they are administered prophylactically or immediately following intoxication. Their relevance to a clinical setting is not established because of the heterogeneity of poisoning cases and the fact that most of the clinical data is derived from human patients.

The traditional approach to antidote development is to find compounds that detoxify either the superoxide radical or the subsequently formed toxic intermediates. Compounds studied so far are SOD or the mimetic enzymes and antioxidants, such as vitamin E, ascorbic acid, deferoxamine, selenium, clofibrate, N-acetylcysteine, riboflavin, and niacin. S-adenosylmethionine (Denosyl) may be another antioxidant that could be considered.

Another approach has been to decrease the reduction-oxidation cycling of paraquat by providing alternative substrates, such as methylene blue, which compete with paraquat for reduction by NADPH. Another approach has been to inhibit the uptake of paraquat into alveolar tissue through polyamine uptake pathways. In vitro studies using the uptake inhibitors putrescine and valinomycin have been successful, but in vivo studies have failed to show antidotal activity.

Other methods employed to reduce the toxic effects of paraquat have included the reduction of pulmonary inflammation and fibrosis through radiotherapy, and the use of various immunosuppressant and cytotoxic drugs, such as cyclophosphamide and steroids. These techniques have thus far failed to produce significant and consistent beneficial effects to the patients.

Lung transplantation for replacement of a fibrotic lung has been done in humans with moderate success when it is performed after paraquat has been completely eliminated from the body. The practicality of this procedure in veterinary medicine is questionable.

Prognosis

The prognosis for animals presented with suspected paraquat poisoning can be determined from the plasma concentration of the compound relative to the time of ingestion. In human medicine, a nomogram is used that relates plasma paraquat levels to prognosis.

Initial plasma concentrations give an indication of prognosis. The urinary concentration of paraquat in the first 24 hours of intoxication also can be used to arrive at a prognosis. Unfortunately, such basal values are not available in animals and have to be extrapolated from humans. In human patients, a urinary paraquat concentration of less than 1 mg/L within the first 24 hours indicates a good prognosis. In patients that die within the first 24 hours, urine concentrations ranged from 10 to 10,000 mg/L, and in those who died later from pulmonary fibrosis the urine paraquat concentrations ranged from 1 to 1000 mg/L.[1]

In animal patients, as in human paraquat ingestions,[7] the presence of gastric and esophageal ulcers indicates a grave prognosis. Early development of renal failure and concurrent acid-base disturbances suggest a poor outlook.[9] The ability of the animal to excrete paraquat depends to a large extent on normal renal function. Various studies have pointed out that the ability of healthy kidneys to excrete paraquat (a polar compound) is so remarkable that toxic concentrations can be attained in the lungs only if there is concomitant renal failure. When such large amounts of paraquat are ingested, however, concurrent multiorgan failure is likely.[9]

Gross and Histologic Lesions

Visible lesions are generally confined to the gastrointestinal tract and lung. Erosive stomatitis and esophagitis are often seen because of the irritating nature of paraquat. Paraquat produces its characteristic, but nonspecific, acute to subacute interstitial pneumonia with fulminating pulmonary edema and hemorrhage. In animals chronically affected, the lungs may be shrunken and fibrotic because of hyperplasia of the alveolar type II cells and the fibroplasia superimposed on the earlier exudative changes. Paraquat also causes proximal renal tubular degeneration and focal centrizonal hepatic degeneration. Diquat, in contrast, causes cerebral hemorrhage and infarcts and renal tubular degeneration and necrosis in addition to ulcerative effects in the gastrointestinal tract.

Differential Diagnoses

In the initial phase, paraquat must be differentiated from other gastrointestinal irritant syndromes marked by abdominal pain, vomiting, and diarrhea; causes of these are caustic agents (e.g., strong acids or alkalis), zinc phosphide, inorganic arsenic or mercury, lead, zinc, pancreatitis, and many viral or bacterial agents.[3] Because the acute and chronic phases of paraquat poisoning include some degree of interstitial pneumonia and fibrosis, this clinical syndrome mimics the signs of many infectious diseases and alpha-naphthyl-thiourea poisoning (rarely reported).

Current Toxicologic Status

The severe consequences of paraquat exposure and its resulting toxic effects mandate that early diagnosis and aggressive treatment, coupled with intensive management, are required if the prognosis for the severely poisoned paraquat patient is to be improved. With the current limited effectiveness of treatment protocols for animal paraquat exposures, a focus on exposure prevention is paramount to prevent continuing companion animal losses from this highly toxic herbicide.[7]

The author would like to recognize the contributions of the authors from the previous editions, Dr. Fred Oehme and Dr. Shajan Mannala.

References

1. Pond MS: Manifestations and management of paraquat poisoning, *Med J Aust* 152:256–259, 1990.
2. Onyema HP, Oehme FW: A literature review of paraquat toxicity, *Vet Hum Toxicol* 26:494–502, 1984.
3. Cope RB, Bildfell RJ, Valentine BA, et al: Seven cases of fatal paraquat poisoning in Portland, Oregon dogs, *Vet Hum Toxicol* 46:258–264, 2004.
4. *Merck veterinary manual*, ed 8, Whitehouse Station, NJ, 1998, Merck & Co.
5. Slade P: Photochemical degradation of paraquat, *Nature London* 207:515, 1965.
6. World Health Organization: *Environmental health criteria 39: paraquat and diquat*, Geneva, 1984, World Health Organization.
7. Cope RB: Helping animals exposed to the herbicide paraquat, *Vet Med* 99:755–762, 2004.
8. Bischoff K, Brizze-Buxton B, Gatto N, et al: Malicious paraquat poisoning in Oklahoma dogs, *Vet Hum Toxicol* 40:151–153, 1998.
9. Shuler CM, DeBess EE, Scott M, et al: Retrospective case series of suspected intentional paraquat poisonings: diagnostic findings and risk factors for death, *Vet Hum Toxicol* 46:313–314, 2004.
10. Smith LL: The mechanism of paraquat toxicity in the lung, *Rev Biochem Toxicol* 26:494–502, 1984.
11. Smith P, Heath D: Paraquat, *CRC Crit Rev Toxicol* 4:411–445, 1987.
12. Meredith T, Vale JA: Treatment of paraquat poisoning: gastrointestinal decontamination. In Bismuth C, Hall A, editors: *Paraquat poisoning*, New York, 1995, Marcel Dekker Inc.
13. Pond MS: Treatment of paraquat poisoning. In Bismuth C, Hall A, editors: *Paraquat poisoning*, New York, 1995, Marcel Dekker Inc.
14. Lewis CPL, Nemery B: Pathophysiology and biochemical mechanisms of the pulmonary toxicant of paraquat. In Bismuth C, Hall A, editors: *Paraquat poisoning*, New York, 1995, Marcel Dekker Inc.

Atypical Topical Spot-On Products

70

Sharon M. Gwaltney-Brant, DVM, PhD, DABVT, DABT

- Topical spot-on products are the newest method of insect control for pets.
- Most products are applied between the shoulder blade or striped down the animal's back.
- Most products are labeled for application every 28-30 days.
- Topical spot-on products may repel or kill fleas, ticks, or mosquitoes.
- Some products prevent flea egg development.
- Most of these products, when used appropriately, present little risk of toxicity to the pet.

Topical spot-on ectoparasiticides are the newest method of insect control for pets, and have taken a large part of the market share formerly held by products such as dips, powders, and sprays. These products are usually designed to be applied between the shoulder blades or striped down the back of the animal, limiting the ability of the animal to lick the product off. Most products have little systemic absorption from the skin, but are distributed over the entire skin surface area of the animal as rapidly as 12 hours following application.[1] This distribution throughout the lipid layers of the skin provides for prolonged effectiveness and resistance to loss of efficacy as a result of bathing or wetting. Most products are designed to be reapplied every 28 to 30 days.

Depending on the formulation, these products have shown efficacy at killing or repelling ectoparasites such as fleas, ticks, mosquitoes, mites, and lice. In addition, some products contain insect growth regulators that prevent the development of flea larvae, effectively interrupting the flea life cycle. Spot-on products are convenient, economical, easy to use, relatively long-lasting, and well tolerated by most dogs and cats. The development of newer insecticides that act against insect-specific biochemical mechanisms has resulted in ectoparasiticides that have a high degree of efficacy and much lower mammalian toxicity compared to formerly used pesticides such as organophosphates and carbamates.

Ectoparasiticides

Dinotefuran

Sources

Dinotefuran (N-methyl-N'-nitro-N''-[(tetrahydro-3-furanyl)methyl)]guanidine) is a neonicotinoid insecticide.[2] It is formulated in combination with pyriproxyfen as a spot-on flea control product, and with pyriproxyfen and permethrin as a spot-on flea and tick control product.[3,4] The manufacturer indicates that the products are not to be used on debilitated, aged, medicated, or pregnant or nursing animals or on puppies younger than 7[4] or 8[3] weeks of age.

Toxic Dose

In 90-day oral feeding studies in dogs, the no observable adverse effect level (NOAEL) was 307 mg/kg/day, and the lowest observed adverse effect level (LOAEL) was 59 mg/kg/day in females based on decreased body weight and 862 mg/kg/day in males based on decreased body weight gain and hemorrhagic lymph nodes.[2] The NOAEL for dogs during a 1-year feeding study was 20 mg/kg/day.[3] Studies of the dinotefuran-pyriproxyfen spot-on formulation at one, three, and five times the recommended topical dose in adult dogs and 50- to 60-day-old puppies resulted in no clinically significant abnormalities in clinical pathologic parameters, behavior, or physical examination.[3] Similar results were obtained in a dose trial at five times the recommended dose on 47- to 55-day-old puppies.

Toxicokinetics

Absorption of dinotefuran following ingestion is more than 90%, and the compound is widely distributed throughout the body.[2] Dinotefuran is primarily excreted via the urine and 84% to 99% is eliminated in the urine within 24 hours of absorption. Dinotefuran undergoes minimal biotransformation in the body, with more than 90% being excreted as the parent compound. Dinotefuran is excreted in the milk and crosses the placenta, with maximum concentrations in milk and fetal tissues occurring 0.5 hours following maternal ingestion; by 24 hours following maternal ingestion, concentrations in milk and fetal tissues are less than detection limits.

Mechanism of Toxicity

Dinotefuran is a contact poison and does not require ingestion by the insect to be effective.[3] Dinotefuran binds irreversibly to insect nicotinic receptors and mimics the effects of acetylcholine, resulting in continuous nerve stimulation, incoordination, tremors, and death of the insect. At levels used in flea control products, dinotefuran does not bind to mammalian acetylcholine receptor sites, which accounts for its low mammalian toxicity.

Clinical Signs

Chronic, high-dose exposures to rats and rabbits have produced neurologic signs consistent with effects on the nicotinic cholinergic nervous system, primarily increased motor activity.[3]

Systemic signs are unlikely at the levels of dinotefuran used in topical spot-on products for pets, even if accidental ingestion should occur. Ingestion of topical products may result in taste reactions such as hypersalivation, gagging, and vomiting. As with other topically applied products, individual dermal hypersensitivity reactions may occur, resulting in agitation, pruritus, or pain at the application site. Serious or systemic signs are not generally expected.

Cats exposed to the canine dinotefuran spot-on combination formulation containing permethrin may present with signs of permethrin toxicosis, including muscle fasciculations, tremors, hyperesthesia, mydriasis, hypersalivation, hyperthermia, and seizures and convulsions.[5]

Minimum Database

Assessment of general health, hydration, and renal function is recommended in all animals showing signs beyond mild gastrointestinal upset or dermal irritation, as other potential causes are likely.

Confirmatory Tests

Hair analysis for dinotefuran can be performed at some laboratories but generally is only useful for confirming exposure to the compound.

Treatment

There is no specific antidote for dinotefuran; treatment for adverse effects is symptomatic and supportive. If the exposure is dermal, treatment includes initial stabilization and bathing with a mild dishwashing detergent. Treatment of ingestion of a topical spot-on dinotefuran product should consist of dilution with milk or water. Hypersensitivity skin reactions could occur with any topical product. In those instances, a bath with a noninsecticidal shampoo and symptomatic care, such as hydrocortisone, antibiotics, or antihistamines, is recommended.

Cats developing signs consistent with permethrin toxicosis subsequent to exposure to a dinotefuran-pyriproxyfen-permethrin product should be managed as outlined in the pyrethroid chapter (see Chapter 73, "Pyrethrins and Pyrethroids").

Prognosis

Because dinotefuran has a low level of mammalian toxicity, serious signs are unlikely and mild signs should resolve with symptomatic and supportive care.

Differential Diagnoses

Differential diagnoses for reactions to oral exposures (drooling, gagging, etc.) include corrosive oral injury, exposure to insoluble calcium oxalate-containing plants, and nontoxicant-related nausea.

Fipronil

Sources

Fipronil (5-amino-1-[2,6-dichloro-4-(trifluoromethyl)phenyl]-4-[(1R,S)-(trifluoromethyl) sulfinyl]-1H-pyrazole-3-carbonitrile) is a phenylpyrazole antiparasitic agent used for fleas and ticks in dogs and cats.[6-8] Fipronil is available as a topical product for flea and tick control and in combination with methoprene for additional control of immature flea stages.[7] For control of fleas, ticks, and chewing lice, fipronil is also available as a spot-on product containing 5.2% cyphenothrin and as a combination product with methoprene and amitraz.[9,10]

Toxic Dose

The reported oral median lethal dose (LD_{50}) in rats for veterinary product formulations is greater than 5000 mg/kg.[11] In chronic feeding studies, the NOAEL for dogs was 0.3 mg/kg/day for females and 1 mg/kg/day for males, whereas dosages of 1 mg/kg/day in females and 2 mg/kg/day in males resulted in signs of neurotoxicity.[6]

Toxicokinetics

Fipronil collects in the oils of the skin and hair follicles and continues to be released over time, resulting in long residual activity.[11,12] Topically applied, the compound spreads over the body within 24 hours via translocation. In oral rat studies, 5% to 25% of the parent compound and metabolites is excreted in the urine, and 45% to 75% is excreted in the feces.[11]

Mechanism of Toxicity

Fipronil is a γ-aminobutyric acid (GABA) agonist.[13] Its mechanism of action in invertebrates is to interfere with the passage of chloride ions in GABA-regulated chloride channels, thereby disrupting central nervous system (CNS) activity.[7,8,11] Blockade of the GABA receptors by fipronil results in neural excitation.[7,11]

Clinical Signs

There is limited published information detailing adverse effects of fipronil in dogs or cats; however, clinical effects from the veterinary product would be expected to be mild. Ingestion of any topical products may cause taste reactions. Also, topical hypersensitivity reactions could occur with any dermal product. Extra-label use of fipronil-based sprays on rabbits has been reported to cause anorexia, lethargy, convulsion, and death.[7,14]

Ingestion or topical overdosage of the canine fipronil-amitraz product may result in signs of amitraz toxicosis, including hypersalivation, vomiting, lethargy, hyperglycemia, bradycardia, and bradypnea (see Chapter 31, "Amitraz").[10]

Cats exposed to the canine fipronil spot-on combination formulation containing cyphenothrin may present with signs of permethrin toxicosis, including muscle fasciculations, tremors, hyperesthesia, mydriasis, hypersalivation, hyperthermia, and seizures and convulsions.[5]

Minimum Database

Assessment of the hepatic function may be required because the liver is the primary site of metabolism of fipronil.

Confirmatory Tests

Some laboratories can test for fipronil in hair and skin samples. These results can only confirm the exposure because toxic levels in tissues have not been determined.

Treatment

There is no specific antidote for fipronil; treatment for adverse effects is symptomatic and supportive. If the exposure is dermal, the treatment would include initial stabilization and bathing with a mild dishwashing detergent. Treatment of ingestion of a topical spot-on fipronil product should consist of dilution with milk or water.

Hypersensitivity skin reactions could occur with any topical product. In those instances, a bath with a noninsecticidal shampoo and symptomatic care, such as hydrocortisone, antibiotics, or antihistamines, is recommended.

Animals showing signs consistent with amitraz overdose following oral exposure to fipronil-amitraz products should be managed as outlined in Chapter 31, "Amitraz."

Cats developing signs consistent with cyphenothrin toxicosis subsequent to exposure to a fipronil-cyphenothrin product should be managed as outlined in Chapter 73, "Pyrethrins and Pyrethroids."

Prognosis

Although published reports of adverse effects of fipronil are limited, in most situations animals are expected to recover within 24 to 72 hours with veterinary care.

Differential Diagnoses

Differential diagnoses for reactions to oral exposures (drooling, gagging, etc.) include corrosive oral injury, exposure to insoluble calcium oxalate-containing plants, and nontoxicant-related nausea.

Imidacloprid

Sources

Imidacloprid (1-[(6-chloro-3-pyridinyl)-methyl]-N-nitro-2-imidazolidinimine) is a neonicotinoid of the chloronicotinyl nitroguanidine class.[15] Imidacloprid is used with pyriproxyfen in topical spot-on products to kill all life stages of fleas on dogs and cats and to prevent and control lice infestations on dogs.[16] The manufacturer states that these products should be used with caution in debilitated, aged, pregnant, or nursing animals, and kittens less than 8 weeks of age or puppies less than 7 weeks of age. Imidacloprid is used in combination with permethrin in dog-only spot-on products that control fleas and ticks. Topical formulations of imidacloprid in combination with moxidectin are used on dogs and cats to prevent heartworms as well as control fleas, ear mites, and intestinal nematodes.[17]

Toxic Dose

Dermal LD_{50} of technical imidacloprid for rats is more than 5000 mg/kg.[15] Dogs fed up to 41 mg/kg of imidacloprid for a year developed increased cholesterol levels and increased concentration of cytochrome P450.[18] Kittens exposed topically to 5.2 times the recommended dose of an imidacloprid-moxidectin combination developed mydriasis, salivation, depression, squinting, and poor appetite.[17]

Toxicokinetics

According to the technical profile of the spot-on formulation, topically applied imidacloprid spreads rapidly over the skin by translocation.[11] The product is not systemically absorbed, but sequesters in hair follicles and glands where it is shed with sebum. Ingested imidacloprid is quickly absorbed from the gastrointestinal tract.[11,13] Within 48 hours, 96% of absorbed imidacloprid is eliminated via urine (70% to 80%) and feces (20% to 30%).[11]

Mechanism of Toxicity

Imidacloprid blocks nicotinergic pathways, which results in a buildup of acetylcholine at the neuromuscular junction.[7,11] Acetylcholine buildup results in insect hyperactivity, then paralysis, and later death.

Clinical Signs

There is limited published information detailing adverse effects of imidacloprid in dogs or cats; however, clinical effects from the veterinary product are expected to be mild. Because the drug is bitter tasting, oral contact may cause excessive salivation.[7,11] Signs of poisoning from imidacloprid are similar to nicotinic signs, including lethargy, vomiting, diarrhea, hypersalivation, initial tremors, muscle weakness, and ataxia.[15]

Animals exposed to oral or topical overdoses of imidacloprid-moxidectin combination products may develop signs consistent with avermectin toxicosis: mydriasis, depression, ataxia, tremors, blindness, and coma (see Chapter 52).[7]

Minimum Database

Assessment of the hydration status and urinary function may be required because the kidneys are the primary sites of elimination of imidacloprid.

Confirmatory Tests

Some laboratories can test for imidacloprid in hair and skin samples. However, these results can only confirm the exposure because toxic levels in tissues have not been determined.

Treatment

There is no specific antidote for imidacloprid; treatment for adverse effects would be symptomatic and supportive. If the exposure is dermal, the treatment includes initial stabilization and bathing with a mild dishwashing detergent. Treatment of ingestion of a topically applied veterinary imidacloprid product should consist of dilution with milk or water.

Hypersensitivity skin reactions could occur with any topical product. In those instances, a bath with a noninsecticidal shampoo and symptomatic care, such as hydrocortisone, antibiotics, or antihistamines, is recommended.

Animals exposed to moxidectin-containing formulations and showing signs consistent with macrocyclic lactone toxicosis (e.g., depression, ataxia, mydriasis, blindness, salivation) should be managed as outlined in Chapter 52, "Ivermectin: Macrolide Antiparasitic Agents."

Prognosis

Although published reports of adverse effects of imidacloprid are limited, in most situations, animals are expected to recover within 24 to 72 hours with veterinary care.

Differential Diagnoses

Differential diagnoses for reactions to oral exposures (drooling, gagging, etc.) include corrosive oral injury, exposure to insoluble calcium oxalate-containing plants, and nontoxicant-related nausea.

Indoxacarb

Sources

Indoxacarb (methyl-(4aS)-7-chloro-2-[methoxycarbonyl-[4-(trifluoromethoxy)-phenyl]carbamoyl]-3,5-dihydroindeno[1,2-e][1,3,4]oxadiazine-4a-carboxylate) is a pyrazoline-type insecticide originally developed for use against insect strains that had developed resistance to organophosphates, carbamates, and pyrethroids.[19] In the United States, indoxacarb is registered for use to control lepidopteran insects on crops, turf grasses, and landscape ornamentals.[20] It is also present in ant and cockroach baits and gels at concentrations of 0.05% to 0.6%, and at 20% for control of termites.[21,22] In the European Union, indoxacarb is approved as a topical spot-on flea control product for dogs and cats, and, in combination with permethrin, as a topical spot-on flea and tick control for dogs only.[23,24] The manufacturer states that the safety of the indoxacarb spot-on product has not been established for dogs or cats less than 8 weeks of age or for dogs weighing less than 1.5 kg or cats weighing less than 0.6 kg.[23]

Toxic Dose

Insect species vary in sensitivity to indoxacarb because of species differences in uptake and absorption rates, bioactivation rates, and sodium channel receptors.[25] Insect sodium channels are sensitive to indoxacarb at nanomolar levels whereas mammalian sodium channels are sensitive to indoxacarb at micromolar concentrations, making indoxacarb more than 1000 times more neurotoxic to insects compared with mammals. The dermal 90-day NOAEL for rodents is more than 2000 mg/kg/day.[26] The oral 90-day NOAEL for dogs is 5 mg/kg/day, and the 1-year NOAEL is 2.3-2.4 mg/kg/day. The oral 90-day LOAEL for dogs is 19 mg/kg/day based on the development of hemolytic anemia; at 18-19 mg/kg/day for 1 year Heinz bodies, anemia, bone marrow hyperplasia, and increased liver weight were reported.

Toxicokinetics

Following application to the skin of dogs and cats, indoxacarb is detectable in the skin and hair coat for at least 4 weeks.[23] The concentration of indoxacarb in the hair is higher than the concentration in the skin.[27] Dermal absorption of indoxacarb following application at recommended label doses is at least 19% in dogs and 34% in cats. Bioavailability of indoxacarb in a polyethylene glycol vehicle administered orally at a dosage of 0.32 mg/kg was 85% in dogs and 82% in cats.[27] In both dogs and cats, indoxacarb is extensively metabolized in the liver to multiple metabolites and eliminated primarily through the feces.[23,27] In mammals, the rapid metabolic degradation of indoxacarb as well as less efficient bioactivation of indoxacarb to its active (toxic) metabolite contribute to the low level of neurotoxicity compared with insects.

Mechanism of Toxicity

In insects, indoxacarb is absorbed via ingestion with lesser amounts absorbed across the insect cuticle, and it is bioactivated by the cleaving of a carbomethoxy group from the parent compound.[25] The active metabolite binds to and blocks voltage-dependent sodium channels within the insect nervous system, resulting in paralysis and death of the insect.

In toxicity studies in dogs, indoxacarb induced Heinz bodies and hemolytic anemia when administered orally at 18-19 mg/kg/day.[26] This effect is suspected to be due to a metabolite of indoxacarb, N-hydroxylarylamine, which causes oxidative damage to red blood cells.[27] Based on in vitro studies, the relative sensitivity of species to the oxidative effect of this metabolite is: rat is more sensitive than dogs, which are more sensitive than humans. Because cats have red blood cells that are more sensitive to oxidative injury, one would expect them to be more sensitive than dogs. Despite humans being less sensitive to oxidative red blood cell injury from the indoxacarb metabolite, several case reports exist of humans who developed methemoglobinemia secondary to ingestion of concentrated forms of indoxacarb.[28-31]

Clinical Signs

When indoxacarb is used as a spot-on flea product, the possibility of hypersensitivity skin reactions is always present, resulting in agitation, pruritus, or pain at the application site. Oral exposure may result in hypersalivation, gagging, or vomiting. Oral exposures to the small amounts of indoxacarb present in ant and cockroach baits is unlikely to cause more than mild gastrointestinal upset. Ingestion of larger amounts may result in signs of methemoglobinemia or hemolysis. Signs include cyanosis, chocolate brown mucous membranes, dyspnea, lethargy, and coma. Seizures secondary to hypoxia may occur. Rhabdomyolysis was not reported in toxicity studies in animals but has occurred in humans with indoxacarb poisoning.[31] Acute renal failure has also been reported in humans, and in most cases was considered to be secondary to hemoglobinemia or myoglobinemia.[28,31]

Minimum Database

For large exposures baseline complete blood cell count and serum chemistry should be obtained. The hematocrit and plasma should be monitored for the development of hemolytic anemia. Should hemolysis develop, renal values should be closely monitored.

Confirmatory Tests

Some laboratories can test for indoxacarb in hair samples, although the utility of these tests in managing the patient is questionable. Additionally, these results can only confirm exposure because toxic levels in tissues have not been determined.

Treatment

There is no specific antidote for indoxacarb; treatment for adverse effects is symptomatic and supportive. If the exposure is dermal, the treatment includes initial stabilization and bathing with a mild dishwashing detergent. Treatment of ingestion of a small amount of indoxacarb product should consist of dilution with milk or water. Hypersensitivity skin reactions could occur with any topical product. In those instances, a bath with a noninsecticidal shampoo and symptomatic care, such as hydrocortisone, antibiotics, or antihistamines, is recommended.

For large oral exposures, early decontamination (emesis induction, activated charcoal administration) may be performed if the patient has no significant clinical signs or other contraindications. Patients developing hematologic abnormalities such as hemolytic anemia or methemoglobinemia may require supplemental oxygen for stabilization. If hemolysis or rhabdomyolysis is present, intravenous fluid support is vital to protect the kidneys from hemoglobin- or myoglobin-induced injury. Blood transfusions may be necessary for managing hemolytic anemia. Methemoglobinemia may be managed with methylene blue, although care must be used in cats so as not to worsen the methemoglobinemia (some clinicians consider methylene blue contraindicated in cats because of the difficulty in correctly titrating the dose).[7]

Prognosis

The prognosis for dermal exposures is very good. Patients developing hemolysis or myoglobinemia secondary to ingestion of indoxacarb are at risk of complications such as acute renal failure and have a more guarded prognosis.

Differential Diagnoses

Differential diagnoses for reactions to oral exposures (drooling, gagging, etc.) include corrosive oral injury, exposure to insoluble calcium oxalate-containing plants, and nontoxicant-related nausea. Differential diagnoses for red blood cell damage include immune-mediated hemolytic anemia, zinc toxicosis, acetaminophen toxicosis, onion or garlic toxicosis, naphthalene (mothball) toxicosis, chlorate toxicosis, and hydroxyurea toxicosis.

Metaflumizone

Sources

Metaflumizone (2-[2-(4-cyanophenyl)-1-[3-(trifluoromethyl)phenyl]ethylidene]-*N*-[4-(trifluoromethoxy)phenyl]hydrazinecarboxamide) is a novel semicarbazone insecticide that is related to pyrazoline sodium channel blocker insecticides such as indoxacarb.[32] Metaflumizone is used alone in topical flea control products for cats and kittens 8 weeks of age and older, and in combination with amitraz in topical flea and tick control products for dogs and puppies 8 weeks of age and older.[33,34] In the United States, both products have been discontinued by the manufacturer as of September 20, 2011, although existing stocks may still be marketed.[35]

Toxic Dose

Metaflumizone has very low acute oral toxicity to mammals, is not irritating to eyes or skin, and was not considered to possess a potential to induce skin sensitization.[36] In dogs, the lowest NOAEL was 12 mg/kg/day in a 1-year study. Metaflumizone was not found to be neurotoxic, genotoxic, oncogenic, or teratogenic, or to cause reproductive dysfunction in studies in rabbits and rats.

In cats a 20% metaflumizone topical product was studied in cats and 8-week-old kittens.[37] Single and repeated doses of one, three, and five times the recommended topical dose had no effect on mortality, body weight, food consumption, clinical findings, physical and neurologic examinations, or clinical pathologic parameters. Some felines demonstrated transient salivation, but this condition occurred in placebo-treated controls as well. Cats dosed orally with 10% of the recommended topical dose developed immediate hypersalivation and head shaking. No other adverse effects were observed following oral administration.

The metaflumizone-amitraz combination product was studied at single and repeated doses of one, three, and five times the recommended topical dosage in dogs and was found to have no effects on clinical findings, heart rate, body weight, food consumption, physical and neurologic examinations, and macroscopic and microscopic pathologic findings.[38] Slight, transient, and clinically insignificant elevations in serum urea nitrogen were noted in some dogs at all dose levels but were not dose-related and were considered to be of nonrenal origin. At dosages three and five times the recommended dosage, mild and transient hyperglycemia was seen in some adult female dogs, and mild, transient elevations in leukocytes, neutrophils, and monocytes were seen in some dogs of either sex. Dogs receiving orally 10% of the recommended topical dose developed immediate salivation and head shaking, and some displayed decreased activity, decreased body temperature, and pale oral mucous membranes within 1-2 hours following ingestion. One dog receiving oral metaflumizone-amitraz developed ataxia, which resolved within 4 hours of ingestion. Oral administration of metaflumizone-amitraz had no effect on clinical pathologic parameters. The signs seen with oral metaflumizone-amitraz are most consistent with the amitraz component of the product, as the alpha-2 adrenergic agonist can cause sedation, hypothermia, and ataxia.[39]

Following its introduction into the marketplace, use of the metaflumizone-amitraz topical product in dogs was associated with the development of autoimmune pemphigus foliaceus in 22 dogs.[40] Although most affected dogs had received several (up to eight) prior applications of the product without incident, a few developed lesions after the first exposure.

Toxicokinetics

Following topical exposure of cats to 40 mg/kg of metaflumizone, plasma levels remained less than quantification levels (<50 ng/mL) in five of six cats, and many samples were less than detection limits of the assay (<1.1 ng/mL).[41] The one quantifiable sample had a plasma metaflumizone concentration of 57.8 ng/mL at 3 days following application. These results suggest that there is minimal systemic absorption of metaflumizone following topical application in cats. Hair sample analysis showed that metaflumizone was widely distributed throughout the hair coat within one day of application, reaching maximum concentration within 24-48 hours of application.

Most dogs treated topically with the minimum recommended dose of 20 mg/kg of metaflumizone and 20 mg/kg of amitraz had detectable (>1 ng/mL) but not quantifiable (<50 ng/mL) levels of metaflumizone.[42] At 42 days after application, metaflumizone was detectable in four of six dogs at levels ranging from 59-138 ng/mL. Hair sample analysis showed that metaflumizone was widely distributed throughout the hair coat within

1 day of application, reaching maximum concentration between 2 and 7 days following application.

Mechanism of Toxicity

The insecticidal action of metaflumizone is through voltage-dependent blockade of sodium channels within the nervous system of susceptible insects.[43] Metaflumizone preferentially binds to the inactivated state of the sodium channel, resulting in near-irreversible blockade and paralysis of the insect.

Clinical Signs

As with most topical insecticides, dermal irritation may occur in some animals following application of products containing metaflumizone. Oral exposure may result in hypersalivation, gagging, or vomiting. Systemic toxicosis has not been reported with metaflumizone exposures. Ingestion of the canine metaflumizone-amitraz product may result in signs of amitraz toxicosis, including lethargy, bradycardia, hypotension, hypothermia, ataxia, and hyperglycemia (see Chapter 31, "Amitraz").[39]

Most dogs developing pemphigus foliaceus following exposure to metaflumizone-amitraz products were more than 6 years of age, female, and more than 20 kg in weight.[40] Lesions usually developed within 14 days following product application. Cutaneous lesions included pustules, erosions, and crusting surrounded by areas of erythema. In one third of the cases, lesions remained localized to the area of product application or extended away from the application site to affect the proximal dorsal trunk; approximately one third of these cases developed systemic signs. In two thirds of the dogs, lesions originated at the application site but eventually erupted at distant sites at body areas typically associated with the development of spontaneous pemphigus foliaceus (i.e., ears, face, nose, etc.); three fourths of these generalized cases developed systemic signs such as lethargy, anorexia, fever, and lameness.

Minimum Database

Animals showing more than mild skin hypersensitivity following topical exposure should have baseline serum chemistry and complete blood cell count assessed. Oral exposure to amitraz-containing products may result in hyperglycemia.

Confirmatory Tests

Some laboratories can test for metaflumizone in hair samples, although the utility of these tests is questionable. Additionally, these results can only confirm the exposure because toxic levels in tissues have not been determined. For dogs suspected of developing pemphigus foliaceus secondary to exposure to the metaflumizone-amitraz product, skin biopsy is warranted to identify the characteristic histopathologic lesions; indirect fluorescent antibody testing of skin biopsies can assist in diagnosis. Additionally, circulating antikeratinocyte antibodies may be detectable in those dogs demonstrating the more generalized form of the disease.[40]

Treatment

There is no specific antidote for metaflumizone; treatment for adverse effects is symptomatic and supportive. If the exposure is dermal, the treatment includes initial stabilization and bathing with a mild dishwashing detergent. Treatment of ingestion of a topical spot-on metaflumizone product should consist of dilution with milk or water. Hypersensitivity skin reactions could occur with any topical product. In those instances, a bath with a noninsecticidal shampoo and symptomatic care, such as hydrocortisone, antibiotics, or antihistamines, is recommended. Animals showing signs consistent with amitraz overdose following oral exposure to metaflumizone-amitraz products should be managed as outlined in Chapter 31.

Treatment for pemphigus foliaceus developing secondary to application of metaflumizone-amitraz products should include bathing of the application site and administration of topical glucocorticoids. For more severe or extensive lesions, oral glucocorticoids and other immunosuppressive drugs such as azathioprine or cyclosporine may be required.[40]

Prognosis

The prognosis for mild dermal hypersensitivity or oral irritation from exposure to metaflumizone-containing products is generally good, as most signs resolve with symptomatic care. Animals showing signs of amitraz toxicosis generally have a good prognosis, assuming prompt veterinary intervention is obtained. Dogs developing localized pemphigus foliaceus secondary to application of metaflumizone-amitraz products usually have a good prognosis for resolution of signs.[44] Not all dogs developing generalized pemphigus foliaceus achieved remission, and some dogs required long-term management with immunosuppressants, as lesions recurred when immunosuppressant doses were decreased.

Differential Diagnoses

Differential diagnoses for reactions to oral exposures (drooling, gagging, etc.) include corrosive oral injury, exposure to insoluble calcium oxalate-containing plants, and nontoxicant-related nausea. Differential diagnoses for amitraz toxicosis include other CNS depressants (e.g., antidepressants, opioids, barbiturates, ethylene glycol, propylene glycol, methanol, ethanol, etc.). Differential diagnoses for metaflumizone-amitraz–associated pemphigus foliaceus include spontaneous pemphigus foliaceus, thermal burns, chemical burns, and dorsal solar thermal necrosis.

Insect Growth Regulators

Methoprene

Sources

Methoprene (propan-2-yl(2E,4E)-11-methoxy-3,7,11-trimethyldodeca-2,4-dienoate) is a synthetic insect growth regulator and is classified as a terpenoid.[45] It is used in topical flea control products to help break the flea life cycle alone or in combination with adulticide products. Methoprene does not kill adult fleas.

Toxic Dose

In dogs the acute oral LD_{50} is 5000 to 10,000 mg/kg.[45] The World Health Organization has approved methoprene as safe for use in drinking water to control mosquitoes because of minimal or no risk to humans, animals, or the environment.[45]

Toxicokinetics

In mammals methoprene is rapidly and completely broken down and excreted, mostly in the urine and feces.[45]

Mechanism of Toxicity

Methoprene is a compound that mimics the action of an insect growth regulation hormone. It is used as an insecticide because it interferes with the normal maturation process. In a normal life cycle, an insect goes from egg to larva to pupa and eventually to adult. Methoprene artificially stunts the insects' development, making it impossible for insects to mature to the adult stages, and thus preventing them from reproducing.[45]

Clinical Signs

There is limited published information detailing adverse effects of methoprene in dogs or cats; however, given the mechanism of action, clinical effects are expected to be mild. Toxicity concerns from overexposure or ingestion of current topical spot-on products come primarily from the adulticidal component of the product rather than methoprene. Ingestion of any topical products may cause a taste reaction as a result of the inert ingredients. Also, topical hypersensitivity reactions could occur with any dermal product.

Minimum Database

Assessment of renal and hepatic function may be helpful because the liver and kidney are the sites of metabolism and elimination of methoprene.

Confirmatory Tests

Some laboratories can test for methoprene in hair and skin samples. However, these results can only confirm the exposure because toxic levels in tissues have not been determined.

Treatment

If the exposure is dermal, the treatment includes initial stabilization and bathing with a mild dishwashing detergent. Treatment of ingestion should consist of dilution with milk or water. Hypersensitivity skin reactions could occur with any topical product. In those instances, a bath with a noninsecticidal shampoo and symptomatic care, such as hydrocortisone, antibiotics, or antihistamines, is recommended.

Prognosis

Given the mechanism of action, prognosis is good in most cases.

Differential Diagnoses

Differential diagnoses for reactions to oral exposures (drooling, gagging, etc.) include corrosive oral injury, exposure to insoluble calcium oxalate-containing plants, and nontoxicant-related nausea.

Pyriproxyfen

Sources

Pyriproxyfen (4-phenoxyphenyl(RS)-2-(2-pyridyloxy)propyl ether) is a broad-spectrum insect growth regulator with activity against a variety of insects.[46] It is used in a variety of flea control topical spot-on products, alone or in combination with adulticidal insecticides, including dinotefuran, fipronil, imidacloprid, and pyrethroids.

Toxic Dose

Pyriproxyfen has very low acute oral toxicity in mammals, with LD_{50} values of more than 5000 mg/kg body weight in mice, rats, and dogs.[46] Dermal toxicity is similarly low. Chronic feeding studies resulted in increased liver weights and alterations of plasma cholesterol levels when doses of more than 120 mg/kg/day were fed to rats. The NOAEL level for dogs is 100 mg/kg/day. Very high doses in dogs and rats resulted in mild anemia.

Toxicokinetics

Pyriproxyfen is poorly absorbed orally with less than 50% of an ingested dose being absorbed.[46] Elimination is primarily (90%) via the feces with 34% to 37% of an administered dose being eliminated in 48 hours. The primary biotransformation route is via hydroxylation. The lipophilic nature of pyriproxyfen results in persistence in skin following bathing or swimming.[3]

Mechanism of Toxicity

Pyriproxyfen acts as a juvenile hormone (JH) mimic, artificially maintaining the regulation of molting after natural JH levels have dropped; this arrests the development of ova and immature flea stages, which ultimately die.[3] Pyriproxyfen interferes with the development of flea eggs, larvae, early pupae, and young adult fleas.

Clinical Signs

There is limited published information detailing adverse effects of pyriproxyfen in dogs or cats; however, given the mechanism of action, clinical effects are mild. Although mild anemia has been associated with very high levels of ingestion of pyriproxyfen,[46] it is extremely unlikely that dogs or cats would be exposed to these levels given the amounts present in spot-on products. Toxicity concerns from overexposure or ingestion of current topical spot-on products come primarily from the adulticidal component of the product rather than pyriproxyfen. Ingestion of any topical products may cause taste reactions, such as drooling, gagging, and vomiting. Also, topical hypersensitivity reactions could occur as with any topically applied product.

Minimum Database

Assessment of general health, hydration, and renal function is recommended in all animals showing signs beyond mild gastrointestinal upset or dermal irritation, as other potential causes are likely.

Confirmatory Tests

Some laboratories can test for methoprene in hair and skin samples. However, these results can only confirm the exposure since toxic levels in tissues have not been determined.

Treatment

If the exposure is dermal, the treatment includes initial stabilization and bathing with a mild dishwashing detergent. Treatment of ingestion should consist of dilution with milk or water. Hypersensitivity skin reactions could occur with any topical product. In those instances, a bath with a noninsecticidal shampoo and symptomatic care, such as hydrocortisone, antibiotics, or antihistamines, is recommended.

Prognosis

Given the very low mammalian toxicity of pyriproxyfen, any signs caused by exposure to this product would be expected to be mild and self-limiting.

Differential Diagnoses

Differential diagnoses for reactions to oral exposures (drooling, gagging, etc.) include corrosive oral injury, exposure to insoluble calcium oxalate-containing plants, and nontoxicant-related nausea.

Acknowledgment

The editors wish to acknowledge the exceptional contribution of Dr. Jill Richardson, who authored this chapter for the second edition of the book. Her contribution served as the foundation for the material appearing in this edition.

References

1. Sabnis S, Zupan J, Gliddon M: Topical formulations of metaflumizone plus amitraz to treat flea and tick infestations on dogs, *Vet Parasitol* 150(3):196–202, 2007.
2. *Dinotefuran: Pesticide Fact Sheet*, Washington, DC, 2004, U.S. Environmental Protection Agency Office of Prevention, Pesticides and Toxic Substances. Retrieved 02/2012 from http://www.epa.gov/opprd001/factsheets/dunotefuran.pdf.
3. *Vectra* [technical monograph], Rutherford, NJ, 2009, Summit VetPharm. Retrieved 02/2012 from http://www.summitvetpharm.com/File/VDP_Tech_Mono_22Jul09_w.pdf.
4. *Vectra 3D* [technical monograph], Rutherford, NJ, 2009, Summit VetPharm. Retrieved 02/2012 from http://www.summitvetpharm.com/File/VDP_Tech_Mono_22Jul09_w.pdf.
5. Boland LA, Angles JM: Feline permethrin toxicity: retrospective study of 42 cases, *J Feline Med Surg* 12(2):61–71, 2010.
6. *Fipronil: Pesticide Fact Sheet*, Washington, DC, 1996, U.S. Environmental Protection Agency Office of Prevention, Pesticides and Toxic Substances.
7. Plumb DC: *Veterinary drug handbook*, ed 6, Ames, Iowa, 2008, Blackwell Publishing.
8. Hainzl D, Cole LM, Casida JE: Mechanisms for selective toxicity of fipronil insecticide and its sulfone metabolite and desulfinyl photoproduct, *Chem Res Toxicol* 11(12):1529–1535, 1998.

9. *Parastar Plus* [package insert], Greensboro, NC, 2011, Novartis Animal Health. Retrieved 02/12 from http://www.parastarpluspet.com/parastar_plus/view/downloads/ParastarPlus_ProductInfoSheet.pdf.

10. *Certifect Summary of Product Characteristics: European Public Assessment Report*, London, England, 2011, European Medicines Agency. Retrieved 02/2012 from http://www.ema.europa.eu/docs/en_GB/document_library/EPAR_-_Product_Information/veterinary/002002/WC500111238.pdf.

11. Hovda LR, Hooser SB: Toxicology of newer pesticides for use in dogs and cats, *Vet Clin Small Anim* 32:455–467, 2002.

12. Birckel P, Cochet P, Bernard P, et al: *Cutaneous distribution of C-fipronil in the dog and cat following a spot on administration*. Proceedings from the Third World Congress of Veterinary Dermatology, September, 1996, Edinburgh, Scotland.

13. Wismer TA: Novel insecticides. In Plumlee KH, editor: *Clinical veterinary toxicology*, St Louis, 2003, Mosby.

14. Webster M: Product warning, Frontline, *Aust Vet J* 77:202, 1999.

15. Gervais JA, Luukinen B, Buhl K, Stone D: Imidacloprid technical fact sheet, National Pesticide Information Center, Oregon State University Extension Services. Retrieved from http://npic.orst.edu/factsheets/imidacloprid.pdf.

16. *Advantage II for dogs* [package label], Shawnee Mission, KS, 2010, Bayer Animal Health.

17. *Advantage Multi for cats* [package label], Shawnee Mission, KS, 2010, Bayer Animal Health.

18. Allen TR, Frei T, Leutkemeier H, et al: *A 52-week oral toxicity (feeding) study with NTN 33893 technical in the dog.* Unpublished Report no. R 4856, 1989, amendment no. R 4856A, 1992, submitted to WHO by Bayer AG, Mannheim, Germany. *INCHEM Toxicological Evaluations: Imidacloprid*, International Programme on Chemical Safety, Geneva, Switzerland, 1989, World Health Organization.

19. Zhao X, Ikeda T, Yeh JZ, Narahasih T: Voltage-dependent block of sodium channels in mammalian neurons by the oxadiazine insecticide indoxacarb and its metabolite DCJW, *Neurotoxicology* 24:83–96, 2003.

20. *Provaunt insecticide* [product label], Wilmington, DE, 2011, E.I. du Pont de Nemours and Company. Retrieved 02/2012 from http://www2.dupont.com/Professional_Products/en_US/assets/downloads/pdfs/PROVAUNT_SL-1603A_0812.pdf.

21. *Arlion insecticide* [product label], Wilmington, DE, 2011, E.I. du Pont de Nemours and Company. Retrieved 02/2012 from http://www2.dupont.com/Professional_Products/en_US/assets/downloads/pdfs/ARILON_SL-1672C_020612.pdf.

22. *Advion insect granule* [product label], Wilmington, DE, 2011, E.I. du Pont de Nemours and Company. Retrieved 02/2012 from http://www2.dupont.com/Professional_Products/en_US/assets/downloads/pdfs/H65697.pdf.

23. *Activyl Spot-on solution* [package leaflet], The Netherlands, 2010, Intervet International BV, Boxmeer. Retrieved 02/2012 from http://www.ema.europa.eu/docs/en_GB/document_library/EPAR_-_Product_Information/veterinary/000163/WC500102510.pdf.

24. *Activyl Tick Plus Spot-on solution for dogs* [package leaflet], The Netherlands, 2010, Intervet International BV, Boxmeer. Retrieved 02/2012 from http://www.ema.europa.eu/docs/en_GB/document_library/EPAR_-_Product_Information/veterinary/002234/WC500120993.pdf.

25. Wing KD, Sacher M, Dagaya Y, et al: Bioactivation and mode of action of the oxadiazine indoxacarb in insects, *Crop Protection* 19:537–545, 2000.

26. *Indoxacarb: pesticide fact sheet*. Washington, DC, 2000, U.S. Environmental Protection Agency Office of Prevention, Pesticides and Toxic Substances. Retrieved 02/2012 from http://www.epa.gov/opprd001/factsheets/indoxacarb.pdf.

27. *Activyl Scientific Discussion*, London, England, 2011, European Medicines Agency, EMA/529995/2010. Retrieved 02/2012 from http://www.ema.europa.eu/docs/en_GB/document_library/EPAR_-_Scientific_Discussion/veterinary/000163/WC500102509.pdf.

28. Park JS, Kim H, Lee SW, Min JH: Successful treatment of methemoglobinemia and acute renal failure after indoxacarb poisoning, *Clin Toxicol* 49(8):744–746, 2011.

29. Chhabra R, Singh I, Tandon M, Babu R: Indoxacarb poisoning: a rare presentation as methemoglobinemia, *Indian J Anaesth* 54(3):239–241, 2010.

30. Prasanna L, Rao SM, Singh V, Kujur R: Gowrishankar: Indoxacarb poisoning: an unusual presentation as methemoglobinemia, *Indian J Crit Care Med* 12(4):198–200, 2008.

31. Jin K: Rhabdomyolysis, methemoglobinemia and acute kidney injury after indoxacarb poisoning, *Clin Toxicol* 50(3):227, 2012.

32. Salgado VL, Hayashi JH: Metaflumizone is a novel sodium channel blocker insecticide, *Vet Parasitol* 150(3):182–189, 2007.

33. *Promeris for cats* [package insert], Fort Dodge, IA, 2006, Fort Dodge Animal Health.

34. *Promeris for dogs* [package insert], Fort Dodge, IA, 2006, Fort Dodge Animal Health.

35. American Veterinary Medical Association: Pfizer discontinuing Promeris, *J Am Vet Med Assoc* 238(12):1542, 2011.
36. Hempel K, Hess FG, Bogi C, et al: Toxicological properties of metaflumizone, *Vet Parasitol* 150(3):190–195, 2007.
37. Heaney K, Lindahl RG: Safety of a topically applied spot-on formulation of metaflumizone for flea control in cats and kittens, *Vet Parasitol* 150(3):233–238, 2007.
38. Heaney K, Lindahl RG: Safety of a topically applied spot-on formulation of metaflumizone plus amitraz for flea and tick control in dogs, *Vet Parasitol* 150(3):225–232, 2007.
39. Hugnet C, Buronrosse F, Pineau X, et al: Toxicity and kinetics of amitraz in dogs, *Am J Vet Res* 57(10):1506–1510, 1996.
40. Oberkirchner U, Linder KE, Dunston S, et al: Metaflumizone-amitraz (Promeris)-associated pustular acantholytic dermatitis in 22 dogs: evidence suggests contact drug-triggered pemphigus foliaceus, *Vet Dermatol* 22(5):436–448, 2011.
41. DeLay RL, Lacoste E, Delprat S, Blond-Riou F: Pharmacokinetics of metaflumizone in the plasma and hair of cats following topical application, *Vet Parasitol* 150(3):258–262, 2007.
42. DeLay RL, Lacoste E, Mezzasalma T, Blond-Riou F: Pharmacokinetics of metaflumizone and amitraz in the plasma and hair of dogs following topical application, *Vet Parasitol* 150(3):258–262, 2007.
43. Song W, Silver KS, Du Y, et al: Analysis of the action of lidocaine on insect sodium channels, *Insect Biochem Mol Biol* 41(1):36–41, 2011.
44. Oberkirchner U, Linder K, Olivry T: Recognizing and treating ProMeris-triggered pemphigus foliaceus in dogs, *Vet Med* 106(6):284–293, 2011.
45. Ramesh C, et al: Pharmacologic profile of methoprene, an insect growth regulator, in cattle, dogs, and cats, *J Am Vet Med Assoc* 194(3):410–412, 1989.
46. Food and Agricultural Organization, World Health Organization: *Pyriproxyfen in drinking water, Guidelines for drinking water quality*, Geneva, Switzerland, 2008, World Health Organization.

Petroleum Hydrocarbons

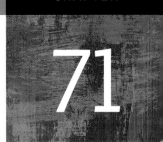

CHAPTER

71

Merl F. Raisbeck, DVM, MS, PhD, DABVT

- The most important toxic effect associated with the petroleum products commonly ingested by small animals is aspiration pneumonia.
- Low viscosity, high volatility, and low surface tension are physical characteristics of hydrocarbons that are more likely to produce respiratory disease.
- Systemic toxic effects in the CNS and to a lesser extent the liver, heart, and kidneys are more likely with aromatic or volatile aliphatic compounds.
- Gastric decontamination, especially with emetics, is contraindicated unless there is a strong probability of some other, systemic toxicant in the gastrointestinal tract. Treatment is symptomatic and supportive in nature.

Sources

Petroleum is a highly complex mixture of hydrocarbons. "Petroleum poisoning" is actually the sum of the toxic effects and interactions of a mixture of disparate compounds. Although crude oil intoxication occurs in large animals and is a serious environmental problem, pets are most frequently exposed to refined petroleum products. These include fuels such as propane, gasoline, kerosene, or diesel oil; solvents such as paint thinner, engine degreaser, or laboratory chemicals; and lubricants such as motor oil, waxes, or asphalt. Petroleum-based solvents are used as "inert" carriers for a number of pesticides, paints, and medications. Petroleum-based chemicals are also the basic feedstock for products as diverse as plastics and pharmaceuticals. In other words, petroleum hydrocarbons represent a very diverse group of chemicals that are very widespread throughout the modern environment.

The precise composition of any specific petroleum product varies with its intended use and the characteristic process or processes used to produce it. For most of the simpler products like gasoline, the refining process consists largely of differential distillation and cracking. The product itself is defined in terms of boiling point rather than any specific chemical composition. Thus, volatility provides one convenient index with which to broadly classify petroleum products. Some products, notably fuels with a high boiling point such as fuel oil, receive little further processing. Others, such as gasoline, are modified with a considerable number of additives such as methanol or manganese, which possess significant toxic properties of their own. Finally, some products, such as the thermoplastics or organohalide solvents, are chemically modified to such an extent that their physical, chemical, and toxic properties are quite distinct from petroleum hydrocarbons as a whole. This last group is not included in this chapter. Conversely, some hydrocarbons of nonpetroleum origin, such as turpentine or linseed oil, are similar enough to be considered with petroleum-based solvents of similar physical-chemical properties.

In people, the most frequent cause of petroleum poisoning involves substance abuse (e.g., using petroleum products to get "high"). Animals usually exhibit a little more common sense, but may still sample motor oil or gasoline out of curiosity if it is available. Inappropriate containers and failure to clean up spills are common sources of exposure to pets. Pets, especially cats, may ingest significant amounts of gasoline or other petroleum products via grooming and transdermally after topical exposure. Gasoline or kerosene is sometimes used in an attempt to remove sticky material, such as tar, from an animal's coat. Many folk remedies contain inappropriate types and amounts of petroleum products. For example, "guard" dogs are sometimes force-fed a mixture of gasoline and smokeless powder to make them more aggressive.

Toxic Dose

The toxicity of a specific petroleum product theoretically varies with its composition. Given the huge number of distinct petroleum constituents in common products, it is impossible to track the toxicity of each individually. Fortunately, however, it is possible to make some broad generalizations about the toxicity of petroleum hydrocarbons on the basis of simple physical-chemical properties such as boiling point. Products with very high boiling points, such as asphalt, mineral oil, or waxes, are relatively nontoxic. As a very loose generalization, more volatile compounds are also more readily absorbed and thus have greater possibility for systemic toxicity. More volatile compounds, such as benzene, also tend to be more readily aspirated and thus are more likely to cause chemical pneumonitis (Table 71-1).

The likelihood of pneumotoxicity is also determined by viscosity and surface tension. Lower viscosity enhances the penetration of the product into smaller and therefore more numerous airways. Low surface tension facilitates the spread of hydrocarbons over larger areas of pulmonary tissues. As little as 0.1 mL of a low-viscosity hydrocarbon such as mineral spirits, when aspirated directly into the trachea of dogs, may produce severe pneumonitis. In contrast, products with a high viscosity, such as motor oil, have a much more limited pneumotoxic potential (Box 71-1).

Hydrocarbon solvents, including petroleum distillates, turpentine, etc., are skin and eye irritants by virtue of their lipid solvent properties and are capable of producing erythema, dermatitis, and epithelial necrosis. Systemic toxicity should be considered following heavy dermal exposure, especially with strong solvents such as gasoline. This is especially important in small animals (e.g., pups or kittens), which have a relatively high body surface area to mass ratio. Again, the relative toxicity of various products by this route of exposure seems to be inversely proportional to molecular weight and proportional to lipophilicity. Toxicity is further enhanced by other factors such as long or matted hair that traps the hydrocarbon against the skin.

Toxicokinetics

Contrary to some older texts, many hydrocarbons are readily absorbed after ingestion. Studies with a number of different radiolabeled hydrocarbons have demonstrated both gastrointestinal and percutaneous absorption and subsequent distribution to all major organ systems. The degree of such absorption was inversely proportional to the molecular weight of the hydrocarbon involved. High-molecular-weight hydrocarbons, such as grease or motor oil, are not absorbed to any significant extent, whereas lower-molecular-weight products, such as gasoline or hexane, are more readily absorbed. Aromatic compounds, such as benzene, are more readily absorbed than aliphatic hydrocarbons of similar molecular weight and thus more likely to cause systemic toxicity.

Regardless of the class of compound or route of exposure, respiration is an important route of elimination for volatile hydrocarbons, once absorbed. Volatile compounds, such as petroleum ether, are largely cleared within 24 hours; less volatile compounds, such as motor oil, may remain in the gastrointestinal tract for a considerably longer time. Most aliphatic hydrocarbons are degraded to some extent by the liver. Metabolism usually involves

Table 71–1	Acute Toxicity of Some Commonly Encountered Hydrocarbons	
Compound	**Dose**	**Clinical Signs**
Acetone	Oral LD_{50}: 5-10 mg/kg	CNS depression, narcosis, coma
Benzene	Oral LD_{50}: 4 mL/kg	CNS depression, narcosis, bone marrow suppression
Carbon disulfide	Oral LD_{50}: 5-10 mg/kg Inhalation LC_{50}: 15 mg/L	Tremor, cyanosis, vascular collapse, coma
Cyclohexane	Oral LD_{50}: >8 mL/kg	CNS depression, ataxia, narcosis, coma
Diesel fuel	Oral LD_{50}: 9 mL/kg	Diarrhea, GI upset, possible aspiration pneumonia
Gasoline	Oral LD_{50}: 18 mL/kg	Moderate topical and GI irritant, aspiration pneumonia
Home heating oil	Oral LD_{50}: 18 mL/kg	Relatively nontoxic; diarrhea, GI upset if dose is sufficient
Isopropanol	Oral LD_{50}: 6-13 g/kg	CNS depression, ataxia, acidosis, coma
Jet fuel A	Oral LD_{50}: >20 mL/kg	Relatively nontoxic; diarrhea, GI upset if dose is sufficient
Lighter fluid	Oral LD_{50}: 25 g/kg	Aspiration pneumonia, CNS depression
Motor oil	Oral LD_{50}: >22 mL/kg	Relatively nontoxic; diarrhea, GI upset if dose is sufficient
Toluene	Oral LD_{50}: 6-8 mL/kg	CNS depression, ataxia, liver and kidney damage
Turpentine	Minimum lethal dose (children): 15 mL/kg	Strong irritant, readily absorbed through skin and by inhalation
Xylene	Oral LD_{50}: 4 mL/kg	Strong topical irritant, CNS depression, tremors, coma

oxidation, rendering the compound more polar and thus more readily excreted, but may also contribute to the pathogenesis of chronic toxic effects. Aromatic hydrocarbons are metabolized to phenols or carboxylic acids; conjugated with sulfates, glucuronides, or glycine; and excreted through urine or bile.

Mechanism of Toxicity

As a general rule, the most acute life-threatening effects of petroleum intoxication result from aspiration pneumonia. Experimental data suggest that the pulmonary injury in aspiration pneumonia results primarily from aspiration and not from gastrointestinal or dermal absorption. Dogs given 250 mL of kerosene by gavage showed no radiographic evidence of pulmonary damage, but substantially smaller volumes (less than 1 mL) given intratracheally caused rapid progression of depression, dyspnea, and death. Vomiting often precedes aspiration; it is not a prerequisite, however, because aspiration can also occur when the hydrocarbon is initially ingested. Thus the lack of emesis in the history does not preclude the possibility of aspiration. Pulmonary function should be monitored carefully following any oral hydrocarbon exposure.

The pneumotoxic potential of any particular hydrocarbon mixture is determined by its volatility, viscosity, and surface tension. Compounds with viscosities of less than 35 Saybolt units (SSU) are very likely to be aspirated, whereas compounds with viscosities of greater than 60 SSU are less likely to cause pneumonia. Gasoline, kerosene, and lighter fluid have viscosities in the 30 to 35 SSU range and are easily aspirated. Mineral oil (150 SSU), motor oil (60 to 500 SSU), and paraffin wax almost never cause pulmonary damage.

At a tissue level, pneumotoxic effects of petroleum hydrocarbons are mediated by the dissolution of the lipid component of cellular membranes in contact with the hydrocarbon. This results in swelling and/or necrosis of the cell that in turn provokes inflammation. In the lung, the end result is edema, bronchospasm, and necrosis of the terminal airways and alveoli within a few minutes to an hour of exposure. There may be hemorrhage into the airways that also compromises respiration. Alteration of pulmonary surfactant is another result of the lipophilicity of petroleum products. Loss of pulmonary surfactant increases the surface tension of the fluid lining of the alveoli and destabilizes the alveoli, resulting in atelectasis and collapse of distal airways. Finally, volatile hydrocarbons may displace sufficient alveolar oxygen to produce acute cyanosis even before pneumonitis becomes apparent.

Later, inflammation, thrombosis, and emphysema extend the functional damage beyond tissues in immediate contact with the hydrocarbon. Bacteria may colonize damaged areas, resulting in further tissue destruction and pneumonia. Uncomplicated lesions typically heal within 2 weeks of the initial crisis, but there is evidence that subclinical effects remain for months or years. A retrospective epidemiologic study in human patients demonstrated an increased incidence of respiratory infections several years following hydrocarbon pneumonitis, and (in a separate study) asymptomatic patients who had experienced hydrocarbon pneumonitis more than 8 years earlier still had detectable functional abnormalities typical of small airway disease.

Systemic effects of the petroleum hydrocarbons involve the central nervous system (CNS) and, to a lesser extent, the liver, kidneys, and heart. Again, the more volatile, lower-molecular-weight hydrocarbons, such as hexane, are more likely to be involved because they are more readily absorbed than heavier products, such as kerosene. For the same reason, aromatic compounds, such as toluene or benzene, are more toxic systemically than naphthalenes, which are in turn more toxic than aliphatics of similar molecular weight. Absorption and subsequent systemic toxicity are also greater when hydrocarbons are inhaled as a vapor rather than ingested.

The principal systemic effect of hydrocarbon intoxication is usually CNS depression. The acute neurotoxic effects of petroleum hydrocarbons apparently result from a direct physicochemical interaction between the hydrocarbon and the neuronal membranes of the CNS. Because this is largely a physical process, clinical signs can become apparent within minutes of toxic exposure and for the most part disappear as soon as the hydrocarbon is cleared from the system. Exceptions to this rule, such as hexane neuropathy, usually require prolonged exposure for metabolic activation and are beyond the scope of this discussion.

Hepatic and renal damage have been reported from a percentage of both experimental and field cases of hydrocarbon poisoning. The mechanism is not clear but probably involves metabolism by the target organ to a toxic intermediate. Some hydrocarbons are also apparently capable of sensitizing the myocardium to endogenous catecholamines, resulting in arrhythmias and even complete cardiovascular collapse.

Clinical Signs

Human patients report a burning sensation in the mouth and pharynx immediately after ingestion of petroleum products such as gasoline. Animals appear to experience much the same sensations: slobbering, champing their jaws, shaking their head, and pawing at their muzzle. This is usually followed by signs of aspiration: choking, coughing, gagging, and varying degrees of dyspnea. Direct damage to the airway components and bronchospasm may result in hypoxia. Cyanosis may also develop immediately as alveolar oxygen is displaced by hydrocarbon vapor. Astute observers may note an odor of the hydrocarbon on the animal's breath. Fever usually occurs in 3 to 4 hours, but may occur in less than 1 hour or as late as 24 hours after exposure.

Pneumonitis is the most common complication following ingestion of volatile, low-viscosity, aliphatic petroleum hydrocarbons (e.g., gasoline). The central nervous and gastrointestinal systems may also be affected, but death, if it occurs, usually results from the pulmonary effects. Respiratory involvement, when present, is progressive over the first 24 to 48 hours and then gradually resolves 3 to 10 days following exposure. Signs referable to the respiratory system usually occur within a few minutes to 1 or 2 hours. Animals that remain asymptomatic for 6 to 12 hours after ingestion are unlikely to develop respiratory illness.

Radiographic abnormalities may lead or lag behind the clinical signs slightly, but animals that eventually develop clinical pneumonitis show readily observable radiographic changes within a few hours of ingestion, thus it is a good idea to radiograph the chest 6 to 12 hours post exposure, before releasing the patient. Radiographic findings are typical of aspiration pneumonia and consist of fine, perihilar densities and extensive infiltrates in ventral portions of the lungs. These changes are worse at 3 to 4 days and then clear over an additional few days. Not all animals with radiographic signs of hydrocarbon aspiration develop respiratory signs, and radiographic changes usually persist past the resolution of clinical signs.

The irritant properties of petroleum products produce gastroenteritis, vomiting, colic, and diarrhea after oral exposure. The severity, and indeed even the presence, of such signs is a function of the dose and the individual hydrocarbon. Heavier, aliphatic hydrocarbons, such as mineral oil, may produce diarrhea and altered gastrointestinal motility but little else. Lighter hydrocarbons, such as gasoline, are more likely to produce colic and vomiting.

The CNS signs of acute hydrocarbon toxicity are similar to those of ethanol inebriation. Intoxicated animals exhibit vertigo, ataxia, and mental confusion. Hydrocarbons produce depression and narcosis in most cases, but tremors and convulsions have also been reported. If the dose is high enough, the animal becomes comatose, and coma may proceed to death without any accompanying respiratory signs. The heartbeat may be irregular as a result of myocardial sensitization, or complete cardiac collapse may occur if the animal is stressed. Myocardial sensitization to the effects of catecholamines may persist for 24 to 48 hours after apparent recovery from the neurologic effects of intoxication.

Minimum Database

A minimum evaluation of possible petroleum hydrocarbon ingestion includes determination of vital signs, careful evaluation of respiratory status including oximetry, auscultation of the chest, and a chest radiograph. The clinical signs and radiographic changes associated with aspiration of petroleum products are indistinguishable from the signs and radiographic changes seen with other forms of aspiration pneumonia. Thus some means of confirming petroleum hydrocarbon exposure is essential to confirm the diagnosis. It is also desirable to identify the particular product involved because its volatility and viscosity affect the prognosis and treatment. This information is most readily available from the history. The owner should be instructed to bring the container or label to the clinic with the animal if the product is not a relatively common one like gasoline. It may also be possible to detect the characteristic odor of petroleum hydrocarbons on the animal's breath, a test often overlooked by clinicians. An inflammatory profile is commonly observed on a complete blood count analysis. Other tests that should be considered include liver and kidney function panels.

Confirmatory Tests

A simple spot test involves mixing vomitus vigorously with warm water. If gasoline or other petroleum distillates are present they will float to the surface. Care must be taken to distinguish between petroleum products and dietary lipids. Most petroleum products lighter than kerosene, if isolated and absorbed onto a paper towel, evaporate relatively quickly and have a characteristic odor. Chemical analysis of ingesta or postmortem tissues is useful forensically but is seldom practical for evaluating the clinical case. If chemical analysis is to be conducted, samples should be taken as quickly as practical and frozen in airtight, glass containers to prevent loss as a result of volatilization.

Treatment

In all cases of uncomplicated (i.e., not contaminated by some other, more toxic substance) petroleum hydrocarbon ingestion, the primary goal should be to minimize the risk of aspiration. If the amount ingested was small, and especially if the hydrocarbon ingested was known to be one of the less volatile, more viscous products, such as motor oil or grease, cage rest and observation may be all that are required. If the volume ingested was substantial and the product involved was one known to cause systemic toxicity (e.g., hexane, toluene, or xylene), gastric lavage may be indicated within the first 4 to 6 hours post exposure. Gastric decontamination may also be indicated, despite the risk of aspiration, *if* the product was contaminated with a highly toxic substance such as a pesticide. If lavage is to be attempted, it is essential to take precautions to prevent possible aspiration of stomach contents. Emetics are contraindicated except as an absolute last resort to clear some other highly toxic constituent, such as a pesticide from the gastrointestinal tract. In any case, the potential systemic toxicity of the ingested product must be weighed against the definite potential for aspiration.

In the past, mineral oil or vegetable oil was recommended to increase the viscosity of petroleum hydrocarbons and thus decrease the risk of aspiration. Oils also produce a mild catharsis, decreasing the period during which the petroleum product might be absorbed. However, retrospective studies in children suggest that such treatment actually increases the likelihood of aspiration pneumonia, and the use of such oils is no longer recommended.

Respiratory effects should be treated symptomatically. The routine use of antibiotics and corticosteroids has been questioned. Hydrocarbon pneumonitis is reported to be largely nonbacterial in origin. In one experimental study in which dogs were given an intratracheal dose of kerosene, parenteral ampicillin and dexamethasone did not reduce either the respiratory rate or the presence of radiographic, gross, or microscopic pulmonary lesions. Corticosteroid use, in another experiment, was associated with increased numbers of positive lung cultures. Corticosteroids are thus considered contraindicated. Antibiotics should only be considered if there is evidence of bacterial pneumonia. Supplemental oxygen, continuous positive airway pressure, and mechanical ventilation should be used as needed. However, because pneumomediastinum, pneumatoceles, and pneumothorax are common complications of hydrocarbon pneumonitis, positive pressure systems must be used with caution. Also, because the lungs are the major route of systemic elimination for many hydrocarbons, closed or semiclosed systems should be purged frequently.

Cage rest is indicated, both for its beneficial effects on the healing process and to minimize the effects of excitement-induced catecholamines on hydrocarbon-sensitized myocardium. Likewise, bronchospasm may be treated with β-2 agonists if the myocardium has been unduly sensitized.

Topical exposures may be treated by gently bathing the animal with warm water and a mild detergent shampoo. If the hair coat is especially heavy or matted, it may be necessary to clip the contaminated areas to prevent systemic absorption and minimize skin damage. Symptomatic treatment of petroleum burns may involve the use of topical antibacterial agents as necessary. Highly viscous hydrocarbons (e.g., tar and waxes) may also be removed with mild detergents. Because they are not readily absorbed they pose only a cosmetic problem or a risk of mechanical irritation and are not as critical to remove. Lipophilic materials (butter, lard, mechanics' hand cleaner) may also be useful in such cases, but the use of hydrocarbon solvents is not recommended.

Prognosis

The prognosis depends on the extent and severity of tissue damage. Animals that remain asymptomatic for 12 to 24 hours require no further follow-up or treatment. If pulmonary lesions are extensive or if the animal is comatose when presented, the prognosis is guarded to poor.

Gross and Histologic Lesions

Systemic toxicity may result in centrilobular hepatic, myocardial, or renal tubular necrosis if the animal survives more than 24 hours after exposure. However, these lesions are not that common, and animals that survive the acute respiratory or neurotoxic effects long enough to develop recognizable lesions usually recover.

If aspiration has occurred, the principal lesions will be found in the respiratory tract. There may be ulcerations in the ventral mucosa of the trachea and larger airways. Pulmonary lesions are bilateral and involve primarily the caudoventral portion. Early lesions include hyperemia, edema, and hemorrhage into the airways. Oil may be grossly visible in the smaller airways. Later, bronchospasm, emphysema, and atelectasis occur. Pneumatoceles, pneumothorax, and subcutaneous emphysema result from airway collapse. Bacterial pneumonia occasionally supervenes and may result in abscesses.

Differential Diagnoses

A large number of infectious diseases and toxins may result in respiratory signs similar to those associated with hydrocarbon aspiration. However, only very acute processes, such as trauma or chylothorax, exhibit a similar rapidity of onset.

Suggested Readings

Bronstein AC, Spyker DA, Cantilena LR Jr, et al: 2009 Annual Report of the American Association of Poison Control Centers' National Poison Data System (NPDS), *Clin Toxicol (Phila)* 48:979–1178, 2010.
Kimbrough RD, Reese E: Acute toxicity of gasoline and some additives, *Environ Health Perspect* 101(Suppl 6):115–131, 1993.
Lifshitz M, Sofer S, Gorodischer R: Hydrocarbon poisoning in children: a 5-year retrospective study, *Wilderness Environ Med* 1478–1482, 2003.

Propylene Glycol

Karyn Bischoff, DVM, MS, DABVT

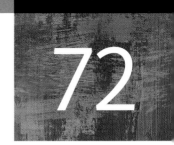

- Propylene glycol (PG) is used as automotive antifreeze, in hydraulic fluid, industrial and pharmaceutical solvent, cosmetics, and as an additive in processed foods.
- Clinical signs following oral exposure are related to propylene glycol's narcotic effects and lactic acidosis: depression, ataxia, muscle twitching, and seizures.
- Increased numbers of Heinz bodies, reticulocytes, and lower packed cell volumes occur in animals, particularly felines, exposed to propylene glycol.

Small animals occasionally have access to automotive solvents. Dogs and cats sometimes obtain access to a garage where there are open containers, or solvents can be found in an outdoor setting when automobile radiators are drained or fluids leak. The most toxic radiator fluid is ethylene glycol (see Chapter 47 on Ethylene Glycol), which animals frequently have access to, and it presents a significant problem to the small animal practitioner.

Propylene glycol is commonly used as a relatively "safe" alternative to ethylene glycol as antifreeze. Propylene glycol has other uses ranging from industrial solvent to food additive. It was once used in semimoist cat foods, some of which contained more than 10% propylene glycol. However, propylene glycol is no longer used in cat foods because cats are particularly susceptible to its adverse effects. Toxicosis from large doses of propylene glycol has been reported in people and various other species.

Sources

Propylene glycol, or 1,2-propanediol, is a stable, colorless, odorless, viscous liquid with a specific gravity of 1.036. It is an excellent solvent because it is freely miscible with water yet dissolves hydrophobic substances. Among the glycols, propylene glycol has the lowest toxicity.[1] Unlike ethylene glycol, propylene glycol does not cause oxalate nephrosis. Propylene glycol is classified by the Food and Drug Administration (FDA) as "generally recognized as safe" except for use in cat foods. Because of these properties, it is used not only as automotive antifreeze, hydraulic fluid, and an industrial solvent, but also as a pharmaceutical solvent for oral, topical, and injectable preparations; an ingredient in cosmetics; and an additive in processed foods for human and animal consumption.

Toxic Dose

The oral median lethal dose (LD_{50}) for propylene glycol in dogs is reported to be as low as 9 mL/kg, although for most laboratory animal species it is approximately 20 mL/kg.[2-5] The toxic concentration in blood in humans is estimated at 100 mg/dL, although metabolic changes have been reported at blood concentrations as low as 12 mg/dL.[6,7] Patients with hepatic or renal disease are at increased risk for propylene glycol toxicosis.[6,7]

Toxicokinetics

Acute propylene glycol toxicosis has occurred in humans, horses, and cattle because of ingestion, parenteral administration, and topical treatment for burns.[2,3,8-16] The condition has also been experimentally produced in cats, dogs, laboratory animals, goats, and chickens.[1,3-5,17-21] Propylene glycol is palatable to dogs.[22] It is absorbed rapidly in the digestive system.[8] Toxic doses can also be absorbed through damaged skin, and toxicosis has been reported in burn patients.[1,16,23,24] Experimental inhalation exposures of 5 mg/dL and greater were associated with adverse effects in dogs.[25]

Oral and pulmonary absorption of propylene glycol are rapid and the volume of distribution is 0.5 L/kg in humans.[25,26] Between 12% and 55% of propylene glycol is excreted in the urine as the parent compound or a glucuronide conjugate in humans, and renal clearance decreases as dose increases.[7,26-30] Remaining propylene glycol is oxidized by two saturable enzymes, hepatic alcohol dehydrogenase and aldehyde dehydrogenase, to D and L isomers of lactic acid.[8] L-lactic acid enters the citric acid cycle and is metabolized rapidly.[10] However, D-lactic acid is not readily metabolized, accumulates in plasma, and produces lactic acidosis.[10,30] Propylene glycol concentrates in the central nervous system in humans.[15] Propylene glycol has narcotic effects similar to those of ethanol, although it is only about one third as potent.[1,2,10,16,23] Dogs eliminate propylene glycol almost completely within 24 hours.[18] The elimination half-life in mature humans is 1.4 to 5 hours, and 10 to 31 hours in infants.[26,29]

Heinz body formation occurs through the interaction of propylene glycol or its metabolite with the sulfhydryl groups on the hemoglobin molecule.[1,31,32] The hemoglobin molecule becomes denatured and adheres to the cell membrane. Cats are particularly sensitive, possibly because their hemoglobin contains eight sulfhydryl groups and because they have less ability to conjugate propylene glycol with glucuronide than other domestic species. Heinz body numbers decrease to reference ranges within 8 weeks of cessation of exposure.[33,34]

Clinical Signs

Clinical signs of acute propylene glycol poisoning in small animals are related to its narcotic effects and to lactic acidosis. Most patients present with central nervous system depression and ataxia after they have ingested large quantities of propylene glycol.[8,26,27,35-39] Seizures have also been reported in human cases.[2,6,8-10] Muscle twitching is sometimes evident in cats.[21] The author is familiar with a case of malicious poisoning with propylene glycol where three dogs were found dead. Parenteral overdosing with propylene glycol has been associated with hypotension in cats and circulatory collapse in dogs and other species.[8,10,18,20,28] Renal failure due to acute tubular injury is reported in people.[6,7] Intravenous infusion of undiluted propylene glycol is associated with hemolysis because of the hyperosmolarity of the compound.[8] Osmotic diuresis and dehydration are also commonly seen with oral and parenteral exposure to propylene glycol.[1,4,19,22]

Topical exposure to propylene glycol has been associated with contact dermatitis due to hypersensitivity in humans.[14] Mucosal irritation has been reported with chronic respiratory exposure in laboratory rodents.[25]

Minimum Database

Clinical pathologic findings in animals with propylene glycol toxicosis are consistent with metabolic acidosis and hyperosmolarity. Animals have an increase in the ion gap, which correlates with blood lactic acid concentrations.[3,8-11,40] Carbon dioxide and carbonic acid concentrations are low.[10] Hypoglycemia has been reported in some animals.[1] Urine has a low specific gravity because of osmotic diuresis and casts are sometimes observed.[11,15] Blood urea nitrogen and creatinine are elevated in people due to proximal convoluted tubular injury.[9] The serum is hyperosmolar after intravenous administration, and the increase in osmolarity correlates with the circulating propylene glycol concentration.[6,8] Hemoglobinuria has been reported in dogs and other species secondary to hemolysis after high intravenous doses of propylene glycol.[3,20,27]

Heinz body formation has been reported in cats and horses secondary to ingestion of propylene glycol.[1,17,31-33,38] Heinz bodies were present in up to 18% of erythrocytes in adult cats and 36% in kittens as a result of dietary exposure.[4,17,31,32] There have been no reports of clinical anemia or methemoglobinemia in cats because of chronic dietary exposure to propylene glycol, although PCVs are mildly reduced.[31,36,41] However, such exposure could predispose feline red cells to more severe oxidative damage by other agents, such as acetaminophen.[17] Experimental dogs fed diets containing 20% propylene glycol had decreased PCVs, increased reticulocyte counts, increased nucleated erythrocyte counts, and evidence of hemolysis.[1,42] Similar changes were seen in experimental dogs with chronic respiratory exposure to propylene glycol.[25]

Confirmatory Tests

Diagnosis of propylene glycol toxicosis is usually based on a history of exposure. Propylene glycol can be detected in urine and serum by gas chromatography.[9,12,23] Poisoning was confirmed using gas chromatography to detect residue in a container found near the three dogs in the terminal case mentioned previously. Importantly, propylene glycol will produce a false positive for ethylene glycol on some commercially available ethylene glycol test kits (refer to Chapter 47, "Ethylene Glycol").

Treatment

Treatment of acute propylene glycol toxicosis is supportive. Intravenous fluids containing sodium bicarbonate should be administered as needed to correct dehydration and acidosis, and any electrolyte abnormalities should be corrective. A horse with propylene glycol toxicosis was treated by gastric lavage to remove remaining material in the stomach, activated charcoal to adsorb propylene glycol, and given isotonic sodium bicarbonate and dexamethasone IV. Blood gas was monitored on an hourly basis.[38] Because of rapid gastrointestinal absorption, gastrointestinal decontamination is unlikely to be beneficial in most cases.

Vitamin C was administered to diminish oxidative damage to erythrocytes in an intoxicated horse.[38] However, experimental administration of vitamin C and vitamin E failed to significantly decrease Heinz body formation in cats fed a diet containing propylene glycol, and N-acetylcysteine was only slightly beneficial.[41] Fomepizole was used in a human patient given excessive doses of propylene glycol intravenously to decrease the rate of metabolism (via alcohol dehydrogenase) and production of lactic acid.[40] Although of possible use in veterinary medicine, fomepizole treatment of propylene glycol toxicosis in cats should be pursued with caution, because it is possible that the parent compound is responsible for the erythrocyte damage seen in this species.

Prognosis

The prognosis is highly variable depending on the exposure dose and time interval between exposure and initiation of treatment. In general, it would be considered guarded to fair.

Gross and Histologic Lesions

There are sometimes no gross or microscopic lesions in animals poisoned with propylene glycol.[18] A foul or garlic-like odor to gastrointestinal contents has been reported in horses and a llama.[38,39] Reported kidney lesions include congestion and tubular necrosis.[5,12,35] Liver lesions have been reported in horses.[35]

Differential Diagnoses

Some toxicants that could mimic this clinical presentation include ivermectin and other macrolide antiparasitic agents, ethylene glycol, methanol, diethylene glycol, 2-butoxyethanol, sedatives and tranquilizers, isopropanol, ethanol, xylitol, and amitraz. Other causes of a hemolytic anemia are zinc, naphthalene-containing mothballs, onions, acetaminophen, copper, and pit viper snakebites.

References

1. Christopher MM, Perman V, Eaton JW: Contribution of propylene glycol-induced Heinz body formation to anemia in cats, *J Am Vet MedAssoc* 194(8):1045–1056, 1989.
2. Yu DK, Elmquist WF, Sawchuck RJ: Pharmacokinetics of propylene glycol in humans during multiple dosing regimens, *J Pharmacol Sci* 74(8):876–879, 1985.
3. Dorman DC, Hascheck WM: Fatal propylene glycol toxicosis in a horse, *J Am Vet Med Assoc* 198(9):1643–1644, 1991.
4. Ruddick JA: Toxicology, metabolism, and biochemistry of 1,2-propanediol, *Toxicol Appl Pharmacol* 21(1):102–111, 1972.
5. Gaunt IF, Carpanini FMB: Long-term toxicity of propylene glycol in rats, *Food Cosmet Toxicol* 10(5):151–162, 1972.
6. Kraut JA, Kurtz I: Toxic alcohol ingestions: clinical features, diagnosis, and management, *Clin J Am Soc Nephrol* 3(1):208–225, 2008.
7. Zar T, Graeber C, Perazella MA: Recognition, treatment, and prevention of propylene glycol toxicity, *Semin Dialysis* 20(3):217–219, 2007.
8. Pastemak G: Ethylene/propylene glycol toxicity. In Goldfrank L, editor: *Case studies in environmental medicine 30*, San Rafael, CA, 1993, DeLima Associates.
9. Cate JC, Hedrick R: Propylene glycol intoxication and lactic acidosis, *N Engl JMed* 303(21):1237, 1980.
10. Christopher MM, Eckfeldt H, Eaton JW: Propylene glycol ingestion causes D-lactic acidosis, *Lab Invest* 60(1):114, 1990.
11. Van de Wiele B, Rubinstein E, et al: Propylene glycol toxicity caused by prolonged infusion of etomidate, *J Neurosurg Anesthesiol* 7(4):259–262, 1995.
12. McConnel JR, McAllister JL, Gross GG: Propylene glycol toxicity following continuous etomidate infusion for the control of refractory cerebral edema, *Neurosurgery* 38(1):232–233, 1996.
13. Levy ML, Aranda M, Zelman V, et al: Propylene glycol toxicity following continuous etomidate infusion for the control of refractory cerebral edema, *Neurosurgery* 37(2):363–371, 1995.
14. Angelini G, Meneghini CL: Contact allergy from propylene glycol, *Contact Dermatitis* 7(4):197–198, 1981.
15. Fligner CL, Jack R, Twiggs GA, et al: Hyperosmolality induced by propylene glycol, *JAMA* 253(11):1606–1609, 1985.
16. MacDonald MG, Getson PR, Glasgow AM, et al: Propylene glycol: increased incidence of seizures in low birth weight infants, *Pediatrics* 79(4):622–625, 1987.
17. Bauer MC, Weiss DJ, Perman V: Hematological alterations in kittens induced by 6% and 12% dietary propylene glycol, *Vet Hum Toxicol* 34(2):127–131, 1992.
18. Hanzlik PH, Newman HW, Van Winkle W Jr, et al: Toxicity, fate and excretion of propylene glycol and some other glycols, *J Pharmacol Exp Ther* 67(12):101–113, 1939.
19. Moon PF: Acute toxicosis in two dogs associated with etomidate-propylene glycol infusion, *Lab An Sci* 44(6):590–594, 1994.
20. Seidenfeld MA, Hanzlik PJ: The general properties, actions and toxicity of propylene glycol, *J Pharmacol Exp Ther* 44:109–121, 1932.
21. Marshall DA, Doty RL: Taste responses of dogs to ethylene glycol, propylene glycol, and ethylene glycol-based antifreeze, *J Am Vet Med Assoc* 197(12):1599–1602, 1990.
22. Glasgow AM, Boeckx RL, Miller MK, et al: Hyperosmolality in small infants due to propylene glycol, *Pediatrics* 72(3):353–355, 1983.
23. Kelner MJ, Bailey DN: Propylene glycol as a cause of lactic acidosis, *J Anal Toxicol* 9(1):40–42, 1985.
24. Lehman AJ, Newman HW: Propylene glycol: rate of metabolism, absorption, and excretion with a method for estimation in body fluids, *J Pharmacol Exp Ther* 60:312–322, 1937.
25. Werley MS, McDonald P, Lilly P, et al: Non-clinical safety and pharmacokinetic evaualtions of propylene glycol aerosol in Sprague-Dawley rats and Beagle dogs, *Toxicol* 287(1-3):76–90, 2011.
26. Brooks DE, Wallace KL: Acute propylene glycol ingestion, *Clin Toxicol* 40(4):513–516, 2002.
27. Arulanantham K, Genel M: Central nervous system toxicity associated with ingestion of propylene glycol, *J Pediatr* 93(3):515–516, 1978.

28. Yu DK, Sawchuk RJ: Pharmacokinetics of propylene glycol in the rabbit, *J Pharmacokinet Biopharm* 15(5):453–471, 1987.
29. Allegaert K, Vanhaesenbrouck S, Kulo A, et al: Prospective assessment of short-term propylene glycol tolerance in neonates, *Arch Dis Child* 95(12):1054–1058, 2010.
30. Pintchuk PA, Galey FD, George LW: Propylene glycol toxicity in adult dairy cows, *J Vet Intern Med* 7(3):150, 1993.
31. Weiss D, McClay CB, Christopher MM, et al: Effects of propylene glycol containing diets on acetamino-phen-induced methemoglobinemia in cats, *J Am Vet Med Assoc* 196(11):1816–1819, 1990.
32. Bauer MC, Weiss DJ, Perman V: Hematologic alterations in adult cats fed 6% or 12% propylene glycol, *Am J Vet Res* 53(1):69–72, 1992.
33. Dzanis DA: Propylene glycol unsafe for use in cat foods, *FDA Vet* 9(1):1–3, 1994.
34. Hickman MA, Rodgers QR, Morris JG: Effects of diet on Heinz body formation in kittens, *Am J Vet Res* 50(3):475–478, 1990.
35. Myers VS, Usenik EA: Propylene glycol intoxication of horses, *J Am Vet Med Assoc* 155(12):1969, 1841.
36. Gross DR, Kitzman JV, Adams HR: Cardiovascular effects of intravenous administration of propylene glycol and oxytetracycline and propylene glycol in calves, *Am J Vet Res* 40(6):783–791, 1979.
37. Martin G, Finberg L: Propylene glycol: a potentially toxic vehicle in liquid dosage form, *J Pediatr* 77(5):877–878, 1970.
38. McLanahan S, Hunter J, Murphy M, et al: Propylene glycol toxicosis in a mare, *Vet Hum Toxicol* 40(5):294–296, 1998.
39. Ivany JM, Anderson DE: Propylene glycol toxicosis in a llama, *J Am Vet Med Assoc* 218(2):243–244, 2001.
40. Zosel A, Egelhoff E, Heard K: Severe lactic acidosis from iatrogenic propylene glycol overdose, *Pharmacother* 30(2):219, 2011.
41. Hill AS, O'Niell S, Rogers QR, et al: Antioxidant prevention of Heinz body formation and oxidative injury in cats, *Am J Vet Res* 62(3):370–374, 2001.
42. Weil CS, Woodside MD, Smyth HF Jr, et al: Results of feeding propylene glycol in the diet to dogs for two years, *Food Cosmet Toxicol* 9(4):479–490, 1971.

Pyrethrins and Pyrethroids

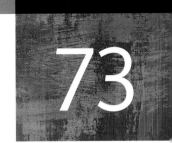

73

Steven R. Hansen, DVM, MS, DABT, DABVT

Reviewed by Safdar A. Khan, DVM, MS, PhD, DABVT

- Commonly used insecticides available in various household, garden, and pet formulations as aerosols, dusts, granules, foggers, shampoos, sprays, collars, dips, and once-a-month concentrated spot-on products for mainly controlling fleas, ticks, lice, and mosquitoes.
- Many combination products include the have a synergist (piperonyl butoxide; MGK-264) or an insect growth regulator (IGR) such as methoprene, pyriproxyfen, hydropene, and fenoxycarb.
- Etofenprox labeled for use in dogs and cats has a similar mechanism of action but is classified as a pyrethroid-like insecticide because it is structurally different from conventional pyrethroids.
- Most EPA-approved products labeled for use on dogs and/or cats represent a relatively low hazard when used per label directions.
- Cats are more sensitive than most other species to pyrethrins and pyrethroids. Very young, aged, anemic, or debilitated animals may be more susceptible to toxic effects.
- Inappropriate use of concentrated spot-on monthly products containing permethrin (36%-65%) in cats can often result in generalized tremors, ataxia, shaking, seizures, and death.
- Clinical signs result from allergic, idiosyncratic, and neurotoxic reactions.
- Treatment is aimed at controlling tremors and seizures in patients with serious neurologic signs, preventing further systemic absorption and topical contact, thermoregulation, and supportive care.

Sources

Natural pyrethrum extract contains a mixture of similar compounds and isomers derived from *Chrysanthemum cinerariaefolium* and related species. The insecticidal activity of pyrethrum has been known since at least the mid-1800s. Today, most agricultural production of pyrethrum extract intended for formulation into insecticidal products occurs in East Africa.[1] Pyrethrin-containing flea and tick control products for dogs and cats have been popular for many years because they can rapidly knock down and kill insects and have a reasonable safety profile. Different pyrethrin formulations may include the presence of an IGR (methoprene) or a synergist like pipernyl butoxide or MGK-264.

Pyrethroid insecticides are synthetic analogues of pyrethrin compounds that have been, and continue to be, developed and formulated to provide enhanced stability and potency on pets and in the environment. Pyrethroids represent a diverse and growing collection of synthetic compounds that have a structure and/or mechanism similar to that of natural pyrethrins. Type I pyrethroids lack an alpha-cyano group. Type II pyrethroids possess an alpha-cyano group. Examples of synthetic type I pyrethroid compounds include allethrin, permethrin, phenothrin, resmethrin, bifenthrin, tefluthrin, and tetramethrin. Examples of type II pyrethroids include cyfluthrin, cyhalothrin, cypermethrin, cyphenothrin, deltamethrin, esfenvalerate, fenvalerate, flumethrin, lambda-cyhalothrin, and tralomethrin.

The United States Environmental Protection Agency (EPA) approves product labels and regulates all insecticidal products. Many pyrethrin and pyrethroid formulations are registered for topical and household use on or around dogs and/or cats for flea and tick control. Other products are registered for environmental and agricultural use for a host of economic and annoyance pests. Products containing pyrethrin or pyrethroid insecticides are readily available through grocery, discount, home improvement, and veterinary locations. Spot-on formulations represent the most popular consumer product form, although some dip, shampoo, spray, mousse, premise, and other formulations remain available. Consumer confusion regarding which products are appropriate for use on dogs, cats, or both results in misuse of dog products on cats with potentially life-threatening consequences.

Toxic Dose

Toxic doses for pyrethrin and pyrethroid compounds vary substantially and in most cases are not known in dogs or cats. The rat acute oral median lethal dose (LD_{50}) for technical-grade pyrethrin isomers is reported to be 260 to more than 600 mg/kg.[2] Acute dermal LD_{50} values for pyrethrins are more than 1350 mg/kg in the rat and more than 4500 mg/kg in the rabbit.[3] Pyrethroids are moderately toxic (EPA category II) because, with the exception of a few compounds, pyrethroids have acute oral LD_{50} values between 50 and 500 mg/kg in laboratory animals. Toxicity of pyrethroids varies similarly; for example, the rat oral LD_{50} for tefluthrin is 22 mg/kg, whereas that for phenothrin is 10,000 mg/kg.[4] Oral LD_{50} of deltamethrin in dogs is greater than 300 mg/kg. No clinical signs were observed when dogs were fed deltamethrin in food at 1 mg/kg per day for 2 years. Although the toxic dose for permethrin in the cat is unknown, clinical evidence clearly demonstrates a marked sensitivity in this species. This sensitivity likely also occurs in response to other pyrethroids. Oral LD_{50} of permethrin in rats ranges from 540 to 2690 mg/kg. The no observable adverse effect level for permethrin in dogs is 5 mg/kg/day for 96 days.

Although valuable information can be gained from insecticide LD_{50} data when considered in the context of a diluted final product, the actual toxicity of the complete formulation in the target species is what is most important. Inert or synergist activity may enhance the toxicity of a formula. Inert ingredients in insecticidal formulations include solvents, such as aromatic and aliphatic hydrocarbons, glycols, and alcohols. Synergists, which are formulated to slow an insect's metabolic processes by inhibiting microsomal enzyme activity, include piperonyl butoxide and N-octyl bicycloheptene dicarboximide (MGK-264). Addition of synergists in different formulations helps increase their insecticidal activity.

Generally, most products registered for use on dogs and cats represent a relatively low hazard when used according to label directions in healthy pets. The EPA requires standardized product toxicity testing to determine which signal word must appear on the label. Signal words, representing the least to the most hazardous compounds, include the terms *Caution, Warning,* and *Danger.* The signal word is determined based on six acute toxicity studies and product composition. These studies include tests for acute oral, dermal, and inhalation toxicity; eye irritation; skin irritation; and skin sensitization. Skin sensitization determines whether a product is capable of causing an allergic reaction and is not considered when determining the signal word. The standard battery of acute toxicity tests is based on rat, rabbit, and guinea pig protocols (not dog or cat protocols). Ultimately the signal word on the label is based on the most sensitive test. Previously defined precautionary statements are determined by the toxic effects noted on each individual test. For example, "Causes eye injury" is an EPA-required statement based on the severity of the eye irritation noted in a study in rabbits.

Most animal-registered products display the signal word *Caution*, which means that the final product formulation exhibited an acute rat oral LD_{50} of less than 500 mg/kg, thereby also requiring the statement "harmful if swallowed." A target animal safety study is conducted in each approved species, which also may trigger specific label requirements.[5]

One specific toxicosis warrants special comment. Based on the public database of the American Society for the Prevention of Cruelty to Animals (ASPCA) Animal Poison Control Center, "spot-on" products that contain the pyrethroid permethrin, which are labeled clearly for use on dogs only, can result in serious toxicosis when used inappropriately on cats. Significant adverse reactions in dogs are rare. Based on these cases, dermal application of 100 mg/kg permethrin (1 mL of 45% permethrin applied dermally to a 4.5-kg cat), if untreated, can result in life-threatening toxicosis. The minimum toxic dose is unknown, but would be expected to be significantly lower. Similarly, case data suggest that some cats that closely cohabitate (direct contact while playing, sleeping, or grooming) with dogs are at risk for permethrin toxicosis when the dog alone was treated appropriately with a permethrin-containing product. Based on data from these and other cases, cats should be considered exceptionally sensitive to permethrin compared with dogs, rats, or humans. Permethrin-based products formulated for dogs can contain anywhere from 0.054% to 65% permethrin. Products formulated for cats should contain less than 0.20% permethrin.

Based on a similar review of public database cases, some cats appear sensitive to properly applied EPA approved spot-on formulations containing 85.7% phenothrin. Clinical signs are generally, but not always, less severe with shorter duration than effects reported following permethrin exposure. Clinical signs reported from most to least frequent included tremors, muscle fasciculation, ear twitching, ataxia, lethargy, trembling, hypersalivation, pruritis, hiding, and agitation.

Veterinarians should take every opportunity to educate clients on the safe appropriate (appropriate dose and species) use of pesticides in compliance with label directions. Many pesticide regulatory documents and other information on pesticides are available on the Internet at http://www.epa.gov/pesticides.

Toxicokinetics

Pyrethrin insecticides are fat-soluble compounds that undergo rapid metabolism and excretion following oral or dermal exposure. In general, pyrethroids are well absorbed orally and via inhalation. As a class, pyrethroids exhibit low systemic toxicity following dermal exposure. Most are rapidly metabolized by ester hydrolysis and via oxidation by microsomal enzymes in the liver. Rapid hydrolysis of ester linkage in the GI tract results in low toxicity. Pyrethroids also undergo intradermal metabolism which likely limits the systemic absorption when applied dermally. They are lipophilic and are therefore rapidly distributed to the CNS and metabolized quickly, limiting the bioaccumulation and chronic toxicity. Pyrethroid insecticides have enhanced stability and potency. Carriers, solvents, and synergists can greatly influence the effect of excess exposure to insecticidal products. For example, some formulations contain large percentages of alcohols and other solvents, which can result in profound depression, especially when applied excessively to cats or small dogs. Synergists, such as piperonyl butoxide and N-octyl bicycloheptene dicarboximide (MGK-264), are included in some formulations to enhance insecticidal activity. It is unclear what impact these compounds have on the metabolism of xenobiotics in dogs and cats, especially in situations of overdose. Local dermal irritation, redness, and itching can be seen in some sensitive animals from formulations with or without the presence of an IGR.

Mechanism of Toxicity

The basic mechanism of action of pyrethrin and pyrethroid insecticides is essentially the same. These compounds affect insects and animals by altering the activity of the sodium ion channels of nerves. Under conditions of normal membrane depolarization, the sodium channels of nerve fibers allow an influx of sodium ions into the nerve axon. Inactivation of the action potential occurs as sodium ion influx decreases. During the peak of the action potential potassium channels open, allowing potassium to move out of the cell. The cell membrane returns to its normal resting state through the action of energy-dependent sodium and potassium pumps. Exposure to pyrethrin or pyrethroid compounds prolongs the period of sodium conductance, which increases the length of the depolarizing action potential, resulting in repetitive nerve firing. Sensory nerve fibers are more susceptible to stimulation because of differences in sodium channel kinetics.[6]

Clinical Signs

Based on the experience of the ASPCA Animal Poison Control Center, clinical signs can result from both appropriate and inappropriate exposure of pets to pyrethrin or pyrethroid insecticides. Such exposures can result in either minor or major clinical signs.

Clinical signs result from immune-mediated hypersensitivity reactions, genetic-based idiosyncratic reactions, and neurotoxic reactions. Although an understanding of the mechanism of the reaction is important when considering a treatment plan, the treatment plan itself is ultimately designed to meet the specific needs of the patient. This concept can be summarized simply as "treat the patient and not the poison."

Minor, usually self-limiting, clinical signs include hypersalivation, paw flicking, ear twitching, hyperesthesia, reduced activity, and single-episode vomiting or diarrhea. Hypersalivation, paw flicking, ear twitching, and hyperesthesia are commonly reported and are caused by topical and oral stimulation of sensory nerves. Vomiting and diarrhea are nonspecific signs. These clinical signs are considered side effects but not adverse, deleterious, or toxic effects. Although these clinical effects are often self-limiting, pet owners can often be greatly alarmed and may describe hyperesthesia as seizure activity.

Topical allergic reactions are relatively common and can be manifested as generalized or local dermal urticaria, hyperemia, pruritus, and alopecia. Such reactions can occur because of sensitivity from the active ingredients or from the carrier (inactive ingredients) and are seen from products with or without the presence of an IGR. Systemic anaphylactic reactions are fairly uncommon but potentially very serious complications and are expressed as circulatory collapse, respiratory distress, and sudden death. Allergic reactions are often the result of minimal or appropriate exposure. Dermal reactions are the most common allergic manifestation and are not considered serious. Anaphylactic reactions are life threatening. Future avoidance of products containing pyrethrin or pyrethroid compounds is recommended for the animal affected.

Idiosyncratic reactions are considered the direct result of pyrethrin or pyrethroid neurotoxic effects, which occur at much lower doses than expected. Typically, these sensitive animals represent a small percentage of a normally distributed population. Standard descriptive toxicology tests use exaggerated doses in an attempt to reveal the likelihood of such occurrences. Future avoidance of pyrethrin or pyrethroid formulations in these animals is important.

True toxic reactions are the result of overdose, inappropriate use or repeated over-application of insecticides.[7-10] Protracted vomiting and diarrhea, marked depression, ataxia, or generalized muscle tremors warrant immediate veterinary examination and treatment. Blindness has also been reported in a significant number of poisoned cats and dogs; this is generally considered reversible and animals will regain their vision as they improve over time. If untreated, marked dermal or oral overdose may result in tremors and, rarely, seizures or death. Cats are especially sensitive to concentrated permethrin-containing products labeled for use on dogs and can develop muscle tremors, ataxia, shaking, seizures, and death within hours. These signs can occur within a few hours to a couple of days of exposure and can last for 2 to 3 days. Seizure activity is unusual following pyrethrin exposure even at exaggerated doses. Future use of these products in accordance with label instructions would not be expected to lead to a recurrence. Exceptions would include the situation in which a very sensitive animal received an exaggerated dose.

Minimum Database

The minimum database includes baseline serum chemistries, complete blood cell count, and urinalysis. These minimal data help to uncover preexisting conditions that can affect the treatment plan and prognosis. Often a suspected poisoning case is actually the result of a preexisting disease process. Very young or very old, anemic, sick, debilitated, or stressed animals may be at higher risk of toxicosis. Heavy flea or tick infestation or other parasitic diseases may also increase individual risk.

Treatment

Minor side effects, such as hypersalivation, paw flicking, ear twitching, hyperesthesia, reduced activity, and single-episode vomiting or diarrhea, are usually self-limiting and require no treatment. If the pet is wet from application of a product, a towel that has been warmed in a dryer works nicely to warm up and dry a small cat or dog. Consumption of water or milk may help dilute and rinse product from the mouth, thereby reducing salivation. Drooling can continue off and on in some cats for a few hours or even for a couple of days and may require dilution with water or milk again. Thorough brushing may remove loose hair and reduce grooming in cats.

Allergic reactions most commonly become manifest as hyperemic and pruritic skin. In these cases, a detergent bath (hand dishwashing product) with copious rinsing in cool water is usually adequate. Topical vitamin E applied to the affected area of skin locally may soothe the skin and reduce inflammation and pruritis. Diphenhydramine, 2 mg/kg IM, IV, or PO q 8 hours for 2 to 3 days, may prove beneficial when topical vitamin E does not yield positive results or systemic corticosteroids may be required to stop self-inflicted trauma. Anaphylactic reactions should be managed aggressively using routine protocols. After bathing, pets must be dried completely to avoid chilling.

Activated charcoal administration is not routinely recommended because benefits often do not outweigh the stress or need for sedation in cats. An exception would be when a topical spot-on product was administered orally to a cat. In this case activated charcoal can be administered orally at 2 g/kg body weight within a couple of hours of exposure in an asymptomatic animal. Overuse of activated charcoal in very small or dehydrated animals should be avoided because of potential of aspiration and adverse effects on sodium homeostasis resulting in hypernatremia, especially in small breed dogs.

In cases where prolonged seizure activity has occurred without early veterinary intervention, achieving adequate seizure control can be challenging and is often the determining prognostic indicator. In most cases, control of marked tremor or seizure activity can be achieved with Robaxin-V (methocarbamol) administered intravenously at a rate of 55 to 220 mg/kg. Administer half the dose rapidly without exceeding a rate of 2 mL/minute, then pause until the pet begins to relax, and then administer the remainder to effect. Repeat methocarbamol as needed. A maximum dose of 330 mg/kg per day should not be exceeded. In serious cases, diazepam will not produce acceptable seizure control. Other agents successfully used to control seizures include barbiturates (watch and correct hypothermia when using barbiturates), isoflurane following mask induction, and propofol. Propofol, 3 to 6 mg/kg IV or 0.1 to 0.6 mg/kg per minute as an IV infusion, can help control severe CNS signs. Care should be used to avoid oversedation, because complete elimination of random muscle trembling is not required or likely.[11,12] There are anecdotal reports indicating that the use of concentrated lipid emulsion therapy in cats with permethrin toxicosis can help reduce the duration or severity of clinical effects. However, no studies are available to show safety or efficacy of this treatment. Lipid solution (20%) can be tried at 1.5 mL/kg IV bolus, then 0.25 mL/kg per minute for 30 to 60 minutes. Repeat in 4 to 6 hours provided no hyperlipemic serum is present. Discontinue if no significant response is observed after giving 3 doses. Lack of efficacy, hyperlipemia, hemolysis, embolism, and infection are possible adverse effects.

Once seizure or tremor activity is controlled, topically exposed animals must be thoroughly bathed with a liquid hand dishwashing detergent and rinsed with copious amounts of water at body temperature. Maintenance of a normal body temperature is extremely important. Severe hyperthermia often results during prolonged tremor or seizure activity. In contrast, hypothermia often results following bathing or sedative administration. Hypothermia is as dangerous as hyperthermia because reduced body temperature enhances nervous activity by slowing sodium channel kinetics. Hypothermia can prolong duration of clinical signs of pyrethrin/pyrethroid toxicosis. Hyperthermia should be treated if >106° F to reduce the risk of heat-induced injury or death. Cooling efforts should be discontinued when body temperature reaches 103.5° F to prevent complications with hypothermia. Adequate nutritional and fluid support also hastens recovery. Administration of atropine should be strictly avoided because atropine is not antidotal and can produce CNS stimulation in excessive doses.

Prognosis

Early, aggressive treatment often results in a full recovery within 24 to 72 hours. Nervous system effects are completely reversible on recovery. Unfortunately, pets, especially cats not receiving early aggressive care, may show signs of status epilepticus and die.

Gross and Histologic Lesions

Pyrethrin and pyrethroid insecticides do not produce identifiable lesions.

Differential Diagnoses

Analysis of hair samples can confirm exposure to specific pyrethroids, especially permethrin. In cats, hair analysis can confirm permethrin exposure when no exposure to permethrin was known or when exposure was reported to be to a feline-approved flea and tick product that contains other insecticides not expected to cause severe neurologic effects.

Pyrethrin or pyrethroid toxicosis must be differentiated from other neurotoxicant exposures, including strychnine; metaldehyde; fluoroacetate (1080); 5-fluorouracil; 4-aminopyridine; caffeine; theobromine; amphetamine; cocaine; tremorgenic mycotoxins; and organophosphate, carbamate, or organochlorine insecticides. Trauma, endocrine abnormalities, and neoplasia also warrant consideration.

Animals found dead must be presented to a veterinary clinic or veterinary diagnostic laboratory for necropsy. Sudden death in cats following exposure to a stressful situation, such as a bath, can result from decompensated cardiomyopathy or cardiac failure secondary to thyroid neoplasia. Other disease processes can similarly complicate diagnosis and treatment.

Case Report 1

A 1-year-old 4.5-kg castrated male domestic shorthair cat was presented to an emergency clinician for treatment. The cat owner had applied a 1-mL 45% permethrin, 5% pyriproxyfen spot-on product EPA registered for use only on dogs. The product had been applied on the cat 4 hours earlier to the dorsal scapular area, where it was thought that the cat could not groom. Within 4 hours of exposure, the cat developed hypersalivation, severe tremors, and seizures. At the time of the call to the ASPCA Animal Poison Control Center, the cat had already been bathed with a hand dishwashing detergent to remove residual permethrin. Subsequently, diazepam, pentobarbital, and methocarbamol were ineffective in controlling seizure activity. The pet owner elected to have the cat euthanized.

The cat in this case report was exposed to a known permethrin dose of 100 mg/kg. The second active ingredient was pyriproxyfen, 11 mg/kg, which is an insect growth regulator of low toxicity. Delayed treatment resulting in progression to intractable seizure activity is the primary reason permethrin-exposed cats die or are euthanized.

Case Report 2

A 5-year-old, 6.8-kg castrated male domestic shorthair cat was presented to a veterinarian for treatment. The cat owner had applied a 2.5-mL 44% permethrin, 8.8% imidacloprid spot-on product EPA registered for use only on dogs. Within 2.5 hours the cat was exhibiting muscle tremors, had a body temperature of 103° F, and had vomited once. Within 4 hours of exposure, the cat had been bathed in a liquid hand dishwashing detergent and was administered methocarbamol. The cat fully recovered.

In this case the cat was topically exposed to 162 mg/kg permethrin and 32 mg/kg imidacloprid. Topical application of imidacloprid alone at this dose would not be expected to cause adverse effects in cats. Topical decontamination and use of methocarbamol resulted in a successful outcome.

References

1. Ray D: Pesticides derived from plants and other organisms. In Hayes WJ Jr, Laws ER Jr, editors: *Handbook of pesticide toxicology*, San Diego, 1991, Academic Press.
2. Casida JE, Kimmel EC, Elliott M, et al: Oxidative metabolism of pyrethrins in mammals, *Nature* 230: 326–327, 1971.
3. Malone JC, Brown NC: Toxicity of various grades of pyrethrum to laboratory animals, *Pyrethrum Post* 9:3–8, 1968.
4. Thomson WT: Agricultural chemicals, *Insecticides*, vol 1, Fresno, CA, 1992, Thomson Publications.
5. Environmental Protection Agency: *Label review manual*, Washington, DC, 1996, EPA Registration Division, Office of Pesticide Programs.
6. Hansen S, Villar D, Buck W, et al: Pyrethrins and pyrethroids in dogs and cats, *Compend Cont Educ Pract Vet* 16(6):707–713, 1994.
7. Boland LA, Angles JM: Feline permethrin toxicity: retrospective study of 42 cases, *J Feline Med Surg* 12:61–71, 2010.
8. Malik R, et al: Permethrin spot-on intoxication of cats: literature review and survey of veterinary practitioners in Australia, *J Feline Med Surg* 12:5–14, 2010.
9. Bradberry S, et al: Poisoning due to pyrethroids, *Toxicol Rev* 24(2):93–106, 2005.
10. Wolansky MJ, Harril JA: Neurobehavioral toxicology of pyrethroid insecticides in adult animals: a critical review, *Neurotoxicol Teratol* 30:55–78, 2008.
11. Volmer P, Khan S, Knight M, et al: Warning against use of some permethrin products in cats (letter to editor), *J Am Vet Med Assoc* 213(6):800, 1998.
12. Richardson J: Permethrin spot-on toxicoses in cats, *JVECCS* 10(2):103–106, 2000.

Ricin

E. Murl Bailey Jr., DVM, PhD, DABVT

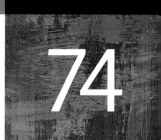

74

- Ricin is the toxic principle isolated from the castor bean plant, *Ricinus communis* (Color Plate 74-1).
- The median oral lethal dose (LD_{50}) is thought to be 20 mg/kg in dogs and cats.
- Clinical signs may be delayed 8 to 24 hours post exposure. Initial signs post inhalation include anorexia and respiratory distress, developing into pulmonary edema. Oral exposures lead to gastrointestinal signs, including diarrhea, abdominal pain, anorexia, and vomiting with or without blood. Seizures are possible.
- Diagnosis is based on history; physical examination findings; biochemical alterations, with increases in ALT, AST, BUN, and creatinine; and ricin residue testing.
- There are no antidotes, and treatment is largely supportive. Patients exposed orally should be decontaminated with emesis induction and dosed with activated charcoal.
- Lesions after oral or intramuscular exposure include hemorrhagic gastroenteritis and hepatic, renal, and splenic necrosis. Fibrino-purulent pneumonia, diffuse necrosis and acute inflammation of airways, alveolar flooding with peribronchial vascular edema, and purulent mediastinal lymphadenitis are seen following inhalation exposures.

Sources

Ricin is a naturally occurring toxin isolated from the castor bean plant (*Ricinus communis*).[1-3] The ricin concentration in the plant is approximately 1% to 5% by weight. Approximately 1 million tons of castor beans are processed annually in the production of castor oil for lubrication and medicinal purposes.[1,4]

Ricin is a large glycoprotein that is a water-soluble white powder in pure form, stable under ambient temperature conditions, but heat labile.[2,5] Heating the compound to 80° C for 10 minutes or 50° C for 50 minutes effectively inactivates the protein. Ricin has a molecular weight of 66 kDa, which is slightly smaller than albumin, and consists of two chains, A and B.[6,7] Two hemagglutinins are associated with ricin, but their significance is unknown.[4]

Ricin is easily obtained in small or large quantities throughout the world. It is a potential terrorist weapon, but not likely a chemical warfare agent because large quantities would be required in an aerosol form.[8-10] It could be used to contaminate food or small bodies of water, but aerosolization would be required in most potential terrorist or weapons of mass destruction activities.[4] Ricin has been used for assassination and suicidal activities in humans.[11] Toxicities have been associated with accidental ingestions of castor beans in humans, dogs, and horses.[12-18] Ricin occurs as a residual product from the plant material after oil extraction, which would require additional purification before use.[2,12,18] The residual "cake" is used in some parts of the world for fertilizer and cattle feed, but the latter is used only after heat treatment.[2,18] Castor oil does not contain ricin and is used for lubricants and as an irritant laxative and rodent repellent.[7,18]

Toxic Dose

The toxic or lethal dose of ricin depends on the species exposed and the route of exposure.[7] There is greater than a 100-fold difference between susceptibility of various species.[13] The oral lethal dose of seed material (assuming 1% to 5% ricin concentration) has been reported for the following species: chicken = 14 g/kg (140 to 170 mg ricin/kg); swine = 1.3 g/kg (13 to 65 mg ricin/kg); rabbit = 0.9 g/kg (9 to 45 mg ricin/kg); and horse = 0.1 g/kg (1 to 5 mg ricin/kg).[2,7] The reported toxic oral doses of pure ricin are mouse = 20 mg/kg (LD_{50}); horse = 1 to 5 mg/kg; dog = unknown, but probably similar to mouse; and in humans it is speculated that the lethal dose is 1.0 mg/kg, but some authors question if ricin is that toxic to humans.[2,7,19]

The intravenous toxic doses of ricin have been reported as being 5 mcg/kg (LD_{50}) for mice, with the minimum lethal dose varying from 0.7 to 2.7 mcg/kg; in humans it is unknown, but 1 to 10 mcg/kg is the suggested toxic dose, and the MLD in the dog is 1.6 to 1.75 mcg/kg.[2,7,20] The inhalation toxic doses are 3 to 5 mcg/kg (LD_{50}) in mice, and 21 to 42 mcg/kg is the reported lethal dose in monkeys.[7,21] The intraperitoneal LD_{50} in mice is 22 mcg/kg.[7] Subcutaneous or intramuscular toxicity of ricin ranges from 24 mcg/kg (LD_{50}) in mice, 33 to 50 mcg/kg in rats (lethal dose), and 70 mcg/kg is apparently a lethal dose in humans, but an individual receiving an estimated 140 mcg/kg survived with hospitalization.[2,7]

Toxicokinetics

Ricin is a large protein molecule, which is poorly absorbed from the gastrointestinal tract.[7] After an oral exposure, most of the ricin is found in the large intestine 24 hours after ingestion, illustrating the limited systemic uptake of the protein.[2] Based on mouse toxicity (LD_{50}) data, approximately 0.025% of the ingested ricin is absorbed following oral administration, but other work has shown that up to 0.27% of the ingested ricin may be absorbed. Once absorbed, ricin most likely distributes throughout the extracellular fluid space in the body.[2,7,22] Ricin appears to be readily absorbed via the inhalation route, but dermal absorption is unlikely to occur through intact skin.[2,7] Intravenously administered ricin distributes primarily to spleen, kidneys, heart, and liver, and intramuscularly administered ricin distributes to draining lymph nodes.[2]

Mechanism of Toxicity

The B chain of ricin binds to galactoside-containing proteins on cell surfaces, which allows for the internalization of the A chain by triggering an endocytotic uptake.[2,7,13] This is the probable cause of the 8- to 24-hour latent period associated with ricin and/or castor bean intoxication because the transport may be slow in some instances.[3,7] The A-chain binds with the 28S RNA subunit of eukaryotic cells, killing the cell through the inhibition of protein synthesis.[7] Ricin has also been shown to disturb calcium homeostasis in the heart, leading to myocardial necrosis and cardiac hemorrhage. Ricin may target Kupffer cells, which gives rise to the hepatotoxicity that is often reported.[2,22] It has been speculated that the lesions seen in ricin and/or castor bean intoxications may be due to effects on endothelial cells, causing fluid and protein leakage along with tissue edema.[2] Inhaled ricin binds to ciliated bronchiolar lining cells, alveolar macrophages, and alveolar lining cells.[7] It is of note that castor beans and leaves also contain a pyridine compound, ricinin, which may cause neuromuscular weakness as a result of an interference with acetylcholine binding at nicotinic receptor sites.[23]

Clinical Signs

The clinical signs associated with ricin exposure vary with the dose and route of exposure. With respiratory and/or inhalation exposures, there may be a preclinical dose-dependent delay of 8 to 24 hours (reported in rats and primates) before the onset of the clinical syndrome.[7,24] Anorexia subsequently develops, and there is a progressive decrease in physical activity, probably caused by developing hypoxemia and the generalized toxic cellular effects of ricin.[7] Respiratory distress starts developing, and there are increased inflammatory cell counts and increased protein from bronchiolar lavage at 12 hours post exposure. At 18 hours post exposure, alveolar flooding and pulmonary edema develop, and at 30 hours post exposure, severe arterial hypoxemia and acidosis are present. In humans a primary allergic syndrome has been reported in workers exposed to castor bean dust, but this type of syndrome has not been reported in animals.[2,7] Postmortem airway and pulmonary lesions associated with inhalation exposure to ricin include marked to severe fibrino-purulent pneumonia, diffuse necrosis and acute inflammation of airways, alveolar flooding and peribronchial vascular edema, acute tracheitis, and marked to severe purulent mediastinal lymphadenitis. The lung lesions are sufficiently severe to cause death. Adrenalitis and hepatic lesions may or may not be present.[25]

Oral exposure to castor beans has been reported in dogs and humans.[12,14-17] It should be noted that the beans must be broken or masticated for the ricin to be released.[12,16] There may be a latent period of 8 to 24 hours following oral exposures to either ricin or castor beans. The gastrointestinal signs, which typically develop, include vomiting with or without blood, depression, diarrhea (with or without blood), abdominal pain, and anorexia.[12,15,16]

In humans there have been cases of intramuscular exposure to ricin and castor beans.[7,11] The initial signs have included localized pain and muscular weakness within 5 hours of exposure. Fifteen to 24 hours after exposure, high body temperatures, nausea and vomiting, tachycardia with normal blood pressures, swollen regional lymph nodes, induration at the injection site, and leukocytosis (26,000/mm^3) have developed in these individuals. Forty-eight hours after exposure, hypotension, tachycardia, and vascular collapse developed in these individuals. At 72 hours, anuria, vomiting blood, complete AV conduction block, and a white blood cell count of 33,200/mm^3 developed in these individuals. Death occurred very rapidly in spite of heroic resuscitation efforts.

Minimum Database

The development of abnormal organ-specific biochemical values may not occur for 12 to 24 hours after exposure. The minimum database to be developed in cases of suspected exposure to ricin or castor beans should include serum alanine transaminase (ALT), serum aspartate transaminase (AST), blood urea nitrogen (BUN), serum creatinine, complete blood cell count, packed cell volume, and total serum protein.

Confirmatory Tests

Analytical methods exist for ricin, and they are now available at some state veterinary diagnostic toxicology laboratories. The analytical method is based on using the alkaloid, ricinine, as a marker.[14]

Treatment

There are no currently available postingestion antidotes for ricin, but pre- and postexposure protocols are being explored. These protocols include prophylactic immunization technologies along with postexposure protocols using liposome encapsulated N-acetylcysteine and lactose glycopolomers.[26-28] Normal therapy for oral exposures should include induction of emesis if indicated, administration of activated charcoal (1 to 5 g/kg in a slurry), a cathartic (magnesium sulfate [250 mg/kg, PO] or sorbitol [70%, 1-3 mL/kg, PO]) unless the animal already has diarrhea, and the placement of at least one indwelling catheter for fluid therapy and other supportive medications. The hypotension, which normally develops, should be treated vigorously as in any emergency situation.[1] Any seizures should be treated with diazepam (0.5 to 1 mg/kg, IV). Sucralfate (0.25 to 1 g, PO, tid) should be used as needed. The affected animals should be fed a soft, bland diet.

Prognosis

It is interesting to note that in 98 dog cases reported over an 11-year period, clinical signs developed in 76% of the cases, but only seven died or 7.1% of total cases or 9% of those cases in which signs developed (three were euthanized for a true case fatality rate of 5%).[12] In more than 751 human cases of castor bean ingestion, 14 died, for a 1.8% fatality rate.[16]

Gross and Histologic Lesions

Lesions caused by ingested ricin or castor beans include hepatic necrosis, splenic necrosis, and renal necrosis, along with hemorrhagic gastroenteritis.[7,17,18] The lesions reported following intramuscular ricin exposure in humans include severe local lymphoid necrosis, gastrointestinal hemorrhage, hepatic necrosis, diffuse splenitis, and mild to moderate pulmonary edema. Similar lesions have been reported in experimental animals.[4,21]

Differential Diagnoses

The differential diagnoses could be many, depending on the locale. Those which should be included are garbage poisoning, any other intoxications resulting in gastrointestinal distress (e.g., zinc phosphide, *Abrus precatorius*—precatory bean, inorganic arsenic, lead, inorganic mercury, thallium, and deoxynivalenol [DON, vomitoxin] and numerous bacterial, viral, neoplastic, and inflammatory gastrointestinal insults.

References

1. Audi J, Belson M, Patel M, et al: Ricin poisoning: a comprehensive review, *JAMA* 294(19):2342–2351, 2005.
2. Bradberry SM, Dickers KJ, Rice P, et al: Ricin poisoning, *Toxicol Rev* 22:65, 2003.
3. Doan LG: Ricin: Mechanism of toxicity, clinical manifestation, and vaccine development. A review, *J Toxicol Clin Toxicol* 42(2):201–208, 2004.
4. Franz DR, Jaax NK: Ricin toxin. In Sidell FR, Takafuji ET, Franz DR, editors: *Medical aspects of chemical and biological warfare*, Washington, DC, 1997, Office of the Surgeon General at TMM Publications, Borden Institute, Walter Reed Army Medical Center.
5. Spivak L, Hendrickson RG: Ricin, *Crit Care Clin* 21:815–824, 2005.
6. Bigalke H, Rummel A: Medical aspects of toxin weapons, *Toxicology* 214:210–220, 2005.
7. Greenfield RA, Brown BR, Hutchins JB, et al: Microbiological, biological and chemical weapons of warfare and terrorism, *Am J Med Sci* 323:326, 2002.
8. Kuca K, Pohanka M: Chemical warfare agents, *EXS* 100:543–558, 2010.
9. Rosenbloom M, Leikin JB, Vogel SN, et al: Biological and chemical agents: a brief synopsis, *Am J Therap* 9:5, 2002.
10. Schep LJ, Temple WA, Butt GA, Beasley MD: Ricin as a weapon of mass terror—separating fact from fiction, *Environ Int* 35:1267–1271, 2009.
11. Passeron T, Mantoux F, Lacour JP, et al: Infectious and toxic cellulitis due to suicide attempt by subcutaneous injection of ricin, *Brit J Derm* 150:154, 2004.
12. Albretsen JC, Gwaltney-Brant SM, Khan SA: Evaluation of castor bean toxicosis in dogs: 98 cases, *JAAHA* 35:229, 2000.
13. Balint GA: Ricin: the toxic protein of castor oil seeds, *Toxicol* 2:77, 1974.
14. Mouser P, Filigenzi MS, Puschner B, et al: Fatal ricin toxicosis in a puppy confirmed by liquid chromatography/mass spectrometry when using ricinine as a marker, *J Vet Diagn Invest* 19:216–220, 2007.
15. Palatnick W, Tenenbein M: Hepatotoxicity from castor bean ingestion in a child, *Clin Tox* 38:67, 2000.
16. Rauber A, Heard J: Castor bean toxicity re-examined: a new perspective, *Vet Hum Toxicol* 27:498, 1985.
17. Roels S, Coopman V, Vanhaelen P, Cordonnier J: Lethal ricin intoxication in two adult dogs: toxicologic and histopathologic findings, *J Vet Diagn Invest* 22:466–468, 2010.

18. Soto-Blanco B, Sinhorini IL, Gorniak SL, et al: Ricinus communis poisoning in a dog, *Vet Hum Toxicol* 44:155, 2002.
19. Lim H, Kim HJ, Cho YS: A case of ricin poisoning following ingestion of Korean castor bean, *Emerg Med J* 26(4):301–302, 2009.
20. Fodstad O, Johannessen JV, Schjerven L, et al: Toxicity of abrin and ricin in mice & dogs, *J Tox Env Health* 5:1073–1084, 1979.
21. Wilhelmsen C, Pitt M: Lesions of acute inhaled lethal ricin intoxication in Rhesus monkeys (Abstract), *Vet Pathol* 30(5):482, 1993.
22. Ishiguro M, Tanabe S, Matori Y, et al: Biochemical studies on oral toxicity or ricin. IV. A fate of orally administered ricin in rats, *J Pharmacobio-Dyn* 15:147–156, 1992.
23. Burrows GE, Tyrl RJ: *Toxic plants of North America*, Ames, IA, 2001, Iowa State University Press.
24. Hong IH, Kwon TE, Lee SK, et al: Fetal death of dogs after the ingestion of a soil container, *Exp Toxicol Pathol* 63:113–117, 2011.
25. Benson JM, Gomez AP, Wolf ML, et al: The acute toxicity, tissue distribution, and histopathology of inhaled ricin in Sprague Dawley rats and BALB/c mice, *Inhal Toxicol* 23(5):247–256, 2011.
26. Griffiths GD, Phillips GJ, Holley J: Inhalation toxicology of ricin preparations: animal models, prophylactic and therapeutic approaches to protection, *Inhal Toxicol* 19:873–887, 2007.
27. Nagatsuka T, Uzawa H, Ohsawa I, et al: Use of lactose against the deadly biological toxin ricin, *ACS Appl Mater Interfaces* 2(4):1081–1085, 2010.
28. Ramasamy S, et al: Ricin (a brief summary), *Br J Pharmacol* 161:721–748, 2010.

Snake Bite: North American Pit Vipers

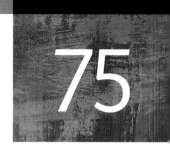

75

Michael E. Peterson, DVM, MS

- Pit viper venoms are a complex combination of enzymatic and nonenzymatic proteins that elicit a wide array of physiological problems.
- Clinical signs can be quite varied and can range from mild to severe localized tissue reactions at the bite site to severe systemic problems.
- A minimum database should include complete blood cell count, serum chemistry panel, urinalysis, and coagulation profile.
- Treatment options, depending on the clinical presentation, may include hospitalization (minimum of 8 hours), IV fluid therapy, antibiotics, and antivenom.
- Prognosis is highly variable and depends on the toxicity of the venom, dose, bite site, and victim's response.

Sources

Two families of poisonous snakes, the Elapidae and Crotalidae, populate many portions of the United States. The Crotalids are represented by the pit vipers and are found throughout most of the United States. Every state except Maine, Alaska, and Hawaii is home to at least one species of venomous snake.

Pit vipers are the largest group of venomous snakes in the United States and are involved in an estimated 150,000 bites annually of dogs and cats.[1] Approximately 99% of all venomous snake bites in the United States are inflicted by pit vipers. In North America, members of the family Crotalidae belong to three genera: the rattlesnakes (*Crotalus* and *Sistrurus* spp.) and the copperheads and cottonmouth water moccasins (*Agkistrodon* spp.).

Pit vipers can be identified by their characteristic retractable front fangs (Color Plate 75-1), bilateral heat-sensing "pits" between the nostrils and eyes (Color Plate 75-2), elliptical pupils, a single row of subcaudal scales distal to the anal plate, and triangular-shaped heads (Figure 75-1). Those members of the *Crotalus* and *Sistrurus* genera (the rattlesnakes) have special keratin rattles on the ends of their tails, with the exception of one subspecies (*C. catalinensis*). *Agkistrodon* species, the copperheads and water moccasins, are found throughout the eastern and central United States. Copperheads are responsible for the majority of venomous snake bites to humans in North America because of their proclivity for living next to human habitation. Water moccasins can be pugnacious and have a greater tendency to deliver venom when they bite. Rattlesnakes (*Crotalus* spp., *Sistrurus* spp.) are found throughout the continental United States and account for the majority of deaths in both human and animal victims. Clinicians should become familiar with their regional indigenous poisonous snake species.

Ninety percent of venomous snake bites occur during the months of April through October. Two thirds of the bites are inflicted by snakes less than 20 inches in length.

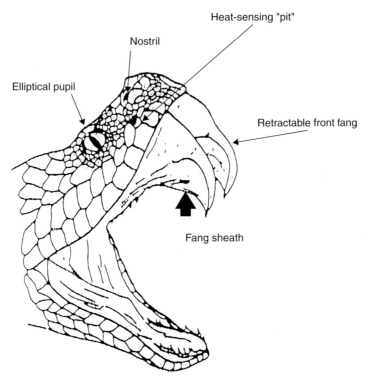

Figure 75-1 Anatomy of a pit viper.

The heat-sensing pit located between the eye and the nostril can differentiate a temperature gradient of 0.003° C at a distance of 14 inches. These snakes can strike approximately one half of their body length at a speed of 8 ft/second. The number of puncture wounds from a single bite can be one to six because several ancillary fangs can rotate forward with the strike. Rattlesnakes do not always rattle before striking.

Based on clinical observations, it was once thought that pit viper venom was more toxic in the hotter months of the year. However, when individual snake venoms were analyzed, no seasonal variation in patterns of venom proteins was evident over any period of time. The venom is not considered more toxic in the summer months; however, snakes show increased aggression and venom yield with environmental warming and an increased photoperiod (as in the spring and summer).[2] The maximum venom yields occur during the hottest months of summer.

Pit vipers control the amount of venom that they inject during a bite. The amount of venom injected depends on the snake's perception of the situation. Initial defensive strikes are often nonenvenomating. Offensive bites meter a given amount of venom into the victim, and agonal bites deliver the entire venom load and are therefore the most dangerous. A decapitated snake head can bite reflexively for up to an hour after decapitation.

Toxic Dose

The severity of any pit viper bite is related to the volume and toxicity of the venom injected and to the location of the bite, which may influence the rate of venom uptake. As a generalization, the toxicity of pit viper venoms ranges in descending order from the rattlesnakes to the water moccasins and then to the copperheads (Table 75-1). The toxicity of rattlesnake

Table 75-1	Venom Yields of North American Snakes		
Snake Species		Dry Weight (mg venom)	LD$_{50}$ IV (mice)
Eastern diamondback (*Crotalus adamanteus*)		200-850	1.68
Western diamondback (*Crotalus atrox*)		175-800	2.18
Mojave rattlesnake (*Crotalus scutulatus*)		75-150	0.23
Eastern coral (*Micrurus fulvius*)		2-20	0.28
Copperhead (*Agkistrodon contortrix*)		40-75	10.92
Cottonmouth (*Agkistrodon piscivorus*)		90-170	4.19

Box 75-1	Examples of Enzymes from Pit Viper Venoms

Arginine ester hydrolase
Proteolytic enzymes
Thrombin-like enzyme
Collagenase
Hyaluronidase
Phospholipase A$_2$
Phospholipase B
Phosphomonoesterase
Phosphodiesterase
Acetylcholinesterase
RNAse
DNAse
5′-Nucleotidase
NAD-nucleotidase
Lactate dehydrogenase
L-Amino acid oxidase

venom varies widely. Nine species and 12 subspecies of rattlesnakes have populations with venoms containing proteins that are immunologically similar to the potent neurotoxin, Mojave toxin. It is possible for pit viper venom to be strictly neurotoxic with virtually no local signs of envenomation. Examples of these venom types are certain subpopulations of rattlesnakes: Mojave rattlesnakes (*C. scutulatus*), canebrake rattlesnakes (*C. horridus atricaudatus*), and tiger rattlesnakes (*C. tigris*).[3-5]

Toxicokinetics

It may take weeks for all venom fractions to be cleared by the body. Because of the complexity of the venom, the victim's metabolic response to the venom components varies with the species of snake, the volume of venom injected, and the species of the bite recipient.

Mechanism of Toxicity

Pit viper venoms are a complex combination of enzymatic and nonenzymatic proteins (Box 75-1). The primary purpose of the venom is not to kill but rather to immobilize the prey and predigest its tissue. The venom is derived from modified salivary glands. The venom is 90% water and has a minimum of 10 enzymes and 3 to 12 nonenzymatic proteins and peptides in any individual snake. The nonenzymatic components, called the "killing fraction," have a median lethal dose (LD$_{50}$) more than 50 times smaller than that of the crude venom.

More than 60 purified polypeptides have been identified in crotalid venoms. Approximately 50 enzymatic crotalid venom fractions have been characterized. Proteolytic trypsin-like enzymes, which are catalyzed by metals (e.g., calcium, magnesium, and zinc), are common constituents of pit viper venom and cause marked tissue destruction. Arginine ester hydrolase is a bradykinin-releasing agent that may adversely affect clotting activity. Thrombin-like enzymes also can mediate increased clotting activity. The eastern diamondback rattlesnake (*C. adamanteus*) venom enzyme, protease H, induces systemic hemorrhage.[6] Five proteolytic toxins from western diamondback rattlesnake (*C. atrox*) venom induce hemorrhage by cleaving laminin and the basement membrane at band A.[7,8] Crotavirin, found in prairie rattlesnake (*C. viridis viridis*) venom, is a potent platelet aggregation inhibitor and prevents platelet-collagen interaction by binding to collagen fibers. Interference with the platelet-collagen interaction has the net effect of blocking collagen-mediated platelet functions, such as adhesion, release reaction, thromboxane formation, and aggregation.[9] The preponderant mechanism of afibrinogenemia seen in a patient after western diamondback rattlesnake (*C. atrox*) envenomation is a reflection of fibrinogenolysis and not a primary consumptive coagulopathy. The fibrinogenolysis results from indirect activation of plasminogen by vascular plasminogen activator.[10]

Differences in venom within a species induced by the age of the snake are highlighted by a study of northern Pacific rattlesnakes (*Crotalus viridis organus*) in which the adult venoms were shown to have approximately fivefold higher fibrinogenolytic protease activity. Two protease bands were identified in juvenile and subadult snakes, and four bands were identified in adult venom using gel filtration.[11] Zinc metalloproteinase with fibrinolytic activity has been isolated from the venom of copperheads (*Agkistrodon contortrix*) and is called *fibrolase*. A specific fibrolase cleavage site is in the alpha chain of fibrin. The complexity of the issue of variation of venom components is highlighted by the differences found in fibrinolysis and complement inactivation of venoms from different blacktail rattlesnakes (*Crotalus molossus molossus*). In a study of 72 individual blacktail rattlesnake venoms, the following conclusion was made: there were no venom differences as a function of geographic distribution; however, individual venom variability was significant enough to be identified as an important clinical reality.[12]

Hyaluronidase, present in most venom, catalyzes the cleavage of internal glycoside bonds and mucopolysaccharides, leading to decreases in the viscosity of connective tissue. Hyaluronidase is commonly called the "spreading factor" since this breakdown facilitates the penetration of other venom components into the tissue. Collagenase is also found in venom, and its major function is to digest collagen, thereby breaking down connective tissue.

The enzyme phospholipase A is distributed throughout pit viper venoms. This enzyme catalyzes the hydrolysis of fatty ester linkages in diacyl phosphatides, which form lysophosphatides and release unsaturated and saturated fatty acids. There are many antigenically different isoenzymes. Some controversy exists about the extent of any neurotoxic effects that these isoenzymes may possess. Many cellular substances may be released by this enzyme, including histamine, kinins, slow-reacting substance, serotonin, and acetylcholine. The extent of the release of these physiologically active compounds most likely depends on the ability of phospholipase A to degrade membranes. The enzyme, phospholipase B, may also be present and is responsible for hydrolyzing lysophosphatides. The phosphodiesterases, such as diester phosphohydrolase, break free the 5'-mononucleotide, thereby attacking DNA and RNA and derivatives of arabinose. L-Amino acid oxidase catalyzes oxidation of L-alpha-amino acids and L-alpha-hydroxy acids. This is the most active of the known amino acid oxidases and has been found in all pit viper venoms studied; it is responsible for the yellow color of the venom. Nicotinamide adenine dinucleotide (NAD)-nucleotidase is found in *Agkistrodon* but not *Crotalus* venom. The enzyme catalyzes hydrolysis of nicotinamide N-ribosidic linkages of NAD, forming adenosine diphosphate riboside and nicotinamide. Other enzymes that are possibly present in viper venom include RNAse, DNAse, 5'-nucleotidase, and lactate dehydrogenase. Direct cardiotoxic effects of venom proteins have been exhibited in some pit viper venoms, particularly the diamondback rattlesnakes.

A key point is that the envenomation syndrome reflects the complexity of the venom. The body has to respond to the effects of multiple venom fractions, metabolize each, and deal with the resultant myriad of metabolites. In addition to the individual pharmacologic properties of these proteins and their metabolites, it has been demonstrated that some components act synergistically in producing specific effects or reactions. The net effect of this interaction of venom with the victim's response is a metabolic stew of toxic peptides and digestive enzymes. Additionally the traditional categorization of pit vipers as having only hematotoxic venoms should be reevaluated because some subpopulations of rattlesnakes possess only neurotoxic venom.

The average rattlesnake needs 21 days to replenish expended venom. The "lethal fraction" peptides are the first to regenerate. This adds yet another variable to any given envenomation.

Clinical Signs

The onset of clinical signs after a snake bite may be delayed for several hours (Box 75-2). In humans it is estimated that 20% of all pit viper bites are nonenvenomating (i.e., dry), with an additional 25% classified as mild envenomations. It is for this reason that so many antidotal treatments are championed, and it also emphasizes the necessity to rely on scientific evaluation for the various treatment modalities proposed.

Every pit viper envenomation is different for many reasons (Box 75-3). The severity of an envenomation is additionally altered by factors such as species of victim, body mass, location of bite, postbite excitability, and use of premedications (e.g., nonsteroidal antiinflammatory drugs in older dogs that may make the dog more susceptible to clotting defects). The snake affects the severity of the envenomation by species and size of snake, age of snake, motivation of snake, and degree of venom regeneration since last use (Color Plate 75-3).

Cats are more resistant, on the basis of milligram of venom per kilogram body mass, to pit viper venom than dogs. However, cats are generally presented to veterinary care facilities in a more advanced clinical condition. This is probably caused by the cat's smaller body size and the proclivity of cats to play with the snake, thereby antagonizing it and inducing an offensive strike, often to the torso. Additionally, cats commonly run off and hide after being bitten before they return home to allow the owner to identify the injury, thus delaying the time from bite to veterinary care. Because dogs generally receive more defensive strikes, have a larger body mass, and more frequently seek immediate human companionship after injury, they are more likely to receive medical attention promptly.

It is possible that a life-threatening envenomation may occur with no local clinical signs other than the puncture wounds themselves. This seems particularly true of those snake species with primary neurotoxic venoms (Box 75-4). Local tissue reactions to pit viper envenomation include puncture wounds, one to six from a single bite, which may be bleeding. Occasionally these fang wounds appear as small lacerations. Rarely, local swelling can obscure puncture wounds from small snakes. Rapid onset of pain may ensue with development of progressive edema. Ecchymosis and petechiation may become evident. Tissue necrosis may occur, particularly in envenomations to areas without a significant subcutaneous tissue mass. The presence of fang marks does not indicate that envenomation has occurred, only that a bite has taken place. It must be reiterated that the severity of local signs does not necessarily reflect the severity of the systemic envenomation.

Systemic clinical manifestations encompass a wide variety of problems, including pain, weakness, dizziness, nausea, severe hypotension, thrombocytopenia, fasciculations, regional lymphadenopathy, alterations in respiratory rate, increased clotting times, decreased hemoglobin, abnormal electrocardiogram, increased salivation, echinocytosis of red cells, cyanosis, proteinuria, bleeding (e.g., melena, hematuria, and hematemesis), obtundation, and convulsions. Not all of these clinical manifestations are seen in each patient, and they are listed in descending order of frequency as seen in human victims.

Severe hypotension results from pooling of blood within the shock organ of the species bitten (i.e., the hepatosplanchnic [dogs] or pulmonary [cats] vascular bed) and fluid loss from the vascular compartment secondary to severe peripheral swelling. This swelling can be great. A 2-cm increase in the circumference of a human's swelling thigh can incorporate one third of the patient's circulating fluid volume.[13] Often this swelling is not edema but extravascularized blood, resulting from damage to blood vessel walls as a result of swelling and rupturing of the endothelial cells of the microvasculature, leaving large gaps in the vessel walls.

The victim's clotting anomalies largely depend on the species of snake involved (Figure 75-2). Coagulopathies range from direct blockage or inactivation of various factors in the patient's clotting cascade to the possible destruction of megakaryocytes in the circulating blood and bone marrow (Box 75-5). A coagulopathy, with prolonged clotting times, develops in approximately 60% of envenomated patients; by far the most common is hypofibrinogenemia. Venom-induced thrombocytopenia occurs in approximately 30% of envenomations with an untreated nadir usually occurring between 72 and 96 hours. Some venom fractions inhibit platelet adhesion. Other pit viper venoms do not affect clotting itself but rather destroy clots once they are formed by initiating aggressive fibrinolysis. Syndromes resembling diffuse intravascular coagulation (DIC) are possible with pit viper envenomations.

Myokymia, a type of fasciculation of various muscle groups, is frequently reported in humans after bites received by timber rattlesnakes (*Crotalus horridus horridus*) and Western diamondback rattlesnakes (*Crotalus atrox*).[14]

> **Box 75-4** Species of Rattlesnakes That Have Populations Containing Neurotoxin
>
> *Crotalus durissus durissus*
> *Crotalus durissus terrificus* var. *cumanensis*
> *Crotalus durissus terrificus* (Brazil)
> *Crotalus horridus atricaudatus*
> *Crotalus lepidus klauberi*
> *Crotalus mitchellii mitchellii*
> *Crotalus tigris*
> *Crotalus vegrandis*
> *Crotalus viridis abyssus*
> *Crotalus viridis concolor*
> *Crotalus scutulatus scutulatus* (venom A)
> *Crotalus scutulatus salvini*
> *Sistrurus catenatus catenatus*

Minimum Database

Monitoring the severity and progression of the clinical envenomation syndrome

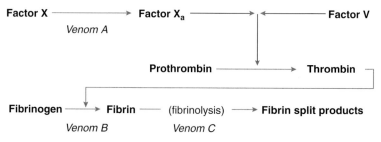

Figure 75-2 Venom effects on clotting mechanisms.

Box 75-5	Pit Viper
Envenomations: Hemostatic Defects	

Consumption coagulopathy
Diffuse vascular damage
DIC-like syndrome
Localized massive clotting
Hyperfibrinolysis
Thrombocytopenia (independent from
    consumption coagulopathy above)
Blood vessel injury

may be difficult. A tool that has proven useful is the envenomation severity score system (Box 75-6). Use of this system more accurately quantifies the severity of the patient's condition over time and allows a more objective assessment of the patient.[15] It is recommended that a severity score be assessed on entry, 6 hours, 12 hours, and 24 hours after initial hospitalization.

A complete blood cell count with differential, including platelet counts, should be obtained; red blood cell morphology along with baseline serum chemistry with electrolytes should be collected. A coagulation profile should be obtained, including activated clotting times, prothrombin time (PT), activated partial thromboplastin time (PTT), fibrinogen, and fibrin degradation products. Urinalysis with macroscopic and microscopic evaluations, including free protein and hemoglobin and myoglobin, should be performed. An electrocardiogram may be indicated in animals with significant envenomations. These laboratory tests should be repeated periodically to monitor the progression of the syndrome and/or the effectiveness of therapy.

Significant rhabdomyolysis may also be seen with large increases in creatine phosphokinase and urine myoglobin levels, particularly in envenomations by snakes with potent neurotoxins (e.g., Mojave, canebreak, and tiger rattlesnakes). Tiger rattlesnake venom (*Crotalus tigris*) has been characterized as having a low protease activity, no hemolytic activity, and toxins that have complete immunoidentity with the potent neurotoxins, crotoxin and Mojave toxin.[3]

Circumferential measurements of the affected body part at, above, and below the bite site at set time intervals aid in objective monitoring of the progression of the swelling secondary to many pit viper bites. Transient (within 48 hours) echinocytosis has been reported in dogs after envenomation, and its presence is an indicator of envenomation. However, absence of this morphological change is not evidence of lack of envenomation.[16]

Hypokalemia has been reported subsequent to pit viper envenomations.[16] In one series, potassium levels of less than 3.5 mEq/L were observed in 11% of 97 pit viper envenomated dogs.[17] It is postulated that this decrease is secondary to the release of epinephrine by the patient, inducing serum insulin elevation and thereby driving potassium into the cells. This is a transient phenomenon, which corrects with intravenous (IV) fluid and antivenom administration.

Confirmatory Tests

There are no diagnostic tests that can definitively confirm that a pit viper bite has occurred.

Treatment

Although many first-aid measures have been advocated for pit viper bite victims, none has been shown to prevent morbidity or mortality.[18] Long-term follow-up of pit viper–envenomated human patients has revealed that the majority of individuals with permanent loss of motion of the affected area or other negative sequelae had received some form of traditional first aid (e.g., cut and suck, constriction bands, and so on).[19] The primary rule of first aid is to do no additional harm. One human study followed 147 patients who had received first aid and 78 who had not; there was no evidence that first-aid treatment had made any difference in the patients' short-term outcome.[20]

First-aid measures to be avoided include ice, incision and suction, tourniquets (which constriction bands quickly become with progressive limb swelling), and hot packs (Box 75-7). Electroshock has been definitively shown to be ineffective in the treatment of pit viper envenomations and should not be attempted.[21,22] Current recommendations for

Box 75-6	Snakebite Severity Score System

Pulmonary System

Signs within normal limits	0
Minimal—slight dyspnea	1
Moderate—respiratory compromise, tachypnea, use of accessory muscles	2
Severe—cyanosis, air hunger, extreme tachypnea, respiratory insufficiency or respiratory arrest from any cause	3

Cardiovascular System

Signs within normal limits	0
Minimal—tachycardia, general weakness, benign dysrhythmia, hypertension	1
Moderate—tachycardia, hypotension (but tarsal pulse still palpable)	2
Severe—extreme tachycardia, hypotension (nonpalpable tarsal pulse or systolic blood pressure <80 mm Hg), malignant dysrhythmia or cardiac arrest	3

Local Wound

Signs within normal limits	0
Minimal—pain, swelling, ecchymosis, erythema limited to bite site	1
Moderate—pain, swelling, ecchymosis, erythema involves less than half of extremity and may be spreading slowly	2
Severe—pain, swelling, ecchymosis, erythema involves most or all of one extremity and is spreading rapidly	3
Very severe—pain, swelling, ecchymosis, erythema extends beyond affected extremity, or significant tissue slough	4

Gastrointestinal System

Signs within normal limits	0
Minimal—abdominal pain, tenesmus	1
Moderate—vomiting, diarrhea	2
Severe—repetitive vomiting, diarrhea, or hematemesis	3

Hematological System

Signs within normal limits	0
Minimal—coagulation values slightly abnormal, PT <20 sec, PTT <50 sec, platelets 100,000-150,000/mm^3	1
Moderate—coagulation values abnormal, PT 20-50 sec, PTT 50-75 sec, platelets 50,000-100,000/mm^3	2
Severe—coagulation values abnormal, PT 50-100 sec, PTT 75-100 sec, platelets 20,000-50,000/mm^3	3

Box 75-6	Snakebite Severity Score System—cont'd	
Very severe—coagulation values markedly abnormal with bleeding present or the threat of spontaneous bleeding, including PT unmeasurable, PTT unmeasurable, platelets <20,000/mm^3		4
Central Nervous System		
Signs within normal limits		0
Minimal—apprehension		1
Moderate—chills, weakness, faintness, ataxia		2
Severe—lethargy, seizures, coma		3
Total Score Possible		**0-20**

Box 75-7	First-Aid Measures to Avoid
1. Ice, cold packs, or sprays 2. Incision and suction 3. Tourniquets 4. Administration of aspirin or tranquilizers 5. Waiting to see how significant the envenomation is before seeking medical care 6. Electroshock 7. Hot packs	

Box 75-8	Pit Viper Envenomation Treatment Outline
1. Aggressive IV fluid therapy 2. Early IV antivenom administration 3. Monitoring of hemostasis and biochemical profiles 4. Antibiotic administration	

first aid in the field are to keep the victim calm, keep the bite site below heart level if possible, and transport the victim to a veterinary medical facility for primary medical intervention. The patient should be hospitalized and monitored closely for a minimum of 8 hours for the onset of signs of envenomation. A severity score sheet should be recorded upon entry and at 6 hours after hospitalization at a minimum for every suspected snake bite victim. This advice cannot be overemphasized because the onset of clinical signs may be significantly delayed. One report in a human victim described resolution of mild swelling over 3 hours, at which time the patient was discharged. The patient returned to the emergency department 12 hours later with severe pain and swelling and a marked coagulopathy.[23] The effects of snake venom are time dependent; any delay in initiating medical treatment is deleterious to the patient and may result in complications that cannot be corrected.

The initial medical response to a snake-bitten patient is to collect the appropriate pretreatment laboratory samples and make circumferential measurements at, above, and below the bite site to allow quantitative monitoring of the progression of swelling. An IV catheter should be placed and a crystalloid fluid drip started.

The only proven specific therapy against pit viper envenomation is the administration of antivenom.[24-27] Coagulation deficits, fluid loss, changes in neurological status, cardiac conduction abnormalities, and the necrotizing effect of the venom can be dramatically reversed when antivenom treatment is initiated appropriately (Box 75-8).

In North America polyvalent antivenom, which is effective against the venoms of all endemic pit viper species, is used. This polyvalent equine origin antivenin (Crotalidae) is made and marketed to the veterinary community by Boehringer-Ingelheim (Ridgefield, CT). The antivenom is produced by inoculating horses with the venoms collected from *Crotalus atrox* (Western diamondback rattlesnake), *Crotalus adamanteus* (Eastern diamondback rattlesnake), *Crotalus durissus terrificus* (South American rattlesnake), and *Bothrops atrox* (Fer-de-lance). Once a horse attains a certain titer, serum is harvested and processed to concentrate the antivenom immunoglobulins. The processes used to extract these proteins result in a final product, which though rich in antibodies, has a very high equine protein contaminant and albumin component, often in the range of 50%. It is these proteins that are primarily responsible for the allergic reactions that can be associated with antivenom use.

Skin testing for allergic reactions to the horse serum is difficult to evaluate in veterinary patients. Human victims of snake bites were often subjected to cutaneous hypersensitivity testing before equine origin antivenom was administered. In one study, none of 12 early (anaphylactic) reactions was predicted by this test.[28] Generally, slow administration of the antivenom initially will identify those patients who may have an allergic reaction.

Antivenom should be reconstituted with the provided diluent; saline may be added to completely fill the vial, ensuring that the antivenom is totally submerged to speed reconstitution. It can be swirled to facilitate reconstitution. This usually takes between 10 and 15 minutes. Warming the vial to body temperature aids in dissolution into the liquid state. Overheating can destroy the proteins and cause foaming, which makes it difficult to collect the antivenom into a syringe. The vial should always be rinsed with saline as a significant amount of residual antivenom remains.[29]

Antivenom should be diluted at a ratio of 1 vial to 100 to 250 mL of crystalloid fluids. In smaller patients, the clinician should adjust the fluid infusion volume to prevent fluid overload of the patient. In one report, antivenom labeled with radioactive iodine (^{131}I) was given IV, and 85% accumulated at the site of envenomation within 2 hours.[30] In contrast there was a 1.4% local concentration when it was given intramuscularly (IM) and a 5.6% local concentration when given SC. Antivenom should not be injected into the bite site, and its uptake can be delayed for up to 12 hours when it is given IM. Administration should begin slowly as an IV infusion. If there is no evidence of an allergic reaction (e.g., nausea, hyperemia of inner pinna, fluffing of tail, and pruritus), the rate of infusion can be increased. The entire initial dose should be given within 30 minutes. The patient then should be reevaluated for further progression of the envenomation syndrome using the appropriate clinical and laboratory measurements.

The dose of antivenom necessary is calculated relative to the amount of venom injected, the body mass of the victim, and the bite site. Bites to the torso, tongue, or intravascular are severe envenomations that require prompt, aggressive antivenom administration. Smaller patients may require higher doses of antivenom because the dose of venom per kilogram body weight of the victim is higher. Multiple vials may be necessary to treat severe envenomations adequately. The average dose in dogs and cats is 1 to 2 vials of antivenom.

The earlier antivenom is administered, the more effective it is. The package insert advises using it within the first 4 hours. However, the product is effective as long as active venom components are found in the bloodstream. Tissue necrosis will not be reversed once it has occurred, but additional damage may be prevented. Antivenom is extremely effective in reversing venom-induced coagulation defects. Coagulation defects can be abated several days after envenomation. If clotting defects continue to be manifest, additional antivenom should be administered. DIC-like syndromes should be treated with additional antivenom. Rattlesnake venom thrombinlike enzymes are not inhibited by heparin, and it should not be administered. Clotting anomalies secondary to envenomations are extremely difficult to reverse with blood products and transfusions.

Antivenom is extremely effective in reversing most rattlesnake venom-induced thrombocytopenias. However, in timber rattlesnake (*C. horridus*) bites, a platelet aggregating protein induces thrombocytopenia, which is resistant to antivenom administration even though PT and PTT are restored.[31] *Crotalus atrox* (Western diamondback rattlesnake) venom was detectable in the victim's urine 6 days after envenomation.[32]

Patients exhibiting allergic reactions to antivenom can still receive it if needed in severe envenomations. It can be given as a slow IV drip and piggybacked with diphenhydramine and possibly epinephrine. Data in both human envenomation and veterinary envenomation databases have not identified a significantly higher reaction rate in patients who have received antivenom previously.[17,19] Some veterinary patients have received antivenom yearly for several consecutive years without higher rates of reactions.[17]

Allergic reactions, though rare, are possible when administering antivenom. These can become manifest in one of three ways: by true anaphylaxis, an anaphylactoid reaction, and delayed serum sickness. The most common reaction to antivenom is an anaphylactoid reaction. This is a complement-mediated reaction to the rapid administration of a foreign protein, such as those seen in rapidly administered blood transfusions. Anaphylactoid reactions can usually be treated by stopping the antivenom infusion, administering diphenhydramine IV (small dogs and cats: 10 mg; large dogs: 25 to 50 mg), waiting 5 minutes, and then restarting the infusion of antivenom at a slower rate. Anaphylaxis is treated by stopping the infusion of antivenom and administering epinephrine, corticosteroids, and crystalloid fluid infusion. Patients taking beta-blockers must be monitored very closely. Beta-blockers may mask the early onset of anaphylaxis, which becomes more difficult to reverse as the reaction progresses. Delayed serum sickness is rare in dogs and cats.[33] This may be because of the smaller volumes of antivenom administered relative to those given to human patients. Onset of delayed serum sickness usually occurs 7 to 14 days after antivenom administration. If it does occur, treatment consists of antihistamines, often type 1 and type 2 inhibitors, and/or corticosteroids.

There is debate about the use of colloidal fluids in pit viper–envenomated patients because leakage of the colloid through damaged vascular walls may pull fluid out of the vascular space and into areas with rich capillary beds, such as the pulmonary tissue.

Broad-spectrum antibiotics are recommended in veterinary patients after envenomation because of the number of pathogenic bacteria found in snakes' mouths and the amount of local tissue damage at the bite site. This is an area of controversy in the therapy of human snake bite victims.[34,35]

Pain is usually controlled with the antivenom. However, in patients in which no or limited amounts of antivenom are administered, pain control may require IV narcotics during the first 24 hours. Fentanyl is preferred and can be administered as a continuous rate infusion (loading dose 2-3 mcg/kg and then 1 mcg/kg per hour). Morphine should be avoided because of its histamine-releasing activity, which may be confused with the onset of anaphylaxis. Nonsteroidal medications compound the risk of developing blood dyscrasias and clotting anomalies.

The use of corticosteroids in the treatment of pit viper envenomation is not recommended. Treatment of pit viper envenomations with corticosteroids has been repeatedly advocated, yet the rationale for their use is obscure, and their ultimate therapeutic value is controversial. Numerous studies have evaluated the effects of treating venomous snake bites with corticosteroids. Most report a worsening of or no improvement in the patient's condition.[35-48] Some studies have shown dramatic increases in mortality with the use of corticosteroids.[49,50] The proposed detrimental effects of corticosteroids are inhibition of the victim's natural defenses against the venom, interference with the antivenom, and potentiation of the venom itself. Also, they potentially confound diagnostic testing, altering coagulation and other objective laboratory monitoring measurements useful in evaluating the clinical progression of the envenomation syndrome. In addition, human clinical trials have shown no beneficial effects of the treatment of pit viper envenomation with corticosteroids.[46] Corticosteroids are of little use in a hypotensive crisis and have little if any effect on the local tissue response to pit viper venom.

Antihistamines have no effect upon pit viper venom. They do not prevent allergic reactions to subsequent antivenom.

Fasciotomy is not indicated in the dog and cat. The rationale for this procedure is to combat damage from compartment syndromes, which are extremely rare in dogs and cats and are not common in humans.[51] The theory used to advocate surgical intervention is that a deep bite injecting venom into the muscle causes that tissue to swell, leading to pressure necrosis when the muscle sheath restricts the ability of the tissue to expand. Fasciotomy is performed to open the muscle sheath, preventing the pressure necrosis. However, most bites are SC, and compartment syndromes are rare. The risks associated with fasciotomy include surgery in the presence of significant coagulopathies, infection, and marked disfigurement after surgery with questionable outcomes.[52] One report that compared antivenom treatment with fasciotomy and debridement revealed 100% survival with antivenom treatment alone, 80% survival in those treated with antivenom and surgery, 30% survival with surgery alone, and 30% survival in the untreated controls.[53] In patients in whom a compartment syndrome secondary to pit viper envenomation may develop, administration of additional antivenom has been demonstrated to lower the IM pressure.[54]

Excision of the snake bite site is generally ineffective and can be complicated by coagulation defects secondary to the envenomation. Allen[55] demonstrated that in cats and rabbits injected with crotalid venoms, excision of the bite area even 5 to 15 minutes after the injection of venom was "useless," and even when a large mass of skin and muscle around the injection site was removed, all the animals died.

Prognosis

The prognosis is highly dependent on the degree of envenomation, location of bite site, and individual animal response. The earlier emergency veterinary care and aggressive treatment options are sought, the better the outcome.

Gross and Histologic Lesions

There are no specific gross and histologic lesions described for snake bite victims. Tissue necrosis is commonly seen at the bite site; hemorrhage and edema are consistent changes observed. Other lesions seen are highly dependent on the extent of the toxicity of the venom (e.g., myocardial lesions, DIC, petechiation, ecchymoses, and renal necrosis).

Differential Diagnoses

Trauma, angioedema (e.g., insect bites and stings), other animal bites, draining abscesses, and penetrating wounds make up the differential diagnoses for snake bites.

Alternative Antivenoms

A newer antivenom (Crotalidae polyvalent immune Fab Ovine, BTG, Brentwood, TN; CroFabAV) was approved for human use by the U.S. Food and Drug Administration in late 2000. This antivenom is a purified and lyophilized preparation of ovine Fab immunoglobulin fragments. The ovine IgG molecules are cleaved to discard the inflammatory stimulating Fc portion of the antibody, retaining only the Fab molecules. The product is affinity purified and contains negligible amounts of extraneous proteins, such as albumin. Advantages of this product include a high affinity for venom antigens, improved penetration into tissue (caused by the smaller size of Fab compared with whole IgG), and decreased antigenic potential, thereby decreasing the risk of possible allergic reactions. Also 99% of the protein in the vial is antibody fragments against pit viper venom, contrasting with 20% in other antivenoms. A disadvantage may be the potential need for repeated administration because the smaller Fab molecules may be more rapidly cleared from the body.

Crotalidae polyvalent immune Fab (ovine) antivenom is prepared from the blood of healthy sheep immunized in groups with one of the following North American crotalid venoms: *Crotalus atrox* (Western diamondback rattlesnake), *C. adamanteus* (Eastern diamondback rattlesnake), *C. scutulatus scutulatus* (Mojave rattlesnake), and *Agkistrodon piscivorus* (cottonmouth or water moccasin). A monospecific antivenom is produced from each sheep group, and these four monospecific antivenoms are then mixed to prepare the final polyvalent antivenom. The four immunizing snakes are all North American species and have been selected to provide the widest immune response to the venoms of pit vipers indigenous to the continent (Western diamondback rattlesnake [*Crotalus atrox*], Eastern diamondback rattlesnake [*Crotalus adamanteus*], Mojave rattlesnake [*Crotalus scutulatus*], and the cotton-mouth [*Agkistrodon piscivorus*]. For example, patients with *C. helleri* envenomation improved following use of the FabAV product, indicating cross reactivity with this snake's venom.[56]

In humans the use of CroFab effectively controlled most of the effects of envenomation, but some patients experienced either a recurrence of coagulopathy or delayed-onset hematotoxicity; usually those patients presented initially with severe coagulopathy.[57] A study in 115 dogs presented with progressive envenomation syndromes from rattlesnake bites showed an average of 1.25 vials of Crofab antivenom was effective in controlling or reversing clinical signs.[58] This antivenom has been successfully used in both feline and equine patients.

An additional newer antivenom (Polyvalent anti-snake Fabotherapic, Fab_2 Equine, Instituto Bioclon, Col. Toriello Guerra, Mexico; Antivipmyn) has been used in Mexico as the primary antivenom for human victims of pit viper envenomations. This antivenom is made by hyperimmunizing horses with the venoms of *Bothrops asper* (Fer-de-lance) and *Crotalus durissus* (central American rattlesnake). The hyperimmunized serum is then ultrafiltered until only Fab_2 antibody fragments are left. However, in each vial only 20% of this Fab_2 is snake venom specific. Results reported in abstract form of a clinical study in 74 dogs bitten by North American pit vipers showed effectiveness with 4 vials of Antivipmyn antivenom in correcting clinical signs of envenomation.[59] Additionally, a peer-reviewed clinical safety evaluation in nonenvenomated dogs was published showing an excellent safety profile after large doses (3 to 6 vials) were administered in a short period of time.[60]

Vaccine Production

In 2004, Red Rock Biologics, Woodland, California, introduced a vaccine for dogs designed to protect them against the venom of North American rattlesnake species, except for the Mojave rattlesnake. The vaccine is also reported to protect dogs against the bite of the copperhead. It is currently recommended to administer the vaccine in two doses 2 to 4 weeks apart and then annually thereafter. To date there are no peer-reviewed studies on the efficacy of this vaccine. It is important to note that the package insert recommends that even if your dog received the vaccine, you should still consider a snake bite as a medical emergency and should immediately seek veterinary care for the pet. Additionally, the manufacturer states that immunization may not preclude the need for antivenom administration.

References

1. Peterson M, Meerdink G: Venomous bites and stings. In Kirk R, editor: *Current veterinary therapy X*, Philadelphia, 1989, Saunders.
2. Gregory-Dwyer V, Bianchi Bosisio A: Righetti: P: An isoelectric focusing study of seasonal variation in rattlesnake venom proteins, *Toxicon* 24:995–1000, 1986.
3. Weinstein S, Smith L: Preliminary fractionation of tiger rattlesnake *(Crotalus tigris)* venom, *Toxicon* 28:1447–1455, 1990.
4. Glen J, Straight R: Mojave rattlesnake *(Crotalus scutulatus scutulatus)* venom: variation in toxicity with geographical origin, *Toxicon* 16:81–84, 1978.
5. Glen J, Straight R, Wolt T: Regional variation in the presence of canebrake toxin in *Crotalus horridus* venom, *Comp Biochem Physiol C Pharmacol Toxicol Endocrinol* 107:337–346, 1994.
6. Anderson S, Ownby C: Pathogenesis of hemorrhage induced by proteinase H from eastern diamondback rattlesnake *(Crotalus adamanteus)* venom, *Toxicon* 35:1291–1300, 1997.
7. Retzios A, Markland F: Fibrinolytic enzymes from the venoms *of Agkistrodon contortrix contortrix* and *Crotalus basiliscus basiliscus*: cleavage site specificity towards the alpha-chain of fibrin, *Thromb Res* 74:355–367, 1994.
8. Bjarnason J, Hamilton D, Fox J: Studies on the mechanism of hemorrhage production by five proteolytic hemorrhagic toxins from *Crotalus atrox* venom, *Biochem Hoppe Seyler* 369(Suppl):121–129, 1988.
9. Liu C, Huang T: Crovidisin, a collagen binding protein isolated from snake venom of *Crotalus viridis*, prevents platelet: collagen interaction, *Arch Biochem Biophys* 337:291–299, 1997.
10. Budzynski A, Pandya B, Rubin R, et al: Fibrinogenolytic afibrinogenemia after envenomation by western diamondback rattlesnake *(Crotalus atrox)*, *Blood* 63:1–14, 1984.

11. MacKessy S: Fibrinogenolytic proteases from venoms of juvenile and adult northern Pacific rattlesnakes *(Crotalus viridis oreganus), Comp Biochem Physiol B Comp Biochem* 106:181–186, 1993.

12. Rael E, Rivas J, Chen T, et al: Differences in fibrinolysis and complement inactivation by venom from different northern blacktail rattlesnakes *(Crotalus molossus molossus), Toxicon* 35:505–513, 1997.

13. Russell F: *Snake venom poisoning*, Great Neck, NY, 1983, Scholium International.

14. Clark R, Williams S, Nordt S, et al: Successful treatment of crotalid induced neurotoxicity with a new polyspecific crotalid Fab antivenom, *Ann Emerg Med* 30:54–57, 1997.

15. Dart R, Hulburt K, Garcia R, et al: Validation of a severity score for the assessment of crotalid snakebite, *Ann Emerg Med* 27(3):321–326, 1996.

16. Brown D, Meyer D, Wingfield W, et al: Echinocytosis associated with rattlesnake envenomation in dogs, *Vet Pathol* 31:654–657, 1994.

17. Peterson M: Veterinary envenomation database 1984-1994. Unpublished data.

18. Stewart M, Greenland S, Hoffman J: First-aid treatment of poisonous snakebite: are currently recommended procedures justified? *Ann Emerg Med* 10:331–335, 1981.

19. McNalley J, Dart R, O'Brien P: Southwestern rattlesnake envenomation database (abstract), *Vet Hum Toxicol* 29:486, 1987.

20. Russell F: First aid for snake venom poisoning, *Toxicon* 4:285–289, 1967.

21. Johnson E, Kardong K, MacKessy S: Electric shocks are ineffective in treatment of lethal effects of rattlesnake envenomation in mice, *Toxicon* 25:1347–1349, 1987.

22. Howe N, Meisenheimer J Jr: Electric shock does not save snakebitten rats, *Ann Emerg Med* 17:254–256, 1988.

23. Guisto J: Severe toxicity from crotalid envenomation after early resolution of symptoms, *Ann Emerg Med* 26:387–389, 1995.

24. Russell F, Ruzic N, Gonzales H: Effectiveness of antivenin (crotalidae) polyvalent following injection of crotalus venom, *Toxicon* 11:461–464, 1973.

25. Brown J: Effects of pH, temperature, antivenin and functional group inhibitors on the toxicity and enzymatic activities of *Crotalus atrox* venom, *Toxicon* 4:99–105, 1966.

26. Snyder C, Knowles J, Pickens J, et al: Snakebite poisoning. In Catcott E, editor: *Canine medicine*, Santa Barbara, CA, 1968, American Veterinary Publications.

27. Smith M, Ownby C: Ability of polyvalent (crotalidae) antivenin to neutralize myonecrosis, hemorrhage and lethality induced by timber rattlesnake *(Crotalus horridus horridus)* venom, *Toxicon* 23:409–424, 1985.

28. Malasit P, Warrell D, Chanthavanich P: Prediction, prevention, and mechanism of early (anaphylactic) antivenom reactions in victims of snakebites, *Br Med J* 292:17–20, 1986.

29. Vohra R, Kelner M, Clark R: Preparation of crotaline F-ab antivenom (Crofab) with automated mixing methods: *in vitro* observations, *Clin Tox* 47:69–71, 2009.

30. Christopher D, Rodning C: Crotalidae envenomation, *South Med J* 79(2):159–162, 1986.

31. Bond R, Burkhart K: Thrombocytopenia following timber rattlesnake envenomation, *Ann Emerg Med* 30:40–44, 1997.

32. Ownby C, Reisbecks S, Allen R: Levels of therapeutic antivenin and venom in a human snakebite victim, *South Med J* 89:803–806, 1996.

33. Berdoulay P, Schaer M, Starr J: Serum sickness in a dog associated with antivenin therapy for snake bite caused by *Crotalus adamanteus, J Vet Emerg Crit Care* 15:206–212, 2005.

34. Kerrigan K, Mertz B, Nelson S, et al: Antibiotic prophylaxis for pit viper envenomation: prospective controlled trial, *World J Surg* 21:369–372, 1997.

35. Clark R, Selden B, Furbee B: The incidence of wound infection following crotalid envenomation, *J Emerg Med* 11:583–586, 1993.

36. Russell F: Snake venom poisoning in the United States: experiences with 550 cases, *JAMA* 233(4):341–344, 1975.

37. Van Mierop L: Snake bite symposium, *J Fla Med Assoc* 63:101, 1976.

38. Arnold R: Treatment of snakebite, *JAMA* 236:1843, 1976.

39. Arnold R: Controversies and hazards in the treatment of pit viper bites, *South Med J* 72:902, 1979.

40. Glen J: Personal communication, Veterans Administration Medical Center, Venom Research Laboratories, Salt Lake City, June 1990.

41. Gennaro J Jr: Observations on treatment of snake bite in America. In Keegan H, MacFarlane W, editors: *Venomous and poisonous animal and noxious plants of the Pacific region*, Tarrytown, NY, 1963, Pergamon Press.

42. Schottler W: Antihistamine, ACTH, cortisone and anesthetics in snakebite, *Am J Trop Med* 3:1083, 1954.

43. Allam M: Comparison of cortisone and antivenin in the treatment of crotaline envenomation. In Buckley E, Porges N, editors: *Venoms*, Washington, DC, 1956, American Association for Advancement of Science.

44. Russell F, Emery J: Effects of corticosteroids on lethality of *Agkistrodon contortrix* venom, *Am J Med Sci* 241:135, 1965.
45. Russell F: Effects of cortisone during immunization with *Crotalus* venom. A preliminary report, *Toxicon* 3:65, 1965.
46. Reid H: Specific antivenin and prednisone in viper bite poisoning: a controlled trial, *Br Med J* 2:1378, 1963.
47. Cunningham E: Snakebite—role of corticosteroids as immediate therapy in an animal model, *Am Surg* 45:757, 1979.
48. Wood J: Treatment of snake venom poisoning with ACTH and cortisone, *Va Med Monthly* 82:130, 1955.
49. Reid H: Snake bite, Part 2. Treatment, *Trop Doctor* 2:159, 1972.
50. Russell F: Shock following snakebite, *JAMA* 198:171, 1966.
51. Mubarak S, Hargens A, Own C, et al: The wick catheter technique for measurement of intramuscular pressure: a new research and clinical tool, *J Bone Joint Surg* 58A:1016, 1976.
52. Garfin S, Castilonia R, Mubarak S, et al: Rattlesnake bites and surgical decompression: results using a laboratory model, *Toxicon* 22:177–182, 1984.
53. Stewart R, Page C: Antivenin and fasciotomy/debridement in treatment of severe rattlesnake bite, *Am J Surg* 158:543–547, 1989.
54. Garfin S, Castilonia R, Mubarak S, et al: The effect of antivenin on intramuscular pressure elevations induced by rattlesnake venom, *Toxicon* 23:677–680, 1985.
55. Allen F: Mechanical treatment of venomous bites and wounds, *South J Med* 31:1248, 1938.
56. Bush SP, Green SM, Moynihan JA, et al: Crotalidae polyvalent immune Fab (ovine) antivenom is efficacious for envenomations by Southern Pacific rattlesnakes *(Crotalus helleri)*, *Ann Emerg Med* 40:619–624, 2002.
57. Ruha AM, Curry SC, Beuhler M, et al: Initial postmarketing experience with crotalidae polyvalent immune Fab for treatment of rattlesnake envenomation, *Ann Emerg Med* 39:609–615, 2002.
58. Peterson ME, Matz M, Seibold K, et al: A randomized multicenter trial of Crotalidae polyvalent immune F_{ab} antivenom for the treatment of rattlesnake envenomation in dogs, *J Vet Emerg Crit Care* 21:335–345, 2011.
59. Seibold K, Wells RJ, Bordeon DJ, et al: Evaluation of an antivenom F(ab')$_2$ in 74 dogs envenomated by North American pit vipers (Abstract), *J Vet Emerg Crit Care* 20(Suppl 1):A13, 2010.
60. Woods C, Young D: Clinical safety evaluation of F(ab')$_2$ antivenom *(Crotalus durissus – Bothrops asper)* administration in dogs, *J Vet Emerg Crit Care* 21:565–569, 2011.

Snake Bite: Coral Snakes

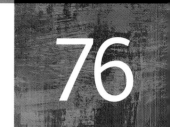

Michael E. Peterson, DVM, MS

- Coral snake venom is primarily neurotoxic, with little local tissue reaction and pain at the bite site.
- Clinical signs can be delayed for several hours and can include generalized weakness, muscle fasciculations, paralysis, and respiratory failure.
- Hyperfibrinogenemia, leukocytosis, elevated creatinine kinase, burring and spherocytosis, anemia, and hemoglobinuria can be observed.
- Treatment options include hospitalization for a minimum of 48 hours, good supportive medical care, and use of antivenom if available.

Sources

Fifty species of coral snakes are found in the New World. Two genera are indigenous to the United States. The two genera are composed of two species and three subspecies. One genus is *Micruroides* (*M. euryxanthus*—the Sonoran coral snake), which inhabits central and southeastern Arizona and southwestern New Mexico. The other genus is *Micrurus*, with three subspecies: *M. fulvius fulvius* (Eastern coral snake), *M. fulvius tenere* (Texas coral snake), and *M. fulvius barbouri* (South Florida coral snake).

The Texas coral snake has a home range extending from southern Arkansas and Louisiana throughout eastern and west central Texas. The Eastern coral snake inhabits eastern North Carolina south to central Florida and west to Alabama, Mississippi, and eastern Louisiana to the Mississippi River. The South Florida coral snake is found in southern Florida and the northern Florida Keys (Figure 76-1).

North American coral snakes are distinctively colored beginning with a black snout and an alternating pattern of black, yellow (occasionally white), and red. They can be differentiated from similar looking nonpoisonous snakes by the coral snake's color bands, which completely encircle the snake's body with the yellow band touching the red band (Color Plate 76-1). This color pattern can be best remembered by the warning that if caution (yellow) touches danger (red), the snake is a coral snake.

Coral snakes have short fixed front fangs and a poorly developed system for venom delivery, thereby requiring a chewing action to inject the venom. Their pupils are always round; they have no facial "heat-sensing" pits, and their heads are not triangular. These snakes are diurnal. Coral snakes are relatively docile, but will respond aggressively if disturbed, delivering a pugnacious bite. In 85% of human bite cases, the snake has to be shaken or pulled off, creating a feeling in the victims reminiscent of separating pieces of Velcro.[1]

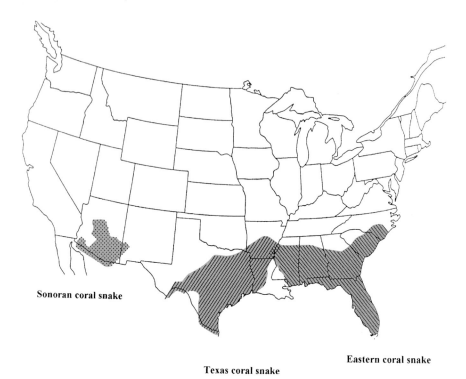

Sonoran coral snake

Eastern coral snake

Texas coral snake

Figure 76-1 Distribution of coral snakes in the United States.

Veterinary patients occasionally are brought in with the snake still attached. Bites by coral snakes are relatively rare. In humans coral snakes account for less than 1% of all venomous snake bites in North America. The majority of coral snake bites occurs during the spring and fall.

The Sonoran coral snake (*Micruroides euryxanthus*) is a small burrowing snake that is relatively innocuous.[2] No human fatalities have been ascribed to this snake. There are no reported cases of dog or cat fatalities caused by envenomation by this snake.

Toxic Dose

The severity of a coral snake bite is related to the volume of venom injected and the size of the victim. Sixty percent of coral snake bites are nonenvenomating. It is suggested that this is because of a relatively primitive venom delivery apparatus.[1] Approximately 4 to 5 mg of venom is a human lethal dose. A large coral snake can deliver a venom volume of up to 20 mg. The length of the snake correlates positively with the snake's venom yield.[3] It is estimated that the human fatality rate caused by coral snake envenomation approaches 10%.[4]

Toxicokinetics

Venom uptake can be delayed for many hours and can take 7 to 14 days to clear the body. One report involving envenomated cats describes clinical improvement by 36 hours, and by 48 hours after the bite, cats were moving their limbs.[5]

Mechanism of Toxicity

Coral snake venom is primarily neurotoxic with little local tissue reaction and pain at the bite site. Several neurotoxins may be involved and in combination act as nondepolarizing postsynaptic neuromuscular blocking agents. The net effect of the neurotoxins is a curare-like syndrome. Additionally the venom induces central nervous system depression, muscle paralysis, and vasomotor instability.

In dogs there have been reports of the venom causing hemolysis with severe anemia and marked hemoglobinuria.[6] The cause of the red blood cell destruction is poorly understood. It is speculated that it is due to the effects of phospholipase A and its interaction with red blood cell membranes.[6]

Initial experimental work has indicated that a profound drop in blood pressure occurs if the venom is rapidly absorbed (such as in an intravenous injection). The rapid drop in blood pressure is caused by decreases in cardiac output and aortic pressure in response to sequestration of venous return in the hepatosplanchnic bed.[7]

Other Elapidae venom components, which can cause significant local tissue destruction, include hyaluronidase, proteinase, ribonuclease, desoxyribonuclease, and phosphodiesterase.[8]

Clinical Signs

The onset of clinical signs may be delayed for as much as 10 to 18 hours.[1,4-6] The mean time from bite to onset of clinical signs in one human report was 170 minutes.[1] There are few if any local signs other than the puncture wounds themselves. Occasionally, local pain and regional paresthesia may occur. The victim then begins to have alterations in mental status, and generalized weakness and muscle fasciculations develop. Progression to paralysis of the limbs and respiratory muscles then follows. These signs are consistent with bulbar dysfunction. The patient is at risk of impending respiratory failure, with pharyngeal spasms, hypersalivation, cyanosis, and trismus (spasms of the masticatory muscles). Aspiration pneumonia is the major complication secondary to marked salivation caused by dysphagia.

Clinical signs of coral snake envenomation reported in dogs are acute central nervous system depression, emesis, excessive salivation, quadriplegia with decreased spinal reflexes in all limbs, and respiratory paralysis. Dogs may exhibit intravascular hemolysis, anemia, hemoglobinuria, and morphological alterations of red blood cells. Also reported in dogs are hypotension and ventricular tachycardia with pulse deficits. Hemolysis has been reported to occur within 72 hours after envenomation.[6] Blood-tinged urine and diarrhea may be present.

Clinical signs of coral snake envenomation reported in cats are acute ascending flaccid quadriplegia, central nervous system depression, and reduced nociception. Additionally, anisocoria, absent spinal reflexes in all four limbs, hypothermia, and loss of the cutaneous trunci reflex have been documented.[5] Anal tone and micturition are typically normal. In one study examining anesthetized cats given 2 mg/kg body weight of Eastern coral snake (*Micrurus fulvius*) venom intravascularly, the cats manifested the following signs: drop in blood pressure, respiratory depression 1 hour postinjection, no spontaneous respirations by 3 hours, and an increase in myoglobin release.[9] Even at this high intravascular dose, hemoglobinuria was not observed in cats. Hemolysis and hemoglobinuria were not evident in three clinical cases of envenomated cats.[5]

In humans clinical signs of envenomation by the Sonoran coral snake are much less marked than with *Micrurus* spp. Clinical signs (e.g., local pain and paresthesia and weakness of the bitten extremity) abated within 24 hours, and the patients were asymptomatic by 4 days after envenomation.[10]

Minimum Database

Baseline laboratory data should include a complete blood cell count, measurement of electrolytes, and serum chemistries. Hyperfibrinogenemia and moderate leukocytosis are reported abnormalities. Creatine kinase can be greatly elevated. Early elevation of creatine kinase is an indicator that envenomation has occurred.[5] In dogs red blood cell morphological changes include burring and spherocytosis.[6] Canine patients in which coral snake envenomation is suggested should be monitored for progressing anemia and hemoglobinuria. Radiographs of the thorax may be indicated because aspiration pneumonia is a major complication of coral snake envenomation secondary to pharyngeal paralysis.

Confirmatory Tests

There are no definitive diagnostic tests to confirm that a coral snake bite and envenomation have occurred.

Treatment

The best field response to coral snake envenomation is rapid transport to a veterinary medical facility capable of 24-hour critical care and assisted ventilation. The wound site should be cleaned with a germicidal soap. Suction is of doubtful benefit. The following first-aid measures should be avoided: incisions, ice, hot packs, and/or electroshock treatment.

First-aid treatment advocated in Australia for elapid bites is the immediate use of a compression bandage. This technique is obviously not applicable to bites of the neck and head. The compression bandage, such as an elastic or crepe bandage material, is rapidly applied to the bitten extremity, starting at the bite site and progressing to encompass the entire limb. The bandage should be wrapped as tightly as one would wrap a sprained ankle. This bandage should not be removed until primary therapy, specifically antivenom, is administered.

The victim should be hospitalized for a minimum of 48 hours for continuous monitoring. Pretreatment blood and urine samples should be collected to establish a clinical laboratory baseline. Of utmost importance is good supportive medical care along with an appreciation and anticipation of events that might develop. This includes care of a paralyzed patient and prevention of aspiration pneumonia. Any evidence of respiratory distress should be aggressively addressed with endotracheal intubation to prevent aspiration. Cardiac and pulse oximetry monitoring should be started. Fluid administration through an intravenous catheter should be given at a maintenance rate. Because the onset of clinical signs can be delayed for hours, extreme vigilance should be maintained in monitoring the patient.

The only definitive treatment for coral snake envenomation is administration of antivenom reactive against coral snake (*Micrurus fulvius*) venom. Antivenom is effective against the venom of all North American coral snakes except the Sonoran coral snake.[11] Currently, there is no approved coral snake antivenom available in the United States. However, studies have shown protective cross-reactivity with either the Australian tiger snake (*Notechis scutatus*)[12] or the Mexican coral snake (*Micrurus*)[12,13] antivenoms in the mouse model. Other South and Central American coral snake antivenoms do not protectively cross-react with North American *Micrurus* species of coral snake venom. At this time the most widely used coral snake antivenom in the United States is Coralmyn (Instituto Bioclon, Mexico) an Fab2 equine origin product. USDA import permits are needed to stock this antivenom; however, they are not difficult to acquire.

The earlier antivenom is administered, the more effective it is. Once clinical signs of coral snake envenomation become manifest, they progress with alarming rapidity and are difficult to reverse. The venom once bound irreversibly damages the postsynapic neuroreceptor. Antivenom treatment is recommended in animals with clinical findings of one or more fang marks from which blood can be expressed or those with a history of the snake hanging by its mouth from the victim regardless of the absence of neurological abnormalities. However, there is one report of apparent coral snake envenomation in a patient without visible fang marks.[14]

The antivenom is produced by inoculating horses with coral snake venom. Once the horse develops the desired antibody titer, serum is harvested and processed to concentrate the antivenom immunoglobulins. The processes used to extract these proteins result in a final product rich in antibodies. Some antivenom manufacturers (e.g., Instituto Bioclon) then remove the Fc portion of the whole IgG antibody, resulting in antivenom consisting of the smaller Fab2 binding fragments.

Antivenom should be reconstituted with the provided diluent. It should not be shaken but can be swirled to facilitate reconstitution. This usually takes between 10 and 15 minutes. Warming the antivenom vial to body temperature aids in dissolution into the liquid state. Overheating can destroy the proteins and shaking can cause excessive foaming, which makes it difficult to collect the antivenom into a syringe.

Skin testing to predict allergic reactions to the antivenom is difficult to evaluate in the veterinary patient. Human victims of snake bites are often subjected to cutaneous hypersensitivity testing before antivenom is administered.[15] A 1:10 dilution of antivenom at 0.02 mL is injected intradermally. A positive reaction, manifested by a wheal surrounded by erythema, occurs within 30 minutes. Drawbacks to skin testing are that it does not guarantee prevention of a severe reaction, has been shown to be not predictive of subsequent reactions, and the time it takes to perform delays prompt administration of antivenom. Generally a slow infusion of the antivenom initially with close monitoring will identify those patients who may experience a reaction with responses, such as nausea, hyperemia of the inner pinna, and pruritus.

Antivenom should be diluted at a ratio of 1 vial to 100 to 250 mL of crystalloid fluids. In smaller patients, the clinician should adjust the volume of fluid infusion to prevent fluid overload of the patient. In one study in which antivenom labeled with radioactive ^{131}iodine was given intravenously, 85% of the antivenom accumulated at the site of envenomation within 2 hours. In contrast there was a 1.4% local concentration when the antivenom was given intramuscularly and a 5.6% local concentration when it was given subcutaneously.[16] Antivenom should not be injected into the bite site, and its uptake can be delayed up to 12 hours when it is given intramuscularly. Administration should begin slowly as an intravenous infusion. If there is no evidence of an allergic reaction (e.g., nausea, hyperemia of the inner pinna, piloerection of tail hair, and pruritus), the rate of infusion can be increased. The entire initial dose should be given within 30 minutes. The patient must then be reevaluated for further progression of the envenomation syndrome using the appropriate clinical and laboratory measurements.

The dose of antivenom needed is calculated relative to the amount of venom injected and the body mass of the victim. Smaller patients require higher doses of antivenom because the dose of venom per kilogram body weight of the victim is higher. The recommended initial dose is 1 to 2 vials of antivenom. Repeated doses are administered as indicated by the progression of the syndrome.[6] Multiple vials may be necessary to adequately treat severe envenomations. The clinician must keep in mind that the dose of antivenom is based on the amount of venom injected in relation to body mass.

Patients with allergic reactions to the antivenom can still receive the antivenom if needed. It can be given as a slow intravenous drip and piggybacked with diphenhydramine and possibly epinephrine. Data in both human and veterinary envenomation databases have not identified a significantly higher reaction rate in patients who have received antivenom previously.[17,18] Some veterinary patients have received equine origin antivenom yearly for several consecutive years.[17]

Allergic reactions though rare are possible when administering antivenom. These may become manifest in one of three ways: true anaphylaxis, an anaphylactoid reaction, and delayed serum sickness. The most common reaction to antivenom is an anaphylactoid reaction. This is a complement-mediated reaction to rapid administration of a foreign protein, such as a blood transfusion. Anaphylactoid reactions can usually be treated by stopping the antivenom infusion, administering diphenhydramine IV or SC (1 to 2 mg/kg IM or SC), waiting 5 minutes, and then restarting the infusion of antivenom at a slower rate.

Stopping the infusion of antivenom and administering epinephrine, corticosteroids, and a crystalloid fluid infusion usually is effective in controlling anaphylaxis. Patients taking beta-blockers must be monitored very closely. Beta-blockers may mask the early onset of anaphylaxis, which becomes more difficult to reverse as the reaction progresses.

Delayed serum sickness is rare in dogs and cats. This may be because of the smaller volumes of antivenom administered compared with human patients. Delayed serum sickness usually occurs 7 to 14 days after antivenom administration. If it does occur, treatment consists of antihistamines, often type 1 and type 2 inhibitors, and/or corticosteroids.

If antivenom is not available or if its administration is delayed, supportive care includes respiratory support. Assisted mechanical ventilation can be used but may have to be employed for up to 48 to 72 hours.[19]

Broad-spectrum antibiotics are recommended in the veterinary patient after envenomation because of the number of pathogenic bacteria found in snakes' mouths. This is an area of controversy in the therapy of human snake bite victims.[20,21] The use of corticosteroids in the treatment of coral snake envenomation is not generally recommended; the justification for their use is tenuous at best. Treatment of Sonoran coral snake envenomation at this time is largely empirical because no specific antivenom is available for this venom.[22] General supportive care and response to clinical manifestations are the mainstays of therapy.

Prognosis

The prognosis is typically guarded and is highly dependent on the site of the bite wound, degree of envenomation, and time interval between the time of bite and seeking treatment.

Gross and Histologic Lesions

There are no definitive gross or histologic changes that can confirm a coral snake bite.

Differential Diagnoses

Differential diagnoses include tick paralysis, botulism, macadamia nut ingestion (dog), bromethalin, ionophore poisoning, delayed neuropathy associated with organophosphate exposure, acute polyneuritis, iatrogenic drug administration, polyradiculoneuritis, and myasthenia gravis.

References

1. Kitchens C, Van Mierop L: Envenomation by the eastern coral snake (*Micrurus fulvius fulvius*): a study of 39 victims, *JAMA* 258:1615–1618, 1987.
2. Lowe C Jr, Limbacher H: *Micruroides euryxanthus*, the Sonoran coral snake, *AZ Med* 8:128, 1961.
3. Fix J: Venom yield of the North American coral snake and its clinical significance, *South Med J* 73:737–738, 1980.
4. Parrish H, Klan M: Bites by coral snakes: report of 11 representative cases, *Am J Med Sci* 253:561–568, 1967.
5. Chrisman C, Hopkins A, Ford S, et al: Acute, flaccid quadriplegia in three cats with suspected coral snake envenomation, *J Am Anim Hosp Assoc* 32:343–349, 1996.
6. Marks S, Mannella C, Schaer M: Coral snake envenomation in the dog: report of four cases and review of the literature, *J Am Anim Hosp Assoc* 26:629–634, 1990.
7. Ramsey H, Taylor W, Boruchow I, et al: Mechanism of shock produced by an elapid snake (*Micrurus f. fulvius*) venom in dogs, *Am J Physiol* 222:782–786, 1972.
8. Ellis M: *Venomous and non-venomous snakes. Dangerous plants, snakes, arthropods and marine life-toxicity and treatment*, Hamilton, IL, 1978, Drug Intelligence Publications Inc.
9. Russell F: Bites by the Sonoran coral snake *Micruroides euryxanthus, Toxicon* 5:39–42, 1967.
10. Weis R, McIsaac R: Cardiovascular and muscular effects of venom from coral snake, *Micrurus fulvius, Toxicon* 9:219–228, 1971.
11. Antivenin *(Micrurus fulvius)* (equine origin) (drug circular), Marietta, PA, 1983, Wyeth Laboratories.
12. Wisniewski M, Hill R, Havey J, et al: Australian tiger snake (*Notechis scutatus*) and Mexican coral snake (*Micruris* species) antivenoms prevent death from United States coral snake (*Micrurus fulvius fulvius*) venom in a mouse model, *J Toxicol Clin Toxicol* 41(1):7–10, 2003.
13. de Roodt A, Paniagua-Solis J, Dolab J, et al: Effectiveness of two common antivenoms for North, Central, and South American Micrurus envenomations, *J Toxicol Clin Toxicol* 42(2):171–178, 2004.
14. Norris R, Dart R: Apparent coral snake envenomation in a patient without visible fang marks, *Am J Emerg Med* 7:402–405, 1989.

15. Malasit P, Warrell D, Chanthavanich P: Prediction, prevention, and mechanism of early (anaphylactic) antivenom reactions in victims of snakebites, *Br Med J* 292:17–20, 1986.
16. Christopher D, Rodning C: Crotalidae envenomation, *South Med J* 79(2):159–162, 1986.
17. Peterson M: Veterinary envenomation database 1984-1994. Unpublished data.
18. McNalley J, Dart R, O'Brien P: Southwestern rattlesnake envenomation database (abstract), *Vet Hum Toxicol* 29:486, 1987.
19. Kerrigan K, Mertz B, Nelson S, et al: Antibiotic prophylaxis for pit viper envenomation: prospective, controlled trial, *World J Surg* 21:369–372, 1997.
20. Moseley T: Coral snake bite: recovery following symptoms of respiratory paralysis, *Ann Surg* 163:943–948, 1966.
21. Clark R, Selden B, Furbee B: The incidence of wound infection following crotalid envenomation, *J Emerg Med* 11:583–586, 1993.
22. Russell F, Lauritizen L: Antivenins, *Trans R Soc Trop Med Hyg* 60:797, 1966.

Sodium

John H. Tegzes, VMD, MA, DABVT

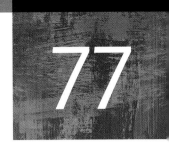

77

- Although hypernatremia is a common clinical pathologic finding in dogs and cats, hypernatremia caused by sodium poisoning is rare. Sodium poisoning can occur as a result of excess sodium exposure or from water deprivation.
- Sources of sodium exposure include modeling dough, homemade and commercial playdough, cooking salt, bottle sterilizing fluids, water softeners, rock salt, sea water, and iatrogenic sources, such as hypertonic saline and sodium bicarbonate.
- Hypernatremia can be a life-threatening clinical problem following exposures to paintballs and single/repeated doses of activated charcoal (with or without sorbitol), particularly in small dogs and cats.
- Plasma osmolality is largely influenced by sodium; an increase in sodium will increase osmolality and cause expansion of the extracellular fluid. As a result, cellular dehydration occurs. The brain is acutely sensitive to sodium changes. If fluid replacement occurs too rapidly, neurons will swell, and cerebral edema may occur.
- Neurologic clinical signs are preponderant after sodium toxicity and include depression, tremors, seizures, and coma.
- Treatment must include the slow, judicious use of fluids while carefully monitoring the animal's neurologic status. In addition, loop diuretics may help to eliminate the salt load.

Sources

Hypernatremia, a common electrolyte abnormality, can occur either as a result of excess salt ingestion, as a consequence of water deprivation, or from a variety of metabolic disorders. Salt poisoning in dogs and cats, however, is rare. In dogs and cats, hypernatremia is most frequently associated with volume depletion secondary to gastrointestinal losses and osmotic diuresis and free water loss caused by conditions such as diabetes insipidus or heat stroke.[1] In addition to an inciting cause, inadequate water intake appears also to be key to the development and maintenance of hypernatremia.[2]

There are few reports of sodium toxicosis in dogs caused by ingestion of excess salt or salt-containing products. The most commonly reported source of sodium chloride exposure in dogs is modeling dough used in crafts and some formulations of homemade or commercial playdough. Other possible sources include cooking salt, bottle sterilizing fluids, water softeners, sea water, salt used to deice roads (rock salt), saline emetics, and the administration of high sodium-containing drugs, such as sodium bicarbonate.[1,3] Paintballs contain a number of osmotically active compounds that can lead to fluid loss within the gastrointestinal tract that can result in hypernatremia.[4,5] And either single or repeated doses of activated charcoal, with or without sorbitol, have also resulted in hypernatremia in small dogs and cats due to fluid movement into the gut.[6]

Toxic Dose

The lethal dose of sodium chloride in dogs has been reported to be 4 g/kg body weight (BW).[3,7] One tsp of table salt is approximately 4.5 g of sodium chloride or 75 mEq of sodium[8]; therefore the toxic dose equates to less than 1 tsp of salt/kg BW. Homemade play-dough formulations can contain close to 8 g of sodium chloride/tbsp and signs of toxicity have been observed in dogs with doses as low as 2 g of sodium chloride/kg BW. There have been numerous cases of paintball toxicities in dogs, though the toxic dose is unknown.

Toxicokinetics

Sodium is readily absorbed by oral and parenteral routes of administration. Excess sodium results in hypernatremia. Hypernatremia exists whenever the serum sodium concentration exceeds 156 mEq/L in dogs and 161 mEq/L in cats.[1] Osmolality is the concentration of ions in a solution. Two tbsp of salt contain approximately 60 g of sodium and will raise the serum osmolality from 280 mOsm/kg to 410 mOsm/kg in a 50-kg adult human (each gram of sodium adds 34 mOsm of solute).[1,9] Because serum osmolality and serum sodium concentrations are proportional, a similar increase in serum sodium would be expected.[9] Salt water has an osmolality of 1000 mOsm/L, and ingestion of small quantities can lead to hyperosmolality.[1,9] In subtoxic sodium exposures with adequate renal function, brisk diuresis will help eliminate the salt load. Only when the sodium intake exceeds the capacity of the kidneys to eliminate it does a net gain of sodium and loss of water occur.[9]

Mechanism of Toxicity

Osmolality of the extracellular fluid is largely influenced by sodium. An increase in sodium will increase plasma osmolality and will cause expansion of the extracellular fluid.[1] Water moves from cells to the extracellular space to reestablish an osmotic equilibrium between the intracellular fluid volume and the extracellular fluid volume.[1] This results in cellular dehydration and vascular expansion. Of all the organ systems, the brain is most susceptible to cellular and tissue shrinkage as a result of its vascular attachment to the calvaria.[9] Vascular damage that occurs may result in hemorrhage, hematomas, thrombosis, or infarction.[10] The water shift that occurs can also lead to extravasation of fluid into the interstitium of the lungs, causing pulmonary edema.[1] In addition, during chronic hypernatremia, which develops over 4 to 7 days, cerebrospinal fluid (CSF) sodium concentrations increase to parallel serum sodium concentrations, and brain intracellular osmolality increases.[11] In the brain, osmoles other than electrolytes are also present, and these prevent the movement of water across the neuronal cell membrane into the hypernatremic CSF and plasma. If blood and CSF sodium concentrations are lowered rapidly because of water consumption or IV replacement, water will move from plasma and CSF into brain cells, causing them to swell and resulting in cerebral edema.[11]

Clinical Signs

Clinical signs caused by salt poisoning may begin with gastrointestinal signs associated with local tissue irritation and inflammation when the exposure is oral.[4,5,9] These include vomiting and diarrhea. Depending on the chronicity of exposure and degree of hypernatremia, signs associated with the central nervous system are most common.[2] These include depression, lethargy, muscular rigidity, tremors, polyuria, polydipsia, myoclonus, hyperreflexia, terminal seizures, and coma.[1,2,4,5,9] Dehydration occurs at the cellular level and may not be obvious clinically.[1] Other clinical signs reported in clinical case reports include dehydration, pyrexia, tachypnea, tachycardia, blindness, irregular heart rhythm, and Q-T prolongation on ECG.[2] In dogs clinical signs become evident when serum sodium concentrations exceed 170 mEq/L.

Minimum Database

Serum sodium and electrolyte measurements are used to determine hypernatremia and other possible electrolyte and acid-base abnormalities. Additionally, measurements to assess dehydration and renal function include the packed-cell volume, blood urea nitrogen (BUN), creatinine, total protein, and urine specific gravity. Physical examination measurements to monitor include the systemic blood pressure, heart rate and rhythm, and capillary refill time.

Confirmatory Tests

In the live animal, serum and CSF sodium concentrations will be elevated[12]; however, hypernatremia occurs for a variety of reasons and is therefore not confirmatory of salt exposure alone. When an animal is evaluated soon after ingesting a large salt load, vomitus and stomach contents can be analyzed for sodium and may indicate elevated concentrations and confirm exposure. Signs of toxicosis can be seen when serum sodium levels exceed 170 mEq/L, and severe neurologic signs can be observed when concentrations exceed 180 mEq/L.[1]

Salt poisoning may be confirmed postmortem by analyzing cerebral sodium levels. Concentrations greater than 1800 ppm on a wet weight basis are sufficient for a tentative diagnosis of sodium toxicosis.[12]

Treatment

It is important that the proper treatment time be taken to correct hypernatremia. If it is corrected too rapidly, it can cause or worsen cerebral edema and elevate intracranial pressure.[1,9] In general, slow correction of hypernatremia is safest. If the animal's neurologic status worsens after fluid therapy is begun, it is likely that cerebral edema is occurring.[1] Slow, judicious administration of D_5W IV is recommended,[1,4,5] so that sodium levels decrease at a rate no greater than 1 mEq/L per hour. Estimated replacement fluid volumes can be calculated using this formula: water deficit = 0.6 × BW in kg × (1 − normal serum sodium/current serum sodium).[1,9] Additionally, saline elimination can be augmented by administering a loop diuretic. Furosemide is a loop diuretic that can be given to dogs and cats at 2.2 to 4.4 mg/kg orally, IV, or intramuscularly one to two times daily.[6]

Prognosis

In humans the prognosis is poor when serum sodium concentrations exceed 170 mEq/L, although humans have survived after initially having serum sodium concentrations greater than 190 mEq/L without major sequelae.[13] In those people who do survive severe hypernatremia, critical care is required until the serum sodium concentration is corrected, and neurologic signs have resolved. Although there are few reports of severe hypernatremia in dogs and cats, there is a report of a dog with severe hypernatremia after ingestion of a figurine made of salt flour. This dog, upon first evaluation, had a serum sodium concentration of 211 mEq/L and later peaked with a serum sodium concentration of 217 mEq/L.[2] The dog expired several hours after initial examination while experiencing neurologic signs, cardiac tachyarrhythmias, and respiratory acidosis.

Gross and Histologic Lesions

Gross lesions reported in dogs after acute salt ingestion include hemorrhage of the stomach, small intestine, and colon. Acute renal and hepatic necrosis have been seen on histopathologic examination.[2] Cerebral edema is commonly reported in various species after salt poisoning.[1,9] Intracranial hemorrhage, hematomas, thrombosis, and infarction have been observed in humans.[10]

Differential Diagnoses

Although hypernatremia is a relatively common clinical pathologic finding, salt poisoning is rare. It is important that the clinician keep all possible causes of hypernatremia in mind. Hypernatremia associated with water loss can be caused by pituitary diabetes insipidus, nephrogenic diabetes insipidus, heat stroke, high environmental temperature, fever, inadequate access to water, burns, diarrhea, vomiting, and osmotic diuresis caused by acute renal failure, chronic renal failure, diabetes mellitus, diuretic use, IV solute administration, and hypoadrenocorticism.[1] Hypernatremia associated with salt gain can be caused by increased salt intake, IV hypertonic fluids, IV sodium bicarbonate, hyperaldosteronism, and hyperadrenocorticism.[1]

References

1. Hardy RM: Hypernatremia, *Vet Clin N Am* 19(2):231–240, 1989.
2. Khanna C, Boermans HJ, Wilcock B: Fatal hypernatremia in a dog from salt ingestion, *J Am Anim Hosp Assoc* 33:113–117, 1997.
3. Campbell A, Chapman M: Salt/sodium chloride. In Campbell A, Chapman M, editors: *Handbook of poisoning in dogs and cats*, Oxford, 2000, Blackwell Science.
4. Donaldson CW: Paintball toxicosis in dogs, *Vet Med* 98(12):995–997, 2003.
5. King JB, Grant DC: Paintball intoxication in a pug, *JVECC* 17(3):290–293, 2007.
6. Plumb DC: *Veterinary drug handbook*, ed 7, Ames, IA, 2011, Iowa State University Press.
7. Lorgue G, Lechenet J, Riviere A: Salt (sodium chloride). In Lorgue G, Lechenet J, Riviere A, editors: *Clinical veterinary toxicology*, Oxford, 1996, Blackwell Science.
8. Moder KG, Hurley DL: Fatal hypernatremia from exogenous salt intake: report of a case and review of the literature, *Mayo Clin Proc* 65:1587–1594, 1990.
9. Feig PU: Hypernatremia and hypertonic syndromes, *Med Clin N Amer* 65(2):271–290, 1981.
10. Simmons MA, Adcock EW, Bard H, et al: Hypernatremia and intracellular hemorrhage in neonates, *N Engl J Med* 291(1):6–10, 1974.
11. Angelos SM, Smith BP, George LW, et al: Treatment of hypernatremia in an acidotic neonatal calf, *J Am Vet Med Assoc* 214(9):1364–1367.
12. Osweiler GD, Carson TL, Buck WB, et al: Water deprivation-sodium salt. In Osweiler GD, Carson TL, Buck WB, et al: *Clinical and diagnostic veterinary toxicology*, ed 3, Dubuque, IA, 1985, Kendall/Hunt.
13. Addleman M, Pollard A, Grossman RF: Survival after severe hypernatremia due to salt ingestion by an adult, *Am J Med* 78:176–178, 1985.

Sodium Monofluoroacetate (1080)

78

Kathy Parton, DVM, MS

- Sodium monofluoroacetate is a potent pesticide used for predator control.
- Clinical signs of toxicosis include vomiting, salivation, urination, defecation, and hyperesthesia. Affected dogs commonly display wild running and barking episodes, and vocalization is a consistent feature in poisoned cats.
- Clinical pathologic changes include metabolic acidosis, hypocalcemia (ionized), and elevations in serum citrate concentrations.
- Treatment includes seizure control with barbiturates, fluids with bicarbonate or acetamide, and symptomatic care. Prognosis for clinically affected patients without treatment is grave.
- Rapid onset of rigor mortis with extensor rigidity is often observed postmortem.

Sodium monofluoroacetate (fluoroacetate, SMFA, and compound 1080) is a pesticide used to control rodents and other pests in the United States and worldwide. Commonly termed *1080*, this compound was identified as an effective rodenticide in the 1940s. Fluoroacetamide (compound 1081) was developed soon afterward as a less toxic alternative to 1080.[1] Both compounds are white, odorless, tasteless, water soluble, and highly toxic poisons.[2] Fluoroacetate also occurs naturally in a variety of plants in Africa (*Dichapetalum cymosum* and *Dichapetalum toxicarium*), Australia (*Acacia georginae*, *Gastrolobium* spp., and *Oxylobium* spp.), and South America (*Palicourea marcgravii*).[1] These and other plants containing fluoroacetate are known to poison livestock. Because these compounds are toxic to carnivores, they have been manufactured for the control of predators, such as the coyote (*Canis latrans*). At the present time, the use of 1080 is restricted to trained, licensed applicators. Although this restriction is intended to control its release in the environment and to target specific predators, unintentional poisoning of nontargeted animals occurs. In the United States the only currently registered use of 1080 is in a livestock protection collar for sheep and goats. There is no currently registered use of 1081 in the United States.[3]

Compound 1080 is also an important toxic metabolite associated with the chemotherapeutic anticancer agent 5-fluorouracil and some fluorinated ethanes that may be toxic when inhaled.[4-6] Clinical signs associated with the adverse effects of 5-fluorouracil and fluorinated ethanes resemble those seen with 1080 toxicity.[5,6]

Sources

Compound 1080 is manufactured in the United States for use in livestock protection collars for sheep and goats to control predators. The Environmental Protection Agency has tightly restricted the use of compound 1080 in these collars. Uses of 1080 and 1081 in rodenticides have been canceled.[3] Evidence suggests that unlicensed operators may use illegally acquired 1080 or 1081 to poison pests or predators.

Poisoning of pets with 1080 or 1081 may result from the ingestion of poisoned rodent carcasses, particularly when the gastrointestinal tract is consumed, because rodents require a relatively high dose of fluoroacetate to be killed. Alternatively, pets may be poisoned intentionally. In New Zealand large quantities of baits containing 0.08% or 0.15% of 1080 are sprayed aerially to control introduced pests, such as the rabbit and brushtail possum (*Trichosurus vulpecula*).[7] Secondary poisoning of cats and dogs results from the ingestion of these dead or dying animals.

Toxicokinetics

Animals have different susceptibilities to 1080 (and 1081) poisoning. The reason for the wide variation in toxicity is not known. Birds are most resistant to poisoning, followed by (in order of increasing sensitivity) rodents, primates, horses, rabbits, ruminants, and carnivores. Because tissue residues are minimal, the ingestion of muscle from a poisoned carcass is unlikely to cause toxicity in carnivores; however, ingestion of any part of the gastrointestinal tract containing 1080 bait can result in poisoning. Compound 1081 has a slower onset of action, and animals may display fewer neurologic signs.[1] The toxic dose of 1080 for dogs or cats is as little as 0.05 mg/kg body weight (Table 78-1). The quantity of 1081 necessary to kill dogs, rabbits, and sheep is two to five times more than the 1080 dose.[1]

Fluoroacetate is readily absorbed in the gastrointestinal tract and lungs and through cuts or abrasions in the skin but is poorly absorbed across intact skin.[1] Compound 1080 is distributed into soft tissues and organs. It was detected in the milk of ewes fed 1080 baits at 0.25 mg/kg body weight.[8] Fluoroacetate is metabolized to toxic fluorocitrate in the liver. Both compounds are excreted in the urine. The elimination half-life is 11 hours for sheep, 5.5 hours for goats, 9.0 hours for possums, 1.1 hours for rabbits, and 2 hours for mice.[8] They are not known to accumulate in any one tissue.[1]

Mechanism of Toxicity

The classic theory of 1080 poisoning is the so-called lethal synthesis effect on the Krebs or tricarboxylic acid (TCA) cycle (Figure 78-1). Fluoroacetate and fluoroacetamide combine with acetyl coenzyme A (CoA) to form fluoroacetyl CoA, which then combines with oxaloacetate to produce fluorocitrate. Fluorocitrate inhibits aconitase and the oxidation of citric acid, resulting in blockage of the TCA cycle, energy depletion, citric and lactic acid accumulation, and a decrease in blood pH.[2] The inhibition of aconitase interferes with cellular

Table 78–1	Toxic Doses of 1080 in Select Species	
Species	**Oral Lethal Dose (mg/kg body weight)**	**LD_{50} (mg/kg body weight)**
Cat	0.3-0.5	0.20 (IV)
Dog	0.06-0.2	0.05-1
Cattle, sheep, and goats	0.15-0.7	0.25-0.5
Horse	0.5-2.75	0.35-0.55
Possum	0.3	
Pigs	0.3	0.4-1
Prairie dogs (*Cynomys ludovicianus*)		0.173
Rabbit	0.8	
Rodents (rats and mice)		2-8

IV, Intravenous; LD_{50}, median lethal dose.

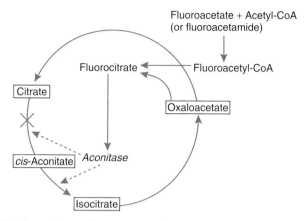

Figure 78-1 Classic theory: fluoroacetate inhibits aconitase in the Krebs-TCA cycle.

respiration and the metabolism of carbohydrates, fats, and proteins.[1,2] Evidence suggests that fluorocitrate is converted to 4-hydroxy-*trans*-aconitate, which binds very tightly to aconitase, thereby inactivating it.[9] The end result is an accumulation of citrate, which binds with serum calcium. The decrease in available ionized calcium has been shown to prolong the QT interval in electrocardiograms in cats.[10] In addition, evidence suggests that fluoroacetate and/or fluorocitrate inhibits other enzymes including succinate dehydrogenase, pyruvate dehydrogenase kinase, and the neurotransmitter glutamate.[8] The accumulation of citrate can have an inhibitory effect on phosphofructokinase and acetylcholine production.[11] Fluorocitrate has been shown to inhibit nitrous oxide production in rats, suggesting that pain and hyperalgesia may be attenuated.[12]

Clinical Signs

Clinical signs may appear 30 minutes to as long as 2 to 4 hours after ingestion, depending on the dose. The variable latent period is a result of the delay in conversion of fluoroacetate or fluoroacetamide to fluorocitrate and its accumulation to toxic levels. Carnivores display central nervous system (CNS) excitation and gastrointestinal hyperactivity. Neurologic signs in dogs include anxiety, frenzied behavior, such as running and howling, and hyperesthesia. Carnivores usually vomit, salivate, urinate, and defecate after ingesting 1080.[1,2] A hypermotile gastrointestinal tract with tenesmus also occurs. Hyperthermia has been reported in dogs.[2] Convulsions begin after a brief period of hyperexcitability. Tonic and clonic convulsions may occur between periods of frenzied and normal behavior. Dogs in the agitated state are not responsive to external stimuli.[12] The anoxia that occurs during convulsions leads to respiratory failure. The animal becomes weaker as the cellular energy supplies decrease. Eventually the animal becomes comatose, and death usually occurs from 2 to 12 hours after the appearance of clinical signs.[1,2]

Cats may have both cardiac dysfunction and neurologic signs. They may become depressed or excited, vocalize, and be hyperesthetic to light and touch. Hypothermia (37° C or 99° F), cardiac arrhythmias, and episodes of bradycardia between convulsions also have been reported in cats.[1,2,13]

Minimum Database

Clinical pathologic findings of hyperglycemia and metabolic acidosis are associated with 1080 poisoning. A twofold increase in serum glucose has been reported.[12] In dogs citrate levels are elevated at least two or more times in serum and heart; however, high levels are not pathognomonic of 1080 ingestion because citrate is a normal substance of cells.[12]

Hypocalcemia also has been associated with 1080 poisonings. Research in cats has shown that ionized calcium rather than total serum calcium is altered.

Confirmatory Tests

A diagnosis of 1080 poisoning is based on the clinical signs, access to the poison, and analysis of the compound in bait or vomitus. Residues of 1080 are most likely to be found in vomitus or stomach contents. A minimum of 50 g of vomitus or stomach contents is required for the analysis. Animals that ingest a minimum lethal dose of 1080 are unlikely to have detectable levels in body tissue. However, detectable fluoroacetate levels in urine and kidneys have been found in dead animals. In experimentally poisoned animals, tissue fluoroacetate levels were considerably below 100 ppb.[14]

Treatment

Because of the rapid onset of clinical signs, it is difficult to treat animals after they have ingested 1080. Often the animal dies before the veterinarian has the chance to examine the animal.

Recent successes in Australia suggest that treating animals with sodium bicarbonate may improve survival.[15] The recommended treatment is to lightly anesthetize the animal with pentobarbital sodium, place an intravenous catheter, and connect it to a saline (0.9% NaCl) drip. Sodium bicarbonate (8.4% wt/vol) is infused during the next 15 to 30 minutes through the giving port at the dose rate of 300 mg/kg (3.6 mL/kg) body weight. Alternatively, half of the calculated dose may be given as a bolus and the remainder infused slowly. The 8.4% sodium bicarbonate solution is approximately equivalent to 1 mEq/mL each of sodium and bicarbonate. Administration of sodium bicarbonate may worsen hypocalcemia and cause hypokalemia.[16] Ionized calcium and potassium levels should be monitored and supplemented as required. Decontamination with activated charcoal and a laxative (e.g., sorbitol) is also recommended. In the anesthetized dog, the activated charcoal should be given through a stomach tube with the animal intubated to prevent aspiration pneumonia. A recent study in rats questions the efficacy of activated charcoal in 1080 poisoning, but the authors suggest further investigation is necessary before recommending colestipol as an alternative sorbent.[16] Anesthesia and fluids are maintained until the animal appears to be recovering (e.g., has no convulsions), usually after about 12 to 24 hours. Animals are generally discharged within 48 hours after initial examination by the veterinarian.

A successful approach (in New Zealand) uses acetamide in 5% dextrose. The treatment replaces glycerol monoacetate (monacetin, glyceryl monoacetate [GMA]), used in the treatment of fluoroacetate poisoning in humans and animals. It may be difficult to obtain GMA from chemical suppliers, and the intramuscular injections are very painful. The GMA and acetamide are believed to decrease citrate levels by competing with fluoroacetate. The dose of acetamide, based on current practice in New Zealand, uses 15 g (approximately 2 tsp) of acetamide in 1 L of 5% dextrose. An emetic is given if clinical signs are absent but this is controversial given the short latent period and the risk of triggering seizures. Decontamination with activated charcoal and laxatives may be indicated whether or not clinical signs are present. If clinical signs are present, the dog is lightly anesthetized with pentobarbital, usually up to 24 hours. The combination of 5% dextrose with acetamide is administered at an initial dose of 20 to 25 mL/kg body weight over a 60-minute period followed by approximately 5 mL/kg per hour for the next 12 to 18 hours as needed. For an average size dog (20 kg) a total of 2 L of 5% dextrose containing acetamide is given.[18] This dose is comparable with experimentally poisoned rats pretreated with acetamide at a dose of 1.25 g/kg that survived after a toxic dose of fluoroacetate was administered.[19] The heart rate may greatly increase with acetamide treatment. If treating a cat with fluoroacetate poisoning, the dose should be reduced by at least 75%. A higher dose (10% solution of acetamide in 5% dextrose at 7 to 10 mL/kg over 30 minutes and then 5 mL/kg every 4 hours for 24 to 48 hours) has been advocated for human treatment but appears to be unnecessary in the dog.

Although researchers in New Zealand are pursuing antidotes for 1080 poisoning, no commercial products have been developed at this writing.[20]

In countries such as New Zealand and Australia, where the risk of exposure to 1080 is high, the use of dog muzzles is the best means of preventing dogs from being poisoned. A well-fitted wire muzzle that prevents the dog from scavenging dead carcasses is money well spent.

Prognosis

The prognosis is poor to grave, depending on the amount of 1080 or 1081 ingested and the severity of clinical signs at initial evaluation. The prognosis is improved with early acetamide or sodium bicarbonate treatment and good supportive care.

Gross and Histologic Lesions

Postmortem findings in carnivores exposed to 1080 are nonspecific. Rigor mortis is rapid in onset. Hypoxia as a result of convulsions may cause general cyanosis, congestion of visceral organs, agonal petechial hemorrhages on the myocardium, and pulmonary congestion. Other findings may include an empty stomach, enteritis, and a flaccid, pale heart in diastole. Histopathologic changes of the brain may include edema and lymphocytic infiltration of perivascular tissue.[2]

Differential Diagnoses

Differential diagnoses associated with convulsions or CNS disorders include strychnine, chlorinated hydrocarbons, lead, hypomagnesemia, hypocalcemia, garbage intoxication (penitrem A and roquefortine), brain injury, cardioglycosides, taxine (Japanese yew), and methylxanthines. Strychnine-poisoned dogs and cats are extremely sensitive to noise and other external stimuli, which is uncharacteristic of fluoroacetate poisoning. The strychnine-poisoned dog is not likely to show frenzied running behavior or vomit, urinate, and defecate when poisoned. Chlorinated hydrocarbons may produce hyperthermia and convulsions, but evacuation of the gastrointestinal tract and urination are not typical clinical signs. Lead poisoning (plumbism) may cause similar CNS signs (convulsions, barking, running fits, and tremors). Lead poisoning is associated with gastrointestinal pain and vomiting, whereas 1080 intoxication results in rapid evacuation of the gastrointestinal tract and bladder. The clinical signs of lead poisoning tend to be intermittent and usually follow a longer course. The other differential diagnoses listed above may cause varying degrees of CNS stimulation, tremors, gastrointestinal signs, or sudden death; however, the frenzied, vocalized excitation seen with 1080 poisoning is uncharacteristic.

References

1. Parton K, Bruere AN, Chambers JP: Fluoroacetate. *Veterinary clinical toxicology,* publication 249, ed 3, Palmerston North, New Zealand, 2006, Veterinary Continuing Education.
2. Osweiler GD, Carson TL, Buck WB, et al: *Clinical and diagnostic veterinary toxicology*, ed 3, Dubuque, IA, 1983, Kendall/Hunt Publishing Co.
3. EPA: *Reregistration eligibility decision (RED) sodium fluoroacetate: prevention, pesticides and toxic substances, EPA 738-5-95-025*, Washington, DC, 1995, Environmental Protection Agency.
4. Arellano M, Malet-Martino M, Martino F, et al: The anti-cancer drug 5-fluorouracil is metabolized by the isolated perfused rat liver and in rats into highly toxic fluoroacetate, *Br J Cancer* 77(1):79–86, 1998.
5. Keller DA, Roe DC, Lieder PH: Fluoroacetate-mediated toxicity of fluorinated ethanes, *Fund Appl Toxicol* 30(2):213–219, 1996.
6. Dorman DC: Neurotoxic drugs in dogs and cats. In Bonagura JD, editor: *Kirk's current veterinary therapy xii*, Philadelphia, 1995, Saunders.
7. Eason CT: International science workshop on the environmental toxicology of sodium monofluoroacetate (1080), *Surveillance* 22(1):24–25, 1995.

8. Eason CT, Miller A, Ogilvie S, Fairweather A: An updated review of the toxicology and ecotoxicology of sodium fluoroacetate (1080) in relation to its use as a pest control tool in New Zealand, *NZ J of Ecology* 35:1–20, 2011.
9. Lauble H, Kennedy MC, Emptage MH, et al: The reaction of fluorocitrate with aconitase and the crystal structure of the enzyme-inhibitor complex, *Proc Natl Acad Sci USA* 93:13699–13703, 1996.
10. Roy (Shapira) A, Taitelman U, Bursytein S: Evaluation of the role of ionized calcium in sodium fluoroacetate ("1080") poisoning, *Toxicol Appl Pharmacol* 56:216–220, 1980.
11. Twigg LE, Parker RW: Is sodium fluoroacetate (1080) a humane poison? The influence of mode of action, physiological effects, and target specificity, *Animal Welfare* 19:249–263, 2010.
12. Sun XC, Chen WN, Li SQ, et al: Fluorocitrate, an inhibitor of glial metabolism, inhibits the up-regulation of NOS expression, activity and NO production in the spinal cord induced by formalin test in rats, *Neurochem Res* 34:351–359, 2009.
13. Bosakowski T, Levin AA: Serum citrate as a peripheral indicator of fluoroacetate and fluorocitrate toxicity in rats and dogs, *Toxicol Appl Pharmacol* 85(3):428–436, 1986.
14. Gammie J: Sodium fluoroacetate poisoning in a cat, *Can Vet J* 21(2):64, 1980.
15. Hugghins EJ, Casper HH, Ward CD: Tissue fluoroacetate residues in prairie dogs dosed with low-level sodium monofluoroacetate, *J Assoc Anal Chem* 71(3):579–581, 1988.
16. Churchill R: *1080 sodium fluoroacetate toxicity in dogs #3796. Control and therapy series*, Sydney, 1996, University of Sydney, Postgraduate Committee in Veterinary Science.
17. Plumb DC: *Veterinary drug handbook*, ed 6, Ames, IA, 2008, Wiley-John & Sons.
18. Norris WR, Temple WA, Eason CT, et al: Sorption of fluoroacetate (compound 1080) by colestipol, activated charcoal and anion-exchange resins in vitro and gastrointestinal decontamination in rats, *Vet Hum Toxicol* 42(5):269–275, 2000.
19. McLaren J: Treatment of 1080 poisoning in dogs, *Vetscrip* XII(2):3, 1999.
20. Gorniak SL, Palmermo-Neto J, Spinosa HS: Effects of acetamide on experimentally induced *Palicourea marcgravii* (St Hill) poisoning in rats, *Vet Hum Toxicol* 36(2):101–102, 1994.
21. Cook CJ, Eason CT, Wickstrom W, et al: Development of antidotes for sodium monofluoroacetate (1080), *Biomarkers* 6(1):72–76, 2001.

Spider Envenomation: Black Widow

79

Michael E. Peterson, DVM, MS

Jude McNally, RPh, DABAT

- Spiders of the genus *Latrodectus* are typically globose black spiders; females have an hourglass red-orange pattern on the abdomen. These spiders are found in every state in the United States except Alaska.
- The spider controls the amount of venom injected into its prey. LD_{50} values range from 0.43 to 1.39 mg/kg. A single bite can be fatal to companion animals. There are virtually no local signs of tissue destruction at the bite site.
- Clinical signs can last up to 7 days; however, weakness and some muscle pain may persist for weeks. These signs include progressive muscle fasciculations, severe pain, cramping of large muscle masses, abdominal rigidity without tenderness, marked restlessness, hypertension, bronchorrhea, regional numbness, and excessive salivation.
- Minimum database includes CBC, serum chemistries, urinalysis, and monitoring of general vital signs including blood pressure.
- Treatment may include the use of Acalatro (*Latrodectus*, equine origin Fab2, Instituto Biclon, Mexico) antivenom given IV.

Sources

Black widow spiders belong to the genus *Latrodectus,* of which there are five primary species residing in the United States. These are *L. mactans, L. variolus, L. bishopi, L. hesperus,* and *L. geometricus.*

Latrodectus mactans is the preponderant species found throughout North America. *Latrodectus variolus* is found in the eastern United States north to Canada. *Latrodectus bishopi,* also known as the red widow, resides in central Florida. The western black widow is *Latrodectus hesperus.* Finally the brown widow of southern Florida is *Latrodectus geometricus.*

Black widow spiders are found throughout the continental United States and north into the southern Canadian provinces. These spiders inhabit funnel-shaped webs in dry, dimly lit, and secluded places. The web is irregularly shaped, has a tattered "cobwebbed" appearance, and is usually found in corners. The spiders are commonly found around houses where outside lights help to attract prey insects. Another spider usually quickly reinhabits web locations if the original inhabitant is displaced.

Male black widow spiders are of little medical importance because they are unable to penetrate mammalian skin because of the small size of their jaws. Female spiders can be 20 times larger than the males. The females can be up to 2 to 2.5 cm long and are capable of life-threatening envenomations. These spiders have several common pseudonyms, including the shoe button and the hourglass spider. The female can be identified by the hourglass pattern, red or orange in color, on the ventral aspect of her shiny, globose black abdomen (Color Plate 79-1). The hourglass becomes more prominent as the spider ages. It is important to recognize the immature female, which has a colorful pattern of red, brown, and beige on the dorsal surface of her abdomen, because she is fully capable of delivering a severe envenomation (Color Plate 79-2). When hatching, these spiders are red, but with each subsequent molt the black color becomes more extensively distributed.[1] With the exception of females protecting a tear-shaped, whitish egg sac, these spiders are usually not aggressive. Black widow spiders bite defensively when the web is disturbed.

Black widow spiders control the amount of venom they inject using striated muscle, which squeezes the venom glands and injects a metered amount of venom into the victim. *Latrodectus* bites do not necessarily indicate envenomation. It is estimated that 15% of bites in humans are nonenvenomating.[2]

Several animal species are extremely sensitive to black widow spider venom. Those of greatest economic importance are camels and horses.[3] Cats are very sensitive to the venom, and deaths are common in envenomated victims. In the dog the toxin provokes severe clinical signs, although they are considered more resistant than cats.[4]

Toxic Dose

A single bite is fully capable of delivering a lethal dose of venom to companion animals. Evidence suggests that the venom has increased toxicity in spiders living in areas with higher environmental temperatures. *Latrodectus* venom is one of the more toxic venoms, exceeding the toxicity of most snake venoms.[3,5] Comparative tests of venoms have demonstrated that the venom of *L. geometricus* (the brown widow) is the most potent of the five species, with a median lethal dose (LD_{50}) of 0.43 mg/kg body weight. The LD_{50} of the black widow venom (*L. mactans*) is 1.39 mg/kg.[3] Although there are antigenic differences in these venoms, the toxic fraction appears to be the same. The differences in median lethal doses of venoms must reflect differences in the volume percentage of the toxic fraction.[3] Although some controversy exists, it appears that venom toxicity is highest in autumn and lowest in spring.[6]

The incidence of black widow spider bites in veterinary medicine is unknown. Diagnosis of *Latrodectus* envenomation in domestic animals is rarely made, primarily because of veterinary unfamiliarity with the clinical manifestations and rarely are bites observed by owners.

Toxicokinetics

Although the toxicokinetics have not been well delineated, some information is known from human cases. The average duration of the syndrome in humans is 3 to 6 days.[7] Untreated patients have exhibited clinical signs for a period of 7 days, but weakness and some muscle pain and malaise may persist for weeks.[8]

Mechanism of Toxicity

Black widow spider venom contains no locally acting toxins that provoke a significant inflammatory reaction at the bite site. There are several toxic components consisting of five or six biologically active proteins. These include a potent mammalian neurotoxin called alpha-latrotoxin, which induces neurotransmitter release from nerve terminals. Initially the neurotoxin stimulates small end-plate action potentials, but later there is a block in neurotransmission, most likely caused by depletion of synaptic vesicle contents at the neuromuscular junction. The complex action seems to result from binding of glycoproteins and/or gangliosides on the neuromuscular synaptic membranes, thus allowing a channel to form for monovalent cation exchange that locks open. This depolarization promotes calcium-independent release of the neurotransmitters acetylcholine and norepinephrine (and others) down concentration gradients and then inhibits their subsequent reuptake.[9] Acetylcholine, noradrenaline, dopamine, glutamate, and enkephalin systems are all susceptible to the toxin.[10]

Clinical Signs

The onset of clinical signs usually occurs during the first 8 hours after envenomation. Local tissue changes are generally absent, and swelling at the bite site is uncommon. Small puncture wounds may be visible, and a mild erythema may develop. These changes are extremely difficult to see in animal victims because of skin pigmentation and dense hair coats.

Systemic manifestations depend on two sets of variables. Spider-dependent variables include the size of the spider, motivation of the spider (e.g., quantity of venom it decides to inject), and time of year (alters venom toxicity). Victim-dependent variables include species and size of victim (e.g., smaller victims receive a potentially higher dose in terms of milligrams of venom per kilogram body weight), location of bite, underlying health problems, and age of the victim (e.g., pediatric and geriatric victims are more severely afflicted).

Envenomated animals often lose up to 20% of their body weight within the first 24 hours after the bite. In contrast, in complete starvation (with water deprivation), at most a 12% weight loss occurs.[4] Initial regional numbness is often observed in dogs. Tenderness in adjacent lymph nodes may precede hyperesthesia, progressive muscle pain, and fasciculations in the affected region. Cramping of the muscles of the chest, abdomen, and lumbar and other large muscle masses is common. Abdominal rigidity without tenderness is a hallmark sign of *Latrodectus* envenomation. The condition is extremely painful in moderate to severe envenomations. Significant respiratory distress may become evident if muscle cramping is marked. Marked restlessness, writhing, and muscular contortions may occur. In humans, strenuous exercise temporarily relieves the pain. Seizures may occur. Hypertension and tachycardia should be anticipated. In high-risk patients (i.e., those with underlying health problems or at either end of the age spectrum), these cardiovascular manifestations may lead to stroke, exacerbation of heart failure, and possibly myocardial ischemia. Signs of motor restlessness may abate over 10 to 20 hours with the possible onset of paralysis. Death is usually due to respiratory or cardiovascular collapse.

Cats are extremely susceptible to *Latrodectus* venom. In one study, 20 of 22 feline victims died subsequent to black widow envenomation; there was an average survival time of 115 hours after the bite.[4] Paralytic signs may appear early and are particularly marked. Severe pain is manifested by howling and loud vocalizations. Excessive salivation and restlessness are common, and vomiting and diarrhea may occur. Muscular tremors, cramping, ataxia, and inability to stand precede complete paralysis. The body becomes adynamic and atonic. A Cheyne-Stokes respiratory pattern may develop, and death ensues.

Envenomated pregnant women and animals have shown significant clinical signs; however, the pregnancies were unaffected. These individuals were treated with antivenom, which had no negative effects on the fetuses or pregnancies.[11]

Minimum Database

The patient's vital signs should be measured frequently during the first 8 to 12 hours in the hospital. Hypertension is a significant threat. Serum chemistries and a complete blood cell count should be obtained. Elevations in creatinine phosphokinase can occur along with leukocytosis and hyperglycemia. Urine production can be decreased, and the urine may have an elevated specific gravity, possibly accompanied by albuminuria.

Confirmatory Tests

There are no diagnostic tests that can definitively confirm that a black widow spider bite has occurred. Cats, however, often vomit up the spider.

Treatment

First aid is essentially of no value in the treatment of *Latrodectus* envenomation. Early identification of bites is difficult unless the event is actually witnessed by the owner. Patients brought in for veterinary care are usually severely envenomated because the diagnosis relies on exhibited clinical signs. Therefore the incidence of "dry" and mild bites is inconsequential, and all diagnosed cases should be treated aggressively. The victim should be hospitalized for a minimum of 48 hours.

The primary treatment for black widow spider envenomation is administration of specific antivenom (Acalatro [*Latrodectus*, equine origin Fab2, Instituto Bioclon, Mexico]) [This antivenom is in final FDA trials for human use and can be imported with a USDA import permit.] This antivenom is supplied in a lyophilized state and reconstitutes rapidly into the supplied diluent. Antivenom should be administered by slow intravenous infusion. Allergic reactions can occur, and anaphylaxis is possible. Diluting the antivenom into a 100-mL saline solution and administering over a 30-minute time frame may decrease the risk of allergic reactions. Close monitoring of patients receiving beta-blockers is important because these compounds can mask the initial signs of anaphylaxis, which is more difficult to control as it progresses. Skin testing may be done, but the results are difficult to interpret and can be unreliable. The inner ear pinna should be monitored while the antivenom is *slowly* administered. If hyperemia develops, the infusion is discontinued, and diphenhydramine (2 to 4 mg/kg SC) is administered. If the allergic manifestations abate, the infusion of antivenom can then be restarted at a slower rate. If the reaction recurs, the infusion is stopped, and consultation is sought. True anaphylactic reactions are rare. A human study of 2062 antivenom-treated patients reported anaphylactic reactions in only 11 recipients (0.54%), none of which were fatal.[12] The veterinary clinician should be prepared to respond to an anaphylactic reaction by having the appropriate drugs, oxygen, and resuscitation equipment available before administering the antivenom. The most common reaction to the antivenom is a complement-mediated anaphylactoid type of reaction, such as occurs with rapid infusion of a foreign protein (e.g., as occurs not uncommonly with rapid blood transfusions). Indicated therapy should not be withheld because of fear of life-threatening reactions to the antivenom. The risks are low if antivenom is used properly. Antivenom treatment provides the most permanent and quickest relief of the envenomation syndrome, usually within 30 minutes of administration. One vial is usually sufficient, but a second vial may be indicated in severe envenomations. Delayed allergic reactions (serum sickness) are rare because of the low volume of foreign protein infused.

Extreme care should be taken with the administration of intravenous fluids. There is a high risk of hypertension developing in these patients as part of the envenomation syndrome. If specific antivenom is not available, 10% calcium gluconate has been recommended in the past to aid in abating the muscle cramping and decreasing the severity of the pain. However, calcium gluconate is no longer recommended for widow spider envenomation. Benzodiazepines are more efficacious than muscle relaxants for treatment of widow spider envenomation. Unlike the antivenom these drugs do not correct the hypertension or respiratory distress often seen with this envenomation syndrome.

Prognosis

The prognosis of *Latrodectus* envenomation is uncertain for several days, and complete recovery may take weeks.

Gross and Histologic Lesions

There are no definitive diagnostic systemic gross and histologic changes reported in dogs and cats.

Differential Diagnoses

Differential diagnoses include acute abdomen, intervertebral disk disease, bromethalin, and rabies (in cats).

References

1. Hunt GR: Bites and stings of uncommon arthropods. I. Spiders, *Postgrad Med* 70:91–102, 1981.
2. Key GF: A comparison of calcium gluconate and methocarbamol in the treatment of Latrodectism (black widow spider envenomation), *Am J Trop Med Hyg* 30(1):273–277, 1981.
3. Rauber A: Black widow spider bites, *J Toxicol Clin Toxicol* 21(4&5):473–485, 1983-84.
4. Maretic Z: Beobachtungen uber Pathologie und Klinik des Latrodektismus in Istrien (1948-1950), *Acta Trop* 8(136), 1951.
5. Kobernick M: Black widow spider bite, *Am Fam Physician* 29:241–245, 1984.
6. Keegan HC, Hedeen RA, Whittemore FW: Seasonal variation in venom of widow spiders, *Am J Trop Med Hyg* 9:477–479, 1960.
7. Russell F: Comparative pharmacology of some animal toxins, *Fed Proc* 26:193, 1967.
8. Rauber AP: The case of the red widow. A review of latrodectism, *Vet Hum Toxicol* 22(2):39–41, 1980.
9. Grasso A, Alema S, Rufini S, et al: Black widow spider toxin: effect on catecholamine release and cation permeability in a neurosecretory cell line (PC12). In Eaker D, Wadstrom T, editors: *Natural toxins. Proceedings of the 6th International Symposium on Animal, Plant and Microbial Toxins*, New York, 1979, Pergamon Press.
10. Knipper M, Madeddu L, Breer H, et al: Black widow spider venom-induced release of neurotransmitters: mammalian synaptosomes are stimulated by a unique venom component (α-latrotoxin), insect synaptosomes by multiple components, *Neuroscience* 19(1):55–62, 1986.
11. Russell FE, Marcus P, Streng JA: Black widow spider envenomation during pregnancy. Report of a case, *Toxicon* 17:188–189, 1979.
12. Sutherland SK: Use of antivenin, *Med J Aust* 2:620–623, 1978.

Spider Envenomation: Brown Recluse

80

Michael E. Peterson, DVM, MS

Jude McNally, RPh, DABAT

- *Loxosceles* spiders inhabit many areas of the United States. They are commonly referred to as violin spiders because of a violin-shaped marking on the dorsum of the cephalothorax (Color Plate 80-1). Pets are often bitten when lying down, trapping the spider between the bedding and themselves.
- A single bite from a brown recluse spider can inflict a lethal envenomation. The initial bite often goes undetected, but it can develop into a severe dermonecrotic lesion characterized by erythema, bullae formation, scabbing, and sloughing of affected tissue, with very slow healing.
- Severe systemic signs are uncommon. The most prevalent is a hemolytic anemia with a negative Coombs' test result.
- The minimum database should include a complete blood cell count, coagulation profile, serum chemistry panel including electrolytes, and urinalysis.
- Treatment can include wound management (cleansing and debridement), a broad-spectrum antibiotic, corticosteroids, antiinflammatory drugs, and analgesics.
- Prognosis is good for animals that show only localized necrotic lesions. Manifestations of systemic clinical signs require aggressive monitoring and treatment and a guarded prognosis.
- Commonly misdiagnosed in areas with no endemic *Loxosceles* species. In humans most mis-diagnosed brown recluse bites are actually methicillin-resistant *Staphylococcus* aureus (MRSA) lesions.

Sources

The venom from spiders of the genus *Loxosceles, the* most famous being *Loxosceles reclusa* (brown recluse spider), can cause serious poisoning. There are 13 species of *Loxosceles* spiders resident in the United States. These spiders inhabit the south and south central states from Georgia through Texas and north to southern Wisconsin. Several other species live in the western United States. At least five species indigenous to the United States have been associated with necrotic arachnidism: *L. reclusa, L. rufescens, L. arizonica, L. unicolor,* and *L. laeta*.[1] *Loxosceles* spiders vary in length from 6 to 20 mm. Their long legs allow them to move rapidly. The range of color found on these spiders runs from gray to orange-red, pale brown, and dusk. They are commonly called violin spiders because of the violin-shaped marking on the dorsum of the cephalothorax, with the neck of the violin pointing toward the abdomen. This feature, however, can be faint depending on the species or when the spider last molted. These spiders can be differentiated from regular brown garden spiders by their eyes; garden spiders have four pairs of eyes, whereas *Loxosceles* spiders have three pairs of eyes.

Loxosceles spiders are nocturnal and are generally active from spring through fall. They are obviously reclusive and live in dark, secluded locations, such as areas with rocks and surface debris. They venture out to prey upon insects and other spiders. These spiders are often found in and around human habitations. They like warm, undisturbed locations, such as storage sheds or behind the clothes washer and dryer. Their webs have a bluish hue.

Females may live 3 to 5 years. These spiders are nonaggressive and bite only when threatened. Domestic pets are usually bitten when they lie down and trap the spider between the bedding and themselves.

Toxic Dose and Toxicokinetics

A single bite can inflict a lethal envenomation. The average female *Loxosceles* spider carries a venom volume of approximately 0.36 mcL. Factors that appear to influence venom volume include the sex of the spider (males of equivalent size generate half of the female volume) and its size (larger, mature spiders can deliver a larger venom volume). Interestingly, prolonged periods of abnormal high or low environmental temperatures induce lower venom volumes.

Mechanism of Toxicity

The primary function of spider venom is to digest an impending meal by enzymatically destroying the victim's tissue. When fractionated by gel electrophoresis, the venom consists of eight major protein bands and four minor bands. Identified fractions include hyaluronidase, esterase, alkaline phosphatase, lipase, and 5'-ribonucleotide phosphorylase. A 32,000-Da protein fraction, sphingomyelinase D, is the primary dermonecrotic factor.[2]

It is thought that sphingomyelinase D exerts its effect by binding to cell membranes and chemotactically influencing polymorphonuclear leukocytes.[2] Histologically the lesions resemble the Arthus and Shwartzman phenomena. These reactions can be inhibited in rabbits by pretreating the victim with nitrogen mustard, which depletes polymorphonuclear neutrophils.

Another important mechanism is the inactivation of serum hemolytic complement. The venom induces rapid coagulation and occlusion of small capillaries, causing subsequent tissue necrosis.

The toxin also prolongs the activated partial thromboplastin time, and depletes clotting factors VIII, IX, XI, and XII.[3]

When serum C-reactive protein and calcium are available, sphingomyelinase D has a direct hemolytic effect. A calcium-dependent platelet aggregation can occur, leading to subsequent activation of the prostaglandin cascade. Serum amyloid protein is required for this platelet aggregation to occur.

The venom also acts on body lipids, freeing fragments into the circulation that subsequently act both as emboli and as inflammatory mediators. It is generally believed that the victim's immune response to *Loxosceles* venom ultimately determines the severity of the ensuing lesion.[3]

Clinical Signs

Clinical diagnosis is difficult because of the initially mild appearance of the lesion.[4] The ensuing severity of the bite is controlled by three factors: the amount of venom injected, the bite site, and the victim's immune status.[1] Dogs are highly susceptible to the effects of the venom.

The victim may not be aware of being bitten by these spiders. There may be a mild stinging sensation for up to 8 hours after the bite. Subsequent pruritus and soreness develop as vasoconstriction causes local ischemia. Edema follows with a classic "bull's-eye" lesion (an erythematous area inside of which is a pale ischemic region that develops a dark necrotic center as the lesion matures). The erythematous margin may progress unevenly as the effects of gravity come into play, leaving an eccentric lesion with the original center located dorsally. Hemorrhagic bullae may develop within 24 to 72 hours with an eschar developing below. The eschar sloughs in approximately 2 to 5 weeks, leaving an indolent ulcer, which usually does not penetrate into the muscle.[1] Lesions in adipose tissue can be extensive. Healing is slow, and these ulcers may persist for months, leaving a deep scar. In humans local swelling and persistent segmental cutaneous anesthesia have resulted from envenomations to the neck and head region.[5]

Systemic signs occur less commonly but can be life threatening. The most prevalent sign is a hemolytic anemia with significant hemoglobinuria, usually beginning within 24 hours after envenomation and persisting for approximately 1 week. This anemia usually gives a negative Coombs' test result. Other early-onset clinical signs include fever, arthralgia, vomiting, weakness, maculopapular rash, and leukocytosis. In humans the systemic syndrome is often described as a severe flu-like condition. Hemoglobinuria can induce renal failure. Disseminated intravascular coagulation and thrombocytopenia are possible sequelae. The systemic reaction is not proportionally related to the local reaction and vice versa.[1]

In humans despite prominent local signs, no fetal injuries were reported in five women who were envenomated during their second or third trimester of pregnancy.

Minimum Database

Pretreatment laboratory values should include a complete blood cell count, coagulation profile (e.g., prothrombin time, partial thromboplastin time, platelet count, and fibrinogen), and a complete serum chemistry panel including electrolytes. The size of the lesion should be measured. Tests with abnormal values or tests used to monitor the onset of hemolysis or hemoglobinuria (e.g., packed-cell volume, red blood cell count, hemoglobin, visual serum evaluation, and urinalysis) should be repeated as indicated to monitor the progression of the syndrome. This is particularly true for tests that reflect systemic manifestations of envenomation.

Confirmatory Tests

No confirmatory tests are commercially available in the United States.

Treatment

There is no specific antidote. Although there is an antivenom (Reclusmyn, Fab2 equine origin, produced by the Instituto Bioclon, Mexico), the advanced stage of the syndrome by the time of diagnosis in veterinary patients generally precludes its effective use. The treatment plan consists of responding to two possible syndromes, local cutaneous lesions and systemic manifestations of envenomation.

Dapsone (4,4′-diaminodiphenylsulfone), a leukocyte inhibitor, has been shown to be effective in treating dermal lesions in animal models.[4] In experimental studies, animals received 1 mg/kg dapsone by mouth for 14 days. The remaining ulcer was then allowed to heal as an open wound. Occasionally a second treatment course of dapsone was indicated. In humans dapsone may induce hemolysis and Heinz body formation in individuals with a deficiency in either glucose-6-phosphate dehydrogenase or methemoglobin reductase. It may be prudent to obtain a pretreatment hematocrit level and retest the patient in 2 or 3 days to monitor for a theoretical drug-induced hemolysis. By the time the maturing dermonecrotic lesion becomes manifest and the animal is brought in for treatment, the clinical syndrome would be past the initial envenomation stage, which has the highest risk of venom-induced hemolysis.

Surgical excision has been advocated in the past, but is no longer an indicated therapy. Results have been generally disappointing, and the procedure is not without complications.

Veterinary patients are frequently not brought to the medical facility until the lesion is well developed and frank necrosis has occurred. Conservative therapy includes several cleanings daily with Burow's solution and hydrogen peroxide. Some debridement may be necessary. One to two atm of hyperbaric oxygen twice daily for 3 to 4 days may be beneficial.[4,6] Broad-spectrum antibiotics are indicated if dapsone is not being administered in the treatment regimen.

Systemic signs of *Loxosceles* envenomation are potentially fatal and should be aggressively addressed. Patients exhibiting such signs should be hospitalized for close observation. Antiinflammatory, antipyretic, and analgesic agents can be useful. Compounds that affect clotting should be avoided. Systemic corticosteroids have a protective effect on the red blood cell membrane, thereby inhibiting hemolysis. They should be used only in the first few days of the syndrome at a rate of 1 to 2 mg/kg per day. Coagulation defects are treated as indicated. Hospitalization and intravenous fluid therapy may be needed to maintain adequate hydration to protect renal function.

Prognosis

The dermonecrotic lesions often take weeks or months to heal, and a scar typically remains at the site. Patients exhibiting severe systemic signs generally have a guarded prognosis.

Gross and Histologic Lesions

There are no definitive systemic gross or histologic lesions reported in dogs and cats.

Differential Diagnoses

In humans MRSA lesions are most commonly misdiagnosed as brown recluse spider bites. Additionally, mycobacterial or other bacterial infection, decubital ulcer, third-degree burn, and pyoderma mimic the dermonecrotic wound of a spider bite. Systemic signs must be differentiated from other causes of hemolytic anemia (e.g., immune mediated, zinc poisoning, acetaminophen, onion poisoning), snake bite, insect sting, and fever of unknown origin.

References

1. Wasserman GS, Anderson PC: Loxoscelism and necrotic arachnidism, *J Toxicol Clin Toxicol* 21(4&5):451–472, 1983-84.
2. Rekow MA, Civello DJ, Geren CR: Enzymatic and hemolytic properties of brown recluse spider *(Loxosceles reclusa)* toxin and extracts of venom apparatus, cephalothorax and abdomen, *Toxicon* 21(3):441–444, 1983.
3. Babcock JL, Marmer DJ, Steele RW: Immunotoxicology of brown recluse spider bites *(Loxosceles reclusa)* venom, *Toxicon* 24(8):783–790, 1986.
4. Rees RS, Campbell D, Rieger E, et al: The diagnosis and treatment of brown recluse spider bites, *Ann Emerg Med* 16(9):945–949, 1987.
5. Smith CW, Micks DW: The role of polymorphonuclear leukocytes in the lesion caused by the venom of the brown spider, *Loxosceles recluse, Lab Invest* 1:90–93, 1970.
6. Rees RS, Altenbern DP, Lynch JB, et al: Brown recluse spider bites—a comparison of early surgical excision versus dapsone and delayed surgical excision, *Ann Surg* 202(5):657–663, 1985.

Strychnine

Patricia A. Talcott, MS, DVM, PhD, DABVT

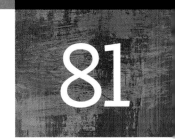

- Strychnine is a highly potent, rodenticide still used in many areas of the United States.
- Dogs are most commonly affected; oral exposures of as little as a few tablespoons of strychnine-laced bait are enough to cause toxicity.
- Clinical signs include early apprehension, anxiety, and salivation, followed quickly by the onset of muscle spasm, severe extensor rigidity, and convulsions.
- Confirmation of poisoning can be made by chemical analysis of vomitus, lavage washings, and stomach contents; strychnine can sometimes be detected in serum, urine, liver, or kidney.
- Treatment aims are directed toward preventing further absorption in asymptomatic patients (emesis or gastric lavage, activated charcoal, and cathartic); preventing or controlling muscle spasms or seizures (pentobarbital, diazepam, or methocarbamol); controlling hyperthermia, hypoxia, and acidosis; and maintaining adequate urine output (intravenous fluids).
- Prognosis is guarded, depending on exposure dose and extent of delay between exposure and medical intervention.
- There are no specific gross or histologic lesions.
- Differential diagnoses include tetanus and poisonings with metaldehyde, penitrem A, roquefortine, 4-aminopyridine, nicotine, caffeine, amphetamines, cocaine, organophosphorus and carbamate insecticides, pyrethrins and pyrethroids, mushrooms, cyanobacteria (blue-green algae), methylxanthines, compound 1080, and chlorinated hydrocarbon pesticides.

Strychnine-containing baits are commonly used outdoors in many parts of the United States by homeowners, farm workers, certified applicators, and animal damage control personnel to control nuisance populations of several species of animals, including ground squirrels or gophers, meadow and deer mice, moles, prairie dogs, rats, porcupines, chipmunks, rabbits, and pigeons. As with other rodenticides (e.g., anticoagulant rodenticides, bromethalin, cholecalciferol, and zinc phosphide), accidental and malicious poisoning of dogs (particularly free-roaming dogs), cats, and other companion animals with strychnine is not uncommon in many areas of the United States, particularly in states where products can still be purchased over the counter.

Sources

Strychnine was first used as a rodenticide in Germany in the early sixteenth century.[1] Poisonings in humans occur in suicide attempts, intentional malicious poisonings, or with its use as an adulterant in heroin and cocaine.[2] Strychnine-containing pesticides have been marketed under a variety of trade names, including Gopher-Go, Milo Bait for Gophers, Gopher Getter, Orco Gopher Grain Bait, Quick Action Gopher Mix, Force's Mole Killer, and Force's Gopher Killer. Many strychnine baits are composed of red- or green-colored grain (e.g., oat, milo, corn, and wheat) containing 0.5% to 1% strychnine sulfate (Color Plate 81-1). Some restricted-use formulations contain much higher concentrations of the alkaloid. Some states allow over-the-counter sales of strychnine-containing products only if strychnine is present at a concentration of 0.5% or less. Liquid formulations have been historically available in other countries (e.g., Canada). All applications are intended to be used underground, either inside artificial burrows made with a burrow builder, or by hand baiting into the main natural burrow runway system, taking care not to cover the bait with soil.

Toxic Dose

The strychnine alkaloid is isolated from the seeds of *Strychnos nux-vomica* and *S. ignatii*. Strychnine sulfate is a white powder that is moderately soluble in water. Strychnine bait is poorly soluble in water and strongly adheres to soil particles. Its environmental persistence is not long, and more than 90% disappears from soil within 40 days. Breakdown in soil depends on the presence and growth of particular microbial or fungal soil organisms.

Strychnine is intensely poisonous to fish, aquatic invertebrates, birds, and mammals (Table 81-1). Most confirmed cases of poisoning occur in dogs; cats are infrequently affected. The reported acute median lethal dose (LD_{50}) of strychnine in dogs and cats is 0.5 to 1.2 mg/kg and 2 mg/kg, respectively. Depending on the size of the animal and the concentration of strychnine present in the bait, ingestion of only a few tablespoons by a dog or cat is sufficient to cause death. Secondary poisoning of dogs and cats resulting from ingestion of strychnine-poisoned rodents can occur but is not commonly reported.

Toxicokinetics

Strychnine is rapidly absorbed from the gastrointestinal tract (small intestine mostly) and mucous membranes. Very little protein binding occurs, and strychnine is readily metabolized by hepatic microsomal enzyme activity to strychnine-N-oxide.[3] Anywhere from 1% to 20% of the original exposure dose is excreted into the urine unchanged.[4,5] Strychnine has a wide tissue distribution, and only small amounts (less than 4 ppm) are ever detected in blood or tissues at any given time. Elimination of strychnine is best described by a linear (Michaelis-Menten) model.[6]

Table 81-1 Reported Oral Lethal Doses of Strychnine

Species	Oral Median Lethal Dose (LD_{50}) (mg/kg body weight)
Cat	2.0
Cow	0.5
Dog	0.5-1.2
Golden eagle	5-10
Horse	0.5
Human	30-60
Mule deer	17-24
Pheasant	8.5-24.7
Pig	0.5-1
Rainbow trout	2.3
Rat	2.2-14
Sage grouse	42.5

Mechanism of Toxicity

Glycine is an important inhibitory neurotransmitter to motor neurons and interneurons in the spinal cord, brainstem, and thalamus, and strychnine effectively blocks the inhibitory action of glycine on the anterior horn of the cells of the spinal cord and that of the endogenous transmitter, preventing it from being released from the Renshaw cells.[7,8] This inhibition ultimately leads to unchecked neuronal activity, producing highly exaggerated reflex arcs. Mild to severe muscle spasms result, generally leading to extreme hyperextension of the limbs and body caused by domination of the more powerful extensor muscle groups. This can ultimately result in a full tetanic convulsion.

Clinical Signs

The primary target organ for strychnine is the central nervous system. Clinical signs generally develop in poisoned patients within 10 to 120 minutes after ingestion. The severity of the signs depends on the exposure dose. Clinical signs in animals exposed to low levels of strychnine may be delayed and mild (e.g., slight ataxia and muscle stiffness), whereas high doses result in rapid onset of severe muscle spasms or seizures. Initial signs commonly observed in strychnine-poisoned dogs include a brief (less than 15 minutes) prodromal phase of nervousness, apprehension, anxiety, increased respiratory rate, and excessive salivation. Ataxia, muscle spasms, and stiffness gradually develop, generally beginning with the face, neck, and limb muscles. This stage rapidly develops into generalized convulsions that are tonic-extensor in nature (i.e., opisthotonos). The neck is usually arched back, the jaw clamped shut, and the face fixed into a "sardonic grin." These episodes may last several minutes intermittently, or they may be continuous. Respiration is obviously impaired during these episodes because of contraction of the diaphragm and the thoracic and abdominal muscles. Many strychnine-poisoned dogs show an increased severity and frequency of these episodes following sensory stimulation (e.g., loud noise, bright light, and touch). This feature, however, is not specific to strychnine and has been observed in other types of poisonings as well (e.g., metaldehyde, penitrem A, roquefortine, chlorinated hydrocarbons, bromethalin). Typically, in the early phases, the patient is conscious and aware of its surroundings. Vomiting is not consistently reported in strychnine-poisoned patients, but it can be seen, particularly if the strychnine bait has been mixed with palatable food items in cases of malicious poisoning. Death is a result of respiratory paralysis, most likely caused by hypoxia from impaired respiration, and can occur as quickly as 10 minutes after ingestion or as late as 24 to 48 hours after ingestion (depending on the degree of medical intervention). Hyperthermia is commonly observed; this is a result of the severe muscle contractions.

Minimum Database

In general, there are few specific blood and serum chemistry abnormalities following strychnine ingestion. At the most, poisoned dogs may display changes compatible with mild dehydration and a mild metabolic acidosis. A complete blood cell count and serum chemistry panel is helpful only in ruling out nonstrychnine causes of seizure activity. Rhabdomyolysis, with subsequent renal failure, has been reported in humans, but has been rarely observed in poisoned dogs and cats.

Confirmatory Tests

In clinical cases, the presence of strychnine can be confirmed by various analytical methods (e.g., thin-layer chromatography, high-performance liquid chromatography, and gas chromatography–mass spectrometry) performed on vomitus or lavage washings (stomach contents postmortem); it is less commonly performed on serum or urine. Because strychnine-poisoned patients may not vomit, the stomach contents are the best tissue to confirm the presence of the alkaloid. The presence of green- or red-dyed grain in the vomitus, lavage washings, or stomach contents postmortem should lead the veterinarian to perform some type of quantitative analysis. However, other types of pesticides have similar appearances (e.g., bromethalin, 1080, zinc phosphide, cholecalciferol). Liver, bile, or kidney can also be used to verify the presence of strychnine in tissue collected postmortem, but these are less likely to yield positive confirmation.

Treatment

The treatment of strychnine-poisoned dogs and cats is initially directed at reducing gastrointestinal absorption of the compound and is followed by appropriate supportive care to reverse the hyperthermia, hypoxia, and acidosis; minimize muscle spasms and convulsive activity; and maintain adequate renal output. Before the onset of seizure activity, emetics can be used to evacuate the stomach. Care should be taken with the use of emetics because this type of sensory stimulation may initiate violent muscle or convulsive activity. A more conservative approach is to perform a gastric lavage once the patient has been adequately sedated and intubated. Administration of activated charcoal followed with a cathartic should follow either procedure (delay a minimum of 45 minutes if emesis was induced). Strychnine is very effectively bound to activated charcoal and should be considered a mainstay in the treatment of poisoned patients.

Typically the more urgent objectives facing clinicians in the treatment of strychnine-poisoned patients are controlling the convulsions and supporting respiration. Because barbiturates have been shown to raise the threshold of spinal reflexes in animals, pentobarbital has been used successfully clinically to control strychnine-induced convulsions. Pentobarbital, like other barbiturate anesthetics, abolishes the spontaneous activity of spinal cord neurons by acting as a γ-aminobutyric acid–mimetic; it should be administered slowly intravenously (IV) at a dose of 3 to 15 mg/kg or to effect.[9] Diazepam, with its muscle relaxant, anxiolytic, and anticonvulsant properties, can also be effective in treating strychnine-poisoned pets (0.5 to 1 mg/kg IV or to effect); it can also be administered as a constant-rate infusion (0.1 to 0.5 mg/kg, diluted in 5% dextrose in water [D5W]; rate of administration per hour should be equal to the maintenance needs of the patient).[9] Methocarbamol can also be used at a dose of 44 to 220 mg/kg IV, generally not to exceed 330 mg/kg/day.[9] Methocarbamol causes skeletal muscle relaxation and a secondary sedative effect. Inhalation gas anesthesia can be used initially to control anxiety or seizure activity. A benefit of this choice is that the clinician can provide a readily available, controlled source of oxygen. However, because of the length of time most patients require sedation (24 to 72 hours, or longer), this choice is highly impractical for the long haul. Respiratory activity should be closely monitored, and some type of respiratory assistance (e.g., mechanical ventilation) should be readily available in animals that are severely compromised.

Intravenous fluids (e.g., Normosol-M and half-strength lactated Ringer's solution in D5W) should be administered to correct hypovolemia, provide continuous maintenance needs, prevent rhabdomyolysis-induced renal disease (rare), and aid in correcting the hyperthermia and mild to moderate acidosis. Bicarbonate can be used to correct the acidosis if traditional fluid therapy is not sufficient; this is not commonly necessary. All forms of sensory stimulation should be minimized, so patients should be kept in a dimly lit, quiet area.

Prognosis

Most poisoned patients are treated continuously and aggressively monitored in the hospital for up to 24-72 hours. Aggressive decontamination procedures, combined with 24-hour intensive care monitoring, significantly lessen the length of hospital stay and hasten recovery. Unfortunately, because of strychnine's rapid onset, most patients are brought to veterinary facilities late in the progression of the disease, and many die before appropriate treatment can be initiated.

Gross and Histologic Lesions

No specific gross and histologic lesions have been described in strychnine-poisoned dogs and cats. Nonspecific changes can include agonal, petechial hemorrhages of the heart and lung, along with generalized congestion of tissues. Some clinicians have noted extensive pancreatic hemorrhage in strychnine-poisoned dogs. Extensive necrosis of the cerebral cortex and brainstem have been reported in humans poisoned with strychnine.[6] The exact cause of this is unclear, but it has been hypothesized that the lesions may be due to poor cerebral perfusion or cortical seizure activity.

Differential Diagnoses

Strychnine poisoning in dogs and cats can mimic a wide variety of other central nervous system disorders. These include tetanus and poisoning with metaldehyde, penitrem A, roquefortine, 4-aminopyridine, theobromine, nicotine, caffeine, amphetamines, cocaine, chlorinated hydrocarbons, organophosphorus and carbamate acetylcholinesterase-inhibiting insecticides, neurotoxic cyanobacteria, bromethalin, compound 1080, and pyrethrins and pyrethroids. Similar clinical signs can occur in pets poisoned with *Taxus* spp. (yew), *Dicentra* spp. (bleeding heart and Dutchman's breeches), *Cicuta* spp. (water hemlock), and some mushrooms.

References

1. Franz DN: Central neurotransmitters. In Gilman AG, Goodman LS, Rall TW, et al, editors: *The pharmacological basis of therapeutics*, ed 7, New York, 1985, Macmillan.
2. Boyd RE, Spyker DA: Strychnine poisoning: recovery from profound lactic acidosis, hyperthermia, and rhabdomyolysis, *Am J Med* 74:507, 1983.
3. Adamson RH, Fouts JR: Enzymatic metabolism of strychnine, *J Pharmacol Exp Ther* 127:87, 1959.
4. Weiss S, Hatcher RA: Studies on strychnine, *J Pharmacol Exp Ther* 14:419, 1922.
5. Sgaragli GP, Mannaioni PF: Pharmacokinetic observations on a cases of massive strychnine poisoning, *Clin Toxicol* 6:533, 1973.
6. Heiser JM, Daya MR, Magnussen AR, et al: Massive strychnine intoxication: serial blood levels in a fatal case, *Clin Toxicol* 30(2):269, 1992.
7. Curtis DR, Duggan AW, Johnston GAR: The specificity of strychnine as a glycine antagonist in the mammalian spinal cord, *Exp Brain Res* 12:547, 1971.
8. Curtis DR, Hosli L, Johnston GAR: A pharmacological study of the depression of spinal neurones by glycine and related amino acids, *Exp Brain Res* 6:1, 1968.
9. Plumb DC: *Veterinary drug handbook*, ed 3, White Bear Lake, Minn., 1999, Pharma Vet Publishing.

Toads

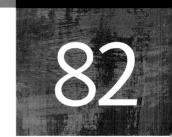

Michael E. Peterson, DVM, MS

Brian K. Roberts, DVM, DACVECC

- Colorado River toad (*Bufo alvarius*) and marine or cane toad (*Bufo marinus*) are the most common toads that cause toxicity.
- Toxic agents include dopamine, epinephrine, norepinephrine, serotonin, bufotenine, bufagenins (digitalis-like compounds), bufotoxins, and indolealkylamines.
- Absorption via the mucous membranes of the oral cavity is rapid.
- The poison affects the heart (arrhythmias), peripheral vasculature, and central nervous system. Clinical signs include hypersalivation, pawing at the mouth, brick-red mucous membranes, hyperthermia, ataxia, collapse, and seizures.
- Clinical pathologic conditions include slightly elevated blood urea nitrogen, hyperkalemia, hypercalcemia, hypophosphatemia, hyponatremia, and hypochloremia (mild). Sinus tachycardia, sinus bradycardia, and ventricular arrhythmias are commonly observed.
- No true confirmatory tests exist. Digoxin levels by immunoassay may support suggested toxicity.
- Treatment consists of flushing the oral cavity with water, controlling seizures, documenting or treating any arrhythmias, and supportive care.
- Differential diagnoses include heat stroke, neuropathies and seizure disorders, other toxins, such as metaldehyde, theobromine, insoluble oxalate-containing plants, pyrethrins and pyrethroids, oleander, and anticholinesterase insecticides.

Sources

There are more than 200 species of *Bufo* toads in the world. These toads have been used for centuries in religious rituals, witchcraft, and healing. Even today toad excretions are used by South American and Mesoamerican tribes as fertility enhancers. In the United States the Food and Drug Administration listed one of the toad excretions, bufotenine, as a schedule 1 substance in 1967 because of "toad licking" and "toad smoking" by drug users.[1]

The two most common *Bufo* species that cause poisonings in small animals in the United States are the cane or marine toad (*Bufo marinus*) (Color Plate 82-1) and the Colorado River toad (also known as the Sonoran desert toad) (*Bufo alvarius*) (Color Plate 82-2).[2] The European *Bufo vulgaris* and the Asian *Bufo gargarizans* are related species that can cause poisonings. Colorado, Arizona, Texas, Hawaii, and Florida are the principal locations in the United States where small animals are exposed to toads and suffer from poisonings. *Bufo* toads were introduced into the southern states from Hawaii for insect and rodent control.[3] The foreign toads have replaced many native species because of their hardiness and proliferative reproductive capabilities.

Exposures usually occur during the summer months in the Southeast and during periods of high humidity or late summer in the Southwest.[2] *Bufo* toad exposures have been reported throughout the year in Florida (Figure 82-1) except in the month of December.[4] Toads are most active after a period of rainfall, especially at dawn, dusk, and evening hours. All *Bufo* species have parotid glands on their dorsum that release toxic substances when the toad is attacked or threatened. These toxins are biologically active compounds.[1]

Toxic Dose

Toxicity truly varies and depends on size and dose. Larger toads have larger parotid glands and therefore have more voluminous excretions. The most severe clinical signs of toxicosis are seen in animals with low body weight that have encountered a large toad for a prolonged period.[4] Although most small animals do not consume *Bufo* toads, severe toxicosis occurs in animals that masticate or hold the toads instead of just biting and then releasing the toad. Exposure to 1 mg/kg of secretions is required for the induction of clinical signs of intoxication.[5]

Toxicokinetics

Toxins secreted from the parotid glands of *Bufo* toads are rapidly absorbed across the mucous membranes and then enter the systemic circulation.[3] The toxins can also be absorbed through the gastric mucosa following ingestion, through open skin wounds, and across the conjunctiva. Once the toxins have entered the systemic circulation, the greatest effects are seen on the heart, peripheral vasculature, and nervous system.[1] *Bufo* toads release many substances that are naturally found in the body, such as the catecholamines, epinephrine, norepinephrine, dopamine, and serotonin; the metabolism of these biologically active compounds occurs in a manner similar to normal physiology. Examples include catecholamine reuptake and metabolism by monoamine oxidase and catechol O-methyltransferase.[6] Elimination of bufagenins, which are the digitalis-like substances, occurs via first-order kinetics, and these substances are excreted through the urine.[6]

Mechanism of Toxicity

The biologically active substances produced by *Bufo* toads include dopamine, epinephrine, norepinephrine, serotonin, bufotenine, bufagenins, bufotoxins, and indolealkylamines.[1,3] All *Bufo* species produce these substances, but there is variation in the quantity of each substance produced by different toads. For instance, *Bufo marinus* and *Bufo viridis* contain the highest known plasma level of endogenous digitalis-like substances, which are collectively

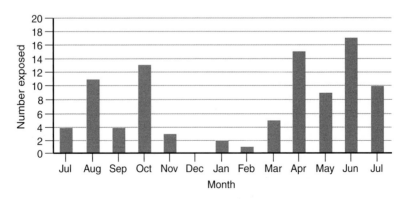

Figure 82–1 Companion animal exposure to *Bufo* toads (July 1997-July 1998).

known as *bufadienolides*.[7] Indolealkylamines have been characterized as similar to the hallucinogen lysergic acid diethylamide.[2]

Bufotenine, or 5-hydroxydimethyltryptamine, has been definitively identified as a pressor, but there is also evidence that this compound may be a hallucinogen or have a "psychedelic" effect.[1,8] The hallucinogenic effects of bufotenine may be secondary to the known systemic pressor activity and oxygen starvation of the optic nerve.[1] Only the Colorado River toad (*Bufo alvarius*) releases 5-methoxydimethyltryptamine from the methylation of serotonin; it acts as a true hallucinogen.[9]

Bufagenins and bufotoxins are cardioactive steroids also known as digitalis-like substances.[7] The bufagenins act like digitalis to inhibit potassium-dependent adenosine triphosphatase, which is the enzyme that allows active transport of sodium out of and potassium into cells.[7] Digitalis-like substances can cause alterations in heart rate and rhythm. Any type of arrhythmia can result from digitalis overdose, especially bradycardia and supraventricular and ventricular tachycardias. Bufotoxins are vasoconstrictors and add to the pressor effect of bufotenine to increase systemic vascular resistance.[1]

Although many of the substances released from *Bufo* toads are known to cause vasoconstriction and an increase in blood pressure, there has been no documentation to support this pressor activity.[3]

Clinical Signs

Dogs are the most common companion animals affected by amphibian toxins. However, cats and pocket pets, such as ferrets, can also be exposed to *Bufo* toads.[4] Most exposed animals have a history of being outside and are then either seen attacking a toad or found by the owner hypersalivating, seizing, or disoriented. Many *Bufo* toads are nocturnal, which is why many exposures occur at dusk or on evening walks. *Bufo* toads are most active during periods of excessive humidity and are often seen in high numbers after a rainstorm.

The first signs of exposure include brick-red mucous membranes, hypersalivation, pawing at the mouth, and vocalizing.[2-5] Many owners describe their dogs as "foaming at the mouth." It is believed that the parotid gland secretions are noxious to mucous membranes and lead to erythema and ptyalism. Within a few minutes the affected animal can become disoriented, circle, stumble, and fall.[4] Many poisoned dogs also exhibit a blank stare or opisthotonic posture. Others become tachypneic and anxious and then vomit. Severe toxicosis results in seizure activity and coma. The elapsed time from exposure to exhibition of signs is only a matter of minutes. Most toxic effects are seen within 30 minutes to 1 hour after contact with a *Bufo* toad.

Physical examination findings may include any or all of the following: erythematous mucous membranes, ptyalism, tachypnea, tachycardia or bradycardia, hyperthermia, and collapse. Much of the data available in companion animal studies denote cardiac arrhythmias, which range from various degrees of bradycardia and heart block to ventricular tachycardia and ventricular fibrillation.[3]

There are also a large number of neurologic abnormalities, such as altered states of consciousness (e.g., disorientation, stupor, and coma) and varying degrees of ataxia, such as circling, falling, leaning, listing, and stumbling. Neurologic examination findings may include nystagmus, midrange or mydriatic pupils with slow pupillary light reflexes, hyperesthesia, conscious proprioceptive defects, and status epilepticus.

Of the described physical findings, erythematous mucous membranes, ptyalism, anxiety or shaking, and tachypnea are most commonly noted (Table 82-1). Neurologic abnormalities are identified in more than half of dogs that are naturally exposed to *Bufo* toads (see Table 82-1). The most common neurologic signs reported are seizure activity, ataxia, stupor, collapse, and nystagmus.[4] Many of the same clinical and neurologic abnormalities described in small-animal exposures have also been identified in human exposures. In a 1986 report a 5-year-old boy was brought to the emergency room in status epilepticus after placing a *Bufo* toad in his mouth.[10] Initial signs of severe hypersalivation and nausea occurred within 10 minutes of exposure and then progressed to delirium and seizure activity. Other findings on examination included slurred speech and left-sided paresis.

Table 82-1	Physical Examination Findings in Animals Exposed to *Bufo* Toads	
Clinical Signs	Number (94 Cases)	Percentage
Neuropathy (seizures, ataxia, nystagmus, coma)	51	54.26
Brick-red mucous membranes	48	51.06
Ptyalism	39	41.49
Anxiety shaking	25	26.60
Collapsed recumbent	17	18.09
Vomiting	11	11.70
Mydriasis and anisocoria	5	5.32

Minimum Database

Currently, there is no information available on minimum database values for animals that have sustained natural oral exposure to *Bufo* toad toxins. In one controlled study, orally exposed and intravenously (IV) exposed dogs under anesthesia showed moderate increases in hemoglobin content, packed-cell volume and icterus index, blood glucose, blood urea nitrogen, alkaline phosphatase, and serum potassium.[3] The study also found decreases in serum sodium, phosphorus, total protein, and white blood cell count.

Patients exhibiting the most serious clinical signs commonly have severe acid-base abnormalities and hemoconcentration. It is common for comatose patients to present with symptoms of hypercapnia and a marked respiratory acidosis. Severe metabolic acidosis secondary to seizure activity or tremors may develop in certain dogs that are severely intoxicated.

Dyspnea secondary to noncardiogenic pulmonary edema has been seen in a few dogs with severe signs of intoxication. It is believed by one of the authors that this edema may be secondary to seizure activity, pulmonary hypertension caused by the pressor effects of the toxins, or acute respiratory distress syndrome. Patients exhibiting any type of increased effort or crackles should undergo thoracic radiographs once stabilization and oxygen supplementation have been instituted.

Confirmatory Tests

There are no routinely available tests to confirm *Bufo* toad poisoning. Reports do exist in human literature for persons exposed to herbal or holistic medicines that contain *Bufo* toad extracts.[11] Intoxicated individuals have elevated serum digoxin levels caused by the digitoxin-like substances ingested from the toad extracts. Therefore it is possible that digoxin serum immunoassays can aid in the diagnosis of *Bufo* toad poisoning in companion animals.

Treatment

The most effective therapy for acute intoxication is thorough flushing of the oral cavity with running water.[2-4] If toxicosis is suggested, the mouth should be flushed as soon as possible unless the affected pet is unconscious or seizing, taking care to flush the mouth in the rostral direction. Owners should be told to perform this procedure at home before traveling to seek veterinary care. The flushing procedure should be repeated at least two to three times for 5 to 10 minutes at a time. Once this is completed, the history should be taken and physical and neurologic examinations performed.

After seizure intervention (when necessary) has been instituted, cardiac rate and rhythm should be documented by electrocardiogram and analyzed. If bradycardia or heart block is detected, atropine at a dose of 0.02 mg/kg may be given IV. Atropine may decrease the amount of salivation and act as a bronchodilator.[2] It is not a true antidote, although some consider it to be one.[3,4] The use of atropine may worsen tachycardia and potentiate ventricular tachycardia. In such circumstances, atropine is not recommended. Sustained tachycardia with heart rates of more than 180 beats/min in dogs or 220 beats/min in cats should be treated with beta antagonists, such as propranolol (0.5 to 0.6 mg/kg given over 5-10 minutes IV), esmolol (0.5 mg/kg IV) followed by a continuous-rate infusion of 50 to 200 mcg/kg/min, or atenolol (0.25 to 1 mg/kg orally).[2,3] Treatment for ventricular tachycardia may be accomplished by using lidocaine as a 2 mg/kg IV bolus, which can be repeated up to three times, followed by a continuous-rate infusion at a dose of 40 to 75 mcg/kg/min. Procainamide can also be used for ventricular tachycardias at a dose of 6 to 8 mg/kg given in an IV bolus, 6 to 20 mg/kg given intramuscularly, or 10 to 40 mcg/kg/min as a continuous rate infusion. If ventricular arrhythmias do not respond to continuous infusion therapies, serum magnesium should be evaluated and corrected using magnesium sulfate at a dose of 0.15 to 0.3 mEq/kg IV given over 5 to 10 minutes. Supraventricular arrhythmias have not been reported, but may occur and respond to beta antagonists or vagal maneuvers.

Because the bufagenins and bufotoxins have effects similar to those of digoxin, treatment with digoxin-specific Fab fragments may be of value. Humans exposed to herbal compounds containing *Bufo* extracts exhibit signs similar to digoxin toxicity, such as bradycardia, hypotension, and various arrhythmias.[11] Treatment with digoxin-specific Fab fragments in these patients has been successful. Digoxin-specific Fab fragments bind to the digoxin-like substances and also block the inhibition of sodium-potassium adenosine phosphatase activity.

Neurologic abnormalities are common, and treatment should be instituted immediately in patients with seizures using diazepam (0.5 mg/kg IV).[4] If seizures or seizurelike activity persists, pentobarbital (3 to 15 mg/kg IV) may be used. In some instances, a continuous-rate infusion of diazepam at 0.2 to 1.0 mg/kg/hr may be necessary. Propofol at a dose of 0.1 mg/kg/min can also be considered as a constant rate infusion for refractory seizure activity. Animals with progressing neurologic signs may benefit from short-acting glucocorticoids, such as prednisolone sodium succinate (Solu-Delta-Cortef) or methylprednisolone sodium succinate (Solu-Medrol) at doses of 10 to 20 mg/kg given slowly IV. Furosemide (2 mg/kg) followed by mannitol (500 to 1000 mg/kg given over 20 minutes) may also be of benefit in animals that have sustained numerous seizures and have a worsening neurologic status.

In severely affected animals, body temperature, blood glucose levels, and hydration should be monitored and corrected. Supportive care with IV fluids (Plasma-Lyte A or lactated Ringer's solution) at maintenance doses of 60 mL/kg/day is recommended for animals that require hospitalization because some of these patients will not eat or drink or may vomit.

Hyperthermic patients require aggressive treatment when core temperatures exceed 105° F. Therapy consists of IV fluids to correct hypovolemia given over 12 to 24 hours, tepid water baths, and alcohol placed on the foot pads. Once the body temperature has decreased to 102° F, external bathing may be stopped. If the patient's temperature remains elevated at more than 105° F despite the aforementioned treatments, a low-dose corticosteroid (dexamethasone sodium phosphate, 0.1 mg/kg IV) may be administered.

Patients that are brought in comatose or with respiratory distress or compromise should have a venous acid-base blood test performed. Dogs with marked signs can have metabolic or respiratory acidosis, hemoconcentration with hematocrit values more than 60%, and noncardiogenic pulmonary edema. In our experience, patients with these documented abnormalities have a guarded prognosis. Correction of metabolic acidosis is generally achieved using a balanced crystalloid IV infusion. Blood pH values of less than 7.1 should be corrected using sodium bicarbonate (0.3 × body weight in kg × base deficit) at one fourth of this calculated dose. The acid-base must be reassessed within an hour after using IV buffers. Patients suffering from respiratory compromise should receive supplemental oxygen (100%) by mask or flow-by until the respiratory problems improve or continuous supplemental oxygen (Fio_2 of 0.4 to 0.6) should be provided. If hypercapnia and respiratory acidosis were diagnosed, then the clinician should consider providing supplemental positive pressure ventilation until the acidosis is corrected and the patient is producing adequate ventilatory effort.

Dogs that have noncardiogenic pulmonary edema should be treated symptomatically with supplemental oxygen, judicious fluid therapy, and furosemide by continuous rate

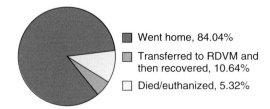

Figure 82–2 Outcome of companion animal exposure to *Bufo* toads (July 1997-July 1998).

infusion (0.0.5 to 1 mg/kg/hr)[12] until signs resolve. Furosemide by continuous rate infusion should be used for as short of a duration as possible because dehydration may occur. Generally the infusion is provided for 4 to 6 hours.

Prognosis

Based on our experience, affected pets have a favorable prognosis (greater than 90% survival rate) (Figure 82-2). Cases with guarded to poor prognostic factors include those with marked hemoconcentration and noncardiogenic pulmonary edema.

Gross and Histologic Lesions

Cerebral edema and hemorrhage were noted in one Philippine study.[13]

Differential Diagnoses

Many other toxicoses and neuropathies can present with signs similar to those of *Bufo* toad intoxication. Primary neuropathies that result in seizures, collapse, and ataxia must be considered when a limited history is provided by the owners in regard to the environment and exposure to toads. Differential diagnoses for animals that are brought in with seizures should include idiopathic epilepsy; inflammatory meningoencephalitis secondary to infectious, immune-mediated, or neoplastic processes; and structural diseases, such as space-occupying masses. In patients whose primary complaint is ataxia, peripheral and central vestibular diseases should be considered.

Because most animals are brought in with acute onset of clinical signs, intoxications with metaldehyde, theobromine, oleander, insoluble oxalate-containing plants, pyrethrins and pyrethroids, and anticholinesterase insecticides must be included in the differential diagnosis until a thorough history of exposure to any of these compounds can be excluded. Caustic materials, such as various acid and alkali materials, cause severe hypersalivation and erythematous mucous membranes and should be excluded. Last, heat stroke in hyperthermic patients should be ruled out.

References

1. Lyttle T, Goldstein D, Gartz J: *Bufo* toads and bufotenine: fact and fiction surrounding an alleged psychedelic, *J Psychoactive Drugs* 28(3):267–290, 1996.
2. Peterson ME: Toad venom toxicity. In Tilley LP, Smith WK, editors: *The five-minute veterinary consult*, Baltimore, 1997, Williams & Wilkins.
3. Palumbo NE, Perri SF: Toad poisoning. In Kirk RW, editor: *Current veterinary therapy VIII*, Philadelphia, 1983, WB Saunders.
4. Roberts BK, Aronsohn MA, Moses BL, et al: *Bufo marinus* intoxication in dogs: 94 cases (1997-1998), *J Am Vet Med Assoc* 216(12):1941–1944, 2000.
5. Sundlof S: Toad poisoning, VEM 5172, *Vet Toxicol* 115–116, 1993.
6. Booth NH, McDonald LE: *Veterinary pharmacology and therapeutics*, ed 6, Ames, 1988, Iowa State University Press.
7. Butler VP, Morris JF, Akizawa T, et al: Heterogeneity and liability of endogenous digitalis-like substances in the plasma of the toad *Bufo marinus*, *Am J Physiol* 271:R325–R332, 1996.

8. Chamakura RP: Bufotenine—a hallucinogen in ancient snuff powders of South America and a drug of abuse on the streets of New York City, *Forensic Sci Rev* 6(1):1–18, 1994.
9. Davis W, Weil AT: Identity of a new world psychoactive toad, *Ancient Mesoamerica* 3(1):51–59, 1992.
10. Hitt M, Ettinger DD: Toad toxicity, *N Engl J Med* 314:1517, 1986.
11. Brubacher JR, Ravikumar PJ, Bania T, et al: Treatment of toad venom poisoning with digoxin-specific Fab fragments, *Chest* 110:1282–1288, 1996.
12. Wall P: Lasix in ARDS. *Proceedings IVECCS VII*, Madison, WI, 2000, Omnipress.
13. Eubig PA: *Bufo* species toxicosis: big toad, big problem, *Vet Med* 96(8):594–599, 2001.

Xylitol

Matthew S. Mellema, DVM, PhD, DACVECC

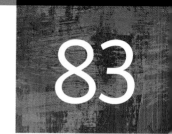

- Xylitol is an artificial sweetener that is found in many food items (e.g, gum, candy), medications (e.g., drugs, children's vitamins), and dental care products (e.g., toothpaste, mouthwash).
- Dogs are most commonly affected, though one must be open to the possibility that other species may be susceptible.
- Good history taking by asking whether anyone in the home is a diabetic, using nicotine gum, or on a low-carbohydrate diet might lead you to suspect xylitol as a suspect in the clinical disease of a pet.
- Hypoglycemia, hypokalemia, hypophosphatemia, and liver failure are potential problems with xylitol.
- Treatment involves monitoring and correcting the above listed problems, along with basic symptomatic and supportive care.

The 5-carbon sugar-alcohol sweetener xylitol is a toxin that has received far greater attention in veterinary medicine in recent years. This sweetener has become almost ubiquitous as a food and drug additive in parts of the world where diabetes is highly prevalent. The widespread usage of xylitol as a sweetener and its presence (known or unknown) in the home environment has led to increased exposure risk to this agent in pets. Dogs are the species in which a toxicologic syndrome has been identified. I am not aware of any published reports of toxicity in cats. However, the editor is aware of a cat who developed severe hypoglycemia and died following ingestion of a xylitol-containing gum. No necropsy was performed to rule out other cause of hypoglycemia. Indeed, xylitol has been studied as a water additive in cats to reduce dental disease, which is of concern as many cat households are also homes to dogs.[1]

Sources

Canine exposures to xylitol are most likely to occur by ingestion of food, candy, gum, or therapeutic/dental care products containing it. However, iatrogenic or unintentional exposures are becoming increasingly more likely as is discussed later in this chapter. The two main sources of xylitol exposures in dogs (foods and dental care products/medications) are discussed individually in the sections that follow.

Foods

Xylitol has become a widespread additive in food products because of its many beneficial properties relative to other sweeteners. It contains only 66% of the calories of sugars with similar levels of sweetness such as sucrose. Xylitol is known to cause very little insulin release when administered to human patients and is absorbed slowly from the gastrointestinal tract. Xylitol's entry into the cell does not require insulin-dependent carbohydrate transport and this property allows it to be used effectively as a cellular energy source in diabetics regardless of whether there is an absolute deficit in insulin production or a decrease in insulin signaling. Use of xylitol is expected to reduce ketogenesis in both diabetics and starving patients, and there is some evidence to support this.[2] These properties make it a very attractive option for those seeking a diet low in carbohydrates and with a low glycemic index.[3] Xylitol can be found as the sweetener in a wide array of food products including the following: (1) low carbohydrate or "low-carb" baked goods and bread products (e.g. Carb Krunchers breads, rolls, and bagels); (2) low-carb desserts such as brownies; (3) low-carb tortillas, pita breads, pizza crusts, and breadsticks; (4) low-carb condiments such as syrups and ketchups; (5) low-carb candies; and (6) low-carb and reduced-calorie chewing gums. One web site alone (The Low Carb Connoisseur: http://www.low-carb.com/) lists some 20 different categories of xylitol-sweetened food products. For this reason, I now consider it essential when taking a history on any dog with acute hypoglycemia or hepatopathy to explicitly ask whether anyone in the home is a diabetic, using nicotine gum, or on a low-carbohydrate diet at present or in the recent past. Although owners may be reluctant at first to answer any questions that tangentially relate to their personal health issues, one can hope that concern for the well-being of their pet will help them overcome such reluctance. Veterinary medicine is faced with the additional challenge posed by the United States Food and Drug Administration (FDA) not requiring that xylitol be listed among the active ingredients in products to which it is added. Fortunately, in the present environment the widely touted health benefits of xylitol in humans has resulted in many manufacturers actively promoting and highlighting the presence of xylitol in their products, but this is not always the case. The Animal Poison Control Center of the American Society for the Prevention of Cruelty to Animals has reported several cases of xylitol exposure and toxicity in dogs with a history of eating xylitol-sweetened food products, including muffins, cupcakes, gum, and cookies.[4]

Medications/Dental Care Products

Both prescription and over-the-counter (OTC) medications may contain xylitol to enhance palatability. The growth of certain bacteria can be inhibited by xylitol and this had led to its widespread use in oral-care products and toothpastes (and the proposed use as a water additive for cats, discussed previously).[5] A similar concern is present in this setting as it was for food products in that the FDA does not require drug companies to list xylitol among the active ingredients. Veterinarians using medications that are off-label for use in dogs must scrutinize and investigate each product to be certain they do not contain xylitol. In my own practice, xylitol has been discovered to be present in a number of important oral products that were in use at the time in canine patients including chlorhexidine-containing oral rinses, the oral moisturizer used to moisten the tongues in our ventilator patients, oral gabapentin solutions, and oral meloxicam suspensions. The author is aware of a canine toxicosis following ingestion of an infant toothpaste that was found to contain 35% xylitol (which was not listed on the label), highlighting the need for veterinarians to be aware that many oral hygiene products can contain very high concentrations of xylitol. It is sometimes necessary to contact a poison control center or the company itself to find the concentration of xylitol present in any particular product.

One of my graduate students, along with personnel from the University of California–Davis Veterinary Medical Teaching Hospital Pharmacy, recently was tasked with spending several days going through the shelves at a local pharmacy (Rite Aid) and a local human hospital pharmacy (Kaiser Permanente) in search of OTC and prescription drugs containing xylitol. The array of medications available OTC that contained xylitol was both large and troubling. Similarly, the pharmacists at the human hospital we collaborated with on this product were extremely helpful in pointing out prescription medications that were known to contain xylitol but that were not labeled as such. These pharmacists were also helpful in pointing out that the energy source in many products used in producing parenteral nutrition was being shifted from dextrose to xylitol with increasing frequency. Veterinarians using total or partial parenteral nutrition in their practices need to be vigilant to ensure the components intended for use in canine patients do not contain xylitol. The full list of medical products that contain xylitol is too lengthy to be given here; rather, it is prudent for veterinarians to determine whether OTC or off-label drugs contain xylitol before use.

An additional concern currently under investigation is the prevalence of xylitol in products manufactured by compounding pharmacies for veterinary use. Many of the palatability-enhanced base solutions used in compounding contain xylitol because of its relative safety and beneficial effects in humans. Compounding pharmacy personnel may be unaware of the risk posed to canine patients unless the veterinarian specifically raises the concern.

Toxic Dose

The margin of safety for xylitol is quite high in species other than dogs. In humans, the principal adverse effect is diarrhea caused by xylitol's slow and incomplete absorption; even this effect requires relatively large amounts to be consumed (>130 g/day).[6] In mice the oral median lethal dose (LD_{50}) is at least 20 g/kg.[7] In dogs, both published and unpublished data suggest that the ingested doses of more than 0.1 mg/kg may lead to hypoglycemia and that doses of more than 0.5 mg/kg are associated with hepatotoxicity.[4] The severity of hepatotoxicity might be idiosyncratic rather than dose dependent because it has been recognized by veterinarians that there are many dogs ingesting xylitol at doses exceeding 0.5 mg/kg that do not exhibit hepatic disease.[8] Xylitol toxicity in cats has not been reported in the literature (one anecdotal report only) or thoroughly investigated to my knowledge. Similarly, nearly all that is known about xylitol toxicity in dogs is based on acute exposures and little is known regarding the toxic potential of more chronic exposure to lower doses. A few chronic xylitol exposure studies have been performed in laboratory animals in the former Soviet Union.[9] It is interesting to note that these studies often observed little or no effect of feeding diets with considerable xylitol content to canine subjects, suggesting that genetic background or other factors may affect susceptibility.

Calculating an exposure dose can be challenging at times. When the exposure is gum, one must look at the label and determine if xylitol is the first sugar alcohol listed. If the answer is yes, one should base the dose on the total amount of sugar alcohols per piece of gum. If the answer is no, one should assume that there is 0.3 g of xylitol per piece of gum. When the exposure is not gum (like baked goods or powdered xylitol), one should assume that 1 cup of xylitol weighs approximately 190 g.[4]

Toxicokinetics

Ingested xylitol is absorbed readily, if incompletely, from the gastrointestinal tract in most species. Peak plasma levels occur approximately 30 minutes after ingestion.[10] Conversion of xylitol to glucose and ultimately glycogen is possible and occurs in the liver when this route of utilization is taken.[11] Ultimately, the liver is thought to be responsible for 80% of the metabolism of xylitol.[12] Xylitol may be converted to D-xylulose intracellularly. It is anticipated, but not yet demonstrated to my knowledge, that D-xylulose can be converted to xylulose-5-phosphate, which is an intermediary in the pentose phosphate pathway that can lead to substrates that may be used in glycolysis. The pentose phosphate pathway is involved in the regulation of insulin release and entry of xylitol metabolites into this pathway seems likely to be involved in the hypoglycemia generating effects of xylitol in dogs.[10] At present, the means by which xylitol toxicity results in hepatic injury is unknown. It has been proposed that adenosine triphosphatase depletion secondary to xylitol metabolism, increased generation of reactive oxygen species, or both may be responsible.[13]

Clinical Signs

Clinical signs of xylitol toxicity in dogs may be related to hypoglycemia or hepatopathy or both.[8] Vomiting is often reported as the first clinical sign. Hypoglycemia may develop within the first hour following ingestion; however, unpublished reports suggest that the onset of hypoglycemia may be delayed for as much as 12 to 48 hours depending on the product ingested, variations in insulin secretion between dogs, or liver failure.[8,13,14] Lethargy may follow the development of hypoglycemia and rapidly progress to ataxia, collapse, and seizure activity.[13] In other dogs, lethargy and vomiting may develop later (9-72 hours following ingestion) followed by signs of hepatic dysfunction with associated coagulopathy. Coagulopathic signs that have been reported in such cases include petechia and ecchymoses as well as gastrointestinal hemorrhage. Gastrointestinal distress such as diarrhea and intestinal gas production can also occur.

Minimum Database

The four most important components to the minimum database in cases of canine xylitol toxicity are serial blood glucose measurement, serum biochemistry profile, a coagulation profile (including partial thromboplastin time [PTT] and activated partial thromboplastin time [aPTT]), and a persistently high index of suspicion on the part of the clinician. It seems likely that the number of cases of xylitol toxicity a clinician uncovers is influenced by how frequently that clinician places it on the list of differentials. Serial blood glucose measurements may reveal hypoglycemia or hyperglycemia. The hyperglycemia may represent the same Somogyi rebound effect, which is observed following the administration of excessive amounts of insulin. Other findings on a chemistry panel in reported cases of xylitol toxicity include hypokalemia and hypophosphatemia, both of which are consistent with insulin's known effects on the distribution of those ions and likely a result of the marked increase in insulin release.

In those cases in which xylitol ingestion has been associated with hepatopathy, the clinicopathologic findings have included markers of hepatocyte injury, markers of cholestasis, and prolonged clotting times. Profound increases in alanine transaminase have been noted in some cases. Increases in bilirubin and alkaline phosphatase have been observed and suggest a degree of cholestasis may be present in these cases. Moderate hypoglycemia and prolongation of PTT and aPTT have been noted and interpreted as resulting from defects in hepatic export and synthesis of glucose and clotting factors, respectively. Hyperphosphatemia has been suggested to be associated with worsening prognosis when evident.

A complete blood cell count may also serve as a component of the minimum database in cases of suspected xylitol toxicity, but the information gained is likely to be nonspecific. Thrombocytopenia has been noted in some reported cases of xylitol toxicity in dogs. Presumably, the decrease in platelet count may be caused by a consumptive coagulopathy with increased use during the formation of platelet aggregates, which ultimately are unstable because of defects in secondary hemostasis (which are themselves caused by hepatic dysfunction).

Confirmatory Tests

Specific confirmatory testing of biologic tissues is rarely attempted in cases of suspected xylitol exposure or intoxication. Xylitol is metabolized quickly and xylitol accumulation in tissue is considered unlikely. However, there are labs that can test for the presence of xylitol in suspect baits/food material and potentially stomach contents from acutely affected animals. The editor is concerned that xylitol is potentially being used to illegally kill coyotes and wolves in areas where anticoyote/antiwolf sentiment exists in the general population. Presumptive diagnosis is based on exposure history and compatible clinicopathologic findings.

Treatment

In acute exposures, the induction of emesis is advised. The use of activated charcoal is rarely recommended because of its limited ability to bind to xylitol. There is no specific therapy at present for xylitol intoxication. Supportive measures are indicated in all but the most mildly affected patients. Hypoglycemia may be managed with parenteral dextrose. Specific treatment protocols have been well described in the literature.[8] For dogs that ingest 0.1 to 0.5 g/kg of xylitol, treatment should consist of hospitalization, monitoring glucose levels every 1 to 2 hours for 12 hours, providing an oral high-carbohydrate diet, and treating for hypoglycemia. Clinical signs associated with hypoglycemia typically occur when serum glucose concentrations fall below 60 mg/dL. Intravenous dextrose bolus of a 25% to 50% dextrose solution 2 to 5 mL/kg can be given as quickly as possible if the patient presents with a clinically significant hypoglycemia. A 2.5% or 5% dextrose constant rate infusion can be started after the bolus to maintain serum glucose levels.[4] Serum electrolyte values should be serially monitored (every 4 to 6 hours) to look for severe or progressive reductions in serum concentrations of potassium and phosphorus.[8] Intravenous fluids supplemented with potassium, phosphorus, and dextrose may be required. Ataxic animals should be confined to reduce injury risk.

Intravenous dextrose administration is also recommended for dogs who have ingested greater than 0.5 g/kg of xylitol, even if their serum glucose is normal at presentation; glucose should continuously be monitored every 1 to 2 hours.[8] The dextrose infusions can be discontinued after 24 hours if no changes in serum glucose concentrations have occurred.[8] For those patients at risk for developing liver disease, administration of liver protectants and antioxidants such as *S*-adenosylmethionine, silymarin, *N*-acetylcysteine, and vitamin E should be considered.[8] In cases of known or suspected xylitol-induced hepatopathy, supportive measures are required to be more extensive. Replacement of coagulation factors with transfusions of plasma, along with vitamin K_1, are indicated in actively bleeding animals or those suspected of having bleeding who also have a progressively declining hematocrit. Plasma transfusion is not definitively indicated in patients with prolonged clotting times in the absence of evidence of hemorrhage but should be highly considered. Nutritional support and intensive monitoring are advised. Recommendations for the use of the above listed hepatoprotective agents are based on consensus rather than scientific evidence; however, it should be noted that no absolute contraindication to their use in this setting is known. The use of hemoperfusion and plasma exchange in this setting is unknown but may serve as a treatment option at centers that can offer this option.[10]

Prognosis

Dogs suffering hypoglycemia alone with minimal liver or other vital organ dysfunction evident have a good prognosis. The presence of hepatic dysfunction warrants a more guarded prognosis. In cases of fulminant hepatic failure, a prognosis of guarded to poor is appropriate, depending on the extent of the manifestations.

Gross and Histologic Lesions

In cases of isolated hypoglycemia, few gross or histologic lesions are expected. In cases in which hepatic failure manifested, severe hepatic necrosis or generalized loss of liver cells with collapse of the liver's architecture was reported.[13]

Differential Diagnoses

Differential diagnoses for isolated hypoglycemia include insulin overdose, insulinoma, liver disease, oral hypoglycemic medication overdose, juvenile hypoglycemia, hypoglycemia of fasted or starved small- and toy-breed dogs, hunting dog hypoglycemia, hypoadrenocorticism (Addison's disease), or idiopathic causes. Rule-outs for acute hepatic necrosis should include other hepatotoxic agents (acetaminophen, aflatoxins, *Amanita* mushrooms, blue-green algae, heavy metals such as iron, copper, and zinc, and sago palms). Infectious causes and causes related to sepsis and the systemic inflammatory response syndrome should also be considered.

References

1. Clarke DE: Drinking water additive decreases plaque and calculus accumulation in cats, *J Vet Dent* 23:2, 2006.
2. Lang KL: Utilization of xylitol in animals and man. In Horecker BL, Lang K, Takagi Y, editors: *International symposium on metabolism, physiology, and clinical use of pentoses and pentitols*, New York, 1969, Springer-Verlag, pp 151–157.
3. Gare F: *The sweet miracle of xylitol*, North Bergan, NJ, 2003, Basic Health Publications.
4. Dunayer EK: New findings on the effect of xylitol ingestion in dogs, *Vet Med* 101(12):791, 2006.
5. Cronin JR: Xylitol: a sweet for healthy teeth and more, *Altern Complement Ther* 9:139–141, 2003.
6. Brin M, Miller ON: The safety of oral xylitol. In Sipple HL, McNutt KW, editors: *Sugars in nutrition*, New York, 1974, Academic Press, pp 591–606.
7. International Programme on Chemical Safety, World Health Organization: *Summary of toxicological data of certain food additives: WHO food additives series no. 12: xylitol*, Geneva, 1977, World Health Organization. Retrieved from www.inchem.org/documents/jecfa/jecmono/v12je22.htm.
8. Piscitelli CM, Dunayer EK, Aumann M: Xylitol toxicity in dogs, Compendium:*CE for Vets*, February 2010, E1–E4.
9. Nesterin MF: Xylitol: experimental and clinical investigations conducted in the USSR (review), *Z Ernahrungswiss* 19(2):88–94, 1980.
10. Kuzuya T, Kanazawa Y, et al: Stimulation of insulin secretion by xylitol in dogs, *Endocrinol* 84(2):200–207, 1969.
11. World Health Organization: *WHO Food Additives Series 12: xylitol*, Retrieved from www.inchem.org/documents/jecfa/jecmono/v18je16.htm.
12. Froesch ER, Jakob A: The metabolism of xylitol. In Sipple HL, editor: *Sugars in nutrition*, New York, 1974, Academic Press, pp 241–258.
13. Dunayer EK, Gwaltney-Brant SM: Acute hepatic failure and coagulopathy associated with xylitol ingestion in eight dogs, *J Am Vet Med Assoc* 229(7):1113–1117, 2006.
14. Dunayer EK: Hypoglycemia following canine ingestion of xylitol-containing gum, *Vet Hum Toxicol* 46(2):87–88, 2004.

CHAPTER

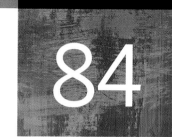

Zinc

Patricia A. Talcott, MS, DVM, PhD, DABVT

- Acute zinc poisoning is not an uncommon poisoning in small-breed dogs, cats, and pet birds.
- Potential sources include zinc-containing pennies, zinc-containing (i.e., galvanized) metal objects, zinc oxide ointment (rare), and zinc-containing lozenges (rare).
- Zinc is readily absorbed by the small intestinal mucosa, widely distributed throughout the body, and excreted in the urine and feces via pancreatic and biliary excretion.
- Acute onset of gastrointestinal distress along with a hemolytic anemia are the common presenting problems.
- Signs include vomiting, depression, diarrhea, anorexia, and abdominal pain. Icterus, hemoglobinemia, and hemoglobinuria are also observed.
- Clinical pathologic changes include a regenerative hemolytic anemia, often accompanied by an inflammatory leukogram and elevated alkaline phosphatase.
- Diagnosis often relies on history of exposure, including supporting evidence of radiodense objects within the gastrointestinal tract; compatible signs associated with a hemolytic event; and serum, liver, kidney, and pancreas zinc concentrations.
- Gross and histologic lesions are generally confined to the kidneys (tubular nephrosis with hemoglobin casts), liver (periacinal to midzonal hepatic necrosis), and pancreas (varying degrees of inflammation, necrosis, and fibrosis). Diffuse intravascular coagulation (DIC) is a potential sequela.
- Treatment is primarily supportive in nature, and the prognosis depends on the ability to control the hemolytic crisis and prevent long-term pancreatic, hepatic, or renal insufficiency, or DIC.
- Metallic foreign bodies should be removed either surgically or endoscopically. Maintenance of adequate hydration, acid-base status, electrolyte balance, and support of renal output via intravenous fluid therapy is important.
- Chelators, such as calcium ethylenediaminetetraacetic acid or D-penicillamine, are of questionable value once the source of exposure has been removed.
- Blood transfusions should be considered in severely anemic patients.

Zinc is an essential trace element in mammals and is a necessary cofactor in the synthesis of more than 200 enzymes, which are involved in gene expression, cell division, and growth.[1] Dietary zinc deficiency can result in dermatitis, poor healing, immunologic deficiencies, poor vision, and abnormal skeletal growth. This chapter focuses on excessive zinc intake or acute zinc poisoning in dogs and cats. Pennies swallowed by dogs and cats seem to be the most commonly reported source of zinc poisoning. Initial signs are often acute in onset and mimic viral, parasitic, or bacterial gastrointestinal distress. A hemolytic event follows, which, if not recognized early, can be fatal. Quantification of serum zinc levels helps to confirm a diagnosis of zinc poisoning antemortem, whereas liver, kidney, and pancreas zinc levels are always abnormally elevated in postmortem samples.

Sources

Almost all cases of zinc poisoning in dogs and cats are a result of oral ingestion. United States copper-coated pennies (standard weight, 2.5 g) minted after 1982 contain 97.5% zinc. Canadian pennies minted from 1997 to 2001 consist of 96% zinc. An undefined percentage of pennies minted in 1982 also contain high zinc concentrations. Small-breed dogs (often less than 25 pounds[2]) seem to be the animals most at risk of showing signs of toxicosis following coin ingestion. Zinc toxicosis in cats is not as common, possibly because of the more discriminating eating habits of felines compared with those of canines. Other zinc-containing metallic objects include nuts from transport cages, plumbing nuts, galvanized cages and nails, staples, fence clips, toys, jewelry, zippers, bra clips, along with a variety of miscellaneous metallic objects. Zinc oxide ointments and creams can be licked from the skin following topical application or may cause problems when a dog chews and swallows the contents of the tube. Problems seen with this type of exposure are generally only gastrointestinal in nature. Other sources of zinc include zinc undecylenate–containing Desenex products, calamine lotion, suppositories, fertilizers, zinc carbonate and gluconate nutritional supplements, zinc acetate throat lozenges, zinc chloride deodorants, zinc pyrithrione shampoos, and zinc sulfide paints.

Toxic Dose and Toxicokinetics

A true toxic dose for metallic zinc in dogs and cats has not been established. The oral median lethal dose (LD_{50}) in dogs has been reported at 100 mg/kg for zinc "salts." Many patients when brought in for treatment have only one or two pennies in their stomach. It is unclear whether this represents a true toxic dose because coins can be vomited or passed in the feces before admission. The approximate normal dietary level of zinc for dogs is in the 80- to 120-ppm range on a dry-weight basis. The oral dose necessary to induce zinc toxicosis appears to depend on the solubility of the zinc salt, the pH of the stomach, and the presence or absence of other food items in the stomach. Phytates present in plant material can bind zinc and form insoluble complexes in an alkaline pH. The acidity of the stomach provides an ideal environment for the quick release of zinc from metallic objects. Zinc oxide in contrast is a much more stable compound in this environment and does not readily disassociate to ionized components. Ingestion usually results in immediate emesis. One report estimated that a toxic dose of zinc in the form of zinc oxide in dogs was 108 g of zinc.[3]

Less than 50% of dietary zinc is absorbed throughout the small intestine. Zinc absorption decreases in the presence of dietary phytates and high dietary levels of phosphate and calcium and increases in the presence of certain amino acids, peptides, or ethylenediaminetetraacetic acid (EDTA).[4] Excess zinc also interferes with the absorption and use of copper and iron. Zinc absorbed in the small intestine is carried to the liver in the portal plasma bound to albumin. Approximately 30% to 40% is extracted by the liver, from which it is subsequently released back into the bloodstream. Circulating zinc is incorporated into various extrahepatic tissues, which have different rates of zinc accumulation and turnover.[4] The most rapid accumulation and turnover of zinc occurs in the pancreas, liver, kidney, and spleen. The liver is the major organ of zinc metabolism, where metallothionein plays a significant role. Under normal dietary conditions, zinc homeostasis is primarily controlled by excretion of zinc into the feces. Bile, pancreatic juice, and mucosal cells are the major routes for endogenous fecal zinc excretion. Small amounts (less than 10%) are excreted in the urine.[4]

Mechanism of Toxicity

The mechanism of zinc toxicity is largely unknown. The major organs affected are the red blood cells, along with liver, kidney, and pancreas; these are the organs that accumulate the highest concentrations of zinc following excessive exposure. Severe intravascular hemolysis is the most consistent abnormality observed. Various theories have been proposed to explain this phenomenon (e.g., inhibition of glutathione reductase and enzymes of the hexose-monophosphate-shunt pathway leading to oxidative damage), but none has been experimentally confirmed.

Clinical Signs

Signs associated with excessive zinc ingestion may occur shortly after ingestion (less than 2 hours), depending on the form and source of the zinc. Signs may be delayed when coins are swallowed. Often the ingestion is not observed. Initial signs are typically caused by the caustic or corrosive properties of the zinc salts and usually involve some gastrointestinal distress, such as vomiting, inappetence, depression, lethargy, and diarrhea. These signs are typically the only ones observed following zinc oxide ingestions. There may or may not be blood present in the feces. This initial phase clinically mimics a viral or bacterial gastroenteritis and can be quite severe. Depending on the exposure dose, within several hours to several days an intravascular hemolysis occurs marked by pale or yellow discoloration of the mucous membranes, tachycardia, hemoglobinemia and hemoglobinuria, with continued anorexia, depression, vomiting, and weight loss. Severe depression, recumbency, seizures, and oliguria and anuria can occur if the hemolytic event goes unrecognized.

Minimum Database

Blood and urine should always be drawn in cases in which zinc toxicity is suggested to perform a complete blood cell count (CBC), serum chemistry panel, and urinalysis. Hemolysis is almost always evident following collection of the serum. Heinz bodies are commonly reported. A normocytic or macrocytic, hypochromic anemia is commonly observed. Evidence of bone marrow regeneration (e.g., increased nucleated red blood cells, basophilic stippling, polychromasia, and elevated reticulocyte count) can be seen later in the disease process. Mild spherocytosis may be observed as well.[2] Leukocytosis, with neutrophilia and a left shift, monocytosis, and lymphopenia are commonly observed. The platelet count is usually normal or slightly decreased. Biochemical abnormalities often include mild hyperproteinemia, mild to marked azotemia, elevated alkaline phosphatase and alanine aminotransaminase activity, and hyperbilirubinemia. Urinalysis often reveals marked proteinuria, hemoglobinuria, and bilirubinuria; glucosuria has also been reported.

Patients should always have a radiographic examination performed for evidence of radiodense objects in the lumen of the gastrointestinal tract. Absence of radiopaque objects should not absolutely rule out zinc toxicosis as a differential because many patients vomit up the objects before admission (or pass them out through the feces).

Confirmatory Tests

Serum zinc concentrations are always elevated in cases of acute zinc poisoning. Blood should be collected in specific vacutainer tubes designed for trace element analysis. Contamination of some blood collection tubes from the rubber stoppers and leaching of zinc from platelets and red blood cells requires that blood be collected with a clean venous stick and stored in the appropriate tube. The blood should be allowed to clot and then spun and separated into a separate tube (another trace mineral vacutainer or small plastic vial) before shipping. Normal serum zinc concentrations generally range between 0.70 and 2 ppm in dogs and between 0.50 and 1.10 ppm in cats.[5] Serum zinc levels often exceed 5 ppm in confirmed cases of zinc toxicity.

Postmortem confirmation is based on compatible gross and histologic lesions and on the presence of elevated zinc levels in liver, kidney, and pancreas. Adequate zinc levels reported for cats in liver and kidney tissue, respectively, are 25 to 80 ppm and 11 to 25 ppm, wet weight.[5] Adequate zinc levels reported in dogs for liver and kidney, respectively, are 30 to 70 ppm and 16 to 30 ppm, wet weight.[5] The approximate normal range for zinc in the pancreas for both dogs and cats is 22 to 60 ppm, wet weight. Any zinc levels notably higher than these, accompanied by an appropriate history, clinical signs, clinical pathologic data, and histologic lesions, are compatible with a diagnosis of zinc poisoning.

Treatment

Efforts to remove zinc-containing foreign objects are highly recommended. The method of removal is a clinical judgment call and can include inducing emesis, endoscopy, or gastrotomy. Once these objects have been removed from the gastrointestinal tract, serum and tissue zinc levels drop greatly, providing that the excretory pathways are working efficiently. In one case in a dog in which the initial serum zinc level was 20 ppm, the level dropped to 6.5 ppm 3 days later (following surgical removal of coins from the stomach, intravenous [IV] fluid therapy, and two blood transfusions), and the level was 4.6 ppm 9 days later (estimated half-life of between 1.8 to 4.2 days). The serum zinc level was back to normal (1.40 ppm) 16 days after initiating treatment. A case describing zinc poisoning in a dog reported a plasma zinc half-life of 7.6 days following removal of the metallic object, blood transfusion, and fluid therapy.[6]

Supportive therapy is essential to a favorable outcome. Various treatment options include controlling the vomiting, blood transfusions to address the anemia, and balanced electrolyte IV fluid therapy to maintain hydration status. Continuous monitoring of the CBC (e.g., packed-cell volume, red blood cells, and platelets) and serum chemistry panel (e.g., blood urea nitrogen, creatinine, liver enzymes, and electrolytes) is essential to assess the patient's response to treatment. Diffuse intravascular coagulation (DIC), along with renal, pancreatic, and liver dysfunction, are possible complications that should be addressed immediately. Anuric renal failure was documented in a 15.4-kg Welsh corgi with a serum zinc concentration of 90 ppm; the dog had ingested an ornamental brass knob from a toilet paper holder.[7]

Chelation therapy has been advocated by some individuals to enhance renal zinc excretion. Considerations to take into account when deciding to use a chelator include the serum zinc concentration, the clinical condition and hydration status of the patient, the degree of excretory organ dysfunction, and whether the zinc-containing object can be removed from the gastrointestinal tract. Calcium disodium EDTA has been the most commonly suggested chelator, and the dose for treating zinc-poisoned pets has been extrapolated from the lead literature (100 mg/kg divided into four SC doses per day and diluted in 5% dextrose in water to reduce local irritation at the site of injection). Penicillamine, 110 mg/kg/day PO divided every 6 to 8 hours for 1 to 2 weeks or longer, has also been suggested (extrapolated from treatment recommendations for lead poisoning). Daily monitoring of the serum zinc concentration should be used to determine the length of chelation therapy. There is very little in the literature that documents any efficacy to chelation therapy, thereby making it a controversial treatment option for zinc-poisoned patients.

Prognosis

The prognosis for acutely poisoned patients is guarded and depends on the severity of the anemia and the extent of any liver, renal, or pancreatic insufficiency. Evidence of DIC is not associated with a favorable outcome. Timely recognition and intervention are the keys to a successful outcome.

Gross and Histologic Lesions

Gross lesions are nonspecific and can include icterus, dark-stained urine, splenomegaly, hepatomegaly, and a firm, coarsely nodular pancreas.[8] Histologic lesions described in dogs and cats include renal nephrosis with hemoglobin casts and centrilobular or peri-acinal to midzonal hepatic necrosis with pigment accumulation. Macrophages within the liver, spleen, and kidney are often engorged with hemosiderin. Varying degrees of pancreatic abnormalities have been described, and the severity of the lesions appears to be time dependent. Reported lesions include necrosis of the pancreatic duct epithelium, interstitial inflammatory infiltrates, and interstitial fibrosis.[8]

Differential Diagnoses

Acute zinc poisoning in dogs and cats must be differentiated from other causes of acute gastrointestinal upset and from an intravascular hemolytic event. The gastrointestinal signs can mimic an acute bacterial, viral, or parasitic infection and a multitude of nonspecific problems, such as hepatic or renal failure or neoplasia. Other causes of an intravascular hemolysis include immune-mediated diseases, onion poisoning, mustard poisoning, copper poisoning, acetaminophen or propylene glycol toxicity, naphthalene toxicity, and rattlesnake bites.

References

1. Sanstead HH: Understanding zinc: recent observations and interpretations, *J Lab Clin Med* 124:322–327, 1994.
2. Gurnee CM, Drobatz KJ: Zinc intoxication in dogs: 19 cases (1991-2003), *JAVMA* 230(8):1174–1179, 2007.
3. Breitschwerdt EB, Armstrong PJ, Robinette CL, et al: Three cases of acute zinc toxicosis in dogs, *Vet Hum Toxicol* 28(2):109–117, 1986.
4. Abdel-Mageed AB, Oehme FW: A review of the biochemical roles, toxicity and interactions of zinc, copper and iron: 1. Zinc, *Vet Hum Toxicol* 32(1):34–39, 1990.
5. Puls R, editor: *Mineral levels in animal health*, Clearbrook, British Columbia, 1994, Sherpa International.
6. Hammond GM, Loewen ME, Blakley BR: Diagnosis and treatment of zinc poisoning in a dog, *Vet Hum Toxicol* 46(5):272–275, 2004.
7. Volmer PA, Roberts J, Meerdink GL: Anuric renal failure associated with zinc toxicosis in a dog, *Vet Hum Toxicol* 46(5):276–278, 2004.
8. Shaw DP, Collins JE, Murphy MJ: Pancreatic fibrosis associated with zinc toxicosis in a dog, *J Vet Diagn Invest* 3:80–81, 1991.

Zinc Phosphide

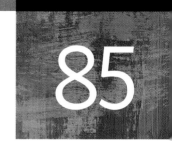

Michael W. Knight, DVM, DABVT, DABT

- Zinc phosphide, a common rodenticide, is dangerous to all animal species. Nontarget intoxication is most commonly noted in dogs.
- Zinc phosphide reacts chemically in the acid environment of the carnivore stomach to liberate phosphine gas, which is a dangerous systemic poison.
- A 10-kg dog could be at significant risk following the ingestion of 10 g (~1 tbsp) of a commercial 2% pelleted bait product.
- In the dog, onset to signs of clinical intoxication often occurs less than 1 hour following ingestion. In severe cases of intoxication, acute, severe gastrointestinal distress and hemorrhage, followed by rapid progression to systemic cellular hypoxia, convulsions, and cardiovascular shock, can develop. Death can occur within hours following high-dose ingestions.
- Treatment involves decontamination efforts early in selected cases, followed by patient stabilization, close systems monitoring, and supportive considerations.
- Although zinc phosphide is very dangerous, a reasonable proportion of dogs exposed to the bait are able to experience successful recovery following ingestion.

Sources

Zinc phosphide (trizinc diphosphide, Zn_3P_2) is a metallophosphide that was initially synthesized in 1740. It was first used as a rodenticide in 1911 to control field rodents in Italy and was introduced into the United States around the time of World War II.[1] Zinc phosphide is a dull to lustrous, gray to black crystal that has a faint, pungent, disagreeable phosphorous odor. Commercial zinc phosphide is available as a paste, tracking powder, or grain-based pellet; generally ranges in concentration from 0.5% to 10%; and in the United States is used primarily for the control of gophers and moles (Color Plate 85-1).[2] When kept in dry, acid-free conditions at up to 40° C (104° F), zinc phosphide is quite stable for at least 2 years, but storage temperatures of more than 50° C (122° F) have been shown to cause significant deterioration of the bait.[3] The average effective bait life when exposed to wet soil is approximately 20 days, although the bait may retain some degree of toxicity for several months in the field, even under substantial rain conditions.[3,4] In a sufficiently acid environment, zinc phosphide is unstable and hydrolyzes to release phosphine (PH_3, hydrogen phosphide, phosphorus trihydride) gas, a dangerous systemic poison.[5]

Other metallophosphide poisons, including aluminum phosphide (e.g., Phosfume, Phostek, Phostoxin, and Fumitoxin; tablets or pellets containing 55% to 60% or more aluminum phosphide) and magnesium phosphide (e.g., Magtoxin), are used primarily as grain fumigants and are less commonly encountered by the veterinary clinician in North America. Veterinary clinical management for these metallophosphides is approached in the same fashion as zinc phosphide, as phosphine is the common offending toxin. Zinc phosphide toxicosis in nontarget animals generally results from accidental ingestion of placed baits. Although various animal relay (secondary) toxicity research trials have reported no relay effect, relay toxicosis has been reported from the field in dogs.[1,6,7]

Toxic Dose

Any observed or suspected exposure to zinc phosphide in a pet should be seriously regarded. The minimum toxic dose, minimum lethal dose, and median oral lethal dose (LD_{50}) of zinc phosphide for the dog or cat have not been reported. Various reported animal LD_{50} values for zinc phosphide include avian spp., 7.5 to 20 mg/kg body weight (BW); rabbit, 8.25 mg/kg BW; rat, 12 to 40 mg/kg BW; goat, 20 mg/kg BW; and pig, 40 mg/kg BW.[1,6,8] Unpublished work indicates that the dose of zinc phosphide producing toxic effects in dogs lies somewhere between 20 and 40 mg/kg BW.[6] In an unpublished trial, a dog dosed with 40 mg/kg of zinc phosphide died following acute convulsive activity approximately 7 to 8 hours later.[9] Fasted dogs may be more tolerant to zinc phosphide intoxication. One source reported that 100 mg/kg of zinc phosphide was lethal in dogs fasted for 24 hours, whereas another source noted that fasted dogs survived 300 mg/kg of zinc phosphide ingestion.[6,9] Using the lowest available canine zinc phosphide toxicity data (20 mg/kg BW) as a guideline, a 10-kg dog could be considered at risk following the ingestion of 10 g of a 2% bait or 6 g of a 3.5% bait. Some pet species that are unable to vomit (rabbits, rats, hamsters, and gerbils) and thus forced to retain ingested bait in the stomach should be considered more susceptible to poisoning. Zinc phosphide should not be used for rodent control near aviary environments as rodents have been reported to carry bait pieces in their cheek pouches into aviaries and into avian feeding dishes.[10]

Toxicokinetics

Zinc phosphide is used as a rodenticide by virtue of its ability to release highly toxic phosphine gas once the bait has been swallowed. A clinically important physical characteristic of zinc phosphide is its relatively poor ability to hydrolyze in a more neutral pH environment.[2,5,6,11] In fact, where zinc phosphide is to be used as a fumigant, an acid or moist environment must be available or supplied for significant hydrolysis and subsequent phosphine liberation to occur.[6] Significant hydrolysis of zinc phosphide with subsequent phosphine liberation occurs in vitro in a pH solution of 4 or less, whereas phosphine generation from zinc phosphide was been reported to be negligible in canine gastric contents at a slightly higher pH of 4.3.[12] This important characteristic of zinc phosphide is in contrast to aluminum phosphide and magnesium phosphide, which are both readily soluble in a neutral pH environment and will hydrolyze in water to release phosphine; thus the preference is for these two metallophosphides over zinc phosphide in grain storage areas.[6,13]

Aluminum phosphide and magnesium phosphide readily hydrolyze in neutral (or acid) pH conditions[13]:

$$2AlP + 6H_2O \rightarrow 2PH_3 \uparrow + 2Al(OH)_3$$

$$Mg_3P_2 + 6H_2O \rightarrow 2PH_3 \uparrow + 3Mg(OH)_2$$

Zinc phosphide requires a sufficiently acid pH environment for hydrolysis to occur[13]:

$$Zn_3P_2 + 6H \rightarrow 2PH_3 \uparrow + 3Zn^{++}$$

Zinc phosphide and other metallophosphides are acutely corrosive and as such often provide a strong, spontaneous vomition effect following ingestion.[2] This characteristic of zinc phosphide can fortunately serve to limit the degree and severity of intoxication in those animal species that are able to vomit.[4,9] Peracute onset of spontaneous, persistent vomiting, often hemorrhagic, is commonly noted in dogs ingesting these baits.[14]

Once phosphine is released from zinc phosphide, little is known regarding the detailed pharmacokinetics of phosphine absorption, distribution, and elimination. Liberated phosphine is readily absorbed into the systemic circulation by inhalation and across the gut wall.[13,15-17] Most absorbed phosphine is eventually excreted via the lung as the parent compound, although some phosphine is slowly and incompletely oxidized to relatively less toxic phosphorus oxides and oxyacids (chiefly hypophosphite and phosphite) and excreted in the urine.[2,6,13] Following a single oral dose of zinc phosphide in humans, phosphine in expired air is negligible after 12 hours, suggesting fairly rapid elimination of parent phosphine from the body.[6] Intact zinc phosphide has also been recovered from the gut wall, blood, liver, and kidney in humans and in animals.[6,13] Absorbed zinc phosphide may remain intact in the body possibly beyond 24 hours, and may play a role in delayed adverse liver and kidney effects that are sometimes noted.[6] Whether dermal absorption of zinc phosphide occurs to any significant degree is unclear but is thought by some to be negligible.[6]

Mechanism of Toxicity

The corrosive action of intact zinc phosphide on the gastric mucosa accounts for the acute spontaneous vomition (often hemorrhagic) noted in dogs.[6,14,18]

The systemic toxicity of zinc phosphide (and other metallophosphides) can be accounted for by the toxicity of phosphine, a colorless, spontaneously flammable, very toxic gas that is released when zinc phosphide comes into contact with the acid environment of the carnivore stomach.[2,9] Phosphine combines with surface moisture to produce direct physical irritant injury to the gastrointestinal and respiratory mucosal surfaces, in addition to causing oxidative injury to the parenchyma.[15,19] Phosphine can freely diffuse into intracellular compartments, and as a highly reactive radical can initiate nucleophilic attack and reduce vital enzyme systems.[15] Although the exact biochemical mechanism of phosphine toxicity is still under investigation, in human aluminum phosphide poisoning cases, acute cardiovascular collapse is a common feature of phosphide intoxication, and severe poisoning often induces multiorgan dysfunction and failure.[15] There is evidence that phosphine interrupts cellular aerobic respiration at the mitochondrial level.[15] It has been shown that inhibition of cytochrome c oxidase complex IV (more dramatic in vitro than in vivo), as well as a decrease in activity of cytochrome complexes I and II in vivo, do occur.[15] This inhibition of the electron transport chain results in decreased adenosine triphosphate (energy) production and electron leakage, with a consequent increase in reactive oxygen species (ROS).[15] Phosphine has been shown to reduce the activity of the metalloenzymes catalase and peroxidase (resulting in reduced ROS scavenging ability), and increasing activity of superoxide dismutase.[15] Through this combined enzyme disruption and reduced ability to scavenge, superoxide ion O_2^- is dismutased to produce hydrogen peroxide, which in turn forms the highly reactive hydroxyl radical •OH, resulting in •OH-associated oxidative stress, lipid peroxidation, damage to cell lipids, proteins, and nucleic acids, and ultimately cell death.[6,15,20,21] This effect is especially significant in tissues of high oxygen demand (heart, brain, kidney, and liver) or of high phosphine concentration (lung).[13] Acute collapse of cell structure and function in individual tissue results in multiple systemic organ failure and cardiovascular shock and collapse.[15,22] Phosphine also denatures mammalian hemoglobin[23] and has been shown to inhibit acetylcholinesterase in vivo in rats, resulting in defined, clinical cholinergic toxicity.[24]

Clinical Signs

During a 10-year period (2001-2011), the American Society for the Prevention of Cruelty to Animals Animal Poison Control Center (APCC) consulted on 773 reliable (agent and exposure history were confirmed or suspected) zinc phosphide ingestion cases involving 1526 dogs that were exhibiting clinical signs at the time of the call.[14] Outcomes on approximately 80% of these cases were lost to follow-up. In case for which outcome was obtained, 171 dogs either died or were euthanized, and 126 dogs experienced full recovery.[14] During this same 10-year period, the APCC consulted on 19 reliable dog cases of aluminum phosphide ingestion.[14]

The most commonly noted signs in this review included (in relative descending order) vomition; generalized lethargy, depression, dullness, and weakness; diarrhea; tremor, agitation, and restlessness; seizure and convulsion; lateral recumbency; abdominal discomfort and pain; and death.[14] Other notable signs or clinical findings included (no particular order) retching, hematemesis, bloody diarrhea, and incontinence; ataxia, circling, anxiety, stiffness and rigidity, paddling, disorientation, hyperesthesia, vocalization, and coma; miosis, mydriasis, blindness, nystagmus, anisocoria, and photophobia; tachypnea, dyspnea, pulmonary edema, and cyanosis; tachycardia, bradycardia, pallor, collapse, and shock; hypothermia and hyperthermia; and discernible bait odor emanating from the patient, icterus, and facial edema.[14]

Notable blood work findings included clinical dehydration, hypoglycemia, hyperglycemia, elevated liver enzymes, hyperbilirubinemia, hypobilirubinemia, and azotemia with elevated blood urea nitrogen and creatinine; elevated lipase and elevated amylase; hyponatremia, hypokalemia, hyperphosphatemia, metabolic acidosis, coagulopathy, thrombocytopenia, and disseminated intravascular coagulation (DIC).[14]

The initial signs of acute vomition may be persistent and hemorrhagic and may be accompanied by signs that the patient is uncomfortable and irritable when handled.[8,14,25] Although most dogs will begin to vomit within 15 to 60 minutes of bait ingestion, onset of initial signs can be delayed up to 4 hours, and rarely up to 12 to 18 hours or longer.[14] With severe intoxications, cardiovascular collapse and death can occur within 3 to 5 hours.[9,14]

As phosphine becomes absorbed, cellular hypoxia develops, leading to cardiopulmonary, circulatory, and neuromuscular compromise. Apprehension, anxiety, discomfort and pacing, weakness and ataxia, labored respiration, struggling, convulsion, collapse, and coma can occur during a relatively short time. Vocalization, frantic behavior, teeth baring, teeth grinding, abdominal straining, and urinary and bowel incontinence may occur.

Auscultation may reveal harsh lung sounds and suspected pulmonary edema; cyanosis may be evident in these cases as well. The abdomen is generally tense and may be distended; blood may be present on rectal examination; a faint odor of rotten fish or garlic may be detected by hospital staff, which indicates a hazard to the staff.[7,9,14,25]

Minimum Database

Obtain the following analyses:[14,15,26,27]

1. An electrocardiogram demonstrates nonspecific effects: ventricular tachycardia, supraventricular tachycardia, ventricular premature complexes, supraventricular and ventricular ectopy, ventricular fibrillation, asystole; atrial fibrillation or flutter bigeminy; prolonged PR interval, widened QRS interval, ST segment changes, and abnormal T waves. Echocardiography may assist in determining ventricular function.
2. Assess blood pressure. Circulatory failure is common in more severe cases.
3. Assess radiographs. Pulmonary edema may be cardiac or noncardiac in origin; pleural effusion and ascites may be noted in more severe cases.
4. Assess CO-oximetry findings.
5. Assess electrolyte levels: acid base and blood gases, systemic metabolic acidosis, and respiratory acidosis. Assess chemistry levels: liver, kidney, muscle (including cardiac).
6. Obtain complete blood cell count, platelets, and methemoglobinemia; hemolysis is possible in severe cases.
7. Assess coagulation profile for increased clotting times; DIC may be noted in more severe cases.
8. Assess urinalysis for color, specific gravity, cell type, protein, glucose, myoglobin, and hemoglobin.
9. Obtain whole blood cholinesterase (optional).

Confirmatory Tests

Gas chromatography and gas chromatography–mass spectrometry are sensitive methods for the determination of phosphine content in patient gastric content and viscera samples.[13,19,28] Dräeger Detector Tubes are also used in the veterinary diagnostic setting.[12,29] The use of silver nitrate–impregnated paper has been used in human metallophosphide poisoning cases as a rapid, qualitative screening tool for the presence of phosphine on gastric contents; diluted gastric content is heated in a flask up to 50° C/122° F for 15-20 minutes, with the impregnated paper positioned over the mouth of the flask; if present, generated phosphine from the sample will blacken the impregnated paper; hydrogen sulfide will also blacken silver nitrate paper and can be further differentiated using lead acetate-impregnated paper.[17,19]

Prior to collecting tissues for histopathologic and toxicologic analyses, gastrointestinal contents, any suspect bait, vomitus, liver, kidney, and lung should be collected in an airtight container for phosphine analysis (beware of phosphine hazard). Zinc levels may be elevated in gastric contents, liver, and kidney, but are not considered to be a reliable indication of zinc phosphide poisoning.[28] Cholinesterase inhibition has been documented in studies of metallophosphide-poisoned rats[24] but, to my knowledge, has not been reported in domestic animal zinc phosphide intoxication cases; heparinized whole blood collection from the live animal or chilled intact eyeball and complete hemisphere of chilled brain postmortem are generally preferred to assess cholinesterase inhibition in animals.

Treatment

Goals

In the as-yet asymptomatic patient suspected to have recently ingested zinc phosphide bait, the clinician's initial consideration is for or against judicious, prompt decontamination intervention, with the obvious objective being to offset or mitigate a potential phosphine effect. Once the clinician has enough logistical details on the case (travel time for the client to the hospital, availability of client transportation, etc.) and because timing is of essence, an initial decontamination decision can be made, with the follow-up objective being to present the patient to the hospital for evaluation and management.

It should also be noted that many dogs vomit spontaneously very soon after an ingestion of zinc phosphide bait because of the corrosive nature of the metallophosphide on the gastric mucosa; in so doing, there is some degree of "auto-decontamination" with some alleviation of the much more serious phosphine effect that can occur.[14] In light of the extreme and serious nature of phosphine toxicity, however, the veterinary clinician should not assume that these "self-decontamination" cases are out of danger. No effective antidote for metallophosphide intoxication exists, and even aggressive clinical management of more severe cases can be unrewarding.

In the symptomatic patient, the clinician's objective is to capture, stabilize, and maintain the patient's respiratory, cardiovascular, neuromuscular, and metabolic systems and to provide ancillary supportive care until the patient recovers.

Prevention of Phosphine Release from Zinc Phosphide

Throughout the course of zinc phosphide ingestion management, and especially during the decontamination phase, every precaution must be taken to prevent collateral human and animal exposure to phosphine gas coming off the patient. Those involved in caring for the exposed patient must remain vigilant to provide adequate, open ventilation. This is critical for veterinary staff when instructing the client at home who will likely be unaware of the associated phosphine hazard, during transport of the patient to the hospital, and finally to veterinary staff in the hospital work area while managing the patient. For example, phosphine gas is spontaneously flammable and heavier than air, and detectable by olfaction (faint fishy to garlic odor). Humans are generally unable to detect phosphine until the ambient concentration reaches approximately 2 ppm, which is above the safe limit for phosphine exposure (the Environmental Protection Agency cites 1 ppm phosphine as the upper limit for a brief, 15-minute exposure, or 0.3 ppm exposure for 8 hours).[18,30] Thus a very large dog that may be recumbent and on the floor of the treatment room could place attending staff and other patients in adjacent floor-level enclosures at risk.

Although little research exists regarding a safe, effective procedure that could minimize phosphine release and subsequent systemic absorption in the veterinary patient following recent ingestion of zinc phosphide bait, several options exist for consideration by the clinician: (1) emetics—apomorphine or oral 3% hydrogen peroxide USP topical solution in dogs, (2) oral pH-altering antacid agents, and (3) oral medical grade mineral oil or vegetable cooking oil.

There is some controversy regarding inducing emesis in an asymptomatic zinc phosphide patient; these concerns legitimately involve the risk of phosphine off-gas, as well as the possible risk of corrosive injury to esophageal mucosa during the emesis procedure.[6,18,30] However, once the phosphine off-gas hazard risk has been properly addressed, the much greater risk to the patient of allowing zinc phosphide bait to remain in the stomach with subsequent release of a dangerous systemic poison relative to the risk of corrosive injury to esophageal mucosa must be weighed by the veterinary clinician.

In cases in which the clinician may opt to instruct the client to induce a dog to vomit at home (outdoors if at all possible), medical-grade USP 3% hydrogen peroxide, topical solution, is recommended at a dose of 1 mL per pound BW,[31] to a maximum of 60 mL total volume in larger dogs. A possible risk using hydrogen peroxide to induce emesis is local hydroxyl radical formation in the gastric lumen subsequent to hydrogen peroxide combining with any available phosphine.[32] The use of table salt or syrup of ipecac to induce vomiting should be avoided because of risks associated with systemic hypernatremia and seizure (salt) and cardiac toxicity (ipecac), but also because ipecac is less prompt and inconsistent as an emetic in pets.[14,27] Finally, care must be taken to prevent accidental ingestion of contaminated vomitus by other pets or animals in the neighboring environment.

In lieu of an emesis procedure, the clinician may opt for attempting to minimize phosphine release by increasing the gastric pH to more than pH 4 (see Toxicokinetics earlier in this chapter). Various proprietary over-the-counter liquid antacid gels containing magnesium hydroxide, aluminum hydroxide, or calcium carbonate are readily available and can be effective in rapidly increasing the pH of the gastric environment. Magnesium hydroxide raises the gastric pH more quickly and higher than does aluminum hydroxide, whereas aluminum hydroxide provides a more sustained pH change.[33] Aluminum hydroxide also decreases phosphorus absorption by forming insoluble phosphates,[33] a desired clinical effect in this case. When available, a combination magnesium hydroxide–aluminum hydroxide liquid antacid gel (e.g., extra-strength forms of Maalox, Gaviscon, or Mylanta) is preferred. Consider dosing an antacid gel at 1 mL/pound BW for these purposes (double the standard dog dose[34]). Antacid tablets are not as effective in this regard, but could be crushed and mixed with a small amount of water or milk for administration.[35] A dilute solution (2% to 5%) of sodium bicarbonate has also been recommended elsewhere to increase gastric pH.[9,25,36] One level teaspoon of baking soda in approximately 3 ounces of water provides an approximate 5% solution and provides approximately 42 mEq sodium; hypernatremia risk should be guarded against if considering this approach. These various pH-altering approaches have not been tested in the clinical setting of zinc phosphide ingestion in animals.

A final, and riskier, intervention measure for consideration is the use of medical-grade liquid mineral oil (liquid paraffin) or vegetable cooking oil as both have been shown in vitro to significantly delay the release of phosphine from aluminum phosphide.[37] This approach has not been tested in the veterinary clinical setting to my knowledge and carries an obvious detrimental concern for aspiration, especially in a veterinary patient that is at imminent risk for vomiting. In the dog, a single, oral dose of medical-grade mineral oil ranges from 2 to 60 mL, depending on the size of the dog.[31] There is also evidence that dietary lipids may enhance systemic absorption of intact zinc phosphide in animals.[6]

Gastric lavage using a dilute (1:5000 or greater) potassium permanganate ($KMnO_4$) solution to attempt oxidation of metallophosphide material to less toxic oxyacids has been recommended, although this recommendation has not been tested for efficacy or safety, and $KMnO_4$ may not be readily available in the United States.[36] Gastric lavage, if deemed appropriate for the case, should be approached with caution, and the patient should be intubated and securely cuffed to minimize risk for phosphine inhalation by the patient, as well as by staff during the procedure. Oral activated charcoal has been recommended for zinc phosphide ingestion intoxication, but efficacy has not been proven.[6,17,18,27] The risk of charcoal aspiration in the severely vomiting patient must be carefully weighed by the clinician.

Symptomatic and Supportive Management

An intravenous (IV) catheter should be placed as soon as possible in the symptomatic patient. Any persistent, nonproductive vomiting should be controlled with an antiemetic of choice. If the patient is in shock, a crystalloid shock dose of 80 to 90 mL/kg/hr as needed for dogs and 40 to 60 mL/kg/hr as needed for cats, or a synthetic colloid shock dose of 20 mL/kg/hr as needed for dogs and 10 to 20 mL/kg/hr for cats as needed should be considered.[38] If additional vascular support is required, consider norepinephrine at 0.05-2 mcg/kg/min[26,39] over dopamine at 1-20 mcg/kg/min or dobutamine at 5-15 mcg/kg/min.[26,31] Systemic metabolic acidosis, often severe, is common in most systemic cases, and respiratory acidosis may be noted. Sodium bicarbonate infusion may be required. Fluid rate should be adjusted to ensure adequate perfusion while guarding against pulmonary overload.

Oxygen supplementation should be instituted in all cases; assisted breathing may be required in severe cases. Steroids have been suggested to assist in checking pulmonary capillary leakage and potentiate responsiveness of catecholamines, and low-dose beta agonists have been recommended to relieve bronchospasm (be aware that albuterol may exacerbate peripheral hypotension).[17,27] Diuretics if used should be administered with caution.[40]

Agitated or seizing zinc phosphide patients may respond to benzodiazepines (diazepam 1-2 mg/kg IV bolus, then 0.5-1 mg/kg/hr) or midazolam 0.2-0.4 mg/kg IV;[31] propofol 1-8 mg/kg IV slowly, then 0.1-0.6 mg/kg/min, titrated to effect (be aware of cardiac effects); a cardiac-safe gas inhalant; a barbiturate (pentobarbital 5 to 15 mg/kg slowly, then constant-rate infusion 0.2 to 1 mg/kg/hr [be aware of potential respiratory depression]); or levetiracetam (20-60 mg/kg BW). Methocarbamol 55 to 220 mg/kg IV, up to a maximum of 330 mg/kg/day, may provide some relief of excessive skeletal muscle activity.[31]

Electrolytes should be monitored frequently and include ionized magnesium and calcium. Myocardial injury as a direct result of phosphine intoxication is a major focus of clinical management in human metallophosphide poisoning cases. A correlation has been made between an acute deficiency of serum magnesium and an increased incidence of cardiac arrest in human metallophosphide case studies,[41,42] and magnesium is crucial to the integrity of myocardial function.[40] There is some evidence that successful correction of magnesium deficiency may result in an increased survival rate in human metallophosphide poisoning cases.[42] The normal reference range for ionized Mg is 0.42 to 0.55 mmol/L in the dog and 0.43 to 0.58 mmol/L in the cat.[43] Because greater than 99% of total body magnesium is intracellular, it may be difficult to determine actual magnesium debt from serum magnesium levels, and a low-normal serum magnesium level may be indicative of a magnesium deficit.[40] The detection of either hypokalemia or hyponatremia should alert the clinician to the possibility of coexisting hypomagnesemia.[40] Mild magnesium deficits may be corrected by IV fluids that contain Mg (Plasma-Lyte, Normosol-R), or magnesium chloride or magnesium sulfate added to 5% dextrose in water (D5W) at an initial dose of 0.75 to 1 mEq/kg BW/day in dogs.[44] For life-threatening ventricular arrhythmias or cardiac arrest, a magnesium dose of 0.15 to 0.3 mEq/kg in the dog (50 to 100 mg/kg) can be diluted in D5W or normal saline and administered slowly IV over 5 to 15 minutes to raise the ventricular fibrillation threshold.[44] Excessive IV Mg therapy may result in hypocalcemia, hypotension, and cardiac conduction abnormalities (arteriovenous and bundle branch blocks), in which case parenteral calcium gluconate may be required.[44]

Cholinesterase inhibition may play some role in metallophosphide poisoning, as aluminum phosphide poisoning in vivo studies in rats has shown a clinically apparent and statistically significant cholinesterase inhibition effect.[24] In these studies atropine and pralidoxime chloride administration increased the survival rate in treated groups.[24] Although the cholinesterase inhibition question has been addressed in human phosphine exposure cases[45] and has received comment in veterinary zinc phosphide poisoning cases in dogs,[12] the question of whether a clinically significant phosphine-associated cholinesterase inhibition effect occurs in zinc phosphide (or other metallophosphide) veterinary cases remains to be determined. If cholinesterase inhibition does occur during zinc phosphide intoxication in domestic animals, research aimed at clinical characterization and management of this aspect of metallophosphide intoxication might increase the chance for survival in the veterinary patient.

In cases in which suspected cholinergic nicotinic or muscarinic effects are apparent in the poisoned patient, the clinician may consider judicious administration of atropine sulfate at 0.05-0.1 mg/kg IV slowly while assessing the cardiopulmonary system. If the patient appears to respond to an initial atropine challenge, then atropine could be carefully titrated as needed to effect, and cholinesterase recovery may be considered using pralidoxime chloride (Protopam) at 10-20 mg/kg IV or intramuscularly (IM) every 8-12 hours for 2-3 treatments.[46] N-acetylcysteine (NAC, the active ingredient in Mucomyst, Acetadote, etc.) is a low-molecular-weight precursor to glutathione that can cross cell wall membranes to replenish intracellular glutathione stores and provide a glutathione substitute, as well as conjugate directly with various detrimental ROS.[22] Reduced glutathione normally present in healthy tissue scavenges a variety of endogenous and exogenous ROS, thereby sparing (and detoxifying) cellular macromolecules to maintain normal cell integrity and function. When glutathione is depleted following tissue injury, ROS bind to cell macromolecules, potentially leading to death of the cell. Research in rodents indicates that glutathione plays an important protective role in phosphine-induced cellular oxidative damage, with exogenous NAC administration providing increased survival time in animals poisoned with aluminum phosphide.[22] It has been proposed that NAC might protect the myocardium and other tissues from cellular hypoxic injury in human metallophosphide poisoning cases and may have significant cytoprotective effects in the face of acute myocardial injury mediated by the formation and release of large quantities of ROS.[22,47]

Several NAC dosing regimens exist in the veterinary literature, with loading doses ranging from 140 to 280 mg/kg BW given IV or per os (PO), followed by a maintenance dose of 70 mg/kg, with dosing intervals ranging from every 4 to 8 hours, and from 3 to 17 treatments, depending on the case.[31] The margin of safety for NAC is quite good (acute IV lethal dose in dogs is 500 mg/kg), and NAC is excreted fairly quickly (elimination half-life of 5.6 hours in humans).[48] NAC general support should begin as soon as possible following the symptomatic veterinary patient's admission.[47]

Melatonin, an indolamine hormone secreted by the pineal gland, has been shown in vitro to block or reduce phosphine-induced oxidative damage in kidney, heart, brain, liver, and lung tissue of rats.[49,50] Melatonin scavenges a variety of detrimental ROS, has the ability to repair damaged biomolecules, and is considered a very effective antioxidant.[51] Melatonin crosses cell membranes with ease and distributes in sufficiently high proportions in the lipid and aqueous phases of the cell, thus effectively protecting macromolecules against oxidative insults in various compartments of the cell, including the membrane, cytosol, mitochondrion, and nucleus.[51] Melatonin given orally to adult dogs at 1 to 1.3 mg/kg resulted in measurable blood levels in 15 minutes, and levels remained greatly elevated for at least 8 hours.[52] Whether zinc phosphide–intoxicated veterinary patients would benefit from melatonin administration remains to be determined. Although melatonin appears to be a relatively safe agent in dogs at relatively high doses,[14] adverse effects of acute melatonin administration may include tachycardia and disorientation.[14,53]

Zinc phosphide veterinary patients generally experience significant pain and discomfort and should receive proper analgesia continuously during hospitalization and throughout recovery. Gastrointestinal mucosal corrosive damage benefits from supportive care with drugs such as a sucralfate (slurry, 1 g PO every 6 to 12 hours), a proton pump inhibitor such as omeprazole (0.5 to 1 mg/kg PO every 24 hours), or an H_2-receptor blocker such as famotidine (0.5 to 1 mg/kg IV, subcutaneously, IM, PO every 12 to 24 hours).[31] If blood work reflects hepatic injury, in addition to NAC support, the patient may be considered for additional liver-protective agents such as S-adenosylmethionine, milk thistle (silymarin) for 10-14 days, B vitamins, vitamin K_1, IV dextrose, and dietary manipulation. Severely affected hepatic patients may benefit from plasma administration.

Prognosis

Dogs remaining asymptomatic for longer than 8 to 12 hours following suspected ingestion of zinc phosphide bait typically experience a favorable prognosis. In those dogs that develop an initial spontaneous vomiting effect, but with no progression of systemic signs over the succeeding 12 to 24 hours, prognosis is generally favorable, although these dogs should be considered for in-hospital supportive care and close monitoring for a minimum of 24 hours, and discharged with a scheduled recheck after 3 to 5 days for possible delayed-onset liver and kidney injury (rare).[14] When moderate to severe multiorgan compromise develops within the first few hours of exposure, a guarded prognosis should be offered initially. Prognosis in symptomatic patients that survive past 24 hours may be upgraded daily. Liver and kidney injury may be delayed from 3 to 5 days in some cases (rare event).[14,27]

Gross and Histologic Lesions

Necropsy generally reveals gross hyperemia of all visceral organs and pulmonary edema. Microscopically, there is typically acute congestion of tissues, vacuolar degeneration, and interstitial edema of the brain myocardium.[7,25] Microscopic studies in humans have demonstrated focal myocardial necrosis with mononuclear infiltrate and fragmentation of fibers, inflammation of mitral and aortic valves, desquamated respiratory epithelium with thickened alveoli and capillary congestion, hepatic fatty infiltrates, central hepatic necrosis with hemorrhage, and medullary congestion and renal tubular epithelial degeneration.[25,36] In a recent equine metallophosphide (aluminum) field case, primary gross necropsy findings included widespread petechial to ecchymotic hemorrhages throughout multiple organ systems (mesentery, subcutis, tracheal mucosa, lung, epicardium, spleen, kidney, adrenal, and skeletal muscle). Microscopic findings included pulmonary edema, hepatocellular lipidosis and centrilobular necrosis, central neuronal edema and necrosis, and severe diffuse adrenal hemorrhage and necrosis.[54]

Differential Diagnoses

Strychnine rodenticide: presents with acute onset and rapidly progresses to tetanic, extensor rigidity (sawhorse stance and sardonic grin) and convulsions. Strychnine cases tend not to vomit and are intensely hyperesthetic to stimuli.

Metaldehyde slug and snail bait: present with acute onset and rapid progression to coarse muscle tremors and seizures. Vomition is common, but gastric corrosion with blood is less likely, and there is less pulmonary involvement.

Tremorgenic mycotoxicosis: results from various penitrem-containing molds growing in compost piles and spoiled food (variety of dairy and carbohydrate food substrates). It presents with very rapid onset and marked neuromuscular effect. Vomiting is possible, but not as pronounced. There is relatively little pulmonary involvement. It generally responds well to management.

Organophosphate or carbamate insecticides: ingestion presents with acute onset and is rapidly progressive. Signs include vomiting and retching, urine and bowel incontinence, pulmonary component with harsh lung sounds, dyspnea, tremor, and seizure. Bloody vomitus is less common. Metallophosphide intoxication may mimic zinc phosphide toxicosis.

4-Aminopyridine (Ampyra, Avitrol): ingestion presents with a clinical picture similar to zinc phosphide, but hematemesis is not expected.

Ingestion of heavy metals (arsenic, thallium, and mercury): presents with acute onset, progressive vomiting with or without blood, painful abdomen, tremor and seizure, and circulatory shock. Respiratory distress may be noted.

Ingestion of sodium monofluoroacetate (1080): presents with acute onset and rapid progression to cellular hypoxia, intense distress, delirium, aimless running, respiratory distress, vomiting, tremor, seizure, collapse, cardiac arrest, and shock. It mimics zinc phosphide intoxication with a clinical picture reflecting cellular hypoxia; it is difficult to manage and typically has a poor to grave prognosis. Sodium monofluoroacetate is a restricted-use pesticide, and is rarely encountered in many practice locations.

Ingestion of 5-fluorouracil (Efudex): presents with acute onset to severe, intractable seizure, vomiting that is often bloody, and abdominal distress. A respiratory component may be present but is generally less intense. Check history for any family member on a topical antineoplastic prescription ointment.

Ingestion of serotoninergic and other central nervous system–stimulant medications and drugs: presents with acute onset of generalized tremor to seizure. Some vomiting may occur, but typically there is no hemorrhage. Pulmonary involvement is much less than zinc phosphide. Generally, patients have a good response to appropriate management. A thorough history typically identifies the source of medication and exposure circumstances.

Ingestion of nonsteroidal antiinflammatory analgesics, such as naproxen, piroxicam, and meloxicam: presents with an onset that is generally not as acute, but significant vomiting occurs early. Hematemesis occurs with high-dose cases, as does moderate abdominal pain, metabolic acidosis, and seizure. The pulmonary effect is much less pronounced. A history often reveals the source.

Ingestion of cycad (sago palm): results in intense, progressive gastrointestinal distress with or without blood, severe hepatotoxicity, tremor, and seizure (see Color Plate 20-4). Management is challenging, and prognosis is usually guarded.

References

1. Witmer GW, Fagerstone KA: The use of toxicants in black-tailed prairie dog management: an overview, *Proceedings of the 10th Wildlife Damage Management Conference*, 2003.
2. Clarkson TW: Inorganic and organometal pesticides. In Hays WJ, Laws ER, editors: *Handbook of pesticide toxicology*, vol II, San Diego, 1991, Academic Press.
3. *Land Protection: Zinc phosphide*, Department of Natural Resources and Mines, Pest Series. The State of Queensland, PA3, May 2002. Retrieved from www.nrm.qld.gov.au/factsheets/pdf/pest/PA3.pdf.
4. Timm R: Zinc phosphide. In Timm RM, editor: *Prevention and control of wildlife damage*, Lincoln, 1983, University of Nebraska, Nebraska Cooperative Extension Service.
5. Index Merck: *An encyclopedia of chemicals, drugs, and biologicals*, ed 11, Rahway, NJ, 1989, Merck & Company.
6. World Health Organization, International Programme on Chemical Safety: *Phosphine and selected metal phosphides, environmental health criteria 73*, Geneva, 1988. Retrieved from http://www.inchem.org/documents/ehc/ehc/ehc73.htm.
7. Stowe CM, Nelson R, Werdin R, et al: Zinc phosphide poisoning in dogs, *J Am Vet Med Assoc* 173(1):270, 1978.
8. *Registry of Toxic Effects of Chemical Substances: Zinc phosphide*, Thomson MICROMEDEX, exp 08/2005.
9. Osweiler GD, Carson TL, Buck WB, et al: *Clinical and diagnostic veterinary toxicology*, ed 3, Dubuque, Iowa, 1985, Kendall/Hunt Publishing Co.
10. Flammer K: Aviculture management. In Harrison GJ, Harrison LR, editors: *Clinical avian medicine and surgery*, Philadelphia, 1986, WB Saunders.
11. Extoxnet, Extension Toxicology Network: *Zinc phosphide pesticide information profile*, June 1996. Retrieved from http://ace.orst.edu/cgi-bin/mfs/01/pips/zincphos/htm.
12. Fessesswork GG, Stair EL, Johnson BW, et al: Laboratory diagnosis of zinc phosphide poisoning, *Vet Hum Toxicol* 36(6):517, 1994.
13. World Health Organization, International Programme on Chemical Safety: *Phosphine and selected metal phosphides, health and safety guide No. 28*, Geneva, 1989. Retrieved from http://www.inchem.org/documents/hsg/hsg/hsg028.htm.

14. American Society for Prevention of Cruelty to Animals: *Antox database 2001-2011.*
15. Anand R, Binukumar BK, Gill KD: Aluminum phosphide poisoning; an unsolved riddle, *J Appl Toxicology* 31:449, 2011.
16. Suman RL, Savani M: Pleural effusion—a rare complication of aluminum phosphide poisoning, *Indian Ped* 36:1161, 1999. Retrieved from http://www.indianpediatrics.net/99nov14.htm.
17. Chugh SN: Metal phosphide poisoning, 2000. Retrieved from www.indegene.com/Int/FeatArt/indIntFeatArt15.html.
18. Rodenberg HD, Chang CC, Watson WA: Zinc phosphide ingestion: a case report and review, *Vet Hum Toxicol* 31(6):559, 1989.
19. Gurjar M, Baronia AK, Azim A, et al: Managing aluminum phosphide poisonings, *J Emerg Trauma Shock* 4(3):378, 2011.
20. Hsu CH, Quistad GB, Casida JE: Phosphine-induced oxidative stress in Hepa 1c1c7 cells, *Toxicol Sci* 46:204, 1998.
21. Pratt SJ: A new measure of uptake: desorption of unreacted phosphine from susceptible and resistant strains of *Tribolium castaneum, J Stored Prod Res* 39:507, 2003.
22. Azad A, Lall SB, Mittra S: Effect of *N*-acetylcysteine and L-NAME on aluminum phosphide induced cardiovascular toxicity in rats, *Acta Pharmacol Sin* 22(4):298, 2001.
23. Lall SB, Peshin SS, Mitra S: Methemoglobinemia in aluminum phosphide poisoning in rats, *Indian J Exp Biol* 38(1):95, 2000.
24. Mittra S, Peshin SS, Lall SB: Cholinesterase inhibition by aluminum phosphide poisoning in rats and effects of atropine and pralidoxime chloride, *Acta Pharmacol Sin* 22(1):37, 2001.
25. Casteel SW, Bailey EM: A review of zinc phosphide poisoning, *Vet Hum Toxicol* 28(2):151, 1986.
26. Soltaninejad K, Nelson L, Khodakarim N, et al: Unusual complication of aluminum phosphide poisoning: development of hemolysis and methemoglobinemia and its successful treatment, *Ind J Crit Care Med* 15(2):117, 2011.
27. Phosphine. In *POISINDEX System* (electronic version). Thomson Reuters (Healthcare) Inc., Greenwood Village, CO. Retrieved 12/12/2011 from http://www.thomsonhc.com.
28. Tiwary AK, Puschner B, Charlton BR, Filgenzi M: Diagnosis of zinc phosphide poisoning in chickens using a new analytical approach, *Avian Disease* 49(2):288, 2005.
29. Morgan S, Niles GA, Edwards WC: Case report-phosphine gas detected in the rumen content of dead calves, *Bovine Pract* 34(2):127, 2000.
30. Pepelko B, Seckar J, et al: Worker exposure standard for phosphine gas, *Risk Analysis* 24(5):1201, 2004.
31. Plumb DC: *Veterinary drug handbook*, ed 6, Ames, IA, 2008, Blackwell Publishing.
32. Nath NS, Bhattacharya I, Tuck AG, et al: Mechanisms of phosphine toxicity, *J Toxicol*, 2011.
33. Boothe DM: Gastrointestinal pharmacology. In Boothe DM, editor: *Small animal clinical pharmacology and therapeutics*, Philadelphia, 2001, WB Saunders.
34. Matz ME: Gastrointestinal ulcer therapy. In Bonagura JD, Kirk RW, editors: *Current veterinary therapy XII, small animal practice*, Philadelphia, 1995, WB Saunders.
35. Papich MG: Medical therapy for gastrointestinal ulcers. In Kirk RW, Bonagura JD, editors: *Current veterinary therapy X, small animal practice*, Philadelphia, 1989, WB Saunders.
36. Metts BD, Stewart NJ: Rodenticides. In Haddad LM, Shannon MW, Winchester JF, editors: *Clinical management of poisoning and drug overdose*, ed 3, Philadelphia, 1998, WB Saunders.
37. Goswami M, Bindal M, Sen P: Fat and oil inhibit phosphine release from aluminum phosphide—its clinical implication, *Indian J Exp Biol* 32:647, 1994.
38. Bateman S: Fluid therapy: the basics. Retrieved from http://www.vet.ohio-state.edu/docs/vm700_11/Notes/basics.html.
39. Barton L: *Refractory hypotension*, IVECCS 2007 symposium, Veterinary Information Network, 2007.
40. Martin LG, Van Pelt DR, Wingfield WE: Magnesium and the critically ill patient. In Bonagura JD, Kirk RW, editors: *Current veterinary therapy XII, small animal practice*, Philadelphia, 1995, WB Saunders.
41. Chugh SN, Jaggal KL, Sharma B, et al: Magnesium levels in acute cardiotoxicity due to aluminum phosphide poisoning, *Indian J Med Res [B]* 94(December):437, 1991.
42. Chugh SN, Kumar P, Sharma A, et al: Magnesium status and parenteral magnesium sulphate therapy in acute aluminum phosphide intoxication, *Magnesium Res* 3/4(7):289, 1994.
43. Jackson CB, Drobatz KJ: Iatrogenic magnesium overdose: 2 case reports, *J Vet Emerg Crit Care* 14(2):115, 2004.
44. Macintire DK: Metabolic derangements in critical patients, *The 21st ACVIM forum proceedings*, Charlotte, NC, 2003.
45. Potter WT, Garry VF, Kelly JT, et al: Radiometric assay of red cell and plasma cholinesterase in pesticide appliers from Minnesota, *Toxicol Appl Pharmacol March* 119(1):150, 1993.
46. Fikes JD: Organophosphate and carbamate insecticides, *Clin North Am Small Anim Pract* 20(2):353, 1990.

47. Acetylcysteine. In: *DRUGDEX System* (electronic version), Thomson Reuters (Healthcare) Inc., Greenwood Village, CO. Retrieved 12/12/2011 from http://www.thomsonhc.com.
48. Food and Drug Administration: N-acetylcysteine, NADA Number 21-539, Rockville, MD, Freedom of Information Office. Retrieved from www.fda.gov/cder/foi/label/2004/21539_N-acetylcysteine_lbl.pdf.
49. Hsu CH, Chi BC, Casida JE: Melatonin reduces phosphine-induced lipid and DNA oxidation in vitro and in vivo in rat brain, *J Pineal Res* 32(1):53, 2002.
50. Hsu CH, Chi BC, Liu MY, et al: Phosphine-induced oxidative damage in rats: role of glutathione, *Toxicology* 179(102):1, 2002.
51. Dun-xian T, Reiter RJ, Manchester LC, et al: Chemical and physical properties and potential mechanisms: melatonin as a broad spectrum antioxidant and free radical scavenger, *Curr Top Med Chem* 2:181, 2002.
52. Ashley PF, Frank LA, Schmeitzel LP, et al: Effect of oral melatonin administration on sex hormone, prolactin, and thyroid hormone concentrations in adult dogs, *J Am Vet Med Assoc* 215(8):1111, 1999.
53. Melatonin. In *DRUGDEX System* (electronic version). Thomson Reuters (Healthcare) Inc., Greenwood Village, CO. Retrieved 12/12/2011 from http//www.thomsonhc.com.
54. Easterwood L, Chaffin MK, Marsh PS, et al: Phosphine intoxication following oral exposure of horses to aluminum phosphide-treated feed, *J Am Vet Med Assoc* 236(4):446, 2010.

Index

Page numbers followed by *f* indicate figures; *t*, tables; *b*, boxes.

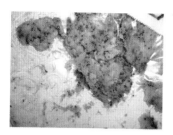

Color Plate 7-1 Bait (tuna) laced with aldicarb. (Photo courtesy of Birgit Puschner)

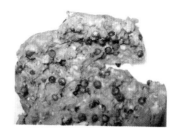

Color Plate 7-2 Bait laced with strychnine. (Photo courtesy of Birgit Puschner)

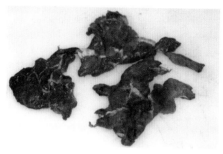

Color Plate 7-3 Meat laced with paraquat. (Photo courtesy of Birgit Puschner)

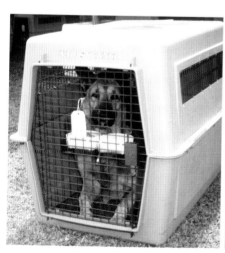

Color Plate 15-1 A German shepherd waits in a kennel at a pet holding area during evacuation processing after the June 10, 1991 eruption of Mount Pinatubo. (Photo courtesy of John Fichensehr)

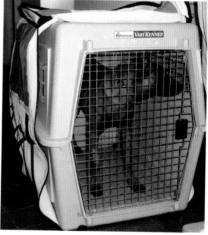

Color Plate 15-2 A military working puppy in an extra-large portable kennel. Large openings allow visual monitoring of the animal and drainage of water during decontamination. (Photo courtesy of Kelley Evans)

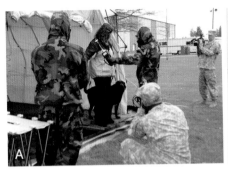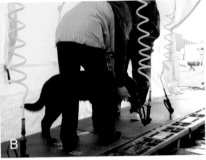

Color Plate 15-3 A, Handler Chris Monroe and animal assisted crisis response dog Pongo undergo mock decontamination by the U.S. Marine Corps' Chemical Biological Incident Response Force (CBIRF) during National Level Exercise 2008. B, Service animals may need to be decontaminated together with their handler or disabled owner. (Photos courtesy of Kelley Evans)

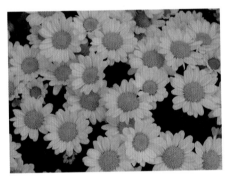

Color Plate 20-1 Chrysanthemum (*Chrysanthemum cinerariifolium*). (Photo courtesy of Forest and Kim Starr)

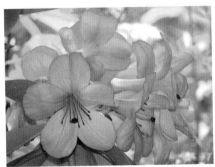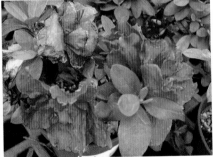

Color Plate 20-2 Heath family (Ericaceae). (Photos courtesy of Forest and Kim Starr)

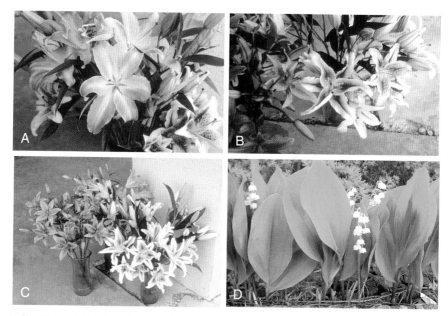

Color Plate 20-3 Lilies. A, Easter lily. B, Tiger lily. C, Day lily. D, Lily of the valley. (Part (*D*) courtesy of Richard Old)

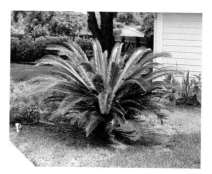

Color Plate 20-4 Cycad (sago) palm.

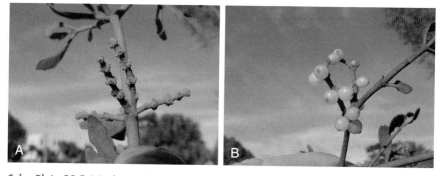

Color Plate 20-5 Mistletoe (*Phoradendron leucarpum*). A, Characteristic stem and leaf pattern. B, Berries. (Photos courtesy of Richard Old)

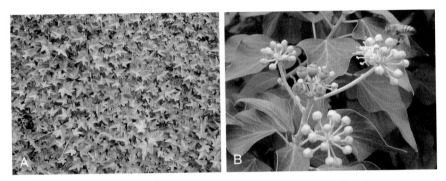

Color Plate 20-6 English ivy (*Hedera helix*). A, Leaves. B, Berries.

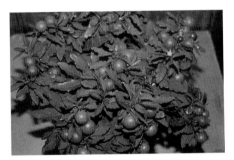

Color Plate 22-1 Christmas or Jerusalem cherry (*Solanum* sp.).

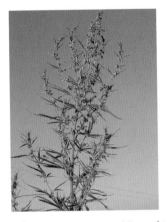

Color Plate 25-1 Marijuana (*Cannabis sativa*). (Photo courtesy of Richard Old)

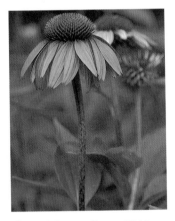

Color Plate 26-1 Coneflower (*Echinacea* sp.)

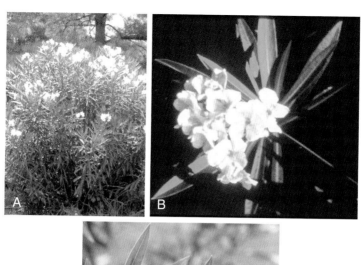

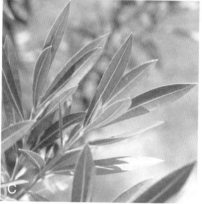

Color Plate 26-2 Oleander (*Nerium oleander*). A, Plant. B, Flower. C, Leaves.

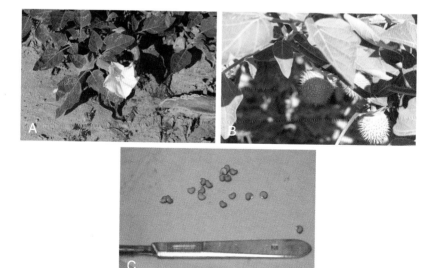

Color Plate 26-3 Jimsonweed, thorn apple (*Datura stramonium*). A, Flower. B, Seed pods. C, Seeds.

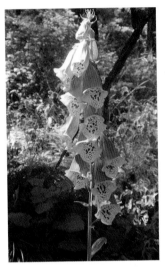

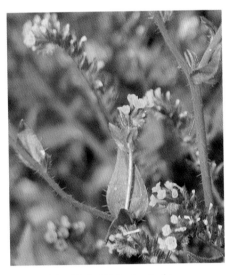

Color Plate 27-1 *Digitalis* sp. (foxglove). (Photo courtesy of Roxolana Elliot)

Color Plate 27-2 *Amsinckia* sp.

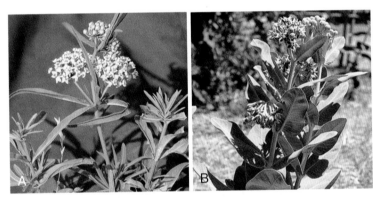

Color Plate 27-3 *Asclepias* sp. A, Narrow leaf. B, Broad leaf.

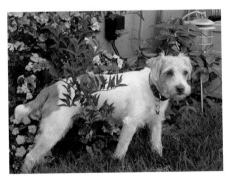

Color Plate 27-4 Image of a dog among *Brunfelsia* (Yesterday-today-and-tomorrow). The dog developed classic signs of *Brunfelsia* poisoning.

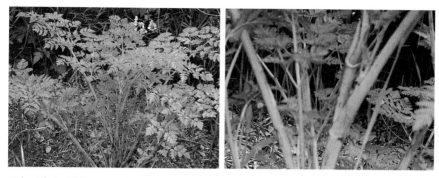

Color Plate 27-5 Poison hemlock (*Conium maculatum*). (Photo courtesy of KH Plumlee)

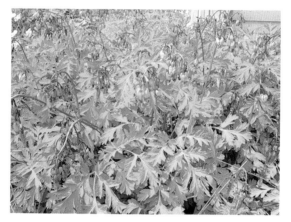

Color Plate 27-6 Bleeding-heart (*Dicentra formosa*). (Photo courtesy of Richard Old)

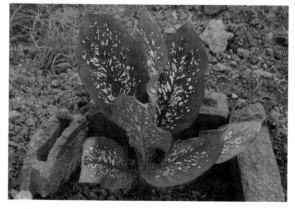

Color Plate 27-7 Dieffenbachia, dumb cane (*Dieffenbachia* sp.).

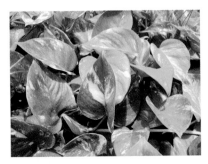

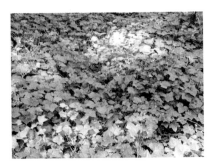

Color Plate 27-8 Golden pothos (*Epipremnum aureum*). (Photo courtesy Forest & Kim Starr)

Color Plate 27-9 English ivy (*Hedera helix*). (Photo courtesy of Richard Old)

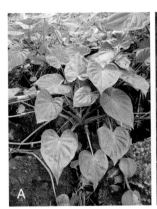

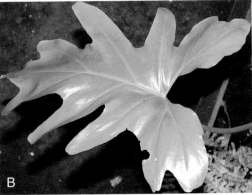

Color Plate 27-10 Philodendron (*Philodendron* sp.). (Photos courtesy of Forest and Kim Starr)

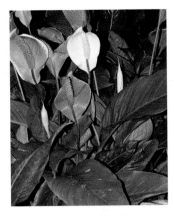

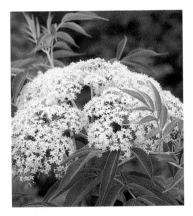

Color Plate 27-11 Peace lily (*Spathiphyllum* sp.). (Photo courtesy of Forest and Kim Starr)

Color Plate 27-12 Elderberry (*Sambucus nigra* L.).

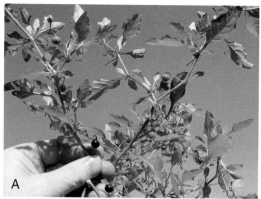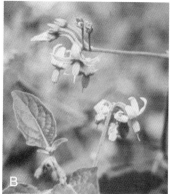

Color Plate 27-13 A, Immature and mature fruit of black nightshade (*Solanum nigrum*). B, *S. americanum* (American nightshade). (Photo courtesy of Richard Old)

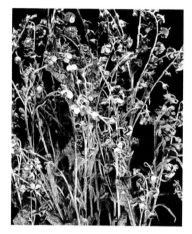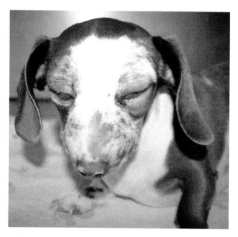

Color Plate 27-14 Houndstongue (*Cynoglossum officinale*) dry senescent plant. (Photo courtesy of Bryan Stegelmeier)

Color Plate 30-1 Facial edema associated with acetaminophen poisoning. (Photo courtesy of Nicole Lindstrom)

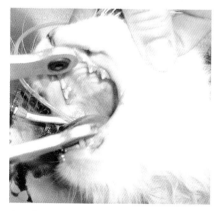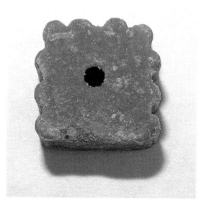

Color Plate 30-2 Cyanotic oral mucous membranes in a cat with acetaminophen intoxication.

Color Plate 36-1 An example of a bromethalin-containing rodenticide. (Photo courtesy of Patricia Talcott)

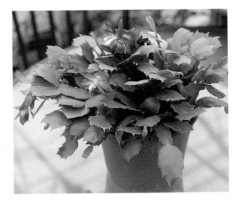

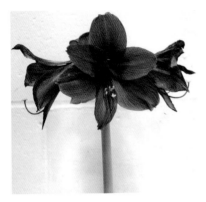

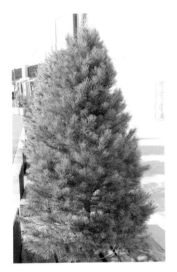

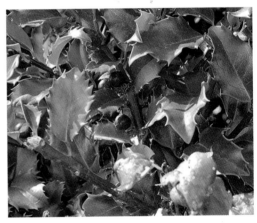

Color Plate 39-1 Amaryllis (*Hippeastrum* cultivar "apple blossom"). (Photo courtesy of TD Brant)

Color Plate 39-2 Christmas cactus (*Schlumbergera truncata*). (Photo courtesy of TD Brant)

Color Plate 39-3 Scotch pine (*Pinus sylvestris*), one of many evergreen varieties that serve as Christmas trees and are used in Christmas decorations. (Photo courtesy of TD Brant)

Color Plate 39-4 English holly (*Ilex aquafolium*) with berries.

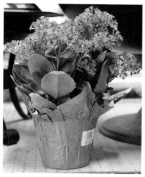
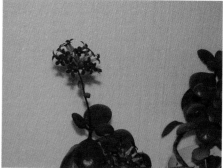

Color Plate 39-5 *Kalanchoe blossfeldiana.* (Photo courtesy of TD Brant)

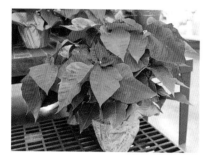

Color Plate 39-6 Poinsettia (*Euphorbia pulcherrima*). (Photo courtesy of TD Brant)

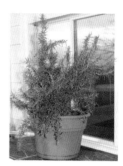

Color Plate 39-7 Rosemary (*Rosmarinus officinalis*). (Photo courtesy of TD Brant)

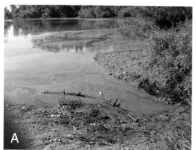
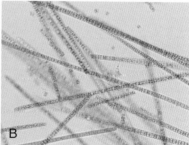

Color Plate 43-1 A, Blue-green algae (cyanobacteria) bloom (Photo courtesy of Mike Corcoran). B, Blue-green algae (*Oscillatoria* sp., photo courtesy of Sandra Morgan).

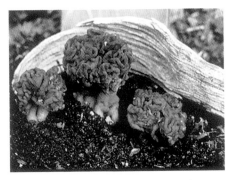

Color Plate 62-1 Mushroom spore surface folded not pitted (*Gyromitra* sp.).

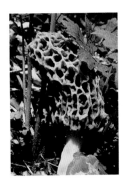

Color Plate 62-2 Mushroom cap pitted not folded (*Mochella esculenta*, common morel).

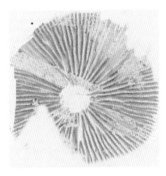

Color Plate 62-3 Spore print.

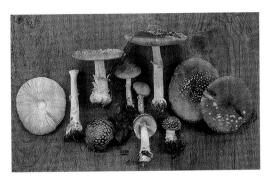

Color Plate 62-4 *Amanita pantherine.*

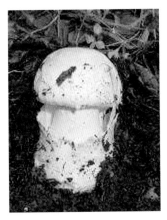

Color Plate 62-5 *Amanita ocreata.*

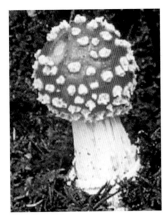

Color Plate 62-6 *Amanita muscaria.*

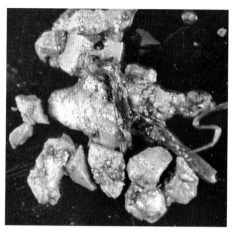

Color Plate 67-1 Carbofuran granules in stomach contents of a dog. (Photo courtesy of Patricia Talcott)

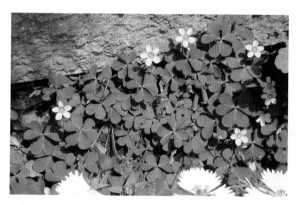

Color Plate 68-1 Soluble oxalate containing shamrock plant (*Oxalis corniculata*). (Photo courtesy of Richard Old)

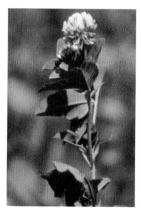

Color Plate 68-2 White clover (*Trifolium repens*).

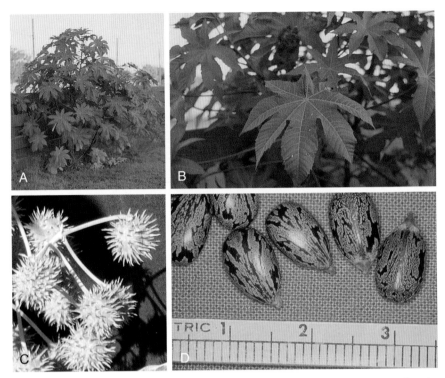

Color Plate 74-1 Castor bean plant (*Ricinus communis*). A, Plant. B, Leaves. C, Seed pods. D, Seeds.

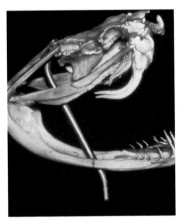

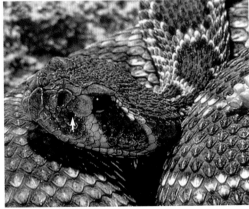

Color Plate 75-1 Pit viper skull retractable front fangs. Note secondary and tertiary fangs. (Photo courtesy of the Arizona Desert Museum, Tucson, Arizona)

Color Plate 75-2 The thermal pit of a rattlesnake. Nostril (*red arrow*), thermal pit (*white arrow*).

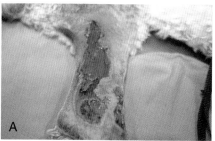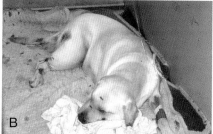

Color Plate 75-3 Rattlesnake envenomated dog. A, Tissue necrosis 72 hours post-rattlesnake envenomation. Note gravity dependent necrosis along fasical planes. B, Note markings for serial circumferential measurements to monitor progression of swelling on rear leg and head. (Photo courtesy of Scott Johnson)

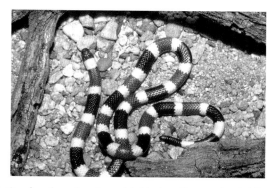

Color Plate 76-1 Coral snake coloration with black, yellow, and red fully encircling bands. (Photo courtesy of the Arizona Poison Drug Information Center, Tucson, Arizona)

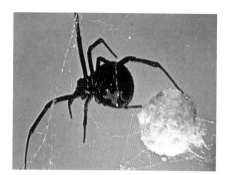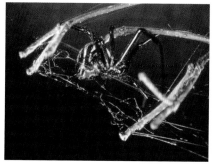

Color Plate 79-1 Mature female black widow spider with egg sac. (Photo courtesy of the Arizona Poison and Drug Information Center, Tucson, Arizona)

Color Plate 79-2 Immature black widow spider, note the coloration. (Photo courtesy of the Arizona Poison and Drug Information Center, Tucson, Arizona)

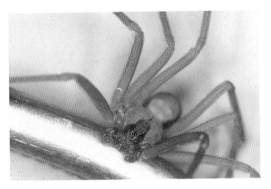

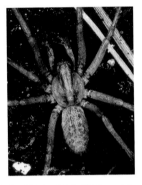

Color Plate 80-1 Brown recluse (*Loxosceles recluse*). Note the violin marking on the cephalothorax and the three sets of eyes. (Photo courtesy of Bill Banner)

Color Plate 80-2 Hobo spider (*Tegenaria agrestis*). (Photo courtesy of Arizona Poison and Drug Information Center, Tucson, Arizona)

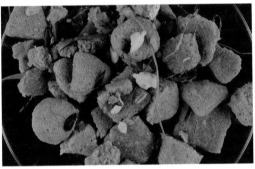

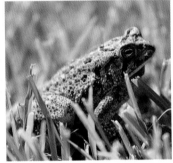

Color Plate 81-1 Strychnine laced grain in bait. (Photo courtesy of Patricia Talcott)

Color Plate 82-1 The cane or marine toad (*Bufo marinus*).

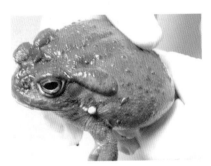

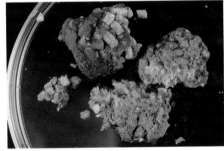

Color Plate 82-2 Colorado River toad (also known as the Sonoran desert toad) (*Bufo alvarius*).

Color Plate 85-1 Zinc phosphide–laced bait. (Photo courtesy of Paul Martin)

Conversion Tables

To Convert	Multiply by	To Obtain
Gallons (gal)	3.785	Liters
Gal	3785	Millimeters
Gal	128	Ounces (liquid)
Grams (g)	0.002205	Pounds
Gram	0.035274	Ounces
Grams per liter	1000	PPM
Grams per liter	10	Percent
Kilograms (kg)	2.2046	Pounds
Liters (L)	0.2642	Gallons
Liters	33.814	Ounces
Liters	2.113	Pints
Liters	1.057	Quarts
Ounces	0.02957	Liters
Ounces	29.573	Milliliters
Ounces	28.35	Grams
PPM	0.001	Grams/L
PPM	1	mg/kg or mg/L
Percent (%)	10	g/kg
Pint	0.473	Liter
Pounds	0.4536	Kilograms
Pounds	453.6	Grams

Liquid Equivalents
1 ft (cubed) of water = 7.5 gal = 62.4 lb = 28.3 L
1 liter (L) = 2.113 pt = 1000 milliliter (mL) = 1.0567 qt = 33.8 fl oz = 0.26 gal
1 US gallon = 4 qt = 8 pt = 16 cups = 128 fl oz = 8.337 lb of water = 3.785 L = 37.85 mL = 256 tablespoons (tbsp)
1 quart = 0.9463 L = 2 pt = 32 fl oz = 4 cups = 64 tbsp = 0.25 gal = 946.4 mL
1 pint = 16 fl oz = 2 cups = 473.2 mL = 32 level tbsp = 0.125 gal = 0.5 qt
1 cup = 8 fl oz = ½ pt = 16 tbsp = 236.6 mL
1 tbsp = 14.8 mL = 3 teaspoons (tsp) = 0.5 fl oz
1 mL = 0.34 fl oz = 0.002 pt
1 tsp = 4.93 L = 0.1667 fl oz = 80 drops
1 US fl oz = 29.57 mL = 2 tbsp = 6 tsp = 0.03125 qt

Temperature Equivalents
degrees Centigrade = (°F − 32) × 5/9
degrees Fahrenheit = (°C × 9/5) + 32

Mixture Ratios
1 mg/g = 1000 ppm
1 fl oz/gal = 75 ppm
1 fl oz/100 gal = 75 ppm
1 pt/100 gal = 1 tsp/1 gal
1 qt/100 gal = 2 tbsp/1 gal

Weight Equivalents

1 ton (US) = 2000 lb = 0.907 metric tons = 907.2 kg

1 metric ton = 106 g = 1000 kg = 2205 lb

1 lb = 16 oz = 453.6 g = 0.4536 kg

1 oz (weight) = 28.35 g = 0.0625 lb

1 g = 1000 mg = 0.0353 oz = 0.001 kg = 0.002205 lb

milligram (mg) = 0.001 g

1 kilogram (kg) = 1000 g = 35.3 oz = 2.205 lb

microgram (mcg) = 10^{-6} g = 0.001 mg

nanogram (ng) = 10^{-9} g = 0.001 mcg

picogram = 10^{-12} g

1 ppm = 0.0001% = 0.013 fl oz in 100 gal = 1 mg/kg = 1 mg/L = 1 mg/g = 0.379 g in 100 gal
    water = 8.34×10^{-6}

lb/gal = 1 mL/L

1 ppb = 1 mcg/kg or 1 mcg/L or 1 ng/g

1 ppt = 1 picogram/g

1% = 10,000 ppm = 10 g/L = 1 g/100 mL = 10 g/kg = 1.33 oz by weight/gal water = 8.34
    lb/100 gal water

1 L ≈ 0.87987699	quart	Imperial 1 quart	≡ 1.1365225 L
1 L ≈ 1.056688	fluid quart	US 1 fluid quart	≡ 0.946352946 L
1 L ≈ 1.75975326	pint	Imperial 1 pint	≡ 0.56826125 L
1 L ≈ 0.2641720523	liquid gallon	US 1 liquid gallon	≡ 3.785411784 L
1 L ≈ 0.21997	gallon	Imperial 1 gallon	≡ 4.54609 L
1 L ≈ 0.0353146667	cubic foot	1 cubic foot	≡ 28.316846592 L
1 L ≈ 61.0237441	cubic inches	1 cubic inch	≡ 0.01638706 L
1 L ≈ 33.8140	customary fluid ounce US	1 customary fluid ounce	≡ 29.5735295625 mL
1 L ≈ 35.1950	fluid ounces	Imperial 1 fluid ounce	≡ 28.4130625 mL

Emergency Hotlines

ASPCA Animal Poison Control Center (24-hour service; $65 fee may apply)	888-426-4435
Pet Poison Helpline (24-hour service; $39 fee may apply)	800-213-6680
Human Poison Control Center (24-hour service; fees may apply to veterinarians)	800-222-1222
National Pesticide Information Center (free—provide technical advice about pesticide products and poisonings)	800-858-7378
Chemical Transportation Emergency Center (free—provide technical assistance for large pesticide spills)	800-424-9300
Adverse Event Reporting/FDA Center for Veterinary Medicine (provide assistance on drugs and animal feeds)	888-332-8387

Common Conversion Factors

Units Given	Units Wanted	Formula for Conversion
mmol/L	mg/dL	$mg/dL = [(mmol/L) \times MW]/10$
mg/dL	mmol/L	$mmol/L = (mg/dL \times 10)/MW$
mmol/L	mEq/L	$mEq/L = mmol/L \times valence$
mEq/L	mmol/L	$mmol/L = (mEq/L)/valence$
%	mg/mL	$mg/mL = \% \times 10$
cm	inches	$inches = cm \times 0.3937$
inches	cm	$cm = inches \times 2.54$
°C	°F	$°F = [(°C \times 9)/5] + 32$
°F	°C	$°C = [(°F-32) \times 5]/9$

MW, molecular weight (the sum of the atomic weights of a molecule or compound).

(From Silverstein DC, Hopper K: *Small Animal Critical Care Medicine,* Elsevier, St Louis, 2009.)

Weight–Unit Conversion Factors

1 lb = 0.4536 kg
1 kg = 2.2046 lb
1 kg = 1000 g
1 kg = 1,000,000 mg
1 g = 1000 mg
1 g = 1,000,000 mcg
1 mg = 1000 mcg
1 oz = 28.35 g
1 g/100 mL = 100%
1 mL water = 1 g

(From Silverstein DC, Hopper K: *Small Animal Critical Care Medicine,* Elsevier, St Louis, 2009.)

Metric Conversions and Abbreviations

Prefix	Number	Weights	Volumes	Lengths
pico	1/1,000,000,000,000	Picogram	Picoliter (pL)	Picometer (pm)
nano	1/1,000,000,000	Nanogram	Nanoliter (nL)	Nanometer (nm)
micro	1/1,000,000	Microgram (mcg)	Microliter (mcL)	Micron (mcm)
milli	1/1000	Milligram (mg)	Milliliter (mL)	Millimeter (mm)
centi	1/100	Centigram (cg)	Centiliter (cL)	Centimeter (cm)
deci	1/10	Decigram (dg)	Deciliter (dL)	Decimeter (dm)
no prefix	1	Gram (g)	Liter (L)	Meter (m)
kilo	× 1000	Kilogram (kg)	Kiloliter (kL)	Kilometer (km)

(From Silverstein DC, Hopper K: *Small Animal Critical Care Medicine,* Elsevier, St Louis, 2009.)